CURRENT PEDIATRIC THERAPY 6

SYDNEY S. GELLIS, M.D.

PROFESSOR AND CHAIRMAN, DEPARTMENT OF PEDIATRICS, TUFTS UNIVERSITY SCHOOL OF MEDICINE; PEDIATRICIAN-IN-CHIEF, BOSTON FLOATING HOSPITAL FOR INFANTS AND CHILDREN, TUFTS—NEW ENGLAND MEDICAL CENTER, BOSTON

AND

BENJAMIN M. KAGAN, M.D.

DIRECTOR, DEPARTMENT OF PEDIATRICS, CEDARS OF LEBANON HOSPITAL DIVISION OF CEDARS-SINAI MEDICAL CENTER; PROFESSOR OF PEDIATRICS, UNIVERSITY OF CALIFORNIA AT LOS ANGELES

W. B. SAUNDERS COMPANY

Philadelphia · London · Toronto

W. B. Saunders Company: West Washington Square
Philadelphia, Pa. 19105

12 Dyott Street
London, WC1A 1DB

833 Oxford Street
Toronto 18, Ontario

Current Pediatric Therapy–6 ISBN 0-7216-4091-5

Library of Congress catalog card number 64-10484.

Print No.: 9 8 7 6 5 4 3 2 1

Preface

For those who may be interested in statistics, the volume introduced by these words contains 335 individual articles describing current therapy for many hundreds of diseases and disorders of childhood. These papers were prepared by 272 contributors, of whom 121 are new to this edition. Some 180 articles are brand new, and all of the others have been carefully scrutinized and, where necessary, revised and updated. A great deal of the writing has been done in the 12 months immediately prior to publication.

All these numbers tell very little about the true content of *Current Pediatric Therapy*. In the present volume, as in previous ones, men and women deeply involved in the care of children as their daily work have contributed their time and effort to a synthesis of clinical experience with the therapeutic methods they have found most useful. The only meaningful measure for a book such as this is the number of times it is consulted in a busy practice. Widespread acceptance of the earlier editions has prompted the preparation of this one.

Once again an attempt has been made to increase the usefulness of the book by urging contributors to confine their remarks to matters concerning therapy. Each of the writers has been asked to assume that readers have already made the correct diagnosis and possess an adequate understanding of the pathophysiology of the disorder.

Previous users will observe several changes of particular importance. The entire section on diseases of the skin has been reorganized and rewritten in recognition of the widely felt need for specific help in this difficult field. The number of individual articles in this section has been reduced, with the dermatoses classified etiologically to save space and avoid duplication. We thank Dr. Alvin Jacobs for wise counsel and strenuous effort on behalf of this revision.

Eight formerly separate articles on pulmonary disorders have been combined into one unified presentation, which has been newly written for this edition, and four papers formerly found in two different parts of the book have been replaced by an organized article on disorders of the female genitalia. A long list of topics covered for the first time includes, for example, total intravenous hyperalimentation, depression and suicide, autism, intractable diarrhea, management of postsplenectomy patients, magnesium deficiency, disorders of purine metabolism, amebic meningitis, toxic reactions to drugs, and trauma.

To the authors of new articles, to those who have written new descriptions of the management of other conditions, as well as to revisors of previously published papers, we extend our warm thanks. They have done their work well. Readers who find their methods useful in difficult situations owe them a special debt. Suggestions from users toward the further improvement of future editions will, as always, be gratefully received. A postpaid card has been bound inside the back cover for convenience in transmitting suggestions.

Special efforts have been made to verify drug dosages and to explain why and how they differ (when they do) from recommendations made by the manufacturers. In addition the roster of drugs which makes up the final section of the book has been rewritten and will, it is hoped, be more useful than ever before. There will continue to be instances in which readers will encounter therapeutic agents that are new or unfamiliar to them, and we again urge a careful review of the indications, precautions, and possible side effects of such drugs before they are prescribed. Our small patients surely deserve no less.

SYDNEY S. GELLIS, M.D.

BENJAMIN M. KAGAN, M.D.

Contributors

JOHN M. ADAMS, M.D., Ph.D.

Professor of Pediatrics, UCLA School of Medicine. Attending Physician, UCLA Medical Center; St. John's Hospital, Santa Monica; Harbor General Hospital, Torrance; Rancho Los Amigos Hospital, Downey, California.
Influenza.

MARGARET E. ADAMS, M.A.

Lecturer in Family Counseling, Lesley College Graduate Centre, Cambridge. Consultant in Social Work to the Interdisciplinary Training Program, Eunice Kennedy Shriver Centre, Walter E. Fernald State School, Waverly, Massachusetts.
Mental Subnormality.

ROBERT M. ADAMS, M.D.

Clinical Assistant Professor, Department of Dermatology, Stanford University School of Medicine, California. Attending Physician, Stanford Medical Center, California.
Topical Therapy: A Formulary for Pediatric Skin Disease.

WILLIAM A. AKERS, M.D.

Clinical Associate Professor of Dermatology, Stanford University School of Medicine, California. Chief, Dermatology Research Division, Letterman Army Institute of Research, Presidio of San Francisco, California.
Urticaria.

DAVID ALLAN, M.D., Ch.B.

Professor of Anesthesia, Northwestern University Medical School, Chicago, Illinois. Head, Division of Anesthesiology, Children's Memorial Hospital, Chicago, Illinois. Medical Director, Respiratory Therapy, Children's Memorial Hospital, Chicago, Illinois.
Anesthesia: Aspects of Significance to the Pediatrician.

JOEL J. ALPERT, M.D.

Professor and Chairman, Department of Pediatrics, Boston University School of Medicine, Massachusetts. Pediatrician-in-Chief, Boston City Hospital and University Hospital, Massachusetts. Lecturer in Pediatrics, Harvard Medical School, Boston, Massachusetts. Consultant in Pediatrics, Children's Hospital Medical Center, Boston; Joseph P. Kennedy, Jr., Memorial Hospital, Boston; Carney Hospital, Boston, Massachusetts.
Acute Poisoning.

MARY G. AMPOLA, M.D.

Assistant Professor of Pediatrics, Tufts University School of Medicine, Boston, Massachusetts. Pediatrician, New England Medical Center Hospital, Boston, Massachusetts.
Phenylketonuria. Amino Acid Disorders.

ALIA Y. ANTOON, M.D., C.H.B., D.C.H.

Assistant Pediatrician, Massachusetts General Hospital, Boston; Shriners' Hospital for Crippled Children and Burns Institute, Boston Unit. Instructor in Pediatrics, Harvard Medical School, Boston, Massachusetts.
Burns.

LEONARD APT, M.D.

Professor of Ophthalmology, Jules Stein Eye Institute, UCLA School of Medicine. Staff, Departments of Pediatrics and Ophthalmology, Cedars of Lebanon Hospital, Los Angeles, California. Consultant, St. John's Hospital, Santa Monica, California. Special Consultant, Los Angeles City Health Department and Bureau of Maternal and Child Health, California.
General Considerations of Eye Disorders. Eyelid Disorders. Conjunctival Disorders. Corneal Disorders. Scleral and Episcleral Disorders. Uveitis. Lacrimal Apparatus Disorders. Ocular Trauma. Retinoblastoma. Strabismus (Squint).

HENRY H. BANKS, M.D.

Professor and Chairman of Orthopedic Surgery, Tufts University School of Medicine, Boston, Massachusetts. Orthopedic Surgeon-in-Chief, New England Medical Center Hospital, Boston, Massachusetts. Director of Orthopedic Surgery, Boston City Hospital, Massachusetts.
Disorders of the Extremities. Diseases of the Hip. Disorders of Bone. Chondrodystrophia Calcificans Congenita.

LEWIS A. BARNESS, M.D.

Professor and Chairman of the Department of Pediatrics, University of South Florida College of Medicine,

Tampa. Attending Physician, Tampa General Hospital, Florida.
Generalized Undernutrition (Marasmus).

MARC O. BEEM, M.D.

Professor of Pediatrics, University of Chicago Pritzker School of Medicine, Illinois. Faculty Position, University of Chicago, Wyler Children's Hospital, Illinois.
Laryngitis and Laryngotracheobronchitis (The Croup Syndromê).

HERMAN BEERMAN, M.D., Sc.D. (Med.)

Emeritus Professor of Dermatology, University of Pennsylvania School of Medicine, Philadelphia. Emeritus Professor of Dermatology, Hospital of the University of Pennsylvania, Philadelphia. Honorary Consultant, Philadelphia General Hospital. Consultant, Graduate Hospital of the University of Pennsylvania and Pennsylvania Hospital, Philadelphia.
Drug Eruptions (Dermatitis Medicamentosa).

A. BARRY BELMAN, M.D., M.S.

Associate in Urology, Northwestern University Medical School, Chicago, Illinois. Attending Pediatric Urologist, Children's Memorial Hospital, Chicago, Illinois.
Urolithiasis.

WILLIAM BERENBERG, M.D.

Professor of Pediatrics, Harvard Medical School, Boston, Massachusetts. Director, Cerebral Palsy Unit and Associate Physician-in-Chief, Children's Hospital Medical Center, Boston, Massachusetts.
Cerebral Palsy.

BERNARD A. BERMAN, M.D.

Assistant Clinical Professor of Pediatrics, Tufts University School of Medicine, Boston, Massachusetts. Chief, Pediatric Allergy, St. Elizabeth's Hospital of Boston, Massachusetts. Pediatric Allergist, Boston Floating Hospital, Massachusetts.
Bronchial Asthma. Drug Allergy.

ALFRED M. BONGIOVANNI, M.D.

Professor of Pediatrics, University of Pennsylvania School of Medicine, Philadelphia. Director of Endocrinology, Children's Hospital of Philadelphia, Pennsylvania.
Undescended Testis.

DAVID S. BRADFORD, M.D.

Assistant Professor, Department of Orthopedic Surgery, University of Minnesota Health Science Center, Minneapolis. Assistant Professor, Fairview Hospital, Minneapolis, Minnesota. Spine Service, Gillete State Hospital for Crippled Children, St. Paul, Minnesota.
Disorders of the Clavicle, Scapula and Spine.

PATRICK F. BRAY, M.D.

Professor of Pediatrics and Neurology, University of Utah College of Medicine, Salt Lake City. Associate Full-Time Neurologist, University of Utah Hospital, Salt Lake City.
Acute Ataxia.

JOHN J. CALABRO, M.D., F.A.C.P.

Professor of Medicine, University of Massachusetts Medical School, Worcester. Chief of Medicine and Director of Rheumatology, Worcester City Hospital, Massachusetts. Consultant in Pediatrics, New England Medical Center, Boston, Massachusetts.
Diseases of Connective Tissue (The So-Called Collagen Diseases).

PHILIP L. CALCAGNO, M.D.

Professor and Chairman, Department of Pediatrics, Georgetown University School of Medicine, Washington, D. C.
Parenteral and Electrolyte Fluid Therapy.

HUGO F. CARAVAJAL, M.D.

Assistant Professor of Pediatrics, University of Texas Medical Branch at Galveston. Staff Physician, Division of Nephrology, Department of Pediatrics, University of Texas Medical Branch at Galveston.
Diabetes Mellitus. Urinary Tract Infections.

JAMES J. CEREGHINO, M.D.

Staff Neurologist, Applied Neurologic Research Branch, National Institute of Neurological Diseases and Stroke, National Institutes of Health, Bethesda, Maryland.
Rabies.

DONALD F. B. CHAR, M.D.

Professor of Pediatrics, University of Hawaii, Honolulu. Director of Student Health Services, University of Hawaii, Honolulu.
Eosinophilic Meningitis. Angiostrongyliasis.

H. PETER CHASE, M.D.

Associate Professor of Pediatrics, University of Colorado Medical Center, Denver.
Parenteral Nutrition in Infancy.

WERNER D. CHASIN, M.D.

Professor of Otolaryngology, and Chairman, Otolaryngology Division, Tufts University School of Medicine, Boston, Massachusetts. Otolaryngologist-in-Chief, New England Medical Center Hospital, Boston, Massachusetts. Visiting Surgeon, Boston City Hospital, Massachusetts. Associate Surgeon (Associate Staff), Massachusetts Eye and Ear Infirmary, Boston.
Malformations of the Nose. Tumors and Polyps of the Nose. Nasal Injuries. Epistaxis. Foreign Bodies in the Nose and Pharynx. Thyroglossal Duct Cysts and Branchial Cysts and Fistulas. Hearing Problems.

VICTOR CHERNICK, M.D.

Professor and Head, Department of Pediatrics, University of Manitoba Faculty of Medicine, Winnipeg, Canada. Paediatrician-in-Chief, Children's Hospital of Winnipeg, Manitoba, Canada.
Disorders of the Lungs and Pleura.

J. JULIAN CHISOLM, JR., M.D.

Associate Professor, Johns Hopkins University School of Medicine, Baltimore, Maryland. Pediatrician, Johns Hopkins Hospital, Baltimore, Maryland. Associate Chief Pediatrician, Baltimore City Hospitals, Maryland,
Pica. Acute Lead Poisoning and Asymptomatic Increased Lead Absorption.

AMOS CHRISTIE, M.D.

Emeritus Professor of Pediatrics, Vanderbilt University School of Medicine, Nashville, Tennessee. Emeritus Staff, Vanderbilt University Hospital, Nashville, Tennessee.
Histoplasmosis.

GREGORY M. CHUDZIK, B.S., Pharm.D.

Assistant Professor of Pharmacy, School of Pharmacy, State University of New York at Buffalo. Clinical Pharmacy Consultant, Children's Hospital of Buffalo, New York.
Adverse Drug Reactions—A Pharmacologic Approach.

HARVEY R. COLTEN, M.D.

Associate Professor of Pediatrics, Harvard Medical School, Boston, Massachusetts. Chief, Division of Allergy, Children's Hospital Medical Center, Boston, Massachusetts.
Angioneurotic Edema.

MORTON COOPER, Ph.D.

Private Practice in Vocal Rehabilitation and Speech Pathology, 10921 Wilshire Boulevard, Los Angeles, California. Formerly, Director, Voice and Speech Pathology, Outpatient Clinic, UCLA Center of the Health Sciences; Clinical Assistant Professor, Head and Neck Surgery Division, UCLA Center for the Health Sciences.
Voice, Speech, and Language Disorders.

MARVIN CORNBLATH, M.D.

Professor and Chairman, Department of Pediatrics, University of Maryland School of Medicine, Baltimore.
Infants Born to Diabetic Women. Hypoglycemia.

HENRY G. CRAMBLETT, M.D.

Professor and Chairman, Department of Medical Microbiology, Ohio State University College of Medicine, Columbus. Professor, Department of Pediatrics, Ohio State University College of Medicine, Columbus. Attending Staff, Children's Hospital, Columbus; University Hospitals, Columbus, Ohio.
Listeria monocytogenes Infections. Typhoid Fever. Salmonellosis. Rickettsial Infections.

JOHN D. CRAWFORD, M.D.

Associate Professor of Pediatrics, Harvard Medical School, Boston, Massachusetts. Chief, Endocrine and Metabolic Unit, Children's Service, Massachusetts General Hospital, Boston. Chief Pediatrician, Shriners Burns Institute, Boston Unit, Massachusetts.
Excessively Tall Stature in Adolescent Girls. Burns.

ALLEN C. CROCKER, M.D.

Associate Professor of Pediatrics, Harvard Medical School, Boston, Massachusetts. Senior Associate in Medicine, Children's Hospital Medical Center, Boston, Massachusetts.
Inborn Errors of Lipid Metabolism. The Histiocytosis Syndromes.

EDWARD C. CURNEN, JR., M.D.

Carpentier Professor of Pediatrics, College of Physicians & Surgeons, Columbia University, New York City. Attending Pediatrician, Columbia-Presbyterian Medical Center, New York City. Consultant in Pediatrics, St. Luke's Hospital, New York City.
Acute Lymphonodular Pharyngitis.

C. W. DAESCHNER, M.D.

Chairman, Department of Pediatrics, University of Texas Medical Branch at Galveston. Professor of Pediatrics, University of Texas Medical Branch at Galveston.
Perinephritis and Perirenal Abscess. Urinary Tract Infections.

GUILO J. D'ANGIO, M.D.

Professor of Radiology, Cornell University Medical School, New York City. Chairman, Department of Radiation Therapy, Memorial Sloan-Kettering Cancer Center, New York.
Lymphoma.

MURRAY DAVIDSON, M.D.

Professor of Pediatrics, Albert Einstein College of Medicine of Yeshiva University, New York City. Director of Pediatrics, Bronx-Lebanon Hospital Center, Bronx, New York.
Chronic Nonspecific Diarrhea Syndrome. Intractable Diarrhea.

VINCENT J. DERBES, M.D.

Professor, Tulane University School of Medicine, New Orleans, Louisiana. Chief, Section of Allergy-Dermatology, New Orleans, Louisiana. Chief of Dermatology, Charity Hospital of Louisiana, New Orleans. Consultant, Southern Baptist Hospital, New Orleans; USPH Hospital, New Orleans, Louisiana.
Treatment of Arthropod Bites and Stings.

MURDINA M. DESMOND, M.D.

Professor of Pediatrics, Baylor College of Medicine, Houston, Texas. Head, Developmental Pediatrics Service, Texas Children's Hospital, Houston. Associate in Pediatrics, Methodist Hospital, Houston; Texas Children's Hospital. Director, Center for Developmental Pediatrics, Texas Children's Hospital, Houston. Consultant, Newborn & Premature Services, St. Luke's Episcopal Hospital, Houston, Texas.
Disorders of the Umbilicus.

DARRYL C. DeVIVO, M.D.

Assistant Professor of Pediatrics and Neurology, Washington University School of Medicine, St. Louis, Missouri. Assistant Pediatrician, St. Louis Children's Hospital, Missouri. Assistant Neurologist, Barnes and allied hospitals, St. Louis, Missouri.
Acute Idiopathic Polyneuritis and Chronic Relapsing Polyneuropathy.

LOUIS K. DIAMOND, M.D.

Professor of Pediatrics, University of California School of Medicine, San Francisco. Professor Emeritus of Pediatrics, Harvard Medical School, Boston, Massachusetts. Attending Pediatrician, Moffitt Hospital, San Francisco, California.
Management of Patient after Splenectomy.

FRANKLIN F. DICKEY, B.S. (Pharmacy)

School of Pharmacy, State University of New York at Buffalo. Director of Pharmacy Services, Children's Hospital of Buffalo, New York.
Adverse Drug Reactions—A Pharmacologic Approach.

HUGH C. DILLON, M.D.

Professor of Pediatrics, University of Alabama in Birmingham, School of Medicine.
Group A Beta-Hemolytic Streptococci Infections.

PAUL A. di SANT'AGNESE, M.D., Sc.D. (Med.), Dr. Med. (Hon.)

Clinical Professor of Pediatrics, Georgetown University School of Medicine, Washington, D. C. Chief, Pediatric Metabolism Branch, NIAMDD, National Institutes of Health, Bethesda, Maryland. Consultant Children's Hospital of the District of Columbia, Washington, D. C.
Cystic Fibrosis.

PHILIP R. DODGE, M.D.

Professor of Pediatrics and of Neurology, Washington University School of Medicine, St. Louis, Missouri. Head, The Edward Mallinckrodt Department of Pediatrics, Washington University School of Medicine, St. Louis, Missouri. Medical Director, St. Louis Children's Hospital, Missouri.
Cerebral Vascular Disorders.

GEORGE N. DONNELL, M.D.

Professor of Pediatrics, and Cochairman, Department of Pediatrics, University of Southern California School of Medicine, Los Angeles. Physician-in-Chief, Department of Medicine, Children's Hospital of Los Angeles, California. Head, Division of Medical Genetics, Children's Hospital of Los Angeles, California.
Disorders of Carbohydrate Metabolism.

JAMES E. DRORBAUGH, M.D., M.P.H.

Director, China Medical Board of New York, Inc.
Birth Injuries.

WILLIAM M. EASSON, M.D.

Professor and Director, Division of Child and Adolescent Psychiatry, University of Minnesota, Minneapolis.
The Autistic Child.

CHESTER M. EDELMANN, JR., M.D.

Professor of Pediatrics, Albert Einstein College of Medicine of Yeshiva University, Bronx, New York. Attending Pediatrician, Bronx Municipal Hospital Center; Hospital of the Albert Einstein College of Medicine of Yeshiva University, Bronx; Lincoln Hospital, Bronx, New York.
The Nephrotic Syndrome. Chronic Renal Insufficiency (Chronic Uremia).

HANS E. EINSTEIN, M.D.

Clinical Professor of Medicine, University of Southern California School of Medicine, Los Angeles. Attending Physician, Mercy Hospital, Bakersfield; Greater Bakersfield Memorial Hospital; Kern County General Hospitals, Bakersfield, California.
Coccidioidomycosis.

LEON EISENBERG, M.D.

Professor of Psychiatry, Harvard Medical School, Boston, Massachusetts. Chief of Psychiatry, Massachusetts General Hospital, Boston.
Reading Disorders.

NANCY B. ESTERLY, M.D.

Associate Professor of Dermatology and Pediatrics, Abraham Lincoln School of the University of Illinois College of Medicine, Chicago. Attending Physician, University of Illinois Hospital, Chicago; Cook County Hospital, Chicago; Hines Veterans Administration Hospital, Illinois.
The Genodermatoses.

AUDREY E. EVANS, M.D.

Professor of Pediatrics, University of Pennsylvania, Philadelphia. Director, Division of Oncology, Children's Hospital of Philadelphia, Pennsylvania.
Lymphoma.

SHIRLEY L. FANNIN, M.D.

Assistant Clinical Professor, U.C.L.A. Director of Pediatric Ambulatory Services, Cedars-Sinai Medical Center, Los Angeles, California.
Alternative Drugs for Selected Parasitic Infections.

MURRAY FEINGOLD, M.D.

Associate Professor of Pediatrics, Tufts University School of Medicine, Boston, Massachusetts. Chief, Genetic and Birth Defect Service, Boston Floating Hospital for Infants and Children, Massachusetts.
Neurocutaneous Syndromes.

CHARLES F. FERGUSON, M.D., F.A.C.S.

Instructor in Otolaryngology, Harvard Medical School, Boston, Massachusetts. Senior Otolaryngologist, Children's Hospital Medical Center, Boston, Massachusetts.
Sinusitis and Rhinitis. Retropharyngeal and Lateral Pharyngeal Abscesses. Foreign Bodies in the Ear. Labyrinthitis. Injuries to the Middle Ear.

COLIN C. FERGUSON, M.D., F.R.C.S. (CAN.), F.A.C.S., F.A.A.P.

Professor of Surgery, The University of Manitoba, Winnipeg, Canada. Surgeon-in-Chief, Health Sciences Children's Centre, Winnipeg, Manitoba, Canada. Consultant, Health Sciences General Centre, Winnipeg, Manitoba; St. Boniface General Hospital, Winnipeg, Manitoba, Canada.
Pyloric Stenosis.

GREGORY C. FERNANDOPULLE, M.D.

Chief Resident, Division of Child Psychiatry, Johns Hopkins University School of Medicine and Johns Hopkins Hospital, Baltimore, Maryland. Fellow, Departments of Pediatrics and Psychiatry, Johns Hopkins University School of Medicine and Johns Hopkins Hospital, Baltimore, Maryland.
Emotional Disorders.

ROBERT M. FILLER, M.D.

Associate Professor of Surgery, Harvard Medical School, Boston, Massachusetts. Chief of Clinical Surgery, Children's Hospital Medical Center, Boston, Massachusetts.
Long-Term Parenteral Nutrition (Hyperalimentation).

LAURENCE FINBERG, M.D.

Professor of Pediatrics, Albert Einstein College of Medicine of Yeshiva University, Bronx, New York. Chairman, Department of Pediatrics, Montefiore Hospital and Medical Center, Bronx, New York.
Salicylate Intoxication.

RICHARD N. FINE, M.D.

Associate Professor of Pediatrics, University of Southern California, Los Angeles. Director, Dialysis and Transplantation Program, Children's Hospital of Los Angeles, California.
Peritoneal Dialysis.

SYDNEY M. FINEGOLD, M.D.

Professor of Medicine, UCLA School of Medicine. Chief, Infectious Disease Section, Veterans Administration Center–Wadsworth Hospital Center, Los Angeles, California.
Infections Due to Proteus, Klebsiella, Pseudomonas and Other Gram–Negative Bacilli. Infections Due to Anaerobic Cocci and Gram–Negative Anaerobic Bacilli.

BURTON W. FINK, M.D.

Associate Clinical Professor of Pediatrics (Cardiology), UCLA School of Medicine. Attending Physician and Director, Department of Pediatric Cardiology, Cedars–Sinai Medical Center, Los Angeles, California.
Congestive Heart Failure. Congenital Heart Disease.

NICHOLAS J. FIUMARA, M.D., M.P.H.

Clinical Professor of Dermatology, Boston University School of Medicine; Boston City Hospital; Boston Dispensary; Massachusetts General Hospital, Boston; University Hospital, Boston, Massachusetts.
Lymphogranuloma Venereum.

DAVID R. FLEISHER, M.D.

Assistant Clinical Professor of Pediatrics, UCLA School of Medicine. Associate Attending Pediatrician, Cedars of Lebanon Hospital, Los Angeles, California.
Constipation.

ROBERT E. FLYNN, M.D.

Assistant Professor of Neurology, Tufts University Medical School, Boston, Massachusetts. Assistant in Neurology, Massachusetts General Hospital, Boston. Chief, Department of Neurology, Division of Medicine, St. Elizabeth's Hospital, Brighton, Massachusetts.
Mental Subnormality.

ERIC W. FONKALSRUD, M.D.

Professor and Chief of Pediatric Surgery, UCLA School of Medicine.
Peritonitis. Diseases of the Pancreas.

IRA M. FRANK, M.D.

Assistant Professor of Psychiatry, UCLA.
Drug Abuse and the Adolescent.

ROBERT I. FREEDMAN, M.D.

Associate Clinical Professor of Medicine (Dermatology), University of Southern California School of Medicine, Los Angeles. Attending Physician, Los Angeles County–University of Southern California Medical Center. Consultant, St. Francis Hospital of Lynwood, California.
Skin Diseases in the Newborn.

GERALD W. FRIEDLAND, M.D., M.R.C.P.E., F.F.R.

Associate Professor of Radiology, Stanford Medical Center–School of Medicine, California. Director of Genito-urinary Unit, Diagnostic Radiology, Stanford Medical Center, California.
Vomiting.

ARNOLD P. FRIEDMAN, M.D.

Clinical Professor of Neurology, Columbia University College of Physicians & Surgeons, New York City. Physician-in-Charge, Headache Unit, Montefiore Hospital and Medical Center, New York City.
Headaches and Migraine.

STEPHEN L. GANS, M.D.

Associate Clinical Professor of Surgery, UCLA School of Medicine. Chief, Pediatric Surgery Service, Cedars of Lebanon Hospital, Los Angeles, California. Attending Surgeon, Children's Hospital of Los Angeles, California. Attending Staff, UCLA Hospital.
Preoperative and Postoperative Care of Patients Undergoing Gastrointestinal Surgery. Disorders of the Anus and Rectum.

RICHARD A. GATTI, M.D.

Guest Researcher, Department of Tumor Biology, Karolinska Institute, Stockholm, Sweden. USPHS Research Career Development Awardee, University of Minnesota Hospitals, Minneapolis.
The Immunodeficiency Diseases.

SYDNEY S. GELLIS, M.D.

Professor and Chairman, Department of Pediatrics, Tufts University School of Medicine, Boston, Massachusetts. Pediatrician-in-Chief, Boston Floating Hospital for Infants and Children (New England Medical Center Hospital), Massachusetts.
Mumps.

GERALD S. GILCHRIST, M.B., B.Ch.

Associate Professor of Pediatrics, Mayo Medical School, Rochester, Minnesota. Consultant, Department of Pediatrics and Division of Hematology and Internal Medicine, Mayo Clinic and Mayo Foundation, Rochester, Minnesota.
The Hemolytic—Uremic Syndrome.

THOMAS H. GLICK, M.D.

Clinical Instructor in Neurology, Harvard Medical School, Boston, Massachusetts. Assistant in Neurology, Massachusetts General Hospital, Boston. Neurologist, Cambridge Hospital, Massachusetts.
Encephalopathy and Fatty Degeneration of the Viscera (Reye's Syndrome).

LOUIS GLUCK, M.D.

Professor of Pediatrics and Obstetrics, University of California, San Diego, School of Medicine, La Jolla. Head, Division of Perinatal Medicine, University Hospital, University of California, San Diego.
Dysmaturity and Postmaturity.

DAVID GOLDRING, M.D.

Professor of Pediatrics, Washington University School of Medicine, St. Louis, Missouri. Director of Pediatric Cardiology, St. Louis Children's Hospital, Missouri.
Hypertension. Hypotension.

NORMAN P. GOLDSTEIN, M.D.

Professor of Neurology, Mayo Medical School, Rochester, Minnesota. Consultant, Department of Neurology, Mayo Clinic and Mayo Foundation, Rochester, Minnesota.
Hepatolenticular Degeneration (Wilson's Disease).

ROBERT A. GOOD, M.D., Ph.D.

Professor of Pathology, Graduate School of Medical Sciences, Cornell University Medical College, New York City. Adjunct Professor and Visiting Physician, The Rockefeller University, New York City. President and Director, Sloan-Kettering Institute for Cancer Research, New York. Director of Research, Memorial Hospital

for Cancer and Allied Diseases and the Memorial Sloan-Kettering Cancer Center, New York.
The Immunodeficiency Diseases.

ALLAN C. GOODMAN, Ph.D.

Assistant Professor of Otolaryngology (Audiology), Tufts University School of Medicine, Boston, Massachusetts. Assistant Professor of Rehabilitation Medicine, Tufts University School of Medicine, Boston, Massachusetts. Director of Audiology, Speech, Hearing and Language Center, New England Medical Center Hospital, Boston, Massachusetts.
Hearing Problems.

ROBERT J. GORLIN, D.D.S., M.S.

Professor and Chairman, University of Minnesota School of Dentistry, Minneapolis. Attending Staff, University of Minnesota Hospitals, Minneapolis; Glenwood Hills Medical Center, Minneapolis; U.S. Veterans Administration Hospital, Minneapolis; Children's Medical Center and Hospital, Minneapolis; Mt. Sinai Hospital, Minneapolis; Hennepin County General Hospital, Minneapolis, Minnesota.
Abnormalities, Injuries and Diseases of the Oral Region.

SARAH E. GORSKI, M.A.

Mental Health Administrator. Instructor, Chicago State University, Department of Mental Health, Illinois State Pediatrics Institute.
Learning Problems.

SAMUEL P. GOTOFF, M.D.

Professor of Pediatrics, Pritzker School of Medicine, University of Chicago, Illinois. Chairman, Department of Pediatrics, Michael Reese Hospital and Medical Center, Chicago, Illinois.
Brucellosis. Tularemia.

WILLIAM A. GOUVEIA, M.S.

Clinical Instructor in Pharmacy, Massachusetts College of Pharmacy, Boston. Director of Pharmacy, New England Medical Center Hospital, Boston, Massachusetts.
Roster of Drugs.

NORMAN GRANT, F.R.C.S.

Consultant Neurosurgeon, Hospital for Sick Children, London, England. National Hospital for Nervous Diseases, London, England.
Venous Sinus Thrombosis. Pseudotumor Cerebri.

SHIRLEY A. GRAVES, M.D.

Assistant Professor of Anesthesiology, University of Florida College of Medicine, Gainesville. Attending Physician, Shands Teaching Hospital and Clinics, Gainesville, Florida.
Near-drowning (Nonfatal Submersion).

IRA GREIFER, M.D.

Director of Pediatric and Children's Kidney Center, Hospital of the Albert Einstein College of Medicine of Yeshiva University, Bronx, New York. Associate Professor, the Albert Einstein College of Medicine of Yeshiva University, Bronx, New York.
The Nephrotic Syndrome.

LAWRENCE S. C. GRIFFITH, M.D.

Assistant Professor of Medicine, The Johns Hopkins University School of Medicine, Baltimore, Maryland. Physician, The Johns Hopkins Hospital, Baltimore, Maryland.
Cholera.

DAVID GROB, M.D.

Professor of Medicine, State University of New York College of Medicine, Downstate Medical Center, Brooklyn.
Myasthenia Gravis.

HERBERT J. GROSSMAN, M.D.

Professor of Pediatrics (Neurology), Abraham Lincoln School of Medicine of the University of Illinois, Chicago. Professor of Neurology and Pediatrics, Rush Medical College, Chicago. Director, Illinois State Pediatric Institute, Chicago; Pediatric Neurology, Presbyterian-St. Luke's Hospital, Chicago, Illinois.
Learning Problems.

PATRICIA BIRD GROSSMAN, M.A., A.C.S.W.

Chief Social Worker, Northern Suburban Special Education District, Highland Park, Illinois.
Learning Problems.

WARREN G. GUNTHEROTH, M.D.

Professor of Pediatrics, University of Washington School of Medicine, Seattle. Cardiologist, University Hospital, Seattle, Washington. Consultant, King County Harborview Hospital, Seattle; Children's Orthopedic Hospital and Medical Center, Seattle; USPHS Hospital, Seattle; Madigan Army Hospital, Tacoma; Rainier School, Buckley, Washington.
Peripheral Vascular Disease.

RONALD L. GUTBERLET, M.D.

Assistant Professor of Pediatrics, University of Maryland School of Medicine, Baltimore. Director of Nurseries, University of Maryland Hospital, Baltimore.
Infants Born to Diabetic Women.

J. ALEX HALLER, JR., M.D.

Robert Garrett Professor of Pediatric Surgery, The Johns Hopkins University School of Medicine, Baltimore, Maryland. Children's Surgeon-in-Charge, The Johns Hopkins Hospital, Baltimore, Maryland.
Gastrointestinal Foreign Bodies. Intussusception. Chest Wall Abnormalities.

JEROME S. HALLER, M.D.

Assistant Professor of Pediatrics (Neurology), Tufts University School of Medicine, Boston, Massachusetts, Assistant Pediatrician (Neurology), New England Medical Center Hospitals, Boston, Massachusetts.
Spasmus Nutans.

KENNETH C. HALTALIN, M.D.

Associate Professor of Pediatrics, University of Texas Health Science Center at Dallas, Southwestern Medical School. Senior Attending Pediatrician, Parkland Memorial Hospital, Dallas, Texas. Active Attending Pediatrician, Children's Medical Center of Dallas, Texas. Consultant in Pediatrics, John Peter Smith Hospital, Fort Worth, Texas.
Escherichia coli Infections. Shigellosis.

SHERREL L. HAMMAR, M.D.

Associate Professor of Pediatrics, University of Hawaii School of Medicine, Honolulu. Director of Medical

Services and Training, Kauikeolani Children's Hospital, Honolulu, Hawaii.
Obesity.

JOHN D. L. HANSEN, M.D., F.R.C.P., D.C.H.

Professor of Paediatrics, University of the Witwatersrand, Johannesburg General and Affiliated Hospitals, Johannesburg, South Africa.
Kwashiorkor (Protein-Calorie Malnutrition).

JAMES B. HANSHAW, M.D.

Professor of Pediatrics and Microbiology, University of Rochester School of Medicine and Dentistry, New York. Pediatrician-in-Chief, The Genesee Hospital, Rochester, New York. Pediatrician, Strong Memorial Hospital, Rochester, New York.
Cytomegalovirus Infections.

HAROLD E. HARRISON, M.D.

Professor of Pediatrics, Johns Hopkins University School of Medicine, Baltimore, Maryland. Chief of Pediatrics. Baltimore City Hospitals, Maryland.
Vitamin Deficiencies and Excesses. Rickets. Tetany.

GAVIN HILDICK-SMITH, M.D., M.R.C.P., F.A.A.P.

Instructor in Pediatrics University of Pennsylvania School of Medicine, Philadelphia.
Fungus Diseases.

HARRY R. HILL, M.D.

Instructor, Departments of Pediatrics and Laboratory Medicine, University of Minnesota Medical School, Minneapolis.
Staphylococcal Infections.

HORACE L. HODES, M.D.

Professor and Chairman, Department of Pediatrics, Mount Sinai School of Medicine, City University of New York. Pediatrician-in-Chief, Mount Sinai Hospital, New York City.
Encephalitis Infections—Postinfectious and Postvaccinal.

JOAN E. HODGMAN, M.D.

Professor of Pediatrics, University of Southern California School of Medicine, Los Angeles. Director, Newborn Service, Los Angeles County–University of Southern California Medical Center. Consultant, Rancho Los Amigos County Hospital, Downey. Huntington Memorial Hospital, Pasadena, California.
Skin Diseases in the Newborn.

HAROLD J. HOFFMAN, M.D., B.Sc. (Med.), F.R.C.S. (Can.), F.A.C.S.

Associate in Surgery, University of Toronto Faculty of Medicine, Ontario, Canada. Senior Surgeon, Department of Surgery, Division of Neurosurgery, Hospital for Sick Children, Toronto, Ontario, Canada.
Brain Abscess. Spinal Epidural Abscess.

PAUL H. HOLINGER, M.D.

Professor of Bronchoesophagology, Department of Otolaryngology, The Abraham Lincoln School of Medicine of the University of Illinois, Chicago. Attending Bronchoesophagologist, Presbyterian–St. Luke's Hospital, Chicago; The Children's Memorial Hospital, Chicago; Eye & Ear Infirmary of the University of Illinois, Chicago; Research & Educational Hospital, Chicago, Illinois.
Disorders of the Larynx. Foreign Bodies in the Air and Food Passages.

CHARLES E. HOLLERMAN, M.D.

Associate Professor of Pediatrics, Georgetown University School of Medicine, Washington, D. C.
Parenteral and Electrolyte Fluid Therapy.

GERALD H. HOLMAN, M.D.

Professor and Head, Division of Pediatrics, University of Calgary, Alberta, Canada. Chief, Department of Pediatrics, Foothills Provincial Hospital, Calgary, Alberta, Canada.
Infantile Cortical Hyperostosis.

PETER R. HOLT, M.D.

Associate Professor of Medicine, College of Physicians and Surgeons, Columbia University, New York City. Chief, Division of Gastroenterology, St. Luke's Hospital Center, New York City.
Lymphatic Obstruction of the Gastrointestinal Tract.

PAUL W. HUGENBERGER, M.D.

Former Lecturer in Orthopedic Surgery, Harvard Medical School, Boston, Massachusetts. Senior Associate in Orthopedic Surgery, Children's Hospital Medical Center & Peter Bent Brigham Hospital. Senior Attending Orthopedic Surgeon, North Shore Children's Hospital, Salem; West Roxbury Veterans Hospital, Boston.
Congenital Muscular Defects. Torticollis.

WALTER T. HUGHES, M.D.

Chief, Infectious Diseases Service, St. Jude Children's Research Hospital, Memphis, Tennessee. Professor of Pediatrics and Microbiology, University of Tennessee Medical Units, Memphis.
Pneumocystis carinii Pneumonitis.

SIDNEY HURWITZ, M.D.

Assistant Clinical Professor of Pediatrics and Dermatology, Yale University School of Medicine, New Haven, Connecticut. Attending Physician in Pediatrics and Dermatology, Yale-New Haven Medical Center; Hospital of St. Raphael, New Haven, Connecticut.
Other Skin Tumors. Diseases of Sweat and Sebaceous Glands.

ALVIN H. JACOBS, M.D.

Professor of Dermatology and Pediatrics, Stanford University School of Medicine, California. Senior Attending Physician, Dermatology and Pediatrics, Stanford University Medical Center, California.
Eruptions in the Diaper Area. Papulosquamous Disorders. Melanin Pigmentary Disorders. Miscellaneous Dermatoses.

L. STANLEY JAMES, M.D.

Professor of Pediatrics, College of Physicians & Surgeons, Columbia University, New York City. Attending Pediatrician, Babies Hospital, New York City.
The Drug-Addicted Newborn Infant.

S. N. JAVETT, M.D., D.C.H., R.C., P. & S.

Honorary Consulting Pediatrician, Transvaal Memorial Hospital for Children, Johannesburg, South Africa.
Acrodynia.

THEODORE C. JEWETT, JR., M.D.

Professor of Surgery, State University of New York at Buffalo. Chief of Surgery, Children's Hospital, Buffalo, New York. Consultant in Surgery, Brooks Memorial Hospital, Dunkirk; Roswell Park Memorial Institute, Buffalo; Meyer Memorial Hospital, Buffalo, New York.
Peptic Ulcer.

DOUGLAS E. JOHNSTONE, M.D.

Clinical Associate Professor of Pediatrics, University of Rochester School of Medicine and Dentistry, New York. Director of Pediatric Allergy Clinic and Training Program, Strong Memorial Hospital, Rochester, New York. Consultant in Allergy, Genesee Hospital, Rochester; Rochester General Hospital; Wayne County Hospital, New York.
Contact Dermatitis.

RODNEY C. JUNG, M.D., Ph.D., F.A.C.P.

Professor of Tropical Medicine, Tulane University School of Public Health, New Orleans, Louisiana. Senior Associate in Internal Medicine, Touro Infirmary, New Orleans, Louisiana. Senior Visiting Physician, Charity Hospital of Louisiana at New Orleans.
Malaria. Chagas' Disease. Amebiasis.

MICHAEL M. KABACK, M.D.

Associate Professor of Pediatrics and Medicine, UCLA School of Medicine. Associate Chief, Division of Medical Genetics, Harbor General Hospital, Torrance, California.
Genetic Disease: Diagnosis, Counseling and Prevention.

GUINTER KAHN, M.D.

Director of Resident Training, Skin and Cancer Unit, Mt. Sinai Medical Center, Miami Beach, Florida.
Vesicolobullous Disorders.

EUGENE KAPLAN, M.D.

Professor of Pediatrics, University of Maryland Medical School, Baltimore. Associate Professor of Pediatrics, Johns Hopkins Medical School, Baltimore, Maryland. Pediatrician-in-Chief, Sinai Hospital, Baltimore, Maryland.
Hemolytic Anemia.

SOLOMON A. KAPLAN, M.D.

Professor of Pediatrics, UCLA School of Medicine.
Hypopituitarism.

SAMUEL KARELITZ, M.D., Ph.B.

Director Emeritus and Consultant, Department of Pediatrics, New Hyde Park Long Island Jewish and Hillside Hospital, New York. Consultant in Pediatrics, Mt. Sinai Hospital, New York City; Huntington General Hospital; Queens General Hospital, Jamaica; Flushing General Hospital, New York. Formerly, Clinical Professor of Pediatrics, New York State Medical School, Downstate Branch, Brooklyn.
Acute Infectious Lymphocytosis.

RAYMOND H. KAUFMAN, M.D.

Ernst W. Bertner Chairman and Professor, Department of Obstetrics and Gynecology, Baylor College of Medicine, Houston, Texas.
Disorders of the Vulva and Vagina. Disorders of the Uterus, Tubes and Ovaries. Tumors of the Uterus, Tubes and Ovaries.

B. H. KEAN, M.D.

Clinical Professor of Medicine (Tropical Medicine), Cornell University Medical College, New York City. Attending Physician, The New York Hospital, New York City; Doctors Hospital, New York City. Director, Parasitology Laboratory, The New York Hospital, New York City.
Toxoplasmosis.

PANAYOTIS P. KELALIS, M.D., M.S.

Assistant Professor of Urology, Mayo Medical School, Rochester, Minnesota. Consultant, Department of Urology, Mayo Clinic and Mayo Foundation, Rochester, Minnesota.
Cystic Disease of the Kidney. Hydronephrosis and Disorders of the Ureter. Malignant Tumors of the Kidney.

C. HENRY KEMPE, M.D.

Professor of Pediatrics, University of Colorado School of Medicine, Denver. Chairman, Department of Pediatrics, University of Colorado School of Medicine, Denver, Colorado.
Smallpox. Vaccinia.

EDWIN L. KENDIG, JR., M.D., Sc.D. (Hon.)

Professor of Pediatrics, Medical College of Virginia, Health Sciences Division, Virginia Commonwealth University, Richmond. Director, Child Chest Clinic, Medical College of Virginia Hospitals, Richmond.
Tuberculosis. Infections with the Unclassified Mycobacteria. Sarcoidosis.

SIDNEY KIBRICK, M.D., Ph.D.

Professor of Pediatrics and Microbiology (Virology), Boston University School of Medicine, Massachusetts. Visiting Physician of Pediatrics, Boston City Hospital, Massachusetts. Consultant on Infectious Diseases, Children's Hospital Medical Center, Boston, Massachusetts.
Varicella and Herpes Zoster, Cat-Scratch Disease.

LOWELL R. KING, M.D.

Professor of Urology, Northwestern University Medical School, Chicago, Illinois. Attending Urologist and Chairman, Division of Urology, Children's Memorial Hospital, Chicago, Illinois. Attending Urologist, Northwestern Memorial Hospital, Chicago, Illinois.
Disorders of the Bladder, Prostate and Urethra.

JEROME O. KLEIN, M.D.

Associate Professor of Pediatrics, Harvard Medical School, Boston, Massachusetts. Associate Director, Department of Pediatrics, Boston City Hospital, Massachusetts.
Bacterial Pneumonia.

PETER J. KOBLENZER, M.D., F.A.A.D., F.R.C.P. (Can.) (Eng.)

Clinical Professor of Dermatology, Temple University Health and Sciences Center, Philadelphia, Pennsylvania. Consultant, Cherry Hill Medical Center, New Jersey; Deborah Hospital, Browns Mills, New Jersey; Zurbrugg Memorial Hospital, Riverside, New Jersey; Rancocas Valley Hospital, Willingboro, New Jersey.
Contact Dermatitis. Nummular Eczema.

ROBERT E. KOEHLER, M.D.

Medical Epidemiologist, Bacterial Diseases Branch, Epi-

demiology Program, Center for Disease Control, Atlanta, Georgia.
Leptospirosis.

MAURICE D. KOGUT, M.D.

Associate Professor of Pediatrics, University of Southern California School of Medicine, Los Angeles. Head, Division of Endocrinology and Metabolism, Children's Hospital of Los Angeles, California. Program Director of Clinical Research Center, Children's Hospital of Los Angeles, California.
Disorders of Carbohydrate Metabolism.

SAUL KRUGMAN, M.D.

Professor and Chairman, Department of Pediatrics, New York University School of Medicine, New York City. Director of Pediatrics, Bellevue Hospital, New York City; University Hospital, New York City.
Rubella (German Measles). Viral Hepatitis.

ROBERT LaPERRIERE, M.D.

Attending Dermatologist, Kaiser Hospital, Sacramento, California.
Scleroderma.

ZVI LARON, M.D.

Professor of Pediatric Endocrinology, Tel Aviv University School of Medicine, Israel. Director, Institute of Pediatric and Adolescent Endocrinology and Israel Counselling Center for Juvenile Diabetics, Beilinson Hospital, Petah Tikva, Israel.
Endocrine Disorders of the Testes.

JOHN K. LATTIMER, M.D., Sc.D.

Professor and Chairman, Columbia University College of Physicians and Surgeons, New York City. Director, Urological Service, Babies Hospital, New York City; Presbyterian Hospital, New York City; Francis Delafield Hospital, New York City; Harlem Hospital Center, New York City.
Exstrophy of the Urinary Bladder. Patent Urachus and Urachal Cyst. Tumors of the Bladder and Prostate.

WILLIAM E. LAUPUS, M.D.

Professor and Chairman, Department of Pediatrics, Medical College of Virginia, Virginia Commonwealth University, Richmond. Pediatrician-in-Chief, Medical Center of Virginia Hospital, Richmond.
Systemic Mycotic Infections.

HAROLD I. LECKS, M.D.

Associate Clinical Professor of Pediatrics, University of Pennsylvania School of Medicine, Philadelphia. Allergist, Children's Hospital of Philadelphia, Pennsylvania. Pediatric Allergist, Philadelphia General Hospital, Pennsylvania.
Allergic Gastrointestinal Disease.

NORMAN E. LEVAN, M.D.

Professor of Medicine (Chairman—Dermatology), Los Angeles County–University of Southern California Medical Center. Senior Attending Physician, Los Angeles County–University of Southern California Medical Center. Consultant, Children's Hospital of Los Angeles, California; United States Naval Hospital, San Diego, California.
Skin Diseases in the Newborn.

RICHARD D. LEVERE, M.D.

Professor of Medicine, State University of New York, Downstate Medical Center, Brooklyn. Chief of Hematology, Downstate Medical Center–Kings County Hospital Center, Brooklyn, New York. Consultant in Hematology, Brooklyn Veterans Administration Hospital, New York.
Disorders of Porphyrin, Hemoglobin and Purine Metabolism.

ELLIN LIEBERMAN, M.D.

Associate Professor of Pediatrics, University of Southern California School of Medicine, Los Angeles. Head, Renal Division, Children's Hospital of Los Angeles, California.
The Hemolytic—Uremic Syndrome.

FIMA LIFSHITZ, M.D.

Associate Professor, Cornell University Medical School, New York City. Chief, Pediatric Research, North Shore Hospital, Manhasset, New York. Chief, Division of Nutrition, Metabolism and Endocrinology, North Shore Hospital, Manhasset, New York. Associate Attending Pediatrician, New York Hospital, New York City.
Malabsorption Syndrome and Intestinal Disaccharidase Deficiencies.

C. D. R. LIGHTOWLER, M.B., B.S. (Lon.), L.R.C.P., F.R.C.S. (Eng.)

Consultant Orthopaedic Surgeon to the South Essex Group of Hospitals, England.
Upper and Lower Neural Tube Dysraphism.

REGINALD LIGHTWOOD, M.D., F.R.C.P., D.P.H.

Consulting Physician, The Hospital for Sick Children, Community of London, England. Consulting Paediatrician, St. Mary's Hospital, Community of London, England. Consultant Paediatrician to International Missionary Training Hospital, Drogheda, Eire.
The Idiopathic Hypercalcemic Syndrome: Infantile Hypercalcemia.

SHUN M. LING, M.D.

Assistant Clinical Professor of Pediatrics, UCLA School of Medicine. Associate Attending Physician, Cedars of Lebanon Hospital, Los Angeles, California.
Parathyroid Disease.

BARBARA M. LIPPE, M.D.

Assistant Professor of Pediatrics, University of UCLA.
Hermaphroditism and Intersex.

SAMUEL LIVINGSTON, M.D.

Director, the Samuel Livingston Epilepsy Diagnostic and Research Center, Baltimore, Maryland. Consultant in Internal Medicine, Sinai Hospital, Baltimore, Maryland. Honorary Consultant in Pediatrics, Sinai Hospital, Baltimore, Maryland. Emeritus Associate Professor in Pediatrics, the Johns Hopkins University School of Medicine, Baltimore, Maryland. Formerly, Director and Physician-in-Charge, the Johns Hopkins Hospital Epilepsy Clinic, Baltimore, Maryland.
Seizure Disorders.

SOL LONDE, B.S., M.D.

Assistant Professor Emeritus, Clinical Pediatrics, Washington University School of Medicine, St. Louis, Mis-

souri. Assistant Pediatrician Emeritus, St. Louis Children's Hospital, Missouri. Associate Pediatrician, St. Louis Labor Health Institute, Missouri.
Hypertension. Hypotension.

WILLIAM B. LORENTZ, M.D.

Assistant Professor of Pediatrics, University of Texas Medical Branch at Galveston, Attending Nephrologist, Division of Nephrology, University of Texas Medical Branch Hospitals, Galveston.
Diabetes Mellitus.

FREDERICK H. LOVEJOY, JR., M.D.

Instructor in Pediatrics, Harvard Medical School, Boston, Massachusetts. Chief Resident in Medicine, Children's Hospital Medical Center, Boston, Massachusetts. Executive Secretary, Boston Poison Information Center, Massachusetts.
Acute Poisoning.

JOHN N. LUKENS, M.D.

Professor of Pediatrics, Charles R. Drew Postgraduate Medical School and UCLA. Director of Pediatric Hematology, Martin Luther King, Jr., General Hospital, Los Angeles, California.
Hemolytic Disease of the Newborn (Erythroblastosis Fetalis). Leukopenia, Neutropenia, and Agranulocytosis.

DONALD M. MacQUEEN, M.D.

Clinical Instructor, New Hanover Hospital, Wilmington, North Carolina.
Allergic Rhinitis.

NOEL KEITH MACLAREN, M.D.

Research Associate, University of Maryland School of Medicine, Baltimore; University of Maryland Hospital, Baltimore.
Hypoglycemia.

M. JEFFREY MAISELS, M.B., B.ch.

Assistant Professor of Pediatrics, The Pennsylvania State University College of Medicine, Hershey. Chief, Division of Newborn Medicine, The Milton S. Hershey Medical Center, Hershey, Pennsylvania.
Congenital Unconjugated Hyperbilirubinemia and Benign Recurrent Cholestasis.

P. E. C. MANSON-BAHR, M.D., F.R.C.P., D.T.M.H.

Senior Lecturer, London School of Hygiene and Tropical Medicine, England. Physician, Hospital for Tropical Diseases, London; Leamen's Hospital, London, England.
Filariasis. Leishmaniasis.

ANDREW M. MARGILETH, M.D.

Professor of Pediatrics, George Washington University School of Medicine, Associate Professor of Pediatrics, Howard University School of Medicine, Instructor of Pediatrics, Georgetown University School of Medicine, Senior Attending Staff Pediatrician, Children's Hospital National Medical Center, Washington, D. C.
Bacterial Infections of the Skin. Warts and Molluscum Contagiosum. Nevi and Nevoid Tumors.

ALAN N. MARKS, M.D.

Assistant Professor of Pediatrics and Psychiatry, Tufts University School of Medicine, Boston, Massachusetts. Child Psychiatrist, New England Medical Center Hospital, Boston, Massachusetts.
Sleep Disturbance.

FLORENCE N. MARSHALL, M.D.

Clinical Associate Professor of Pediatrics, New York Hospital-Cornell University Medical College, New York City. Attending Pediatrician, Hôpital Albert Schweitzer, Deschapelles, Haiti; New York Hospital, New York City.
Tetanus.

BENEDICT F. MASSELL, M.D.

Associate Professor of Pediatrics, Harvard Medical School, Boston, Massachusetts. Research Director, House of the Good Samaritan, Children's Hospital Medical Center, Boston, Massachusetts.
Rheumatic Fever.

ALLEN W. MATHIES, JR., M.D., Ph.D.

Professor of Pediatrics, University of Southern California School of Medicine, Los Angeles. Head Physician, Communicable Disease Service, Los Angeles County–University of Southern California Medical Center.
Food Poisoning.

JOHN M. MATSEN, M.D.

Associate Professor of Pediatrics, Laboratory Medicine and Pathology, and Microbiology, University of Minnesota School of Medicine, Minneapolis. Director, Clinical Microbiology Laboratories, University of Minnesota Hospitals, Minneapolis.
Staphylococcal Infections.

S. MICHAEL MAUER, M.D., C.M.

Assistant Professor of Pediatrics, University of Minnesota Medical School, Minneapolis. Attending Pediatrician, Associate Director of Pediatric Hemodialysis, University of Minnesota Hospitals, Minneapolis.
Renal Vein Thrombosis.

GEORGE H. McCRACKEN, JR., M.D.

Associate Professor of Pediatrics, University of Texas Southwestern Medical School at Dallas. Attending Pediatrician, Parkland Memorial Hospital, Dallas; Children's Medical Center of Dallas, Texas.
Neonatal Sepsis, Meningitis and Pneumonia. Postneonatal Meningitis and Sepsis of Unknown Cause. Tetanus.

WALLACE W. McCRORY, M.D.

Professor and Chairman, Department of Pediatrics, Cornell University Medical College, New York City. Pediatrician-in-Chief, New York Hospital, New York City.
Glomerulonephritis.

ROBERT L. McLAURIN, M.D.

Professor of Surgery (Neurosurgery), University of Cincinnati Medical College, Ohio. Attending Staff and Director, Children's Hospital of Neurosurgery, Cincinnati General Hospital (Neurosurgery), Ohio. Consultant, Veterans Administration Hospital, Cincinnati, Ohio.
Head Injury. Cerebral Edema. Epidural Hematoma and Subdural Hematoma and Effusion. Intracranial Hemorrhage. Acute Infantile Hemiplegia.

RICHARD H. MEADE, III, M.D.
Associate Professor of Medicine, Tufts University School of Medicine, Boston, Massachusetts. Senior Physician, New England Medical Center Hospital, Boston, Massachusetts. Assistant Chief, Infectious Disease Service, Boston Floating Hospital, Massachusetts.
Lymphangitis. Lymph Node Infections. Osteomyelitis and Suppurative Arthritis.

HARRY MEDOVY, M.D., F.R.C.P. (Can.)
Professor of Pediatrics, University of Manitoba, Winnipeg, Canada. Consultant in Pediatrics, Children's Hospital of Winnipeg, Canada.
Pylorospasm. Pyloric Stenosis.

K. F. MEYER, M.D., Ph.D.
Director, G. W. Hooper Foundation, University of California, San Francisco. Emeritus Professor of Experimental Pathology and Microbiology University of California, San Francisco. Emeritus Lecturer, History of Health Sciences, University of California, San Francisco.
Plague.

JEROME H. MODELL, M.D.
Professor and Chairman of Anesthesiology, University of Florida College of Medicine, Gainesville. Attending Staff, Shands Teaching Hospital and Clinics, Gainesville, Florida.
Near-drowning (Nonfatal Submersion).

C. H. MOK, M.B.B.S., D.C.H.
Assistant Medical Superintendent, Austin Hospital, Victoria, Australia.
Visceral Larva Migrans.

RALPH E. MOLOSHOK, M.D.
Clinical Professor of Pediatrics, The Mount Sinai School of Medicine of the City University of New York, New York City. Attending Pediatrician, The Mount Sinai Hospital, New York City.
Familial Dysautonomia.

THOMAS S. MORSE, M.D.
Associate Professor of Surgery, Ohio State University College of Medicine, Columbus. Director of Outpatient Surgical Services, Children's Hospital, Columbus, Ohio.
The Injured Child—Evaluation and Initial Management.

EDWARD A. MORTIMER, JR., M.D.
Professor, University of New Mexico School of Medicine, Albuquerque. Chief of Pediatrics. Bernalillo County Medical Center, Albuquerque, New Mexico.
Nasopharyngitis (The Common Cold). Otitis Externa. Otologic Infections. Viral Respiratory Disease.

HUGO W. MOSER, M.D.
Professor of Neurology, Harvard Medical School Boston, Massachusetts. Neurologist, Massachusetts General Hospital, Boston. Assistant Superintendent, Walter E. Fernald State School, Waverley, Massachusetts. Codirector, Eunice Kennedy Shriver Center for Mental Retardation, Inc., Waltham, Massachusetts.
Mental Subnormality.

H. DAVID MOSIER, JR., M.D.
Professor of Pediatrics, University of California, Irvine, College of Medicine. Head, Division of Endocrinology and Metabolism, Department of Pediatrics, University of California, Irvine, College of Medicine. Attending Physician, Children's Hospital Medical Center, Long Beach, California.
Gynecomastia.

ARTHUR J. MOSS, M.D., M.B., M.S.
Professor and Chairman, Department of Pediatrics, UCLA School of Medicine.
Congestive Heart Failure. Congenital Heart Disease.

HARRY MOST, M.D., D.Sci. (Med.), D.T.M. and H. (Eng.)
Professor and Chairman, Department of Preventive Medicine, New York University Medical Center, New York City. Visiting Physician, Bellevue Hospital, New York City; University Hospital, New York City. Consultant, Booth Memorial Hospital, New York; Lenox Hill Hospital, New York City; Veterans Administration Hospital, New York City; Creedmoor State Hospital, New York City; Willowbrook State School, New York City.
Hookworm. Tapeworm.

HARRY LOUIS MUELLER, M.D.
Associate Clinical Professor of Pediatrics, Harvard Medical School, Boston, Massachusetts. Chief, Division of Allergy, Department of Medicine, Children's Hospital Medical Center, Boston, Massachusetts.
Stinging Insect Hypersensitivity.

ANDRÉ J. NAHMIAS, M.D., M.A., M.P.H.
Professor of Pediatrics, Chief, Infectious Disease and Immunology Division, Emory University School of Medicine, Atlanta; Grady Memorial Hospital, Atlanta; Henrietta Egleston Hospital for Children, Atlanta, Georgia.
Herpes Simplex Infections.

J. LAWRENCE NAIMAN, M.D.
Associate Professor of Pediatrics, Temple University School of Medicine, Philadelphia, Pennsylvania. Chief of Hematology, St. Christopher's Hospital for Children, Philadelphia, Pennsylvania.
Polycythemia.

THOMAS F. NECHELES, M.D., Ph.D.
Associate Professor of Pediatrics, Tufts University School of Medicine, Boston, Massachusetts. Chief, Pediatric Hematology, New England Medical Center Hospitals, Boston, Massachusetts.
Hemorrhagic Disorders. Congestive Splenomegaly, Splenic Cytopenia and Trauma to the Spleen.

ROBERT C. NEERHOUT, M.D.
Professor of Pediatrics, UCLA School of Medicine. Chief, Division of Pediatric Hematology–Oncology, UCLA Center for the Health Sciences and the Gwynne Hazen Cherry Memorial Laboratory, Los Angeles, California.
Aplastic and Hypoplastic Anemia.

CATHERINE NEILL, M.D., F.R.C.P. (Lon.)
Associate Professor of Pediatrics and Cardiologist, The Johns Hopkins University School of Medicine, Baltimore, Maryland. Pediatrician and Cardiologist, The Johns Hopkins Hospital, Baltimore, Maryland.
Bacterial Endocarditis.

JOHN D. NELSON, M.D.

Professor of Pediatrics, University of Texas Health Science Center at Dallas, Southwestern Medical School. Senior Attending Pediatrician, Parkland Memorial Hospital, Dallas, Texas. Active Attending Pediatrician, Children's Medical Center of Dallas, Texas.
Escherichia coli Infections. Pertussis.

JAMES C. NIEDERMAN, M.D.

Associate Clinical Professor of Epidemiology and Medicine, Yale University School of Medicine, New Haven, Connecticut. Associate Physician, Yale–New Haven Medical Center, Connecticut.
Infectious Mononucleosis.

DONOUGH O'BRIEN, M.D., F.R.C.P.

Professor of Pediatrics, University of Colorado Medical Center, Denver. Attending Staff, University of Colorado Medical Center, Denver.
Parenteral Nutrition in Infancy. Magnesium Deficiency.

EDWARD J. O'CONNELL, M.D.

Assistant Professor of Pediatrics, Mayo Medical School, Rochester, Minnesota. Consultant, Department of Pediatrics, Mayo Clinic and Mayo Foundation, Rochester, Minnesota.
Recurrent Bacterial Parotitis.

R. D. PAGTAKHAN, M.D., M.Sc.

Assistant Professor, Faculty of Medicine, University of Manitoba, Winnipeg, Canada. Assistant Director, Respiratory Service, Children's Hospital of Winnipeg, Manitoba, Canada. Director, Cystic Fibrosis Clinic, Children's Hospital of Winnipeg, Manitoba, Canada.
Disorders of the Lungs and Pleura.

MARCEL PATTERSON, M.D.

Professor of Internal Medicine, University of Texas Medical Branch at Galveston. Chief, Division of Gastroenterology, University of Texas Medical Branch at Galveston.
Ulcerative Colitis and Regional Enteritis.

HOWARD A. PEARSON, M.D.

Professor of Pediatrics, Yale University School of Medicine, New Haven, Connecticut. Attending Physician, Yale–New Haven Hospital, Connecticut.
Thalassemia.

HART deC. PETERSON, M.D.

Associate Professor of Pediatrics and Neurology, Cornell University Medical College, New York City. Associate Attending Pediatrician and Neurologist, New York Hospital, New York City.
Degenerative Diseases of the Central Nervous System.

LAWRENCE K. PICKETT, M.D.

William H. Carmalt Professor of Clinical Surgery and Pediatrics, Yale University School of Medicine, New Haven, Connecticut. Attending Surgeon, Yale–New Haven Hospital, Connecticut. Chief, Section of Pediatric Surgery, Yale University School of Medicine, New Haven, Connecticut.
Disorders of the Esophagus. Gastritis. Malformations and Malrotations of the Stomach and Intestine.

DONALD P. PINKEL, M.D.

Medical Director, St. Jude Children's Research Hospital, Memphis, Tennessee. Attending Physician, St. Jude Children's Research Hospital, Memphis; St. Joseph Hospital, Memphis, Tennessee.
Acute Leukemia.

LUIS MARCELO PRUDENT, M.D.

Sarda Hospital, Cap. Federal., Buenos Aires, Argentina.
The Drug-Addicted Newborn Infant.

DAVID H. H. PULLON, M.B., M.R.C.P., F.R.C.P.E., F.R.A.C.P., D.C.H.

Pediatrician, Waikato Hospital, Hamilton, New Zealand.
Amebic Meningoencephalitis.

EDWARD F. RABE, M.D.

Professor of Pediatrics (Neurology), Tufts University School of Medicine, Boston, Massachusetts. Chief, of Pediatric Neurology, New England Medical Center Hospitals (Boston Floating Hospital for Infants and Children), Massachusetts. Consultant, Paul A. Dever State School, Taunton, Massachusetts.
Hypsarhythmia and Infantile Spasms Hypoxic Encephalopathy and Acute Toxic Encephalopathy. Congenital Hypotonia.

JOSEPH L. RAUH, M.D.

Associate Professor of Pediatrics, University of Cincinnati College of Medicine, Ohio. Director, Adolescent Medical Services, Cincinnati General Hospital and Children's Hospital Medical Center, Ohio.
Emotional Problems of the Adolescent. Menstrual Disorders. Premarital Counseling for the Adolescent. Pregnancy in Adolescence.

ALAN B. RETIK, M.D.

Associate Clinical Professor of Urology, Tufts University School of Medicine, Boston, Massachusetts. Associate in Surgery, Harvard Medical School, Boston, Massachusetts. Director of Pediatric Urology, Boston Floating Hospital for Infants and Children; Massachusetts Hospital School for Crippled Children, Canton, Massachusetts.
Vesicoureteral Reflux. Neurogenic Vesical Dysfunction. Disorders of the Penis and Testes. Hernia and Hydrocele.

HARRIS D. RILEY, JR., M.D.

Professor of Pediatrics and Head of the Department, University of Oklahoma School of Medicine, Oklahoma City. Pediatrician-in-Chief, Children's Memorial Hospital, University of Oklahoma Health Sciences Center, Oklahoma City.
Measles (Rubeola).

DAVID L. RIMOIN, M.D., Ph.D.

Professor of Pediatrics and Medicine, UCLA School of Medicine. Chief, Division of Medical Genetics, Harbor General Hospital, Torrance, California.
Genetic Disease: Diagnosis, Counseling and Prevention.

ALAN M. ROBSON, M.D., M.R.C.P.

Associate Professor of Pediatrics, Washington University School of Medicine, St. Louis, Missouri. Director of Pediatric Nephrology, St. Louis Children's Hospital, Missouri.
Hypertension. Hypotension.

ALEJANDRO RODRIGUEZ, M.D.

Associate Professor of Pediatrics and Psychiatry, Johns Hopkins University School of Medicine and Johns Hopkins Hospital, Baltimore, Maryland.
Emotional Disorders.

FRED S. ROSEN, M.D.

James L. Gamble Professor of Pediatrics, Harvard Medical School, Boston, Massachusetts. Chief, Division of Immunology, Children's Hospital Medical Center, Boston, Massachusetts.
Angioneurotic Edema.

LEON ROSEN, M.D., D.P.H.

Clinical Professor of Tropical Medicine and Medical Microbiology, University of Hawaii School of Medicine, Honolulu. Head, Pacific Research Section, National Institute of Allergy and Infectious Diseases, Honolulu, Hawaii.
Eosinophilic Meningitis. Angiostrongyliasis.

JON E. ROSENBLATT, M.D.

Assistant Professor of Medicine, UCLA School of Medicine. Assistant Chief, Infectious Disease Section, Veterans Administration Center–Wadsworth Hospital Center, Los Angeles, California.
Infections Due to Proteus, Klebsiella, Pseudomonas and Other Gram-Negative Bacilli.

JAMES P. ROSENBLUM, M.D.

Assistant Clinical Professor, Department of Psychiatry, UCLA School of Medicine. Associate Attending Physician, Department of Psychiatry, Cedars of Lebanon Hospital, Los Angeles, California. Adjunct Attending Physician, Department of Psychiatry, Mt. Sinai Hospital, Los Angeles, California.
Psychosomatic Illness.

JACK H. RUBINSTEIN, M.D.

Professor of Pediatrics, University of Cincinnati College of Medicine, Ohio. Director, University Affiliated Clinical Program for the Mentally Retarded and Children's Neuromuscular Diagnostic Clinic, Cincinnati, Ohio. Attending Pediatrician, Children's Hospital, Cincinnati; Cincinnati General Hospital, Ohio.
Craniostenosis, Crouzon's Disease and Apert's Syndrome. Hypertelorism and Hypotelorism.

FINDLAY E. RUSSELL, M.D.

Professor of Neurology, Physiology and Biology, University of Southern California, Los Angeles. Director, Laboratory of Neurological Research, Los Angeles County–University of Southern California Medical Center.
Snakebite.

HARRY J. SACKS, M.D.

Clinical Professor of Pathology, University of Southern California Medical School, Los Angeles. Director, Department of Clinical Pathology, Cedars-Sinai Medical Center, Los Angeles, California.
Hemolytic Reaction to Transfusion of Incompatible Blood.

JOSEPH W. ST. GEME, JR., M.D.

Professor and Chairman, Department of Pediatrics, UCLA School of Medicine; Harbor General Hospital, Torrance, California.
Ornithosis (Psittacosis).

FREDERICK J. SAMAHA, M.D.

Associate Professor, University of Pittsburgh School of Medicine, Pennsylvania. Chief, Pediatric Neurology, Children's Hospital of Pittsburgh, Pennsylvania.
Muscular Dystrophy and Related Myopathies.

JAY P. SANFORD, M.D.

Professor of Internal Medicine, University of Texas Southwestern Medical School at Dallas. Senior Attending Physician, Parkland Memorial Hospital, Dallas, Texas. Consultant Physician, St. Paul Hospital, Dallas; Presbyterian Hospital of Dallas; John Peter Smith Hospitals, Fort Worth, Texas.
Rat Bite and Rat-Bite Fever.

ARTHUR D. SCHWABE, M.D.

Professor of Medicine, UCLA School of Medicine. Chief, Division of Gastroenterology, UCLA School of Medicine.
Familial Mediterranean Fever (Benign Paroxysmal Peritonitis, Familial Paroxysmal Polyserositis, Armenian Disease).

ROLAND B. SCOTT, M.D., F.A.A.P.

Professor of Pediatrics, College of Medicine, and Center for Sickle Cell Anemia, Howard University. Senior Pediatrician, Freedmen's Hospital; Senior Attending Pediatrician, D. C. General Hospital; Children's Hospital, Washington, D. C.
Sickle Cell Disease.

ALFRED W. SENFT, M.D., D.T.M.&H., M.P.H.

Associate Professor, Division of Biological and Medical Sciences, Brown University, Providence, Rhode Island. Attending Physician, Roger Williams Hospital and Miriam Hospital, Providence, Rhode Island. Consultant, Falmouth Hospital (Courtesy Staff), Falmouth, Massachusetts.
Schistosomiasis.

BORIS SENIOR, M.D.

Professor of Pediatrics, Tufts University School of Medicine, Boston Massachusetts. Chief, Pediatric Endocrine-Metabolic Service, New England Medical Center (Boston Floating Hospital for Infants and Children), Boston, Massachusetts.
Thyroid Disease. Adrenal Disease.

HARVEY L. SHARP, M.D.

Associate Professor of Pediatrics, University of Minnesota Medical Center, Minneapolis.
Cirrhosis and Tumors of the Liver. Chronic Aggressive Hepatitis. Congenital Abnormalities of the Gallbladder and Bile Ducts.

SHEILA SHERLOCK, M.D.

Professor of Internal Medicine, Royal Free Hospital School of Medicine (University of London), London, England. Consultant Physician, Royal Free Hospital, London, England.
Portal Hypertension.

MADOKA SHIBUYA, M.D.

Assistant Professor of Pediatrics, Cornell University Medical College, New York City. Attending Pediatrician, New York Hospital, New York City.
Glomerulonephritis.

SYDNEY SHORE, M.D.

Chief of Otolaryngology, Scripps Clinic and Research Foundation Hospital, La Jolla; Children's Hospital, San Diego; Sharp Memorial Hospital, San Diego; Scripps Memorial Hospital, La Jolla; El Centro Community Hospital, California.
The Tonsil and Adenoid Problem.

CALVIN CHIA JUNG SIA, M.D.

Associate Clinical Professor of Pediatrics, University of Hawaii School of Medicine, Honolulu, Active Staff, Kauikeolani Children's Hospital, Honolulu; Kapiolani Maternity Hospital, Honolulu, Hawaii.
Leprosy.

MURRAY SIDMAN, Ph.D.

Professor of Psychology, Northeastern University, Boston, Massachusetts. Director, Behavioral Sciences Unit, Eunice Kennedy Shriver Center for Mental Retardation, Inc., Waltham, Massachusetts.
Mental Subnormality.

SHELDON C. SIEGEL, M.D.

Clinical Professor of Pediatrics, UCLA School of Medicine. Co-director, Pediatric Allergy Clinic, UCLA Center for Health Sciences.
Atopic Dermatitis. Serum Sickness. Anaphylaxis.

BRADLEY E. SMITH, M.D.

Professor and Chairman, Department of Anesthesiology, Vanderbilt University Hospital, Nashville, Tennessee. Chief Anesthesiologist, Vanderbilt University Hospital, Nashville, Tennessee.
Resuscitation of the Newborn.

FRANK E. SMITH, M.D.

Assistant Professor, Pharmacology and Medicine, Baylor College of Medicine, Houston, Texas. Associate Attending Physician, Methodist Hospital, Houston; Ben Taub General Hospital, Houston, Texas. Attending Physician, Houston Veterans Administration Hospital, Texas.
Trichuriasis. Balantidiasis. Giardiasis. Ascariasis. Enterobiasis.

ROBERT M. SMITH, M.D.

Director of Anesthesia, Children's Hospital Medical Center, Boston, Massachusetts.
High Fever.

MYRON M. SOKAL, M.D.

Attending Physician, North Shore Hospital, Manhasset, New York.
The Drug-Addicted Newborn Infant.

ADRIAN SPITZER, M.D.

Associate Professor of Pediatrics, Albert Einstein College of Medicine of Yeshiva University, Bronx, New York. Attending Pediatrician, Bronx Municipal Hospital Center; Hospital of the Albert Einstein College of Medicine, Bronx; Lincoln Hospital, Bronx, New York.
Chronic Renal Insufficiency (Chronic Uremia).

ALEX J. STEIGMAN M.D., Sc.D. (Hon.)

Professor of Pediatrics, Mount Sinai School of Medicine, New York City.
Active and Passive Immunization.

BENNETT M. STEIN, M.D.

Professor, Neurological Surgery, Tufts University School of Medicine, Boston, Massachusetts. Chairman, Neurological Surgery, New England Medical Center Hospital, Boston, Massachusetts.
Hydrocephalus. Brain Tumors. Spinal Diseases.

GUNNAR B. STICKLER, M.D., Ph.D.

Professor of Pediatrics, Mayo Medical School, Rochester, Minnesota. Head, Section of Pediatrics, Mayo Clinic and Mayo Foundation, Rochester, Minnesota.
Cystic Disease of the Kidney. Hydronephrosis and Disorders of the Ureter. Malignant Tumors of the Kidney.

E. RICHARD STIEHM, M.D.

Professor of Pediatrics, University of California, Los Angeles.
Purpura Fulminans. Disseminated Intravascular Coagulation.

H. HARLAN STONE, M.D.

Associate Professor of Surgery, Emory University School of Medicine, Atlanta, Georgia. Director of Pediatric Surgical, Trauma, and Burn Services, Grady Memorial Hospital, Atlanta, Georgia. Attending Surgeon, Emory University Hospital, Atlanta; Henrietta Egleston Hospital for Children, Atlanta, Georgia.
Lymphedema. Lymphangioma.

D. EUGENE STRANDNESS, JR., M.D.

Professor of Surgery and Chief, Peripheral Vascular Division, University of Washington School of Medicine, Seattle, Washington. Surgeon, University Hospital and Veterans Administration Hospital, Seattle, Washington.
Peripheral Vascular Disease.

RONALD G. STRAUSS, M.D.

Fellow, Division of Hematology Research, Children's Hospital Research Foundation, University of Cincinnati College of Medicine, Ohio.
Amyloidosis.

LEO R. SULLIVAN, M.D.

Assistant Professor of Pediatrics (Neurology), Tufts University School of Medicine, Boston, Massachusetts. Pediatric Neurologist, New England Center Hospital, Boston, Massachusetts.
Depression and Suicide. Paralysis of the Facial Nerve. Brachial Palsy. Injury to the Sciatic Nerve Following Intragluteal Injections.

PHILIP SUNSHINE, M.D.

Associate Professor of Pediatrics, Stanford School of Medicine, California. Director of Nurseries, Stanford Medical Center, California. Director of Pediatric Gastroenterology, Stanford Medical Center, California.
Vomiting.

SIDNEY J. SUSSMAN, M.D.

Associate Professor of Pediatrics, Temple University Medical School. Director, Ambulatory Services, Project Director, Model Cities Comprehensive Health Care

Program, St. Christopher's Hospital for Children, Philadelphia, Pennsylvania.
Mycoplasma Pneumonial Infections.

ORVAR SWENSON, M.D.

Professor of Surgery, Northwestern University Medical School, Chicago, Illinois. Surgeon-in-Chief, Children's Memorial Hospital, Chicago, Illinois.
Hirschsprung's Disease.

LARRY H. TABER, M.D.

Assistant Professor of Pediatrics, Baylor College of Medicine, Houston, Texas. Attending Physician, Ben Taub General Hospital, Houston; Children's Hospital, Houston; The Methodist Hospital, Houston, Texas.
Meningococcal Disease.

HUGO R. TAPIA, M.D.

Instructor of Medicine, Mayo Medical School, Rochester, Minnesota. Consultant, Division of Nephrology and Internal Medicine, Mayo Clinic and Mayo Foundation, Rochester, Minnesota.
Hepatolenticular Degeneration (Wilson's Disease).

PETER K. THOMPSON, M.D.

Instructor, Department of Obstetrics and Gynecology, Baylor College of Medicine, Houston, Texas.
Disorders of the Vulva and Vagina. Disorders of the Uterus, Tubes and Ovaries. Tumors of the Uterus, Tubes and Ovaries.

WILLIAM H. TOOLEY, M.D.

Professor of Pediatrics and Member of the Cardiovascular Research Institute, University of California, San Francisco. Chief, Children's Chest Disease, University of California, San Francisco.
Idiopathic Respiratory Distress Syndrome.

LUTHER B. TRAVIS, M.D.

Associate Professor of Pediatrics, University of Texas Medical Branch at Galveston. Director and Attending Nephrologist, Division of Nephrology, University of Texas Medical Branch Hospital, Galveston, Texas.
Diabetes Mellitus.

DENNY L. TUFFANELLI, M.D.

Associate Clinical Professor, University of California, San Francisco.
Scleroderma. Discoid Lupus Erythematosus.

J. THOMAS UNGERLEIDER, M.D.

Associate Professor of Psychiatry, UCLA Center for the Health Sciences.
Drug Abuse and the Adolescent.

JOHN P. UTZ, M.D.

Professor of Medicine, Medical College of Virginia, Richmond. Chairman, Division of Immunology and Infectious Diseases, Medical College of Virginia, Richmond.
Systemic Mycotic Infections.

ROBERT A. VICKERS, D.D.S., M.S.D.

Professor, University of Minnesota School of Dentistry, Minneapolis. Attending Staff, University of Minnesota Hospitals, Minneapolis; Hennepin County General Hospital, Minneapolis, Minnesota.
Abnormalities, Injuries and Diseases of the Oral Region.

FRED Q. VROOM, M.D.

Associate Professor, Department of Medicine (Neurology), University of Florida, Gainesville.
Periodic Paralysis. Myositis Ossificans.

JACK WAINSCHEL, M.D.

Assistant Clinical Professor of Neurology, University of Southern California School of Medicine, Los Angeles. Consultant in Neurology, Los Angeles County–University of Southern California Medical Center. Attending Staff, Methodist Hospital of Southern California, Arcadia.
Snakebite.

STANLEY L. WALLACE, M.D.

Clinical Professor of Medicine, New York University Medical Center, New York City. Attending Physician, Jewish Hospital of Brooklyn; Bellevue Hospital, New York City. Consultant in Rheumatology, Veterans Administration Hospital, Brooklyn; U. S. Naval Hospital, St. Albans; Queens Hospital Center, Brooklyn; Greenpoint Hospital, Brooklyn, New York.
Disorders of Porphyrin, Hemoglobin and Purine Metabolism.

ALAN A. WANDERER, M.D.

Clinical Assistant Professor of Pediatrics, University of Colorado Medical School, Denver. Attending Staff, National Jewish Hospital at Denver, Colorado.
Hypersensitivity to Physical Factors.

PAUL F. WEHRLE, M.D.

Hastings Professor of Pediatrics, University of Southern California School of Medicine, Los Angeles. Director of Pediatrics, Los Angeles County–University of Southern California Medical Center.
Hemophilus influenzae Infections.

LOUIS WEINSTEIN, M.D., Ph.D.

Professor of Medicine, Tufts University School of Medicine, Boston, Massachusetts. Lecturer in Medicine, Harvard Medical School, Boston, Massachusetts. Chief, Infectious Disease Service, New England Medical Center Hospital, Boston, Massachusetts. Associate Physician, Medical Service, Massachusetts General Hospital, Boston.
Diphtheria.

PAUL J. WIESNER, M.D.

Chief, Operation Research Section, Venereal Disease Branch, State and Community Services Division, Center for Disease Control, Department of Health, Education and Welfare, Atlanta, Georgia.
Syphilis.

GEORGE F. WILGRAM, M.D., Ph.D.

Clinical Professor of Medicine, Tufts University School of Medicine, Boston, Massachusetts.
Diseases of the Hair and Scalp.

ISAAC WILLIS, M.D.

Assistant Professor of Dermatology, Johns Hopkins University School of Medicine, Baltimore, Maryland. Attending Dermatologist, Johns Hopkins Hospital, Baltimore; Baltimore City Hospitals; Good Samaritan Hospital, Baltimore, Maryland.
Photodermatoses.

DAVID M. WILSON, M.D.

Assistant Professor of Medicine, Mayo Medical School, Rochester, Minnesota. Consultant, Division of Nephrology and Internal Medicine, Mayo Clinic and Mayo Foundation, Rochester, Minnesota.
Hepatolenticular Degeneration (Wilson's Disease).

HEINZ J. WITTIG, M.D.

Professor, Department of Pediatrics, University of Florida College of Medicine, Gainesville, Florida. Director of Pediatric Allergy, University of Florida College of Medicine, Gainesville, Florida.
Allergic Rhinitis.

JAMES A. WOLFF, M.D.

Professor of Pediatrics, College of Physicians & Surgeons, Columbia University, New York City. Attending Pediatrician, Babies Hospital, New York City.
Anemias of Iron Deficiency, Blood Loss, Renal Disease and Chronic Infection. Megaloblastic Anemia.

WALTER P. WORK, M.D.

Professor and Chairman, Department of Otorhinolaryngology, University of Michigan Medical Center, Ann Arbor.
Salivary Gland Tumors.

HARRY T. WRIGHT, JR., M.D.

Associate Professor of Pediatrics, University of Southern California School of Medicine, Los Angeles. Attending Physician and Research Associate, Division of Virology, Children's Hospital of Los Angeles, California.
Enterovirus Infections. Acute Aseptic Meningitis Syndrome.

SUMNER J. YAFFE, M.D.

Professor of Pediatrics, School of Medicine, State University of New York at Buffalo. Associate Chairman, Department of Pediatrics, School of Medicine, State University of New York at Buffalo.
Adverse Drug Reactions—A Pharmacologic Approach.

JAMES N. YAMAZAKI, M.D.

Clinical Professor of Pediatrics, UCLA School of Medicine. Attending Physician, Neurology Division, Children's Hospital of Los Angeles, California.
Radiation Injury.

MARTHA DUKES YOW, M.D.

Professor of Pediatrics, Baylor College of Medicine, Houston, Texas. Attending Physician, Ben Taub General Hospital, Houston; Children's Hospital, Houston; the Methodist Hospital, Houston, Texas.
Meningococcal Disease.

SEYMOUR ZIMBLER, M.D.

Associate Professor, Tufts University School of Medicine, Boston, Massachusetts. Vice Chairman Department of Orthopedics, Tufts University School of Medicine, Boston, Massachusetts.
Bone Tumors.

Contents

4
RESPIRATORY TRACT

5
CARDIOVASCULAR SYSTEM

6
DIGESTIVE TRACT

7
BLOOD

8
SPLEEN AND LYMPHATIC SYSTEMS

9
ENDOCRINE SYSTEM

14
BONES AND JOINTS

15
MUSCLES

16
SKIN

Alvin H. Jacobs, Editor

17
THE EYE

18
THE EAR

20
ALLERGY

21
ACCIDENTS AND EMERGENCIES

22
UNCLASSIFIED DISEASES

23
DISEASES PECULIAR TO THE NEWBORN

24
MISCELLANEOUS

1

Nutrition

Generalized Undernutrition
(Marasmus)

LEWIS A. BARNESS, M.D.

Marasmus is usually due to a combination of food (calorie) insufficiency and social and emotional deprivation. An attempt should be made to treat all aspects simultaneously. Provision should be made for education of the parents and stimulation and care of the child.

Dietary treatment is based on suitable modification of normal daily requirements. For the first year these are approximately 100 calories per kilogram; after the first year, the formula is as follows:

Age in years × 100 + 1000 = Calories required

The diet should consist of 8 to 15 per cent of the calories as protein, 35 to 45 per cent as fat, and 35 to 45 per cent as carbohydrate. If specific vitamin deficiencies are detected, therapeutic doses of vitamins should be administered. Otherwise, the recommended daily dietary allowances of vitamins should be administered.

Because these infants and children frequently are famished and have a voracious appetite, care in early repair is necessary. Ordinarily, giving the child 75 per cent of the estimated caloric requirement the first day or two will result in no diarrhea or vomiting. If the child tolerates this, the caloric intake is increased to 100 per cent of the estimated requirement for three to five days, and then the child is fed *ad libitum*.

Weight gain is usually prompt. However, failure to gain weight regularly after the onset of adequate dietary intake is not cause for alarm, since shifts in the body water may occur over a three- to six-week period. However, failure to gain should prompt one to reinvestigate the possibility of excess losses, infections or inadequate emotional support.

Marasmus secondary to anorexia nervosa may respond not only to the usual psychiatric measures, but also to total intravenous hyperalimentation. If at all possible, other causes of marasmus should not be treated by intravenous hyperalimentation until the oral route has been tried.

Obesity

S. L. HAMMAR, M.D.

Obesity is one of the most frequent serious nutritional problems encountered in the practice of pediatrics. The current approaches to management of obesity in the older child and adolescent have been almost totally unsuccessful in producing long-term weight control. Girls from the lower strata of our society appear to be particularly vulnerable to obesity, which is often evident by six years of age (Stunkard et al.). Once obesity has developed, successful weight reduction and maintenance are rare. At least 85 per cent of patients who become obese during childhood and adolescence will remain obese as adults (Abraham and Nordsieck). For most adolescents, obesity has serious behavioral and social consequences which are as difficult to manage as the weight problem. If this complex public health problem is to be controlled, greater attempts must be directed toward prompt identification of susceptible individuals and prevention of excessive weight gain during infancy and early childhood.

INFANCY AND EARLY CHILDHOOD

Critical periods for developing obesity appear to be during the rapid cell proliferation and early growth phases of infancy and early childhood. Excessive nutrition during this period may produce increased numbers of adipose cells, which make the individual perpetually susceptible to obesity (Hirsch and Knittle). Prevention should begin in the prenatal clinic, when expectant parents with a family incidence of obesity can be identified. Efforts should be directed not only toward attempting to change family eating patterns but also toward sensitizing parents to appropriate feeding and activity patterns of their expected infant. The relationship between genetic and environmental factors in predisposing to obesity is not clear, but large mothers frequently produce large infants. These babies often grow rapidly and can be readily overfed. Consequently, they require closer surveillance of their growth patterns and closer supervision of their early feeding patterns. Careful monitoring of growth in length and weight utilizing a standard growth chart is essential and a habit which should be ingrained early in obesity-prone families.

Breast feeding or the use of an iron-supplemented proprietary formula is a recommended method of meeting the nutritional requirements of the large, obesity-prone infant. If breast feeding is not continued for the whole first year of life, which is usually the case in the United States, the use of one of the lower caloric-density proprietary formulas, which have recently been introduced commercially, can be instituted following weaning. These formulas provide approximately 16 calories per ounce, are higher in protein content and have substituted vegetable fats for animal fats. Their use is preferable to substituting skim milk or half-skim milk in the diet after four to six months of age. Using skim milk significantly reduces the caloric intake, but it also effectively removes from the diet the source of essential fatty acids which are important during the active growth period. Further, in order to meet the caloric requirements necessary for adequate growth, the intake of infant solids may have to be increased quantitatively more than the infant is able to consume. By increasing solids, sodium, potassium and chloride are also increased, expanding the renal solute load and water demands.

The mother will need specific guidance in the introduction and selection of solid foods. The social pressure to institute solid foods early and the erroneous impression that this will increase satiety and promote sleeping throughout the night are significant factors which require much parental education and supportive counseling. The introduction of solid foods should be delayed until late in the first year of life; when solids are added, they should be carefully selected. Some fruits and vegetables are relatively low in calories, whereas cereals, eggs, meats, mixed dinners, wet pack cereals and desserts are high contributors to the caloric intake and should be excluded from the diet of large, rapidly gaining infants. Homogenized milk should be avoided during the first year of life. Serious efforts should be made to avoid prolonged bottle feeding. These infants should be weaned from the bottle by 12 months of age. The baby should not be put to bed with a bottle. Allowing the infant to become accustomed to sucking on his bottle in bed not only adds unnecessary calories to the diet but is now believed to increase dental caries and contribute to middle ear infections (Hemenway and Smith). Pacifiers may be substituted at times to satisfy the infant's sucking needs. The visiting public health nurse is often a resource that can provide psychologic support for the mother and help establish and reinforce proper eating patterns for the infant. Many mothers feel guilty about restricting the food intake of their infants, but a plump baby is not an indication of good mothering or of a healthy baby.

During the second year of life, 16 ounces or a pint of milk per day is an adequate intake together with appropriate table foods. Snacks should be controlled carefully. Toddlers usually need snacks, but these foods should be nutritionally sound. Pieces of cheese, lunch meat, frankfurters, Vienna sausage and fresh fruits and vegetables are snack items which are nutritious. Products such as potato chips, cookies, cheese puffs, candy, sweetened fruit drinks and soft drinks are high in calories, nutritionally poor and should be strenuously avoided.

The importance of proper activity is often overlooked during early childhood. Establishing and promoting patterns conducive to energy expenditure are as important as limiting dietary intake. Excessive confinement in restrictive playpens should be discouraged, and regular periods of daily exercise such as walks and outdoor play activities should be encouraged as a part of the weight control program of these children.

THE OBESE SCHOOL-AGE CHILD

The management of obesity in the school-age child requires a high degree of parental responsibility, understanding and cooperation. Motivation on the part of the child to lose weight is often minimal and short-lived. Dietary instruction should involve both the mother and child; the mother, however, will usually have to be responsible for food selection and purchasing. She can help limit the size of food portions by filling the plates in the kitchen rather than serving the meals family style. Desserts, when served, should be limited to those which are lower in calories. The availability of snack foods and sweets should be restricted. During school the child should carry a packed lunch from home, over which the mother has closer control, rather than eating the school lunch or purchasing lunch elsewhere. Spending money should be carefully monitored by the parents.

The parents' attitude toward the child's weight problem requires careful investigation and discussions. The child's obesity at this age often becomes the focus of parental and sibling criticism; he is subjected to teasing and ridicule and scapegoated by other family members. Mealtime becomes a nightmare of belittling, nagging, caustic comments and discriminatory restrictions. The importance of carefully evaluating the family's interrelationships and attitudes cannot be overemphasized. At this stage, a child's obesity usually becomes a total family problem and requires the mutual support and cooperation of all family members in treatment. Often the excuse is used that it is not possible to prepare a special diet for the obese child or that nonobese siblings or the hard-working father requires more food and will not tolerate food restriction.

Candy, sweets and desserts are often used by parents as a reward for good behavior or as a means of bribing children to eat less desired foods such as vegetables at mealtime. The use of sweets as positive reinforcers should be vigorously prohibited.

Most children get very hungry by late afternoon. Again, the choice of snack items is important. The use of fresh fruits and vegetables should be encouraged in preference to "junk" foods.

Regular periods of physical activity should be prescribed. The family should be encouraged to plan frequent recreational activities and to assist the child in developing skills in swimming, sports and hobbies.

THE OBESE ADOLESCENT

Like diabetes or epilepsy, obesity is a chronic disease which, for the adolescent, has serious behavioral and social implications. The goals in working with an obese adolescent should be not only to produce a weight loss if possible but, more importantly, also to help the patient understand his disease and the environmental forces which influence his weight control, and make the best possible adaptation and personal adjustment to his life situation. To lose weight successfully requires extremely high motivation, intelligence, some compulsiveness and the ability to set long-range goals. Not every obese adolescent is a candidate for weight reduction.

Ideally, this problem lends itself to a team approach. As a minimum, an obese adolescent should receive a thorough and comprehensive medical evaluation before a treatment program is initiated. Ninety-five per cent of adolescent obesity is exogenous; rarely are endocrine disorders, central nervous system tumors or other organic abnormalities responsible. The young adolescent with longstanding childhood obesity usually has advanced skeletal maturation and moderately accelerated pubertal development (Bruch, Forbes). A careful review of previous height-weight data and growth patterns, a bone age evaluation and an assessment of pubertal stage will help confirm a diagnosis of exogenous obesity.

Even though the patient is clinically euthyroid, a test of thyroid function is often helpful in convincing parents and teenager that hypothyroidism has been considered and ruled out. In adolescents with a family history of diabetes, a glucose tolerance test will identify those with carbohydrate intolerance and chemical diabetes for whom aggressive weight reduction is extremely important.

The initial medical examination should also include a behavioral assessment or psychologic status and an exploration of dietary intake, eating habits, activity patterns and family dynamics. It is important to develop a thorough understanding of the psychologic characteristics and life situation of obese teenagers in order to identify those for whom a weight reduction program is inappropriate or who merit further psychiatric investigation. Often the obese teenager is responding to parental, family or outside pressure to lose weight; his own motivation to lose weight may be minimal. The patient's goals for weight loss are often unrealistic. Most obese adolescents show signs of depression and extremely low self-esteem. However, teenagers with significant complaints of chronic fatigue, sleep problems, frequent crying spells and suicidal thoughts should be referred for psychiatric consultation before attempting weight reduction. Characteristically, many obese teenagers are immature, passive and overly dependent on their parents. Those who are unable to assume responsibility for their own diet or weight reduction program are poor candidates for treatment.

Dietary habits and nutrition knowledge must be carefully reviewed. Having the patient keep a seven-day food diary (including weekend) is an excellent tool for obtaining information regarding normal eating habits. It is also a good test of motivation. A teenager who will not keep a food record for a brief period of time is not a candidate for weight reduction. The patient should be asked to record the types of foods and approximate quantities eaten for breakfast, lunch, dinner and snacks. For easy record keeping, forms can be mimeographed and given to the patient at his initial visit. These records are reviewed with the patient at the next visit and assist the physician in designing the diet program. It is also helpful to have the patient keep a seven-day activity record, noting the approximate times spent studying, watching television, playing and sleeping.

Treatment. DIETARY MANAGEMENT. Providing good nutritional education and knowledge regarding proper food selection and caloric food values is essential for weight control. It is also laborious and time consuming. The long-term results in maintaining weight losses appear to be better in adolescents given intensive nutritional instruction than in those managed in a more flexible manner (Hammar et al.). There is no evidence that any one type of weight reducing diet is superior to another (Wilson). Crash diets are only temporary measures, difficult to maintain for long periods and expensive, and they do not permanently change the patient's dietary patterns. Most adolescents can adhere to crash diets for only a few days, after which they become too hungry and revert to their regular eating habits. Starvation regimens should not be used for weight reduction in children or adolescents. The diet should be well balanced and nutritionally adequate. The diet should be flexible and allow for variety to prevent monotony. If an adolescent experiences extreme hunger in the late afternoon or evening, part of his lunch or dinner allotment can be used for these snack periods. The food likes and dislikes of the individual must be considered in designing the diet. A positive approach in diet instruction, which emphasizes foods which can and should be eaten, rather than those which cannot, should be used. A diabetic exchange diet is sound and fairly easy for teenage patients to follow. A 1200 calorie diet is an absolute minimum for growing adolescents. It is difficult to meet nutritional requirements for growth on diets less than 1200 calories, and the teenager is constantly hungry. Low calorie soft drinks and snacks of fruits and vegetables help to reduce hunger. Ideally, an effective diet should induce approximately a 1- to 2-pound weight loss per week. The patient should be counseled to expect plateaus or periods during which no weight loss occurs.

The adolescent should be provided with a calorie counter. Requesting the patient to calculate his caloric intake one or two days per week will reinforce his knowledge of caloric values.

The use of anorexigenic drugs is discouraged. Their effectiveness is usually short-lived since tolerance is quickly induced, and the potential for drug abuse is inherent. In addition, the use of drugs tends to perpetuate the adolescent's magical thinking and search for a pill which will solve his weight problem.

Some form of regular exercise should be prescribed as a part of the treatment program. The type of physical activity should be the adolescent's choice. Walking the dog for 30 minutes each evening, swimming or using such programs as the Royal Canadian Air Force exercises are often acceptable. Exercises alone will do little to produce weight loss but are an important aspect of changing the obese adolescent's activity pattern.

Frequent follow-up visits are necessary for support and counseling. These visits should occur a minimum of every two weeks. Since most obese adolescents have adjustment difficulties, the physician should use his patient contact regarding the diet as an entree for discussing other important problems in the teenager's life such as peer relationships and problems with parents. Criticism, threats and rebukes regarding an adolescent's failure to adhere to the diet do little good and irreparably damage the physician-patient relationship. The adolescent must be encouraged to accept total responsibility for his diet and treatment. If he is not motivated for treatment or does not view his weight as a problem, this should be openly recognized and discussed. Parents should be advised to reduce their pressure for weight loss until the adolescent desires professional assistance.

GROUP THERAPY. Many obese adolescents can be treated more effectively in groups. In many communities, commercial organizations, such as Weight Watchers or TOPS, are available and may be an appropriate referral source for obese individuals. Some have special groups for adolescents. These offer the advantage of providing an accepting climate as well as a social outlet for the obese girl. In addition, they can provide more intensive support and nutritional education than can a busy physician. The major disadvantage is the cost. At the present time, some schools have established special clubs or self-improvement groups for obese youngsters. The school nurse or counselor is usually a good source of information regarding the availability of such groups. It is recommended that every adolescent receive a medical-psychologic evaluation before being referred for group treatment.

Recently, behavioral modification techniques have been applied to the treatment of obesity (Bernard, Stuart, Stunkard). The results of regimens which incorporate techniques such as counting each bite of food, eating only under controlled situations or using positive reinforcers for pounds lost have been promising with adults but appear to be less successful with adolescents. To adhere to such a program, adolescents must be highly motivated, moderately compulsive and have constant parental support and reinforcement.

SUMMARY. In treating adolescent obesity, the following factors must be kept in mind:

1. Successful weight control requires maturity, intelligence and the ability to delay gratification and set long-range goals. Passive, dependent, immature adolescents, or those with subnormal intelligence are poor candidates for a weight reduction program.

2. The environment plays a critical role in promoting and perpetuating the obese state. Hereditary or familial predisposition to obesity cannot be altered but at best only controlled by the availability of food. Obesity is in most instances a lifelong chronic disease. Early recognition and intervention are the only effective means of preventing adolescent obesity.

3. The obese adolescent usually occupies a unique role within the family structure, often being a source of embarrassment, a focus of family conflicts and a scapegoat. These firmly ingrained family attitudes and methods of relating are refractory to change and tend to undermine any attempts to disturb the status quo. Intensive family counseling may be required to help the adolescent.

4. The social pressures on the obese adolescent are usually underestimated. These result in social isolation, withdrawal from the peer group, inactivity and damaged self-esteem, making rehabilitation difficult.

5. For many obese adolescents eating becomes an obsessive source of comfort and relief from depression. When this source is restricted or removed, other means of satisfaction must be sought.

6. The primary objective of treatment should be to help the adolescent achieve a satisfactory adjustment, and the second is to help him achieve a normal body weight if possible. Not every obese adolescent is a candidate for weight reduction.

References

Abraham, S., and Nordsieck, M.: Relationship of Excess Weight in Children and Adults. *Public Health Rep.*, 75:263, 1970.

Bernard, J. L.: Rapid Treatment of Gross Obesity by Operant Techniques. *Psychol. Rep.*, 23:663, 1968.

Bruch, H.: Obesity in Relation to Puberty. *J. Pediat.*, 19:365, 1941.

Forbes, G. B.: Lean Body Mass and Fat in Obese Children. *Pediatrics,* 34:308, 1964.

Hammar, S. L., Campbell, V., and Woolley, J.: Treating Adolescent Obesity, Long-Range Evaluation of Previous Therapy. *Clin. Pediat.*, 10:46, 1971.

Hemenway, W. G., and Smith, R. O.: Treating Acute Otitis Media. *Postgrad. Med.*, 47:110, 1970.

Hirsch, J., and Knittle, J. L.: Cellularity of Obese and Nonobese Human Adipose Tissue. *Fed. Proc.,* 29: 1516, 1970.

Stuart, R. B.: Behavioral Control of Overeating. *Behav. Res. Ther.*, 5:357, 1967.

Stunkard, A.: New Therapies for the Eating Disorders, *Arch. Gen. Psychiat.*, 26:391, 1972.

Stunkard, A., d'Aquili, E., Fox, S., and Filion R.: Influence of Social Class on Obesity and Thinness in Children. J.A.M.A., 221:579, 1972.

Wilson, N. L. (ed.): *Obesity*. Philadelphia, F. A. Davis Co., 1969.

Kwashiorkor

(Protein-Calorie Malnutrition)

JOHN D. L. HANSEN, M.D.

Kwashiorkor (like nutritional marasmus) is a severe and late form of protein-calorie malnutrition. Management therefore depends on the stage at which the malnutrition becomes manifest. *Early* protein-calorie malnutrition affects most children in underdeveloped populations who present to the doctor with failure to thrive or with unrelated complaints of all kinds but particularly of infections and diarrhea. It is diagnosed by finding the weight and height to be below the third percentile. The well-known signs of kwashiorkor, such as the skin lesions and edema, are usually not evident at this point.

These children must be regarded as being at risk as far as their nutritional status is concerned. Increasing the protein and calorie intake in the form of milk or other suitable supplements produces rapid improvement in growth and well-being. Dietary advice or assistance given with the specific treatment for the presenting complaint reduces the incidence of kwashiorkor and marasmus and leads to a significant reduction of preschool mortality and morbidity.

Treatment. Once kwashiorkor or marasmus has developed there are four main principles in therapy: resuscitation, dietary therapy, anti-infective therapy and follow-up care.

RESUSCITATION. This is of the utmost importance in the first 24 hours. Many children, although edematous, are nevertheless relatively dehydrated from diarrhea and suffer from electrolyte imbalance and acid-base disturbance. Half-isotonic Darrow's solution (sodium, 60 mEq. per liter; potassium, 17 mEq. per liter; chloride, 50 mEq. per liter; lactate, 25 mEq. per liter) with 2.5 per cent dextrose is recommended as a standard fluid for correcting these abnormalities. It may be given orally in small frequent feedings to a total of 100 to 150 ml. per kilogram daily, the smaller amounts being applicable to severely edematous patients. If there is vomiting or dehydration the quantity should be increased by 50 to 100 ml. per kilogram and the fluid given intravenously.

If the hemoglobin value is less than 6 Gm. per 100 ml., whole blood, 20 ml. per kilogram, should form part of the intravenous fluid regimen. Plasma in the same dosage is also useful in peripheral circulatory failure. Sodium bicarbonate, 4 ml. per kilogram of 4 per cent solution, should be used to correct acidosis if present, and extra glucose should be added (as much as 10 per cent) in the event of hypoglycemia.

Potassium and magnesium depletion may be severe, and additional oral supplements of these two ions should be started immediately and continued for at least two weeks (potassium, 4 to 5 mEq. per kilogram daily, and magnesium, 2 to 3 mEq. per kilogram daily).

DIETARY THERAPY. This type of therapy must not be rushed, and milk or another suitable source of protein should be prescribed in small frequent feedings from the second day. Milk is usually used, and a suitable regimen is to start with 60 to 90 ml. per kilogram daily divided into small feedings at frequent intervals. This supplies 2 to 3 Gm. of protein per kilogram daily. If more fluid is needed, a supplement of half-isotonic Darrow's solution can be given. Tube feeding may be necessary at first. Over the next few days, milk can be gradually increased to a maximum of 120 ml. per kilogram daily or 4 Gm. of protein per kilogram daily. On this regimen, skimmed, full cream or other modified milks are all well tolerated except in instances in which there is lactose intolerance (see later).

Within a week, mixed feeding may be introduced to complement the milk and to provide sufficient calories to equal the increase of appetite and well-being. In ambulatory outpatient cases simple advice that the recommended quantities of milk or other protein be added to the basic home diet (usually a cereal) is all that is needed and probably best understood by the parent.

Sometimes diarrhea is aggravated or brought on by the addition of milk to the diet. If the stools are sour smelling and acid in reaction, the patient probably has lactose intolerance. For the most part the children make good progress despite this complication and it can be ignored. Occasionally the diarrhea is so severe that it becomes necessary to use a lactose-free formula, such as one of the soya bean (Mull-Soy) or hydrolyzed casein mixture (Nutramigen) milks. Other sources of animal protein, e.g., egg, meat, fish or cheese, are all effective and can be used in place of milk.

In many parts of the world animal protein sources are either expensive or unavailable. Cure is achieved by giving suitable mixtures of vegetable protein, e.g., Incaparina in South and Central America and Pronutro in Africa. Beans or peas (the legumes) and ground nuts added to cereals, such as wheat, maize or rice, are also effective. A suitable mixture is two parts maize (corn) meal with one part bean or pea flour. A small amount of animal protein in the diet at least for the first week gives a more efficient result than does vegetable protein alone.

A vitamin preparation containing vitamin D, 400 I.U. daily, and vitamin A, 1500 units daily, is advisable because of a high incidence of rickets and xerophthalmia in areas in which kwashiorkor occurs. Folic acid, 5 mg. daily, is indicated for megaloblastic anemia, and iron, e.g., ferrous sulfate, 4 to 5 mg. per kilogram, for hypochromic anemia.

ANTI-INFECTIVE THERAPY. Infections must be actively treated by specific drugs. As a routine antibacterial cover, procaine penicillin, 300,000 units intramuscularly daily, and a sulfonamide, such as sulfadiazine or sulfadimidine (120 mg. per kilogram daily for five days),* are effective and cheap. Broad-spectrum antibiotics

* Manufacturer's precaution: Sulfadiazine and sulfadimidine are contraindicated in infants under two months of age except in the treatment of congenital toxoplasmosis as adjunctive therapy with pyrimethamine.

should be used only if specially indicated. Tuberculosis, malaria, hookworm and other tropical parasites must be dealt with actively. *Giardia lamblia* infestation is a frequent cause of malabsorption and diarrhea. Treatment is discussed on page 677.

FOLLOW-UP CARE. The duration of treatment for the hospitalized child is usually about three weeks. By this time there is a dramatic improvement in his general condition with complete resolution of edema and skin lesions. Cure has been initiated. However, the child will still be underweight for age, and follow-up care and observation are necessary for three or more months to ensure consolidation of cure and normal growth. Education of the mother in sound nutrition in relation to her economic status and environment can be most usefully done during follow-up visits.

Prophylaxis. The potential for kwashiorkor is greatest in areas of poverty, ignorance and population explosion. The attending physician should be aware of these facts. He can do much to counteract them by appropriate advice to parents and his support and use of all agencies and ancillary personnel that deal specifically with such problems. These include family planning clinics, maternal and child welfare clinics, clinics for preschool children, social welfare and health and nutrition projects. Individual, community and national effort is needed to deal with what is probably the biggest public health problem of our time.

Vitamin Deficiencies and Excesses

HAROLD E. HARRISON, M.D.

Deficiencies of vitamins are rarely encountered in children in the United States at this time. The usual diets of infants and children in this country can supply all of the needed vitamins if a vitamin D–fortified milk is included. Vitamin concentrates are therefore not required unless the diet is severely limited owing to allergy, food intolerance or food faddism. (See Table 1.)

FAT-SOLUBLE VITAMINS

Vitamin A and Carotene. The recommended dietary allowance for infants is 1500 units per day; and for older children and adults up to 5000 units per day. These are liberal amounts and are available in diets containing pigmented vegetables, butterfat, fortified skimmed milk and egg yolk. In children with fat malabsorption, such as those with cystic fibrosis, larger amounts of vitamin A are needed, and 10,000 to 20,000 units in a water-miscible base should be given.

TABLE 1. Recommended Daily Allowances of Vitamins*

VITAMIN	INFANT (0–12 months)	CHILD (5–10 years)	ADOLESCENTS (10–15 years)
A (I.U.)	1500	3500	5000
D (I.U.)	400	400	400
E (I.U.)	5	10	15
Thiamine (mg.)	0.25	1	1.2
Riboflavin (mg.)	0.4	1	1.4
Niacin (mg.)	7	14	18
Pyridoxine (mg.)	0.25	0.9	1.4
Folate (mg.)	0.05	0.2	0.4
B_{12} (μg.)	1.5	4	5
Ascorbic acid (mg.)	35	40	50

* Adapted from *Recommended Dietary Allowances*, 7th ed. National Academy of Sciences, 1968. These are not minimum requirements but allowances which take into consideration biologic variability and increased needs in some individuals.

HYPERVITAMINOSIS A. Excessive administration of vitamin A can produce severe toxicity. This can be acute in the infant following ingestion of several hundred thousand units of a vitamin A concentrate, or chronic due to continued high doses of vitamin A, 20 or more times the recommended daily allowance. The treatment is cessation of vitamin A administration and symptomatic treatment for the anorexia, irritability and vomiting which may be prominent symptoms.

Excess carotene is not converted to vitamin A sufficiently rapidly to produce vitamin A toxicity, but does accumulate in the plasma, producing carotenemia, a yellowish discoloration of the skin. Treatment is discontinuance of the excessive carotene intake.

Vitamin D. An adequate daily allowance for infants and children is 400 I. U. Vitamin D deficiencies can occur, since most foods given to young infants are low in vitamin D, including human milk. This is understandable if we remember that the natural source of vitamin D for man is exposure of the skin to short-wave ultraviolet radiation with resultant conversion of skin 7-dehydrocholesterol to cholecalciferol (vitamin D_3). The prevention and treatment of vitamin D deficiency is discussed in the section on rickets.

HYPERVITAMINOSIS D. Since inactivation and excretion of vitamin D are slow processes, excessively large doses of vitamin D accumulate in the plasma, the adipose tissue and, to a lesser extent, the liver. There is thought to be a wide spectrum of sensitivity to vitamin D, with some individuals developing toxicity at doses perhaps only 10 times the recommended daily allowance, whereas others may tolerate doses of 100 times or more the daily allowance before hypercalcemia results. The toxicity is due to hypercalcemia and hypercalciuria. Treatment is directed at reducing the excessively high concentrations of calcium in body fluids. Immediate discontinuance of vitamin D is of course essential, and reduction of calcium intake to as low a level as possible is also important. Since the hypercalcemia of vitamin D intoxication is sensitive to adrenal corticosteroids in amounts which are customarily used to suppress inflammatory reactions, prednisone, 2 mg. per kilogram up to 60 mg. per day, is given to these patients. Reduction of hypercalciuria by calciuresis is also effective. This is accomplished by the combination of a diuretic, such as furosemide* or ethacrynic acid,† and replacement of the water, sodium and potassium lost in the urine, so that maximal diuresis is maintained without sodium deficiency and dehydration or hypokalemia. The thiazide diuretics cannot be used for this purpose, since they increase tubular reabsorption of calcium and reduce urine calcium output. A successful regimen has been furosemide,* 1 mg. per kilogram intravenously repeated at 6- to 8-hour intervals, with intravenous infusion of a solution composed of equal parts of 5 per cent D/W and saline or Ringer's lactate, plus potassium chloride, 20 mEq. per liter. This is given in an amount equal to urine volume plus estimated evaporative water loss. Following reduction of the acute hypercalcemia, sodium phosphate orally can be added in a dosage equivalent to 1 Gr. of phosphorus per day, 300 ml. of Neutra-phos solution, in divided doses and continued until serum calcium concentrations remain in the normal range.

Vitamin E (α-Tocopherol). Tocopherol is an essential nutrient for man, but there is uncertainty concerning the clinical evidences of tocopherol deficiency. The requirement of infants is 2 to 10 I. U. per day (1 I. U. $\doteq$ 1 mg. synthetic *dl*-α-tocopherol acetate). Prematurely born infants fed cow's milk may need added vitamin E. The only other known need for vitamin E supplementation is in patients with steatorrhea whether due to cystic fibrosis or other causes of fat malabsorption. Such patients should receive supplements of the fat-soluble vitamins A, D and E. There is no known toxicity of large doses of vitamin E.

Vitamin K. Vitamin K_1 in a total dosage of 1 mg. is injected immediately after birth to prevent hemorrhagic disease resulting from prothrombin deficiency. There is no further need for vitamin K supplementation except in patients with fat malabsorption due to biliary atresia, cystic fibrosis, specific lipase deficiency or intrinsic abnormalities of intestinal mucosal fat transport.

Vitamin K Toxicity. Excessively large amounts of vitamin K_3 (menadione), which in the past were given to the newborn, particularly the prematurely born infant, were found to cause increased red cell hemolysis and consequent hyperbilirubinemia. There is no basis for giving these large doses; if vitamin K is used as previously indicated, this complication does not occur.

WATER-SOLUBLE VITAMINS

Thiamine (B_1). Deficiency of thiamine is extremely unlikely in infants and children in the United States. Breast fed infants of mothers with thiamine deficiency may develop a deficiency with neuropathy and cardiac failure. A generous daily thiamine requirement is 0.2 mg. for infants up to one year of age, increasing to 1 mg. for adolescents.

For treatment of thiamine deficiency, 5 to 10 mg. per day are customarily given. This can be administered intravenously as a slow infusion in saline or 5 per cent D/W in the acutely ill patient with cardiac failure; otherwise, oral administration is satisfactory.

Riboflavin (B_2). The daily requirement for riboflavin in infancy is about 0.4 to 0.5 mg. per day, and cow's milk feedings supply several times this amount. Clinical ariboflavinosis is extremely rare.

Niacin. Deficiency of this vitamin results in pellagra, which was once not an uncommon problem particularly in the southeastern portion of the United States. It is now very rare. The niacin requirement is partly dependent on the quantity of tryptophan in the diet, which is adequately supplied by animal proteins. If diets are extremely restricted in protein, all of the requirements should be given as niacin, 5 mg. per day in infants increasing to 10 mg. per day for older children. In the treatment of niacin

* Manufacturer's precaution: Furosemide should not be given to children until further experience is accumulated.

† Manufacturer's precaution: Until further experience in infants is accumulated, therapy with oral and parenteral forms of ethacrynic acid is contraindicated.

deficiency, 100 mg. per day are given as niacinamide, which avoids the unpleasant side effects of niacin.

Pyridoxine (B_6). Deficiency of this vitamin has occurred in infants fed heat-processed cow's milk feedings in which the pyridoxine was destroyed by excessive temperature. This is no longer a problem, owing to controls on heat processing of prepared infant feedings. There is an inborn error of metabolism, pyridoxine dependency, in which extremely large amounts of pyridoxine are required to prevent manifestations of pyridoxine deficiency, particularly convulsions. Another form of pyridoxine dependency is thought to exist in the hemopoietic system, so that anemia develops unless larger than usual amounts of pyridoxine are given. The normal daily requirement of pyridoxine is 0.2 mg. for infants, increasing to 1.8 mg. per day for adolescents. For the treatment of pyridoxine dependency with convulsions in infants, 50 mg. of pyridoxine is injected immediately, and 10 to 25 mg. per day is given orally thereafter. Ten mg. of pyridoxine per day is the customary regimen for pyridoxine-responsive anemia.

Folacin. This is also a rare deficiency in childhood at the present time, except as a complication of intestinal malabsorption or extensive operative removal of the small intestine. Megaloblastic anemia due to folate deficiency was once seen as the result of giving prepared milk feedings low in both folate and vitamin C, or goat's milk, which is low in folic acid. Folic acid antagonism by the anticonvulsant drugs, Mysoline and Dilantin, has been suggested as another cause for increased folate requirement. The normal infant requirement for folacin is met by 0.05 mg. daily, increasing to 0.4 mg. in the adolescent. For the treatment of folate deficiency, 5 mg. per day are given orally.

Cyanocobalamin (B_{12}). Deficiency of vitamin B_{12} is usually a conditioned one, due to lack of gastric intrinsic factor, which can be congenital or acquired, or to failure of absorption of the B_{12}–intrinsic factor complex in the distal intestine. B_{12} deficiency has occurred in patients with hypoparathyroidism and steatorrhea. It has occurred in breast fed infants of mothers with B_{12} deficiency. The requirement in infants and children is generously met by 1 microgram per day. In patients unable to absorb B_{12}, however, it should be given by intramuscular injection in a dosage of 30 to 50 micrograms per month.

Ascorbic Acid (Vitamin C). Vitamin C deficiency, scurvy, is also now extremely uncommon in the United States. Scurvy can be prevented by as little as 10 to 15 mg. of ascorbic acid per day, but the recommended daily allowance for infants is 35 mg. per day, increasing up to 60 mg. per day in adolescents. Extremely large amounts of vitamin C are used to acidify the urine in patients on mandelamine therapy for the control of chronic urinary tract infections and also sometimes to prevent respiratory infections. There is no objective evidence at the present time to support the latter use, but these large doses of several grams per day in adults have not been productive of major toxicity. Scurvy can be quickly treated by large doses of ascorbic acid, 100 to 500 mg. per day, until the patient is symptom-free; thereafter, ordinary maintenance doses are continued.

Parenteral Nutrition in Infancy

DONOUGH O'BRIEN, M.D., *and*
H. PETER CHASE, M.D.

In the last five years intravenous alimentation has been increasingly used in the postoperative care of infants after major gastrointestinal surgery and in the nutritional support of infants small for gestational age.

In principle, such a solution should be simple to prepare, sterile, not injurious to the venous intima and capable of affording an adequate nutritional intake in a physiologic volume of water. Hypertonic solutions of glucose alone have been used in the past; they must be administered slowly into a large vein to avoid thrombosis, and sudden changes in the rate of flow may lead to hypoglycemia or hyperglycemia. Because of this, fructose and invert sugar, an equimolar mixture of fructose and glucose, have been extensively used as alternatives. The use of other carbohydrates, such as xylitol, is also being explored.

To increase caloric intake in relation to volume, cottonseed oil emulsates were at one time popular. However, these led to occasional toxic reactions with a bleeding diathesis, fever, hepatosplenomegaly and pigmentary deposits in the Kupffer cells. Soybean oil emulsates, however, have now been reintroduced in Sweden and Canada. They appear to cause fewer complications, but Intralipid is still approved by the Food and Drug Administration for experimental use only.

Most recent experience has been gained with a mixture of casein hydrolysate in hypertonic glucose with added minerals, vitamins and electrolytes. The only nutritional omission is unsaturated fatty acids, which should theoretically provide 2 per cent of the calories. The incorporation of ethyl linoleate into the parenteral solution as an emulsate is being studied; in the meantime, essential fatty acids and trace mineral needs may be contained by giving intravenously 3 ml. of fresh-frozen plasma per kilogram every four days. For all the apparent simplicity of this program, it should be undertaken only when it is the only feasible means of nourishing the infant and this only with good laboratory and pharmacy support together with a trained clinical team.

Preparation and Composition of the Basic Solution. The solution described here can be easily dispensed in any well-equipped hospital pharmacy. Ideally, it should be prepared in

TABLE 1. Equipment for Preparation of Basic Solution

Laminar air flow table unit, Model C, $1100 (Abbott Clear Air Control, Inc., Norristown, Pennsylvania).
Swinnex-25, Millipore filter units. Type GS (0.22μ). (Millipore Corporation, Bedford, Massachusetts 01730.)
Sterile 250-ml. vacuum bottles for intravenous use. (Travenol Laboratories, Inc., Morton Grove, Illinois 60053.)
Plexitron transfer sets for mixing sterile solutions. (Travenol Laboratories, Inc.).

48-hour batches, since changes in sodium, potassium and other components may be required. A laminar flow table should be used to preserve sterility. If such a unit is not available, solutions may be assembled with sterile disposable syringes with Millipore filter attachments. The following materials and solutions are required to manufacture the base solution.

If the base intravenous solution is administered at the rate of 125 ml. per kilogram per 24 hours, the infant will receive the daily amounts of nutrients shown in Table 3. The pH is approximately 7.3.

Management. In ward preparation for intravenous alimentation the following materials have to be assembled:

- 250-ml. bottles of base solution.
- No. 2C0200 Plexitron solution administration set with filter (Travenol). Change every other day.
- Silastic tubing, 0.025 in. I.D., 0.047 in. O.D. (Dow Corning Corp., Midland, Michigan).
- No. A1030/23 Intramedic liver stub adaptors, 23 ga. (Clay-Adams, Inc.).

The surgical staff should be requested to insert the catheter into the region of the junction of the superior vena cava and the right atrium via the right external jugular vein, and the position should be confirmed by fluoroscopy. This should be carried out with sterile conditions, and the catheter should then be passed through a subcutaneous tunnel from the right parietal area. The catheter opening on the skin should be sealed with Neosporin ointment and dressed with dry sterile gauze. Care of the area should be carried out by the physician and inspected and re-dressed at least every 48 hours. The catheter should be changed every 30 days. The solution should be administered at a rate of 125 ml. per kilogram given evenly throughout the 24-hour period. Initially, however, a half-strength solution in 5 per cent dextrose should be used. We have found it necessary to

TABLE 2. Composition of Base Intravenous Solution per 250-ml. Bottle*

ITEM	AMOUNT
5% casein hydrolysate in 5% dextrose, containing 3.5 mEq. of sodium, 1.8 mEq. of potassium, 2.5 mEq. of calcium and 1 mEq. of magnesium (Travamin, Travenol Labs. Morton Grove, Ill.) or 8.5% FreAmine (McGaw Labs.), 60 ml.; 20% dextrose, 45 ml., and dextrose 5% with 0.45% sodium chloride, 45 ml.	150 ml.
50% dextrose solution (Travenol Laboratories.)	100 ml.
50% magnesium sulfate in 2-ml. ampules (Abbott Laboratories, North Chicago, Ill.).	0.08 ml.
20% calcium gluconate in 10-ml. ampules (Endo Laboratories, Inc., Garden City, N. Y.).	2.0 ml.
Potassium phosphate in 10-ml. ampules, containing 3 mEq. of potassium and 65 mg. of phosphorus per ml. (Travenol Laboratories).	1.0 ml.
Sodium hydroxide in water for injection.	3.0 ml.
M.V.I. injectable vitamins (USV Pharmaceuticals Corp., Tuckahoe, New York).	1.0 ml.
Sodium heparin, 1000 U.S.P. units per ml. (Organon, Inc., West Orange, N. J.).	0.05 ml.
Folvite folic acid solution in 10-ml. ampules (Lederle Laboratories, Pearl River, New York 10965). Dilute 1:100 before use.	0.01 ml.
Ducobee–1000, 1000 μg. of vitamin B_{12} per ml. in 10-ml. ampules (Breon Laboratories, N. Y.).	0.4 ml.
Imferon, 50 mg. per ml. in 2-ml. ampules (Lakeside Labs., Milwaukee). Omit in infants less than three months of age.	20 μl.

* Amigen and Hyprotigen are other commercial casein hydrolysates; the latter is a 10 per cent solution. Products should be checked for electrolyte content. Note also that only 50 per cent of nitrogen is as free amino acid; the remainder is in peptide form. Freamine is a free amino acid mixture now under consideration by the Food and Drug Administration.

TABLE 3. Daily Amounts of Nutrients Supplied by 125 ml./kg./24 hours of Base Solution

NUTRIENT	I.V. ADMINISTRATION/24 HOURS	MINIMAL DAILY REQUIREMENT*
Total water	2.3 liters/m.2	2–2.5 liters/m.2
Total calories	126 Kcal./kg.	100–120 Kcal./kg.
Total amino nitrogen	476 mg./100 Kcal. (300)**	290 mg./100 Kcal.
Threonine†	118 mg./kg. (102)**	45–87 mg./kg.‡
Valine	193 mg./kg. (108)**	85–105 mg./kg.
Methionine	81 mg./kg. (135)**	33–45 mg./kg.
Isoleucine	162 mg./kg. (177)**	102–119 mg./kg.
Leucine	256 mg./kg. (231)**	76–229 mg./kg.
Phenylalanine	124 mg./kg. (144)**	47–90 mg./kg.
Tryptophan§	22 mg./kg. (39)**	15–20 mg./kg.
Lysine	193 mg./kg. (231)**	110–160 mg./kg.
Histidine	81 mg./kg.	16–34 mg./kg.
Linoleic acid (ethyl linoleate)		300 mg./100 Kcal.
Sodium	2.7 mEq./kg.	1–3 mEq./kg.
Potassium	2.4 mEq./kg.	2–5 mEq./kg.
Magnesium	0.33 mEq./kg.	0.2 mEq./kg.
Calcium	0.9 mEq./kg.	1.2 mEq./kg.
Phosphorus	26 mg./100 Kcal.	25 mg./100 Kcal.
Iron	0.4 mg./100 Kcal.	1 mg./100 Kcal.
Copper	50 μg./100 Kcal.	60 μg./100 Kcal.
Iodine	< 1 μg./100 Kcal.	5 μg./100 Kcal.
Vitamin A	433 I.U./100 Kcal.	250–750 I.U./100 Kcal.
Ascorbic acid	22 mg./100 Kcal.	8 mg./100 Kcal.
Thiamine (B_1)	2.2 mg./100 Kcal.	25 μg./100 Kcal.
Riboflavin (B_2)	430 μg./100 Kcal.	60 μg./100 Kcal.
Pyridoxine (B_6)	67 μg./100 Kcal.	35 μg./100 Kcal.
Nicotinamide	4 mg./100 Kcal.	0.25 mg./100 Kcal.
Pantothenic acid	1.1 mg./100 Kcal.	0.3 mg./100 Kcal.
Vitamin D	43 I.U./100 Kcal.	40 I.U./100 Kcal.
Vitamin E	0.22 I.U./100 Kcal.	0.3 I.U./100 Kcal.
Folic acid	6 μg./100 Kcal.	4 μg./100 Kcal.
Vitamin B_{12}	174 μg./100 Kcal.	150 μg./100 Kcal.

* Figures for minimal daily requirement are based on those for oral feeding using the *International Codex Alimentarius.*

† Figures for total amino acid contents.

‡ From Holt, I. E., and Snyderman, S. E.: The Amino Acid Requirements of Children; in W. I. Myhan (ed.): *Amino Acid Metabolism and Genetic Variation.* New York, McGraw-Hill Book Co., 1967.

§ Additional nicotinamide is derived from tryptophan in Aminosol.

** Figures in parentheses are for 30 ml. of FreAmine soy hydrolysate per 125 ml. solution.

use a constant infusion pump. The system should not be used for drawing routine venous samples. Prophylactic antibiotics should not be given. Meticulous clinical microbiologic and biochemical monitoring is imperative, particularly in the first days of the regimen. Urine osmolality, glucose, serum osmolality and levels of sodium, potassium, chloride, carbonate, calcium, magnesium and glucose should be monitored at least on alternate days until tolerance is stabilized. Body weight and total urine volume should be recorded daily.

Complications. INFECTION. An indwelling intravenous catheter carries a risk of septicemia and bacterial endocarditis. Sepsis may not develop until the catheter has been in place for a week or more. It is wise to culture the flora of skin, upper respiratory tract, bowel and urine at weekly intervals. If there is clinical evidence of infection, first decide whether this is associated with the catheter or is a separate event. In the latter case, specific treatment for the causative organism is initiated. In the former case the catheter should be removed, the tip cultured and a new one inserted. The organisms most often involved are from the normal body flora and are *S. aureus, Streptococcus viridans,* Proteus, Klebsiella and *E. coli.* Saprophytes, such as Candida and Aspergillus, and low pathogens, such as Serratia, may also be involved. In small infants the incidence of infection can be reduced by inserting a small Silastic catheter into the right temporal vein and threading it down into the right atrium.

Pulmonary Embolism. Fronds of clot may develop from the external surface of the catheter around the tip. These may become infected or may detach to produce pulmonary emboli. Embolism is suggested by evidence of infection, with increased respiration and pulse rates, cyanosis and radiologic changes. The treatment is to heparinize the patient and to change the catheter. For major emboli, embolectomy is a possibility, but the likelihood of success is very small.

Control of Glucose Metabolism. Patients receiving intravenous nutrition frequently have been undernourished for a period of time, and glucose intolerance is a complication of undernutrition. It is thus usually necessary to increase the glucose concentrations in two- to four-day increments until the 23 per cent concentration is tolerated.

Effective utilization of the glucose load can be increased by adding 1 unit of regular insulin to the infusate for each 5 Gm. of glucose, and by giving up to 5 mEq. of potassium per 100 Kcal. The latter procedure requires that serum potassium be monitored. Serum and urine glucose levels must also be regularly checked to ensure that there is no osmotic overload. In particular, in the first 48 hours it is wise to monitor the blood glucose level with Dextrostix at least every 4 hours.

Hypoglycemia is also a complication which is most liable to occur if the rate of glucose administration is allowed to fluctuate. Therapy, when discontinued, must be done so gradually. Under certain conditions it may also be necessary to reduce amino acid concentration to keep up glucose levels, especially when Hyprotigen is used.

Amino Acids. Acidosis, ammonia intoxication and a distortion of normal serum amino acids with elevated levels of methionine and, less importantly, of threonine, valine and glycine, result from conventional solutions. The actual nitrogen content of hydrolysates may vary significantly, and the potential effects of infusing peptides are not yet understood.

Calcium and Vitamin Metabolism. The known actions of vitamin D are to enhance calcium absorption from the intestine and to mobilize calcium from bone. Because the calcium is being given intravenously and it is not desired to mobilize bone calcium, it might be argued that vitamin D need not be given intravenously. There is evidence that calcium may be precipitated by the phosphate buffer in the hydrolysate and that hypercalcemia may develop if other buffers are used. Until intravenous needs of calcium and vitamin D are more clearly understood, they should continue to be added to the solution.

Anemia. The constant infusion of a hypertonic solution may result in a mild hemolytic anemia. This should be monitored by weekly determination of hemoglobin values, hematocrit values and red blood cell counts. The appearance of anisocytosis and otherwise distorted red cells of serum haptoglobin saturation with hemoglobin are sensitive indications of hemolysis. Occasional transfusions of packed cells may be required.

Psychologic Problems. Older children and adults who have been encouraged to eat in order to maintain their nutritional status may become severely depressed at having failed when intravenous nutrition is initiated. Psychiatric help to allow them to vent their feelings is generally wise. Parents should be encouraged to hold infants receiving intravenous nutrition so that normal emotional attachments can develop.

References

Gradini, H.: A Review: Current Status of Parenteral Amino Acid Therapy. *Pediat. Res.*, 7:169, 1973.

Piedes, R. S., et al.: Intravenous Supplementation of L-Amino Acid and Dextrose in Low Birth Weight Infants. *J. Pediat.*, 82:945, 1973.

Symposium on Total Parenteral Nutrition. American Medical Association, 1972.

Long-Term Parenteral Nutrition
(Hyperalimentation)

ROBERT M. FILLER, M.D.

Dudrick and coworkers first demonstrated that the intravenous infusion of a fat-free, amino acid and glucose solution could support normal growth and development, and four years ago Filler and coworkers reported the successful long-term use of this solution in 14 critically ill infants. The success of the method depends on the infusion of glucose as a source of calories and a protein hydrolysate as a source of nitrogen. Because this hypertonic material cannot be introduced into peripheral veins, special equipment and techniques are required for administration. As a result, serious problems not ordinarily seen with routine intravenous therapy may arise. Intelligent use of this life-sustaining system therefore requires the careful selection of patients for therapy, persistent attention to the minute details of procedures which minimize the dangers, and constant surveillance for the development of complications.

INDICATIONS

Total intravenous alimentation is reserved for those infants and children whose lives are threatened because feeding by means of the gastrointestinal tract is impossible, inadequate or hazardous. The common conditions for which this treatment has been used include the following: chronic intestinal obstruction due to adhesions or peritoneal sepsis, complicated omphalocele and gastroschisis, bowel fistulas, inadequate intestinal length, chronic nonremitting severe diarrhea, extensive body burns and enteritis arising during tumor therapy. The goal of treatment depends on the patient's underlying condition. In some instances, such as in those infants with chronic nonspecific diarrhea, placing the gastrointestinal tract at rest for a prolonged period is curative. In others, the restoration and maintenance of adequate nutrition will permit corrective surgery. The decision to begin a program of total intravenous alimentation requires mature clinical judgment. Such a decision can be made readily in an infant with complicated omphalocele or one in whom a large portion of the midgut has been resected because of volvulus. In other patients the decision may be more difficult. For example, in a child with chronic diarrhea and malnutrition, one must be certain that customary therapy has failed before beginning total intravenous therapy. One must cautiously weigh the need for improved nutrition to save life and reduce morbidity against the possibility of serious complications. Intravenous alimentation should not be used in those children in whom nutrients can be safely delivered and absorbed from the gastrointestinal tract by careful oral feedings, gavage or gastrostomy.

METHODS

The intravenous infusate of 20 per cent glucose, 3.5 per cent protein (as amino acids and polypeptides) and appropriate vitamins and minerals must be prepared aseptically, preferably by a trained pharmacist using a laminar flow hood. The sodium, potassium and chloride concentrations in the infusate are usually adjusted to the needs of the individual patient at the bedside. To avoid peripheral venous inflammation and thrombosis, this hypertonic infusate must be delivered through a central venous catheter. For this purpose, a silicone rubber catheter is passed through the internal or external jugular vein to the superior vena cava. This procedure is best carried out in an operating room or cardiac catheterization laboratory where adequate exposure, proper instruments and strict aseptic conditions are available. To minimize blood stream contamination, the venous catheter is tunneled from the vein entry point to a skin exit site 2 to 4 inches away. In the infant, it is brought out on the scalp, whereas in the older child the exit site may be the neck or upper extremity. Central venous intubation by percutaneous subclavian vein puncture has also been used. The silicone rubber venous line may be left in place until the completion of therapy unless it becomes accidentally dislodged or septic complications develop. We have had a single catheter in place for as long as 90 days.

The proper position of the catheter in the vena cava must be confirmed. This is easily accomplished radiographically by the use of a radiopaque catheter or one filled with contrast material.

An antibacterial ointment and sterile dressing are applied to the skin exit site. To avoid accidental displacement, a coil of catheter is included in the dressing. Every three days the dressing is removed aseptically, the skin cleansed with an antiseptic and a sterile dressing and antibacterial ointment reapplied. Povidone-iodine (Betadine) ointment is now used routinely for its effectiveness against both bacteria and fungi. Before the infusion is started, a Millipore filter (0.22 μ) is placed inline to remove particulate matter and microorganisms which may have contaminated the solution. A calibrated burette is placed in the circuit to monitor the volume delivered. An injection tubing may also be added to the circuit so that antibiotics or other intravenous drugs can be administered intermittently.

The infusate must be delivered at a slow uniform rate to insure proper utilization of the glucose and amino acids. In the infant and small child, this is most readily accomplished by the use of a constant infusion pump.

METABOLIC OBSERVATIONS AND RESPONSES

Clinical measurements which are essential to evaluate the child's metabolic response include daily body weight and accurate volume of urine and other body fluid losses. The important laboratory tests include qualitative urinary sugar analysis, blood sugar concentrations and serum electrolyte content and osmolarity. The urine sugar content is monitored at each voiding. In the stable patient, the other tests are obtained every three days for the first two weeks, and thereafter only as indicated. These determinations will indicate the child's nutritional progress and readily detect the occurrence of osmotic diuresis, abnormal fluid retention or electrolyte and acid-base abnormalities. Since hyperammonemia and abnormal liver chemistries have been noted in some patients, a periodic check of these parameters is also indicated.

Weight change during the period of intravenous feeding will vary with the patient's overall clinical status. Weight gains comparable to those of normal infants may be expected in those children who are not malnourished or in whom sepsis is not a part of their clinical problem at the time intravenous feedings are instituted. A significant weight gain in the first two weeks of therapy is not usually seen in those infants and children who are severely depleted at the start of treatment.

Despite the variations in weight curves, positive nitrogen balance has been noted in *all* patients studied in detail. In infants on the intravenous diet providing 0.65 Gm. nitrogen per kilogram per day (equivalent to 4.05 Gm. protein per kilogram per day), a persistent positive balance of nitrogen of 100 to 300 mg. per kilogram per day has been observed. Fecal loss of nitrogen is usually negligible since stools are infrequent and scanty during periods of intravenous feeding. Urinary amino acid losses have been found to be negligible and not sufficient to produce osmotic diuresis except in infants under 1 kilogram and in those children with severe renal disease.

In most patients the large quantity of intravenous glucose (27 Gm. per kilogram per day) is well tolerated without the addition of exogenous insulin. Blood sugar levels remain in the normal range, but urinary sugar content usually varies between 0 and 3+ by the Clinitest method. Quantitative glucose excretion studies have shown that this represents less than 1 per cent of the total glucose infused. Urinary sugar levels are generally highest during the first day or two of treatment, and during this period a temporary decrease in hourly infusion rate or use of a more dilute solution may be necessary. In the patient in whom the urinary glucose spill has been negligible during many days of therapy, the onset of glycosuria is often the first sign of blood stream infection.

COMPLICATIONS OF CENTRAL VENOUS CATHETER

The presence of a catheter in the superior vena cava for prolonged periods may cause venous thrombosis with obstruction to flow or pulmonary embolus. The use of silicone rubber catheters, instead of the plastic polyethylene or polyvinyl plastic catheters which cause more tissue reaction, minimizes this danger and results in far less inflammation along the subcutaneous catheter tract.

Accidental withdrawal of the venous line has been a common problem. This complication is ordinarily recognized by the occurrence of swelling near the venotomy site. It may be confirmed by x-ray visualization of the catheter tip. If the tip is not in the superior vena cava, the catheter should be completely removed and a new line inserted at another site. This event is more frequent when using a soft silicone rubber catheter, which is difficult to secure. Perforation of the vena cava has been reported with central venous catheters made of stiff plastic.

The most serious complication of this method of feeding is sepsis. Long-term indwelling venous cannulas have been a well-documented source of blood stream infection. Organisms may enter the blood stream along the catheter tract or with a contaminated intravenous solution. The catheter, a foreign body in the blood stream, may act as a focus for bacterial growth even if organisms enter from a distant septic site. Sepsis should be suspected when fever or glycosuria occurs without any apparent cause. To minimize the risk of sepsis, the following measures should be emphasized. Catheters should be inserted under aseptic conditions in an operating room. Silicone rubber catheters rather than polyethylene or polyvinyl catheters should be used because they cause less tissue reaction and are less likely to produce a thrombus which will support the growth of microorganisms along the wall of the intubated vein. The skin exit site for the catheter should be placed in an area which can be aseptically and meticulously cleansed. In an infant, the scalp area behind the ear is satisfactory, whereas the umbilicus is not. Proper dressing changes at the catheter exit site every three days should not be omitted. Use of the central venous catheter for blood sampling (except for blood culture or emergency central venous pressure measurements) should be avoided. Nutrient solutions should be prepared aseptically in the hospital pharmacy preferably in a laminar flow hood, not on the open ward. Intravenous bottles and tubing should be changed daily. A bacterial filter should be placed in-line to remove any organisms which may have contaminated the solution. Since the high sugar content of these infusates supports the growth of yeast, the external surface of the intravenous tubing should be washed with Betadine solution twice a day to remove any traces of nutrient solution which may have inadvertently dripped from the bottle onto the tubing. Betadine ointment should also be applied to all joints in the circuit to prevent entry of microorganisms at these points. Antibiotics need not be used unless warranted by the child's primary illness. The intravenous infusion should be supervised only by specially trained individuals who are alert to all the hazards.

Adherence to these precautions does not completely eliminate the possibility of infection. Sepsis still occurs in about 15 per cent of children treated for more than one week. *Candida albicans* is the most common offending organism. However, with early recognition of sepsis and prompt withdrawal of the venous catheter, mortality and serious morbidity can be avoided.

References

Dudrick, S. J., et al.: Long-term Total Parenteral Nutrition with Growth, Development, and Positive Nitrogen Balance. *Surgery,* 64:134, 1968.

Filler, R. M., Eraklis, A. J., Rubin, V. G., and Das, J. B.: Long-term Parenteral Nutrition in Infants. *New England J. Med.,* 281:589, 1969.

Filler, R. M., and Eraklis, A. J.: Care of the Critically Ill Child: Intravenous Alimentation. *Pediatrics,* 46: 456, 1970.

2

Mental and Emotional Disturbances

Mental Subnormality

HUGO W. MOSER, M.D.,
ROBERT E. FLYNN, M.D.,
MARGARET E. ADAMS, M.A., *and*
MURRAY SIDMAN, PH.D.

In spite of much effort and public interest, treatment of the subnormal child is still unsatisfactory. Not only do we lack fundamental knowledge about the cause, pathogenesis, prevention and specific therapy of mental subnormality, but also there is a tragic failure to apply the established therapeutic principles. This latter problem, in our opinion, exists because the care of the retarded child is society's responsibility, and it involves in an important and continuing way disciplines such as psychology, special education and vocational rehabilitation, with which physicians usually have only limited contact.

The shortcomings of society affect particularly members, such as the retardates, who are unable to fend for themselves. Even though there are hopeful signs of change, lack of funds and inertia in social systems have caused the treatment of the institutionalized retardate to become a national disgrace. Although community services for mildly and moderately retarded people are improving, they are still in the pilot stage and fragmented. The overall national picture of what active and effective therapeutic measures are available to counter the many problems associated with subnormality is still extremely bleak.

These considerations have led us to use the team approach for the diagnosis and treatment of the retardate within the framework of a state regional evaluation center and residential institution. The team approach is necessary because no one person can possess all the skills required for evaluation and therapy. Location of the professional team in a state regional facility obviates a handicap that is otherwise encountered frequently, namely, the geographical separation of the professional team from most of the subnormal children it serves. Such a geographical separation fosters an artificial and harmful division between evaluation and therapy, in which the professionals evaluate, whereas most therapy is left to understaffed residential and community facilities. Even in terms of evaluation this is unwise, because skilled therapy applied for several months or years may bring out capacities in a child that could not have been detected during initial evaluation. More important, such a separation is an injustice to the child and an inefficient utilization of professional talent. If the child is admitted to a residential institution, most of which are located at great distances from the metropolitan area, the child is separated not only from many professional resources but, even more damaging, from his own family. It is our view that close cooperation between professionals and the state is essential: The cost of comprehensive services is so high that private resources cannot provide them; furthermore, the structure and distribution of services are almost as important as their quality. Professionals must work with the state to improve all three.

Mentally subnormal people can be divided into two general categories: those who function at subnormal levels because they are socioculturally disadvantaged and those with congenital or acquired abnormalities of the nervous system. The first group is much larger and is associated with mild or moderate levels of mental subnormality. However, because of higher rates of prematurity, infection, malnutrition and exposure to toxins and trauma, the incidence of brain damage in the socioculturally disadvantaged is greater than in the general population. The second group, i.e., patients with congenital or acquired subnormality of the nervous system, encompasses all the severely and profoundly retarded patients, an unknown portion of those who are moderately retarded and a small fraction of those who are mildly retarded.

Treatment of mental subnormality due to sociocultural disadvantage is of great importance. It is part of the task being undertaken by comprehensive health care centers now being established within disadvantaged regions. The physician's role here is to provide good medical care in a way that does not differ greatly from what is done for the child who functions normally; efforts to deal with subnormal performance fall mainly in the province of the educators and workers in the behavioral and social sciences. In the remainder of this chapter we will focus mainly on the treatment of the moderately, severely and profoundly retarded children because this group presents the more specialized aspects of subnormality that confront pediatric care.

THE MULTIDISCIPLINARY TEAM

The diagnostic and therapeutic team that we use includes the pediatrician, psychiatrist, neurologist and, on an ad hoc basis, other medical specialists, social worker, nurse, psychologist, educator, speech and hearing consultant, rehabilitation counselor, physical therapist, occupational therapist and recreational therapist. This model differs from that in the usual outpatient hospital clinic in that it has, as full-time members, professionals from disciplines other than medical, such as the educator, rehabilitation counselor and recreation therapist.

Of greater significance, however, is the definition of roles within this interdisciplinary framework. It is essential to reach the rather delicate balance between a conglomerate of professionals and the organizational structure in which the physician-director exercises direct supervision of all phases of diagnosis and therapy. Overall direction of our clinic rests with the chief physician. He is part of a team that screens all patients shortly after they are admitted to the clinic. At this early screening conference, responsibility for further diagnostic and therapeutic programs is assigned to the team member whose expertise relates most closely to the patient's main problem. This may be, among others, the psychologist, educator, rehabilitation counselor, public health nurse or social worker.

The chief physician reviews progress at three- to six-month intervals or when so requested by members of the team. The team member to whom the patient is assigned otherwise assumes full responsibility for the diagnostic and therapeutic program, using members of other disciplines for consultation when appropriate. Such a team is not easily achieved. It requires maturity, responsibility and a clear idea of professional identity on the part of staff members who in more traditional settings may have functioned only in subsidiary capacities, as well as skilled physicians who are able to recognize and, when appropriate, defer to the expertise of other disciplines.

To illustrate this interdisciplinary team concept, the remainder of this chapter will be concerned with describing the role of the physician in this type of medical setting, and the contributions made by the disciplines of social work and psychology to the care of subnormal children. We realize that the latter resources are not routinely available to physicians practicing in other settings, but we feel strongly that in discussing this ideal—if not attainable—paradigm, we can best demonstrate the essential principles governing the treatment of this disability. Social work and psychology are chosen from the wide array of professional disciplines previously listed because the former's traditional concern for the family is a prerequisite of effective therapy, and because the latter has been conspicuously successful in devising a modality of treatment with the severely subnormal child.

THE PHYSICIAN'S ROLE

It is evident that the physician is responsible for the care of all illnesses that strike the retardate. In most instances the therapeutic approach does not differ from that used for patients with normal intelligence. It is, however, essential to discuss four aspects of medical therapy that are influenced by the child's being of subnormal intelligence: pharmacologic therapy of seizures and of the overactive or destructive child, management of emotional problems in the mentally retarded child, a treatment program for congenital malformations and acquired deformities and correction of metabolic or endocrine disturbances.

There are at this time no pharmacologic agents that specifically improve memory or intelligence. Nevertheless, pharmacologic agents may help in a child's mental development by removing factors that interfere with learning. The most important example of this is the achievement of seizure control. Repeated and frequent seizures inevitably interfere with the learning process, and they are managed as in patients with normal intelligence. However, care must be taken to avoid sedation from excessive dosage, because this in turn interferes with learning.

Pharmacologic agents are of value in the management of the hyperkinetic child—a state that affects almost exclusively preadolescent boys. The short attention span and overactivity inevitably interfere with the learning process and may exhaust parents and teachers. Drugs in this instance are only part of an overall treatment plan, the essence of which, as Eisenberg has emphasized, is environmental manipulation. Dextroamphetamine,* 10 to 30 mg. per day, and methylphenidate,† 30 to 60 mg. per day, often are the most effective pharmacologic agents. Other useful medications are the sedative diphenhydramine and chlorpromazine.‡ Phenobarbital, except as an anticonvulsant, is contraindicated because of the frequency with which it produces paradoxical excitation. Aggressive or self-destructive behavior is also a common, but usually intermittent, manifestation of older retarded men and women. Unless it is part of a psychotic reaction, such behavior does not appear to be strongly influenced by even very large doses of tranquilizers, such as 2000 to 3000 mg. of chlorpromazine. In our experience, such destructive behavior is handled more effectively by the behavioral management described in the following paragraphs.

Retardates suffer from the same types of emotional problems as do people with normal intelligence; in fact, because of secondary stresses to which they are exposed, emotional problems are more frequently encountered. Mental subnormality does not diminish the person's emotional needs, and we have often been impressed by the degree of awareness of interpersonal relationships and the depth of feeling-tone displayed by people whose IQ measurement places them among the moderately or occasionally even severely retarded. The psychiatric approach does not differ qualitatively from that applicable to patients with normal intelligence, except that it is carried out at a simple and more concrete and nonverbal level. Group therapy is quite effective. The psychiatric therapy of childhood schizophrenia or autism is a matter of controversy, as are all other therapeutic approaches. None has as yet proved consistently effective.

The therapeutic approach to patients with congenital malformations of the nervous system requires that a comprehensive and long-range therapeutic program be established as soon after birth as possible. It is our strong recommendation that the possibility or probability that a child may later be retarded not deter the physician from undertaking such a program. This recommendation is made for the following reasons: (1) Prognosis as to the intelligence and neurologic function of a young infant is often in error. We have repeatedly seen children in whom surgery for myelomeningocele was not performed because the presence of brain damage was diagnosed in infancy, and then have found the children to be of normal intelligence. Also, the width of the cerebral mantle, as estimated when a pneumoencephalogram or ventriculogram is performed in a hydrocephalic child, has been shown to correlate poorly with the degree of intellectual function that may be achieved after surgical shunts are performed. (2) Nursing care of patients with untreated meningomyelocele or hydrocephalus is extremely difficult. Tissue breakdown and infections are almost impossible to avoid. Furthermore, the existence of the uncorrected deficit almost inevitably means that the child must be admitted to a residential institution, and this is almost always to the child's disadvantage. With present nursing care and antibiotics, patients with uncorrected deficits survive for years and even decades; their grotesque appearance and other aspects of their care cause serious management and emotional problems for family and ward personnel. (3) Surgical procedures have been greatly improved. For these reasons we recommend that whenever possible, these malformations be surgically corrected. These programs, of course, require close and continued coordination between the pediatrician, neurosurgeon, plastic surgeon, orthopedic surgeon, psychiatrist and neurologist, as

---

* Manufacturer's precaution: Dextroamphetamine not recommended for hyperkinetic behavior disorders in children under three years of age.

† Manufacturer's precaution: Methylphenidate not recommended in children under six years of age. Parenteral form not recommended in children.

‡ Manufacturer's precaution: Chlorpromazine not recommended for children under six months of age except when lifesaving.

well as other members of the interdisciplinary team.

The specific therapy of conditions such as phenylketonuria, galactosemia, maple syrup urine disease and cretinism is discussed in other sections of this book. In most instances, for treatment to be optimal it must be begun in early infancy, at the presymptomatic stage, and the management of the metabolic problems of such patients is best left under the supervision of physicians with special interest and experience in these matters. However, care must be taken that attention is also directed to the emotional, social and educational needs of these patients.

Counseling. GENETIC COUNSELING. Recent advances in genetics have made this type of counseling of great importance. In many instances, the family can now be given precise estimates of the risk that future offspring will also be affected. Accurate diagnosis is a prerequisite of genetic counseling, and a considerable number of biochemical and cytogenetic investigations may first have to be completed. Genetic counseling should not be attempted until all data are available, and allowance should be made for the frequency with which parents may misunderstand or misinterpret the physician's advice. This may be tested by having the parents relate their impressions of the physician's advice to a social worker or nurse.

FAMILY COUNSELING. The physician is, and will remain, the principal professional person to whom the family turns for advice when there is a subnormal child. Often this is a serious burden because problems are invariably difficult, in respect to both diagnosis and management, and in many cases they require the services of other professionals who may not be readily available. Furthermore, as mentioned earlier, the overall medical, educational and social services that a subnormal child needs are not yet equal to the task. Counseling the family about their problem is an important aspect of help, and it is not essentially different in principle from that in any other chronic disease.

Certain principles of management are specifically relevant to the subnormal child: (1) Whenever feasible, retardates belong in their own homes, and their lives should be structured to resemble those of normal children as much as possible. Intelligence quotients in themselves are not meaningful prognostications as to ability to make a successful occupational adjustment; patients with formal IQ's in the 30's have held jobs successfully. Provided proper teaching methods are used and a suitable milieu is offered, able-bodied severely and profoundly retarded patients can learn to look after their own basic needs (e.g., dressing, eating, toilet training). (2) Placement in a large institution almost inevitably leads to deterioration in intellectual and social functioning because of the depersonalized care that currently prevails in state-supported facilities.

Whenever possible, the referring physician should know the institution to which the child is being admitted. The following criteria may help him in evaluating it: (*a*) an overall patient census of 500 or less, (*b*) dormitory units that contain no more than eight patients (the present trend is toward single or double rooms, (*c*) accessibility of the institution to the family, and its encouragement and facilitation of the family's desire to have the child remain part of the family unit, (*d*) most important and most difficult to judge, a general atmosphere in which the child is treated as an individual and the atmosphere is rehabilitative rather than custodial and (*e*) a qualified professional and consultant staff.

SOCIAL ISSUES FOR THE FAMILY AND COMMUNITY RESOURCES

An axiom of treatment for any childhood disability is that the family be closely involved in the total therapeutic endeavor. In the case of mental subnormality, this concept is often the principal focus, because this handicapping condition creates social byproducts that not only demand an exceptional capacity for protective nurturing from the family but also constitute a substantial threat to the family's cohesiveness and viability. For this reason any therapeutic regimen, be it primarily medical, psychologic or educational, must take into account these associated social difficulties. It is the purpose of this section to discuss the contribution of social work in helping to ameliorate this aspect of the total problem complex.

Retardation makes its sharpest impact on the family when they learn that their newborn baby has an innate physical anomaly that is inseparably associated with marked intellectual dysfunction. This creates a series of complex psychologic and social stresses for the family which must be handled with promptness and insight if the parents are to weather the emotional crisis that the child's birth has precipitated. Ideally, after the physician has broken the news and discussed the physiologic components of the child's condition and his developmental prognosis, the parents should be introduced to a social worker to discuss what practical help is available. Aside from relieving the parents' realistic anxiety about how they will manage their painful and unpredicted situation, the introduction of a person with a social as opposed to a clinical orientation to the problem helps neutralize the unreal crisis atmosphere evoked by the child's defect. The concern with the practical features of the family's life (Is the mother going to take the baby home when she leaves the hospital? What difference will the special care he requires make to the overall economy of the family? What should other siblings or relatives be told about his current status and prognosis?) shifts the emphasis from the overwhelming abnormality of the situation and introduces the implication that, even though painful and disturbing, the problem is within the manageable limits of reality and, with help, can be successfully contained by the family. Further, by involving the family in plans for the child beyond the immediate context, the social worker implicitly links the present clinical setting with the ordinary normal milieu of home and reinvokes the familiar and competent parental roles. Should residential placement be required because of serious medical problems, it will be easier for the family to adjust to this step if it has been carefully discussed and planned rather than being arranged impromptu in an atmosphere of acute emergency.

The whole question of whether a seriously defective child should be institutionalized or cared for at home is highly controversial and carries many social implications which make it a very difficult measure both to recommend and to accept. Several factors need to be considered. First, the child's condition should not be the sole criterion for placement, and equal care should be given to weighing the social and psychologic factors in the family in order to determine the extent and nature of the stresses caused by his handicap, how these match with the family's resources, and what the different consequences will be for *the family* if the child is separated from them or cared for at home. For example, the mother's psychologic investment in pregnancy and the resultant maternal set to nurture a newborn child may have to be worked through by caring for even a very defective baby before the long-term separation of placement can be tolerated. Too drastic an interruption of this mothering cycle can have adverse effects on the entire family; for example, there may be unconscious displacement of affect belonging to the retarded child onto the normal siblings in the shape of excessive protective anxiety or pressures to excel to compensate for the loss. Such a critical decision must always rest finally with the parents, and the most effective contributions any professional can offer in this painful situation are factual information about realistic alternatives (which are always much more limited than the parents realize or hope for) and helping the parents evaluate the overall and long-term implications of their decision for the child, themselves and the rest of the family.

The techniques by which social workers handle these important emotional factors cannot be described in this brief presentation, nor is it to be implied that they are the exclusive prerogative of this discipline. What is emphasized here is the overriding need for an open-minded approach on the part of all professions toward the family's problems, for an awareness that the critical event of the defective child has wider ramifications than the immediately obvious clinical one and for solutions that will meet as many of the complex difficulties of the situation as possible. Beyond this attitude of imaginative compassion, which is the basis of all therapy for the stricken family, help ideally includes the offer of concrete services to assist them in day-to-day living around this handicapped new member. For example, guidance by the visiting nursing service on caring for the child can provide both psychologic and practical support; a homemaker service can alleviate normal household pressures; nursery school and day care may provide compensatory attention for an older preschool sibling, provided it is not interpreted as ejection from home because of the newcomer; sustained medical surveillance will keep normal anxiety at a lower level. Counseling from the social worker following the child's birth and return home or after placement is also of immense value in giving parents an outlet for voicing and revoicing their feelings of bewilderment, disappointment and anger about the child, and also in helping them to reevaluate their plans for him in the light of his gradual development and their growing acceptance of his disability and its meaning for them.

We have been talking at considerable length about the revelation crisis concerning an obviously defective newborn child because this event crystallizes in its purest form the psychologic and social trauma that retardation presents for the family, and the pattern of help required in this situation applies, with some modification, to subsequent phases of retardation. The family with a moderately impaired child experiences another crisis four or five years following his birth when he faces the social hurdle of education within the next two years, without having acquired the social maturity and skills needed to meet the extra demands that school will impose. If there is delay in toilet training and speech, poor comprehension which poses disciplinary problems and hyperactive destructive behavior that disrupts family life, parental anxiety about the child's future will be heightened. Often a very disturbed parent-child relationship develops, creating an overlay of psychologic maladjustment and acute management problems besides the basic intellectual disability.

A child with this type of disability imposes on the whole family excessive and realistic strains that urgently demand prompt and well-coordinated intervention. To reinforce the treatment modalities of other disciplines (drug therapy to control the physiologic basis of hyperactivity, psychologic and educational techniques to modify behavior), the social worker must intervene on behalf of the harassed family. Assistance should include counseling to help them sort out their feelings toward the child so that their handling becomes less conflict-ridden and more consistent, and actual practical help to reinforce their efforts. A day training program for the child, even if it accepts him only one day a week, breaks into the cycle of hopeless frustration; homemaker or babysitter service will give the parents relief as well as freeing their time and energy for other children; and temporary residential care (such as is being provided by some state institutions) is a very excellent therapeutic measure which allows the parents to distance themselves from the child and see his problems in perspective. Many parents feel that they have failed miserably when they cannot manage their child. To counteract this understandable but distorted perception there should be a real effort to emphasize the positive points in the situation. Pinpointing even minimal developmental gains or training achievement introduces a note of hopefulness and perspective which parents desperately need; it is also helpful to the physician because it accords with his basic function of promoting health and neutralizes the feeling of professional defeat that is often evoked by the more intractable features of mental subnormality.

When a child is wreaking havoc in the home, longer-term placement may be the appropriate treatment, but before initiating plans it is important to know whether this step is a response to acute emergency strain that would be better relieved by the less drastic step of supportive services from the community. If placement is the more desirable treatment, it is of vital importance that both the family and the professional adviser regard it as a time-limited therapeutic measure designed to improve the child's social functioning so that he can eventually return to normal life in the community, either by rejoining the family or by transferring to a foster or group home. This point is being heavily emphasized in order to counteract the deeply entrenched traditional approach to residential placement as a life sentence in a custodial institution segregated from the community at large. As with the newborn seriously impaired child, placement must be considered from a variety of angles, particularly the fact that removing one child from his home breaks into the family's cohesiveness and integrity and may threaten the psychologic security of the other children. Sending the handicapped child away from home can seriously shake the siblings' confidence in the family as a totally reliable nurturing system; when he has lived with them for three or four years and is felt to be a peer, his removal is felt more personally.

Thus far we have dealt with the crisis experience of families who have a retarded child with a marked degree of handicap, in most cases associated with organic impairment. Another aspect of subnormality that has strong social ramifications is represented by the mildly retarded latency child whose disability presents itself as school failure, with or without additional behavior disorder. The strain in this situation derives from the marginal character of the handicap, which creates confusion about the child's role and makes it difficult for the parents to know where to place their expectations for him. Further, the child invariably comes for professional help at a point when he is thoroughly enmeshed in a complex of situations involving social failure—in poor school performance, in limited social relationships, and in not meeting parental expectations. The dominant problems in these circumstances relate as much to social interaction and functioning as to lower intelligence; help must be simultaneously directed toward relieving the pressures of the child's current existence by mobilizing special educational, social and recreational resources and in some cases psychotherapy, and toward improving family attitudes and relationships. Since the mildly retarded child usually comes from a socially deprived environment, his specific difficulties must be seen as a salient manifestation of the total family's problems; direct help for him must often be accompanied by more generalized intervention on behalf of the total family unit in order to ensure that it remains viable and able to contain him and his handicap.

BEHAVIORAL MANAGEMENT OF THE SEVERELY RETARDED CHILD

Once a child has been diagnosed as retarded, a new set of problems arises. From that time on, his parents, relatives, teachers and friends watch him with more than ordinary concern. Expectations are always tempered by the suspicion that he is not really capable of meeting them. Ordinary rules of behavioral management are suspended because they are thought to be inapplicable to the retarded child, particularly the severely retarded child.

As a consequence of this abandonment of normal behavioral management procedures, the severely retarded child is likely to display serious behavior problems by the time he reaches chronologic adolescence. In addition to the expected slow (or no) learning and the absence of spoken communication, he may be destructive to himself or to his environment, prone to temper tantrums, hyperactive, inattentive, withdrawn and dependent upon others even for the simplest self-care.

His parents are likely to be confused, exhausted, despairing, hostile, guilty and ready to abandon the child to an institution. But the same problems exist within most institutions, which are usually understaffed with competent child-care specialists, poorly designed and permeated with the custodial philosophy having as its basic principle that ordinary rules of behavioral management do not apply to the retarded.

In most instances this situation is avoidable and, if it has been allowed to develop, is treatable, although not easily.

It has been our experience that all retarded children, regardless of any ultimate low ceiling on their development, are responsive to the most basic behavioral laws. As with all of us, their behavior is governed by its consequences, both positive (reward) and negative (punishment). The effectiveness of any positive behavioral consequence depends on the level to which a child has been deprived of it. Thus, if mealtime provides a child with an otherwise rare opportunity for social contact and for manipulation of his social and physical environment, he learns not to feed himself but rather to make someone else feed him, and he prolongs the feeding period by whatever means are available to him—spilling or throwing food and utensils, playing and general negativistic behavior. It would be a mistake to assume that this is behavior of a retardate. It is, in fact, exquisitely adaptive. The child succeeds in satisfying three needs simultaneously – food, social contact and environmental manipulation.

To prevent such a feeding problem, it is necessary to follow these principles: (1) Provide food *only* as a consequence of self-feeding. Depending upon the degree of retardation, special "shaping" procedures may be necessary to teach the child the basic skills involved in self-feeding. (2) Limit the duration of mealtimes. It may be necessary even to allow the child to miss a meal or two until food itself becomes a sufficiently strong consequence to override the other rewards of mealtimes, particularly if the feeding problem is a longstanding one. This does not hurt the child, and the ultimate benefits to all concerned more than justify the seemingly strict show of consistency. (3) Provide the child with opportunities other than mealtimes for social contact and environmental manipulation. It is important, however, to provide these opportunities only as a consequence of appropriate behavior. Otherwise, the basic problem simply shifts from meals to other times, as will be described.

Whenever problem behavior arises, the first question to ask the parent, and to teach the parent to ask himself, is, "What happens immediately after the problem behavior occurs?" In the answer to that question are found the consequences that generate and maintain the undesired behavior. Temper tantrums, destructiveness and self-injury, when their consequences are examined closely and objectively, are almost always manipulative, in that they produce parental attention of some sort—soothing caresses, first-aid, housecleaning or repairs carried out near the child, replacement of toys or even punishment.

Since the severely retarded child is ordinarily considered incapable of learning normal forms of attention-producing behavior, he is not taught such behavior. But the need nonetheless exists, and a vicious cycle begins. The parent, seeing no normal behavior to which he can attend, tends to react only to emergency situations. The child quickly learns that behavior such as screaming, head banging, window breaking or toy destruction brings the solicitous parent running. The tragedy of the situation is that the parent himself, out of love and solicitude, generates the behavior in the child that makes love difficult or impossible. Even when in desperation he turns to punishment, the unwanted behavior persists, because even punishment becomes rewarding if that is the child's only method of gaining attention.

An objective observer of aggressive and destructive behavior by retarded children is often amazed by the absence of the emotional tone that one usually associates with such behavior. This is because the behavior is, in fact, not emotionally determined. It is learned, maintained by its consequences and often coldly and openly manipulative. It is remarkable how rarely the chronic window smasher cuts himself. In a very real sense the existence of such behavior is a hopeful sign. It demonstrates that the child is capable of learning, that he is responsive to his environment. By identifying the controlling consequences one achieves a kind of communication with the child, because such consequences reveal his otherwise unfulfilled needs. The problem of treatment, then, is not to eliminate these consequences, i.e., attention, but to make them contingent upon constructive behavior.

The parent must become an objective observer, not just of the child, but of himself. What does he do when the child misbehaves? He must then do these same things when the child behaves appropriately. It is often not easy for the parent to describe his own behavior objectively and operationally, and if the child's problem behavior has been allowed to persist for a long time, it may even be difficult for the parent to find desirable behavior to which he can react. The physician, less involved in the day-to-day emotional stress of the parent–retarded child relationship, can be of assistance here. By being gently insistent, he can get a parent to state exactly what he does when the child misbehaves, can show him that his response is maintaining the misbehavior and can suggest likely forms of desirable behavior to which the parent can shift his attention.

The rule that behavior is generated and maintained by its consequences can be applied to the hyperactive or otherwise poorly attentive child. Although hyperactivity, unlike destructiveness, may be a physical symptom often associated with retardation, it can be modulated or eliminated by teaching, and providing appropriate consequences for, competing forms of behavior. Hyperactivity need not be aimless or random behavior. It can be channeled into directed and purposeful activity if teaching methods are used that proceed slowly enough to maintain a high level of success by the child, and if the child's rewards for successful learning are substantial. Our experience has been that we lose the hyperactive child's attention when we set tasks for him that he cannot perform. We regain his attention immediately when we again set a task that he has shown he can do, and for which rewarding consequences are provided. Again, the consequences most important to the child must consistently be contingent upon directed activity, not on seemingly aimless hyperactivity. The parent or teacher need not worry that his standards are set too high. The child's behavior tells him whether he is moving too fast. Any recurrence of undirected hyperactivity is a signal to slow down and find out where the teaching process has gone astray.

Most physicians, of course, have neither the time nor the training to be teachers of retarded children, or even to instruct the parents of retarded children in effective teaching methods. It is even difficult for the physician to recommend other sources because effective teaching programs for retarded children, especially those with behavior problems, are even less available than they are for normal children. To suggest to parents that their hyperactive child can be treated through effective training methods, and then to be unable to recommend a source of such help, can be more destructive than helpful. Unless the parents are intelligent enough to work out practical procedures themselves once they have become acquainted with general principles such as those just described, the physician is in an unenviable position. At the very least, however, we recommend that he assume the responsibility for becoming informed of recent developments in methods and principles of behavior modification and that he use his position of prestige and community leadership to promote the establishment of new, and the improvement of existing, institutions for the effective behavioral management and instruction of retarded children.

Emotional Disorders

ALEJANDRO RODRIGUEZ, M.D., *and*
GREGORY FERNANDOPULLE, M.D.

ENURESIS

Patients may be divided into two broad groups: Those from "dirty families" and those from "clean families." Those from "dirty families," who have never been toilet trained and in whose homes sanitary conditions are at a very low level, are usually brought in after a crisis, such as a behavior problem at school, and we learn, incidentally, that the child is also a bedwetter. There is very little shame attached to the bed-wetting per se. Three useful steps in management are (1) a simple form of conditioning therapy using rewards, such as stars on a chart and a material gift at the end of each week, (2) any placebo at bedtime, and (3) some environmental manipulation if practicable.

Children from "clean families" have often been toilet-trained too early by neurotic-compulsive mothers, and the matter of who controls whom is now at issue. Parents do not like to talk about bed-wetting because of the social stigma attached. More than one interview may be necessary to talk the parents and the child into a compromise on the issues involved. For the specific problem, ask the parents to buy an alarm clock for the child, who is taught to set it at about the time he wets at night so that he can empty his bladder. Imipramine (Tofranil), 25 to 50 mg. at bedtime, is useful, especially for children over six and particularly if depression is associated with the enuresis. (With younger children, placebos are just as useful, and we prefer not to use imipramine ordinarily in this age group; the manufacturer does not recommend imipramine for children under six years of age.) A system of rewards as outlined for the first group sometimes helps these children as well. Often the children and families do very well with some supportive psychotherapy lasting at least two or three months. Nocturnal fears, especially of going to the bathroom, may need to be explored.

ENCOPRESIS

This symptom, unlike enuresis, disappears during adolescence. We classify the families according to the same system as for enuresis: those who feel social shame and those who do not. Success in therapy depends on how early the children are seen.

In younger children of both types of family, stool softeners (for two to three weeks) and rewards are used. Parental counseling is also useful for both groups. With more sophisticated patients, play therapy appears to be useful; in others, such forms of environmental manipulation as having the parents spend more time with the children, giving more attention to any maternal shortcomings, and helping with school work, appear to have some effect.

In older children, this symptom is a clue to more serious psychiatric disturbances. Mental retardation and severe personality conflicts between child and parents or siblings should be investigated. Play therapy is less successful. Separation, perhaps hospitalization for a few weeks, helps to overcome the problem.

HYPERACTIVITY

Hyperactivity is often part of the more complex syndrome known as "minimal brain dysfunction." Impulsivity, temper tantrums, inability to be satisfied under any circumstance, low frustration tolerance, and a short attention span, sometimes associated with a learning difficulty, point to this syndrome. These patients most often are referred by the schools.

Hyperactive children are also likely to have visual-motor impairment, electroencephalographic abnormalities, poor coordination and minor congenital anomalies.

Stimulants (dextroamphetamine and methylphenidate) constitute the most commonly used and single most effective form of treatment. Approximately 80 per cent of patients with obvious hyperactivity will show a clear benefit, such as decreased restlessness, increased attention span, improved school work and better social and emotional behavior. Over 50 per cent show profound behavior changes. A small number (1 per cent) of hyperactive children are made worse by stimulants; not infrequently these are borderline or psychotic children.

Most children with "minimal brain dysfunction" respond favorably to either dextroamphetamine or methylphenidate. Dextroamphetamine (Dexedrine) * has the advantages of being longer acting and of being available in spansule and elixir forms. Methylphenidate (Ritalin) † has less of an effect on appetite and is less costly. It is given in a single daily (morning) dose of 20 mg., or 10 mg. may be given in the morning and 10 mg. at noon. Its effect begins in half-an-hour to 2 hours and lasts 3 to 5 hours, depending on the severity of the condition.

Dextroamphetamine can be started in a 5-mg. dose twice a day or a single (morning) dose of 10 mg. For longer-lasting action, 10-mg. spansules can be used, and the elixir is useful for children under six years of age. Half a teaspoon morning and noon is the recommended dosage. For school-age children, a single daily dose of tablets is best on school days, with half that amount being administered on other days for going to church, going visiting and other such activities.

Regardless of which medication is employed, a trial period is necessary to determine whether the drug works in the particular child. Give a morning dose on each school day and have the child's teacher report any improvement over a week or two. Adjust the dosage if necessary and repeat the trial. If the results seem

* Manufacturer's precaution: Dextroamphetamine (Dexedrine) is not recommended for hyperkinetic behavior disorders in children under three years of age.

† Manufacturer's precaution: Methylphenidate (Ritalin) is not recommended in children under six years of age.

inconsistent or variable, make sure that the pills are actually being taken. Alternating a week of therapy with a week without therapy should make the results obvious. Do not use more than 40 mg. per day of methylphenidate, or more than 20 mg. per day of dextroamphetamine.

The most common temporary side effects of stimulant therapy are headaches, moodiness, stomachaches, and talkativeness. Insomnia may occur if a noontime dose is used, and irritability accompanies it. Very rarely, a hallucinatory episode can occur as a response to stimulants. Reducing the dose for a few days usually alleviates the side effects, which are almost never enough of a problem to warrant discontinuing the medication.

The only long-term side effect of importance is growth suppression, which has been reported particularly with dextroamphetamine. Children who are being maintained on this drug will grow at approximately 60 to 75 per cent of their normal rate, and they show a distinct growth rebound when the drug is stopped. Suppression of appetite and consequently of weight gain are most prominent during the first year on dextroamphetamine. It is advisable to keep careful charts of height and weight. The long-term effects of stimulants on sleep and on pulse rate have yet to be determined.

Besides actual side effects, certain problems can develop with continued use of stimulants. Parents decide to stop giving the medication because of a fear of side effects, or after a long period of no negative school reports, or because it is too expensive, or because it is not effective at the prescribed dose (or at least it does not seem to be effective). Moreover, the medication may in fact become ineffective because the child appears to take it but actually does not, or because tolerance develops and a higher dose becomes necessary but is not prescribed.

We recommend a therapeutic hiatus at the beginning of each school year to determine whether medication is still necessary. It may be necessary to continue therapy into the early teens. At times a change of environment, such as to a more organized style of life, appears to reduce the irritations that produce hyperactivity. When considering a continuation of stimulant therapy, be sure to distinguish between the child who has actually not improved and the one whose parents or teachers can accept him only when he is sedated and thus apply considerable pressure to continue the use of stimulant therapy.

We prefer to start older children on some medication other than the stimulants, chiefly in order to avoid problems of drug abuse later. Phenothiazine derivatives, such as thioridazine (Mellaril)‡ and chlorpromazine (Thorazine) §, will reduce restlessness and anxiety in dosages of 25 to 50 mg. three times a day. Psychotic, borderline psychotic and mentally subnormal hyperactive children will often respond better to these tranquilizers than to stimulants. Side effects include drowsiness, weight gain, extrapyramidal reactions (uncommon at the usual dosage level), tardive dyskinesias over the long term and, occasionally, increased photosensitivity and pigment deposits.

Diphenhydramine (Benadryl) is a generally safe alternative to stimulants that is especially useful for young children. We recommend 150 to 300 mg. as a night-time sedating dose, even if the child is taking a stimulant each morning.

Diphenylhydantoin (Dilantin) is not recommended; its effect on hyperactivity appears to be nil. Phenobarbital often aggravates hyperactivity. For hyperactive children who also have seizure disorders, stimulants themselves have anticonvulsant properties, and combining a stimulant with diphenylhydantoin is better than the usual combination of diphenylhydantoin and phenobarbital.

Ancillary Measures. Parents of hyperactive children need to be reassured about the potential benefits of stimulants and their recognized value in the treatment of this condition. Distraught parents, particularly, will benefit from a clarification of the intertwined biologic and emotional aspects of the problem. It reassures parents to tell them that the immaturity, much of the behavior difficulty and the restlessness are biologically based.

The long-term prospects are also discussed. In the past, many pediatricians have simply reassured parents that their children will outgrow hyperactivity. In the light of recent studies, it is now advisable to be less reassuring, but it is still true that restlessness will decrease in the last preteen years. The associated learning disability usually persists, but by itself, this is usually not an insurmountable handicap.

For management of the child at home, advise parents that short-term limited discipline works best. Requiring 5 minutes in a chair, or in the bedroom, or outside, as need be, is effective discipline for infractions of household rules, obstructive behavior, and so forth. For temper

---

‡ Manufacturer's precaution: Thioridazine (Mellaril) is not recommended for children under two years of age.

§ Manufacturer's precaution: Chlorpromazine (Thorazine) is not recommended for children under six months of age except when lifesaving.

outbursts, 3 to 5 minutes of isolation is recommended, using a stove timer or a clock to demonstrate the end point.

Parents often feel better when they are told that depending primarily on physical punishment is seldom effective with hyperactive children. By trial and error, responsive and flexible parents soon find a short period of restriction to be the most useful type of discipline. Many parents shout too much at their hyperactive children. It is recommended that they try consciously to restrict this and try to adopt a "disciplinary posture", such as moving toward the child when enforcing a rule. Specific household chores to be carried out at specific times are always helpful.

Plan with the parents to capitalize on the child's areas of strength so that he can taste success. Swimming, bicycling or roller skating are activities in which even children with fine motor incoordination can excel; baseball and basketball are not. A newspaper route or some other part-time job can give a measure of status to the academically dull child. At the same time, plan with the parents and the school to bolster the child in his particular areas of weakness. If social behavior is poor, recommend summer camp, recreational activities and clubs. If academic achievement suffers, tutoring or remedial education will be needed.

Convince the parents to tolerate more restlessness than usual and to consciously attempt to channel the child's activity; for example, carry a writing tablet in the car for drawing during rides. Parents must also be urged to lessen social restrictions on hyperactive children. Parents become sensitive to complaints of their neighbors and will try to keep the child in the house for long periods. It would be better to allow the child to play outside and tell the neighbors to keep their own children away if they find his hyperactive behavior objectionable. Of course, some amount of restraint is still required, for these children will throw stones at people and engage in other undesirable behavior.

Parents whose children are criticized at school believe that their child-rearing is held suspect; frequently they feel a need to retaliate, but at heart they do feel guilty about their home management and they will attempt to punish the child at home for infractions at school. The pediatrician can call a truce and, if possible, point out to both parents and teachers the child's inherent limitations, thereby alleviating some of the blame and guilt. Other family issues frequently arise, such as disagreements between parents about disciplinary measures and overprotectiveness. Because hyperactive children show a high degree of immaturity and consequent academic, athletic and social failure, they need closer parental dependency ties than most children during the preschool and elementary school years. These ties are appropriate for both parents; problems arise when one parent responds in an exaggerated way but the other does not.

Individual psychotherapy is not generally useful, but a therapeutic relationship may help with other difficulties that these children are prone to experience.

Special Education. Hyperactive children do best in a one-to-one learning situation or close to it. If small classes are not available, a slower-learning "track" may help, especially for the less intelligent and those with a concurrent learning disability. Parents strongly influence the academic performance of their children. Middle-class parents traditionally tutor their children and convey to them the significance of learning. Parents of children with learning difficulties can also be successful tutors, but the task requires more flexibility. The simplest and most profound concept that a parent can teach is the joy of learning, which is taught mainly by example. In cases of delayed acquisition of reading skills, the parent can read to the child for 5 to 15 minutes every day. In time the child will want to verbalize words or parts of words from the daily stories, a procedure which is best not forced.

Many children with learning handicaps appear to benefit from school-based remedial instruction. It speeds up improvement, but its benefits often wash out. Some children with profound reading impairment who do not benefit from reading assistance require a bookless curriculum. They need a supportive, informative, nonstressful educational program that will not humiliate them and that will give them a sense of success and a compensatory avenue. If the hyperactive child with impaired learning ability is not retarded and is at least moderately motivated to learn, in all likelihood he will develop adequate academic skills for basic adult needs. In his junior high school years he will be better at learning concepts than he was in the elementary school years.

CRUELTY

Cruelty is premeditated deriving of pleasure by hurting other people or animals. It has to be differentiated from impulsive behavior, which always arises from a stimulus to which the child responds. Cruelty may be a symptom reinforced by parents as an expression of their own impulses. Management requires a detailed history from the patient and the parents, and a statement of their values and attitudes. Reinforcements being provided, consciously or not, by the parents need to be discouraged. If the behavior continues, a change of environment (school or neighborhood) may be useful. Individual treatment in the form of play therapy has been used with success. The condition may at times be part of the "minimal brain dysfunction" syndrome.

STEALING

This is a difficult symptom to evaluate at an early age. It is even more difficult among poor families, where the sense of individual ownership is not clearly delineated and children have common beds, pillows, books, toys and clothes. In the well-to-do, stealing among families becomes a real crime, and parents have a realistic fear of being ostracized. Part of management is helping parents and children return stolen articles in the case of shoplifting.

Stealing coins at home is a common problem. We encourage parents to count coins openly and place them on a table or cupboard so that the child understands that the parents know how much money there is. Parents often resent this nuisance, and it then becomes necessary to lock up all the cash. A youngster who repeatedly steals may need individual therapy or merely a few things to call his own. At times we have found stealing to be part of an effort to get more attention, and teaching parents how to spend more time with their children alleviates the problem.

LYING

In early childhood, lying is difficult to distinguish from fantasy; habitual lying becomes significant after the age of six or seven, when a good part of the child's conscience has been formed. Accompanying symptoms such as stealing, school problems, somatic complaints and so on, may also need investigation. Habitual lying could also appear as part of "minimal brain dysfunction." The system of punishment in use at home also needs investigation, since lying can be a device to avoid uncomfortable situations.

SETTING FIRES

Being fascinated with fire is a universal phenomenon. Once a child has acquired motor coordination, lighting matches gives him great pleasure. When he learns that setting fires annoys adults, he uses this weapon when things do not go his way. We recommend that parents carry pocket lighters and put away all matches. Persistence of the behavior in older children should suggest mental retardation. Play therapy in which the child may "set fires" with dummy matches might be helpful. However, external control of all possible sources of matches is extremely important to prevent fire hazards.

BREATHHOLDING ATTACKS

These brief events can provoke acute anxiety from the parents. Children who engage in this behavior have often been conditioned by the parents, and there may be a dependency-control struggle involved. The sudden cessation of respiration following a crying outburst frequently produces loss of consciousness and rarely may lead to convulsions.

Explain to the parents (if they are sufficiently educated) that there is a physiologic "cut-off" point at which carbon dioxide accumulation stimulates the respiratory center and the child will breathe even if he tries not to. Offer the parent a device, such as a cold sponge, to apply to the child's face. This often reduces the parent's anxiety and also restarts breathing in many instances. In "normal" children, these attacks disappear spontaneously by the fourth year, when the child has less of a need to control his environment for secondary gains. Persistence of breathholding attacks beyond four years is an indication for psychiatric evaluation.

Medication has little place in management. In hyperactive patients we have used dextroamphetamine,‖ 2.5 to 5 mg. twice a day, to reduce hyperactivity as well as the crying spasms that often bring on breathholding spells.

TEMPER TANTRUMS

Commonly encountered in toddlers and children, temper tantrums in one form or another may continue as a way of life into old age. Outbursts usually consist of screaming, kicking, cursing, breaking things and rolling on the floor; younger children often vomit or pass urine. The child is usually out of control, and parents respond too often by getting out of control themselves, thus reinforcing the child's behavior. In fact, parents help their children learn to throw tantrums by their own violent acts. Children who are retarded or have serious or chronic illness are also victims of this disorder.

Help the parents to provide a consistent, reasonable form of response and urge them to minimize their own tantrums. Recommend

‖ Manufacturer's precaution: Dextroamphetamine is not recommended for hyperkinetic behavior disorders in children under three years of age.

that situations be avoided in which the child is likely to throw a tantrum, such as a shopping trip on which the child will demand all sorts of toys and fly into a rage when refused.

PSYCHOTIC REACTIONS

Disorders of thought, affect and communication are perhaps the most common of the various forms of psychotic disorders. Some children cannot distinguish reality from fantasy. Some withdraw from the environment; in others, fears and identity crises are common. Impaired emotional relationships with other people are frequently noticed. Hallucinatory phenomena, both auditory and tactile, are also seen.

Acute transitory reactions usually present with evidence of trauma, toxic or febrile illness, recent or anticipated loss or separation, or some other triggering event. Phenothiazine derivatives in doses of 25 to 100 mg. daily according to age and weight will calm these patients; lesser tranquilizers, such as diphenhydramine, 50 to 100 mg. daily, are just as useful for the less severely disturbed; a hypnotic at bedtime, such as chloral hydrate, 250 to 500 mg., may be used in combination. Counsel the parents to remove any possible exciting factor, and advise that most such episodes are not only transitory but unique.

In the case of disorders having a prolonged and insidious onset, gradual isolation is a common presenting symptom. It is usually accompanied by a decline in school performance, withdrawal from social activities, head-banging, rocking, fears, somatic complaints and ritualistic behavior. These episodes could be interspersed with acute episodes, especially if the child has to endure panic-inducing situations. Most of these children benefit from at least a short-term close evaluation in a hospital. Medications allay many of the symptoms; we use phenothiazine tranquilizers in doses of 50 to 200 mg. per day, or haloperidol,** 1 to 5 mg. per day. At times an antidepressant must be used as well, and we prefer imipramine†† in doses of 25 to 75 mg. daily.

The parents should be told about the prolonged nature of the illness and, hence, the need for long-term adjustment and management, so that their expectations will be reasonable. School authorities may have to be persuaded to allow patients to be tutored at home part of the time. We recommend a gradual increase in social activities, and we discourage long-term hospitalization except in special circumstances such as severe illness or an impossible family setting. Day-care centers are ideal as a way of taking the load off the parents, at least for part of the day. Electroconvulsive therapy has no value in children.

HABITUAL MANIPULATIONS

Twisting and pulling the hair is a problem often exacerbated by parents, teachers and peers commenting on a child's physical appearance; the child finds the habit an excellent device to control the environment. In younger children (up to age six or seven) or retarded children, educating the parents to spend more time with their children helps to break the pattern of isolation. At times parents need specific instructions about more varied ways of interacting with their children.

Thumb-sucking, nail-biting and ear-pulling are all battlegrounds of dissension between children and adults. Less isolation and more stimulation will relieve the symptoms, which are cured completely by maturation.

MASTURBATION

The number of children referred because of masturbation has been greatly reduced since the misconception that masturbation produces insanity has passed into history. The few children who are still brought to the hospital are guilty of masturbating in public, a behavior which is still socially unacceptable.

Parents find it difficult or embarrassing to identify the problem in front of the child. We usually ask the patients what they would think of a friend who engaged in some unacceptable behavior, as a means of introducing a discussion about confining certain behavior to more private settings. As with so many other emotional disorders, these children are isolated and basically need more interaction with other children and with their parents.

TICS

Tics are "habitual spasms that are sudden, quick, involuntary and frequently repeated movements of circumscribed groups of muscles, serving no apparent purpose." Some are due to organic causes, while others are functional, but both types can present in the same fashion. There is a need to eliminate any possible organic cause, general or localized.

In children under the age of six years, identification with an adult who has the same habit is the most common cause of tics. Obtain-

---

** Manufacturer's precaution: Haloperidol is not recommended for use in the pediatric age group because safety and efficacy have not been established.

†† Manufacturer's precaution: Administration of imipramine for pediatric conditions other than enuresis is not recommended for children under 12 years of age.

ing a detailed history will uncover this relationship; at some later time, raise the possibility in a manner that will not injure the child's self-respect. The use of the third person ("I know a boy who used to blink because his uncle used to blink") is a nonthreatening way to interpret findings to children, and a useful and successful one.

Children over six years present with an assortment of tics, such as grimacing, jerking the hands or clearing the throat. Explaining the involuntary nature of the disorder to parents or others concerned will relieve most of the associated anxiety and reduce the social shame. Dextroamphetamine, 5 to 15 mg. daily (not recommended for children less than three years of age), or methylphenidate, 10 to 30 mg. daily (not recommended in children under six years of age), reduces hyperactivity and eliminates many tics. At times one tic is replaced by another, and still later by another, leading one to suspect more serious psychopathology.

The Gilles de la Tourette syndrome includes tics (often jerky movements of the head), coprolalia and barking sounds; the electroencephalogram sometimes shows features characteristic of the convulsive disorders. Haloperidol,‡ 0.5 to 2 mg. daily, is the drug of choice; at times dextroamphetamine (not recommended for children under three years) or methylphenidate (not recommended for children under six years) may have to be added to reduce hyperactivity, the dosage being determined by the child's age and weight. Manifestations of convulsive disorders require the addition of diphenylhydantoin, 50 to 100 mg. daily.

The Autistic Child

WILLIAM M. EASSON, M.D.

The autistic child looks at the world in his own unique way, he communicates in a manner that is often very different and he interprets our communication to him in his own private fashion. Frequently the autistic child is hypersensitive and overreacts to certain perceptions while he appears not to recognize other stimuli.

Constitutional factors seem to be etiologically important in most cases of autism and many of these children show evidence of neurologic immaturity, "soft" neurologic signs or frank neurologic limitations; quite often the autistic child develops convulsions in later childhood. Children who are born with special perceptual limitations, such as blindness, deafness or mental retardation, are especially liable to grow up in their own private world and to react in an autistic fashion.

The pediatrician must help every autistic child use all his capabilities and the resources of his family and his community to become socially acceptable, then socially productive and, as a long-term goal, socially independent. The treatment goals must always be realistic and reasonable. Long-term, financially costly psychotherapy and even the best inpatient programs have only minimal therapeutic success with most autistic children. Many effective treatment programs seem to work because they develop a warm, predictable environment where the autistic child is encouraged and rewarded to modify his behavior gradually so that he becomes more tolerable, and where he is trained to use his skills so that he can cope with social expectations.

It is very easy to see only the seemingly bizarre behavior of the autistic child and nothing else, but the physician must place his major treatment emphasis on the youngster's strengths and potentials. The autistic child is usually physically sturdy and energetic and he may be trained to use this physical energy in work tasks or athletic activities rather than in periodic, disruptive explosiveness. The emotionally driven autistic child can work out his tensions and, at the same time, develop his muscles by using this energy in bicycling around the neighborhood block, throwing a basketball or raking leaves. The special sensitivities and interests of the autistic child may have, in the past, made him more vulnerable psychologically, but in a controlled treatment program these same sensitivities may be used to help him develop social skills and even acceptance. The autistic youngster who is hypersensitive to sound may also have a special talent for music; his memory for music, his alertness to the musical beat and his capacity to hear a tune in a different fashion may be developed into a socially rewarding talent. The autistic child who is fascinated with moving engines may be helped to channel this interest toward automotive, electronic or horologic training in a sheltered vocational workshop. When the autistic patient is severely compulsive, this compulsiveness may be used in a socially acceptable fashion if the youngster can, for example, be placed as a stock boy who can stack and arrange endlessly. Each autistic child must be thoroughly evaluated, after which

‡ Manufacturer's precaution: Haloperidol is not recommended for use in the pediatric age group because safety and efficacy have not been established.

a program is planned to meet his individual skills.

Parental Considerations. The physician must use the strengths of the parents and the family to help the autistic youngster. His first task may be to make life tolerable for the parents. Often they are emotionally battered by the time they see the doctor. The mother has been overwhelmed and exhausted by this child who is so different. Both father and mother may be scared of the child and fear that they might damage him even further. This special child often becomes the focus of marital conflict. The physician must help these burdened parents develop lives of their own. They have to replenish their own emotional reserves so that they can be stronger, more flexible parents and adults and find parenthood rewarding again. When the autistic child is young, it is difficult but often possible to get a babysitter so that the parents can get away temporarily. When this child approaches adolescence, it is usually impossible to get home supervision; the physician can often support the parents best by helping them place the autistic child temporarily in a residential unit or hospital while they have a well-earned rest or vacation. During periods of increased or extended family stress, the parents may need tranquilizers, mood elevators, or night-time sedation. The physician also has to help these parents be realistic in what they do for the autistic child. The welfare of the other children in the family must not be forgotten. Sometimes parents, in their anguish or guilt, mortgage their future and the future of their other children to get what they feel is the "best" treatment for the autistic child. By sacrificing the family in this way, the parents may be destroying what little home life the autistic child has, and often this extreme sacrifice usually has little guarantee of therapeutic success.

Treatment Program. In planning the treatment program for the autistic child the physician and the parents must know what is available in the local community and in the state. Often it is very helpful if the parents can join a group of other parents of autistic children. There they can see that these parents are normal, rational people who have had to cope with what often becomes an overwhelming family problem. If there is not a local parents' group, the parents should contact the National Society for Autistic Children (61 Central Avenue, Albany, New York 12206), where they will receive information about facilities and programs available and be given contacts with other parents of autistic children. Sometimes families with autistic children develop programs jointly with parents of neurologically handicapped children, but these youngsters are usually much more handicapped physically than the autistic child. The physician and the parents should certainly consult the director of local school special education programs. Trainable retarded children show many autistic features, and if there are not special school classes for autistic children, they can often be placed in educational and treatment programs for the trainable retarded to develop necessary social and academic skills. The pediatrician will wish to consult any local child psychologist or psychiatrist who might be experienced in working with autistic or profoundly psychotic children.

In this fashion the doctor and the parents can use all the resources available to them to set up a gradual long-term treatment program to modify the autistic child's behavior and train him in socially acceptable skills and social independence. This plan, which will have to be maintained for many years and modified as the child changes, is carried out at home, at school and, at times, possibly in an inpatient institution, or some combination of these. When the autistic child shows increasingly disruptive tension, the physician can prescribe tranquilizers, but like any medication for the autistic child, these tranquilizers have to be prescribed on a very individual basis. The autistic patient may react unpredictably to any drug; he can develop a temperature of 104° F. in response to a penicillin shot or to a few aspirin tablets, while he may show absolutely no sign that he has a massive peritonitis. An autistic child may become deeply tranquilized with only a minimum dose of chlorpromazine or he may take massive doses with no outward effect; the same patient may show opposite and extreme reactions at different times.

Institutionalization. Over the years the progress of the autistic child is liable to be slow, uneven and erratic. Periodically he may show sudden exacerbations of disturbed behavior or he may go through a period of rapid social improvement. As the child grows and shows changing capabilities, the treatment plan will have to be modified in response to the patient and the changing resources of the family and the community. Even with the most intensive, best supported treatment, many autistic children never become completely acceptable socially. As this child gets older, he becomes much more difficult to keep at home; he is too big and uncontrolled and his parents are getting older and physically less able. Eventually the parents and the physician must consider institutional placement. Hospitals, which are largely custodial, tend to accentuate the autistic tendencies of any patient and the autistic child is especially liable to become even more withdrawn and autistic in such an environment. The doctor and the parents should look for an inpatient setting with adequate staffing and facilities to continue the treatment program that has been established. As the autistic child grows older, he may still benefit from treatment and eventually be able to leave the institution and return to society.

By working closely with the autistic child and his family, the pediatrician can help the autistic youngster to some extent. Perhaps even more important, he will help the parents and the other children in the family. Pediatricians who are especially interested in ongoing research, evaluation and management of autistic children should consult the newly published *Journal of Autism and Childhood Schizophrenia.*

Psychosomatic Illness

JAMES P. ROSENBLUM, M.D.

Among those disorders which have been thought to be in large measure psychosomatic, asthma, eczema, ulcerative colitis and regional ileitis are well recognized.

Why do we call such illnesses "psychosomatic"? It should be remembered that an infant's response to stimuli, be they pleasant or unpleasant, is a physiologic one. Through a series of stages, the healthy adult will have learned a different response; namely, the stimuli will evoke a feeling response (rather than a physiologic one) which will enable him to recognize what is happening and to attempt to cope with the situation.

When, however, for whatever reason, the individual carries with him into physical adulthood the childhood pattern of continuously responding physiologically to such stimuli, the result of such repeated assaults upon the organs will be the development of some form of psychosomatic illness.

Which of many forms such an illness will take will depend on a number of factors: some are genetic predisposition, trauma, constitutional "weakness" and so forth.

Because the inter-relationship between psyche and soma is extremely complex, such conditions frequently do not consist of a single entity. Furthermore, the precipitating causes are sometimes quite difficult to determine.

A recent study of 25 children with asthma revealed that in about 50 per cent of the cases emotional stress and/or parental behavior appeared to have strongly influenced the onset of attacks. In the other 50 per cent no such correlation was discovered. It is not clear whether this is because there was no correlation or whether the correlation did exist but was less evident.

At all times and under all circumstances, a careful and thorough history is vitally important. The relationships between the patient and significant people in the immediate environment, such as parents, siblings, other relatives, baby-sitters, friends and teachers, are of paramount importance for investigation. In addition, valuable information can be adduced from observation of the reactions of those who are being interviewed; this includes the patient (both when being questioned alone and when his or her parent or parents are being questioned in the child's presence) and the parent or surrogates, as the case may be. For the physician, the ability to observe these reactions is as important (if not more so) as the sorting out of the overtly presented "facts." The "give-aways" which reveal the underlying feelings of significant participants are seen in facial and body movements of which the communicants are usually totally unaware.

Since the illnesses in question here usually have a large psychic component to their pathogeneses, psychiatric help should be sought whenever possible. However, there are often circumstances which render this infeasible. Therefore, the pediatrician will do well to deal with the emotional factors that he recognizes in the interactions between the patient and significant people in the environment. Tension can often be markedly reduced merely by making those involved consciously aware of interpersonal problems and of their importance vis-a-vis the illness. This may require frequent reinforcement over a long period of time. Sometimes it may not be sufficient only to make the patient or those involved with him aware of these problems. It may be necessary to teach them new, less destructive ways of dealing with these problems.

In addition to primary emotional difficulties, secondary emotional conflicts usually arise in anyone with chronic illness. One common problem where an illness has been prolonged is that the patient and/or his parents come to relish the "secondary gains" of invalidism. The physician should be alert to this. Insight into this problem is generally difficult to convey, even to the most intelligent. By small steps, however, and through frequent repetition, insight can often be developed. The results are worth the effort.

The physician needs to show as much sympathy (if not more) toward a patient with a problem of psychic origin as he would show if the patient had been injured in an accident. At the same time, he must be truthful with the child. No doubt he ought always to be so, but in these cases it is even more important because of the probable underlying, as yet undiscovered, anxiety. Finally, he must be patient and not appear rushed. This overall approach, as opposed to the "phony" sounding "everything is going to be all right", will convey a sense of real assurance. The reassurance that everything will be taken into consideration, every avenue explored and utilized where useful, is itself an important part of the therapeutic armamentarium in these cases.

Reference

Purcell, K., et al.: The Effect on Asthma in Children of Experimental Separation From the Family. *Psychosom. Med.* 31:144, 1969.

Pica

J. JULIAN CHISOLM, Jr., M.D.

The habit of pica is prevalent in one- to three-year-old children. Its psychologic and physiologic dynamics are not well understood. The behavior is variously attributed to inadequate mothering, stress and nutritional deficiencies. Some have speculated that many toddlers have an innate need to chew on hard crunchy substances. Studies in behavioral psychology indicate that adjunctive behavior such as pica can be readily induced in animals by a combination of restricting overall caloric intake and presenting the food in very small amounts throughout the day so that hunger is never really satisfied at any single feeding. In children, the use of food as an oral pacifier may also play a role. The use of lead acetate in centuries past to sweeten wine and other alcoholic beverages has led to the unsubstantiated speculation that old lead pigment paints and putty may have a sweet taste to which certain children are attracted.

Permissiveness toward pica varies considerably on a cultural basis. Indeed, instances have been encountered in which clay-eating, earth-eating and starch-eating mothers and grandmothers deliberately fed these items to younger children. Clinical experience suggests that a child may indulge in pica when under the care of only one or two of the several adults (mother, father, aunt, uncle, babysitter, grandparents and so forth) who share the responsibility for his care. Because the etiologic factors are not clearly understood and may be multiple in any given case, the clinical management of pica is largely empirical and should be individualized.

There is no general agreement on a definition of pica. The term is used here to mean the repetitive search for and ingestion of nonfood items. The range of items eaten may be wide. The amount and duration may vary considerably from the child who indulges in pica for a few months only to the severely brain-damaged child in whom pica may be voracious and virtually uncontrollable, and persist for years.

This author has found the approach of Lourie and his coworkers to be the most useful from the practical viewpoint. Conceptually, pica is viewed as a response to stress in the young child. The stress, in turn, may be potentiated by a lack of mothering. For example, the working mother, who is unavailable to her child during working hours, may not be able to provide an adequate substitute during her absence. The arrival of a new infant can divert a mother's attention from her toddler. She may be embroiled in marital conflict or other social, emotional or financial difficulty. She may be inadequate, owing to emotional immaturity or disturbance. Conflicts with grandparents may disturb her relationship with her child. Some of the greatest difficulty is encountered in very young, immature and impulsive parents unable to control either their own or their child's behavior.

It can be appreciated that a variety of etiologic factors may conduce to pica in the toddler and that, for the most part, behavioral, social and financial rather than medical problems are the important ones. For these reasons, it has been our policy for the past 20 years to refer all clinical cases of lead poisoning and those asymptomatic children with confirmed blood lead concentrations greater than 50 to 60 micrograms per 100 Gm. of whole blood to the Medical-Social Service Department for evaluation. Among the allied health professions, the orientation and training of medical-social service workers best fits them to collaborate with the pediatrician in the long-term management of children with plumbism and pica. It is the medical-social worker who is usually most adept in eliciting the needed types of information cited above. Within the clinic setting, they best provide the continuity of care during the several preschool years in which follow-up may be needed.

As soon as a diagnosis is made, each case is reported to the Health Department (for investigation of environmental sources) and to the Medical-Social Service Department (for consultation with the family). After about one week, a conference between pediatrician and the medical-social worker is held. All information is reviewed and evaluated and a tentative plan for management is agreed upon. (Steps are, of course, taken to correct nutritional deficiencies and to institute regular mealtimes without nibbling in the home.) If it is considered that the prospect for controlling pica is remote (i.e., severely mentally defective child, highly unfavorable family situation or grossly dilapidated dwelling), the family is urged to move into modern (public) housing. Placement of older preschool siblings in day care centers may permit the parent to devote greater attention to the toddler. Sometimes placement of the toddlers themselves in such facilities, even for a few hours each week, can be helpful. The medical-social service worker assists in all of these areas and helps to mobilize the family resources in a way which can reduce stress in the home and its reflection in the child's behavior. The medical-social service worker may also find it necessary to meet with grandparents, aunts and uncles if they appear to play a dominant role in the child's rearing.

The effectiveness of the approach employed in each case is evaluated through serial measurements of blood lead concentration and the indices of lead toxicity (i.e., erythrocyte protoporphyrin, delta-aminolevulinic acid dehydrase test). If these show the expected slow but steady decrease toward normal during the succeeding months and years, management may be considered adequate. Recurrences of plumbism indicate the need to reevaluate both the environment and family dynamics. Since pica is often clandestine and since it may occur when the child is not with the parent, abdominal x-rays positive for radiopaque foreign material are often helpful in demonstrating to the parents the actuality of pica in their child. We have found this maneuver quite helpful: The findings often come as quite a surprise to the mother. Whether this approach is actually therapeutically effective or whether it simply provides for close supervision until the habit abates is not known. However, the extent to which the management plan for pica is effective is probably determined by the commitment of mother, pediatrician and medical-social worker to the care of the child and the assistance and support given to the mother in coping with her varied problems.

References

Cooper, M.: *Pica*. Springfield, Illinois, Charles C Thomas, Publisher, 1957.

Falk, J. L.: Theoretical Review, The Nature and Determinants of Adjunctive Behavior. *Physiol. and Behav.*, 6:577–588, 1971.

Lourie, R. S., Layman, E. M., and Millican, F. K.: Why Children Eat Things that are not Food. *Children*, 10:143, 1963.

Millican, F. K., Layman, E. M., Lourie, R. S., and Takahashi, L. Y.: Study of an Oral Fixation: Pica. *J. Am. Acad. Child Psychiat.*, 7:79, 1968.

Sobel, R.: The Psychiatric Implications of Accidental Poisoning in Childhood. *Pediat. Clin. N. Am.*, 17: 653–685, 1970.

Sleep Disturbance

ALAN N. MARKS, M.D.

Almost all small children present some sleep problem. Most of these problems represent an interaction between the child's developing personality and needs and the personality and attitudes of the parents. Children differ widely in their sleep needs. Usually the wiry and active child needs less sleep than the obese, placid, relatively inactive child. It is absurd to set rules concerning the duration of sleep required at different ages. Some sleep difficulties are man-made rather than child-made. They arise from overrigid methods of management.

The majority of sleep problems are transient and irritating. Medication is usually not indicated. The short-term use of small doses of chloral hydrate can be prescribed to promote some peace and quiet in the family. Understanding the source of the child's anxiety, the parental concerns and the current family situation is often sufficient to enable the pediatrician to provide supportive guidance until the disturbances subside.

Sleep disturbances may occur from the imminent approach of bedtime to the time of awakening. These disturbances have been reviewed and classified according to the most common age of appearance. This system provides a developmental context for understanding the disturbance.

FIRST YEAR

Two major concerns of the family during the first year of the child's life are sleeping through the night and night awakening. Over 70 per cent of babies sleep through the night by the age of three months. The factors which promote sleeping through the night (settling) are unknown, but it is generally believed that settling is related to the process of CNS maturation. Infants who have suffered some perinatal insult, such as anoxia, settle later. Environmental conditions, such as feeding schedule, sleep arrangements and minor illness, do not seem to be related to the age of settling. A high level of maternal anxiety reflected by inconsistent handling or insufficient nonfeeding play does delay settling. Once the process of settling has occurred, waking normally recurs in 50 per cent of infants between five and nine months. During the second half of the first year, environmental factors, such as changed sleeping arrangements, separations, minor trauma and new family members, have been reported to be associated with wakenings. These disruptions are usually transient, though severe trauma may result in more prolonged disturbances. After six months of age, parental concern and anger over poor sleeping habits may precipitate more complicated problems. Therefore, during the first year of life, if the baby's physiologic needs are met adequately, empathetic understanding and guidance from the pediatrician to allay excessive parental anxiety should lead to resolution of the sleep disturbance.

SECOND YEAR

During the second year of life, sleep disturbances often reflect infantile anxiety. At this age psychologic and cognitive components are added to the physiologic requirements of sleep. With the strengthening of the child's ties to significant people and to the happenings of the external world, he clings to wakefulness. A reluctance to go to sleep is a common disturbance of this age.

To allay the anxiety associated with going to sleep, presleep habits or rituals develop as well as the taking of teddy or blanket to bed. In a minority of cases the rituals seem to stem from conflicts centering around overzealous attempts at early discipline (e.g., toilet training, limit setting). Children of this group are easily overexcited by parents or upset by frightening daytime experiences. They may develop a transient fear of going to sleep because of the "bad dream" experience. When the child develops a clear-cut distinction between dreams and reality, this type of disturbance disappears.

THIRD TO FIFTH YEAR

It is rare to find a child in this group who is not experiencing some difficulty over sleep, whether it is tardiness in falling asleep, night wakening, nightmares projecting fears of ghosts and wild animals, inability to sleep alone or in the dark or ritualistic presleep behavior. Most of these difficulties are transient and respond to minimal supportive intervention. If refractive, the sleep disturbance often represents one symptom of a more profound conflict that necessitates psychiatric evaluation.

AGE SIX TO ADOLESCENCE

During this stage there is an amelioration of most sleep disturbances. On occasion, sleep disturbances may arise de novo or may carry over from an earlier age. The minor disturbance may persist through adolescence into adulthood.

Voice, Speech, and Language Disorders

MORTON COOPER, Ph.D.

Children of all ages may experience voice, speech and language disorders. Some of these children, depending on the severity of the problem, the age of the child and other relevant considerations, may need the assistance of a voice therapist, a speech therapist, an audiologist or other specialists as recommended by the pediatrician.

A child's speech and language development proceeds through stages which may overlap or run concomitantly. These stages include crying, babbling, lallation, echolalia and jargon. By the end of the first year of age, the child usually is beginning to use words. From this point, the child's vocabulary increases rapidly, and gradually speech becomes more intelligible as more sounds are correctly articulated.

If speech and language are not developing normally, that is, if the child is not speaking by 2 to 2½ years or if he is not basically intelligible by 3½ to 4 years, speech and language evaluations are advisable. The child may be diagnosed as having delayed language and/or an articulation disorder (sound substitution, distortion, omission or addition). Other tests (hearing, psychologic, physical and so forth) may also be appropriate.

Table 1 may be used as a guide for speech sound development, although speech sounds may appear earlier or later than indicated in the table. Speech sounds correctly produced in isolation or in single words do not constitute correct speech; the pediatrician must listen to the child's spontaneous, connected speech. Table 1 also indicates language development as depicted by sentence length.

In referring the child for speech therapy

TABLE 1. Speech and Language Development

AGE	SPEECH (*Sound Development*)*	LANGUAGE (*Sentence Length in Words*)†‡
1		1
1½		1.2
2		1.8
2½		3.1
3	All vowels and diphthongs; *m, n, ng, p, f, h, w*	4.1
3½	*y*	4.7
4	*b, d, k, g, r*	5.4
4½	*sh, ch, s*	5.4
5		5.7
6	*t, th* (unvoiced), *v, l*	6.6
7	*th* (voiced), *z, zh, j*	7.3
8		7.6

* Sounds listed by age at which 75 per cent of children tested produced sounds correctly in all positions in words, except in consonant blends (Templin).

† McCarthy (ages 1 to 2½).

‡ Templin (ages 3 to 8).

for articulation disorders, the pediatrician must take into account factors other than the sound development. These include the child's reaction to his speech, the parents' reaction to the child's speech and the importance that the parents (and the family) place upon correct speech.

Speech and language disorders may be either functional or organic in origin. Functional causes may include lack of speech stimulation, acceptance of gesture language by parents, inadequate speech models, bilingual influence, an environment which penalizes speech, an older sibling speaking for the child, an accident or illness and any incident or continuing situation which creates psychologic trauma. Organic causation may be neurologic, such as a hearing loss (slight or severe), mental retardation, brain damage, aphasia and cerebral palsy, or it may involve structural deviations, such as cleft palate, submucous cleft and tonguetie. (Tonguetie, although infrequently encountered, should be treated surgically as early as possible, before the child is one to two years of age, to avoid any interference with normal speech development.)

The length of speech or language therapy depends on the severity of the disorder, age of the child, parental support, motivation and the child's emotional and psychologic reactions to the speech or language problem, among other factors. Organic involvement requires early diagnosis, long-term speech and language therapy, special school programs and extensive parent counseling.

In speech and language therapy with a child who has delayed language (functional or organic causation), the child must learn that using language is enjoyable and is the only realistic means of controlling his environment. The therapist may begin with an initial babbling of bilabial sounds, such as *b, p, w,* combined with physical movement (jumping, clapping and so forth), which will encourage the child to participate and imitate. Any attempt at speech imitation by the child is rewarded by appreciative verbal approval. Language used in the therapy session must be direct and simple, with constant repetition. The therapist may initiate a structured framework to develop such concepts as colors, animals, family and community helpers. As therapy progresses, concepts may be combined, such as talking about environmental objects and colors, e.g., "blue car," "brown shoes." When the child's language begins to develop, introduction of familiar words with initial bilabial sounds may be instituted with auditory, visual and tactile stimulation. Throughout the therapy program the parents are guided by the therapist to reinforce the same type of program into the home environment.

Various approaches can be used by the therapist in the treatment of articulation disorders. After determining which sounds are incorrectly produced, the therapist may choose that sound which the child can most easily produce correctly. Success is essential at the initial stage of therapy so that the child develops a positive attitude toward therapy and its goals.

Personalizing the speech sounds for the younger child within a construct of speech activities geared to correct production of the sound helps the child remember the sound. The reward of a move on a speech game board, a picture he can paste in a book or a bell he can ring further reinforces the child's use of the correct sound in words, phrases and sentences. Carry-over of the speech sound into spontaneous speech can be accomplished by structuring situations that approximate those in the child's world. Doll families, manipulative toys, story telling and puppets are some of the ways in which to move the child toward his final goal of carry-over of correct speech production into his everyday life. For the older child, speech activities emphasize the positive aspects of acceptable sound production and stress a more direct approach to therapy with the use of tape recordings, advanced speech materials and reading.

Some children may have the problem of stuttering. Stuttering is an interference with the normal flow of speech, actual (physical) or anticipated (psychologic), and a reaction to the interference which involves an attempt to avoid the interference. Stuttering usually involves noticeable or excessive dysfluencies, such as repeating, hesitating, prolonging or blocking on speech sounds. Stuttering may be due to psychologic tension which has been created by an attempt to avoid the normal dysfluencies that are present in normal speech.

Stuttering usually develops in two stages. In the primary stage, the child appears to be without self-awareness or self-concern for the dysfluencies in his speech. In the secondary stage, the child either becomes aware or is made aware of the dysfluencies, seeks to minimize or prevent them and attempts to produce perfect speech. Complicating factors of the secondary stage may include facial grimaces and other contorted body movements by which the child tries to prevent stuttering.

For a child in the primary stage of stuttering, play therapy encourages positive speech experiences and affords the child an opportunity to express directly his feeling state and to structure a more relevant self-image. The use of direct speech therapy depends on the therapist's discretion. For a secondary stutterer, the therapist needs to develop a close relationship with the child, to meet the child's specific needs and to work with the child on his own individual manner of stuttering. This approach allows the child to understand how he stutters, why he stutters and how to cope with the stuttering.

An essential part of the therapy program is parent counseling. The parent (s) should be given information regarding the problem and suggestions to attenuate the emotional and psychologic tensions which may contribute to or which may be activated by stuttering.

The following suggestions are for parents of primary stutterers: (1) As the child speaks, listen attentively and help the child to enjoy talking. (2) Provide experiences which the child can describe, such as visits to the park, museum, zoo and library. (3) Plan times to play, read and talk to the child. (4) Guide the child toward self-discipline but avoid strict discipline. (5) Be accepting of the child and his efforts, praising him whenever possible. (6) Do not refer to the child as a stutterer or discuss the child in his presence. (7) Do not interrupt or correct the child when he is speaking. (8) The child should not be provided with words to complete his thoughts when he hesitates. (9) The child should not be pressured unrealistically in speech, in school work or in other activities. (10) Do not force the child to perform or participate in events which are threatening to him.

In addition to these suggestions, parents of secondary stutterers should accept the child, his behavior and his speech; they need to provide reassurance, understanding, support and love, which in turn helps the child accept himself. The child needs to be encouraged to develop himself and his talents and to become a self-sufficient individual according to his age and his capabilities.

Voice disorders in children may be either functional or organic. Functional dysphonias seen most frequently include nasality, falsetto and functional misphonia (tired or weak voice with hoarseness present), which is the most prevalent type. Organic dysphonias most often encountered are nodules, polyps and papillomas.

Voice problems are evidenced by negative vocal symptoms—visual, auditory and/or sensory. Visual symptoms may be inflammation, edema or growths on the vocal folds. Auditory symptoms may include hoarseness, nasality, breathiness, limited vocal range, voice breaks and reduced volume. Sensory symptoms may include throat clearing, a sore, tight or strained throat, a feeling of a foreign substance in the throat, voice produced with effort and progressive vocal fatigue.

Childhood dysphonias are most frequently caused by vocal misuse and abuse, such as use of incorrect pitch, tone focus, volume and breath support; imitation of inadequate vocal models or inappropriate vocal models (vocal image); group singing in an incorrect pitch range; voice change at puberty; and poor vocal hygiene, such as shouting, screaming or talking constantly above noise. Contributing factors may be a cold or upper respiratory infection if pitch and tone focus are affected; medical conditions, such as allergy, postnasal drip, hay fever, sinusitis and infected tonsils; emotional and psychologic problems; and a hearing loss.

Most childhood dysphonias may be alleviated or eliminated through vocal rehabilitation. Vocal rehabilitation essentially eliminates vocal misuse by retraining the individual's voice in the use of pitch, tone focus, quality, breath support, volume or rate. The practice of good vocal hygiene is instituted to minimize or eliminate vocal abuse.

The habitual pitch level (pitch the child is using) may be above (too high) or below (too low) the optimal or natural pitch level (pitch the child should use). With the exception of falsetto, most children with dysphonias are using too low a pitch level. The child is taught to use the natural or optimal pitch level.

Tone focus (sound resonance) may incorrectly emphasize nasal resonance (from nasopharynx), oral resonance (from oropharynx) or laryngeal resonance (from laryngopharynx); the last is the most frequently heard resonance in dysphonias, except in nasality. Proper tone focus involves a balanced oro-naso-laryngopharyngeal resonance, which the child must develop.

Voice quality is determined by the vocal folds which produce the sound and by the resonating areas which modify the sound. Impaired vocal folds may create a hoarse or a breathy voice; excessive nasal resonance may cause nasality. Correct pitch level and proper tone focus usually result in the resolution of a deviant voice quality.

Breath support may stress clavicular breathing, upper chest breathing or midsection breathing. Midsection breath support has been found to be the most effective for speech.

Incorrect volume may be too loud or too soft; inappropriate rate may be too fast or too slow. Vocal rehabilitation establishes appropriate volume and rate.

During vocal rehabilitation as the voice is being retrained, the child usually requires brief or extended *vocal* psychotherapy to help him adjust to the new voice and the new vocal image. The vocal image involves the positive or negative feelings and reactions toward a voice and determines the type of voice a child likes (and will use) or dislikes (and will not use). Children usually have a positive vocal image toward the old voice and a negative vocal image toward the new voice. Vocal psychotherapy allows a vocal catharsis, an expression of feelings and reactions toward the old and new voices. The extent of vocal psychotherapy, which varies from one child to another, is dependent on the strength of the old vocal image. If the child does not become adjusted to and accepting of the new voice and the new vocal image, he will not use the new voice, and vocal rehabilitation will not be successful. In a few selected cases, psychotherapy may be necessary alone or in conjunction with vocal rehabilitation.

In conclusion, the pediatrician's role in the management of voice, speech and language disorders is that of (1) recognizing disorders of speech, language and voice, (2) counseling the parents regarding the child's problem, (3) referring the child to appropriate specialists, (4) serving as a coordinator of the various specialists assisting the child, in some cases and (5) providing continual support for the rehabilitative programs.

References

Cooper, M.: Speech Disorders and Problems (Speech and Language Development). *Pediat. News,* 4:16, 27, 37, 57, 1970.

Cooper, M.: Modern Techniques of Vocal Rehabilitation for Functional and Organic Dysphonias; in L. E. Travis (ed.): *Handbook of Speech Pathology and Audiology.* New York, Appleton-Century-Crofts, 1971.

Cooper, M.: Speech Disorders and Problems (Voice Disorders). *Pediat. News,* 5:48–49, 1971.

Cooper, M.: Speech Disorders and Problems (Stuttering). *Pediat. News,* 5:55–56, 1971.

Cooper, M.: Speech Disorders and Problems (Aphasia). *Pediat. News,* 6:21, 1972.

Cooper, M.: *Modern Techniques of Vocal Rehabilitation.* Springfield, Illinois, Charles C Thomas, Publisher, 1973.

McCarthy, D.: Language Development in Children; in L. Carmichael (ed.): *Manual of Child Psychology,* 2nd ed. New York, John Wiley & Sons, Inc., 1964.

Templin, M. C.: *Certain Language Skills in Children: Their Development and Interrelationships.* Minneapolis, University of Minnesota Press, 1957.

Learning Problems

PATRICIA BIRD GROSSMAN, M.A., A.C.S.W., SARAH C. GORSKI, M.A., *and* HERBERT J. GROSSMAN, M.D.

WHOSE PROBLEMS?

The very term "school adjustment problem" connotes maladaptation or even failure, but this failure is never one-sided and must be considered from different perspectives. School difficulties reflect not only an impairment in the student's capacity to adjust to the educational environment, but also the school's inability to meet the child's educational needs. The teacher is often frustrated because her best efforts to teach and help the child seem fruitless. The child may see the situation as a convergence of puzzling, frightening demands, often confusing, sometimes overwhelming. Parents, trying to help the child and "cooperate" with the school often feel bewildered and inadequate at a time when the child is most in need of parental stability and support. It is very important for the pediatrician to be aware of these different perspectives and the feelings they engender so that he may assess the situation correctly and support feelings appropriate to the common goal: helping the student move toward a positive school experience.

School problems are often described in terms of academic and/or behavioral difficulties. Academic difficulties center around a slow rate of mental development (mental retardation), perceptual handicaps and specific learning disabilities. Behavioral disorders may include hyperactivity, bizarre behavior, "acting out," impulsivity and short attention span. Other maladaptive behaviors such as withdrawal, depression, depressive equivalents, immaturity and inappropriate dependency are often seen. These are just as serious as the more disruptive actions.

Most of these children suffer from a combination of academic and emotional problems. It is extremely rare to find a child with serious academic problems who does not have feelings of failure, depression and anxiety. Conversely, children with serious emotional problems do not have the free psychic energy needed for learning.

It should be stressed that children with these difficulties do not necessarily present serious school adjustment problems. Some children are able to adapt (however minimally) to school expectations and certain teachers and school systems are able to adjust their requirements in order to help the child in coping with the school environment.

WHAT CAN THE SCHOOL DO?

Traditionally, schools had few options in dealing with children who presented problems. The school could carry the child along with "social promotions", encourage the parent to seek tutoring or private schools or push the child to drop out as soon as he reached the legal age for such termination. Over the past 20 years, schools have taken more responsibility for setting up alternatives to meet the needs of the special child. Special education classes have been established, using certain diagnostic criteria for eligibility. Classes for the mentally retarded, socially maladjusted, physically handicapped, hard of hearing and blind have proliferated. More recently, programs have been developed for children with learning disabilities. These children are described as having average intelligence but lower than average academic functioning. They may or may not have a specific perceptual handicap.

Admission to these special classes is based on psychologic evaluation, teacher assessment and medical and social information. Historically and legally, a diagnostic "labeling" has been required for admission to special classes. More sophisticated diagnostic assessment has led to greater awareness of the complexity of these problems and a growing dissatisfaction with the "labeling" process. Educators are currently looking for other methods of grouping children. One method is to assess the child's needs in terms of specific academic and behavioral goals and plan the educational program to meet these objectives.

In addition to special classes, schools are developing other alternatives to help children within the regular school setting. Itinerant teachers provide individual instructions to children with learning disabilities, slow learners and children with behavioral problems. These teachers also assist the classroom teacher in setting and implementing appropriate educational plans. Resource rooms can provide a part-time learning experience under the direction of an educational specialist. Guidance and counseling, speech therapy, remedial reading, psychologic and social work services are becoming an integral part of the school program in many places.

REFERRAL TO THE PEDIATRICIAN

A child with a "school adjustment problem" is often referred to the pediatrician. Referral may come directly from the teacher, school nurse or principal; more often the parents are directed to seek help from their physician. A vaguely worded referral may state that the child is having a problem in school and request a "complete evaluation", which leaves the pediatrician wondering (1) what the problem is, and (2) what he is expected to evaluate. More specific referrals may ask for a "complete neurologic examination and an EEG", again leaving the pediatrician in the dark regarding the child's behavior, symptomatology and the school's concerns. A more appropriate referral is the one in which both school and parents describe the child's behavior and academic performance in detail, list their questions and outline how they expect the pediatrician to aid in solving the problem. If this information is not clear in the initial referral, the pediatrician should request further clarification from the school.

When the problem has been delineated by parents and school, the physician must determine what diagnostic steps to pursue. One of the most important and most frequently forgotten steps is an interview with the student. The physician is in a unique, nonthreatening position to help the student voice his concerns and complaints. He may be right!

The medical and developmental history should be reviewed in conjunction with an assessment of the child's current adaptation at home, with peers and in school. The physical examination should include vision and hearing screening. Further studies and diagnostic procedures (neurologic, psychiatric, psychologic, electroencephalographic) should be undertaken if indicated. Following the medical assessments, the pediatrician has the responsibility of collating and evaluating the information and transmitting this, with his recommendations, to the student, the parents and the school.

This medical diagnosis may or may not be of value in determining an appropriate educational plan. It is important for the pediatrician to know how his medical assessment will be used by the school. It can be used appropriately to provide additional understanding of the child; medical information should not be used as the primary point of reference for educational programming.

Schools and parents may request the pediatrician to prescribe some medication to calm the child or increase his attention span. It is important for the physician to have adequate, detailed behavioral observations from home and school when medication is being considered or administered. While some children show marked improvement in behavior with certain drugs, these drugs are at best an adjunct in total management. Drug therapy is not a substitute for a carefully conceived, conscientiously implemented program of management. Of great importance is the pediatrician's availability for a longitudinal relationship with the school and the parents. It may be desirable and sometimes necessary for the pediatrician to take the initiative in encouraging this type of relationship and subsequent communication.

Reading Disorders

LEON EISENBERG, M.D.

A reading disorder exists whenever there is a significant discrepancy between a child's actual performance on a standardized reading test and the normative expectations for his age and school placement. By convention, a discrepancy of two years or more signifies a severe reading disorder. This standard is obviously inapplicable in the first several grades of school when aberrant function is detected only at a level below the floor of the test.

Reading retardation is the functional expression of inadequate learning, the cause of which is highly varied. Efforts at prevention and treatment require specification of causes when causes can be identified.

Major causes may be listed under two generic headings: sociopsychologic and psychophysiologic. Among the former are: (1) *Deficiencies in teaching*—insufficient school attendance, as in the case of children of migrant workers, or poor quality of teaching, as is so often the case in overcrowded schools in blighted urban areas and in poorly staffed schools in rural communities. (2) *Deficiencies in intellectual stimulation,* characteristic of children who enter school from illiterate homes, never having been read to or exposed to books and lacking the background perceptual stimulation and hearing vocabulary which are the prerequisites for reading. Because these experiences are assumed to be the common property of six-year-old children, the necessary experiential supplementation is not provided to the deficient child before reading instruction is attempted. (3) *Deficiencies in motivation,* secondary to social pathology or to individual psychopathology. The former is a major problem among underprivileged children whose neighborhood experience and family values are such that school is seen as irrelevant to life performance; the latter is found in psychiatrically disturbed children who may be resisting parental pressure for success by failing to learn or who may be so preoccupied with anxiety or obsessional ideas that they are unavailable for classroom learning.

Psychophysiologic sources of reading retardation include: (4) *General debility*—the chronically ill or malnourished child. (5) *Sensory defects.* Visual impairment is rarely decisive until acuity is reduced below 50 per cent; auditory imperfection far short of deafness may, however, be an important and too easily overlooked source of difficulty. (6) *Mental deficiency.* Impairment in intelligence will result in failure to learn to read along with failure to master other academic subjects. (7) *Brain injury.* Perceptual deficits and specific intellectual disabilities even in the presence of adequate general intelligence may lead to reading failure. (8) *Specific reading disability,* which may be defined as the failure to learn to read with normal proficiency despite conventional instruction, an adequate home, proper motivation, intact senses, normal intelligence and freedom from detectable neurologic defect.

When the primary cause is absence from school or poor quality of teaching, the remedy obviously is in assuring every American child a full academic year of instruction of high quality. For children whose problem is in the area of intellectual disadvantage and motivational inadequacy, the solutions lie in rectifying the underlying sources of this social pathology (unemployment, slum housing, discrimination) and in steps to supplement early life experience by developing a network of child development centers. When the problem is related to psychiatric disorder, efforts to provide psychiatric care would seem justified; relief of the emotional disturbance is frequently followed by a spurt in learning.

Adequate pediatric examination and prescription of rehabilitative measures are the steps of choice in a child with chronic illness or sensory defect. It has been suggested, particularly in France and the Soviet Union, that speech and hearing therapy for the child with problems in auditory perception is helpful in improving the ability to read.

Careful studies of poor readers have demonstrated problems in relating spatially displayed symbols (i.e., static visual presentation) to temporally displayed symbols (i.e., sounds or flashing lights) in children with no obvious hearing defect. Moreover, difficulties in blendings sounds to form a word as well as in visual perception of complex figures point to developmental neuropsychologic abnormalities as factors underlying these disorders in reading.

A wide variety of instructional methods are currently under intensive study: perceptual training, kinesthetic methods, operant conditioning techniques (as exemplified by the automated typewriter) and others. Such instruction is best given individually or in small groups. Its success is highly dependent on the ability of the teacher to evoke an enthusiastic and cooperative response from the child. The need for special instruction is likely to extend over years. Several recent follow-up studies have suggested that the outcome, as measured in terms of being able to read (but not enjoying reading), is better than has been generally assumed.

The physician's role is primarily a diagnostic one. A screening procedure, such as the Gray Oral Reading Test (available from the Psychological Corporation, 304 East 45th Street, New York, New York 10017) should be administered to school-age children as a standard part of the periodic health examination. When a problem is detected, discussion with school authorities or referral to a competent clinical psychologist is indicated. The physician should familiarize himself with the adequacy of remedial reading services in his community. As a citizen, he can provide leadership in securing the resources to guarantee adequate treatment, early in school, for all children at risk.

References

Birch, H. G., and Gussow, J. D.: *Disadvantaged Children.* New York, Grune & Stratton, Inc., 1970.

Chall, J.: *Learning to Read: The Great Debate.* New York, McGraw-Hill Book Company, 1967.

Eisenberg, L.: Reading Retardation: Psychiatric and Sociologic Aspects. *Pediatrics,* 37:352, 1966.

Naidoo, S.: *Specific Dyslexia.* London, Sir Isaac Pitman & Sons Ltd., 1972.

Rutter, M., Tizard, J., and Whitmore, K.: *Education, Health and Behaviour.* London, Longmans Green & Co. Ltd., 1970.

Emotional Problems of the Adolescent

JOSEPH L. RAUH, M.D.

Adolescence is a rapidly changing, perplexing, seemingly irrational time of life. Many pediatricians avoid adolescents and find difficulty in helping adolescents cope with their problems. They are attracted to Mark Twain's view of the adolescent—namely, that when a child reaches the age of 13 he should be placed in a barrel and fed through the bung hole. Twain further stipulated that when the youth reached the age of 16, the bung hole should be plugged up. However, the pediatrician can effectively manage most of the emotional or "feeling" ills of adolescents if he understands their developmental processes and tasks, has a basic, sound, comfortable approach to the adolescent and knows when and how to use psychiatric consultation and management.

UNDERSTANDING ADOLESCENTS

Developmental Tasks. Much of the emotional growth of an adolescent is reflected in the process of his behavioral experimentation. Basic to this behavior, which is often paradoxical, irritating and self-destructive, are a number of essential developmental tasks. A knowledge of these tasks is needed to understand and treat the emotional problems of this age group. These tasks are as follows: (1) the establishment of emotional and psychologic independence from the parents and other adults; (2) the final arrival at self-definition, which results in the development of a stable self-concept (identity); (3) the development of self-motivation and self-determination; (4) the establishment of an appropriate set of values to be used as a guide for adult behavior and the self-control to implement and adhere to the ethical system selected; (5) the development of empathy and reciprocity in interpersonal relationships; (6) the development of new intellectual capacities; (7) the ability to function satisfactorily with age mates and to behave appropriately in relating to the peer group; (8) the acquisition of training that will develop the skills for achieving economic independence.

Trust. The need to trust peers and distrust adults is part of establishing emotional independence, the first developmental task. The adolescent often distrusts his parents and other adults who act like parents. The physician must establish a private, confidential, nonjudgmental attitude and relationship with his adolescent patient. He must listen more than he talks, not overreact to the more irritating acting-out behavior of teenagers and look for "messages" or clues that suggest what is really bothering the patient.

Above all, he must be able to "shift gears" when the adolescent comes to see him. For instance, the adolescent patient may take more time than the infant requiring a well-baby checkup. Very young children don't talk, allowing the doctor to examine the patient, talk to the parent and be done in 15 minutes. Adolescents will talk and express feelings if the doctor allows time and will listen and then talk to the parent at some other time. This is not to say that the adolescent does not need limits set on the doctor-patient relationship, as is the case with patients of all ages.

The doctor-adolescent relationship can be used to understand and treat many emotional problems if it is based on trust, confidentiality and compassionate neutrality.

Messages. Adolescents can be quick, dramatic and blunt in communicating their feelings. They say what they mean, but for reasons different from those that adult thinking perceives and interprets. For instance, a boy who is anxious over his recent drug experimentation may first refer to this problem by asking about drug reactions in general or about a prescribed medication; a girl who is worried about her sexuality and wants to talk about birth control will suddenly ask for medication for mild menstrual cramps or irregular periods. The physician can understand the many milder situational problems that confront adolescents by searching for the meaning of messages his adolescent patients give—verbally and nonverbally. The physician's recognition of these messages and availability to listen to them are often all that is needed. Milder, fairly acute adolescent adjustment problems do not require complicated psychiatric formulations for effective management. However, more serious pleas for help, especially suicidal thoughts, talk and behavior, often require psychiatric consultation and therapy.

PSYCHIATRIC CONSULTATION

Pediatricians are not the only specialists in medicine who may feel uncomfortable with adolescents. Psychiatrists may also be anxious about seeing teenagers and may shun them. Therefore, it behooves the pediatrician or general physician to establish a professional relationship with a psychiatrist who is at ease with this age group and skilled in dealing with the more difficult and chronic emotional problems of some adolescents.

Whom to Refer? The psychotic adolescent usually requires immediate hospitalization and psychiatric assistance. Psychotic behavior is not difficult to recognize. Even if it is relatively transient, associated, for example, with a drug overdose or reaction or with an acute anxiety or panic state, the patient should have psychiatric consultation to determine the cause and extent of the problem. Chronic problems which are not responsive to a good doctor-adolescent relationship over a period of several weeks or months should be referred. This is especially true of psychosomatic problems—for example, anorexia nervosa or ulcerative colitis—and management problems with diabetes, asthma and epilepsy, where psychologic factors are interfering with medical therapy. Psychiatric consultation is enhanced by explaining the process carefully to the patient and then asking the consultant to answer certain questions about the patient and his problems. Adolescents often are especially sensitive to seeing a "shrink"; the very thought immediately threatens his self-concept or identity. Yet the referral from the pediatrician who has already established a solid relationship will be accepted and positively used by the patient.

EMOTIONAL ILLNESSES

Depression is very common during adolescence and may be overlooked if subtle pleas for help are not recognized. Depression during adolescence often presents with symptomatology strikingly different from that of the adult patient. For example, the boy who has recently had two or three inexplicable motorbike or car accidents or the girl who has had venereal disease or an out-of-wedlock pregnancy may be expressing a depressive emotional reaction by acting-out, self-destructive behavior. Since depression can be severely self-destructive at this age, it is wise to seek psychiatric assistance early. Often the depression is the result of a traumatic experience which happened before adolescence—especially loss of a parent through death or separation, resulting in prolonged, unresolved grief. Such a situation usually requires some interpretive psychiatric treatment, although it may be brief and set in the context of general management by the pediatrician.

Hospitalization. Admission to the hospital can be crucial to the management of many adolescent emotional problems. Suicidal threats or behavior, hysterical conversion reactions, severe neurotic conflicts, panic reactions and drug reactions, severe home deprivation or rejection and psychosis are some of the major problems helped by hospitalization. The seriousness of the problem and the need for sophisticated psychiatric services and personnel will help determine whether the patient belongs in a psychiatric unit or in a general medical adolescent unit. Certainly, nonpsychotic patients who have reasonably good impulse control can be managed in an "open" hospital setting. Age-oriented adolescent activities such as recreation, occupational therapy, school and social opportunities with peers are essential regardless of the medical orientation of the hospital area.

Drug Therapy. The use of mood modifiers or tranquilizers should be avoided for the milder, situational emotional problems. Adolescents need to feel that their body is intact. This is part of their developing a stable self-concept. The use of psychoactive drugs may threaten the teenager's feeling of body intactness. More importantly, the physician must ask himself whether the advantages of a pharmacologic agent outweigh the risk of its being abused by the patient. What message is the physician communicating to the patient when he prescribes a mood modifier? Is the physician hypocritical when he condemns acid, speed and narcotics and, at the same time, prescribes a legitimate mood modifier?

The phenothiazines (chlorpromazine hydrochloride and others) are of value in the more severe anxiety states as well as with psychotic patients. Doses vary considerably: 10 to 25 mg. of Thorazine three or four times a day may be adequate for a mildly agitated patient, but other adolescents, especially those with psychotic problems, may require as much as 400 mg. daily. Adolescents vary in their body mass as a result of their particular state of development. Adult doses may be needed for the more physically mature patients.

Imipramine hydrochloride (Tofranil)* may be useful in the treatment of the depressed adolescent. Dosage should be initiated at a low level, 10 to 25 mg. three to four times a day orally, and be increased gradually over several weeks. In some patients, relatively high doses of 300 to 400 mg. a day may be necessary for amelioration or remission of depression. When such doses are used, hospitalization is strongly recommended. Often treatment must continue for at least two weeks before improvement is noted, regardless of dosage. There are many side effects, including hypotension or hypertension, confusion, restlessness, agitation, bone marrow depression and liver dysfunction, as well as anticholinergic effects such as urinary retention.

Adolescents with enuresis, in which organic causes have been ruled out, may be helped with Tofranil at bedtime. The dose is 25 mg. orally every night and may be increased to 50 mg. if the lower dose is not effective. Treatment should continue for three months. Although the manufacturer does not list enuresis among the indications for Tofranil, this medication has worked well in our experience. Parenteral administration of Tofranil for adolescents is not recommended.

Valium (diazepam) is indicated in the treatment of the acutely agitated adolescent. It is an effective sedative with a wide margin of safety.† It is especially helpful with the intoxicated adolescent, especially if he is high on alcohol or if there is a withdrawal reaction from mild to moderate narcotic addiction. The physically mature adolescent may be given 20 to 50 mg. intramuscularly. Smaller patients should receive 10 to 20 mg. This can be repeated every 4 to 6 hours, as necessary. The adolescent who is hallucinating following LSD ingestion may be similarly treated with Valium or Thorazine. Valium is also useful in the short-term treatment of agitation and skeletal muscle spasm due to acute trauma, and in certain cerebral palsy problems where more muscle relaxation is needed. Oral doses of 5 to 10 mg. three to four times daily are recommended for the adolescent with these problems.

Crisis Intervention. Most communities have several types of crisis intervention services available to adolescents. Many of these use the telephone as the vehicle for identifying the patient in crisis and providing help for him. Some telephone answering services rely on volunteers to talk to the adolescent in distress and then refer him to an agency or a psychiatrist for professional counseling. A more effective (and more expensive) method is to use trained, supervised health professionals to serve as psychotherapists on the telephone.

"Rap" or group sessions are very common today and can be quite effective in the management of acute emotional problems and medico-

* Manufacturer's precaution: Imipramine is not recommended for children under 12 years of age.

† Manufacturer's precaution: Safety and efficacy of injectable diazepam in children under 12 years of age have not been established.

social problems such as drug abuse, venereal disease and sexuality problems. The effectiveness of a group is always related to the training, experience and dedication of its leaders. Screening of the professionals involved is recommended before referring patients to such services.

Social Services. Social work in its myriad forms is very important in the management of emotional problems. Caseworkers can provide extensive family information about patients, see many patients in a clinic or private practice setting as well as in the hospital and, most importantly, see parents and keep them informed of their adolescent's developmental tasks, problems and progress while the physician sees the patient. Family service agencies should be utilized for patients and parents if the particular agency is experienced and comfortable with teenagers. Many other community agencies can be helpful in management. Most noteworthy are the Big Brother and Big Sister agencies, professionally run group homes for displaced adolescents and summer camps where staff is available to manage the mildly disturbed adolescent.

Depression and Suicide

LEO R. SULLIVAN, M.D.

Depression is a frequent disease in childhood, manifested by depressed mood, self-deprecatory feelings, aggressive behavior, sleep disturbances, difficulty with socialization, loss of interest in usual activity, somatic complaints, change in usual energy level and change in appetite and weight. Depressed children often present complaints of headaches, refusal to go to school, enuresis and sleep disturbances. When asked, the severely depressed child frequently will admit thoughts of suicide. Some children will even admit making attempts at suicide which were not necessarily appreciated as such by those around him.

Depression is a self-limited disease with a high familial incidence. Many cases improve spontaneously without specific treatment. In children, depressive episodes are usually of shorter duration than in adolescents and adults, i.e., lasting days to weeks rather than months. Mania is rarely seen in children.

Treatment is indicated in all moderate to severely depressed children. Treatment involves (1) environmental manipulation, (2) adjustment of school expectations where these are inappropriate and (3) judicious use of medication. The drug of choice for children who are primarily depressed and not severely agitated is Elavil. Initially, for a child under 25 kilograms, 10 mg. of Elavil are given at bedtime. Frequent side effects are lethargy and sleepiness. These usually pass in 24 to 48 hours and the drug should be continued. The medicine is then increased in 10-mg. increments, dividing the dose between morning and night, or morning, noon and night, to the point where the child's symptoms have improved or side effects occur. Side effects most commonly seen are dry mouth, photophobia, lethargy and urinary retention. Most children under 25 kilograms can be adequately treated with 30 to 60 mg. of Elavil per day in divided doses. Children over 25 kilograms are started initially with one 25-mg. tablet at bedtime and increased stepwise as outlined above. Larger children usually respond to 75 to 150 mg. of Elavil per day.

In a child who is primarily aggressive, agitated and acting out, the initial drug of choice is Mellaril*—10-mg. tablets for the child under 25 kilograms and 25-mg. tablets for the child over 25 kilograms. Initially, one tablet should be given two or three times a day. The drug is increased in a stepwise fashion as previously outlined for Elavil. With either Mellaril or Elavil, one may initially see a satisfactory response to medication with a secondary breakthrough. Such children may respond to a combination of Mellaril and Elavil, or a combination of Elavil and Thorazine (chlorpromazine). Thorazine doses are similar to the doses of Mellaril and Elavil. Depressed children should definitely not be given barbiturates or Ritalin, since these drugs have been shown to worsen depression.

It is important to note that at the present time Elavil is not recommended for children under 12 years of age. However, we have used this medication for several years in depressed children in the first decade of life without difficulty, and with very pleasing results. Also to be noted is that the recommended doses here for Mellaril and Elavil are greater than those listed by the manufacturers. It is our and other people's experience that the doses of Elavil and Mellaril listed in the *Physician's Desk Reference* are inadequate to treat the moderate to severely depressed child.

Additional points of importance in the use of medication to treat the depressed child

* Manufacturer's precaution: Mellaril is not recommended for children under two years of age.

are that one is totally at the mercy of the child's parents or guardian's cooperation. Obviously, if there are any reservations about the reliability or dependability of these individuals, the child should be hospitalized for treatment. Also, it is important for the physician to see the patient at frequent intervals during the initial stages of therapy. One cannot rely on observations of the child's mood made by the parents or guardians. The physician must personally see and form his own impression as to how the child is responding to medication. Children respond to antidepressant medications usually within a week to 10 days.

The retarded depressed individual with tricyclic antidepressants may initially become agitated. The parents should be prepared for this eventuality.

Any child who seriously is contemplating suicide obviously needs in-hospital management. As indicated above, medication is only part of the treatment regimen; along with the medication, it is of utmost importance that the family and patient be counseled. Environmental and family stresses should be removed and attempts in general should be made to place the child in a more favorable environmental situation.

Treatment is usually continued for a minimum of six weeks. In the school-age child, treatment is often continued for the entire school year and then slowly discontinued for the summer. Depression being a cyclical disease, it is important that these children be watched at frequent intervals in the future for recurrence of symptoms.

3

Nervous System

Head Injury

ROBERT L. McLAURIN, M.D.

Head injuries occur frequently in the pediatric age group, but fortunately only few are of sufficient seriousness to leave permanent residual effects. In general, the pediatrician's responsibility is in making a decision about which injuries require hospitalization and possible neurosurgical care.

There are three basic mechanisms responsible for most head injuries: the head may be struck by a relatively small, rapidly moving object, the stationary head may be suddenly accelerated or the moving head may be suddenly decelerated. The first mechanism results in tearing of the penetrated tissues. The others, acceleration and deceleration, cause damage to intracranial contents by movement of the brain against bony prominences and by tearing of vascular channels. Some knowledge of the mechanism of injury, therefore, can be of assistance in evaluating the possible damage.

Injuries to the head may cause damage to the coverings of the brain, to the brain itself or to blood vessels; the latter, in turn, may lead to hematomas and secondary brain compression. This article deals only with injuries to the coverings (the scalp, skull and meninges) and direct injury to the brain. It is apparent that in most cases these occur simultaneously, but for purposes of evaluation and treatment they should be considered as separate aspects of the same injury.

SCALP INJURIES

Most injuries of the scalp result in laceration or in bleeding into the subgaleal space causing a cephalohematoma. Lacerations should not be dealt with lightly but should be surgically cleansed and closed at the earliest possible time. Fortunately, the high degree of vascularity of the scalp helps prevent infection and avascular necrosis of the skin. Nevertheless, meticulous surgical technique is of value and suturing should be done without burying foreign material. Adequate preparation of the skin adjacent to the laceration includes shaving an area extending at least 1 inch from the laceration. Antibiotics are not used unless the laceration has remained open for more than 4 hours or unless there is extensive soft tissue damage and wound contamination. There is no specific treatment needed for subgaleal hematomas which are not compounded by adjacent lacerations. Such hematomas may persist for several days but invariably subside spontaneously. Tapping of hematomas is not only unnecessary but risks the introduction of organisms. Subgaleal hematomas probably do not ever become calcified, but occasionally hematomas occurring beneath the periosteum in association with skull fracture may calcify. The latter can usually be distinguished in infancy and childhood because they do not cross the cranial sutures where the periosteum is attached.

SKULL INJURIES

Fractures of the skull may be classified as linear, diastatic, basal and depressed; each has its own significance. The most common fracture is the simple linear fracture in one or more bones of the cranial vault. Those occurring in the frontal and parietal bones are usually of no clinical significance. The linear fractures which require careful observation are those occurring in the temporal area and crossing the middle meningeal artery, those crossing the sagittal plane with potential injury to the underlying sagittal sinus and its tributaries and those in the occipital bone extending to the foramen magnum. This last fracture usually results from falls on the back of the head and may be accompanied by injury to the brain stem. Thus, undisplaced linear fractures in these three locations must be treated with respect, and a period of hospital observation is usually indicated.

Another type of linear fracture with potential hazard is one in which the fracture line is greater than 3 mm. in width. Such a fracture implies a rather severe impact to the skull and also suggests that the underlying dura mater is also torn, since there is firm fixation of the dura to the suture lines, especially in infancy. This type of fracture may require surgical repair of the meningeal defect if there is evidence of underlying brain damage. It is also imperative that such a fracture be followed by a radiogram three months later to be certain that the fracture line is not becoming progressively wider, as occurs with the development of a leptomeningeal cyst.

The term diastatic fracture is usually applied to separation of the cranial bones along a suture line as a result of mechanical force. This is more likely to occur in infants and toddlers and the fracture itself is simply an index of the severity of the impact. The most frequent sutures involved are the sagittal and lambdoid, and since both of these are closely related to subjacent major venous channels, the possibility of intracranial bleeding must be suspected. No specific treatment of the fracture is necessary unless there is significant inward or outward displacement of a bony plate. Over a period of several weeks the bones become reapproximated and the suture line resumes a normal appearance.

The third type of fracture of clinical significance is the basal fracture. Since this fracture is usually accompanied by a tear of the dura, which is closely adherent to the skull base, and since the fracture usually communicates with an air-filled space (the mastoid, middle ear, paranasal sinus or nasal cavity), the fracture is, by definition, compound. Most fractures involving the temporal bone and characterized by cerebrospinal fluid otorrhea, heal sufficiently in 24 to 72 hours to stop the fluid leakage. Therefore, in this clinic for the past 10 years, antibiotics have not been routinely employed and no increase in intracranial sepsis has occurred. If, however, the child has a purulent upper respiratory infection at the time of injury or if the drainage persists longer than 48 hours, antibiotics are used. Penicillin G, 300,000 to 600,000 units per 24 hours, is employed, since the contaminating organism is usually Pneumococcus. Basal fractures involving the anterior fossa and paranasal sinuses are more likely to result in persistent CSF drainage lasting from several days to indefinitely. For this reason, antibiotic treatment is to be given as soon as the drainage is recognized or suspected, and continued until it ceases. If cerebrospinal fluid drainage from the nose persists for 7 to 10 days after the injury, surgery is recommended to close the dural defect.

The final type of fracture requiring special management is the depressed fracture. Such a fracture usually results from impact of a relatively small object against the head, and there may be an associated scalp laceration. There is no convincing evidence that all depressed fractures need to be corrected surgically, but the following criteria are used to determine whether evaluation is necessary: (1) if the wound is compounded and the fragments are severely comminuted, removal of the fragments is part of adequate débridement; (2) if the depressed fracture is accompanied by local neurologic deficit corresponding to the fracture site, elevation of the depressed fragment should be done immediately; and (3) if the inner table depression is greater than 3 mm. over the sensorimotor strip or greater than 5 mm. over other portions of the cerebral surface, as measured on tangential x-ray views, elevation of the depressed element, repair of the dural tear and restoration of the normal cranial contour are indicated. Thus, with the exception of compound injuries, emergency treatment of depressed fractures is not necessary.

BRAIN INJURY

The usual method of classifying brain injuries includes concussion (mild closed head injury) and contusion (severe closed head injury). The criterion for concussion is generally considered to be loss of consciousness, but in the pediatric age group there are many injuries which are not accompanied by definite loss of consciousness but which are followed by lethargy, pallor, confusion and vomiting which may last for several hours. The principles of management of such a situation include close observation for possible intracranial bleeding and control of vomiting. Thus, hospitalization is recommended for any child who has had a definite period of unconsciousness or in whom the sequelae last more than 2 hours. Observation is concerned mainly with the level of consciousness, and the patient should be watched at hourly intervals for the first 6 hours after injury; the frequency of observation is then decreased if the patient appears stable. In addition to observation of consciousness the observer should also note pupillary symmetry and response to light, and symmetry of movement of the extremities. Changes in vital signs (pulse, blood pressure, respiration) are of little importance in the management of the child with a simple concussion. They are late manifestations of intracranial complications and are usually not required for evaluation of associated bodily injuries in patients with concussion only. It is, therefore, unwise to use valuable nursing time for taking and recording vital signs at frequent intervals; it is more advantageously used in observation of conscious level. If vomiting persists more than 2 to 3 hours, Phenergan (12.5 to 25 mg. suppository) or Compazine (2.5 to 5 mg. suppository) should be given. The patient should remain on nothing by mouth until approximately 4 hours have elapsed from the time of injury or from the most recent episode of vomiting. He may be started on clear liquids in small amounts with progression to regular diet over 8 to 12 hours if tolerated. The total period of hospitalization for a simple concussion may be overnight or, at most, two days if vomiting is controlled and the patient remains alert and responsive. There is no evidence that limitation of subsequent activity has any beneficial effect.

Contusion of the brain is a much more serious injury, is apt to be associated with other bodily trauma and may be followed by prolonged or permanent neurologic deficits. It is usually accompanied by unconsciousness lasting from ½ hour to an indefinite period. As with concussion, however, the most important aspects of neurologic observations concern consciousness, pupillary function and motor responses. Vital signs are of less importance except as they may be used to evaluate other aspects of bodily injury.

In addition to neurologic observation certain specific therapeutic measures are indicated. If the child remains comatose following hospitalization, care of respiratory function is of paramount importance, since pulmonary complications account for the greatest mortality in comatose patients. Endotracheal intubation is usually indicated in deeply comatose patients because of the lack of cough reflex. The endotracheal tube should be attached to a device for assisted or controlled respiration, until a period of observation has established that adequate exchange can be maintained without the device. Close observation of blood gases should be made and an effort made to keep the patient mildly hypocarbic ($paCO_2 \pm 30$ mm.), since elevation of pCO_2 leads to vascular dilatation and aggravation of intracranial hypertension which may already be present from cerebral bruising. Meticulous care of the respiratory system should be maintained by frequent suctioning and constant humidification. Antibiotics are not routinely used unless pulmonary complications occur.

Nasogastric suction should also be a routine part of the management of a child comatose from cerebral contusion. Aspiration of gastric contents may easily occur otherwise, leading to chemical pneumonitis. The gastric suction should be measured carefully and the volume replaced as normal saline in addition to other fluid requirements. Fluids and electrolytes are administered entirely parenterally during the first week of post-traumatic coma. If there are no fluid losses other than gastric secretion and insensible loss, the daily volume should not exceed 150 ml. per square meter. Administration of nitrogen substances are not a necessary part of nutritional replacement during the first few days after injury.

After severe cerebral contusion, prophylactic anticonvulsant medication should be used. Since a minimum sedative effect is advisable, Dilantin is used in daily divided dosages totaling 3 to 8 mg. per kilogram. Hyperthermia is treated most effectively by means of a cooling blanket. For lesser degrees of temperature elevation, aspirin by rectum may be employed. For control of intracranial pressure, glucocorticoids have been recommended, but there is no good evidence of their effectiveness against traumatic cerebral edema. Hypertonic agents (urea, mannitol,* glycerol) may be used for short-term control of pressure only. Lumbar puncture has no role in the diagnostic or therapeutic management of acute head injury and may indeed contribute hazard.

Cerebral Edema

ROBERT L. McLAURIN, M.D.

The normal intracranial compartments include the intra- and intercellular spaces of the nervous tissue, the intravascular space and the cerebrospinal fluid component. Cerebral edema, by definition, is an increase of the total water content within the cells or the extracellular

* Manufacturer's precaution: Use of mannitol in pediatric patients has not been studied comprehensively.

space. It has incorrectly come to be used synonymously with cerebral swelling, which includes an increase of the intravascular compartment. The present discussion will include consideration of the vascular factor as well as treatment of increased brain water.

The vascular compartment is responsive to CO_2 and may be reduced by lowering of arterial $paCO_2$. In any condition, therefore, in which there is intracranial hypertension, it is imperative that the $paCO_2$ be maintained at normal or hypocarbic levels. Since this is dependent on ventilatory function, particular attention must be directed toward adequate ventilation. Respiratory function may be depressed by elevated intracranial pressure and a vicious circle may be created. Thus, if there is depression of conscious level accompanying the cerebral swelling, attention must be directed toward maintaining a clear airway and sufficient pulmonary exchange to prevent accumulation of CO_2. If cerebral swelling has occurred to the point of causing progressive neurologic deterioration, it may often be reversed by mechanical hyperventilation. Hyperventilation is achieved by a 25 to 50 per cent increase over the patient's normal minute volume. Initially the hyperventilation should be done with 100 per cent O_2, and this can then be reduced to maintain the arterial oxygen tension between 100 and 200 mm. Hg. The $paCO_2$ may be maintained in the 20- to 25-mm. range with a corresponding vasoconstriction of the cerebral vessels and reduction of the total intracranial mass. Respiratory alkalosis will occur during hyperventilation but is usually of no consequence in the presence of normally functioning kidneys. In addition to causing vasoconstriction, artificial hyperventilation prevents the compounding of cerebral swelling with edema, which can result from a combination of hypoxia and hypercapnia.

The pathogenesis of true cerebral edema is still uncertain, but a better understanding of the principles of treatment may be obtained if certain basic concepts are recognized. It is necessary to recognize that there are several kinds of cerebral edema and these may be classified as either cytotoxic or vasogenic. In the former, there is increase of intracellular water, in the gray or white matter, without enlargement of extracellular spaces and without breakdown of the blood-brain barrier. Examples of this type of edema are seen in lead encephalopathy and water intoxication. In vasogenic edema there is damage to the blood-brain barrier and there is extravasation of protein-rich fluid into the extracellular space, especially of the white matter. Examples occur in the vicinity of brain tumors, following head trauma and with inflammatory lesions. Management of all forms of cerebral edema is based on attempts to reduce the water content, and several methods are available.

While overhydration per se does not lead to cerebral edema, hypotonicity of the body fluids does lead to cellular overhydration of the brain. This is due to the fact that since water crosses the cell membrane more easily than do electrolytes, there is a consequent imbibing of water by the cells and cellular swelling. Thus, fluid therapy in the child with cerebral edema should be directed toward maintaining normal serum osmolality. While the total volume administered should be a normal daily maintenance (1500 ml. per square meter) to ensure adequate renal function, it should not be a salt-poor solution which leads to an excess of free water. The ultimate of cerebral cellular overhydration is seen in water intoxication, which must then be treated with hypertonic solutions.

The most rapid method of reducing cerebral edema and lowering intracranial pressure is by using hypertonic agents. Such agents create an osmotic gradient between the intravascular and extravascular compartments and thereby reduce the extravascular water content. These substances are probably most effective in the presence of a stable blood-brain barrier and are relatively less effective in areas of vasogenic edema. The substances most frequently employed for this purpose are urea and mannitol.

Although diuresis is not a necessary occurrence in the effectiveness of osmotic agents, it does routinely occur. For this reason, an indwelling catheter should always be inserted to prevent bladder distention and to allow accurate assessment of output.

Urea is administered intravenously as a 30 per cent solution and is given in dosages of 0.5 to 1.5 Gm. per kilogram of body weight. It should be given rapidly, over a period of 15 to 30 minutes. Lowering of intracranial pressure usually occurs within about 30 minutes, and the effect is maintained for 4 to 6 hours. This dosage can be repeated as often as every 6 to 8 hours for several times, but repeated use may lead to systemic dehydration and hypertonicity. Thus, serum osmolality should be determined at least every 12 hours and should not be allowed to exceed 320 milliosmoles per liter. Urea should not be used if renal insufficiency is suspected. In general, the osmotic agents should be considered as effective short-term treatment and should rarely be relied on for intervals longer than 48 hours. There is not general agreement as to whether there is a "rebound" after the effect of urea ceases. While rebound is less likely to occur in cytotoxic edema, it may occur in vasogenic edema owing to the accumulation of the substance in the extravascular space. Nevertheless, this rebound effect is seldom troublesome.

Mannitol* has increased in popularity as an osmotic agent during the past few years because it is less expensive than urea and possesses other favorable characteristics. Mannitol is a hexahydric alcohol which is rapidly excreted by the kidney and produces a diuresis. The molecular weight is larger than that of urea, and therefore a greater weight must be administered to achieve a similar osmotic effect. It is given intravenously in a 20 per cent solution and in amounts of 1.0 to 2.0 Gm. per kilogram over 30 to 45 minutes. The effective decline of intracranial pressure is 5 to 8 hours and it has been found that equilibrium between brain and serum mannitol does not occur until 6 hours after administration. As with urea, mannitol can be used repeatedly for limited times, but the same hazards are present with repeated administration, i.e., systemic dehydration, hemoconcentration, hypotension, tachycardia and so forth. These effects, however, can be rapidly counteracted by infusion of isotonic glucose solution. Mannitol, like urea, is contraindicated in the presence of impaired renal function.

Glycerol, a trivalent alcohol which is not metabolized completely when given in large doses, may also be used as an osmotic agent. It acts promptly, can be given repeatedly over a prolonged period of time and is not toxic. The dosage is 0.5 to 2.0 Gm. per kilogram given through a nasogastric tube. While the substance is of advantage in dealing with chronic types of cerebral edema, it is not as effective as urea or mannitol in treating acute edema.

The above agents are principally used for short-term management of acutely elevated intracranial pressure. The corticosteroids have become extremely useful in treating certain types of edema over a more protracted period. It is believed that the steroids act by restoring or stabilizing the blood-brain barrier. For this reason, steroids would be thought to be most effective against vasogenic edema but, in fact, there is no good evidence that they prevent or decrease edema resulting from mechanical trauma. There is definite evidence, however, that they are effective against edema due to inflammation or adjacent to a mass lesion. The most commonly used drug is dexamethasone. Lowering of intracranial pressure may be recorded within 1 to 2 hours after administration, but the clinical effect is usually noted within 6 to 8 hours and reaches a maximum at 18 to 24 hours. The effect of a single loading dose lasts for 10 to 12 hours, and it is customary to follow such a dose with maintenance doses at 6- to 8-hour intervals. In the child whose weight exceeds 50 kilograms, an initial intravenous dose of 10 mg. is followed by maintenance intramuscular doses of 4 mg. If the body weight is between 20 and 50 kilograms, the doses are halved; and when the body weight is less than 20 kilograms, doses of 2 mg. initially and 1 mg. thereafter are used. Because of the increased likelihood of gastric ulceration during steroid therapy, antacids are routinely administered through a nasogastric tube in any comatose patient. Preparations containing aluminum hydroxide are administered every 4 hours. There seem to be no other significant complications of dexamethasone therapy, since the salt-retaining effect of this steroid is not marked. If the acute stage of cerebral edema is followed by the need for more prolonged treatment, it is frequently possible to decrease the maintenance dose administration to 12-hour intervals. If corticosteroids are used for periods less than seven days, the dose does not have to be tapered but can be discontinued abruptly. If administration has been longer than seven days, the dose should be tapered over a period of one week to allow resumption of normal adrenocortical function, which will have been suppressed during therapy.

As previously indicated, corticosteroids are of doubtful value in the treatment of post-traumatic edema despite their popularity in such situations. They are of unquestionable help in treating edema which surrounds a tumor or which is adjacent to an abscess or hematoma, since these are clear examples of vasogenic edema. They are also effective as an adjunct in the treatment of swelling due to heavy metal intoxication, e.g., lead encephalopathy, and should be part of the standard treatment of that condition. Steroids are also effective against the edema which leads to pseudotumor cerebri, an entity which is poorly understood pathophysiologically but which is characterized by generalized swelling of the cerebral tissue and consequent intracranial hypertension. Finally, the cerebral edema which follows withdrawal or decrease of steroids after prolonged use responds appropriately to an increase of dosage.

* Manufacturer's precaution: Use of mannitol in pediatric patients has not been studied comprehensively.

Hypothermia has been used in the past to assist in control of cerebral edema, but more recent experience has led to the conclusion that it simply retards but does not prevent edema. For this reason, and because of the complications of hypothermia, this device is seldom used. However, it is important to maintain normothermia in the patient with cerebral edema or swelling, since the intracranial dysfunction seems to be aggravated during hyperthermia.

Mechanical decompression of the swollen brain is another means of treatment which presently has very limited application. Subtemporal and suboccipital craniectomy, with opening of the meninges, has been used in the past, but the pharmacologic agents have largely replaced these procedures. The exception to this is acute massive post-traumatic brain swelling which rarely may be managed effectively by extensive bilateral craniectomies; in this condition the edema is not being treated but the brain is given room to expand, thereby preventing fatal transtentorial herniation.

Epidural Hematoma and Subdural Hematoma and Effusion

ROBERT L. McLAURIN, M.D.

Accumulation of blood or fluid in a localized area over the surface of the brain leads to several pathophysiologic events. An understanding of these events is helpful in planning management. A surface hematoma or effusion is an added mass within the limited intracranial space and in certain instances progressively enlarges. By virtue of its mass it raises intracranial pressure and, if unilateral, it displaces the brain toward the opposite side and downward through the tentorial incisura. If the mass is bilateral, the lateralward displacement does not occur. Intracranial pressure is further increased by edema which occurs beneath the surface lesion, and progression of the edema may be responsible for neurologic deterioration despite a static size of the surface mass. In addition, there may be obstruction to the surface circulation, and reabsorption of cerebrospinal fluid leading to hydrocephalus. In the case of effusions associated with meningitis, there may be further interference with CSF circulation by the basic inflammatory process.

EPIDURAL HEMATOMA

Epidural hematoma, usually the result of traumatic laceration of the middle meningeal artery, is a true surgical emergency. When the diagnosis is made, the patient is usually losing consciousness and showing signs of uncal herniation with pupillary asymmetry and respiratory irregularity leading to decerebrate rigidity and respiratory failure. The objective of management at that stage is to maintain respiration, to attempt to minimize intracranial pressure and herniation and to proceed as quickly as possible to surgical decompression. If the diagnosis is suspected from the classic history of a minor injury with unconsciousness followed by a lucid interval followed by neurologic deterioation, all within a few hours, time should not be used to obtain x-rays of the skull. While the operating room is being made ready, measures should be taken to retard the intracranial pathophysiology. The most important measure to accomplish this is the rapid intravenous administration of urea (1 Gm. per kilogram) or mannitol* (½ Gm. per kilogram). While these are being given, a catheter should be inserted into the bladder. If the conscious level has deteriorated sufficiently and respiratory function is being affected, the child should be intubated and hyperventilated. This maneuver assures adequate oxygenation and also produces hypocarbia, which further improves intracranial pressure by vasoconstriction. If seizures have occurred during the stage of neurologic deterioration, Valium† should be administered. There is no indication for steroids under these conditions. Definitive treatment, of course, consists of craniotomy to release the rapidly expanding arterial hematoma, and location and coagulation or clipping of the bleeding meningeal vessel. If irreversible brain stem damage has not been done, the prognosis for survival and recovery is excellent.

SUBDURAL HEMATOMA

Whereas extradural hematomas are usually acute lesions, subdural hematomas, because they are most often of venous origin, are usually chronic. In the occasional instance of an acute subdural hemorrhage, the treatment is the same as that for extradural hematomas. One significant difference is that in infancy, subdural bleeding may be of sufficient volume to render the patient hypovolemic. Therefore, hypotension may occur in the early phase or anemia may occur later; in the former situa-

* Manufacturer's precaution: Use of mannitol in pediatric patients has not been studied comprehensively.

† Manufacturer's precaution: Safety and efficacy of injectable Valium in children under 12 years of age have not been established. Oral Valium is not for use in children under six months of age.

tion blood replacement should be done by transfusion, while in the latter situation the use of whole blood or iron depends on the severity of the anemia.

The clinical picture of chronic subdural hematoma varies according to the age of the patient but is most common in infancy where it presents as intracranial hypertension with macrocrania and, frequently, with seizures. Management, therefore, includes control and prevention of seizures, followed by investigation of the cause of increased intracranial pressure. Seizure control in this age group is best done by phenobarbital in doses of 5 mg. per kilogram per day. If the intracranial hypertension has led to vomiting prior to diagnosis, dehydration may be present and should be corrected by appropriate fluid replacement. The objective of definitive treatment is, of course, removal of the subdural hematoma or control of intracranial pressure regardless of the persistence of some fluid and blood in the subdural space. Diagnosis is usually confirmed by insertion of a 21-gauge needle through the lateral border of the anterior fontanelle or through the coronal suture (at least 1.5 cm. from the midline), and treatment begins as the fluid is removed for diagnosis. Subdural hematomas in infancy are usually bilateral; bilateral subdural tapes are therefore always necessary. Fluid should not be aspirated from the subdural space. Fluid containing blood and xanthochromic supernatant is allowed to drip from the needle until it stops. When this occurs, the subdural fluid is equilibrated with atmospheric pressure, but it does not indicate that the subdural accumulation has been completely eliminated; indeed, if significant macrocrania is present, some craniocerebral disproportion is bound to be present and the subdural space cannot be completely collapsed. There is no limit to the amount of fluid which may be drained at one time, but it rarely exceeds 50 ml. Subsequent taps are performed only when there is evidence of build-up of pressure as judged by fontanelle tension or by clinical signs such as vomiting, lethargy or irritability. The intracranial pressure may become elevated again within 24 hours or it may require several days; occasionally, it does not recur. If hypertension does not recur, no further taps are necessary. This method of treatment is based on the principle that fluid in the subdural space is itself not harmful unless accompanied by intracranial hypertension. Moreover, membrane removal is not done, since it is untenable that subdural membranes are capable of restricting cerebral growth which normally is not restricted by the scalp, skull and dura mater.

Rarely, intracranial pressure cannot be controlled by tapping alone. If, after 8 to 10 taps, fluid accumulation and pressure continue to recur, a shunt procedure on the subdural space may be necessary. Shunting may be done into the pleural or peritoneal spaces or into the vascular system. Shunting of ventricular fluid to other body compartments is the method of treatment necessary in those rare cases of hydrocephalus.

SUBDURAL EFFUSION

Subdural effusion occurs in some cases of meningitis and occasionally may be responsible for increased intracranial pressure. Treatment is similar to that described above, i.e., subdural tapping only in response to intracranial hypertension. Since effusion is not chronic, craniocerebral disproportion does not occur and reaccumulation is therefore uncommon.

Intracranial Hemorrhage

ROBERT L. McLAURIN, M.D.

Intracranial hemorrhage includes bleeding into the substance of the brain or into one or more of the meningeal compartments–epidural, subdural or subarachnoid. The bleeding may be a direct result of trauma, it may occur spontaneously from a vascular abnormality (aneurysm, angioma, arteriovenous malformation) or it may result from a coagulation defect. While there is no constant relationship between the location of hemorrhage and its cause, some relationships do occur with sufficient frequency to be of diagnostic value. Thus, trauma most frequently leads to surface bleeding, aneurysms commonly rupture into the subarachnoid space and arteriovenous malformations and angiomas usually bleed into the brain substance.

The first goal of management is to define the cause and primary location of hemorrhage. History is especially important in relation to injury and to bleeding tendencies. When vascular deformity is responsible, there is usually no historical assistance in the pediatric age group, since the hemorrhage is likely to be the first which has occurred. Examination is of limited etiologic help but may provide evidence of head trauma or of other areas of spontaneous bleeding. On the other hand, examination may provide considerable help as to the location of hemorrhage. Subarachnoid blood leads to signs of meningeal irritation without localizing neurologic signs, since blood diffuses rapidly and evenly throughout the CSF compartment. Acute or progressive focal neurologic deficit may occur with localized hematomas (which are primarily unilateral) either within or compressing the brain. Infantile subdural hematomas, being chronic and usually bilateral, may cause signs of intracranial hypertension only, manifested by macrocrania. Seizures are more likely to be present with localized surface hematomas. Transillumination of the skull may occur in infants of less than six months of age who harbor subdural hematomas. Cranial bruit may accompany arteriovenous malformation but does not occur with aneurysm.

More definitive diagnostic studies are usually necessary. Lumbar puncture is of limited value, but it differentiates meningeal signs due to blood from those due to infection. The presence of blood in the CSF does not mean that the primary source of bleeding was in that compartment; bleeding may have occurred within the brain substance and ruptured into the ventricular or subarachnoid space. Spinal tap has no therapeutic value and may contribute to brain herniation through the incisura if a supratentorial hematoma is present. If the diagnosis has otherwise been confirmed, therefore, or if hemorrhages are present on funduscopic examination, lumbar puncture is not recommended.

Subdural taps are used to detect the presence of blood in that space and can be done with ease up to about two years of age. The needle is introduced at least 1.5 cm. from the midline and must penetrate through the dura mater. Aspiration should not be done, since liquefied hematoma, if present, will spontaneously flow from the needle. Thus, when the diagnosis is made, therapy is automatically begun by release of the hematoma contents. If the infant is in extremis and subdural fluid is not obtained, the needle may be inserted through the cortex and brain substance to the lateral ventricle. This may allow life-saving intracranial decompression for a brief period of time as well as detect evidence of blood within the ventricular system.

Angiography is the most definitive diagnostic study and should be performed in all cases of post-traumatic hemorrhage with localized neurologic deficit. In this situation, the exact location, intra- or extracerebral, and the size of the hematoma can be determined. In addition, it should be done in all cases of spontaneous hemorrhage with neurologic localization and in cases of subarachnoid bleeding unexplained by trauma or blood dyscrasia. In the latter circumstance, the presence of a vascular anomaly may be determined.

After diagnostic determination of the location of an intracranial hematoma, therapy is directed toward its removal as expeditiously as possible. If neurologic deterioration is progressing rapidly, it may be arrested temporarily by relief of intracranial pressure. As stated previously, ventricular tapping may cause transient relief of pressure, but this can be done by needle only in the first few years of life because of subsequent fusion of cranial sutures. Moreover, it provides relief for only 30 to 60 minutes in most instances. A more prolonged reduction of pressure can usually be achieved by dehydrating agents such as hypertonic mannitol or urea solutions. Mannitol* is given intravenously in a 20 per cent solution in amounts of 1.0 to 2.0 Gm. per kilogram over a period of 20 to 30 minutes. The pressure reduction occurs within 30 minutes and may be maintained for 4 to 6 hours. Urea is administered in a 30 per cent solution in dosages of 0.5 to 1.5 Gm. per kilogram with the same duration of effectiveness. Both of these agents can be repeated after 6 to 8 hours but should not be used in lieu of hematoma evacuation; after hematoma removal, it is seldom necessary to repeat them.

Maintenance of an adequate airway during neurologic deterioration is of the utmost importance, since any increase of pCO_2 is immediately reflected in the intracranial pressure due to its vasodilatory effect. Ideally, the pCO_2 should be maintained at 25 to 30 mm. Hg, and this may require use of tracheal intubation or tracheostomy with mechanical respiratory assistance or control. Removal of the hematoma is accomplished by whatever is appropriate in relation to the patient's age and the location and age of the blood clot. Hematomas become liquefied after 10 to 12 days and can then be removed by needle. The chronic subdural hematoma of infancy is illustrative of this lesion. It is noteworthy that sufficient bleeding may occur into the infant's subdural space to cause hypovolemia, and blood replacement may be necessary. Acute meningeal hematomas usually require burr holes or craniotomy for removal, and intracerebral hematomas should be removed only through a craniotomy approach.

Anticonvulsant therapy should be part of the treatment of any intracranial hemorrhage other than subarachnoid. Phenobarbital (5 mg. per kilogram per day) should be started immediately and continued or replaced with Dilantin (3 to 8 mg. per kilogram per day) until there is no clinical or electroencephalographic evidence of seizure tendency.

* Manufacturer's precaution: Use of mannitol in pediatric patients has not been studied comprehensively.

Hydrocephalus

BENNETT M. STEIN, M.D.

The term hydrocephalus has been broadened through custom to encompass a variety of intracranial abnormalities associated with an excessive amount of cerebrospinal fluid (CSF). The presence of hydrocephalus is established in children by plotting an abnormally steep head growth curve. The rate of development of hydrocephalus depends chiefly on the site and completeness of blockage to the flow of CSF. In order to institute appropriate therapy, the subarachnoid and ventricular spaces must be thoroughly defined. This is accomplished by the instillation of air into either the subarachnoid space or the ventricles. If the blockage occurs in the region of the aqueduct, then both routes must be used in order to define both sides of the block.

Treatment. In all cases in which an unequivocal diagnosis of hydrocephalus has been made, surgery is the proper therapy. The mainstay of treatment has been the shunting of CSF from the ventricular system to some extracranial absorptive space, usually the vascular or abdominal compartments (Shulman). The former shunt is termed the ventriculojugular or ventriculoatrial shunt, while the latter is the ventriculoperitoneal shunt. These may be used for all forms of hydrocephalus regardless of the site of blockage.

Recognizing that the two common causes of hydrocephalus are blockage in the region of the aqueduct (aqueductal stenosis, noncommunicating hydrocephalus) or blockage of the extraventricular absorptive areas (communicating hydrocephalus), it is apparent that in the latter circumstance, CSF could be shunted from the lumbar CSF space. This has been accomplished through the placement of a lumboureteral shunt with the sacrifice of one kidney. This shunt is infrequently used since it requires (1) the sacrifice of a kidney and (2) the meticulous control of serum electrolytes which are copiously lost in the urine. Alternatively, a lumboperitoneal shunt could be used.

In either the ventriculoatrial or ventriculoperitoneal shunt, the positioning of the cranial end is similar. The objective is to place the open end of the catheter in the largest portion of the ventricular system in the nondominant hemisphere away from the choroid plexus. Through either an occipital entry or a frontal entry anterior to the coronal suture, the tube is positioned in the right frontal horn. A variety of tips have been used for the ventricular end; most of these have a number of small holes acting as filters, while others have flanged tips which are designed to keep them free from the ventricular walls or choroid plexus.

In the case of the ventriculoatrial shunt, the distal end of the catheter is placed into the jugular vein via the common facial vein and threaded into the right atrial region. The position is verified by filling the tubing with 3 per cent saline to make it a conductor and, by use of the electrocardiogram, the exposed end of the tube then becomes a unipolar electrode. At the point where maximal upward deflection of the P wave is noted, the tube is secured. Radiographic check indicates that this places it well within the right atrium. If radiographic techniques are relied upon to determine the site of the atrial catheter, rapid exposures should be used in order to define the distal tip and compensate for the cardiac motion. Optimum position is between T4 and T7.

In the case of the ventriculoperitoneal shunt, the distal end is placed in the peritoneal cavity, either at McBurney's point, through a paramedian point or into the suprahepatic space. Tubing measuring in the range of 8 to 12 inches is placed within the peritoneal cavity. The extra length of tubing gives it greater mobility and prevents obstruction by omental adhesions.

Two basic systems of one-way valves are used in these shunts, all of which are Silastic. One is associated with a valve at the distal end, and the other with a valve near the cranial end. A flushing device often is incorporated into the system. The opening pressures of these valves are predetermined; however, a moderately wide range of variation must be accepted since the length of the distal tubing and the position of the child produce a siphoning effect on the system.

Each of these shunt systems has distinct advantages (Little et al.). The ventriculoatrial shunt has a greater longevity and is probably not as susceptible to blocks of the distal end. Its disadvantages lie in (1) migration, due to the growth of the child, of the distal tip into the superior vena cava where it may become thrombosed and (2) a greater incidence of sepsis. Although microemboli from the atrial end of the shunt entering the pulmonary circulation have been described, the dire consequence of pulmonary hypertension has not been a major problem in this shunt. The advantages of the ventriculoperitoneal shunt lie in its ease of placement and revision, as well as its inherent compensation for growth because of the long distal end. Disadvantages include (1) a tendency to occlusion of the distal end, and (2) in rare instances the long abdominal portion of tubing may result in an intestinal volvulus requiring surgical correction. Beyond the difficulty of keeping the distal end patent, the more common problem in both shunts is blockage of the ventricular end, which occurs in spite of various new designs in ventricular catheters.

Our policy is to insert a ventriculoperitoneal shunt in the infant because of the ease with which it can be revised to compensate for the growth of the child. When the child's growth curve levels off around the age of two and the shunt requires revision, it is then converted to the more stable and reliable ventriculoatrial shunt. In the older child the primary shunt used is the ventriculoatrial.

In the follow-up treatment of the child with a shunt, certain options are available:

1. In the presence of aqueductal stenosis it is unlikely that the child will ever be independent of a shunt. If a ventriculoatrial shunt has been installed at an early age, elective revision is used whereby the distal end of the shunt is repositioned into the optimal cardiac position, regardless of the state of the child or the shunt. This tends to prevent the formation of thrombi about the tip and occlusion of the superior vena cava, which could prevent surgical repositioning of the shunt (Becker and Nulsen).

2. Some children who have been adequately shunted develop patent subarachnoid spaces over their hemispheres. On the basis of this transformation, in special cases of aqueductal stenosis, a third ventriculostomy may be carried out in order to convert a shunt-dependent child with irrevocable hydrocephalus into one in which the CSF flows into the basal cisterns and over the surface of the brain into normalized absorptive pathways.

Complications. Common complications include (1) obstruction of the shunt system due to disconnection or occlusion by debris at the ventricular end, clotting at the cardiac end or adhesions at the peritoneal end. Initial proper positioning of these shunts with elective revisions as indicated will minimize these complications. An extremely difficult problem is encountered when the ventricular system has been so adequately shunted that it becomes normal or small in size. The narrowing of the cavity compromises the flow of CSF into the ventricular end of the shunt. Because of the expansion of cerebral mantle associated with this process, the child has very little compensatory ability to deal with sudden rises of intracranial pressure associated with blockage of the shunt. In such cases the child may deteriorate rapidly, herniate and irrevocably damage the brainstem in a relatively short time before surgical therapy can be instituted. There is no adequate therapy currently available to prevent this complication of shunt occlusion, which usually occurs in older children. (2) Because of the foreign-body nature of the shunt, even though the Silastic is relatively inert, sepsis can be a major problem, affecting about 15 per cent of shunts (Shurtleff et al.). When the atrial shunt is involved, the sepsis often spreads to the blood stream. The infection is frequently due to *Staphylococcus epidermidis,* although other organisms may be involved. Therapy consists of intravenous methicillin in a dose of 100 to 150 mg. per kilogram per day for 48 hours,* followed by shunt removal and replacement of a new shunt. Antibiotics are continued for at least 14 days postoperatively. Concurrently, intraventricular methicillin* in a dose of 3 mg. per kilogram per day is given (Perrin and McLaurin). The routine administration of prophylactic antibiotics in shunts has not been universally utilized. (3) A somewhat higher incidence of seizures is associated with cranial shunts; however, the problem is not of sufficient magnitude to warrant prophylactic anticonvulsants. (4) Subdural effusions may occur following a shunt, especially if the preoperative ventricular dilation was severe. The treatment is surgical drainage with or without temporary occlusion of the shunt (Illingworth).

In certain selected cases, a direct attack on the cause of hydrocephalus may be utilized. Membranes occluding the aqueduct can be punctured and a Silastic tube left in situ to prevent reocclusion of the aqueduct. Virtually all cases are successfully treated by this means alone. The Dandy-Walker syndrome has been treated by direct surgical attack, with only 50 per cent of the cases responding favorably. A procedure directed at the reduction of CSF formation is choroid plexectomy. The technical difficulties and the necessity for removing large portions of choroid plexus in deep areas of the brain have made this procedure impractical.

The prognosis in hydrocephalic children depends on the maintenance of shunt function. Under most circumstances there is no way to equate the prognosis with the degree of hydrocephalus, although the duration of the hydrocephalus prior to surgical relief, complications

---

* Manufacturer's precaution: The number of times methicillin (Staphcillin) has been given intravenously to infants and children is not large enough to permit specific intravenous dosage recommendations. Also, intraventricular use of methicillin is investigational.

of shunt malfunctions, sepsis and associated congenital defect of the brain bear a direct relationship to the prognosis. All aspects being considered, the prognosis is for a 40 or 50 per cent yield of competitive children who have been treated by the measures outlined here (Foltz and Shurtleff). The ultimate aim is to produce a situation in which the child is independent of a shunt. In certain selected cases, such an objective may be realized.

References

Becker, D. P., and Nulsen, F. E.: Control of Hydrocephalus by Valve-Regulated Venous Shunt. *J. Neurosurg.*, 28:215–226, 1968.

Foltz, E. L., and Shurtleff, D. B.: Five-year Comparative Study of Hydrocephalus in Children With and Without Operation. *J. Neurosurg.*, 20:1064–1079, 1963.

Illingworth, R. D.: Subdural Haematoma after the Treatment of Chronic Hydrocephalus by Ventriculocaval Shunts. *J. Neurol. Neurosurg. Psychiat.*, 33: 95–99, 1970.

Little, J. R., Rhoton, A. L., and Mellinger, J. R.: Comparison of Ventriculoperitoneal and Ventriculoatrial Shunts for Hydrocephalus in Children. *Mayo Clin. Proc.*, 47:396–401, 1972.

Perrin, J. C. S., and McLaurin, R. L.: Infected Ventriculoatrial Shunts. *J. Neurosurg.*, 27:21–26, 1967.

Shulman, K.: *Workshop in Hydrocephalus*. Philadelphia, University of Pennsylvania Press, 1965.

Shurtleff, D. B., Christie, D., and Foltz, E. L.: Ventriculoauriculostomy–Associated Infection. *J. Neurosurg.* 35:686–694, 1971.

Brain Tumors

BENNETT M. STEIN, M.D.

Brain tumors in children often present with signs and symptoms of raised intracranial pressure. The mechanism of this pressure elevation is based on two factors: (1) the progressive space-taking nature of the lesion and/or (2) obstruction of the cerebrospinal fluid by the tumor. In understanding the development of the neurologic syndrome associated with brain tumor, cognizance is taken of the three intracranial components—(1) brain tissue, (2) cerebrospinal fluid, (CSF) and (3) vascular space—residing within the relatively fixed volume of the skull. Because of their high water content, each of these spaces is incompressible and must yield to the expansion of a brain tumor by displacement. Shift of a cerebral hemisphere results in distortion of midline structures and herniation of the uncus into the tentorial notch, with compression and irrevocable damage to the midbrain leading to coma and death. In the posterior fossa, cerebellar tonsil herniation leads to medullary compression and death. Therapy in brain tumors is directed toward preventing these intracranial shifts by compensating for the tumor mass by reducing the volume of the CSF and vascular spaces. The ultimate aim is to reduce the mass of tumor.

Where direct attack on the tumor must be delayed, temporizing means may be utilized to sustain the patient. These include the following:

1. Elevation of the head approximately 30 degrees from the horizontal in order to facilitate venous drainage from the cranial cavity.

2. Maintenance of an unobstructed airway. Compromise of the airway will lead to elevation of the pCO_2 and the Valsalva effect, which elevate intracranial pressure by increasing the vascular volume. If necessary, the patient should be intubated or a tracheostomy performed.

3. A child with raised intracranial pressure should be placed on intravenous balanced electrolyte solutions at maintenance level. It is a mistake to give nonelectrolyte solutions, such as D_5W, or to overdehydrate the child.

4. The intravenous dehydrating agents urea or mannitol are used exclusively in the acute situation to alleviate raised intracranial pressure. These drugs have a rapid and sustained action for 4 to 6 hours. In the case of urea, a rebound of intracranial hypertension may follow. Most often a single bolus of the drug is given and subsequent infusions have a diminishing effect and may produce serious electrolyte and fluid disturbances. Mannitol* is preferred and is given in doses of 1.5 to 2 Gm. per kilogram intravenously in a rapid infusion.

5. Steroids have the ability to minimize the development of cerebral edema in areas adjacent to intracranial tumors. In addition, they may decrease edema which already exists. A definite clinical improvement may therefore be noted in many cases of intracranial tumor following steroid therapy. The advantage of steroids over the intravenous dehydrating agents is that they can be used over a longer time. Our therapeutic regimen does not take into account the age or weight of the patient but rather relies on a prearranged dose. Dexamethasone is given in an initial intravenous bolus of 8 to 10 mg., followed by a high maintenance dose of 10 to 16 mg. per 24 hours over the first 48 to 72 hours when edema is at a maximum. If the situation warrants, steroids are gradually tapered, until they are stopped from one to two weeks following inception. Prolonged use of steroids will lead to a cushingnoid state. Short-term use of steroids, especially with posterior fossa tumors, will in approximately 10 per cent of cases lead to a significant gastric hemorrhage, which is

* Manufacturer's precaution: Use of mannitol in pediatric patients has not been studied comprehensively.

managed by suspension of the steroids, gastric aspiration, antacids, ice water irrigations and, if the situation demands, gastric resection. A non-dose-related complication of steroids, especially where temporal lobe pathology is encountered, is the induction of a psychosis, which is relieved by the cessation of steroids.

6. Hyperventilation may be used for the short-term reduction of intracranial pressure, especially in the operating room when relaxation of the brain is required. In the medical management of brain tumor, severe and prolonged hyperventilation may lead to a significant reduction of cerebral blood flow and therefore cause more damage than benefit.

In their distribution and biologic behavior, intracranial tumors are different in children than in adults (Matson). Major differences include a high percentage of posterior fossa tumors in children, and the presence of two intracranial tumors which are rarely seen in adults: the cystic astrocytoma and the medulloblastoma of the cerebellum. According to their site of origin, tumors are divided into those occurring in the subtentorial or posterior fossa region and those occurring supratentorially.

Posterior fossa tumors cover a wide range of biologic activity and surgical accessibility. The general approach to these tumors is through a suboccipital craniotomy with removal of the bone over the cerebellar hemispheres and of the posterior arch of C1 in order to decompress the upper cervical spinal cord which may be compromised by tonsillar herniation. The fact that many of these operations are done in a sitting position should alert one to the postoperative complication of subdural effusion, especially in cases of advanced hydrocephalus. In addition, if the dura of the posterior fossa is left open, the closure of muscle tissue directly over the cerebellum leads to an aseptic meningitis associated with a high CSF white count, low sugar, meningismus and signs of raised intracranial pressure. This syndrome, when associated with negative cultures, is best treated by steroids.

One of the few curable central nervous system tumors is the *cystic cerebellar astrocytoma* (Geisinger and Bucy). Anything short of total removal of these tumors is unacceptable, since they are invariably located within the cerebellum, do not involve the brainstem and have a well-developed capsule. They do not respond to radiotherapy, and if residual tumor is left the rate of recurrence is significant. In spite of the massive size of these tumors, children usually recover normal cerebellar function following tumor removal.

At the other end of the spectrum of posterior fossa tumors is the *medulloblastoma,* a highly malignant tumor generally arising in the vermis. Apparent total resection of this tumor will not result in greater longevity than will a partial or biopsy resection of the tumor. On the other hand, radiotherapy is extremely effective in treating these tumors. Because of the inability to diagnose preoperatively the nature of a posterior fossa tumor, these lesions are operated on for two purposes: (1) to establish a diagnosis and (2) to resect a sufficient portion to open CSF pathways which have been blocked by the tumor. To radiate without unblocking the CSF pathways may lead to further swelling of the tumor and the demise of the child.

Radiotherapy to medulloblastomas must be directed at the entire neuraxis, since these tumors have a propensity for seeding throughout the nervous system. Surgical treatment and radiotherapy result in a 50 per cent five-year survival rate (Bloom et al.). The initial response is often dramatic, with the child being completely competitive and functional.

The *ependymoma of the fourth ventricle,* which is a tumor of intermediate growth characteristics, has a lesser tendency to seed throughout the nervous system but does behave in a malignant fashion. Therapy is directed toward removal of as much tumor as possible with postoperative radiation directed to the tumor site. If CSF cytology shows the presence of neoplastic cells, entire neuraxis radiotherapy is utilized. The survival rate approaches that for the medulloblastoma. Because many of these tumors involve the brainstem as well as the cerebellum, the posttherapeutic course is not as gratifying as that of the previously described posterior fossa tumors.

The infiltrating *brainstem glioma* is generally a benign type of tumor but is inoperable because of its location. Neuroradiographic techniques, including angiography and pneumoencephalography, provide a pathognomonic appearance, so that surgery plays no role in the management of these lesions. Radiotherapy directed at the tumor mass is indicated. Nevertheless, most of these children die within two years of the diagnosis of the tumor.

Pineal tumors have been generally considered to be nonoperable lesions. However, the variety of pathology in this region, including a 25 per cent incidence of encapsulated benign tumors, warrants surgical exploration. Our recent experience with a small series of cases in which no morbidity or mortality was incurred from an aggressive approach has dictated our therapy in these lesions. Exploration is carried out, and if the tumor is encapsulated, attempts are made to remove all of the lesion. If the tumor is malignant or invasive, a biopsy is made and radiotherapy directed to the lesion. Certain tumors of the atypical teratoma variety have a propensity to seed throughout the nervous system. In such instances with a positive CSF cytology, whole neuraxis radiotherapy is indicated.

Generally, tumors in the supratentorial space respond less dramatically to surgery and/or radiotherapy.

One of the most responsive tumors is the *craniopharyngioma.* This tumor occurs in the suprasellar region and involves the optic nerves and chiasm, resulting in visual failure. Surgical resection early in the growth of this tumor prevents irreversible hypothalamic damage and will often reverse severe visual loss. The aim is a total resection of these benign and encapsulated tumors. Evacuation of the cyst and partial removal of the tumor is often followed by recurrence, even after radiotherapy, and opening of the tumor capsule without resection may result in the flow of the high-cholesterol-content fluid into the CSF, resulting in arachnoidal obstruction and secondary hydrocephalus. These children, prior to surgery, are treated with steroids. Following surgery, they must be managed by careful attention to their metabolic state (Matson and Crigler). Concomitant diabetes insipidus is managed by injections of aqueous Pitressin† or Pitressin tannate in oil. Postoperative patients are followed by meticulous charting of their fluid intake and output and by daily or twice daily weights, serum and urine electrolytes and osmolalities. This necessitates the availability of a well-staffed and well-equipped surgical metabolic unit.

If total removal of these tumors is accomplished, the recurrence rate is extremely low and the child will show gratifying recovery of vision although the diabetes insipidus may be permanent.

Infiltrating *astrocytomas of the optic nerves or chiasm* occur predominantly in childhood. If the tumor is confined to the optic nerve, surgical resection is indicated to prevent further growth, albeit slow, of the tumor into the chiasm where it becomes nonresectable. Lesions involving both nerves or the chiasm usually can be diagnosed without surgical exploration through refined pneumoencephalographic techniques. In such cases, surgery plays no role and radiation proves to be of benefit.

† Manufacturer's precaution: Pitressin is not approved for intravenous use.

Solid or cystic tumors of the cerebral hemispheres are usually astrocytomas. Even in the case of a cystic encapsulated tumor, the opportunity for total resection does not approach that of a similar tumor in the posterior fossa. The reason for this is that many of these tumors in the hemisphere grow to a large size and therefore involve vital motor, speech or sensory areas. Partial resection of such tumors followed by radiotherapy has resulted in long-term survivals of 20 or more years. At the other end of the spectrum are malignant tumors of the astrocytoma variety, where surgical resection followed by radiotherapy has a palliative effect, with survivals measured in terms of one to three years.

Tumors of the third ventricle also occur predominantly in children. Because of histologic variety, these tumors should be surgically confirmed, and in some cases a total or partial resection may be carried out. The use of radiotherapy following such surgical procedures depends on the nature of the tumor. The result of treatment in each of these cases is highly variable.

In general, the therapeutic prognosis in treatment of brain tumors in children ranges from the extremely optimistic in cases of cystic cerebellar astrocytoma and craniopharyngioma, to dismal in the case of malignant astrocytoma. In most cases the nature of the lesion cannot be determined without histologic examination, and therefore surgery plays a role in management of almost all childhood brain tumors. Encouraging results in some malignant tumors, such as the medulloblastoma, are seen following radiotherapy, and there is some indication that a combination of radiotherapy and chemotherapeutic drugs, such as BCNU (bis-chlornitrosourea)‡ and CCNU [1-(2-chloroethyl) 3-cyclohexyl-1-nitrosourea]‡ may have a further palliative effect on these tumors (Fewer et al.).

References

Bloom, H., Wallace, E., and Henk, J. M.: The Treatment and Prognosis of Medulloblastoma in Children. *Amer. J. Roentgen.*, 105:43–62, 1969.

Fewer, D., Wilson, C. B., Boldrey, E. B., Enot, K. J., and Powell, M. R.: The Chemotherapy of Brain Tumors. *J.A.M.A.*, 222:549–552, 1972.

Geisinger, J., and Bucy, P.: Astrocytomas of the Cerebellum in Children; Long-Term Study. *Arch. Neurol.*, 24:125–135, 1971.

Matson, D.: *Neurosurgery of Infancy and Childhood.* 2nd ed. Springfield, Illinois, Charles C Thomas, Publisher, 1969.

Matson, D., and Crigler, J.: Management of Craniopharyngioma in Childhood. *J. Neurosurg.*, 30:377–390, 1969.

‡ *Note:* BCNU and CCNU are investigational.

Brain Abscess

HAROLD J. HOFFMAN, M.D.

Brain abscesses are not an uncommon disease of childhood and their incidence has not decreased during the antibiotic era. About one-third of these abscesses are due to direct extension of adjacent infection in the middle ear or the nasal sinuses. About one-third occur secondary to congenital cyanotic heart disease, and the remaining one-third are associated with bacteremias, penetrating wounds of the brain and cranial dermal sinuses.

Brain abscesses begin as a localized area of nonsuppurative encephalitis. The patient may have a headache, some focal neurologic deficit and a history in keeping with the bacterial origin of the brain abscess. At this stage, if the patient is treated with large doses of appropriate antibiotics, the process may be arrested and not proceed to form a true brain abscess. In the case of a known organism, such as one obtained from ear culture in otitis media or from blood culture in septicemia, a specific antibiotic can be used. However, in most cases the organism is unknown or open to speculation, and we recommend using a combination of ampicillin in a dose of 400 mg. per kilogram per day intravenously, and gentamicin in a dose of 3 mg. per kilogram per day intravenously.* Blood levels of gentamicin should not exceed 12 micrograms per ml. A brain scan will frequently be positive at this early stage and the efficacy of treatment can be followed by repeated scans.

If the process is not arrested, the abscess progresses to an area of suppuration which is not encapsulated and is known as an acute brain abscess. At this stage the patient may begin showing signs of raised intracranial pressure. If the acute brain abscess is in a nonvital area of the brain, such as the cerebellum, it should be treated by surgical excision. However, because the zone between normal brain and abscess is ill-defined at this stage, it is preferable to treat acute brain abscesses in any other site by burr-hole aspiration. At the time of the initial aspiration the pus should be smeared and cultured. With the brain needle still in the abscess, 50 mg. of cephaloridine in 1 ml. of saline, 2 ml. of Steripaque (micronized barium sulfate) and 1 ml. of air are instilled. Immediate skull x-rays will show the site and size of the abscess, and if cross-table techniques are used, the air will move to one end of the abscess and the Steripaque to the other. Within a day the macrophages in the abscess wall pick up the Steripaque and allow follow-up films of the abscess after the air is absorbed. Usually several aspirations are necessary, and this is determined by the quantity of pus obtained and the appearance of the abscess on x-ray. With a resolving abscess, little if any pus is obtained and radiographically the wall has a collapsed and wrinkled appearance. Some acute abscesses may require only one or two aspirations whereas others may require several. The timing of each aspiration is determined by the patient's clinical state and the x-ray appearance. With each aspiration, 50 mg. of cephaloridine should be instilled. Systemic antibiotics are continued for two weeks after the last aspiration.

The patient with an acute brain abscess will have associated cerebral edema. This should be managed with dexamethasone in a dose of 0.2 mg. per kilogram orally or intramuscularly every 6 hours. If the edema leads to clinical deterioration despite aspiration of pus, 20 per cent mannitol† should be administered intravenously in a dose of 1.0 to 3.0 Gm. per kilogram over 20 to 30 minutes. In this situation the mannitol may provide only a temporizing effect and the abscess may have to be excised despite its nonencapsulated stage. However, at this point, excision can be done more safely because the organism has been cultured and the exact size and site of the abscess have been established radiologically. Systemic antibiotics should be continued for three weeks after excision of a brain abscess. At the time of surgery, whether burr-hole aspiration or excision, in addition to instillation of cephaloridine, the entire wound should be liberally irrigated with a solution of 30,000 units of bacitracin in 60 ml. of saline.

The acute brain abscess goes on to encapsulation to form a chronic brain abscess, which is treated by excision when located in the cerebellum, in either frontal lobe or in the nondominant temporal lobe, unless the abscess is gigantic, such as are the infantile brain abscesses, in which case aspiration is the more feasible form of treatment. Elsewhere, particularly in the parietal lobe and in the case of multiple brain abscesses, the abscess is treated

* The drug dosages recommended are based on information available in the literature and personal experience and may or may not agree with those recommended by the manufacturer.

† Manufacturer's precaution: Use of mannitol in pediatric patients has not been studied comprehensively.

by repeated aspirations through a burr hole. The method of treating chronic brain abscesses, using either aspiration or excision, is the same as that outlined for acute brain abscesses.

Once the culture reports are available both the systemic and intracavitary antibiotic management may require revision. If the cultures are negative, systemic ampicillin and gentamicin and intracavitary cephaloridine are continued. If the cultures yield a sensitive gram-positive coccus, *E. coli* or *Proteus mirabilis*, ampicillin is continued alone, the gentamicin being discontinued. If the cultures yield an enterobacterium or a species of Proteus other than *P. mirabilis*, gentamicin in a dose of 50 mg. is instilled into the abscess at the time of each aspiration. With a penicillinase-producing staphylococcus, the systemic antibiotics are changed to methicillin, 400 mg. per kilogram per day, and the instillation of cephaloridine into the abscess is continued. With a Bacteroides brain abscess, chloramphenicol‡ in a dose of 100 mg. per kilogram per day (not to exceed 4 Gms.), or clindamycin in a dose of 30 mg. per kilogram per day, is used. In the case of penicillin allergy, the ampicillin or methicillin must be changed to cephaloridine in a dose of 70 mg. per kilogram per day, or cephalothin in a dose of 200 mg. per kilogram per day. Patients with brain abscesses at any stage are prone to seizures, and these should be prevented by prophylactic anticonvulsant medication such as diphenylhydantoin in a dose of 10 to 30 mg. per kilogram per day in three divided doses.

Once the abscess has been dealt with, the focus from which it arose should be vigorously treated to prevent any further problems. This would include a mastoidectomy in the case of an otogenic abscess, corrective heart surgery in the case of an abscess secondary to cyanotic heart disease and excision of a dermal sinus.

References

Heineman, H. S., Braudo, A. I., and Osterholm, J. L.: Intracranial Suppurative Disease. J.A.M.A., 218: 1542, 1972.

Hoffman, H. J., Hendrick, E. B., and Hiscox, J. L.: Cerebral Abscesses in Early Infancy. *J. Neurosurg.*, 33:172, 1970.

McGreal, D. A.: Brain Abscess in Children. *Canad. M. A. J.*, 86:261, 1962.

‡ Manufacturer's precaution: Chloramphenicol is not recommended for intravenous or intramuscular pediatric use. Chloramphenicol sodium succinate has been approved for intravenous pediatric use.

Spinal Epidural Abscess

HAROLD J. HOFFMAN, M.D.

Spinal epidural abscesses are surgical emergencies which require immediate recognition and treatment. They usually occur in a patient who has had some cutaneous staphylococcal infection which had been regarded as minor.

The patient has no doubt had a bacteremia and presents several days or weeks later with a high fever, high white cell count, general malaise, severe back and nerve root pain and rapidly progressive paraparesis which can proceed to paraplegia very quickly. A more chronic type of epidural abscess occurs in association with a congenital dermal sinus which ends blindly in the epidural space and thus allows organisms entrance from the skin surface. The staphylococcus is also the common organism of this type of abscess, but with dermal sinuses in the lumbosacral region, coliform organisms can colonize along the dermal sinus to produce an epidural abscess. Chronic granulomatous types of epidural abscesses can be seen in association with tuberculosis, fungal infections and syphilis. Anterior epidural abscesses can be seen in association with vertebral osteomyelitis.

A lumbar puncture should not be done at the site of a suspected epidural abscess because this would allow bacteria access to the subarachnoid space. This would necessitate cisternal puncture for myelography.

Once a diagnosis is made, an immediate decompressive laminectomy is indicated. These abscesses can track long distances in the epidural space and the entire area must be opened to provide adequate decompression. Preoperatively the patient is started on a systemic antibiotic, which, in the case of the usual staphylococcal abscess, is methicillin in a dose of 400 mg. per kilogram per day.* At the time of surgery the wound is liberally irrigated with several hundred milliliters of a solution containing 200 micrograms of cephaloridine per milliliter. Systemic antibiotics are maintained for three weeks postoperatively.

In the case of an anterior epidural abscess (usually staphylococcal) secondary to vertebral osteomyelitis, a costotransversectomy is per-

* The drug dosages recommended are based on information available in the literature and personal experience and may or may not agree with those recommended by the manufacturer.

formed for drainage of the abscess. This can then be combined with a detergent perfusion system in which an afferent drain and efferent drain are left at the site of the abscess and 500 ml. of saline containing 50 mg. of cephaloridine and 30 ml. of Alevaire are irrigated through the drains every 8 hours. If Alevaire is unavailable, normal saline can be used. This perfusion should be continued until the efferent solution is clear; this will usually occur within three to seven days. Light suction should be continuously applied to the efferent drain. Systemic methicillin is given in the same manner for the posterior epidural abscesses.

If an unknown organism or a gram-negative organism is the causative bacterium, then instead of methicillin, a combination of ampicillin, 400 mg. per kilogram per day, and gentamicin, 3 mg. per kilogram per day, is given intravenously.

In the case of penicillin sensitivity, cephaloridine, 70 mg. per kilogram per day, or cephalothin, 200 mg. per kilogram per day, is used instead of methicillin or ampicillin.

References

Durity, F., and Thompson, G. B.: Localized Cervical Extradural Abscess. *J. Neurosurg.,* 28:387, 1968.

Fleming, P. C., Huda, S. S., and Bobechko, W. P.: Cephaloridine and the Penicillins in the Treatment of Staphylococcal Osteomyelitis and Arthritis. *Postgrad. Med. J.,* 46 (Suppl.):89, 1970.

Grant, F. C.: Epidural Spinal Abscess. J.A.M.A., 128: 509, 1945.

Cerebral Vascular Disorders

PHILIP R. DODGE, M.D.

The patient with a subarachnoid hemorrhage should be kept at bed rest in an effort to reduce the systemic blood pressure. Sedatives, analgesics and antihypertensive agents may be given. Surgical evacuation of an intracerebral clot may be lifesaving. Aneurysms may be treated by carotid ligation in the neck or by direct surgical attack. Arteriovenous malformations, when their size and location permit, are excised. The results of surgery depend on the site and size of the lesion and on the surgeon's skill.

The value of surgery in childhood carotid occlusions is questionable, but experience with adults suggests that it may occasionally be effective if accomplished within a few hours of the apoplectic incident and before irreversible cerebral damage has occurred. There is no evidence to support the use of anticoagulants in the treatment of occlusive cerebral vascular disease in children, although studies in adults suggest that they are of use in the syndrome of carotid artery insufficiency and possibly in cases of thrombosis in evolution. Fibrinolysin therapy with urokinase may prove to be of value in thrombosis of arteries and veins when used early in the course of disease, but this treatment is experimental.

The established medical treatment of occlusive vascular disease is supportive and directed toward preventing further brain damage. Systemic hypoxia secondary to aspiration, impaired ventilation and shock may further damage cerebral tissue, accentuate brain swelling and increase an already elevated cerebrospinal fluid pressure. The risk of aspiration is increased in the patient with altered consciousness or with other neurologic defects that impair swallowing and coughing.

The practice of restraining children on their backs and leaving them unattended is deplorable, because it invites disaster. The comatose or stuporous patient should be positioned on his side in a slightly head-down position. This facilitates drainage of secretions from the lungs and assures that vomitus will not be aspirated. Tracheostomy or an endotracheal tube is indicated if maintenance of an adequate airway is difficult.

Seizures must be controlled because they increase metabolic requirements, produce fever and may accentuate the neural deficits. Diazepam (Valium injectable, undiluted), administered slowly intravenously in a dose of approximately 5 to 8 mg. per square meter, to be repeated in 1 hour if necessary, is now widely used in the treatment of seizures.* If barbiturates or other respiratory depressants have been administered previously, the initial dose should be reduced. Phenobarbital, 7 mg. per kilogram (200 mg. per square meter), and, if seizures persist for 15 minutes, diphenylhydantoin sodium, 7 mg. per kilogram (200 mg. per square meter), should be given slowly intravenously. The diphenylhydantoin comes dissolved in 40 per cent propylene glycol and 10 per cent alcohol but should be diluted with 10 ml. of sterile distilled water before injection. Half of this dose may be repeated if the seizures continue.

Paraldehyde, 0.5 ml. per kilogram (14 ml. per square meter) in 15 to 30 ml. of mineral oil, administered rectally, and general anes-

* The safety and efficacy of injectable diazepam (Valium) in children under 12 years of age have not been established.

thesia may be necessary in exceptional circumstances. (Note: This dose exceeds manufacturers recommendations, but under these circumstances I have found this large dose to be necessary.)

A daily dose of phenobarbital, 2 to 4 mg. per kilogram (50 to 100 mg. per square meter), and diphenylhydantoin, 6 to 8 mg. per kilogram (150 to 200 mg. per square meter), should then be used throughout the acute illness or for longer periods if seizures recur. Fever must be controlled with salicylates, sponging, exposure or a cooling mattress.

Proper hydration helps to combat fever, but the amount should be rigidly restricted to 1200 ml. per square meter daily by all routes during the first two or three days. A multiple electrolyte solution (sodium, 40 mEq.; potassium, 35 mEq.; chloride, 40 mEq.; lactate, 20 mEq.; and phosphate, 15 mEq. per liter; and 5 per cent glucose) has proved generally satisfactory for intravenous therapy when renal function is good.

Hypertonic solutions (mannitol† or urea) are used in emergency situations when there is impending herniation at the tentorium or foramen magnum. The dose of these agents should be calculated to increase the blood osmolality by about 10 to 15 per cent. Dexamethasone, 0.5 to 1 mg. per square meter every 4 hours intramuscularly to minimize cerebral edema, may also have a place in therapy. The dose should be tapered as soon as the period of maximal edema has passed. Equivalent amounts of other steroidal preparations may be used. Protective measures against gastrointestinal hemorrhage are indicated (such as milk and alkali by mouth or by tube) if treatment is prolonged. We have not found it necessary to use hypothermia in these cases.

Proper positioning in the acute phase is important to prevent contractures that delay rehabilitation. Passive exercises should be instituted as soon as the patient's general condition permits, with progression to active exercises as soon as the patient can cooperate.

Venous Sinus Thrombosis

NORMAN GRANT, F.R.C.S.

Thrombosis of major intracranial venous sinuses, such as the sagittal, cavernous and lateral sinuses, occurs as a complication of dehydration, debility, polycythemia, meningitis and penetrating injuries of the skull, and by spread from neighboring sepsis such as that of mastoiditis or orbital cellulitis. It may result in an acute rise in intracranial pressure from rapidly developing cerebral venous congestion and edema. This is an entirely different picture from that of pseudotumor cerebri, in which despite exceedingly high intracranial pressure, the patient may remain alert and uncomplaining.

Dehydration and sepsis must be treated by the appropriate fluids and antibiotics. Dexamethasone in the dose of 0.2 to 0.4 mg. per kilogram initially, reduced to 0.1 to 0.2 mg. per kilogram every 6 hours, should be used to diminish edema. Because of its damaging effect on the already compromised brain, pyrexia over 101° F. should be aggressively treated by exposure, fanning, tepid sponging and, if necessary, the use of a drug such as promazine. Rheomacrodex, which is Dextran of average molecular weight 40,000, may be given intravenously in an attempt to reduce the viscosity of the blood and so improve the venous outflow. This is given either in 5 per cent dextrose or in normal saline, the volume delivered being the total fluid requirement for 24 hours. Anticonvulsants are used should there be seizures. Anticoagulants are not indicated in this situation, where there is the possibility of hemorrhagic infarction of the brain.

Pseudotumor Cerebri

NORMAN GRANT, F.R.C.S.

Pseudotumor cerebri is a syndrome in which there is raised intracranial pressure in the absence of a space-occupying lesion or obstruction of the cerebrospinal fluid circulation. Although no explanation for the raised intracranial pressure has been found, there are several agents which have been unequivocally incriminated in producing the syndrome, and these must be considered in reaching a diagnosis and in recommending effective treatment.

The most common single precipitating condition remains otitis media, which may operate through thrombosis of the major lateral venous sinus, although this is by no means invariably present. Tetracycline, chlorotetracycline, nalidixic acid, steroid hormones, Vitamin A in deficiency or excess, iron deficiency anemia and hypocalcemia have been recorded as producing pseudotumor cerebri. When ster-

† Manufacturer's precaution: The use of mannitol in pediatric patients has not been studied comprehensively.

oid hormones have been blamed, it has usually been found that the child has been on long-term steroid treatment for such conditions as asthma or arthritis, and that the dose of steroid has been either inadvertently or deliberately reduced. Under these circumstances, the original dose should be reinstated and a more gradual tapering program instituted over a period of three months. In situations where a particular drug is implicated, it should of course be withdrawn. Such measures as are recommended in the absence of specific etiological factors should be carried out if withdrawal of the drug does not produce prompt regression of the symptoms and signs.

The mainstay of treatment is lumbar puncture. This should be carried out daily until the lumbar cerebrospinal fluid pressure is 100 mm. H_2O or less. It is perfectly safe to withdraw fluid in sufficient quantity to reduce the pressure to half its initial level or to 100 mm. H_2O, whichever is lower. This presupposes that adequate investigations have been carried out to exclude the possibility of an intracranial space-occupying lesion causing distortion of the brain or blockage of the cerebrospinal fluid pathways. If such a lesion were present, lumbar puncture could be extremely hazardous.

Frequently only a few lumbar punctures are required to return the cerebrospinal fluid pressure to persistently normal levels. Should this fail to be the case, further measures are available. The cerebrospinal fluid pressure can be reduced by giving glycerol by mouth. Glycerol operates as an osmotic diuretic and its effect lasts for approximately 8 hours. Pure glycerol is unpleasantly sweet and is made more palatable by mixing it with an equal volume of pure lemon juice. If necessary, it can be given by nasogastric tube. The dose is 1 ml. per kilogram every 8 hours. Throughout the period of administration of glycerol, it is necessary to continue daily lumbar punctures, since it is not unusual for the patient to swing from high pressure into low pressure with persistence of similar symptoms. Glycerol has the disadvantage of providing the patient with a source of calories and this is undesirable in those who are already obese. Dexamethasone has become popular in treating pseudotumor cerebri. Although it can prove effective, there is no evidence that it is any more effective in the majority of patients than are the simpler measures outlined above. A good case can be made for reserving the use of such a powerful and potentially dangerous drug for resistant cases. It should then be given aggressively in the dosage used for treating cerebral edema of traumatic or neoplastic origin. An initial dose of 0.2 to 0.4 mg. per kilogram orally or intramuscularly should be followed by 0.1 to 0.2 mg. per kilogram every 6 hours until symptoms and signs begin to regress and the lumbar pressure returns to normal. The drug may then be tapered off over two weeks. If treatment with dexamethasone is prolonged, there are the attendant hazards of steroid overdose and gastrointestinal hemorrhage. Acetazolamide has been shown to cause a significant if short-lived fall in the rate of production of cerebrospinal fluid. In resistant cases of pseudotumor, it may be used to effect a lowering of the cerebrospinal fluid pressure. The dosage is 25 to 50 mg. per kilogram per day.

The main cause for concern in pseudotumor cerebri is the ill effect which persistent papilledema may have on visual acuity. This complication is rare in childhood. However, should papilledema fail to subside in spite of the measures advocated, it is necessary to consider the surgical maneuvers available. Insertion of a ventriculoatrial shunt using a low pressure valve such as a Dahl-Wade-Till or a low pressure Holter valve is fortunately rarely necessary. Technically the procedure is not easy because the lateral ventricles are usually of normal size or smaller than normal, making the insertion of a catheter difficult and its subsequent functioning erratic. Even less likely to be required are the time-honored procedures of subtemporal craniectomy or occipital craniectomy.

If there is coexistent acute otitis media, this should be treated with appropriate antibiotics. Chronic otitis media does not demand treatment until the pseudotumor has settled. Interference with the lateral sinus in an attempt to find and remove a thrombus is likely to be unsuccessful and may make the situation worse.

Once effectively treated—and this may take from days to several months—pseudotumor is exceedingly unlikely to recur.

Neurocutaneous Syndromes

MURRAY FEINGOLD, M.D.

NEUROFIBROMATOSIS (VON RECKLINGHAUSEN'S DISEASE)

The numerous café au lait spots require no treatment, although cosmetically they may be of some concern to the patient. Surgical removal of cutaneous tumors is usually not indicated unless they are growing exceedingly rapidly and the question of malignancy is raised. Spinal cord compression occurs secondary to tumors of the spinal nerves and requires extensive resection. Other masses that may be present include tumors of the brain (usually meningiomas and gliomas), mediastinum, gastrointestinal tract and cranial nerves. These tumors may undergo sarcomatous degeneration, which is associated with a very poor prognosis. There is an increased incidence of pheochromocytoma in patients with neurofibromatosis. Occasionally there are bony abnormalities, including cystic bone lesions and pseudoarthroses, that may require orthopedic treatment.

Seizures should be treated with anticonvulsants (see Seizure Disorders). Mental retardation occasionally occurs and special schooling is helpful. Retardation is generally mild to moderate. If hyperactivity is present, methylphenidate hydrochloride (Ritalin) * may be of some benefit. The initial dose is usually 5 mg. at breakfast and, if needed, another 5 mg. in the early afternoon. The dosage may be increased up to 30 mg. in 5-mg increments. If the hyperactivity is not controlled with this dosage, another medication, usually some type of amphetamine,† can be tried.

Genetic counseling is an important part of therapy. The parents should be informed that this condition is inherited as an autosomal dominant trait and that if one of the parents has the disease, there is a 50 per cent chance, with each pregnancy, that the child will be affected. If neurofibromatosis is due to a mutation, it is very unlikely that the parents will have another affected child. However, the affected child will then have a 50 per cent chance of having an affected child of his own. Before the parents are told that a mutation has occurred, they should be examined very carefully for café au lait spots.

STURGE-WEBER SYNDROME (ENCEPHALOTRIGEMINAL ANGIOMATOSIS)

Plastic surgery offers very little help in removing facial angiomatoses. Cosmetics are available which may help conceal the port-wine stain. However, it is debatable whether they should be used on children because of the emotional involvement incurred by calling attention to the lesion each time the cosmetic is applied. In our experience this mode of therapy has not been particularly successful. Glaucoma occurs secondary to outflow occlusion of the angle or hypersecretion of the aqueous humor, and this is only occasionally correctable. Seizures are also part of the syndrome, and controlling them may be difficult (see Seizure Disorders). When anticonvulsants have been unsuccessful, cortical resection or hemispherectomy has been done with some success. Orthopedic treatment and physical therapy may be helpful if hemiplegia is present. Associated hyperactivity can be treated with methylphenidate hydrochloride (Ritalin) or other amphetamines.

At the present time the exact mode of inheritance is not known, and recurrence in the same family is very rare.

TUBEROUS SCLEROSIS

Seizures frequently occur and are difficult to control. They are usually of the major motor, focal, psychomotor and petit mal types; however, infantile spasms occur during infancy. Adrenocorticotropic therapy should be started, although the response is not particularly good. It may be necessary to try a variety of seizure medications until the proper one is found.

The cerebral glial nodules may impinge on vital brain structures and cause symptoms. Increased intracranial pressure may also result. Surgical removal of such tumors may be helpful in selected cases. Tumors may also be present in the lung, heart, and kidney and should be removed if complications occur secondary to them.

The degree of mental retardation varies but is usually moderate to severe. Special schooling may be helpful.

Genetic counseling is an important part of the treatment. Although tuberous sclerosis is inherited as an autosomal dominant trait, the majority of cases are the result of a mutation. Therefore, when providing genetic counseling it is mandatory that both parents be examined for manifestations of the disease, especially depigmented spots. Some clinicians believe that if a parent of an affected child has a documented depigmented spot (skin biopsy may be necessary to differentiate the depigmented spot from vitiligo), it is likely that they also have the disease, and their chance of having another child with tuberous sclerosis is therefore 50 per cent.

ATAXIA-TELANGIECTASIA

There is no treatment for the cerebellar ataxia, choreoathetosis, nystagmus and telangiectasia associated with this disease. Control of

* Manufacturer's precaution: Methylphenidate hydrochloride (Ritalin) is not recommended in children under six years of age. The parenteral form is not recommended in children.

† Manufacturer's precaution: The use of amphetamine for treatment of hyperkinetic behavior is not recommended in children under three years of age.

the sinopulmonary infections is very difficult. Immunoelectrophoresis shows a deficiency of IgA and IgE. There is some preliminary work concerning the use of frozen plasma in an attempt to increase the IgA, but it is too early to determine its effectiveness. Occasionally there may be a decrease in IgG, for which we give gamma globulin (0.6 ml. per kilogram intramuscularly approximately every six weeks), although some believe it is not very helpful. Aggressive physical therapy, including pulmonary toilet, may decrease the severity of the bronchiectasis. Other complications that should be looked for and treated when found include growth hormone deficiency and malignancies, mainly of the lymphoreticular system.

The parents should be informed that ataxia-telangiectasia is inherited as an autosomal recessive trait and that their chance of having another child with this syndrome is one in four with each pregnancy.

LINEAR SEBACEOUS SYNDROME

Seizures should be treated with the usual anticonvulsant medications (see Seizure Disorders). Plastic surgery has little to offer for correction of the multiple sebaceous nevi that are present on the face. The congenital anomalies of the eye and brain are usually not treatable. Mental retardation is generally profound, but if not severe special schooling may be of some help. Occasionally a correctable congenital heart lesion is present and surgery should be considered after the overall status of the child is evaluated and discussed with the parents.

The exact mode of inheritance is not known.

Acute Ataxia

PATRICK F. BRAY, M.D.

Writing about a subject like ataxia where so much depends on exactly what one sees and how one interprets it reminds me of the descriptions of the Loch Ness monster: The observers, impressed with the importance of what they've seen, elaborate like the seven blind men feeling the elephant, and the reader is often left dubious or confused.

Expert observers will see a patient with a movement disorder and may disagree strongly on what it is they're observing. For example, it is not uncommon to have several neurologists see the same patient and then conclude that the patient has ataxia, or choreoathetosis or myoclonus or hypotonic muscle weakness or even myoclonic seizures. For this reason I believe the reader should not be too rigid about his definition of terms. Instead, he should consider the spectrum of involuntary movements which can masquerade as ataxia and think about all of the diseases that can cause incoordination and movement disorders.

Strictly speaking, we can say that ataxia is the hallmark of damage to the cerebellum or to its incoming or outgoing pathways. The usual findings on examination are an unsteady, broad-based (drunken) gait, disability with tandem (heel-to-toe) walking, intention tremor (on finger-to-nose or heel-to-shin movements), dysmetria (missing the intended mark), impaired performance of rapid alternating movements (dysdiadochokinesia), associated hypotonia with pendular reflexes and exaggerated rebound and impaired check mechanisms. Often one sees associated dysarthric speech and nystagmus, especially when the lesion involves the cerebellum itself.

A careful differential diagnosis is essential not only in terms of treatment but also in terms of prognosis and in some cases the risk of recurrence in a sibling. We will consider disease conditions and syndromes in their approximate order of incidence and discuss their management pari passu.

INTOXICATIONS

Acute or chronic overdosage with many drugs, especially those which act upon the nervous system, including sedatives, tranquilizers and anticonvulsants, usually produce ataxia. In addition, those rare poisons which slowly produce a peripheral neuropathy, e.g., lead, mercury, arsenic, thallium and, rarely, the "weed killers" such as 2,4-D, can cause weakness which may be manifested as incoordination. Most physicians promptly suspect intoxications when they see ataxic young children and begin their search for a cause. Treatment, of course, involves discontinuation of exposure to the poison and institution of remedies to diminish absorption and hasten excretion. The treatment of specific intoxications is covered elsewhere in this text.

INFECTIONS

Acute viral infections of the central nervous system are often ushered in with fever and ataxia, along with other systemic symptoms. Some believe that this happens more often in the case of postexanthematous encephalomyelitis. Assuming that one can be reasonably sure that there is not an intracranial mass lesion, a lumbar puncture provides helpful diagnostic supporting data. Pleocytosis, with or without mild elevation of the protein concentration, along with a collection of paired sera for antibody titers and attempts to recover the virus, may offer specific diagnostic information.

For all practical purposes, no specific therapy for these diseases is available, other than supportive care and the treatment of cerebral edema and seizures.

DISORDERS OF POSSIBLE INFECTIOUS ETIOLOGY

Acute Cerebellar Ataxia, Opsoclonus or Polymyoclonus. This uncommon syndrome is seen in infants or young children and is characterized by the abrupt onset of severe incoordination, wild chaotic eye movements (opsoclonus), diffuse myoclonic activity of the skeletal muscles, irritability and sometimes vomiting. The striking clinical picture is also described in the literature under the headings "myoclonic encephalopathy" and the syndrome of "dancing eyes and dancing feet," adding to the semantic confusion.

The myoclonic activity may be mistaken for true seizures, but the electroencephalogram is nearly always normal. An antecedent upper respiratory infection occurs in about a third of the patients, but fever is usually absent. The differential diagnosis usually involves viral encephalitis and posterior fossa brain tumor. Cerebrospinal fluid (CSF) examination is usually normal, but a mild pleocytosis occurs in a minority of cases. Several microbial agents have been incriminated in selected cases. Recently, a number of different workers, including ourselves, have been impressed with the association between this syndrome in infants and occult neuroblastoma (Bray et al.). Because the latter tumor is amenable to cure if it is detected early, especially in infants, we strongly recommend that all patients with this syndrome be surveyed for an inapparent neural crest tumor arising from the adrenal gland or anywhere along the paraspinal sympathetic chain. The survey should include a chest x-ray, intravenous urogram, plain x-rays of the spine, an accurate measurement of vanillylmandelic acid (VMA) excretion and a bone marrow aspiration (with examination for malignant cells). In some cases, visceral angiography and isotopic scans of the chest, adrenal region and the retroperitoneal area may be necessary to locate the neoplasm.

If a tumor is detected, it should be treated with surgical excision, radiation and appropriate chemotherapy (vincristine* or cytosine arabinoside). The movement disorder can be treated effectively in many cases with a course of corticotropin [adrenocorticotropic hormone (ACTH)]. For reasons that are not clear to me, most clinicians have found that adrenal cortical steroids per se are not as effective as corticotropin in alleviating the acute myoclonic movements. If benefit is going to result from corticotropin (ACTH) therapy, it will usually occur with a dose of 40 units of ACTH gel given intramuscularly three times a week. Higher doses can be tried but they may be of no greater value. If improvement occurs, slow tapering of the dose should be started after 7 to 10 days of treatment. Tapering the dose to nothing may require weeks or a few months. If prednisone is used, a full dose of 1 mg. per pound per day can be instituted with the same general rules for tapering the dose as those given for ACTH. Although there is little doubt about the dramatic effect of the adrenal steroid therapy on the movement disorder, doubt exists about whether these agents reduce long-term neurologic morbidity.

This dramatic movement disorder is usually self-limited, and most patients recover normal motor function in a few weeks or months. However, I have been impressed with the acute and sometimes persistent damage to the mental and intellectual function in about one-third of the patients. The latter observation suggests that the responsible mechanism may involve a diffuse encephalopathy even though attention is usually focused initially on the incapacitating loss of coordination.

Acute Labyrinthitis. This disorder is uncommon in the 1970s because its usual antecedent, purulent otitis media or mastoiditis, has diminished in incidence owing to widespread antimicrobial therapy. The patient usually prefers to lie quietly because movement causes vertigo and vomiting. Nystagmus and loss of hearing are common and an abnormal caloric response to ice water instilled in the ear is seen in severe cases.

Intensive antimicrobial therapy, appropriate for the causative agent, is used along with surgical drainage of the middle ear if necessary.

Infectious Polyneuritis (Landry-Guillain-Barré Syndrome). Often patients with this uncommon disorder appear ataxic although, in fact, their incoordination is due to muscle weakness. The key clinical findings which establish the diagnosis include absent or depressed deep tendon reflexes, mild distal sensory loss, elevated CSF protein and normal cell count and slowing of nerve conduction velocities. The

* Manufacturer's precaution: Vincristine is recommended only for treatment of acute leukemia in childhood.

cause of this syndrome is usually obscure. It probably results from multiple factors, but circumstantial evidence (including occasional elevation of CSF gamma globulin and beneficial response to adrenal steroids in some cases) suggests an immunologic or infectious basis. As a specific example, this syndrome is well known as a complication of infectious mononucleosis.

The acute phase of the illness is managed with special nursing and good supportive medical care, preferably in an intensive care unit. Many patients recover slowly in 7 to 10 days with no specific therapy. Others, with bulbar or respiratory muscle weakness, need tracheostomy and assisted ventilation. In order to follow the patient's course accurately, it is helpful to keep a portable device (Vitalor†) at the bedside to measure vital capacity. This, along with the measurement of blood gases, is helpful in deciding when mechanical respirators are needed. Early consultation with ENT and chest specialists should be sought in the proper management of this life-threatening disease.

If the patient is getting steadily worse, I recommend a trial of adrenal steroid therapy. In general, I suggest the same dosage plan and treatment schedule here as that outlined above for acute cerebellar ataxia. This benefits some patients and fails to help others. As with any disease which naturally remits, the value of therapy in a given case of infectious polyneuritis may be unclear, but one repeatedly sees occasional patients where the weakness recurs when adrenal steroids are withdrawn only to improve again with reinstitution of steroid therapy. This sequence of events occurs more commonly in adults with peripheral neuropathy than in children.

TUMOR

Brain tumors in the posterior fossa are quickly considered in children who develop ataxia, especially when the more common intoxicants and infectious causes are eliminated from consideration. Such patients usually have changes in behavior and disposition, as well as headache, vomiting and other focal neurologic signs. Additional diagnostic studies should include skull x-rays, electroencephalogram and brain scan. Decisions about lumbar puncture, angiography and pneumography should be made by neurologic or neurosurgical consultants. Treatment of brain tumors consists of judicious surgical procedures, radiation therapy and, in special cases, chemotherapy.

† Manufactured by McKesson, Toledo, Ohio.

Children with intraspinal tumors may present with "ataxia," usually due to spastic weakness. Occasionally a slowly growing cord tumor is mistaken for "cerebral palsy" or "muscular dystrophy." A high index of suspicion, along with spine x-rays and myelography, leads to accurate diagnosis. Treatment is surgical, with or without radiation and chemotherapy.

TRAUMA

As in the case of syphilis in the prepenicillin era, one must always consider head trauma and hematoma formation with a host of presenting neurologic signs, including ataxia. Following an acute head injury the patient is often acutely ataxic; the reason for this is frequently obscure. The latter disability usually disappears unless hemorrhage in the midbrain or brain stem is sufficient to cause permanent damage to the cerebellar outflow tract. Subdural hematoma over the brain convexity in older children may cause some focal incoordination, usually due to spastic weakness. Much less often, true ataxia is seen in patients with posterior fossa subdural hematoma. The latter lesion is often overlooked because of its rarity and because it may only cause symptoms of increased intracranial pressure. Once the diagnosis is established, evacuation of a loculated blood clot is strictly a surgical problem.

DEGENERATIVE DISEASES

Nearly all of the disorders are very rare and none of them is amenable to specific treatment. However, often they do present with ataxia. Strictly speaking, these conditions follow a subacute or chronic course, but because ataxia does not escape detection for long, a few paragraphs of discussion seem warranted. Discussion will be limited to the key diagnostic procedures and to the important aspects of family counseling.

Multiple Sclerosis. Ataxia is commonly seen in early multiple sclerosis and is often associated with other focal deficits. Accurate measurement of CSF gamma globulin (IgG) is the only useful laboratory test and is elevated in about three-fourths of the cases.

Leukodystrophies. Metachromatic leukodystrophy often first appears as ataxia in a young child who has just learned to walk. The CSF protein is elevated at some time during the course of the disease and metachromatic material can be demonstrated in a urine sediment stained with methylene blue. Measurement of the leukocyte arylsulfatase-A content is a more reliable test, however. This enzyme is markedly depressed in affected patients. The carrier state can also be detected with this same laboratory method, levels falling between those seen in the homozygote and those in the unaffected controls. Because the disease is inherited as an autosomal recessive trait, its appearance in other siblings occurs commonly.

Subacute Sclerosing Panencephalitis. This rare and late complication of measles causes myoclonic seizures, ataxia, dementia and death. The diagnosis can be suspected on the basis of extreme elevations of CSF gamma globulin along with markedly elevated antibody titers to measles virus in the CSF.

Rare Hereditary Metabolic and Degenerative Disorders. Ataxia and similar movement disorders may occur regularly or intermittently with some of the extremely rare hereditary diseases, including ataxia-telangiectasia, Hartnup disease, acanthocytosis, Wilson's disease, X-linked primary hyperuricemia and Friedreich's ataxia.

CHOREOATHETOSIS

Because patients with this syndrome may be classified as ataxic, one must consider both rheumatic chorea and Huntington's chorea in any patient with an atypical movement disorder and in whom a definitive diagnosis has not been established. With rheumatic chorea one looks for evidence of carditis (murmur, abnormal electrocardiogram) or elevated "acute phase reactants," including an antistreptolysin O titer. This syndrome is usually self-limited and the chorea disappears in three months. When the chorea is disabling it can often be ameliorated with phenobarbital (16 to 32 mg. every 6 to 8 hours) or reserpine (0.02 mg. per kilogram per day in divided doses). In addition, long-term penicillin prophylaxis should be instituted (see Rheumatic Fever).

The diagnosis of Huntington's chorea is made on the basis of its relentlessly progressive course, the associated dementia, a positive family history and atrophy of the caudate nucleus seen with pneumoencephalography.

Choreoathetosis secondary to neonatal hypoxia is seen often enough to create a puzzling diagnostic picture. Not uncommonly the movement disorder becomes increasingly obvious in the maturing child, giving rise to the vexing question of whether one is dealing with a progressive disease or a static disorder which is simply attracting more attention. Surgical relief with pallidotomy does not usually produce permanent relief. However, sedative agents, such as those suggested for rheumatic chorea (chlorpromazine,* reserpine and haloperidol)† are worth a therapeutic trial.

Reference

Bray, P. F., Ziter, F. A., Lahey, M. E., and Myers, G. G.: The Coincidence of Neuroblastoma and Acute Cerebellar Encephalopathy. *J. Pediat.,* 75:983, 1969.

Degenerative Diseases of the Central Nervous System

HART DeC. PETERSON, M.D.

Any of the individual degenerative diseases of the central nervous system is very likely a rare occurrence in the practice of a typical pediatrician or general physician. Some examples of the group as a whole, however, are not unlikely. The general principles of management of these chronic, usually progressive disorders do not vary widely from case to case. Specifics of management are mentioned under diagnostic headings.

After diagnosis is reached, the nature and implications of the disorder must be presented to the parents. The physician's ultimate goal is to secure a mature understanding by the parents of the disease and its implications for the child. After sympathetic presentation of the diagnosis and prognosis, the physician should present a positive program for management of the child. The parents should understand the goals of therapy. Active involvement in a treatment program, even with modest objectives, is frequently gratifying to parents.

Neuromuscular Function. Active exercise should be continued as long as possible. Weak or atrophic limbs should not be put at rest, since this may accelerate disability. When active exercise becomes limited, passive and assistive exercises should be carried out. Every effort should be made to avoid contractures, which interfere with nursing care. Occasionally, bracing is of assistance. Orthopedic procedures, such as Achilles tendon lengthening, may improve function if the disorder is arrested or only slowly progressive.

Respiratory Function. Difficulty with swallowing due to pharyngeal dysfunction com-

* Manufacturer's precaution: Chlorpromazine is not recommended for children under six months of age except when lifesaving.

† Manufacturer's precaution: Haloperidol is not recommended for use in the pediatric age group because its safety and efficacy have not been established.

monly leads to aspiration with secondary pneumonitis and atelectasis. A tracheostomy facilitates tracheal suction. If care is taken, all lung segments can be drained by postural means. Moist air is of value in promoting removal of secretions.

Bladder Functions. If catheters are used, urinary infection eventually develops. Acute infections should be treated according to the bacterial flora, and every effort should be made to do without the catheter. Urinary acidification may be of value in retarding or preventing recurrent infection.

Bowel Function. Constipation may be prevented by using stool softeners, such as dioctyl sodium sulfosuccinate, or laxatives, such as milk of magnesia or cascara preparations.

Skin Hygiene. Every effort should be made to avoid decubitus ulcers because they are ready portals for infection and greatly increase nursing requirements. Frequent changes of position, especially when sensation is reduced, are of value. A lamb's wool mattress or alternating pressure mattress, along with frequent massage, retards development of decubitus ulcers.

Behavior. Children with cerebral dysfunction occasionally show hyperactive, distractible, aggressive behavior. This behavior can sometimes be improved with tranquilizing drugs, such as chlorpromazine* or milder tranquilizers, such as hydroxyzine. Occasionally such a child may be remarkably improved by dextroamphetamine,† 2.5 to 10 mg. once or twice per day, or methylphenidate,‡ 5 to 10 mg. one to three times per day.

Convulsions. Convulsions should be treated with the usual anticonvulsants (see Seizure Disorders).

Death. Some children with central nervous system degenerative disease progressively deteriorate despite every effort in their behalf. Sensitive recognition of the point at which death is shortly inevitable and prolongation of life has become a technical exercise is the doctor's responsibility. The family may be informed, but the physician should assume responsibility for the decision not to extend meaningless existence by heroic measures.

* Manufacturer's precaution: Chlorpromazine is not recommended for children under six months of age except when lifesaving.

† Manufacturer's precaution: Dextroamphetamine is not recommended for hyperkinetic behavior disorders in children under three years of age.

‡ Manufacturer's precaution: Methylphenidate is not recommended for children under six years of age. The parenteral form of methylphenidate is not recommended in children.

Genetic Counseling. Many of these diseases have established patterns of inheritance. When this is known, parents should be made aware of the risk of producing future children with the disease. In a few disorders, such as the gangliosidoses and mucopolysaccharidoses, prenatal diagnosis of the fetus is possible and permits selective therapeutic abortion, where legal. Prenatal diagnosis requires an experienced team with varied skills, including amniocentesis by an experienced obstetrician, expertise in tissue culture, ability to carry out the specific diagnostic test required and the ability and willingness to provide treatment on the basis of the diagnosis established.

ATAXIA-TELANGIECTASIA

The neurologic deterioration in this condition is not treatable. Recurrent sinopulmonary infections should be managed according to their bacterial flora (see Infectious Diseases). This disease is inherited as an autosomal recessive.

LEUKODYSTROPHIES; SCHILDER'S DISEASE

No specific treatment is available for any of these progressive disorders. The physician's efforts should be directed toward minimizing the impact of neural injury on the child and his family. If a diagnosis can be made, genetic counseling of the parents may be possible.

Sudanophilic Leukodystrophy (Schilder's Disease). Inheritance of this disorder is variable. Its occasional association with Addison's disease may require steroid replacement therapy (see Addison's disease, in Adrenal Disorders).

Pelizaeus-Merzbacher Disease. This disorder is usually inherited as a sex-linked recessive trait. Because this disorder is only very slowly progressive, efforts at preserving independence with wheelchairs and other orthopedic devices are especially worthwhile. Passive joint movements help avoid contractures and facilitate nursing care.

Krabbe's Disease (Globoid Cell Leukodystrophy). This disease is frequently inherited as an autosomal recessive.

Spongy Degeneration of the White Matter (Canavan's Disease). This disease is frequently inherited as an autosomal recessive.

Metachromatic Leukodystrophy (Sulfatide Lipidosis). No specific therapy alters the course of this illness. It is frequently inherited as an autosomal recessive.

DISSEMINATED SCLEROSIS (MULTIPLE SCLEROSIS)

No specific treatment is available for this disorder. Steroids may be useful when acute optic neuritis is present (see Neuromyelitis Optica), but their value is otherwise not established.

DYSTONIA MUSCULORUM DEFORMANS (TORSION SPASM)

Although the cause of this disease is not known, dramatic reversal of all its manifestations by lesions of the basal ganglia has been reported. This form of therapy is by no means invariably successful and even in experienced hands carries distinct risks.

FRIEDREICH'S ATAXIA (HEREDITARY SPINAL ATAXIA)

Specific treatment is not available for this disorder. Exercise should be encouraged as tolerated. Surgical measures to correct foot deformity or to arrest scoliosis are appropriate only when the disease is slowly progressive. Dementia may be anticipated in many cases. Inheritance is variable but may sometimes be determined by study of the family.

HEPATOLENTICULAR DEGENERATION (WILSON'S DISEASE)

See page 345.

HEREDITARY OPTIC ATROPHIES

No specific treatment is available for this group of disorders. Inheritance varies from family to family. If mental function is adequate, rehabilitation therapy should be started promptly when the diagnosis is reached.

HEREDITARY SENSORY NEUROPATHY (HEREDITARY PERFORATING ULCER OF THE FOOT, HEREDITARY SENSORY RADICULAR NEUROPATHY)

Great care must be taken to protect the feet from unappreciated injury. Amputation of the feet may nevertheless become necessary. Nerve deafness develops in some cases. Some cases are sporadic, but others can be identified as dominantly transmitted.

HEREDITARY SPASTIC PARAPLEGIA

No specific treatment is available for this disorder. The pattern of hereditary is variable but sometimes may be determined by individual family study. Ambulation may be prolonged by the use of crutches and by bracing. Passive exercises to prevent joint contracture facilitate nursing care.

HYPERTROPHIC INTERSTITIAL POLYNEURITIS (DÉJÉRINE-SOTTAS DISEASE)

No specific treatment is known for this disease. The inheritance is frequently dominant but may be recessive. Although the course may be quite slow, vocational counseling should anticipate eventual limitation of ambulation and manual dexterity.

KINKY HAIR DISEASE

This disease is transmitted as a sex-linked recessive. To date it has not been successfully treated, but a newly identified defect in copper absorption provides a theoretical basis for treatment.

LAURENCE-MOON-BIEDL SYNDROME

No specific treatment is available for this syndrome. Obesity is a problem in these children and may limit their activities if it is not controlled. Progressive decrease of vision can be anticipated in many cases and should be a factor in educational planning for these mentally retarded children.

This disease is usually inherited as a recessive characteristic and will affect 25 per cent of births of heterozygous parents.

NECROTIZING ENCEPHALOPATHY WITH PREDILECTION FOR THE BRAIN STEM (WERNICKE-LIKE ENCEPHALOPATHY: LEIGH'S DISEASE)

No specific treatment is available for this recessively inherited disorder.

NEUROMYELITIS OPTICA

No specific treatment is available for this disorder. During acute episodes of optic nerve inflammation, prednisolone, 2 to 3 mg. per kilogram daily for two weeks, or ACTH injections, 25 to 30 units daily for two weeks, may reduce swelling and secondary pressure injury to the optic nerve. Either regimen should be discontinued gradually over about four weeks.

PERONEAL MUSCULAR ATROPHY (CHARCOT-MARIE-TOOTH DISEASE)

Although no specific therapy is available for this disorder, its frequently very slow progression justifies a substantial therapeutic effort. Regular mild exercise of weak muscles should be encouraged, since disuse of a partially atrophic muscle may accelerate disability. If there is sensory loss, the patient must learn to protect partially anesthetic extremities from inadvertent injury.

The patient should be guided in his long-term planning to avoid occupations that put a premium on ambulation, manual dexterity or extremity strength. Inheritance of this disorder is variable but frequently dominant.

SYRINGOMYELIA

Laminectomy and drainage by placement of a catheter or wick within the cystic cavity have been frequently tried. Low dose x-irradiation also has been employed. Neither form of therapy has been of convincing benefit.

References

Daubs, D. M., et al.: Menkes's Kinky Hair Syndrome. *Pediatrics,* 50:188, 1972.

Nadler, H.: Prenatal Detection of Genetic Disorders. *Advances in Human Genetics,* 3:1–37, 1972 (Harris, H., and Hirshhorn, K., eds.).

Rawson, R. D., Liversedge, L. A., and Goldfarb, G.: Treatment of Acute Retrobulbar Neuritis with Corticotrophin. *Lancet,* 1:1044, 1966.

Cerebral Palsy

WILLIAM BERENBERG, M.D.

Cerebral palsy is not a single disease entity but rather a group of conditions differing in type and severity and resulting from a variety of cerebral insults. Associated with the damage to the motor pathways, (pyramidal and extrapyramidal), there may coexist any or all of a host of other aftermaths (e.g., seizures and problems of intelligence, vision, hearing, speech and emotion). There is no single drug or system of therapy which will produce a cure. Each patient's deficits and needs must be assessed and dealt with on an individual basis. The following recommended guidelines for the pediatrician neither constitute a specific system of treatment nor are by any means all-inclusive.

The primary therapeutic objective is the prevention of cerebral palsy. Prematurity remains the number one cause but, unfortunately, too little is known regarding measures needed for its prevention. Prenatal virologic insults can now be met only partially by such measures as immunization against rubella prior to conception. The neuromotor consequences of the cytomegaloviruses and other prenatal viral challenges remain to be conquered. The welcomed era of the pediatrician as a fetologist, in partnership with the obstetrician, demands our participation in the interpretation of studies of amniotic fluid and, when indicated, in interference with pregnancy. Maternal and, consequently, fetal malnutrition demands closer collaborative attention. Maternal exposure to radiation, inadequately controlled diabetes during pregnancy and a growing list of identifiable causes require concerned preventive attention to the fetus in utero. Also, increased attention must be paid to a host of other agents, such as lead, silver, mercury and strontium, which may play significant roles in the causation of cerebral palsy.

The pediatrician must join with his obstetrical colleagues in fetal monitoring and decision making during the critical period of obstetric anesthesia, labor and delivery.

After birth, the neonatal attendant must be particularly aware of bilirubinemia, hypoxia, hypoglycemia, polycythemia, intracranial hemorrhage and other peri- and postnatal challenges to the neurologic integrity of the newborn.

In the postnatal period, one must remain alert to the prevention of head injuries, early therapy of meningitis, avoidance of lead poisoning, efficient management of cardiopulmonary arrest, appropriate treatment of cerebral edema and a growing list of significant cerebral insults.

The importance of early recognition and therapy has long been debated. Its principal virtue appears to reside in improvement in achieving parental acceptance of the catastrophe and subsequent appropriate adjustment. In patients with pyramidal tract involvement and progressive muscle spasticity, early use of physical therapy may ameliorate although not necessarily prevent contractures and ensuing deformities. In the hypotonic group with extrapyramidal disease, the value of conventional physical therapy is debatable. A wide variety of systems of therapy based on using, overcoming, or modifying primitive reflexes and postural patterns await final definition of value. Well-designed studies, adequately controlled and appropriately matched, are sufficiently meager to defy positive conclusions.

It must be emphasized, however, that few if any cerebral palsied infants will fail to progress with or without specific therapy. For example, all infants with hemiplegia will walk independently close to the average age for ambulation provided they are not sufficiently retarded mentally so that they would not have walked in any event. The proficiency of their gait may indeed be improved by heel cord or thigh adductor muscle stretching, the use of night casts or braces or actual surgery if there is a threat of hip subluxation.

Pediatricians following young infants at high risk should be alert to neurologic consequences that require early therapeutic intervention. Significantly hyperbilirubinemic infants should be observed closely not only for hypotonia and subsequently athetosis but also for sensorineural hearing loss, which should be treated early by lip reading techniques, by auditory amplification and especially by appropriate interpretation of their failure to relate to environmental stimuli. In premature infants, major attention should be paid to persistent lower extremity hyperreflexia, muscular spasticity, ankle clonus, extensor plantar responses and other pyramidal tract signs of the spastic diplegia often associated with prematurity. Early physical therapy is frequently indicated in these infants.

The provision of sensory stimuli is most important for all immobile infants and children. Sensory stimuli are the major educational building blocks of infancy. Hot and cold, smooth and rough, light and heavy, fragile and unyielding and near and far are but a few of the critical discriminations which mobile toddlers learn for themselves. For the immobile child, these must be prescribed by the pediatrician as learning experiences at an early age. Instead of reacting with "nothing can be done now," the pediatrician ought to ask himself what the child would normally be doing at this age in terms of sensory input and prescribe the same, albeit on a passive basis.

At a variety of appropriate ages, the primary physician might utilize, with consultation, a number of the following professional therapeutic adjuncts:

Neurosurgery. In the neonate, young infant and postmeningitic, subdural hematomata should be treated vigorously by repeated tapping and subsequent membrane removal if indicated. Revision of vascular malformations must be considered, especially in the hemiplegic cerebral palsied. In older children with extrapyramidal dystonic cerebral palsy, chemopallidectomy or cryosurgery offers some potential for amelioration.

Orthopedic Surgery. The orthopedic surgeon is a critical member of the therapeutic team. Physical therapy should be conducted under his supervision. Casts are frequently employed to maintain extremities in a position necessary to avoid contractures and other deformities. Braces are used to promote or improve gait or to avoid deformity in any extremity. The type of brace should depend on the patient's needs and not be stereotyped to the surgeon's prejudice. Myotomy, tenotomy, tendon transplant, arthrodesis and neurectomy are of value in selected cases with the spastic variety of cerebral palsy. Unless threatened by an impending catastrophe, such as subluxation of the hip, these surgical measures should be deferred to an age when maximal improvement may result and at least to such age when a patient will cooperate postoperatively. Postoperative casting and patient cooperation with physical therapy are prime prerequisites for surgical success and cannot be anticipated in very young or retarded children.

Physical Medicine. Physicians versed in this specialty may be of great value in employment of phenol nerve block and the use of a variety of specially constructed braces and adjunctive devices as well as in the supervision of physical and occupational therapeutic regimens.

Psychiatry. The parents of the child with cerebral palsy often need formal psychiatric help during their period of attempted adjustment. The siblings of these children occasionally revolt against or suffer from the consequence of a significantly handicapped child in the household. The patient himself is most apt to need formal help if he is handicapped to a small degree either physically or mentally. Particularly during adolescence, children who have minor but cosmetically significant deficits often face catastrophic psychiatric conflicts. The child who intellectually lacks insight or whose severe motor defects have never permitted the aspiration of normal acceptance is less prone to this emotional crisis than is the child who was promised normality and can never achieve it. Total, objective and honest prognosis is the best psychiatric prophylaxis although formal intervention may ultimately be required.

Psychology. The psychologist selected to evaluate and guide the child with cerebral palsy must be specially equipped to use techniques designed to permit accurate assessment despite motor, visual or auditory defects or a combination of these. He must also be sensitive to the frequent occurrence of specific learning disabilities.

Nursing. An informed nurse is of significant help in teaching parents of cerebral palsied children such things as techniques of feeding, lifting, transportation and toilet training as well as cast supervision.

Physical Therapy. As indicated previously, the therapist is of extreme therapeutic value in the prevention of contractures, as well as in gait training and the development of balance and coordination.

Occupational Therapy. Efforts in this area should be coordinated into the overall therapeutic regimen of aiding motor development and skills. Early objectives include self-care skills such as self-feeding, dressing and relating to environmental needs. Later efforts may be directed toward development of special skills.

Nutrition. The pediatrician should be aware of the increased energy expenditure associated with active athetosis or severe muscular spasticity and the fact that many such children are in negative nitrogen balance. Immobile children with lesser degrees of activity may, on the other hand, become unduly obese owing to the lack of exercise and excessive intake.

Speech. Speech therapy is of little value in the development of speech if nonexistent in a retarded child, but it is of value in improving the character and quality of impaired or dysarthric speech.

Hearing. Since most hearing deficits in cerebral palsy are of a sensorineural variety, aids result chiefly in amplification without increase in range and are of limited value. Lip reading, speech indoctrination and special education are of primary value.

Eye. The eye problems of the cerebral palsied include disorders of motility, strabismus and hemianopia and should be dealt with in conventional fashion. The correction of strabismus, even if of solely cosmetic value, is an important adjunct in the effort to decrease as many deficits as possible in a multihandicapped child. The appreciation of hemianopia is of particular significance in decision making when confronted with a request for medical approval for driving privileges.

Seizures. Drug therapy in this area parallels that recommended for seizure control generally. (Refer to Seizure Disorders, p. 78.)

Drug Therapy. There are no drugs of proved or specific value in the treatment of cerebral palsy. Valium (diazepam), in doses of 2.5 mg. two times a day in children up to five years of age, and in doses of 5.0 to 10.0 mg. two or three times a day in older children, is of limited value in the partial relief of spasticity. This drug should not be given to children under six months of age.* It should be avoided in the presence of congenital glaucoma and discontinued if the patient becomes excessively drowsy. It should be withdrawn if it produces paradoxic hyperexcitability or increased muscle spasticity. The phenothiazines and barbiturates may potentiate its action. At present, the use of L-dopa† is without clear-cut value in the treatment of the spastic or athetoid variety of cerebral palsy, but is still under hopeful review, particularly in treatment of the dystonic type. Since this drug has not yet been released for general use in pediatric patients, no specific dosage can be recommended.

It must be reemphasized that all, none or a mixed variety of the therapies just described may be appropriately prescribed for a child with cerebral palsy, since treatment depends on individual assessment of each child's particular deficits and needs.

* Manufacturer's precaution: Safety and efficacy of injectable Valium in children under 12 years of age have not been established. Oral Valium is not for use in children under six months of age.

† Manufacturer's precaution: Safety of L-dopa in children under 12 years of age has not been established.

Spinal Diseases

BENNETT M. STEIN, M.D.

If meningomyeloceles and similar forms of dysraphism are excluded from discussion, treatable disorders of the spinal region in children are uncommon. Degenerative diseases and other myelopathies due to noncompressive lesions may produce severe neurologic deficit, but present a therapeutic dilemma since there is little beyond supportive therapy that can be offered.

TRAUMA

Dislocations and fractures of the spinal canal produce sudden neurologic deficit which may or may not indicate total loss of spinal cord function (Tuell). In spite of devastating injury the cauda equina and, to a much lesser extent, the spinal cord have the ability to recover if the compressive aspect of the injury is alleviated. In general, the therapeutic aims are twofold: (1) immediate release of the spinal compression and (2) stabilization of an unstable spine.

A predisposing factor in spinal cord injury is a congenital maldevelopment of the odontoid process or its ligaments. Minor trauma may then produce a dislocation between the first and second cervical vertebrae. In other areas of the cervical spine, fracture dislocation, especially following diving accidents, is common at the C5–C6 or C6–C7 region. Compression of the vertebral bodies due to a fall on the buttocks may produce compromise of the spinal cord or the cauda equina. In cases of fracture or fracture dislocation, immediate attention is given to correcting the deformity through skeletal traction, accomplished by placing tongs or other traction apparatus into the skull and applying weight. If a spinal block or progressive neurologic deficit is noted or x-rays indicate the displacement of bone elements into the spinal canal, immediate decompressive surgery is indicated. This is usually accomplished through a posterior laminectomy, although in certain cases in the cervical region the same aim can be accomplished through an anterior cervical approach with a fusion performed at the time of operation. For the odontoid dislocations, posterior fusion is usually carried from the occipital bone to the upper cervical vertebrae. In certain instances, occipital mobility may be maintained, with fusion limited to the upper cervical vertebrae. It is extremely important to produce adequate stabilization in these latter lesions, since any dislocation in this region may produce sudden death due to spinal cord and medullary compression (Forsyth et al.).

Penetrating missiles usually produce immediate spinal cord injury, and in most cases surgery is not indicated, since the damage is irrevocable. In other cases, in which a progressive neurologic deficit follows penetrating trauma, a hematoma must be considered and surgical decompression accomplished. High doses of steroids are also helpful.

MASS LESION

Spinal masses may be categorized as follows: (1) extradural lesions, (2) intradural lesions and (3) intramedullary lesions. The more common lesions in children lie extradurally. These may be neoplastic, such as neuroblastoma, or inflammatory, such as epidural abscess, the latter being quite rare. Neoplastic lesions have a tendency to involve not only the extradural space but extend out through a neural foramen in dumbbell fashion, producing a large mass in the thoracic or abdominal cavity. The most critical lesion is the intraspinal lesion, and immediate attention is turned to this in order to accomplish decompression of the spinal cord or cauda equina. The extraspinal mass is usually removed at a second operation. Many of the malignant tumors respond to surgery plus radiotherapy or chemotherapy and the prognosis in many instances is excellent not only for return of neurologic function but also for long-term survival.

Bacterial epidural abscesses are characterized by a fulminating course with severe neurologic deficit, tenderness over the spine and fever, and are difficult to diagnose. If recognized, immediate surgery is indicated. The abscess is incised and drained and catheters are left in the region for appropriate antibiotic irrigations. In most instances the dura prevents spread of this abscess into the spinal canal and there is no necessity for intrathecal therapy. The patient should have an excellent recovery, provided systemic antibiotics are continued for four to six weeks or longer if the infection is not controlled.

Tuberculous involvement of the spine with neural compression is treated by decompression, usually via an anterior approach, and use of appropriate drugs.

Whereas intradural neurofibromas and meningiomas are more frequent in the adult while rare in children, except in neurofibromatosis, the more likely lesions in this compartment are dermoids and lipomas of the cauda equina (Hirt et al.). Both lesions are benign, slow-growing and often static in their expansion; however, they become interwoven in the roots of the cauda equina and total removal in either instance may be difficult or impossible. Fortunately, even subtotal removals are associated with quiescence of the lesion and long-term follow-up without progressive neurologic deficits.

Intramedullary lesions include the astrocytoma, ependymoma and syringomyelia, which is a nontumorous cystic expansion within the central portion of the spinal cord. With microneurosurgical techniques, many of the intramedullary tumors may be removed in toto. In some instances a two-stage operation is indicated. The initial stage is a splitting of the dorsal portion of the spinal cord over the tumor with closure of the wound. Subsequently, reoperation will often reveal deliverance of the tumor from within the spinal cord, and an easy removal may be accomplished. In cases in which removal is subtotal, postoperative radiotherapy directed to the site of the tumor is indicated. In the case of total tumor removal and to a lesser extent in those with subtotal removal followed by radiotherapy, the long-term results are encouraging.

In the case of syringomyelia, the aim is to prevent progression of the disease, and remission of the neurologic disorder is usual following surgery. A number of techniques have been developed to treat this condition. They consist of drainage of the syringomyelia cavity into the subarachnoid space or plugging of the obex, the latter based on a theory that the cavity is promoted through flow of the CSF via the obex into the central canal of the spinal cord.

MISCELLANEOUS

Degenerated and herniated discs as well as *lumbosacral spondylolysis* with or without spondylolisthesis are uncommon conditions in children (Turner and Bianco). In many instances the herniated disc or, more commonly, the spondylolysis will present with hamstring spasm and an abnormal gait. Radiating sciatic-like pain may or may not be present. Other neurologic deficits, such as diminished reflexes or weakness, may not be seen. Following diagnosis through spine x-rays and myelography, treatment consists of removal of herniated discs and, in the case of spondylolisthesis, fusion of the involved spinal portion. These procedures have produced excellent results in about 85 per cent of cases.

Diastematomyelia is a condition associated with block vertebrae, hemivertebrae, wedge vertebrae and a central bony spicule with a splitting or duplication of the spinal cord. Theory has it that the bone spicule impedes the natural migration of the spinal cord in relationship to the vertebral bodies. A progressive neurologic deficit may thereby result. Therapeutic aims are twofold: (1) to remove the bony spicule and form a common dural tube around the divided spinal cord, releasing any obstruction to the normal migration of the cord, and (2) to stabilize or correct spinal deformities. The results have been gratifying, and in some cases neurologic deficits have been reversed (Meacham).

The *tethered cord syndrome* may or may not be associated with meningomyelocele or lipoma of the cauda equina region. This condition is characterized by a thickening of the filum terminale and a low-lying spinal cord. The patients often have deficits, such as incontinence, localized to the lower sacral roots. The anatomic defect may be visualized at myelography. The surgical aim is to section the filum terminale to allow proper migration of spinal cord. Postoperatively, a significant number of patients have improved bladder function.

VASCULAR DISORDERS

With improved spinal angiography, the recognition of treatable arteriovenous vascular anomalies of the spinal cord has increased. The therapeutic result is predicated on the anatomic configuration of these lesions. Diffuse vascular malformations which are centered within the spinal cord are generally not amenable to surgery. However, those associated with tortuous veins and limited arterial contributions lying on the dorsal surface of the spinal cord can be safely removed by microsurgical techniques (Krayenbuhl et al.). Following such successful surgery, remission of neurologic deficits may be expected. In other instances, a progressive neurologic disorder is arrested.

References

Forsyth, H. F., Alexander, E., Jr., Davis, C., Jr., and Underdal, R.: The Advantages of Early Spine Fusion in the Treatment of Fracture Dislocation of the Cervical Spine. *J. Bone Joint Surg., 41-A:*17–36, 1959.

Hirt, H. R., Zdrojewski, B., and Weber, G.: The Manifestations and Complications of Intraspinal Congenital Dermal Sinuses and Dermoid Cysts. *Neuropadiatrie,* 3:231–247, 1972.

Krayenbuhl, H., Yasargil, M. G., and McClintock, H. G.: Treatment of Spinal Cord Vascular Malformations by Surgical Excision. *J. Neurosurg.* 30:427–435, 1969.

Meacham, W. F.: Surgical Treatment of Diastematomyelia. *J. Neurosurg.,* 27:78–85, 1967.

Tuell, J. I.: Fracture-Dislocation of the Cervical Spine in Small Children. *J. Bone Joint Surg.,* 39-A:459–460, 1957.

Turner, R. H., and Bianco, A. J.: Spondylolysis and Spondylolisthesis in Children and Teen-agers. *J. Bone Joint Surg.* 53-A:1298–1306, 1971.

Upper and Lower Neural Tube Dysraphism

C. D. R. LIGHTOWLER, F.R.C.S.

In the last decade of the 19th century, 153 babies in every 1000 live births in the United Kingdom died in the first year of life. In 1965 this figure had been reduced to 19 deaths per 1000 live births. Of these 19 deaths, 21 per cent were due to congenital abnormalities. This dramatic reduction reflects the large-scale prevention of common crippling and fatal diseases and the more efficient and speedier treatment of many others. The improvement in treatment has caused other problems, because children with congenital malformations who would previously have died are now surviving to require lifelong complicated and expensive treatment. Not least among these children are patients with neural tube malformations: spina bifida, anencephaly and cranium bifidum.

SPINA BIFIDA

This is the most common single major congenital malformation. Clinically, spina bifida can be grouped into three entries: viz., open meningomyelocele, simple meningocele and closed meningomyelocele and spina bifida occulta. Open meningomyelocele is the most frequent of these (approximately 85 per cent) and is the most difficult to treat medically and ethically.

Open Meningomyelocele

The most common site for the presentation of this lesion is at the lumbar or lumbosacral level, but thoracolumbosacral, thoracolumbar, sacral and thoracic lesions occur. Cervical lesions are rare and are often found to be part of an occipital encephalocele.

When the patient is seen in the first day of life there is an obvious defect in the back, with an oval glittering area of red in the center. This is the dysplastic portion of the cord. The width of the neural portion varies and if it is small the membrane attaching it to the skin may take the form of a floppy sac. This may later fill with cerebrospinal fluid and become tense. The deep surface of the plaque is found to be covered by meninges, separating it from the intact anterior wall of the canal. Accompanying these appearances, the child may have hydrocephalus, lower limb deformities and loss of sensation and motor power in the lower limbs. When the child is seen soon after birth, abnormal neurologic function may not be present. If the child is not treated, the lesion may become infected, the limb movements, where present, will cease or hydrocephalus will progress. Ninety-four per cent of children left untreated died early of meningitis, progressive hydrocephalus or complications of paraplegia. Of the remainder, 4 per cent lived as permanent invalids and 2 per cent managed some form of life after multiple operations.

This dreadful prognosis was greatly improved with the advent of antibiotics and shunt procedures. The three-year survival rate for children so treated was 30 per cent, and these survivors were almost invariably totally paraplegic. The exceptions to this were those children whose lesions were not extensive.

Sharrard et al. showed that early closure of the lesion improves the prognosis for the patient and prevents the progressive paralysis of the lower limbs. Because the leak of cerebrospinal fluid is prevented by this treatment, many of these patients develop hydrocephalus early, and this has to be treated. The major problem facing the doctor is which child to treat, for to treat them all will produce an intolerable financial burden on most countries; yet, to withhold treatment from many of these unfortunate children will produce a higher proportion of totally paraplegic infants. Each case must be judged on its own merits by the attending physician, and he alone must make the decision. It is a reasonable policy to treat all such patients with the utmost vigor except those with gross permanent multisystem defects. It is probably better on humanitarian grounds to offer no active treatment to those patients who within hours of birth are found to have any of the following problems:

1. Severe flaccid paraplegia.
2. Kyphosis.
3. Severe clinical hydrocephalus.
4. Other gross congenital defects.

If the child with these problems survives unexpectedly, then active treatment should be started later.

Primary Operative Closure. As soon as the child is born, the lesion should be covered with a sterile nonadherent dressing and the child transferred to a neonatal care unit. The lower limb neurologic function should be assessed as accurately as possible. As a matter of emergency, within the first 24 hours, the defect should be closed under general anesthesia with intubation. Blood is required for the procedure. Normal precautions for controlling the baby's temperature must be taken. The aim of the procedure is to cover the neural tissue with dura and skin. The dura is dissected up from the wall of the spinal canal, and by undercutting the skin edges, using relaxing incisions if necessary, the lesion is covered. Rotational flaps are rarely necessary. This operation may be made difficult by an abnormally thick neural plaque or by the presence of kyphosis. The neural plaque can be shaved down, if stimulation produces no movements and if there are no nerves issuing from the defect. Bony procedures may be necessary to deal with the kyphosis. Postoperatively the child is nursed prone in an incubator and antibiotics administered if the aspirated fluid shows established infection to be present. Healing is usually sound in 7 to 10 days. Cerebrospinal fluid may leak under the flaps and from the wound postoperatively in children with severe hydrocephalus. This can be avoided by performing a ventriculoatrial shunt prior to closure of the defect, but this has the disadvantage of allowing drying and destruction of the neural plaque. These bypass procedures may be required soon after closure in patients with severe hydrocephalus, but if possible the shunt should be delayed to reduce the risks of infection and the need for subsequent revision.

Subsequent Management. It is reasonable to discharge the child after four weeks. This may seem early, but it helps parental acceptance and eases pressure on the nursing staff. The postoperative management is a matter of personal preference, but regular follow-up of the patients is essential. The children should be reviewed in combined clinics staffed by representatives from all the disciplines managing the child. Review at three months, six months, nine months and one year and then every six months until the patient stops growing is a reasonable routine, but any discipline may need to see the child more often. It is recommended that one person keep the general state of the patient constantly under review. It does not matter who this is, but he must be a combination of enthusiasm and tact to obtain the teamwork required for the best patient care. Each child will require about one operation a year for the first five years of life, and about half of them will require valve revision at least every five years.

The types of problems suffered by these children are orthopedic, urologic and neurosurgical.

ORTHOPEDIC. Paralysis of the lower limbs is the most obvious problem and this may vary from complete paraplegia and a chair life, to weakness of feet and toes. The variable paralysis produces a wide spectrum of orthopedic conditions, such as dislocated hips with fixed flexion, hyperextension of the knees and a variety of foot problems such as talipes equinovarus and vertical talus. Tendon transfers, osteotomies and soft tissue procedures help correct these deformities mainly by overcoming the deforming forces. There is no place in the treatment of these children for serial plastering except postoperatively. Even after the most complicated of procedures many children will require splinting and crutches to allow any form of walking. Kyphosis, scoliosis and lordosis, singly or in combination, present further orthopedic problems. Although spinal osteotomy may help, the condition tends to relapse and the child remains severely handicapped.

GENITOURINARY. The renal tract provides a constant problem in these patients, socially and medically. The bladder contracts abnormally, bladder sensation is missing and sphincter control is absent or incoordinated with vesicular contractions. Dribbling incontinence occurs and urinary tract infections are common, giving rise to chronic pyelonephritis, hydronephrosis and hypertension in later childhood. These children require frequent urine cultures, since the infections are usually silent, repeated intravenous pyelograms, cystograms and isotope renograms. Long-term antibiotics are essential and the child or his parent must learn to express the bladder manually to prevent infection. Early urinary diversion to a ileal conduit offers some degree of protection and may help eliminate the social problem of odor. This procedure is not without problems, such as recurrent crusting, bleeding and stenosis, and since this operation does not eliminate infection, many surgeons favor the conservative management.

NEUROSURGICAL. About 50 per cent of these children have hydrocephalus. Insertion of unidirectional valves can now allow normal head growth and prevent visual loss and spasticity. These operations are not without complications; revisions, either prophylactically or because of infections, blockage or breakage of parts of the shunt system, are frequently required. No child with a shunt is free from the risk of sudden illness and death, and many are mentally retarded in spite of this treatment.

Other Complications. Patients with meningomyelocele suffer from many other handicaps, such as indolent ulceration especially over buttocks and over the kyphosis from constant sitting. Their limbs are cold, their bones fracture easily and their wounds heal slowly. Growth of the patient is frequently stunted and many of these children are obese.

With the most advanced surgical and medical treatment, the prognosis for patients with meningomyelocele remains poor. The expense to society or parents is tremendous, and this is in sharp contrast to the necessarily limited earnings of the 70 per cent of patients who are able to work.

Simple Meningocele

The lumbosacral and sacral areas are the most common sites for presentation of these lesions, but any region of the spine may be affected. The lower limbs show no abnormality and the anus is not patulous. Simple meningoceles should be treated operatively, but if the sac is well covered by skin, urgent surgery is not necessary. If the lesion is repaired in the first 48 hours the mortality is very low and the future innervation of the lower limbs and bladder should be normal provided there is no complicating lesion such as a lipoma or diastematomyelia. The skin is dissected from the dural sac, which is opened to ensure there are no neural elements in it. The sac is then removed, the neck being ligated and the skin closed. Hydrocephalus sometimes occurs in these patients and postoperatively a watch should be kept for it.

Closed Meningomyelocele and Spina Bifida Occulta

In these lesions the skin is intact but may show abnormal pigmentation, hair formation or a dermal sinus. The vertebral arches are unfused, but the meninges do not bulge. There may be other swellings such as lipomata or cysts. The nerve roots and cord may be abnormal and produce appropriate symptoms and signs. Pressure on these structures, tethering or infection may also produce symptoms and signs in the lower limbs or spine.

Spina bifida occulta produces no abnormal neurologic signs and therefore requires no treatment. It is normally discovered accidentally when the patient has a roentgenogram. Lipomata and dermoid cysts should be removed from those patients in whom there is paralysis. The operation may be indicated even if there is no neurologic abnormality because of the risk of paralysis occurring later.

Diastematomyelia should be treated by laminectomy and removal of the bony spur whenever there is progressive paralysis. Lipomatous bands; arachnoid adhesions and abnormal nerve roots should be explored when they produce symptoms and signs.

ANENCEPHALY

In this condition the posterior parts of the skull bones fail to develop and unite and the brain is rudimentary and malformed. The condition is incompatible with life, but it is important because of the increased risk of central nervous system abnormalities in other siblings.

CRANIUM BIFIDUM

This is a lesion similar to spina bifida, except brain tissue and not spinal cord is involved in the lesion. The lesion is usually occipital, and when it consists of meninges and cerebrospinal fluid only, the results of closure of the sac are excellent. Hydrocephalus occurs frequently and should be treated along the same lines as hydrocephalus associated with spina bifida.

In encephalocele the prognosis is poor because the cranium is small and closure is impossible without resection of brain tissue. The brain itself may also be abnormal. Surgery is indicated as an aid to management and the survivors are rarely mentally normal.

References

Lightowler, C. D. R.: Meningomyelocele: The Price of Treatment. *Brit. Med. J.,* 2:385–387, 1971.

Lorber, J.: Congenital Malformations of the Central Nervous System. *British Journal of Hospital Medicine,* 8:37–48, 1972.

Sharrard, W. J. W.: *Paediatric Orthopaedics & Fractures.* London, Blackwell Scientific Publications Ltd., 1971.

Acute Infantile Hemiplegia

ROBERT L. McLAURIN, M.D.

This clinical entity is a neurologic result of an underlying disease process. The immediate management, assuming there is no life-threatening respiratory obstruction due to accompanying coma, consists of differential diagnosis. In general, hemiplegia which occurs abruptly in the absence of seizures is due to vascular occlusion or rupture. Hemiplegia that begins in a more gradual manner, over periods of hours, may result from expanding mass lesions or inflammatory diseases. The third major category includes those hemiplegias that follow seizures. Proper therapy, therefore, is largely dependent on diagnostic accuracy, and the following discussion summarizes the diagnostic steps.

Taking the history may be important in eliciting evidence of congenital heart disease, prior episodes of hemiparesis, family or past history of seizures, preexisting upper respiratory infection, antecedent symptoms of intracranial hypertension, or recent trauma. The age of the patient is important, since the great majority of postconvulsive hemiplegias occur before two years of age, while the onset of paralysis due to other causes is distributed much more evenly throughout the pediatric age group. The causes of arterial occlusion include, most commonly, embolism and focal arteritis, the latter occurring either idiopathically or in the wake of nasopharyngeal infection. Vasospasm associated with migraine may also cause abrupt hemiparesis which usually clears within minutes or a few hours. Venous thrombosis in children is usually the result of cortical thrombophlebitis, which in turn is secondary to infections involving the upper respiratory passages or ears. Although seizures may occur at the onset of vascular occlusions, a history of prior seizures suggests that the seizure has been the primary event or that an arteriovenous malformation exists.

Examination may provide etiologic clues. A rapidly clearing hemiparesis suggests migraine or a postictal state. Disproportionate involvement of the face and arm with relative sparing of the leg indicates the probability of middle cerebral artery occlusion. Fever may indicate that febrile convulsions have occurred or that infection is present and may be associated with an occlusive vasculitis, either arterial or venous. Nuchal rigidity accompanying the hemiparesis indicates either inflammation, as may occur with cortical thrombophlebitis, or blood in the CSF suggesting rupture of a vascular anomaly. Evidence of trauma about the head should be sought, as well as signs of infection. If papilledema is present, the etiologic process is an expanding lesion of considerable duration. Signs of congenital heart disease, the source of emboli, should be noted.

Special diagnostic studies include skull x-rays, spinal puncture, electroencephalography, isotope scan and arteriography, although each of these is not necessary in every case. X-rays should be a routine part of the evaluation, since they may demonstrate evidence of recent trauma, signs of intracranial hypertension or abnormal intracranial calcification. Lumbar puncture is indicated only if there are signs of meningeal inflammation. Examination of the CSF should include careful evaluation for evidence of recent or remote bleeding or inflammatory cells. Measurement of pressure should be done routinely, if possible, but spinal punctures should be avoided if there has been prior evidence of intracranial hypertension such as papilledema. Electroencephalography, like spinal tap, should not be done routinely and is seldom indicated as an emergency diagnostic study. It should be performed whenever the evidence suggests a postconvulsive onset of the paralysis, since it may distinguish between an epileptogenic focus and a generalized underlying seizure disorder. Brain scanning with isotopes likewise has only limited application; it will not necessarily distinguish between the cause of hemiplegia and the residual effect of the disease process on the blood-brain barrier.

Arteriography is the most definitive diagnostic study, particularly in those cases in which hemiplegia was not preceded by status epilepticus. Several types of disease may be uncovered. Arteriovenous malformation of the cerebral circulation will be demonstrated, or the presence of a hematoma can be detected. Focal narrowing or irregularity of the cervical carotid artery indicates a focal arteritis which may be secondary to tonsillitis or cervical adenitis. Occlusion of a major branch of the cerebral circulation may be seen, or mycotic aneurysms, secondary to bacterial endocarditis, may be noted.

While etiologic diagnosis is the most important part of early management, there are several general therapeutic measures which should be noted. Since depressed consciousness or coma may accompany the acute hemiplegia, there may be associated depression of respiratory function. It is particularly important that normal oxygenation be maintained, since cerebral hypoxia will compound the neurologic deficit which may be due to infarction. Thus, monitoring of blood gases should be done at regular intervals in the comatose patient and respiratory assistance or control may be necessary to maintain normal gas exchange.

Anticonvulsant therapy is important and is not limited to those patients whose hemiplegia followed convulsions, since seizures may occur in the course of any disease causing sudden hemiplegia. Diazepam* (5 to 10 mg.) or sodium phenobarbitol (5 mg. per kilogram) intravenously or intramuscularly is used to stop the seizures of status epilepticus and should then be continued for about three days. Meanwhile, Dilantin (3 to 8 mg. per kilogram per day) is begun and continued for long-term therapy. If the hemiplegia did not follow convulsions, Dilantin should be started immediately and continued through at least the acute phase.

Corticosteroids may be of value when focal arteritis is suspected, although this therapy is unproved. Dexamethasone may be used in dosages of 2 to 4 mg. every 8 hours, with tapering after three to four days; in addition to its effect on the local arterial disease, it will help prevent intracranial hypertension from cerebral swelling. Attempts have been made to restore circulation in occluded cerebral vessels by surgical means, but this has not proven to be of significant benefit.

The patient should be started on a program of physical therapy and rehabilitation as soon as possible after the acute phase of the illness has subsided. This will include passive manipulation of the paralyzed extremities initially, followed by active retraining and use of mechanical devices. Speech training should be started early in those older children whose speech function has been affected.

* Manufacturer's precaution: The safety and efficacy of injectable diazepam in children under 12 years of age have not been established.

Seizure Disorders

SAMUEL LIVINGSTON, M.D.

EPILEPSY

Antiepileptic Drugs. The physician should see the patient at regular intervals to regulate the dosage of his medication, to examine him for untoward drug reactions and to discuss socioeconomic problems when present. He should also examine the patient for signs or symptoms of a specific cause for the seizure disorder which may have been overlooked or were not present at the time of the initial visit.

It is our general policy to have each patient return in two to three weeks after the initial administration of therapy primarily to determine his tolerance to the prescribed antiepileptic regimen. The frequency of subsequent visits depends on the magnitude of the patient's problems and the type of anticonvulsant medication with which he is being treated. We see every patient, including those who have been rendered free of seizures, at least once every six months during the entire time he is taking anticonvulsant medication.

INITIATION OF TREATMENT. Treatment should be instituted as soon as the diagnosis has been established. This is a most important aspect of the treatment of epilepsy for the following reasons. First, it has been our experience that in most cases the degree of success in the control of seizures is related to the duration of the epilepsy: the longer the duration, the less likely a satisfactory result will be obtained. Second, it is exceedingly important to institute measures to prevent a recurrence of seizures, not only because of the seizures but also because of injuries and emotional disorders which are sometimes associated with the occurrence of seizures.

The problem of whether the physician should assign a diagnosis of epilepsy to a patient who suffers a seizure of undetermined etiology remains controversial. In such instances, we assign a diagnosis of epilepsy to patients in whom the electroencephalographic examination reveals abnormalities such as those seen in overt epilepsy. However, in patients in whom the EEG examination reveals normal findings, we make a tentative diagnosis of epilepsy and continue with this diagnosis unless the passage of time proves that the seizure was a manifestation of some other disorder. We would like to reemphasize that such patients should be observed very closely for a prolonged period of time for signs or symptoms of a specific cause for the seizure disorder, particularly an intracranial neoplasm.

Our general policy is that daily medication be prescribed to patients with one seizure of undetermined cause in essentially the same manner as to those who have experienced recurrent epileptic seizures. *We do not utilize this plan of treatment, however, in infants and young children whose first convulsion was the type that we classify as a simple febrile convulsion.* Our recommendations for the treatment of simple febrile convulsions are described later in this article.

SELECTION OF DRUG. The selection of the drug of first choice for the treatment of any case of epilepsy should be based on the type of seizure and the toxicity of the drug.

Table 1 lists, in order of our preference, the various drugs which were being used at The Johns Hopkins Hospital Epilepsy Clinic at the time of this writing for the control of epileptic seizures.

COMBINED THERAPY FOR PETIT MAL EPILEPSY. Many patients with pure petit mal epilepsy subsequently develop other types of epileptic seizures, particularly grand mal attacks. Based on studies carried out in our clinic, we recommend the following therapeutic regimen for the treatment of patients with pure petit mal epilepsy.

TABLE 1. Drugs Currently Used at The Johns Hopkins Hospital Epilepsy Clinic for Control of Epileptic Seizures*

MAJOR MOTOR (*Grand Mal*)	PETIT MAL	MYOCLONIC	PSYCHOMOTOR (*Temporal lobe*)
Phenobarbital	Zarontin	Ketogenic diet‖	Tegretol‡
Mysoline	Tridione		Mysoline
Dilantin	Paradione	Valium**	Dilantin
Mebaral†	Celontin	ACTH and corticosteroids (for infants with hypsarhythmia)	Phenobarbital
Tegretol‡	Milontin		Mesantoin§
Bromide (for young children)	Dexedrine	Bromide	Phenurone§
Peganone	Diamox	Phenobarbital	
Gemonil	Atabrine		
Mesantoin§			
Diamox (for menstrual seizures)			

* Arranged in order of our preference, based on relative effectiveness and toxicity of drugs.

† We use this drug almost entirely as a substitute barbiturate for patients whose seizures are benefited by dosages of phenobarbital that produce side reactions, such as marked drowsiness or hyperactivity.

‡ Tegretol is available in 200-mg. tablets. Attention is directed to the package insert, which recommends that this drug be used for pain associated with true trigeminal neuralgia. Our nine years of experience with Tegretol have demonstrated that it is an exceedingly effective agent for the control of epileptic seizures, particularly psychomotor (temporal lobe) seizures.

§ These drugs possess potent anticonvulsant properties, but because of marked toxicity, they should be prescribed only to patients whose seizures are refractory to all other antiepileptic drugs.

‖ This diet is included in this table because of its value in controlling this type of epilepsy.

** Manufacturer's precaution: Safety and efficacy of injectable Valium have not been established in children under 12 years of age. Oral Valium is not for use in children under six months of age.

SPECIAL NOTE: The drugs employed for the control of autonomic and other miscellaneous epileptic seizures are the same as those recommended for the control of major motor seizures.

Treatment should be started with the conventional dosage of phenobarbital (Table 2). It is important to note that phenobarbital is prescribed as a prophylactic measure against the development of grand mal seizures and not for the purpose of controlling the petit mal spells. Treatment should be continued with phenobarbital alone for approximately one month, during which time the physician will have the opportunity to determine the patient's tolerance to the prescribed dosage and also to ascertain whether it adversely affects the frequency of the patient's petit mal spells. After one month of phenobarbital therapy, we perform a blood level determination to ensure that the phenobarbital blood concentration falls within the range that we have found to be of therapeutic value in most patients. If the blood level determination reveals subtherapeutic levels, we increase the daily dosage of phenobarbital until the blood concentration reaches "clinically effective" levels. Information relative to barbiturate blood levels is presented in a subsequent section of this article. If the patient does not tolerate this drug satisfactorily, another major motor anticonvulsant, such as Mysoline or Mebaral, should be prescribed, commencing with the conventional dosage (Table 2). We have not achieved sufficient experience relative to Mebaral or Mysoline blood concentrations to define the "average" therapeutic blood level range for either medication. Since Dilantin

TABLE 2. Average Dosages of Antiepileptic Drugs*

DRUG	AGE *(Years)*	STARTING DOSAGE *Mg.*	STARTING DOSAGE *Times/Day*	MAXIMAL DOSAGE *Mg.*	MAXIMAL DOSAGE *Times/Day*
ACTH and corticosteroids‖					
Atabrine	Under 6	50	1	50	3
	Over 6	50	2	100	3
Bromides	Under 3	160	2	320	3
	3 to 6	320	2	640	3
	Over 6	320	3	1000	3
Celontin‡	Under 6	150	3	300	4
	Over 6	300	2	600	4
Dexedrine	Under 6	2.5	1	2.5	3
	Over 6	2.5	2	7.5	3
Diamox	Under 6	125	3	250	3
	Over 6	250	2	250	4
Dilantin†	Under 2	15	3	30	3
	2 to 4	30	2	50	4
	4 to 6	30	3	100	3
	Over 6	100	2	100	4
Gemonil	Under 6	50	3	100	3
	Over 6	100	3	200	3
Mebaral	Under 2	32	3	50	4
	2 to 4	32	4	82	3
	4 to 6	50	4	100	3
	Over 6	100	3	200	3
Mesantoin‡	Under 6	50	3	200	3
	Over 6	100	3	400	3
Milontin‡	Under 6	250	2	500	3
	Over 6	500	2	1000	4
Mysoline	Under 2	25	2	50	4
	2 to 4	50	3	125	4
	4 to 6	125	3	250	4
	Over 6	250	3	500	4
Paradione	Under 6	150	2	300	3
	Over 6	300	2	600	3
Peganone‡	Under 6	250	3	750	4
	Over 6	500	3	1000	4

TABLE 2. Average Dosages of Antiepileptic Drugs*—Continued

DRUG	AGE (Years)	STARTING DOSAGE Mg.	Times/Day	MAXIMAL DOSAGE Mg.	Times/Day
Phenobarbital	Under 2	16	3	32	3
	2 to 4	16	4	32	4
	4 to 6	32	3	48	3
	Over 6	32	4	65	3
Phenurone‡	Under 6	250	3	1000	3
	Over 6	500	3	2000	3
Tegretol§	Under 6	100	1	100	3
	6 to 12	100	2	100	4
	Over 12	100	3	200	4
Tridione	Under 6	150	2	300	3
	Over 6	300	2	600	3
Valium¶ **					
Zarontin	Under 6	250	2	250	4
	Over 6	250	3	500	4

* This table includes only the antiepileptic drugs used in our clinic.

|| The patient should receive a daily intramuscular injection of 25 to 30 units of corticotropin (Acthar Gel) for four to six weeks, depending upon seizure response. If complete control of seizures and normalization of the electroencephalogram are obtained, no further therapy is indicated unless there is a recurrence of clinical seizures.

If after six weeks of treatment with ACTH clinical control of seizures is attained but the electroencephalogram remains abnormal, steroid therapy (cortisone or prednisone) should be instituted and continued for a prolonged period in an attempt to normalize the electroencephalogram.

If there is no clinical response to six weeks of ACTH therapy, the patient may be given a trial of oral steroid therapy, administered daily for at least two months.

It is important that oral steroid therapy be discontinued gradually.

‡ The maximal dosages of these drugs for children over six years old exceeds manufacturers' recommendations.

† We only rarely prescribe Dilantin for infants.

§ Tegretol is available in 200-mg. tablets. Attention is directed to the package insert, which recommends that this drug be used for the pain associated with true trigeminal neuralgia. Our nine years' experience with Tegretol has demonstrated that it is an exceedingly effective agent for the control of epileptic seizures, particularly psychomotor (temporal lobe) seizures.

¶ The effective dosage of Valium varies considerably from patient to patient. In our clinic, we start treatment with this drug as follows: children under one year of age—1 mg. every 3 hours for five doses daily; young children—2 mg. every 3 hours for five doses daily; older children—5 mg. every 3 hours for five doses daily. The daily dosage is increased, if necessary, by one dosage per week, depending on clinical response and the patient's tolerance to the drug. The appearance of marked drowsiness indicates that the maximal tolerable dosage has been surpassed.

The maximal daily dosages we have employed are as follows: children under one year of age—15 mg.; young children—30 mg.; older children—50 mg.

** Manufacturer's precaution: Safety and efficacy of injectable Valium in children under 12 years of age have not been established. Oral Valium is not for use in children under six months of age.

often increases the frequency of petit mal spells, we give this drug as the major motor anticonvulsant only as a last choice.

It has been our experience that petit mal spells are occasionally controlled with phenobarbital and, obviously, in such instances this drug should be continued as the sole therapeutic agent.

After a satisfactory major motor anticonvulsant dosage schedule has been established, a specific antipetit mal agent should be added to the therapeutic regimen. Our antipetit mal drugs of choice are Zarontin and Tridione, respectively. The dosages of these drugs are presented in Table 2. If the petit mal seizures do not respond to these drugs, the physician has no alternative but to prescribe less effective antipetit mal medications (Table 1).

The combined medications should be continued in full dosage until the patient has been free of clinical petit mal episodes for at least four years and until an EEG examination performed after this period of freedom from attacks does not reveal the classic EEG discharge of petit mal epilepsy.

We withdraw the antipetit mal agent gradually over an interval of 6 to 12 months, depending on the amount of medication the patient had been taking. It is important that all patients receive the full dosage of the prophylactic major motor anticonvulsant until they reach 14 years of age, since in our experience the peak incidence of the development of major convulsions subsequent to petit mal epilepsy is from 10 through 13 years of age. We gradually withdraw the major motor anticonvulsant over the course of one year in those patients who have not developed major motor seizures by the time they reach 14 years of age.

Toxicity of Drugs. Treatment should be started with the drug which is known to be the least toxic. As noted in Table 1, our drugs of choice for the control of major motor seizures are phenobarbital, Mysoline and Dilantin, respectively. Each of these drugs possesses significant anticonvulsant properties and is of considerable value in controlling major motor (grand mal) seizures.

Our drug of first choice for major motor epilepsy is phenobarbital, because the toxic reactions associated with its use are singularly few. When this drug is properly administered, the only major side effects are drowsiness, which is usually dose-related, and hyperactivity simulating the hyperkinetic syndrome, which is not dose-related and is encountered primarily in young children. These reactions are not serious and both are reversible.

Dilantin is our third choice because of the large number of adverse reactions associated with its use. Some of these side reactions are frequent and disturbing, e.g., gingival hyperplasia; some are irreversible, e.g., hypertrichosis; others may be a threat to the patient's life and have, on occasion, terminated fatally, e.g., Stevens-Johnson syndrome, hepatitis with exfoliative dermatitis.

We believe that the use of Dilantin as the drug of first choice for the control of grand mal seizures is specifically contraindicated in infants, females (particularly adolescents) and children receiving orthodontic treatment.

Infants. The recognition of Dilantin intoxication due to overdosage is frequently exceedingly difficult in infants. Ataxia and/or diplopia are frequent signs that the maximal tolerable dosage of this drug has been surpassed. It is obvious that a 16-month-old child with grand mal epilepsy who is receiving Dilantin would be unable to describe diplopia to the physician. Also, if this child is just beginning to walk and shows unsteadiness of gait, one may have considerable difficulty in determining on clinical grounds whether the unsteadiness is a manifestation of Dilantin overdosage or merely a result of the child's not yet having mastered the walking technique.

Girls, Particularly Adolescents. It is needless to state that gingival hyperplasia and hypertrichosis are cosmetically unattractive in any person.

We have been called upon many times to change the antiepileptic regimen in persons who had been rendered seizure-free with Dilantin but in whom the drug produced marked gingival hyperplasia. These patients, mostly adolescent girls, stated that they would rather have seizures than suffer the embarrassment and emotional distress caused by the swollen gums. In addition, pronounced hyperplasia frequently causes displacement of the teeth, which is also esthetically objectionable and necessitates extensive orthodontic and periodontic procedures in many instances.

Hypertrichosis that is marked and occurs on exposed surfaces presents a very serious cosmetic problem, particularly in females. It has been our experience that the abnormal growth of hair persists in all patients after discontinuance of Dilantin.

Children Receiving Orthodontic Treatment. Many patients to whom Dilantin had been prescribed while they were undergoing orthodontic therapy have been referred to our clinic for regulation of their antiepileptic regimens. In most of these children, the gingival hyperplasia was so marked that it extended over the orthodontic appliances. These patients complained of a constant oral malodor and also of almost continually bleeding gums. Obviously, it was virtually impossible for these patients to keep their mouths free from residual food particles and other irritants that lodged between the hyperplastic tissues and the braces. The braces probably acted as an additional local irritant.

Management of Side Effects of Antiepileptic Drugs. *Drowsiness.* In our experience, drowsiness occurs with practically all antiepileptic agents when the dosage is increased to sufficiently high levels. However, this reaction is frequently encountered in patients receiving conventional dosages of Mesantoin, Mysoline and Paradione. The addition of stimulating drugs, such as Dexedrine or Ritalin,* to the therapeutic regimen is helpful in counteracting drowsiness in some patients.

Nystagmus, Diplopia and Disturbances of Equilibrium (Ataxia). These reactions are encountered most frequently with the hydantoinates, especially Dilantin. They are generally dose-related and can usually be alleviated or minimized by a reduction in the dosage.

* Manufacturer's precaution: Ritalin is not recommended in children under six years of age. The parenteral form is not recommended in children.

There is currently some controversy as to whether Dilantin causes irreversible cerebellar changes. We were the first to report the persistence of ataxia for prolonged periods of time (up to six months) following discontinuance of Dilantin therapy. Subsequent to our report, some evidence has been presented that Dilantin taken in high toxic dosage over an extended period of time produces histologic changes in the cerebellum of both animals and humans. In a series of investigations designed to determine whether irreversible cerebellar damage in man is due to Dilantin or to the seizures per se, Dam studied the cerebellum of pigs, monkeys and humans following Dilantin administration. He reported that the number of Purkinje cells in pigs and monkeys was the same in intoxicated animals as in controls. In the cerebellum of 32 patients with major motor epilepsy treated with various amounts of Dilantin, he did not find systematic change in the number of Purkinje cells as a function of the dose or the duration of treatment. However, when plotted as a function of the incidence of major motor seizures, patients with frequent attacks revealed fewer Purkinje cells than those with infrequent episodes. Dam concluded that Dilantin intoxication did not cause a loss of Purkinje cells in pigs or monkeys, nor was it responsible for the loss of Purkinje cells in patients with grand mal convulsions. It should also be borne in mind that investigators, such as Spielmeyer, described degeneration of Purkinje cells in epileptic patients many years before the anticonvulsant properties of Dilantin were discovered.

Our clinical experience and the results of postmortem examinations in our patients are in accord with Dam's findings, and we believe that irreversible cerebellar damage in patients treated with Dilantin is more likely related to the seizures than to the medication.

Hyperactivity. Although phenobarbital is generally considered a sedative, it causes hyperactivity in many patients, particularly young children. Hyperactivity indicates an idiosyncrasy to the drug and is not related to the dosage.

Gingival Hyperplasia. In our experience, this reaction occurs primarily in association with Dilantin. We have only occasionally encountered hyperplasia of the gums with the other hydantoinates (Mesantoin, Peganone). Dilantin-induced gingival hyperplasia occurs much more frequently in the younger person than in the adult. Based on observations made in our clinic, we estimate the incidence of this disturbance to be at least 40 per cent.

Gingival hypertrophy, in most patients, appears two to three months after the initial administration of the drug and reaches its maximal severity in 9 to 12 months. There is no relationship between the occurrence and severity of gingival hyperplasia and the Dilantin dosage or serum concentration.

Secondary inflammatory changes frequently occur in association with the primary hyperplasia induced by Dilantin. These secondary lesions can usually be eliminated or at least minimized by fastidious oral physiotherapy. Some physicians have stated that gingival hyperplasia caused by Dilantin can be eliminated by massaging the gingivae and maintaining meticulous oral hygiene. However, our experience, and also that reported by prominent dental specialists, is that *neither of these methods appreciably reduces the magnitude of the primary hyperplastic tissue.* It has also been our experience that the primary hyperplastic lesion remains essentially unaffected by reductions in the dosage of Dilantin.

Obviously, the best and most satisfactory treatment of the primary lesion would be withdrawal of the drug, following which the hyperplastic tissue disappears spontaneously in mild to moderate cases, usually within 3 to 12 months. However, in some patients with severe gingival hyperplasia, withdrawal of Dilantin results in a considerable, but not complete, regression of the gingivae to normal. Treatment in patients in whom discontinuance of Dilantin is not feasible consists of removal of the hyperplastic tissue by gingivectomy. The decision regarding this procedure must be individualized for each patient and depends on the magnitude of the hyperplastic tissue and its effect upon mastication, speech and esthetics. It must be noted that gingivectomy is not a final solution to the problem since, if the patient continues therapy with this drug, the gingival hyperplasia invariably recurs and progresses to its previous intensity, usually within six months. Therefore, repeated gingivectomies may be necessary in patients who must continue taking Dilantin.

Skin Rashes. A drug should be discontinued immediately at the first appearance of any type of cutaneous reaction. When this is done, it is important that the patient be protected with some other antiepileptic agent, since sudden withdrawal may precipitate a recurrence of seizures or major motor status.

Drug rashes, especially those associated with hydantoinates, are frequently accompanied by lymphadenopathy, fever and hematopoietic disturbances, particularly leukopenia.

If the rash is mild, the drug may be readministered after the cutaneous reaction has completely disappeared and there is no evidence of lymphadenopathy, fever or hematopoietic disturbance. Continued use of the drug in patients with purpuric rashes, exfoliative dermatitis and other serious skin reactions is inadvisable.

Blood, Liver and Kidney Disturbances. Periodic physical examinations and at least monthly blood, urine and liver function tests should be performed on all patients receiving drugs which are known to have adversely affected the hematopoietic, genitourinary and hepatic systems.

Complete blood cell counts should be performed on all patients receiving drugs such as Mesantoin, Paradione, Phenurone, Tegretol, Tridione and Zarontin before the institution of therapy and at least at monthly intervals thereafter. If no abnormalities occur within 12 months, the period between counts may be extended. It is our general policy to discontinue the drug in patients in whom the total white cell count drops below 3500, or in whom there is a definite percentage reduction in the neutrophils, or in whom the platelet count drops below 125,000. The drug may be readministered when the blood cell count returns to normal. In such cases, however, cell counts should be made twice a week for a month or so thereafter. The parents or the patient should be instructed to report immediately any sign or symptom of possible damage to the hematopoietic system, such as fever, sore throat, easy bruising, petechiae, ecchymosis or epistaxis.

Periodic urine examinations and kidney function tests, such as blood urea nitrogen determinations, should be performed on patients receiving drugs such as Tridione, Paradione and Phenurone.

Before the institution of therapy and at regular intervals thereafter, liver function tests should be performed on patients receiving drugs, such as Phenurone, that in some cases have adversely affected the hepatic system. The parents or the patient should be advised to report immediately to the physician the appearance of jaundice, dark urine, general malaise, fever, gastrointestinal upset or any other disturbance which may be indicative of hepatitis. Drugs such as Phenurone should be given with caution to any patient with a history of liver damage.

OTHER PRINCIPLES IN TREATMENT. *Treatment Should Begin with One Drug.* Other drugs should be prescribed, if necessary, only after the maximal tolerated dosage of the starting drug has failed to produce a satisfactory clinical response. If the maximal tolerated dosage of the first drug fails to control satisfactorily the seizures, but does reduce the frequency or severity, it should be continued at that same dosage and a second drug should be added to the therapeutic regimen. The dosage of the second drug should be increased as needed to tolerance. However, if the maximal tolerated dosage of the first drug fails to help the patient, it should be gradually withdrawn simultaneously with the administration of the second drug. If during the withdrawal of the first drug and the addition of the second drug a satisfactory combination of dosages of both drugs is found, the patient should continue with both drugs. Occasionally, it may be necessary to prescribe the maximal tolerated dosage of more than two drugs in order to obtain good control of seizures.

There are three principal reasons for instituting treatment of an epileptic patient with one drug: (1) Since there are only a few really good drugs available for the control of seizures, and since the dosage necessary to control epileptic seizures varies from patient to patient, the physician should give each drug a thorough trial before resorting to another drug. (2) If two drugs of completely different chemical structure were initially prescribed and the patient were to manifest some untoward reaction, such as drowsiness or a cutaneous eruption, the physician might have considerable difficulty in determining which of the two drugs was responsible for the unfavorable reaction. (3) If treatment is initiated with one anticonvulsant, the possibility of a drug interaction—whereby one therapeutic agent causes the abnormal metabolism (acceleration or impairment) of another—is precluded.

The Medication Should Be Taken Daily. Several investigators have advocated administering the total daily dosage of antiepileptic drugs, such as phenobarbital and Dilantin, in a single dose, preferably at bedtime. We are not convinced that the administration of antiepileptic medication in this manner is superior to or even as effective as when it is given in divided doses throughout the day, particularly in children. Moreover, Svensmark and Buchthal have demonstrated that the maintenance of constant serum concentrations of phenobarbital and Dilantin in children requires the administration of these drugs in divided doses throughout the day.

We cite two difficulties we have encountered in some of our patients who received the total daily dosage of their medication at bedtime: (1) some were so drowsy and sleepy that they were unable to perform their routine activities for the greater part of the following morning, and (2) others either forgot or neglected to take their medication at bedtime and experienced a recurrence of seizures the following afternoon or evening; the latter patients had received no antiepileptic medication for almost 48 hours.

We generally recommend that the total daily dose of anticonvulsant medication be administered in two to four equal portions throughout the course of the day at times which do not interfere with the patient's customary affairs, such as with meals, upon returning home from school and at bedtime.

The Dosage of Anticonvulsant Medication Varies from Patient to Patient. The proper dosage of antiepileptic medication for any patient is that which controls his seizures without producing untoward reactions which interfere with his general well-being. The average daily starting and maximal dosages of anticonvulsant drugs employed in our clinic are given in Table 2. Obviously, the ideal goal in the treatment of epilepsy is to attain complete control of seizures; however, the drug dosage necessary for complete control of seizures may, in some patients, produce unpleasant reactions, such as drowsiness, which are more of a handicap to the patient than are the seizures.

ANTICONVULSANT BLOOD LEVEL DETERMINATIONS. Clinical response is the most important criterion in titrating the dosage of antiepileptic medication. However, we have found blood level determinations to be very helpful in the management of most patients, and of inestimable value in those patients who do not respond to average or high doses or who manifest signs or symptoms of toxicity while receiving small or conventional dosages of anticonvulsant agents. Over the past 12 years, we have performed thousands of antiepileptic drug (phenobarbital and Dilantin) blood level determinations, and our experience has convinced us that this procedure represents one of the most, if not the most, significant advancements achieved in the management of the epileptic patient.

Our findings relative to phenobarbital and Dilantin blood level determinations indicate that there is a good relationship between the blood concentration and signs of intoxication, but that the correlation of the blood level to the drug dosage and seizure control is inconsistent, particularly with Dilantin. Our studies reveal that the usual therapeutic and tolerable blood serum levels of phenobarbital and Dilantin are, respectively, 10 to 30 micrograms per ml. (1 to 3 mg. per 100 ml.) and 10 to 25 micrograms per ml. (1 to 2.5 mg. per 100 ml.).

We have also observed that there is a more consistent relationship between the blood concentration and signs of intoxication in patients taking Dilantin than in those receiving phenobarbital. Our studies of Dilantin blood levels have demonstrated that most patients can tolerate concentrations below 25 micrograms per ml. However, in some patients, levels of 25 micrograms per ml. are associated with nystagmus, ataxia and diplopia; as the level exceeds 30 micrograms per ml., drowsiness and lethargy are encountered; extreme lethargy and sometimes comatose states are observed in association with levels above 50 micrograms per ml. Based on our investigations of phenobarbital blood concentrations, we have determined that generally a level not exceeding 30 micrograms per ml. is unassociated with toxic reactions; when the level approaches 50 micrograms per ml., the patient frequently becomes drowsy; levels above 70 micrograms per ml. are associated with marked drowsiness and in some instances with a comatose state.

Because of the lack of space, we shall limit our presentation of indications for antiepileptic drug blood level determinations to those that we have found to be not only exceedingly important but also pragmatic in the management of the patient with epilepsy:

1. To establish whether a patient is taking his medication as prescribed. In a large number of cases referred to us as "refractory," a blood level determination revealed either no anticonvulsant material in the blood or so low a concentration with respect to the prescribed dosage that we were convinced that the patients were taking their medication on an irregular basis or not at all. Subsequent to supervised drug administration, each of these patients presented satisfactory serum levels. Therefore, we recommend obtaining a blood level determination in every patient before assuming that any antiepileptic agent prescribed in maximum dosage is ineffective.

2. To establish more rapidly the optimal dosage of drugs, such as Dilantin, which do not consistently yield a predictable serum concentration in relation to a specific mg. per kilogram of body weight dosage.

3. To make precise adjustments in the dosage schedule of patients who manifest evidence of intoxication while receiving small or conventional doses of a drug. Signs of Dilantin overdosage are observed in some patients in association with small or average dosages, and this condition has been reported in the case

of congenital deficiency of the hepatic parahydroxylation enzyme system, liver disease, coexisting disease of the central nervous system, intercurrent infection, impairment of elimination mechanisms and interaction of drugs.

4. To determine the offending agent in a patient on a multiple drug program who presents evidence of drug intoxication (e.g., ataxia in a patient receiving Dilantin and Mysoline), and also to determine if the failure of a multiple drug regimen is due to drug interaction, whereby one medication is responsible for the accelerated metabolism of another.

5. To ensure the maintenance of theoretically adequate serum concentrations in patients who are receiving a drug for prophylactic purposes, e.g., in a patient with petit mal epilepsy who is taking phenobarbital to prevent the development of major motor seizures.

6. To investigate the possibility of drug toxicity in a patient who exhibits symptoms which may also be manifestations of another disorder, e.g., a neurodegenerative disease in a patient receiving Dilantin.

7. To investigate the feasibility of once-daily administration of drugs with long plasma half-lives, such as Dilantin, to patients in whom a daily divided dosage schedule is undesirable or absolutely unacceptable.

Several procedures, such as spectrophotometry, thin layer chromatography and gas-liquid chromatography, are available for the quantitative determination of anticonvulsant blood level concentrations. Gas-liquid chromatography, particularly the on-column methylation technique, appears to be the method of choice, since it is easier, less time consuming and less expensive than the other means of analysis. Kupferberg recently described a gas-liquid chromatographic procedure for the simultaneous determination of multiple anticonvulsant drug (Dilantin, Mysoline, phenobarbital) levels. The availability of gas-liquid chromatographic determinations is increasing rapidly, as evidenced by the fact that 69 laboratories in 44 cities in the United States were performing this examination in 1971.

The Medication Should Be Taken for a Prolonged Time. It is our general policy to continue antiepileptic medication in full dosage for at least four years after the last seizure. We do make exceptions to this general plan of duration of therapy, the principal one being that if the four-year period of freedom from seizures should coincide with the usual age at onset of puberty, the medication should be continued in full dosage throughout the adolescent period. This is particularly important in girls.

The Medication Should Be Discontinued Very Gradually. A sudden withdrawal of anticonvulsant medication, particularly phenobarbital, is a frequent cause of recurrence of seizures or grand mal status. Therefore, when the physician decides to withdraw anticonvulsant medication in a patient who has been rendered seizure-free, he should reduce the dosage of the medication very gradually.

The period necessary for complete withdrawal is governed by the severity of the patient's previous seizure state and also by the dosage of the medication that the patient has been taking. In patients who had a mild form of epilepsy that was controlled by an average dosage of medication, we generally withdraw the medication by a gradual reduction of the dosage over one to two years. In patients who had severe epilepsy and were taking large amounts of medication, we extend the period of withdrawal of medication to three or four years. It should be noted that we generally withdraw antipetit mal drugs over a period of 6 to 12 months, as previously described.

If there is a recurrence of seizures during or subsequent to withdrawal, the patient should be restarted immediately on the same dosage of medication that had previously controlled the seizures, and the physician should consider continuing this medication in full dosage for the rest of the patient's life.

It has been our experience, by and large, that the EEG has but little to offer relative to prognostic implications. In our clinic, we rarely, if ever, utilize information obtained from an EEG examination as a complete indicator of a patient's progress, except in petit mal epilepsy, in which there is almost invariably a direct relationship between the disappearance of the classic bilaterally synchronous spike-wave discharge and the control of clinical spells, and in myoclonic epilepsy of infancy (infantile spasms, minor motor epilepsy), in which we have noted the absence of the typical hypsarhythmic pattern concurrent with cessation of attacks in many patients.

Over the past 30 years, we have performed serial EEG examinations on thousands of epileptic patients, and exclusive of those with petit mal epilepsy and some with infantile myoclonic attacks, we have not observed a direct relationship between normalization of the EEG and clinical improvement in a significantly large number of our patients. In many, the EEG became more abnormal even though the patient had fewer or no seizures; in others, the EEG continued to reveal abnormalities despite the fact that the patient had remained free of seizures for a period of years. It should be noted that in many children the EEG tends to revert to normal during adolescence, regardless of their clinical progress.

We concur with the finding of Holowach and coworkers that the results of EEG examinations are not predictive of prognosis following termination of drug therapy, and also with their recommendation that "in most cases the existence of important electroencephalographic abnormalities, including clear-cut paroxysmal findings, need not interdict withdrawal of drug therapy in patients with well controlled epilepsy."

Anticonvulsant Drug Interactions. Dilantin is the anticonvulsant most frequently involved in the reported cases of drug interaction in humans, most of which described an impairment of metabolism presumably due to inhibition of hepatic microsomal enzyme systems. Conversely, evidence has been presented that phenobarbital, a potent inducer of liver microsomal enzyme activity, increases the rate of metabolism of Dilantin and diminishes its blood concentration and pharmacologic effects in both experimental animals and humans; however, the consensus at present, including our own opinion, is in agreement with Diamond and Buchanan, whose investigation, in which plasma assays were followed over a two-month controlled period, failed to demonstrate any stimulation of Dilantin metabolism by phenobarbital. We have not encountered acceleration of Dilantin metabolism with resultant pejoration of seizure control in any of the thousands of our patients who have taken Dilantin and phenobarbital simultaneously. It is of interest to note that some patients have presented an elevated Dilantin serum level in association with the administration of phenobarbital. Tegretol has been reported to cause a decline in the Dilantin blood concentration and plasma half-life in several patients, but our observations in a large number of patients receiving both of these drugs concomitantly did not reveal an adverse effect on seizure control.

The following drugs have been reported to inhibit Dilantin metabolism with resultant intoxication and/or elevation of plasma levels, and their use should be avoided, if possible, or scrupulously supervised in patients receiving Dilantin: Analexin (phenyramidol), no longer commercially available in the United States; Antabuse (disulfiram); Chloromycetin (chloramphenicol)*; Dicumarol (bishydroxycoumarin); isoniazid [isonicotinic acid hydrazide (INH)], alone or in combination with para-aminosalicylic acid (PAS); and Ospolot/Conadil (sulthiame), currently limited to investigational purposes in this country. We have prescribed sulthiame to a large group of patients receiving Dilantin, and have not observed signs of Dilantin intoxication or an adverse effect on seizure control in any case.

In addition, Butazolidin (phenylbutazone), Compazine (prochlorperazine), Darvon (propoxyphene),† Fluothane (halothane), Librium (chlordiazepoxide), Ritalin (methylphenidate), Sulfabid (sulfaphenazole), Thorazine (chlorpromazine),‡ Valium (diazepam) and Zarontin (ethosuximide) have also been reported to impair Dilantin metabolism, but the evidence for drug interaction resulting in an adverse clinical effect is generally lacking or so meager as to disallow the formation of definite conclusions. We have administered Compazine, Librium, Ritalin, Thorazine, Valium and Zarontin to hundreds of patients in conjunction with Dilantin therapy, and have not encountered clinical proof of altered Dilantin metabolism in any instance. Nevertheless, the physician should bear in mind that Dilantin intoxication may result from the concurrent administration of any of the previously cited drugs with Dilantin.

Isolated reports of Dilantin-induced acceleration of metabolism of Dicumarol and digitoxin have appeared in the literature. While the precise clinical significance of these drug interactions has not been established, the physician should be aware that therapeutic regimens consisting of Dilantin and Dicumarol and/or digitoxin may be potentially hazardous. We also direct attention to the case "with a nearly fatal outcome" reported by Viukari and Aho, in which a direct interaction of both digoxin and Dilantin on the membrane NaK–ATPase enzyme system resulted in catastrophic clinical consequences.

It has also been reported that Dilantin can stimulate the metabolism of endogenously produced steroids (e.g., cortisol) and those administered exogenously (e.g., dexamethasone, vitamin D) in humans.

The development of osteomalacia, rickets and hypocalcemia in epileptic patients has

* Manufacturer's precaution: Chloramphenicol is not recommended for intravenous or intramuscular pediatric use. Chloramphenicol sodium succinate has been approved for intravenous pediatric use.

† Manufacturer's precaution: Safety of propoxyphene in children has not been established.

‡ Manufacturer's precaution: Chlorpromazine is not recommended for children under six months of age except when lifesaving.

been attributed to the acceleration of vitamin D metabolism by anticonvulsant drugs, notably Dilantin, and is currently a topic of great interest and controversy. Although it is an attractive hypothesis, we do not believe that liver enzyme induction by anticonvulsant drugs with a resultant relative lack of vitamin D activity has been unequivocally proven in any of the published reports. Many other factors may have played a role in the development of the rachitic skeletal and chemical changes in the reported cases.

We have not encounterd chemical, clinical or radiologic evidence of rickets in any of the 22,000 patients seen and followed in our clinic since 1936, approximately 15,000 of whom were referred to us on an antiepileptic regimen that consisted of Dilantin, phenobarbital or Mysoline, taken singly or in combination in high dosage for prolonged periods of time. Attention is directed to the fact that part of the initial evaluation at our clinic has always included a skull roentgenogram series, a fasting glucose determination, serum urea nitrogen, calcium and phosphorus levels, liver function tests and, for the past three years, a Sequential Multiple Analysis 12. In view of our findings over many years, we hesitate to accept at this time the evidence so far presented in the literature that anticonvulsant drug therapy plays a significant role in the causation of the chemical and/or skeletal changes associated with rickets.

Since hundreds of thousands, and probably millions, of epileptic patients have been treated throughout the world for prolonged periods of time with an antiepileptic program consisting of Dilantin, phenobarbital and Mysoline in various combinations, it is incredible that, if anticonvulsant drug therapy were responsible for the reported rachitic bone and chemical changes, no such case, to our knowledge, had been described prior to that of Schmid in 1967. We believe that all one can opine, relative to the cases in which it was postulated that the antiepileptic medication was responsible for the chemical and radiographic evidence of rickets, is that the disease occurred coincidentally in patients receiving anticonvulsant drug therapy.

Dietary Treatment. The *ketogenic diet regimen* is an excellent form of therapy for patients with myoclonic seizures, and is also of value in major motor (grand mal) epilepsy. However, we have found it to be essentially ineffective in patients with petit mal or psychomotor epilepsy. The ketogenic diet is most effective in children between the ages of two and five years. Details relative to our methods of prescribing and managing the ketogenic diet regimen are presented in a previous publication.

A new ketogenic diet was introduced in 1971 by Huttenlocher and associates. Ketosis is usually achieved after a two-day fast, and is maintained by the administration of a diet containing 60 per cent of the total calculated caloric maintenance as *medium chain triglycerides (MCT).* The remainder of the caloric intake is given as 19 per cent carbohydrate, 10 per cent protein and 11 per cent dietary fat. We are currently evaluating a group of patients on this diet and our findings will be reported at a later date. Indications for using the MCT diet are similar to those for the standard ketogenic diet regimen.

Surgical Treatment. The primary treatment for a patient with an epileptic disorder is medical, consisting in anticonvulsant therapy, psychotherapy and social and occupational rehabilitation. It is worth emphasizing that medical treatment should be given an adequate trial in all cases of epilepsy and considered unsuccessful only when all appropriate therapeutic agents have been administered alone and in combination without beneficial results. Surgical investigation should be considered in patients who have not responded to medical therapy and are incapacitated by their seizure disorder. Obviously, if the seizures are symptomatic evidence of a progressive cerebral lesion, such as tumor, abscess or hematoma, surgery is the method of treatment.

Surgical excision of an epileptogenic focus does not terminate the treatment. It is only an intermediate stage, and medical therapy must be continued after the operation just as intensively as before. Anticonvulsant medication should be started as soon as the patient has regained consciousness, and continued until the patient has been free of seizures for at least four years.

The Socioeconomic Aspects of Epilepsy. This is a very important phase of the overall management of the epileptic patient and one that is very much neglected. It would be impossible to discuss adequately this exceedingly important subject here. However, the reader may refer to recent publications for details concerning problems such as education, automobile driving, employment and marriage.

BREATHHOLDING EPISODES

Breathholding episodes most often appear during the first two years of life, but rarely before six months of age. These attacks tend to disappear spontaneously after three or four years of age and rarely recur after six years of age.

The convulsive movements associated with breathholding episodes are almost always short and innocuous and require no immediate care. The administration of daily antiepileptic therapy, in our experience, is of no value in prevention of the recurrence of breathholding episodes. We have also had similar experience with the use of the tranquilizing drugs.

The treatment of breathholding attacks consists primarily in parent-child guidance and reassurance. We inform the parents of the harmlessness of the attacks, reassure them that their child does not have epilepsy and direct our treatment toward a solution of a parent-child conflict, if such a situation is apparent.

FEBRILE CONVULSIONS

There is a diversity of opinion regarding the diagnosis, treatment and prognosis of convulsions that occur in association with an elevation of temperature during early childhood.* We classify convulsions occurring in young children in association with fever, excluding, of course, convulsions that occur in children with a demonstrable intracranial infection, such as meningitis or encephalitis, or with diseases that adversely affect the central nervous system (rubeola, shigella gastroenteritis and others) or other disorders toxic to the brain, into either epileptic seizures precipitated by fever or simple febrile convulsions.

A diagnosis of an epileptic disorder in a child who suffers with seizures in association with an elevation of temperature is strongly indicated by the presence of one or more of the following findings: prolonged seizures, focal convulsions, febrile convulsions in a child over six years of age or specific electroencephalographic abnormalities. *We recommend that this group be treated with daily antiepileptic medication in the same manner as patients with epileptic seizures unassociated with fever.*

We make a diagnosis of a simple febrile convulsive disorder in children who present the following: generalized seizures of brief duration, seldom lasting longer than five minutes, occurring soon after an elevation of temperature; no clinical or laboratory evidence of an infection of the brain; and a normal electroencephalogram after the patient has been afebrile for a week or so. We believe that the exceedingly high familial incidence of simple febrile convulsions can be used as an additional, supportive criterion in categorizing febrile convulsions and also in prognosticating the outcome in young children who have convulsions in association with an elevation of temperature.

Simple febrile convulsions usually appear initially between 9 and 15 months of age; they seldom occur in infants under six months and rarely begin after five years of age. They are almost always associated with an extracranial infection, such as tonsillitis or otitis media.

The treatment of an isolated simple febrile convulsion does not require special consideration, since the seizure is so brief that it would be terminated before any therapeutic measure could be instituted.

Phenobarbital and aspirin may be prescribed at the first signs of an infection and continued for at least 24 hours thereafter. This sort of therapy, however, is generally of no avail, since the convulsion is frequently one of the first manifestations of the febrile disorder. On the other hand, this therapy may serve some useful purpose, because it provides the parents with "something to do" and may relieve some of their anxiety.

It has been our experience that the administration of daily anticonvulsant medication is generally ineffective in preventing the recurrence of simple febrile convulsions. We believe that when the physician is confronted with a child who has experienced his first simple febrile convulsion, he should advise the parents of the good prognosis. We do not believe, however, that he can be completely dogmatic and tell the parents that there is absolutely no chance of epilepsy developing later in life. We recommend that these patients be observed periodically by the physician. If the patient should have a recurrence of seizures other than that typical of simple febrile convulsions, or if the convulsions should recur more frequently than four times a year or after six years of age, or if subsequent electroencephalographic examinations reveal electrical aberrations diagnostic of epilepsy, the physician should change the diagnosis to that of an epileptic disorder and treat the patient accordingly.

PROLONGED SEIZURE ACTIVITY OF EPILEPTIC ORIGIN

In our clinic, we employ the term prolonged seizure activity to designate epileptic manifestations of long duration, as follows: (1) status epilepticus, including major motor (grand mal) status, myoclonic status, petit mal status and prolonged psychomotor seizure, and (2) prolonged major motor (grand mal) seizure.

* The following evaluation and recommendations regarding the diagnosis, prognosis and treatment of febrile convulsions are based on the findings of three separate investigations conducted during the past 40 years at The Johns Hopkins Hospital Epilepsy Clinic.

When the physician is confronted with a patient with a prolonged major seizure or major motor status, he should direct his treatment toward two goals: the general care of the patient and the administration of anticonvulsant therapy to terminate the seizure. If the patient had been treated earlier for the convulsive episode, the physician should consider the nature and dosage of the previous therapy so that he does not prescribe unduly large dosages of the same medication or of drugs of similar chemical structure.

When a physician is called on to administer immediate therapy to a child in an active convulsion, the past history may supply pertinent information relative to the type of therapy which should be used at that time. In those instances where there is a history of previous convulsive episodes, it is reasonable to assume that the current seizure will follow the same pattern as did the previous ones. On the other hand, in those patients for whom there is no previous history of seizures, it is obvious that it would be impossible for the physician to have any idea regarding the precise nature of the seizure in question, i.e., whether it is more likely one of a prolonged convulsion or the beginning of major motor status. In such instances, he should treat the seizure state as a prolonged convulsion.

In the case of a physician called to treat a patient who is suffering with major motor (grand mal) status, but who is in an unconscious interseizure state at the time the physician arrives, we emphasize that although the patient had experienced seizures just previously, the physician should administer general care and not antiepileptic drugs at this time.

General Care of the Patient. This aspect is exceedingly important and is one that is frequently neglected. The patient should be allowed to remain, if possible, at the place where the seizure occurred until the active spell has subsided. The patient should be placed in such a position that he cannot hurt himself by knocking his body against hard objects.

Tight clothing, especially around the neck, should be loosened or removed.

If the seizure occurs while the patient is in bed, he should be observed so that he does not fall to the floor. Such falls can also be prevented by placing protective guard-rails or boards on the sides of the bed. All pillows should be removed from the bed. There are reports of patients who presumably died of suffocation caused by the head being buried in a soft pillow or mattress.

If possible, the patient should be kept on his side so that mucus and saliva will flow more freely from the mouth. Since patients are unable to swallow during convulsive episodes, mucus or saliva may flow down into the lungs and cause respiratory distress; therefore the patient should not be placed or be permitted to lie flat on his back for any length of time. Another reason it is important to keep the patient on his side rather than on his back is that vomiting sometimes occurs during a seizure; if a patient were on his side, the vomitus would more likely be expelled from the mouth than flow into the lungs. Occasionally food or vomitus may so choke the air passages that suction becomes necessary. If anoxia becomes apparent, as often happens in greatly prolonged or frequently repeated convulsions, oxygen should be administered by inhalation.

We would like to emphasize that, in most instances, placing an object between the teeth of a patient having a seizure is an unnecessary procedure and sometimes can do more harm than good. Nevertheless, this procedure should be carried out in patients who bite their tongue or cheeks or show evidence of respiratory difficulty. Any firm, blunt, nondamaging object of the right size and not too hard, such as a padded tongue depressor, a folded leather belt or a leather glove, can be inserted between the patient's teeth. Extreme care should be taken when any object is inserted into the mouth of a patient with carious teeth because such teeth are easily broken and can cause respiratory difficulties if aspirated.

As with any other unconscious patient, it is necessary to maintain fluid intake. Catheterization may be necessary if the patient does not void spontaneously. Hyperthermia, if present, should be dealt with appropriately.

Prolonged Major Motor (Grand Mal) Seizure. Administer Valium intravenously slowly over a period of two minutes in a dosage not exceeding 10 mg. If the convulsion does not stop within five minutes after the administration, we administer paraldehyde by intramuscular injection in a dosage of 1 ml. per year of age. The total dosage of paraldehyde should not exceed 5 ml., regardless of the age of the patient. (See Table 2 for precautions on use of Valium.)

If the convulsion continues, the intravenous Valium injection should be repeated 20 to 30 minutes after the administration of paraldehyde, and if the convulsion is not terminated within five minutes, the intramuscular injection of paraldehyde should be repeated.

If the convulsion persists despite the administration of Valium and paraldehyde, intravenous barbiturates, such as phenobarbital sodium or Amytal sodium, may be administered 30 minutes after the second injection of paraldehyde. If the convulsion still continues, the administration of thiopental sodium or ether by an anesthesiologist should be considered.

Most seizures can be terminated almost immediately by the intravenous injection of the quicker-acting barbiturates. We prefer, however, to initiate treatment with Valium and paraldehyde, since the barbiturates, particularly the quicker-acting ones, when administered by the intravenous route, sometimes cause acute respiratory depression and even death. The quicker-acting barbiturates should be administered intravenously only under hospital conditions where oxygen therapy and other means of resuscitation are readily available.

It should be noted that although the administration of intravenous Valium is designated by most investigators as being relatively free of serious side effects, and we also have not encountered serious toxic effects, we are aware of serious cardiopulmonary side reactions; two occurred in adults who died of cardiac arrest, and six were in children who suffered severe respiratory depression that necessitated emergency therapeutic measures. In several of these cases, there is a question of whether Valium was solely responsible for the adverse reaction.

Major Motor (Grand Mal) Status. The principal aspect of the treatment of major motor status is the general care of the patient, since if this condition persists, the patient may sink deeper and deeper into a coma and become dehydrated and exhausted, and death may ensue.

Our current method for the immediate treatment of major motor status is initially to administer Valium intravenously slowly over two minutes in a dose not exceeding 10 mg., immediately followed by the subcutaneous injection of phenobarbital in a dose of 65 mg. per year of age, but not exceeding a total dose of 325 mg. regardless of the age of the patient. (See Table 2 for precautions on use of Valium.) The phenobarbital is administered not for the purpose of controlling the convulsive reaction in progress, but as prophylaxis against the occurrence of subsequent active seizure phases of the grand mal status episode.

Intravenous Valium may be repeated in 20 to 30 minutes after its initial administration, if necessary. If the convulsions do not stop within five minutes after the second injection of Valium, we then administer paraldehyde intramuscularly in a dose of 1 ml. per year of age, but not exceeding a total dose of 5 ml., regardless of the age of the patient. If the seizures are not controlled, the same dose of paraldehyde may be repeated, but not sooner than one hour.

Beginning six hours after the initial subcutaneous injection of phenobarbital, we administer the maximal daily dose of phenobarbital recommended in Table 2 and continue with this dose thereafter, depending on the patient's tolerance and seizure control. The medication should be given orally, if possible; otherwise, it should be given subcutaneously.

When possible, we recommend that blood barbiturate levels be determined daily to make sure that tolerable levels are not exceeded. Information relative to therapeutic and toxic blood concentrations of phenobarbital is presented in the section of this chapter entitled anticonvulsant blood level determinations (p. 85).

Much more harm can be done to a patient with major motor status, particularly when treated with the longer-acting barbiturates, by overtreating than by undertreating. Patients with major motor status frequently go into a deep comatose state, which could be worsened by the depression of the central nervous system caused by the cumulative effect of frequent injections of large doses of barbiturates.

Mention has been made in the literature of a possible synergistic action of Valium and barbiturates. We have administered Valium and phenobarbital concomitantly to many children and have not encountered evidence of a synergistic relationship, nor did Calderon-Gonzalez and Mireles-Gonzalez observe serious complications in children who had received significant amounts of phenobarbital just prior to or in immediate association with the intravenous administration of Valium.

Myoclonic Status. The most effective drug for the control of myoclonic status is Valium administered intravenously slowly over 2 minutes in a dose not exceeding 10 mg. This dose may be repeated in 20 to 30 minutes, if necessary.

Petit Mal Status and Prolonged Psychomotor Seizure. These forms of prolonged seizure activity are, in our experience, generally refractory to antiepileptic medication. Both petit mal status and prolonged psychomotor seizures are usually self-limited. It is important that patients with these disorders be kept under close surveillance to prevent them from doing harm during the attacks.

References

Berman, W.: Dietary Treatment of Epilepsy. *Pediat. Annals* (in press).

Buchanan, R. A., Kinkel, A. W., Goulet, J. R., and Smith, T. C.: The Metabolism of Diphenylhydantoin (Dilantin) Following Once-Daily Administration. *Neurology,* 22:126, 1972.

Calderon-Gonzales, R., and Mireles-Gonzales, A.: Management of Prolonged Motor Seizure Activity in Children. *J.A.M.A.,* 204:544, 1968.

Dam, M.: Diphenylhydantoin: Neurologic Aspects of Toxicity; in D. M. Woodbury, J. K. Penry and R. P. Schmidt (eds.): *Antiepileptic Drugs.* New York, Raven Press, 1972.

Diamond, W. D., and Buchanan, R. A.: A Clinical Study of the Effect of Phenobarbital on Diphenylhydantoin Plasma Levels. *J. Clin. Pharmacol.* 10:306, 1970.

Holowach, J., Thurston, D. L., and O'Leary, J.: Prognosis in Childhood Epilepsy: Follow-up Study of 148 Cases in which Therapy had been Suspended after Prolonged Anticonvulsant Control. *New England J. Med.,* 286:169, 1972.

Huttenlocher, P. R., Wilbourn, A. J., and Signore, B. S.: Medium-chain Triglycerides as a Therapy for Intractable Childhood Epilepsy. *Neurology,* 21:1097, 1971.

Kupferberg, H. J.: Quantitative Estimation of Diphenylhydantoin, Primidone and Phenobarbital in Plasma by Gas-Liquid Chromatography. *Clin. Chim. Acta,* 29:283, 1970.

Kutt, H.: Diphenylhydantoin: Interactions with Other Drugs in Man; in D. M. Woodbury, J. K. Penry and R. P. Schmidt (eds.): *Antiepileptic Drugs.* New York, Raven Press, 1972.

Livingston, S.: Treatment of Grand Mal Epilepsy; Phenobarbital versus Diphenylhydantoin Sodium. *Clin. Pediat.,* 7:444, 1968.

Livingston, S.: Breathholding Spells in Children: Differentiation from Epileptic Attacks. *J.A.M.A.,* 212: 2231, 1970.

Livingston, S.: Management and Prognosis of Febrile Convulsions in Children; in S. Spitzer and W. W. Oaks (eds.): *Emergency Medical Management.* New York, Grune & Stratton, Inc., 1971.

Livingston, S.: *Comprehensive Management of Epilepsy in Infancy, Childhood and Adolescence.* Springfield, Illinois, Charles C Thomas, Publisher, 1972.

Livingston, S., and Livingston, H. L.: Cutaneous Reactions of Antiepileptic Drugs. *Hosp. Med.* (in press).

Livingston, S., and Livingston, H. L.: Gingival Hyperplasia: Be Ready for this Drug-Induced Problem. *Consultant* (in press).

Schmid, F.: Osteopathien bei antiepileptischer Dauerbehandlung. *Fortschr. Med.,* 85:381, 1967.

Svensmark, O., and Buchthal, F.: Diphenylhydantoin and Phenobarbital: Serum Levels in Children. *Am. J. Dis. Child.,* 108:82, 1964.

Viukari, N. M. A., and Aho, K.: Digoxin-Phenytoin Interaction. *Brit. Med. J.* 2:51, 1970.

Hypsarhythmia and Infantile Spasms

EDWARD F. RABE, M.D.

This syndrome consists of an electroencephalographic abnormality (hypsarhythmia) and a bizarre seizure called infantile spasm, consisting of lightning generalized flexion or extension myoclonic jerks. The EEG abnormality consists of multiple asynchronous very high voltage spikes, occurring at some time in every lead, interspersed with recurrent, usually asynchronous high voltage slow waves at 1½ to 3 cycles per second interrupted occasionally by sudden decreases in voltage to almost isoelectric levels lasting 1 to 2 seconds. The abnormality is most marked in sleep. Thus, all comparisons of serial tracings should be made during sleep.

This seizure type responds most consistently to steroid or to adrenocorticotropic hormone (ACTH) and variably, if at all, to benzodiazepines, barbiturates or hydantoins. As soon as the diagnosis is established, ACTH is given intramuscularly in a daily dose of 40 units. Because 55 per cent of infants with this syndrome develop other types of seizures or have them concomitantly, phenobarbital tablets are given in a total daily dose of 6 mg. per kilogram, divided into two doses. The aims of ACTH therapy are to obliterate the peculiar irritability seen initially in the syndrome, to control seizures, to return the EEG to normal and to accelerate global development to a normal rate. Each of these parameters should be monitored at closely spaced intervals, and then at longer intervals as improvement is noted.

Disappearance of the initial irritability occurs within 48 hours of onset of treatment. Within 7 to 10 days, a decrease in the number of seizures will be noted, and the EEG, in approximately 40 per cent of cases, will show a decrease in the frequency of asynchronous spikes and high voltage slow waves as well as an increase in the amount of normal rhythm for age and state of consciousness. The infant will become more alert. When these events are noted, the intramuscular ACTH dose is changed to 80 units every other day. The patient is then followed at two-week intervals and then at monthly intervals. When a plateau of changes is reached in serial EEGs, frequency of seizures and global performance (similar events at three observations over two months), the

ACTH is gradually decreased at two-month intervals by 20 units per dose. The change at 20 units every other day is to 10 units every other day, three times a week, for one month; then 5 units every two days, three times a week, for one month; and then the medication is discontinued. During this time, phenobarbital is continued and if another seizure type intervenes and the EEG changes (for example, to a focal or hemispheric spike), appropriate conventional anticonvulsant therapy is instituted.

If during the period of reduction of ACTH, the previous improvement is reversed (i.e., massive myoclonic jerks recur or increase in number, and/or the EEG pattern regresses and/or irritability and obtundation recur), the ACTH dose is immediately increased to 80 units every other day and continued at this level until a performance plateau is reached as described above, and again the ACTH is systematically lowered.

Expectations for therapeutic results are affected by several important factors. The syndrome is primarily the response of the infantile brain to many known and some unknown events. Thus, the cases are divided into idiopathic and symptomatic ones. Furthermore, since the syndrome usually begins between three and six months of age, one can reliably determine if the global performance is significantly retarded or only mildly or questionably retarded at the onset of the symptoms. In idiopathic, symptomatic, severely or mildly retarded patients, ACTH therapy causes a reduction or obliteration of seizures, a rapid change in the EEG to normal or to another distinct abnormality and disappearance of irritability. On the other hand, symptomatic severely retarded infants cannot be induced to develop normally with ACTH therapy. Mildly or questionably retarded idiopathic or symptomatic patients usually attain a normal level of performance if ACTH therapy is given within six weeks of onset of symptoms.

It has been stated that this syndrome should be regarded as a medical emergency with diagnosis and treatment occurring as early as possible. Early versus late therapy does not seem to affect the outcome of the severely retarded symptomatic cases. It is unclear whether early as opposed to late treatment differentially affects the mildly or questionably retarded patients. Until this is clearly known, this syndrome, in general, should be treated as a medical emergency.

With increased sensitivity to seek these cases, physicians are bound to see variations of the syndrome which need to be commented upon. Massive myoclonic jerks with normal neurologic performance and normal EEGs occur, and such patients need no therapy since the condition has an excellent prognosis. Hypsarhythmia without infantile spasms but with other seizure forms occurs. It has a worse prognosis than hypsarhythmia with infantile spasms. The effect upon the global development of ACTH and steroids in hypsarhythmia without infantile spasms is not clearly defined, but until data on this subject appear, these patients should be treated in the same manner as those with hypsarhythmia and infantile spasms.

Spasmus Nutans

JEROME S. HALLER, M.D.

The clinical entity of spasmus nutans, consisting of head nodding, nystagmus and head tilt, is considered a benign and relatively transient disorder of young children without residua. In spite of recent attempts to classify it as an inherent brainstem dysfunction, and of past attempts to incriminate inadequate ambient light, nutrition and parental stimulation, the disorder remains etiologically unclassified.

Because the symptomatology might express more serious disorders, the physician must exclude diseases or anomalies of the eye and visual system and of the brainstem-cerebellar pathways. Thus, one should demonstrate normal vision, normal-appearing retinae and full conjugate eye movements, the absence of signs of other cranial nerve or cerebellar dysfunction and the absence of signs of pyramidal tract involvement.

With the relative assurance of a disease-free state, the best mode of therapy is "tincture of time."

Headaches and Migraine

ARNOLD P. FRIEDMAN, M.D.

Chronic recurring headaches in children, as in adults, fall into two broad diagnostic categories. The first group presents characteristics so commonly together that they can be diagnosed primarily on the basis of the patient's history, as in migraine and muscle-contraction ("tension") headache. In the second group, diagnosis is based primarily on associated physical and laboratory findings rather than on history. These include headaches associated with intracranial disorders, systemic disease and more localized disorders, such as nephritis or pulmonary disease, as well as emotional disturbances or trying environmental or life situations. Treatment of this latter group is primarily directed toward the underlying disorder. This may entail operative therapy, chemotherapy, removal of offending allergic factors or formal psychotherapy. The associated headache is generally of secondary importance and can usually be alleviated or minimized by analgesics.

The most common types of chronic recurrent headache are the vascular headache of the migraine type and muscle-contraction or tension headache.

MIGRAINE HEADACHE

Migraine is polysymptomatic in nature and is characterized clinically by periods of increased and decreased activity. The principal features of the migraine attack are not always pain. Ophthalmologic, sensory, motor or mental symptoms may be prominent, with or without headache. In early childhood, motion sickness and cyclical vomiting may frequently be present. A family history of migraine is present in approximately 65 per cent of patients with migraine. There are no reliable figures as to the frequency of migraine in children. In Sweden, studies of headaches in children indicated that 3.9 per cent had classic migraine, which represents only about 10 per cent of the total migraine population.

As a broad generalization, vascular headaches of the migraine type are recurrent attacks of pain in the head, commonly unilateral in onset and usually associated with anorexia and sometimes nausea and vomiting. In some patients they are preceded by or associated with sensory, motor and mood disturbances. However, there are an infinite variety of migraine attacks which may occur in many complex patterns and settings.

In *classic migraine,* the prodromes usually are sharply defined neurologic manifestations of a visual, sensory or motor nature, or a combination of these.

The prodromes of *common migraine* are not sharply defined and may precede the attack by several hours or days. They include psychic disturbances, gastrointestinal manifestations and changes in fluid balance. The actual headache episode is frequently longer than in the classic type, lasting from many hours to days.

Cluster headache occurs in a series of closely spaced attacks which may be followed by remissions of months or even years. In cluster migraine the onset is sudden; it frequently occurs nocturnally, each attack lasting 20 to 90 minutes, and associated symptoms are a prominent feature of the attack. These include conjunctival injection, lacrimation, nasal congestion and a Horner's syndrome which occurs on the same side as the headache in about 20 per cent of patients. This type is rare in childhood.

Hemiplegic and ophthalmoplegic migraine is a rare type, but one that usually begins in childhood or young adulthood. The pain is moderate, ipsilateral and accompanied by extraocular muscle palsies involving the 3rd cranial nerve (internal and external ophthalmoplegia) and other oculomotor nerves. Often the paralysis becomes evident as the intensity of the headache diminishes, usually three to five days after onset of a persisting headache.

The hemiplegic migraine complex is characterized by neurologic deficits, hemiparesis or hemiplegia. The neurologic phenomena of both types may persist for some time after subsidence of the headache. The 3rd cranial nerve may be permanently injured if the attacks of ophthalmoplegic migraine are frequent.

Another type of migraine called *basilar artery migraine* has been reported by Bickerstaff. Its prodromal symptoms include visual loss and a variety of brainstem symptoms, including vertigo, ataxia, dysarthria, and paresthesias, followed by severe throbbing occipital headaches with vomiting. This type of migraine occurs in young women and girls, and often has a striking relation to menstruation.

A migraine patient may have the attacks replaced by periodic episodes of other bodily disturbances called "migraine equivalents." These are presumed to be related directly or indirectly in mechanism to migraine itself, and may include abdominal pain associated with nausea, vomiting and diarrhea (abdominal migraine); pain localized in the thorax, pelvis or extremities; bouts of fever; attacks of tachycardia, including paroxysmal auricular tachycardia; benign paroxysmal vertigo; and cyclical edema. Psychic disturbances, including confusion, lethargy and disorders of sleep, mood and behavior, have been reported as psychic equivalents of migraine.

The patient susceptible to migraine has been described as tense, meticulous and obsessional in nature. Many have these characteristics, but there are no published control group studies of similar age, sex, social and economic background. The significance of these factors in the migraine patient has been overemphasized and is still open to question. It must be emphasized that stress in itself does not necessarily precipitate migraine but rather, the significance of the stressful event.

On occasion, nonspecific stimuli not necessarily stressful for the average person can produce a migraine attack. These include fatigue, bright or flickering lights, a mild hypoglycemic state (missing a meal stimulates production of noradrenalin and other biochemical changes), ingestion of food products containing tyramine or monosodium glutamate, exposure to high altitudes, meteorologic changes, drugs, chemical agents, and factors which change the endocrinal hormonal balance during the menstrual cycle.

The clinical course of childhood migraine is somewhat similar to that of adults. However, careful questioning of the child and the parents will reveal differences from the adult pattern. Often the attacks are less severe and of shorter duration; nausea, vomiting and abdominal complaints may be more prominent than the headache itself; the prodromes are shorter, with visual aura most prominent in classic migraine.

The taking of a detailed history is most important; it establishes contact with the child, indicates the probable diagnosis and provides essential information. The physical examination (neurologic and medical) should be thorough and should include blood tests, urinalysis, electroencephalography and psychologic tests. The results may confirm the first impressions or may suggest the need for further study. Interviews with at least one parent are valuable, since this is often a source of pertinent information. These procedures supply the basis for institution of treatment and of preventive measures.

Treatment is twofold: symptomatic, i.e., pharmacologic, and prophylactic, with the main emphasis on an adequate psychologic and social adjustment in the child, necessarily starting with an understanding by the parents of their role in the problem.

Symptomatic Treatment. Drugs for a migraine attack should be used only when need has been definitely established. For many of the drugs currently used in the treatment of migraine, data on optimal permissible dosages for children are inadequate. Caution is therefore essential in prescribing drugs for chronic recurrent headache. Each drug and each child must be considered individually. Table 1 may be used as a guide for therapy.

Ergotamine tartrate, the drug of choice for migraine in adults, is contraindicated in younger children, and must be used with caution in older ones. In most children a simple non-narcotic analgesic (acetysalicylic acid), alone or with a sedative (amobarbital), will control the headache attacks. If nausea or abdominal pain is prominent, addition of an antiemetic–trimethobenzamide (Tigan) * or chlorpromazine (Thorazine)–and an antispasmodic (atropine) is advisable. However, the phenothiazine derivatives tend to induce extrapyramidal stimulation, and this must be kept in mind. A tranquil environment is of therapeutic value, and the need

* Manufacturer's precaution: The injectable form of trimethobenzamide (Tigan) is not recommended for children.

TABLE 1. Drugs Used in Symptomatic Treatment of Headache and Migraine*

DRUG	USED AS	DOSAGE	COMMENTS
Acetylsalicylic acid	Analgesic	60 mg. per year of age up to 600 mg.	Repeat at 6-hour intervals
Amobarbital	Sedative	16 mg. (less than 5 years) 32 mg. (5 years)	
Trimethobenzamide†	Antiemetic	150 mg. (2–8 years; 30–60 pounds) 200 mg. (8–12 years; 60–90 pounds) 250 mg. (over 12 years; over 90 pounds)	3 to 4 times a day
Chlorpromazine	Antiemetic	10 mg. (less than 5 years)‡ 10–25 mg. (5–10 years) 25 mg. (after 10 years)	Repeat at 4- to 6-hour intervals Repeat at 4- to 6-hour intervals Repeat at 4- to 6-hour intervals
Atropine	Antispasmodic	0.2 mg. (less than 5 years) 0.3 mg. (5–10 years) 0.5 mg. (after 10 years)	
Ergotamine tartrate	Vasoconstrictor	1 mg.	1 mg. (2 mg. in adolescents) is the maximal dose for any one attack. Contraindicated in younger children

* The author gratefully acknowledges the assistance of Dr. Arnold Gold in preparing the drug dosage.

† Manufacturer's precaution: The injectable form of trimethobenzamide (Tigan) is not recommended for children.

‡ This dosage is slightly larger than manufacturer's recommendations; administration to children less than six months of age is contraindicated except in life-threatening situations.

for it should be impressed on parents. The aim of treatment should be so directed that the child maintains his usual environmental relations. In some children, ergotamine tartrate, combined with 50 mg. (9.75 grain) of caffeine and an antiemetic for nausea and vomiting, may have to be used to interrupt an attack of migraine; even rectal administration may occasionally be necessary but should not be used indiscriminately because of its psychologic connotations. It is of great importance that the drug or drugs be given early in the course of an attack (prodromal period) and in adequate dosage.

Prophylactic Treatment. The results of drugs in the prophylaxis of migraine have been notably unrewarding. Diphenylhydantoin sodium (Dilantin) is worth a trial in the small number of children whose family history is heavily weighted with migraine or epilepsy, or both, and whose electroencephalogram is abnormal, with spiked patterns. The dose range of diphenylhydantoin is 9 mg. per kilogram of body weight per day, administered in capsules. Usually the initial symptoms of Dilantin overdosage are disturbed equilibrium or diplopia, or both. Vomiting may occur, most frequently when Dilantin is taken "on an empty stomach," particularly before breakfast. In many cases this reaction can be controlled if the drug is taken during or immediately after meals.

Methysergide, a serotonin antagonist, has been found to be effective in reducing the number and severity of headaches in adults. However, its use in children is not advised because of possible side effects.

An infrequent precipitant of migraine is sensitivity to an allergen. In such cases, the allergen should be eliminated, or the child desensitized.

Adequate relaxation, improved sleeping habits and correction of any existing physiologic abnormalities help to reduce the frequency of attacks.

Psychotherapy is the preferred form of prophylactic treatment. It is of paramount importance to orient the parents to the child's problems, as well as to their relation to the problem. Parents should be helped to understand some of the precipitating circumstances of their child's headache and the importance of avoiding any overt anxiety. Their warm and realistic attitude is equally important. In fact, the familial incidence of migraine may in part be due to this factor of exposure, rather than to heredity. Possible conflict-inducing relations in the home, school and social environment should be explored with skill and tactful probing, both with the child and the parents. An adequate picture of the child's significant personal relations and the manner in which these have influenced and contributed to his headache problem will provide the framework for further treatment. It should be made clear to the child that the migraine attacks do not indicate a serious disease, and the importance of incapacities produced by the headache should be minimized. Except when the headaches are incapacitating, the child should attend school and social functions and not limit his activities.

When parents learn that others are faced with the same problem, they tend to feel less isolated and guilty. As they become able to talk about their feelings for their children and about their own headaches and those of their child, they will become increasingly willing to change their attitudes. The parents must be led to realize the importance of playing down the manifestations of their own headaches in the child's presence; it is one of the most significant aspects of prophylactic therapy.

The goals of treatment will depend on the frequency, duration and severity of the headache, as well as on the associated personality disturbance. More intensive psychotherapy will be necessary for children in whom neurotic symptoms are outstanding or headaches are frequent and overwhelming. In many instances, one or both parents may also need psychotherapy.

MUSCLE-CONTRACTION HEADACHES

Tension headaches (muscle-contraction headache) may occur in children and young adults. These headaches are produced by prolonged tension in which sustained contraction of the muscles of the scalp and neck occurs. Tension headaches are characterized by a steady dull discomfort or tightness varying widely in intensity and frequency. They may be localized to the back of the head and neck or to the frontal area, or cover the entire head. Treatment is primarily directed toward relieving and understanding the situational and environmental stress that produces the tension. Drugs should be used sparingly and limited to the nonnarcotic analgesics for the severe type of tension headache.

Acute Idiopathic Polyneuritis and Chronic Relapsing Polyneuropathy

DARRYL C. DEVIVO, M.D.

Three assumptions are helpful in discussing the management of children with the acute and chronic forms of idiopathic polyneuritis: (1) Other forms of polyneuropathy have been appropriately excluded, including those conditions derived from toxins, deficiency states, predisposing immunologic disturbances, identifiable infections and underlying endocrine, metabolic or heredofamilial diseases. (2) The clinical picture is consistent with the diagnosis in question: that is, the findings generally ascend symmetrically, are mainly motor with variable sensory involvement and are associated with areflexia; the CSF examination shows an elevated protein content after the first day or so, usually with little or no cellular response; and the nerve pathology demonstrates perivenular inflammatory infiltrates and segmental demyelination in the acute-subacute process and hypertrophy of peripheral nerve with "onion-bulb" formation in the chronic processes. (3) The chronically progressive or relapsing forms of polyneuropathy are in part derived from acute idiopathic polyneuritis (Landry-Guillain-Barré syndrome).

Management of acute polyneuritis is facilitated by an understanding of the temporal profile of the illness. A minor febrile illness involving the respiratory or gastrointestinal system is an identifiable harbinger in 50 per cent or more of the cases. One to three weeks later weakness appears and evolves over several days, usually beginning with subjective complaints of numbness and tingling followed by overt signs. The illness is usually monophasic, peaking by three weeks in 85 per cent of cases and followed by gradual recovery.

The mainstay of treatment under these circumstances is supportive with attention focused on the adequacy of ventilation. Many patients will develop respiratory insufficiency at the height of their illness, requiring intubation or tracheostomy and assisted ventilation. Insufficiency can be anticipated by recording the vital capacity twice daily and by assessing the strength of voice, the ability to blow out a match and the breathing rate. Blood gases should be monitored closely before and after intubation to avoid the disastrous complications of hypoxia. Ventilators designed to generate either a fixed volume or pressure may be employed. The physician should be familiar with the advantages and disadvantages of both instruments and be prepared to adjust them appropriately to ensure adequate ventilation. Extreme restlessness and anxiety and lability of vital signs may suggest hypoxia, fright or autonomic nervous system involvement. In the latter situation, one can anticipate ileus, urinary retention, disturbed temperature regulation with associated loss of sweating, tachycardia, hypertension or orthostatic hypotension. Ileus may require nasogastric suction and avoidance of oral alimentation. Urinary retention is uncommon and, when present, always raises the question of a postinfectious myelitis. Catheterization may be necessary, although this can be avoided in most cases. The Credé maneuver is helpful in emptying the bladder, offsetting the laxity of weak abdominal musculature. Because cardiovascular complications may occur precipitously, cardiac monitoring and vital signs every 4 hours are necessary until the disease process stabilizes and the patient shows evidence of recovery. Hypotension requires fluid replacement and vasopressors.

Attention should be directed toward good skin care, continual repositioning, postural drainage and pulmonary suctioning if intubation or tracheostomy has been necessary. Physical therapy, including passive and active range of motion exercises, and bivalve casts to maintain normal joint position should be initiated after the condition has stabilized. Adequate nutrition should be maintained orally or by tube feeding unless contraindicated. Alternatively, a balanced electrolyte solution containing glucose is necessary to ensure adequate fluid intake. Five per cent dextrose in Isolyte M,* 1600 ml. per square meter body surface area per 24 hours, is usually appropriate. Precise intake and output should be recorded with daily checks of urine specific gravity and periodic evaluation of serum electrolytes, because the inappropriate antidiuretic hormone syndrome can occur.

Early evidence of pulmonary infection should be detected. Chest x-rays should be obtained to evaluate the initial placement of the endotracheal tube and repeated weekly, or more frequently, for continuing evaluation. Pulmonary secretions should be cultured periodically so that appropriate antibiotics may be initiated promptly when signs of pneumonia

* Available from McGraw Laboratories.

appear. Fever should be interpreted as a sign of infection, although it may reflect disturbed temperature regulation or dehydration.

Anxiety frequently occurs in these patients, particularly early in the course of their illness, and may be counteracted with diazepam (Valium).† Usually diazepam in a dose of 2 mg. two or three times a day is sufficient in the small patient, although larger doses, up to 10 mg. three times a day, may be employed with careful monitoring of vital signs.

The use of glucocorticoids, adrenocorticotropic hormone (ACTH), or immunosuppressive agents such as azathioprine during the acute phase of the illness remains a controversial issue. Clear evidence justifying their use is not available. However, in the chronically progressive or relapsing forms of polyneuropathy, there is evidence to support the efficacy of glucocorticoids in certain cases. Prednisone is given orally each morning in a dose of 60 mg. per square meter. This dose is continued for two to six weeks until there is evidence of improvement or until significant side effects intervene. In the more chronic disorders, glucocorticoids may be given for three months before being abandoned as ineffective. If the patient responds to this dosage, it can subsequently be slowly tapered to a lower maintenance dose or converted to an alternate-day schedule. An alternate-day schedule facilitates longer periods of treatment without associated complications from the medication. A high protein, low carbohydrate, low salt isocaloric diet and the generous use of antacids minimize the side effects of steroids. Selected reports suggest that immunosuppressive agents such as azathioprine may be of benefit in the chronic forms of polyneuropathy which have proven refractory to glucocorticoids, although the total number of cases reported remains small. When glucocorticoids are used, potassium supplementation is advisable. Two mEq. per kilogram body weight per day, usually in two divided doses, is given in the form of potassium chloride syrup.

Some patients develop high CSF pressure and papilledema probably related to very high CSF protein concentrations. In some patients, vision may be compromised, requiring repeated therapeutic lumbar punctures. If this fails to control the pressure, a lumboperitoneal shunt procedure is advisable. Continued physical therapy and use of braces are helpful aids in offsetting footdrop, counteracting contractures and increasing stability in the erect position.

† Manufacturer's precaution: Safety and efficacy of injectable diazepam in children under 12 years of age have not been established. Oral diazepam is not for use in children under six months of age.

References

Austin, J. H.: Recurrent Polyneuropathies and Their Corticosteroid Treatment. *Brain,* 81:157, 1958.

DeVivo, D. C., and Engel, W. K.: Remarkable Recovery of a Steroid Responsive Recurrent Polyneuropathy. *J. Neurol. Neurosurg. Psychiat.,* 33:62, 1970.

Matthews, W. B., Howell, D. A., and Hughs, R. C.: Relapsing Corticosteroid-Dependent Polyneuritis. *J. Neurol. Neurosurg. Psychiat.,* 33:330, 1970.

Tasker, W,. and Chutorian, A. M.: Chronic Polyneuritis of Childhood. *J. Pediat.,* 74:699, 1969.

Yuill, G. M., Swinburn, W. R., and Liversedge, L. A.: Treatment of Polyneuropathy with Azathioprine. *Lancet* 2:894, 1970.

Familial Dysautonomia

RALPH E. MOLOSHOK, M.D.

Many of the clinical manifestations of familial dysautonomia are caused by a deficit in autonomic homeostatic function probably due to a deficit in the synthesis of a neurohumoral substance of importance to the transmission of nervous impulses. Thus, the patient exhibits difficulty in the maintenance of body temperature and blood pressure, impaired neuromuscular coordination and gastrointestinal function, emotional lability, absent or diminished deep tendon reflexes and corneal anesthesia. In addition, most patients present with acute episodic life-threatening crises characterized by varying degrees of pulmonary disease, intractable vomiting and dehydration, severe hyperpyrexia, acute hypertension or convulsive manifestations.

There is no specific treatment for this condition, and therapy is largely symptomatic. Inasmuch as these children adjust poorly to environmental change and stress, a stable routine of daily activity may prove helpful. The use of tranquilizing drugs has been of benefit to some children. Feeding and swallowing difficulties may be encountered in the young infant and may necessitate the use of gavage feedings to maintain nutrition and prevent aspiration.

The occurrence of unexplained fever is treated with antipyretics and sedation, but may require sponging or a hypothermic mattress for severe hyperpyrexia. Vomiting crises may occasionally be aborted by the use of chlorpromazine* † and phenobarbital* but may require

* It has been my experience that the individual tolerance for these medications is so variable that each patient must be considered different and "titrated" as →

parenteral fluids for the maintenance of hydration.

Corneal complications have been decreased with the use of artificial tear solutions (Tearisol, three to six times daily, depending on environmental conditions), inspection routinely for foreign bodies and the use of protective sunglasses when the patient is exposed to sun and wind. Corneal ulcers tend to present more difficulty in healing in the child with dysautonomia and should be treated in consultation with an ophthalmologist. Eyelid suture may be indicated if other means of management prove ineffective.

Hypertensive crises are generally associated with hyperpyrexia and may be complicated by severe oliguria and convulsive phenomena. Intensive sedation and anticonvulsive therapy may be required. Tongue and cheek biting during episodes of acute illness may be a particularly troublesome complication and may lead to severe self-mutilation. Sedation and chlorpromazine may provide some relief, but at times prosthetic dental devices have been employed. Kyphoscoliosis has been seen in more than half the children who have reached the adolescent period and has proved to be extremely refractory to a variety of therapeutic regimens.

Anesthesia for surgical procedures is associated with an increased risk because of extreme lability of blood pressure and a diminished responsiveness to variations in blood pH, pCO_2 and pO_2. The anesthesiologist should be aware of these factors, and the patient must be carefully monitored. Because accidental drownings in a few patients have been ascribed to a lack of appropriate response to hypoxia and pCO_2, diving and underwater swimming should be interdicted.

The administration of Urecholine to a small group of children with familial dysautonomia has been reported to have a favorable effect on some of the manifestations of this syndrome. There was an increase in eye moisture, reduction in gastric distention and vomiting, improvement in esophageal motility and better bladder control. In the patients treated, the effective dose has been 0.2 to 0.4 mg. per kilogram per day administered subcutaneously in four divided doses with about 4 hours between doses. It is preferable to give Urecholine ½ hour prior to meals and with an antacid. There is usually a three- to four-day lag period before the patient demonstrates the optimal effect. After two weeks of four subcutaneous injections a day, oral medication may be instituted. A 5-mg. tablet by mouth appears to be equivalent to 1 mg. subcutaneously, but absorption may not be reliable. However, an oral dose at mid-day allows greater flexibility, especially if the child is of school age.

Although the therapy of dysautonomia is nonspecific, the physician can render the family a great deal of support and comfort by thoroughly familiarizing himself with the varied manifestations of this condition. Living with the dysautonomic child imposes a great burden upon the parents, who are aware of the serious prognosis and are faced with the care of a chronically handicapped child with repeated life-threatening crises. A sympathetic, artful physician can provide needed reassurance.

to the dose of tolerance. Generally, the smaller children have been started on 2.5 mg. of chlorpromazine intramuscularly or 5 to 10 mg. by rectal suppository. The dose may be repeated at 6-hour intervals if necessary and increased if well tolerated. Many of the children in the 6- to 12-year-old age range have been given 25 mg. by suppository or 5 to 10 mg. intramuscularly at the outset of the episode of vomiting. Early morning nausea is a manifestation of several of the children, and their parents have learned to administer a suppository before the child rises from bed in the morning. However, in some instances this produces the undesirable effect of exaggerating the postural hypotension which these children are very apt to experience.

With regard to phenobarbital, 30-mg. doses are usually prescribed parenterally for smaller children and 45 to 60 mg. for older children, with the dose repeated at 6-hour intervals as necessary.

† Manufacturer's precaution: Chlorpromazine is not recommended for children under six months of age except when lifesaving.

Paralysis of the Facial Nerve

LEO R. SULLIVAN, M.D.

Idiopathic Bell's palsy, acutely, may be helped by adrenocorticotropic hormone (ACTH) injections, 40 units per day for three days, tapering to discontinuation over a two-week period. If signs of improvement are evident at the time of the first examination, steroids are probably not indicated. Instead of ACTH, one can use prednisone, 1 mg. per pound per day for a total of 10 to 14 days.

If the child is unable to close his eye fully, methylcellulose drops should be administered three times a day to prevent corneal injuries. This is continued until the eye can be fully closed. Complete recovery is the rule in the vast majority of children with idiopathic Bell's palsy.

Nerve stimulation and nerve conduction studies have not universally been shown to be helpful and are not used routinely.

Obviously, one has to rule out underlying causes such as otitis media with secondary compression of the facial nerve, the rare neoplastic lesion and facial palsies secondary to hypertension in renal disease.

Differential diagnosis is aided by testing the discrete functions of the facial nerve to determine the exact site of disease.

Brachial Palsy

LEO R. SULLIVAN, M.D.

Brachial palsies can be divided into Erb's paralysis, which involves proximal arm muscles, and Klumpke's paralysis, which involves the lower arm and hand. More severe lesions can also occur, involving both upper and lower brachial plexus. Frequently associated with lower brachial plexus injuries is an ipsilateral Horner's syndrome. Patients with lower brachial plexus injuries should undergo fluoroscopy to observe movement of the diaphragm on that side.

Neonates with brachial plexus injuries should have x-ray examinations to rule out fractures of the clavicle or abnormalities of cervical vertebrae. In addition, they should be closely observed for abnormalities of their breathing patterns. Children with such breathing abnormalities are more prone to aspiration or infection. The lower extremities of newborns should also be carefully observed to rule out any associated spinal cord injuries secondary to traction during delivery. There is no specific treatment for the injured nerves per se. Full range of passive motion exercises for the involved arm is essential to prevent contractures.

In the young child, the arm can be abducted and externally rotated with the elbow flexed and the hand pinned to the bed, or an airplane splint may be used. However, it is essential for the parents to remove the splint and perform full range of passive motion exercises two or three times a day. With lower brachial plexus injuries, the arm can be pinned across the chest with the hand near the opposite shoulder. Surgical exploration of the area of injury is generally of little use.

In older children, brachial plexus palsies are almost exclusively secondary to some form of trauma. Treatment is that which would be directed to the specific trauma involved, one exception being lower brachial plexus palsy secondary to thoracic outlet syndrome. These children usually have associated paresthesias and pain on the ulnar side of the hand, and manipulation of the arm over the head reveals diminished to absent arterial pulse in that arm. Therapy in such instances involves shoulder shrugging exercises and, where indicated, surgical intervention.

Injury to the Sciatic Nerve Following Intragluteal Injections

LEO R. SULLIVAN, M.D.

Injuries caused by the injection of neurotoxic substances into or in close proximity to the sciatic nerve are best treated by prevention. Once the material has been injected into the area of the nerve, if the problem is diagnosed immediately, 50 to 100 ml. of physiologic saline can be injected to flood the subgluteal space, thereby possibly lessening the concentration of neurotoxic material. Unfortunately, the problem is usually not diagnosed at the time of injection, but only hours to days later. At this point, there is no specific therapy available. Repeated detailed neurologic examinations should be performed in search of signs of improvement. Also, a regular program of physiotherapy to maintain freedom of movement at the hip, knee and ankle should be instituted.

A lower-leg brace with a foot spring can be employed for the footdrop which is frequently present. One should wait a minimum of six months before considering exploratory surgery. If some degree of recovery has occurred during that period, one might wait even longer, since recovery has been reported even up to three years after injury.

Indications for surgery would be the development of a deep granuloma above the sciatic nerve, or the total absence of any recovery after six months of observation. Long-term prognosis is poor for patients who do not show signs of recovery during the first six months.

Hypoxic Encephalopathy and Acute Toxic Encephalopathy

EDWARD F. RABE, M.D.

Hypoxic encephalopathy is seen in the neonate following difficult delivery and is presumably due to a combination of hypoxic and stagnant hypoxia. Other events preceding hypoxic encephalopathy include temporary cardiac arrest during anesthesia, prolonged tonic and clonic seizures in epilepsy, severe asthmatic attacks and carbon monoxide poisoning. The pathologic result of these events is brain swelling and, frequently, systemic hypotension.

Acute toxic encephalopathy (ATE) of undetermined origin is a disease which must be differentiated from acute meningoencephalitis of bacterial or viral origin, postinfectious meningoencephalitis, hypertensive encephalopathy, subarachnoid hemorrhage, water intoxication, hypernatremia, postictal stupor or coma following a prolonged convulsion or poisoning due to lead, thallium, prochlorperazine, barbiturates, organic thiophosphates in insect sprays or other poisons. Patients with this syndrome develop acute brain swelling frequently aggravated by hypoxia from depressed respirations and hypotension. Some patients with acute toxic encephalopathy also have symptoms and signs of acute liver malfunction as indicated by elevated concentrations of serum transaminases and serum ammonia, hypoglycemia and liver biopsy showing diffuse fatty degeneration. This combination of signs and symptoms has been termed Reye's syndrome.

Since brain swelling, hypoxia and hypotension are seen in hypoxic encephalopathy and acute toxic encephalopathy with or without fatty degeneration of the viscera, and since much of the treatment of these three entities is supportive and similar, their management will be considered together.

Infants and children with brief periods of hypoxia followed by obtundation or stupor and no hypotension will recover with supplemental moist oxygen administration through a scrupulously maintained airway.

Patients with severe acute hypoxia lasting more than 3 minutes usually develop coma and maintain this state for hours to over a week. Patients with ATE rapidly progress down the scale of consciousness to coma. At this stage, both types of patients show brain swelling. Those with hypoxic encephalopathy, in addition, have predictable areas of neuronal fallout while patients with ATE at this stage usually do not.

Treatment aims should include the provision of adequate oxygen through a patent airway, maintenance of a normotensive and normothermic state, reduction of brain swelling, stopping and preventing the recurrence of seizures and maintaining a normal fluid and electrolyte balance; in short, initiating and continuing meticulous supportive care.

Maintenance of an adequate airway requires constant attention to positioning the patient so that the neck is slightly hyperextended. Frequent monitoring of blood pO_2, pCO_2 and pH should be carried out. If pharyngeal secretions accumulate, shallow or irregular respirations appear or pO_2 and pH fall while pCO_2 rises, a tracheostomy should be done and a cuffed tube inserted. To this, a respirator can be attached with an "on demand" or automatic setting. Inhalation of moistened oxygen is mandatory. Persistent maintenance of adequate ventilation is important, since hypoxia and acidosis can cause an increase in intracranial vascular volume, adding further to the increased intracranial pressure from brain swelling.

Normothermia is best obtained by an automatically controlled "cooling" blanket upon which the patient lies. The blanket perfusion is adjusted so that it maintains a body "core" temperature of 97 to 99° F. The thermistor for the blanket is placed in the retrocardiac esophagus.

Blood pressure is monitored by measurement every 10 to 15 minutes. If falling pressure is observed, Levarterenol bitartrate (Levophed Bitartrate) is given intravenously by adding 1 ml. of 0.2 per cent solution to 250 ml. of 5 or 10 per cent glucose. This solution is administered at a rate of 0.5 ml. per minute. If this medication extravasates into the surrounding tissue, the area is infiltrated with 3 to 5 ml. of a solution containing phentolamine 0.5 to 1.0 mg. per ml. Alternately, metaraminol bitartrate (Aramine), which is similar to but longer acting than Levophed, can be used. This is given intravenously in a solution containing 1 mg. (1000 micrograms) in 25 ml. of 5 per cent dextrose in a single dose of 10 micrograms (0.01 mg.) per kilogram. The same solution can be given as a constant infusion at a rate to maintain blood pressure at a desired level.

Reduction of brain swelling is attained with the concomitant use of two agents–dexamethasone (Decadron), which decreases the blood-brain barrier permeability, and a hypertonic solution, which produces a transient osmolar gradient between brain fluid and plasma. Dexamethasone is given intravenously in four equally divided doses in 24 hours. During the first day, a total of 12 mg. is given, followed by daily decrements of 2 mg. per day. When a daily dose of 4 mg. is reached, one must decide whether to continue the reduction or, because the patient is still clinically not well, whether to continue the dose at this level until the patient has improved.

The most commonly used intravenous hypertonic solution is mannitol,* a hexahydric alcohol. This is given intravenously as a 20 per cent solution in a dose of 1.5 to 2 Gm. per kilogram of body weight over a 2-hour period. Since it is not metabolized by the body and is excreted by the kidney, adequate fluid intake and monitored urinary output must be assured. If clinical benefit accrues from one infusion and relapse occurs later, a repeat dose may be given in 8 to 12 hours. Although glycerol has been used intravenously to produce transient hyperosmolality, it is known to cause intravascular hemolysis. At present, it is not recommended for intravenous use.

Seizures may occur early or during the later course of hypoxic or toxic encephalopathy. To stop these, sodium phenobarbital is given intramuscularly in a single dose of 6 mg. per kilogram (125 mg. per square meter for patients weighing over 25 kilograms). This usually suffices, but if not, it may be repeated in 10 minutes if the tonic and clonic seizures persist. Diazepam (Valium)† in a single dose of 0.2 mg. per kilogram (5 mg. per square meter in patients weighing more than 25 kilograms) may be used in a single dose, and if needed, this may be repeated in 15 to 20 minutes. Following the control of the seizures by either drug, intramuscular phenobarbital in a single dose of 6 mg. per kilogram (125 mg. per square meter for patients weighing more than 25 kilograms) should be given every 8 hours for one day, then a dose of 3 mg. per kilogram per dose (75 mg. per square meter) every 8 hours during the next day, then 3 mg. per kilogram per dose (75 mg. per square meter) every 12 hours thereafter until the improved clinical condition permits stopping the medication.

Daily fluid requirements should be maintained with 5 per cent glucose containing a hypotonic mixture of multiple electrolytes such as Normosol-M in D5-W solution (Abbott). It is given in a total daily amount of 1200 ml. per square meter. In those instances when ATE with fatty degeneration of the viscera is suggested by appropriate laboratory findings, a 10 per cent glucose solution can be prepared by adding 110 ml. of 50 per cent glucose to 1 liter of Normosol-M solution D5-W. In addition to the basic 24-hour fluid volume, any 24-hour volume of urine in excess of 700 ml. per square meter should be replaced.

In patients with the clinical picture of ATE plus signs of impaired liver function (elevated transaminase, elevated serum ammonia, occasional hypoglycemia, liver biopsy showing fatty degeneration) there is current speculation as to the most fruitful method of modifying the basic therapy of ATE. Although no definite conclusions are available to recommend any method of treatment, certain procedures may be recommended to attempt to correct some of the disturbed physiology.

If the initial blood glucose is less than 40 mg. per 100 ml., or if the patient is less than five years of age and the glucose is less than 50 mg. per 100 ml., glucose in a hypotonic multiple-electrolyte solution should be the intravenous solution used the first 24 hours of therapy. If blood ammonia is in excess of 150 micrograms per 100 ml. (method of Seligson and Harahara), saline cleansing enemas should be given containing Neomycin in a concentration of 500 mg. per 150 ml. of normal saline, and oral Neomycin should be given in a dose of 250 to 500 mg. every 4 hours by gastric tube. If coma persists and the patient's symptoms are worsening, exchange transfusion with fresh heparinized blood in a volume to replace 70 to 75 per cent of the circulating volume should be performed. Exchange increments of 20 to 50 ml. should be used depending on the total volume to be exchanged. Post-exchange intravenous protamine should be given in a dose of 1 mg. for each milligram of heparin in the transfused blood. A repeat transfusion may be given in 12 hours if persistent clinical improvement is not noted. The value of this therapy remains to be proved.

Other forms of therapy, such as peritoneal dialysis or insulin plus glucose infusions, have little to recommend them at present. In one careful study of peritoneal dialysis, serum ammonia concentration was not affected.

* Manufacturer's precaution: Use of mannitol in pediatric patients has not been studied comprehensively.

† Manufacturer's precaution: Safety and efficacy of injectable diazepam in children under 12 years of age have not been established. Oral diazepam is not for use in children under six months of age.

Encephalopathy and Fatty Degeneration of the Viscera

(Reye's Syndrome)

THOMAS H. GLICK, M.D.

Rational management of this syndrome has been limited by a meager understanding of its pathogenesis, and no therapeutic regimen has thus far been proven effective. Nevertheless, as in any patient with progressive obtundation, assiduous attention to details of intensive care is fundamental, and no current formula can substitute for careful monitoring of critical parameters. An intravenous fluid line, central venous catheter or, better yet, pulmonary artery catheter, nasogastric tube and indwelling urinary catheter are placed, and cardiac monitoring begun. Endotracheal intubation is performed prophylactically with the onset of coma, or even earlier, in the delirious phase, if control of hyperventilation is elected. In the presence of severely depressed pCO_2, a slow, partial correction by controlled ventilation of the curarized patient may possibly be beneficial. A brachial or radial arterial line and a catheter in the internal jugular vein (which can be threaded from a peripheral arm vein) are used in monitoring central nervous system as well as systemic lactic acidemia, hyperammonemia and arteriovenous oxygenation, data which aid in assessing the course of illness and effect of therapy. The placement of specialized monitoring lines should, of course, depend on the gravity and progression of the clinical state, as well as on availability of the pertinent tests.

In case of relative hypovolemia with low central venous pressure (CVP), volume is replenished with 5 to 10 per cent glucose in normal saline and/or colloid, such as albumin, to ensure good perfusion, but caution should be exercised against fluid overload. Free water load in particular is minimized in view of incipient cerebral edema and the risk of water intoxication as hyperosmolarity is corrected. Ringer's lactate is avoided. In the event of severe acidosis, slow infusion of bicarbonate may be necessary, especially for pressor response. Intrathecal bicarbonate has been advocated for CSF acidosis with pH less than 7.25, but its use requires detailed physiologic calculations and lumbar puncture may be hazardous in the advanced stages of illness. Serum potassium should ordinarily be maintained in the high-normal range.

A high index of suspicion for gastrointestinal or other bleeding is essential, especially if steroids are used. Antacids via nasogastric tube are given prophylactically. Vitamin K [phytonadione (AquaMEPHYTON), 2 to 10 mg. intravenously (slowly), then 2 to 10 mg. intravenously or intramuscularly per day, as needed] may suffice to correct the prothrombin time. However, in case of severe coagulation derangement or clinical bleeding, fresh frozen plasma (10 ml. per kilogram body weight in 90 minutes, followed by 5 ml. per kilogram every 4 to 6 hours) and/or fresh whole blood are transfused, since all liver-dependent clotting factors are typically depressed.

A corticosteroid [dexamethasone (Decadron), 1 to 4 mg. every 6 hours intravenously], although not of proved benefit, is routinely given to diminish impending cerebral edema. Glycerol and other osmotic diuretics with the disadvantage of volume depletion are not ordinarily required. Decerebration in this syndrome does not necessarily signify tentorial herniation; surgical decompression or ventricular taps are not recommended.

Hypoglycemia occurs most frequently in infants and young children, but requires careful monitoring of blood glucose by Dextrostix and laboratory determination in all cases. In the event of hypoglycemia, 1 to 2 ml. per kilogram of 50 per cent glucose solution is infused initially, followed by maintenance infusions of 10 to 20 per cent glucose in normal or half-normal saline. Blood glucose is kept well above hypoglycemic levels, e.g., 120 to 140 mg. per 100 ml. in all patients. Seizures are not necessarily related to hypoglycemia. Dilantin is administered prophylactically; phenobarbital and other agents can be used in treatment if needed. (See Seizure Disorders, p. 78.)

In view of evidence implicating ammonia intoxication in the pathogenesis of this syndrome, a standard hepatic encephalopathy regimen is routinely instituted. This includes cleansing enemas, followed by enemas with 500 mg. neomycin per 150 ml. normal saline given every 6 hours, and neomycin by nasogastric tube in a dosage of 15 to 25 mg. per kilogram every 6 hours.

Among the various measures aimed at the correction of the "toxic-metabolic" basis of coma (as yet not adequately defined), only exchange blood transfusion, "total body washout" and peritoneal dialysis, as well as glucose and insulin administration, have commanded widespread attention, and none has thus far been proven effective in a controlled trial. Staging the neurologic condition is valuable in management and essential for evaluation of therapy. Despite the high mortality rate, variation in the natural course of illness requires a cautious approach to experimental therapy, and most groups have undertaken exchange transfusion or other major intervention only after signs of decortication or even decerebration have appeared.

Exchange transfusion has been used with apparent success at several medical centers, but the favorable experience has not thus far been reproduced at other, comparable centers. Although more rapid and complete exchange has been advocated, a conservative technique involves the exchange of fresh heparinized blood in fractional volumes of 20 to 50 ml., with the total exchange calculated to replace approximately 75 per cent of blood volume. Heparin is neutralized with protamine at the end of each exchange. Exchange may be repeated every 12 to 24 hours in the comatose patient, but it should be noted that clinical improvement, if it occurs, is often delayed for 12 to 24 hours.

"Total body washout," using cardiopulmonary bypass, hypothermia, and virtually complete hemodilution, represents a possibly advantageous extension of the principle of exchange transfusion. Although still highly experimental, modifications of this technique should be considered in hospitals with appropriate technical capability.

Peritoneal dialysis has been cited for advantages in metabolic regulation and fluid balance, as well as use in clearance of hypothetical toxins, but, like exchange transfusion, its efficacy has not yet been adequately demonstrated. Recent evidence suggests failure to remove ammonia. Peritoneal dialysis cannot be widely recommended unless additional evidence of its efficacy is forthcoming.

The use of glucose and insulin has been suggested to suppress the mobilization of possibly toxic free fatty acids. The regimen·consists of intravenous infusion, at rates up to 60 ml. per hour, of glucose solutions containing up to 1 unit of regular insulin per 5 Gm. of glucose, with close monitoring of blood glucose, since hypoglycemia has been induced. Although evidence of beneficial effect is not persuasive, trials of glucose and insulin therapy can be justified at any state of illness, the earlier the better, after correction of preexisting hypoglycemia. Additional modalities, such as steroids and levodopa,* have not shown promise as the principal therapeutic approach.

* Manufacturer's precaution: Safety of L-dopa in children under 12 years of age has not been established.

4

Respiratory Tract

Malformations of the Nose

WERNER D. CHASIN, M.D.

In the newborn, a most serious problem requiring immediate recognition and attention is choanal atresia. When the choanae fail to open, the neonate, an obligatory nose breather, has difficulty in accommodating to mouth breathing. The child becomes cyanotic, breathes adequately only while crying and cannot coordinate mouth breathing with sucking and feeding. The diagnosis is made by finding an obstruction in the back of the nose with a probe or catheter. The diagnosis can be verified with x-ray contrast studies. The immediate but temporary management requires the insertion into the oral cavity of a small metal or plastic airway, securing it with tape to the sides of the face. Alternatively a Goodel airway or a rubber nipple, the tip of which has been cut off, may be similarly inserted and secured. The patient should then be immediately referred to an otolaryngologist. The simplest surgical procedure to correct the stenosis consists of a transnasal opening of the atresia under the surgical microscope, and stenting the newly made choanal openings with plastic tubing that simultaneously serves as a nasal airway. The stents are removed after six weeks. If a partial stenosis recurs, the child will have to undergo a transpalatal repair of the choanal narrowing. This can wait until the the child is four or five years old.

Malformations of the external nose commonly include the deformity associated with harelip, hemangioma, dermoid, encephalocele or meningocele, glioma and septal deformity.

The nasal component of the harelip deformity is repaired as part of the initial surgery to correct the cleft lip, though secondary cosmetic nasal procedures are often required when the child is older.

Hemangiomas, if they show no tendency to regress spontaneously, might be managed with cryotherapy, injection of sclerosing solutions, systemic steroids or surgery. The more serious but rare pulsating arterial angioma, which tends to expand and destroy bone, must be managed by aggressive surgery to prevent a fatal outcome. Radiation therapy is now rarely used to treat benign hemangiomas because of delayed skin cancer formation and possible disturbance of the growth centers of the nasal and facial bones.

Before removing an external nasal tumor, radiologic examination must be carried out to determine whether the growth communicates with the cranial cavity. Meningoceles or meningoencephaloceles, which can be suspected from the observation that they are soft, compressible, and reducible, should be surgically corrected by a team composed of otolaryngologist and neurosurgeon. Gliomas may also require this team approach, although some do not retain a connection with the anterior cranial cavity. Dermoids can be removed surgically without fear of communication with the cranial cavity. Septal deformities usually do not require early repair unless there is severe nasal obstruction.

The manifestations of congenital syphilis of the nose are ushered in by the appearance of snuffles at three to four weeks of age. The saddle-nose deformity due to syphilitic destruction of cartilage and bone does not become manifest until later in childhood. Timely diagnosis and appropriate antiluetic treatment may prevent the later destruction of the nose and may obviate the need for more extensive cosmetic procedures later on.

Tumors and Polyps of the Nose

WERNER D. CHASIN, M.D.

External nasal tumors, which include hemangiomas, lymphangiomas, dermoids, gliomas, encephaloceles and meningoceles, have been described in the section on Malformations of the Nose. Malignant melanoma is fortunately rare and would require aggressive surgical management coupled with tumor chemotherapy. Papillomas can be removed surgically, although those which occur in the nasal vestibule have a tendency to recur.

Intranasal polyps are uncommon in children. Their presence almost always signifies a concomitant sinusitis. A unilateral polyp must be differentiated from an encephalocele or meningocele by appropriate radiologic studies. The surgical removal of the encephalocele must be performed by an otolaryngology-neurosurgery team. Although most intranasal polyps are manifestations of chronic allergic ethmoid sinusitis, a unilateral polyp often arises from chronic maxillary sinusitis. These polyps, though unilateral, may become so large that they descend into the nasopharynx and obstruct it completely, thereby causing bilateral nasal obstruction. This antrochoanal polyp is removed surgically under general anesthesia, and the maxillary sinus must also be cleaned to prevent recurrence of the polyp.

Although chronic ethmoid sinusitis is not uncommon in children, especially when due to allergy, the formation of polyps as a result of this sinusitis is uncommon in children compared with adults. Chronic sinusitis due to cystic fibrosis does result in nasal polyposis so frequently that this cystic fibrosis should be ruled out in any child with nasal polyposis.

The treatment of nasal polyps involves foremost the management of the underlying sinusitis by the use of antibiotics according to culture, irrigations, allergic evaluation and management, and by treatment of cystic fibrosis when found, coupled with the intranasal removal of the polyps. Polyps which are removed without attention to the underlying sinusitis will recur.

The nasopharyngeal angiofibroma is a sex-linked, extremely vascular teratoma found exclusively in males. This tumor produces nasal obstruction, recurrent and severe epistaxis and, sometimes, headaches. It must not be mistaken for an enlarged adenoid because adenoidectomy could result in fatal hemorrhage. The angiofibroma, which may be limited to the nasopharynx or extend into the sinuses, pterygomaxillary fossa or base of the skull, is managed either by surgery, external irradiation, radioactive implants or a combination of these modalities.

Malignant growths of the nose in children are fortunately uncommon. When present, they are managed by surgery, by external radiation therapy or by a combination of these, depending on the nature of the malignancy.

Nasal Injuries

WERNER D. CHASIN, M.D.

The nose is the most frequently injured part of the face. The effects of childhood nasal trauma are deformity and partial or total nasal obstruction due to deviation of the nasal septum. Less common but more serious complications are cerebrospinal fluid rhinorrhea due to a fracture involving the cribriform plate in the medial part of the nasal roof and an unrecognized hematoma of the nasal septum. The latter, due to a combination of vascular deprivation of cartilage and secondary infection, may result in a dissolution of the cartilaginous portion of the septum, producing a saddle-nose deformity, which requires for its correction the use of graft materials and other cosmetic surgery.

External nasal deviation in the newborn usually includes a dislocation of the septal cartilage from its normal pocket groove in the bony part of the floor of the nose. The pediatrician may be able to reduce this deformity by grasping the nose firmly between the thumb and index finger, pulling it upward and, in this stretched position, pushing it to the midline. If a click is heard or felt, the reduction may have been successfully accomplished. When this maneuver fails, an attempt is made to grasp the septum between the blades of a small and straight hemostatic clamp, the blades of which have been padded with either moist cotton, adhesive tape or segments of thin rubber tubing. The hemostat is inserted with one blade passing through each nostril. The blades are then closed so that the tips of the blades rest inside the lower half of the nasal bones. While he lifts the nasal framework outward and upward with the hemostat, the physician pushes the nose laterally across the midline, again feeling and listening for a click. If these measures fail, the patient should be referred to an otolaryngologist.

Nasal injuries in older children include hematoma, abrasion, laceration and avulsion from injuries and animal bites. The soft tissue injuries may be associated with fractures of the nasal skeleton. Hematomas and abrasions resolve and heal without treatment. External lacerations should be repaired with fine 5–0 or 6–0 nylon or polyethylene sutures with a swedged needle to minimize the size of the needle puncture marks. Sutures are removed in five days. A complex laceration or one in which some skin has been lost requires plastic surgery techniques to minimize the inevitable scar, and patients with such wounds should be referred to an otolaryngologic plastic surgeon. Conspicuous scars about the nose and face cause parents and children great concern quite out of proportion to the actual size or functional significance of these scars. Lacerations of the internal mucosal surfaces, unless they are quite extensive, require no suturing. They may be left untreated or stented by the insertion of a small strip of petrolatum-impregnated gauze. Avulsed and amputated portions of the external nose should be saved, cleaned with 70 per cent isopropyl alcohol and reattached by a careful suturing technique. These parts usually will take, and the cosmetic result is superior to a subsequent grafting procedure.

Fractures of the nasal bones can be reduced for up to 7 to 10 days after the injury. Radiograms should include lateral views and an occlusal view with the x-ray beam projecting the nasal pyramid onto a small film which the patient holds in the mouth. When a great deal of soft tissue swelling is present, the reduction is best delayed for a few days so that the nasal skeleton can be better palpated during the reduction procedure. A septal hematoma, recognized by the presence of a bilateral, soft, compressible bogginess of the nasal septum (usually not discolored like a cutaneous hematoma), must be drained to prevent the formation of a septal abscess and resultant saddle-nose deformity. Although most nasal fractures can be corrected satisfactorily by closed manipulations, comminuted fractures or those which cannot be easily reduced may require an open reduction and stenting. An open reduction is performed under general anesthesia and requires a brief hospitalization.

Septal fractures may be difficult to correct perfectly and may later require a submucous resection procedure if there is enough deviation to cause significant nasal obstruction.

The physician must ever bear in mind the possibility of associated fractures in a case of nasal injury. Untreated fractures of the medial portion of the maxilla can result in permanent narrowing of the nasal chamber and require immediate open reduction. Fractures of the infraorbital rim can be recognized by the palpation of a step deformity of the rim; this is verified by x-rays. These fractures may require an open reduction. Fractures of the orbital floor (blow-out fractures) may require surgical attention to prevent the delayed development of enophthalmos and diplopia.

Epistaxis

WERNER D. CHASIN, M.D.

The causes of nosebleed include self-inflicted damage with the finger, crusting of mucosa from whatever cause, allergic rhinitis, external injury and, less commonly, blood dyscrasias and hereditary hemorrhagic telangiectasia. In the majority of cases of childhood epistaxis, the bleeding source is a small vessel which has been torn or has burst and which is situated on the anterior inferior portion of the septum known as Little's area. In children, bleeding from the posterior region of the nasal cavity or from the nasopharynx is uncommon and should arouse a suspicion of a more serious cause such as blood dyscrasia or angiofibroma of the nasopharynx. Bleeding after blunt external trauma to the nose signifies a fracture of bone or cartilage. Cartilage fractures must be detected by physical examination alone, since they are not visualized on radiograms.

The majority of nosebleeds in children cease spontaneously or can be halted by simple means. Compression of the entire nose between the index finger and thumb for 5 minutes often works. When this measure fails, a small piece of cotton, preferably moistened with 1/8 or 1/4 per cent Neo-Synephrine, can be twisted into the appropriate nasal chamber and external compression applied as in the first step. To this maneuver may be added the insertion of a moistened piece of cotton or paper high under the uppermost central portion of the upper lip above the incisor teeth. This tamponades a branch of the labial artery which ascends in the nasal floor to "feed" the vessel which has burst in Little's area.

If these measures fail, a more tightly fitting anterior pack consisting of 1/2-inch petrolatum-impregnated gauze must be inserted into the bleeding nasal chamber and, if necessary, also into the nonbleeding side to offer counterpressure against the flexible cartilaginous nasal septum. To minimize the discomfort involved in anterior packing of the nose, the nasal mucosa is first topically anesthetized with a pledget of cotton that has been wrung almost dry after being saturated with 10 per cent cocaine solution, 2 per cent tetracaine with 1:1000 adrenalin or 2 per cent Xylocaine with 1:1000 adrenalin. Wringing out the cotton reduces the possibility of anesthetic overdose. Local anesthetics reach the general circulation as rapidly by mucous membrane absorption as by intravenous administration.

When adequate anterior packing also fails the physician will have to resort to anteroposterior packing, wherein the choana on the appropriate side is occluded and a firmer anterior pack is inserted. Unless the bleeding clearly originates from the nasopharynx, the posterior plug need not be larger than 2 by 3 cm. in size, since it is required to occlude only one choana. A larger pack is difficult to insert, is uncomfortable and can cause respiratory obstruction as it forces down the soft palate and uvula. A larger pack is required in the case of nasopharyngeal bleeding due to postadenoidectomy hemorrhage or to control bleeding from an angiofibroma, where it becomes necessary to tamponade the nasopharynx rather than the nasal chamber.

Two preliminary steps will minimize the physical and psychologic discomfort of anteroposterior packing:

1. A careful and kind explanation to the child of the exact maneuvers which are to follow.

2. Sedative medication, preferably given intravenously for faster onset of action.

A number 10 French rubber or plastic catheter is inserted through the bleeding side of the nose and is drawn out through the mouth. A hemostat is clamped so that it grasps both ends of the catheter loop not quite at the tips, so that the child cannot pull out the catheter. The posterior pack which can consist of two 2- by 2-inch gauze sponges rolled up, should have tied tightly to its center three 30-cm. strands of a braided, relatively thick string. Suture material is too thin and tends to cut into the soft tissues of the nose and palate. Two of the strands are tied to the oral end of the catheter. The hemostat is released and removed. The child is asked to take a deep breath and, during this moment, while the physician or his assistant pulls forward the nasal end of the catheter, the physician helps to push the posterior pack against the posterior pharyngeal wall and up behind the soft palate out of sight. The third strand hangs down behind the palate, its outer end remaining outside the mouth. The two nasal strands are detached from the catheter and the latter is laid aside. While either the physician or his assistant exerts a constant forward pull on the nasal strings, the physician packs strips of ½-inch petrolatum-impregnated gauze into the nose, filling first the posterior half of the nasal cavity and then completing the packing of the anterior region. The idea is to tamponade the entire nasal chamber, and the only function of the posterior choanal pack is to keep the anterior pack confined to the nose so that it does not fall into the nasopharynx, thereby nullifying its tamponading effect. The two nasal strings are now tied about a rolled piece of gauze resting on the outside of the nostril so that the posterior pack cannot fall back. The third string, which serves as the handle for the subsequent removal of the posterior pack via the mouth, either can be taped to the cheek, or can be cut off flush with the uvula where it can be subsequently grasped with a hemostatic forceps.

A child who has required anteroposterior packing should be hospitalized. The pack is left in place for a minimum of three days after all bleeding has ceased. During this hospitalization, the child may be evaluated for a possible blood dyscrasia.

If the anteroposterior packing procedure fails, the child might require a surgical procedure involving arterial ligation of the anterior ethmoidal, external carotid or internal maxillary artery, or a combination of these, depending on the precise location of the bleeding site.

Cauterization of the bleeding source in the nose should be attempted only when (1) the bleeding point can be seen precisely and (2) the bleeding can be stopped temporarily so that the cauterizing chemical is not washed away immediately by the flow of blood. The commercially available silver nitrate stick, 6 inches long, is well suited for such cauterization. Random cauterizations of large areas of nasal mucosa are destructive, can result in adhesions and usually fail to stop the bleeding. After the spot cauterization, the parent is instructed to apply either petrolatum or borafax ointment into the nostril to soften the eschar which invariably forms and which is so tempting to the child's index finger.

Foreign Bodies in the Nose and Pharynx

WERNER D. CHASIN, M.D.

Nasal foreign bodies include any object small enough to pass through the nostril. Other orifices, including the ears, should also be checked. The foreign substance elicits a purulent, often fetid rhinorrhea, which is usually the presenting symptom. Success in removal depends on:

1. Accurate assessment of the size and shape of the foreign body so that proper instruments are chosen.
2. Maximum shrinkage of the nasal mucous membranes to permit adequate visualization and space for instrumentation and extraction.
3. Adequate local or, if necessary, general anesthesia.

Four drops of 10 per cent cocaine solution, 2 per cent Xylocaine with 1:1000 adrenalin or 2 per cent tetracaine with 1:1000 adrenalin are instilled into the appropriate nasal chamber after it has been suctioned using a number 5 Baron suction tip. If the nasal secretions are not first aspirated, the anesthetic and vasoconstrictor will be diluted and become ineffective. To assess the size and shape of the foreign body, an x-ray may be helpful. A curved, blunt probe is passed over and behind round objects (pearls, beads, marbles) and the object is fished forward along the floor of the nose. To remove other foreign substances, a 3-inch Hartmann ear forceps is a useful instrument.

Foreign bodies in the oral cavity are not common. Pins, fishbones and other pointed objects must be sought for in the tonsils, in lingual tonsils just above the epiglottis and in the pyriform sinus. Upon occasion a pointed foreign substance may, as a result of sneezing or swallowing, be carried up into the nasopharynx where it becomes imbedded in the adenoid.

Whenever possible, pharyngeal foreign bodies should be removed in a hospital setting where a laryngoscope, laryngoscopic suction and a variety of forceps are available. Should a foreign body be loosened during attempts at removal, it may fall into the larynx causing laryngospasm and acute respiratory obstruction.

Nasopharyngitis
(The Common Cold)

EDWARD A. MORTIMER, JR., M.D.

One of the most ubiquitous infections that plague man is the common cold. Many different viruses can produce this syndrome. It is significant because of its frequency, its responsibility for loss of time from work and school and its tendency to predispose to secondary bacterial infections such as otitis media, sinusitis and pneumonia. Unfortunately, there is no way to prevent colds, no method by which the course may be shortened or any means by which secondary bacterial infections may be prevented. Thus, therapy is only symptomatic.

Symptomatic therapy may comprise efforts to reduce the mild malaise often associated with the common cold plus attempts to relieve nasal symptoms and keep passages open. Relief of the mild systemic symptoms may be achieved temporarily by aspirin; the dose is 60 mg. per year of age in children, not to be given more than four times in 24 hours and for no more than two days. Care must be exerted to avoid inducing dangerous salicylism by the administration of aspirin to a child whose intake of fluids has diminished markedly, by the administration of excessive doses or by therapy for a protracted period of time. The dangers of salicylism are such that many physicians prefer to use acetaminophen (Tempra or Tylenol), supplied as a liquid in a dropper bottle with 100 mg. per ml. The dose is 60 mg. per year of age every 4 to 6 hours. The dropper is marked at the 0.6-ml. (60 mg.) dose. Tempra and Tylenol are also supplied as tablets and syrup. Tenlap, a third commonly used preparation of acetaminophen, is available as syrup.

Nasal obstruction sufficient to interfere with feeding and sleeping in young infants may be relieved partially by humidification, by the employment of an infant's nasal aspirator bulb obtainable at most pharmacies, or by 1 to 3 drops of 1/8 per cent phenylephrine (Neo-Synephrine) in each nostril before feeding – particularly if the nares have been aspirated first. In older children, 1/4 per cent phenylephrine may be employed. Such nasal vasoconstrictors should not be used more than three or four days because of rebound phenomena and dependence.

Recurrent colds are a particularly vexatious problem to parents and physicians. Some children seem to have "one cold after another." They are not prevented by antibiotics or by adenotonsillectomy; and they are not associated with immunologic deficiencies, so gamma globulin is useless. They are not induced by chilling and are unrelated to allergy. In children with a seemingly excessive number of colds, the physician must remember that six per year is more or less average in the preschool years, decreasing to three in the teens. Reassuring and supporting the parents, avoiding the expense of unnecessary antibiotics and adenotonsillectomy, and symptomatic therapy for infections are the only measures of use.

Sinusitis and Rhinitis

CHARLES F. FERGUSON, M.D.

Proper care of the initiating respiratory infection may abort acute sinusitis, because the latter is always preceded by a nasal infection (rhinitis), which is the source of entry of the organism. Measures to be employed are adequate rest, isolation from further exposure, since resistance is already low, good ventilation, and humidification to avoid excessive dryness of the atmosphere. In chronic sinusitis or chronic rhinitis, investigation should be directed toward *underlying allergies* (nasal smears, blood eosinophilia, skin tests, elimination of environmental or dietary allergens), *cystic fibrosis* (including plate or sweat tests), *Kartagener's syndrome* (chest and sinus x-ray films) or deficient *gamma globulin* (blood levels with electrophoresis).

Treatment of *acute* sinusitis is based on improved ventilation and drainage and systemic drug therapy. Cultures should always be taken and sensitivity tests performed.

Improved Ventilation and Drainage. 1. Increase the humidification by a vaporizer in the room.

2. Give a mild vasoconstrictor, such as 0.25 per cent Neo-Synephrine, Vasocort or Paredrine. In the child above six years of age, Afrin may be used as a long-acting spray once every 12 hours. It produces more prolonged vasoconstriction. Synthetics are better than ephedrine or epinephrine because they usually produce less "rebound edema." Antibiotic sprays or drops should be avoided, since the concentration of antibiotic is ineffective, contact with the organism is only momentary and the dangers of development of allergy or resistant organisms are great. Continued use of any vasoconstrictor is to be deplored. Sprays are more easily applied than drops, and may be used every 3 to 4 hours during the *acute stage only.* A cotton pledget moistened with the vasoconstrictor and left in the nose 4 or 5 minutes may open passages better so that later spraying is more effective. Gentle spot suction cleans the airway, and the Davol Aspirator is especially helpful in babies.

3. *Oral decongestants,* such as Sudafed, Triaminic or Actifed, may be useful if local therapy is difficult or if the mucosa is unduly irritated. Relatively large doses seem necessary. Disophrol Chronotabs, one every 12 hours, may be beneficial in older children or young adults. They are not recommended for children under 12 years of age.

4. *Hot compresses* may be helpful.

5. *Proetz displacement* treatments using an antibiotic solution (2 million units of penicillin and 500 mg. of streptomycin in 10 ml. of saline with a few drops of Neo-Synephrine added) may promote faster resolution. The patient lies supine with the head extended. The solution is dropped into one side of the nasal cavity, and as the patient closes his nasopharynx by constantly repeating "k, k, k" or "chocolate," intermittent suction is applied to one nostril, with the other occluded. This causes removal of secretions from the sinuses and displacement of the antibiotic solution into them. Obviously, cooperation is necessary, so that this treatment is not too satisfactory in the younger age group.

6. *Puncture* of the antrum through an inferior meatal approach with irrigation to remove secretions, and the instillation of a solution of 2 million units of penicillin and 500 mg. of streptomycin, may quickly clear up a purulent antrum infection. This treatment may have to be repeated once or twice.

Systemic Drug Therapy. 1. Give a broad-spectrum *antibiotic,* such as erythromycin, lincomycin* or ampicillin. (After the culture has been reported, if necessary shift to the best drug available.)

2. If the patient is uncomfortable, analgesics such as aspirin, codeine or Demerol may be indicated.

3. *Corticosteroids* have been used in cases of acute sinusitis, but they are not necessary and possibly not desirable.

In *chronic* cases, adenoidectomy may remove the focus of chronic infection as well as improve nasal ventilation and aeration of the sinuses, resulting in better drainage of secretions. Today radical sinus surgery is rarely

* Manufacturer's precaution: Lincomycin is not indicated in the newborn (up to one month of age).

indicated. Removal of nasal polyps in cases of cystic fibrosis may have to be performed to keep the airway adequate. External trephine of the floor of the frontal sinus will occasionally be indicated to drain an acute empyema. If an orbital abscess has localized from an acute ethmoiditis in an infant, incision and drainage in the lower lid may have to be done when fluctuation has occurred. Treatment of underlying allergies in any case of chronic rhinitis and sinusitis is of extreme importance. An associated anemia or hypothyroid state should be properly treated. Vaccine therapy in chronic nasal or sinus infection may be of occasional value. If so, an autogenous vaccine is usually the best. The empiric use of gamma globulin in doses of 0.1 ml. per kilogram of body weight every three or four weeks may give good results when more specific therapy fails, although there seems to be little rationale for such use.

Acute Lymphonodular Pharyngitis

EDWARD C. CURNEN, JR., M.D.

In 1962, Steigman et al. described a symptom complex, attributed to infection with Coxsackie virus A10, which they designated "acute lymphonodular pharyngitis." Most but not all of the patients were children seen during the summer and early fall. Characteristic findings were temperature elevations ranging from 100 to 105° F., mild headache, malaise, anorexia and sore throat. Small, raised, discrete, solid, white or yellowish nodular lesions surrounded by a zone of erythema were observed on the soft palate, anterior pillars and posterior pharynx. Two children also had conjunctival nodules.

The self-limited febrile illness resembled herpangina except for the lesions, which were not vesicular and did not progress to ulceration. The lack of subsequent similar reports to date suggests that this may be a relatively uncommon manifestation of infection by a Coxsackie virus, or one which perhaps is overlooked. The course appears to be unaffected by antimicrobial agents, which are not indicated. As in other infections by Coxsackie viruses, treatment is symptomatic.

Reference

Steigman, A. J., Lipton, M. M., and Braspennickx, H.: Acute Lymphonodular Pharyngitis: A Newly Described Condition Due to Coxsackie A Virus. *J. Pediat.*, 61:331, 1962.

Retropharyngeal and Lateral Pharyngeal Abscesses

CHARLES F. FERGUSON, M.D.

The true *peritonsillar abscess* (i.e., localized in the supratonsillar fossa), with marked swallowing difficulty, excessive salivation, drooling and trismus, is rare under 10 years of age. The proper diagnosis is usually *lateral pharyngeal abscess,* when the infection is not localized in or above the fossa directly involving the pillars or palate, but is *posterior* to the pillars in the lateral wall. This is the common abscess of childhood. Under two to three years of age, the most common localized infection is the *retropharyngeal abscess,* located on the posterior pharyngeal wall. If situated low down, this abscess (or adenitis) may cause serious laryngeal obstruction. Any beginning abscess should be suspected as soon as possible in the course of the upper respiratory tract infection, so that adequate therapy may be instituted early, and the patient carefully observed.

Always culture the throat and obtain sensitivity tests (before administration of antibiotics, if possible).

Start antibiotic therapy in adequate doses early. Penicillin or ampicillin in large doses is preferable, since most cases are due to the beta hemolytic streptococcus. If a resistant staphylococcus is suspected, methicillin (as Staphcillin) or sodium oxacillin (as Prostaphlin) should be used. Therapy should be continued at least 10 days *after* infection appears to be completely controlled.

Local heat should be given in the form of hot compresses or poultices to the neck, and hot saline irrigations, if the patient is old enough or cooperative enough to tolerate them.

Only if fluctuation develops should *incision and drainage* be performed. Today, most cases, adequately treated, will resolve without surgery. Digital palpation is not without risk and should be done only when possible emergency treatment can immediately be carried out. [Serious carotid reflex (? vagal) stimulation, with cessation of respiration, has occurred, and actual rupture of the abscess is always a possible danger.]

Incision and drainage can safely be performed under general anesthesia if careful intubation is used early during induction. The patient should already be in extreme Trendelenburg position, with suction and laryngoscope in immediate readiness. A cruciate incision over the most fluctuant area, together with simultaneous suctioning, followed by spreading the incision with a hemostat accomplishes the drainage. For a few days the edges of the incision may have to be spread daily (without anesthesia) to avoid pocketing of pus, since no packing can be used. Rapid sealing of the opening may occur, especially if the incision is too small or heals too rapidly. Since such abscesses tend to recur unless tonsils and adenoids are removed, this procedure is strongly advocated soon after complete recovery from the initial infection has occurred.

The Tonsil and Adenoid Problem

SYDNEY SHORE, M.D.

One should follow the dictates of common sense and advise tonsillectomy and adenoidectomy only when definite indications exist. It is not always necessary to perform a tonsillectomy at the time of adenoidectomy. The reverse also holds true.

Indications for Tonsillectomy. The most common indication is recurrent severe tonsillitis, five or more episodes yearly in two successive years, confirmed clinically (ideally by throat culture). Indications in children with rheumatic disease or asthma are essentially the same. Another indication is peritonsillar abscess. Not only extremely toxic and painful, it is indicative of future tonsillar difficulty.

Tonsillar cryptitis may indicate tonsillectomy. The tonsils are often not enlarged and during acute episodes may not appear typically inflamed with exudate. However, symptoms of sore throat and malaise with fever are present, and careful throat culture often yields beta-hemolytic streptococci. Such patients may respond to proper antibiotics, but a later culture when the patient is asymptomatic again yields beta-hemolytic streptococci. The infection is deep-seated in the crypts where antibiotics cannot completely eradicate the disease. Rarely, tonsillar cryptitis may exist without positive throat cultures and be a cause of fever of undetermined origin. If complete medical evaluation is negative but the tonsils have a soft, moist appearance and there is significant cervical adenopathy, one may consider diagnostic tonsillectomy.

An unusual indication is gross tonsillar hypertrophy. Such a child may present with a typical muffled "hot potato" voice or have difficulty in swallowing and fail to gain weight. If such tonsils become acutely inflamed and swollen, they can cause significant respiratory obstruction.

A rare indication for tonsillectomy may be marked halitosis and choking or gagging on pieces of whitish debris from the tonsil crypts, but only if significantly disturbing to the patient.

THROAT CULTURES. Look for coagulase-positive *Staphylococcus aureus* as well as beta-hemolytic streptococci. The production of penicillinase will prevent a good response to penicillin.

Indications for Adenoidectomy. Perhaps the most common indication is recurrent acute otitis media with nasopharyngoscopy revealing enlarged adenoids encroaching on the eustachian tubal openings. There may be persistent serous otitis between episodes or, indeed, chronic serous otitis without frequent acute otitis, with the only symptom being decreased hearing. Allergy should be considered. Advise adenoidectomy when a child has five bouts of acute otitis media yearly in two successive years or chronic fluid in the middle ear that fails to clear medically. They often require myringotomy as well and even polyethylene tubes to prevent fluid reaccumulation.

Gross adenoidal hypertrophy, without ear infection, may indicate adenoidectomy. These children breathe through the mouth, snore, and often have typical adenoidal facies, with a dull appearance and tendency to drool. Severe malocclusion may develop. They often complain of sore throat on arising since breathing through the mouth leads to excessive oral dryness. The obstruction may result in chronic nasal discharge and even sinusitis.

Adenoids may not be grossly enlarged, yet be the seat for repeated acute or chronic infection. Diagnosis is often difficult. The child may be toxic and complain of pain in the roof of his mouth. There may be purulent nasal or postnasal discharge. If five or more episodes occur yearly in two consecutive years, adenoidectomy should be considered.

Remember that the tonsils or adenoids may be the seat of a malignancy. The isolated symptom of cough is rarely due to tonsils or adenoids.

Mortality Rate. The most common figure quoted is 300 deaths per year in the United States directly related to tonsil and adenoid surgery, a minute percentage of all tonsillectomies and adenoidectomies performed. The risk of mortality, or significant morbidity, is virtually nil when the operation is performed under proper conditions. Benefits derived by careful patient selection are most gratifying. However, tonsillectomy and adenoidectomy are not panaceas for nonspecific upper respiratory infection.

Disorders of the Larynx

PAUL H. HOLINGER M.D.

Disorders of the larynx manifest themselves by two principal groups of symptoms: phonatory, consisting of hoarseness, an abnormal or absent cry; and stridor and dyspnea, indications of respiratory obstruction.

The quality of the cry is a significant clue to the nature of a laryngeal anomaly. A weak, breathy or aspirate cry suggests a vocal cord paralysis; a muffled sound suggests a retropharyngeal abscess or a thyroglossal duct cyst; a high-pitched squeak or even an absent cry during obvious crying efforts suggests a laryngeal web, cyst or laryngocele; and a "seal bark", a subglottic edema.

CONGENITAL ANOMALIES

Laryngomalacia

So-called congenital laryngeal stridor is a transient form of stridor in infants which is associated with an abnormal flaccidity of the laryngeal tissues. The epiglottis may be tubular to accentuate the stridor. Accurate diagnosis of the condition requires direct laryngoscopy to eliminate other causes of stridorous, noisy respiration in infants. Laryngomalacia is rarely severe enough to require surgical intervention, although in extreme cases tracheostomy may be necessary if an infant labors so hard at breathing that he becomes cyanotic and totally exhausted during feedings. After tracheostomy, weight gain is usually rapid. The condition gradually disappears spontaneously by one-and-one-half to two years of age.

Congenital Subglottic Stenosis

This clinical picture is a difficult one to evaluate. Infants with this condition constitute the largest group of congenital laryngeal anomalies requiring tracheostomy under one year of age. Furthermore, congenital subglottic stenosis is responsible for the prolonged need of a tracheostomy, some infants requiring the tube until two or three years of age. The condition consists of thickening of subglottic structures and sometimes of the true cords themselves to cause persistent respiratory obstruction. Minimal laryngeal inflammation precipitates a tracheostomy. Instruction of parents in home care of the tracheostomized infant is essential to avoid long periods of hospitalization. Occasional direct laryngeal dilatations permit reevaluation of the process. Steroids do not appear to be effective. Extubation depends on normal laryngeal growth and is generally accomplished during the latter part of the second year.

Congenital Webs

Congenital webs of the larynx most frequently consist of membranes across the anterior half or two-thirds of the vocal cords, but supraglottic and subglottic webs are included in this category. Supraglottic webs consist of a fusion of the false cords above an apparently normal glottis. These may be slit in the midline under direct laryngoscopy; they are then dilated with laryngeal bougies several times at intervals of once or twice a week to maintain their patency. Glottic webs constitute a somewhat more difficult problem. Some are membranous, others a true fusion of the anterior half or two-thirds of the cords. Simple, rapid dilatation with laryngeal bougies suffices to improve the glottic chink and the voice in those with a small web. A more definitive procedure consists of a thyrotomy, an incision to separate the edges of the fused cords and the insertion of a tantalum plate between the cords. This is necessary only in those with severe fusion of a large portion of the membranous cords. It is preceded, of course, by a tracheostomy. The metal plate remains in the midline of the larynx for six weeks to two months to permit epithelialization of the cut edges of the cords, and then the plate and tube are removed.

Congenital Cysts and Laryngoceles

These become clinically perceptible when swollen by air forced into them when coughing or when they become filled with mucus. Symptoms of extreme dyspnea in the newborn with an absent, diminished or muffled cry suggest this anomaly; a lateral x-ray film of the neck shows a circumscribed, cystic deformity of the laryngeal airway. On direct laryngoscopy the cyst is seen in the aryepiglottic fold or extending from the ventricle. Aspiration with a large-bore needle will relieve acute obstruction in the type of cyst involving the aryepiglottic fold. Aspiration should be repeated when obstructive symptoms recur, which may be two or three times in the early months of infancy and less frequently later. Resection through an external pharyngotomy or laryngotomy is rarely necessary. Incision and removal of the frayed edges usually suffice for infants having a ventricular cyst, although a tracheostomy may be required preliminarily.

Hemangiomas

The association of laryngeal obstruction with lymphangiomas and hemangiomas of the head and neck in infants presents a serious problem of diagnosis and treatment. When these processes involve the larynx by direct extension into the mucosa of the pharynx and larynx, a tracheostomy during the first few days of life indicates a situation in which the prognosis must be guarded. The condition appears to increase in severity until the sixth month is reached, when spontaneous regression usually begins. Tracheostomy is eventually necessary in the majority of infants in whom hemangiomas involve the larynx. Radiation is to be avoided if at all possible, but if laryngeal destruction accompanies the advancing hemangiomatous process, the administration of small amounts of x-ray therapy (600 to 800 r to the midlarynx) may be advisable. This may permit carrying the infant over the acute phase and should not be repeated. Infection must be adequately controlled and, if possible, the thyroid should be shielded.

Laryngeal Paralysis

Paralysis of the larynx in infants is rarely accorded the significance it deserves. In bilateral paralysis, obstruction is severe, both cords lying flaccid in the midline. The cry is clear, but respiratory obstruction is severe with a crowing, inspiratory stridor. A tracheostomy is almost always necessary, and the ultimate prognosis is poor. Mental retardation, cerebral birth injuries, meningoceles and hydrocephalus are often the neurologic lesions of which the laryngeal problem is only one aspect. Arytenoidectomy or transposition procedures are reserved for later in life when the larynx has increased in size sufficiently to make such procedures effective enough to permit extubation.

Unilateral paralysis is more common on the left than on the right and is frequently associated with congenital cardiovascular lesions. It should be identified preoperatively if surgery of a congenital heart or great vessel anomaly is to be done, because it is responsible for some of the more severe postsurgical respiratory problems in these infants. Occasionally it is a complication following cardiovascular surgery or operations for correction of an esophageal atresia and tracheoesophageal fistula, and increases the postoperative respiratory and swallowing difficulties. Right cord paralysis may be an isolated finding in an otherwise normal infant, but more frequently is seen in association with other neurologic defects such as pharyngeal or facial paralyses.

Tracheostomy is rarely necessary in unilateral left or right cord paralysis except to assist tracheobronchial aspiration in the postoperative period after some of the extensive procedures used to correct major anomalies of other systems. Thus the prognosis is dependent on the cause of the anomaly responsible for the paralysis. In unilateral paralysis the prognosis regarding voice is fair, since ultimately compensatory action of the unaffected cord is often adequate to provide a serviceable voice. In bilateral paralysis in infants the prognosis is usually poor because of the underlying extensive neurologic etiology.

TRAUMA

Both internal and external laryngeal trauma involve the infant and child's larynx. Self-induced are the *screamer's nodes* of children of all ages. Lack of discipline, emphasis on competitive sports and high noise levels against which children shout or scream result in vocal cord thickening with persistent hoarseness. Mirror examination of the larynx is often successful even in four- or five-year-olds, but if not, direct laryngoscopy must be made to be certain of the diagnosis. Voice correction therapy is helpful and usually adequate, calling attention of the child to his voice abuse. With therapists available in an increasing number of schools, teachers are becoming aware of this problem and are more discerning of it because the family has become accustomed to the abnormal voice: "He's always talked like that." If the nodules are unusually large and affect reading and recitation in class, direct laryngoscopy under general anesthesia and removal of the nodules with cup forceps are indicated. This should always be preceded and followed by voice therapy to ensure maximum benefit.

Flash *burns* of the larynx or *edema* associated with inhalation of hot gases or smoke in fires often requires a tracheostomy. Destruction of tissue, and obstruction by tracheobronchial serum exudates and products of infection make these the most difficult of tracheostomies to manage. Occasional bronchoscopic aspiration is indicated because of inspissation of charred bronchial exudates that act as major bronchi obstructions.

Fractures of the larynx incurred in sports or automobile accidents are increasingly numerous and require prompt correction. Children that play or are allowed to move about without restraints in the front seats of cars are most subject to these tragedies. In the event of collision or sudden braking, they incur multiple facial injuries as well as direct trauma to the larynx. Although a tracheostomy is lifesaving, the crushed larynx should be corrected promptly in a position of function through appropriate intralaryngeal splinting, just as fractures of legs and arms are reduced and splinted. Extubation cannot be done if the larynx heals with the cartilages completely crushed and distorted. Thus, in multiple-injury accidents necessitating tracheostomy, a careful evaluation of the degree of laryngeal involvement should be made as soon after the accident as practical. This includes x-ray studies and direct inspection. In the presence of laryngeal collapse, the insertion of appropriate intralaryngeal supporting polyethylene tubing or replacement of cartilage by open reduction is essential.

NEOPLASMS

Neoplasms of the larynx in infants are relatively rare with the exception of laryngeal *papillomatosis*. These are warty tumors usually originating on the vocal cords; they may grow rather rapidly to occlude the airway as multiple tiny tumors or more rarely as solitary pedunculated masses. They may extend onto the pharyngeal walls or grow downward into the trachea and bronchi; they require frequent removal and often a tracheostomy. Maintenance of the airway during anesthesia may be critical, and preliminary removal of a major obstructing papilloma without anesthesia may obviate a tracheostomy, the residual papilloma then being removed under general anesthesia after the airway has been established.

Repeated surgical removal with cup forceps is the most effective surgical treatment. Other forms of therapy, such as chemical or thermal cautery or x-ray treatment, should be avoided. X-ray therapy causes destruction of growth factors of the larynx and results in chronic laryngeal stenosis. Bovine papilloma vaccine has been used, but often produces sterile abscesses at the site of injection and has not been successful in eliminating the papilloma. An autogenous papilloma vaccine is under investigation. It has been effective in controlling or eliminating the recurrences in some, particularly during the course of its administration. A larger series and more time, however, will be required to evaluate its ultimate place in the management of this distressing condition.

Foreign Bodies in the Air and Food Passages

PAUL H. HOLINGER, M.D.

In a review of 3000 consecutive cases of foreign bodies in the air and food passages, 70 per cent were infants and children under 14 years of age; 10 per cent were infants under one year of age, 20 per cent were one to two years of age, 25 per cent were children two to four years of age (55 per cent under four years of age) and 15 per cent were between four and 14 years of age. In 33 per cent of the 3000 cases, the foreign bodies were in the tracheobronchial tree. Nuts and other vegetal material (dried beans, crisp bacon, popcorn, "flower" of an orange, raw carrots) were in approximately 15 per cent of infants and children who aspirated these materials that required endoscopic removal. From these percentages, it would seem obvious that the most important treatment would be to prevent the accident; i.e., in families with children under five years of age, nuts, nut candies, nut cookies and popcorn should not be in the house, and crisp bacon and raw carrots should not be included in the diet some pediatricians recommend.

Specific therapy consists of endoscopic investigation when the diagnosis is suspected or when symptoms or findings suggest tracheal or bronchial obstruction even though the history is not conclusive. Small caliber endoscopes should be used to keep laryngeal reaction at a minimum and to permit deep investigation of the small branch bronchi into which fragments of these vegetal foreign bodies descend. Newer techniques of anesthetics and "ventilation" bronchoscopes permit the use of general anesthetics with closed systems for respiration in older children. However, bronchoscopy without sedation or anesthesia is preferred in infants with acute respiratory obstruction due to the foreign body. Meperidine hydrochloride, 0.5 mg. per kilogram of body weight, is sufficient to permit good bronchoscopic working conditions with maximal safety for most problems involving peanuts in the under-three-years age group.

The degree of reaction to both the foreign body and the endoscopic procedure used to remove it depends on the age of the infant, the size of the bronchoscope, the duration of sojourn of the foreign body and the operating time necessary to remove it. If postoperative laryngeal edema is apparent, suspected or anticipated, the use of a high humidity tent is mandatory. If symptoms increase to necessitate oxygen, a tracheostomy must be considered. However, this is rarely needed if the operating time has been less than 15 minutes; it is better to discontinue the procedure if it takes longer and to wait four or five days for laryngeal reaction to subside rather than to prolong it and be forced to do a tracheostomy.

Twelve per cent of the objects removed from children in these age groups were metal objects, such as common pins, screws, nails, tacks, valve caps, pieces of wire, 22-caliber shells, pencil tops and other hardware. In general, these create less reaction in the trachea or larynx than do the vegetal foreign bodies. The mechanical problems created by their size, shape and location are best studied prior to removal if a duplicate of the object is available to the endoscopist, and the parents should be instructed to bring one, if possible, when the child is brought to the hospital. The use of the multiplane fluoroscope and the image intensifier has been of inestimable help in bronchoscopic removal of metallic foreign bodies.

In 56 per cent of the 3000 consecutive cases mentioned, the foreign bodies were removed from the esophagus. Most common in infants and children (17 per cent) were coins and discs (buttons, slugs, tokens, campaign pins) and safety pins (10 per cent). Although a few safety pins were in the bronchi or esophagus of adults, most were in infants less than 18 months of age. Again, treatment begins with prophylaxis: all safety pins should be closed – never left open in the bed or on a table. The most common site of lodgment is in the cervical esophagus, open, point up. The usual chest x-ray may be deceiving, suggesting that the pin could be removed with a hemostat and a tongue depressor. However, the point and keeper are in the pyriform sinuses and the spring well within the esophagus itself from which it is removed by careful rotation and extraction, point trailing. Failure to rotate it results in laceration of the lateral pharyngeal wall and possible perforation of the carotid artery. Other esophageal foreign bodies are items such as small toys, skate keys, can opener keys and meat lodged in a benign esophageal stenosis. The use of tenderizers to digest the meat has been suggested, but in occasional instances this has also digested the esophageal walls with a fatal result.

Treatment of these foreign bodies is endoscopic removal under direct vision.

Handling Foreign Body Problems. Some do's and don'ts regarding foreign bodies will answer many questions that arise most frequently in foreign body problems.

1. If signs and symptoms suggest the presence of a foreign body, do not accept the absence of a foreign-body history. The infant may have swallowed or aspirated the object in a brief moment during which he was unobserved.

2. Do not say, "Wait and see if it will pass," if symptoms have subsided after an initial episode of coughing and choking; this may be merely the symptomless interval phase of a dangerous foreign body problem.

3. Do not rely on the interpretation of a single film in establishing the presence or absence of a foreign body. Even though it is thought that a child has swallowed a coin, no metallic object may show on the film, but a film of the lateral view may reveal the tracheal compression caused by a button or a plastic disc in the cervical esophagus.

Aspirated Foreign Bodies. Do a physical examination of the chest; inspiration and expiration films are only confirmatory studies. The presence of a wheeze may precede positive x-ray findings.

Do not slap the child on the back. A peanut lodged in the bronchus will cause cough, wheezing and dyspnea. But if it is dislodged, though it may be expelled, it may also get caught in the larynx to cause immediate, total obstruction.

Swallowed Foreign Bodies. Obtain lateral roentgenograms of the neck, chest and abdomen in addition to the anteroposterior views.

Do not use barium or cotton soaked in barium. This complicates the subsequent attempt at removal, covering the field with a white paste and necessitating the removal of the strands of cotton from the original foreign body before it can be satisfactorily manipulated for extraction. If a radiopaque substance must be used, substitute Gastrografin or an iodized oil (Lipiodol, Iodochloral) for the barium.

Foreign Bodies in the Stomach and Intestines. Most foreign bodies pass spontaneously if they reach the stomach. Take films (anteroposterior and lateral views) for the record and repeat every third day to note progress. Do not conduct fluoroscopy repeatedly beyond x-ray tolerance.

Insist on a normal diet to allow the normal bowel contents to carry the foreign body onward. Do not give apomorphine to patients with gastric foreign bodies in an effort to expel the object by vomiting. The object may lodge in the esophagus or lacerate it upon return, necessitating endoscopic removal or surgical repair, whereas it will almost invariably pass by bowel if permitted to proceed without outside interference.

Consider bobby pins and needles in the stomach and duodenum as separate entities. In children under two years of age they should be removed at once, perorally by magnets.

Do not give cathartics, excess roughage or "paper, cotton and string" diets in an effort to aid the passage of an object through the intestinal tract. Such "diets" increase the likelihood of obstruction or perforation through mechanical block and increased peristalsis.

Laryngitis and Laryngotracheobronchitis

(The Croup Syndrome)

MARC O. BEEM, M.D.

Acute inflammations of the larynx and adjacent trachea are characterized by hoarseness and coughing, often associated with stridor and respiratory distress especially in children between one and three years of age. Infection is the most common cause of this condition, and of the infectious causes, the great majority are viral. Virtually any of the large number of viruses that infect the respiratory mucosa may involve the laryngotracheal segment with sufficient intensity to result in the croup syndrome. However, this is particularly true of the influenza and parainfluenza viruses as well as of the measles virus. Bacteria play a minor role as primary pathogens in acute respiratory illness in general, and the croup syndrome is no exception. In the unimmunized child, it is necessary to consider *Corynebacterium diphtheriae* as a possible cause of illness. Although hemolytic streptococci and *Hemophilus influenzae* are recognized as the major causes of acute epiglottitis, their role in inflammation of the glottis, subglottis and trachea is questionable. Acute epiglottitis differs from the croup syndrome in that it occurs in a somewhat older age group of children, there is dysphagia associated with the altered phonation and respiratory distress and an enlarged, inflamed epiglottis can be visualized. It is important that acute epiglottitis be differentiated from the croup syndrome, since the bacterial cause and frequently fulminant course of acute epiglottitis dictate immediate antimicrobial therapy (ampicillin, 100 to 150 mg. per kilogram per day intravenously) and early consideration of tracheostomy. However, that which is true of inflammation of the epiglottis does not hold for the glottis and subglottis and the routine administration of antimicrobial therapy to patients with croup is not indicated.

Respiratory mucosa damaged by viral infection is readily colonized by bacteria, but these do not ordinarily make a significant contribution to the illness and, again, this does not constitute a basis for the routine administration of antimicrobial therapy. In patients whose clinical condition is too critical to allow time for deliberate evaluation or who develop signs of significant bacterial superinfection, such as increased fever, polymorphonuclear leukocytosis or copious purulent sputum, ampicillin, 50 to 100 mg. per kilogram per day, may be administered by mouth or parenterally in four doses. If the clinical condition of the patient permits, antimicrobial therapy may be more precisely directed on the basis of bacteriologic culture and, where possible, examination of stained smears of sputum.

Acute inflammation of the larynx and adjacent trachea may produce respiratory obstruction that is due to inflammatory edema, laryngospasm and exudate. This is evidenced by inspiratory stridor and, as the degree of severity increases, suprasternal, costal and subcostal inspiratory retractions. Placing the child in a well-humidified atmosphere plays a central role in the treatment of this problem. This may be quickly accomplished in the bathroom by running hot water from the shower or faucet and, for longer periods, by using a steam vaporizer or cold nebulizer. The necessity of reaching the lower respiratory tract with particulate water has not been demonstrated, but it is clear that inspired air should be saturated with water vapor at body temperature. This degree of humidification cannot usually be achieved unless the output of the steamer or vaporizer is concentrated by tent or canopy about the head of the child. Parents should be given specific instructions about equipment and procedures to be used and, when steam devices are employed, about precautions to avoid accidental burns.

Ipecac may be useful in lessening respiratory obstruction that is predominantly due to laryngospasm. Care should be taken to prescribe syrup of ipecac (U.S.P.). This is given in subemetic doses of 1 drop per month of age up to two years, and 1 ml. per year of age in older children. Full effect may not be achieved unless vomiting occurs, and for the hour after administration of medication the child should be observed in order to avoid accidental aspiration. If relief has not been obtained and provided vomiting has not occurred, the dose may be repeated. Although administration of steroids has been advocated in some quarters, the true value of this is yet to be demonstrated and no particular regimen of steroid administration can be recommended. Anxiety and agitation accentuate the severity of evident respiratory obstruction, and management of children with croup should be planned to avoid unnecessary stimulation and disturbances. The general dictum that sedation should be used with great caution in children with respiratory distress holds in these cases. However, a single dose of chloral hydrate (10 mg. per kilogram) or paraldehyde (0.15 ml. per kilogram) may be useful, particularly in order to quiet the child so that baseline observations can be made on the extent of anatomic obstruction and the ability of the child to cope with it. Orders for continuing administration of sedatives are contraindicated.

The child with severe respiratory distress should be observed closely in a tent with an oxygen-driven nebulizer that provides maximum humidification and an ambient oxygen concentration of 35 to 40 per cent. Distress that is rapidly progressing in severity or that is so severe that the child is unable to rest may require intervention by intubation or tracheostomy to bypass the obstruction. The decision for such a procedure is optimally made before the child becomes agitated or cyanotic, since sudden cardiorespiratory arrest may occur under these conditions and there is a clear technical advantage to performing either intubation or tracheostomy as a deliberate procedure under optimum conditions.

Endotracheal intubation is a useful alternative to tracheostomy but may be technically difficult and is best performed by an experienced operator. Intubation for sufficient time to avoid the need for tracheostomy is possible if the tube used can be of large enough caliber to permit adequate suctioning of the lower airway and if it can be kept in place. As with tracheostomy, there are also complications of prolonged endotracheal intubation and the choice between these alternative procedures may depend on the particular preferences and skills of the available consultants. The nursing care requirements following either procedure are equally exacting and are beyond the scope of this discussion.

ACUTE BRONCHITIS

Although allergy and, less frequently, chemical and physical irritants occasionally play a primary or contributing role in acute bronchitis, most cases are due to infection with one of the numerous viruses that may involve the respiratory mucosa and affect, in varying degrees of severity, the entire respiratory tract. In the patient with acute bronchitis, there is particularly intense involvement of this portion of the respiratory tract. Bacteria act infrequently as primary pathogens in acute bronchitis. Infection due to *B. pertussis* may be suspected on clinical grounds, the diagnosis supported by the demonstration of lymphocytosis and isolation of the organism, and appropriate therapy given. Otherwise, routine or empirical antimicrobial therapy of acute bronchitis is not warranted. A wide variety of bacterial species may become implanted upon virus-damaged respiratory mucosa, including *H. influenzae, Streptococcus pneumoniae (Diplococcus pneumoniae), S. aureus* and numerous other species that may act as opportunistic pathogens. These most frequently represent colonists rather than invaders and, again, routine administration of antimicrobials has not been found to be helpful in abbreviating the course or severity of these infections. In cases where fever, leukocytosis or progressive course suggest bacterial superinfection, optimal antimicrobial therapy can be based only on appropriate bacteriologic studies. If given on an empirical basis, ampicillin, 50 to 100 mg. per kilogram per day in four doses, would be appropriate for the organisms most likely to be encountered.

The chief functional disorder in acute bronchitis is that of the mucus-producing, clearing and shielding actions of the tracheobronchial mucosa. Measures taken to support this also provide symptomatic relief, and they consist almost entirely of protection of the mucosa from air that is physically irritating and damaging. Coldness, dryness and a burden of dust or irritating chemical substances are common to winter air and adversely affect the inflamed mucosa. Counter measures to be taken during the acute phase of bronchitis include minimizing exposure to outside air and avoidance of strenuous exercise. It is desirable that ambient air be maximally humidified, although it is debatable whether it is necessary to provide moisture that will reach the lower respiratory tract in particulate form. Either a steam vaporizer or cold nebulizer can be employed. In the use of the former, it is important to take appropriate precautions against accidental burns, and with either apparatus, effectiveness often depends on construction of a hood or tent to concentrate the vapor output about the head of the patient.

Since secondary infection is promoted by retention of secretions in lower airways, coughing to clear this and variation of position should be encouraged. Relief of excessive coughing and maintenance of fluid mucous secretions are usually accomplished by the above measures. It is questionable whether cough medicines are of benefit beyond a possible placebo effect on parent and child, since increase in volume of lower respiratory secretions is not really desirable and successful suppression of the cough reflex can compromise clearing of the lower airways.

CHRONIC BRONCHITIS

It is doubtful that the entity of chronic bronchitis exists in childhood. In the child with such an infection, a careful search must be made for an underlying abnormality, such as cystic fibrosis, sinusitis, immunologic deficiency state or bronchiectasis, so that management appropriate to the underlying disorder may be instituted.

BRONCHIOLITIS

Acute bronchiolitis is a respiratory illness with clinical manifestations caused by inflammatory narrowing of the caliber of the small respiratory passages. It is a disease of early infancy; almost 90 per cent of patients are less than a year of age, and 75 per cent are less than six months of age. Although bronchiolar inflammation may be caused by a number of agents, noninfectious as well as infectious, most cases are infectious and the majority of these, in turn, are caused by viruses. Adenovirus and parainfluenza virus cause a minor portion of cases of bronchiolitis. Most cases, particularly those occurring in winter epidemics, are caused by the respiratory syncytial virus.

Infections with this respiratory virus occur in annual winter-spring epidemics. In the young, diffuse infection of the respiratory tract appears to be the rule. Although this may be manifest by nothing more than a cough and runny nose, symptomatic involvement of the lower respiratory tract is common. This involvement is seldom localized to the larynx and trachea (hence, the croup syndrome is infrequently encountered in respiratory syncytial virus infections) but usually extends diffusely into the bronchi and bronchioles. The ensuing disorder may be conceptualized as a function of the intensity of the inflammatory reaction and of the size of the respiratory passages. Where this relationship is such that the bronchiolar lumen remains patent though narrowed, the greater inspiratory than expiratory diameter of the bronchiole results in air-flow obstruction that is relatively greater on expiration than inspiration, and in the trapping of air in the alveoli. With complete obstruction of the lumen there is resorption of air from alveoli distal to this point. The resulting physical signs include those of air trapping and a spectrum of abnormal auscultatory findings present in all lung fields. Diminished breath sounds are heard where the air trapping is of a high degree and there is little respiratory exchange, prominent wheezes where this is less intense and medium to fine rales in areas where inspiratory effort brings air into passages and spaces previously collapsed. Thus, physical signs and x-ray findings may range from those of air trapping to bronchopneumonia and usually include elements of both.

Since bronchiolitis is a basically benign, self-limited viral respiratory infection, therapy is limited to supportive measures and the detection and treatment of complications.

Respiratory distress is the foremost problem encountered. The increase in rate and effort of respiration required to overcome the ventilatory handicap imposed by this disease may be fatiguing and inadequate to maintain normal oxygenation of the blood. Infants with respiratory rates over 50 per minute or those showing fatigue, irritability, unwillingness to eat or cyanosis should receive oxygen therapy. Ambient concentrations of 40 per cent will suffice in most instances, but some infants will require the maximum concentration attainable. Because oxygen therapy is the most important supportive measure available, close attention should be given to the details of administration in order to be certain the desired concentration is attained and provided without interruption. Maximum humidification of the oxygen is essential and can be assured by concomitant provision of cool mist. Very high concentrations of fine particles, such as exist when the output of ultrasonic nebulizers is confined in a small space, such as an Isolette, are to be avoided, since they may produce a volume and fluidity of lower respiratory secretions that a seriously ill infant handles with difficulty.

In addition to hypoxia, the most severely ill infants may have carbon dioxide retention. The resultant respiratory acidosis is usually accompanied by both dehydration and metabolic acidosis; the extent of dehydration and acidosis should be ascertained and appropriate fluid and electrolyte therapy given.

Although the cough may be a troublesome reminder of the infant's illness, therapy directed at this is best restricted to provision of a well-humidified atmosphere. Phenobarbital, 15 mg. twice a day, is sometimes helpful for the infant with paroxysmal coughing and vomiting. Frequent feedings of small quantities of formula or a maintenance sugar-electrolyte solution can achieve oral maintenance of fluid and electrolyte needs for the few days in which this is a major problem.

Because the basic pulmonary lesion is inflammatory in nature, bronchodilators are without effect. The infant with bronchospastic disease simulating bronchiolitis may be identified by his response to a test dose of aqueous adrenalin and treated accordingly. Otherwise, bronchodilators should be avoided.

Antimicrobial therapy is reserved for infants with a demonstrated bacterial complication or those in whom such a complication cannot reasonably be ruled out. Temperatures of 101° F. and leukocyte counts of 17,000 with 60 per cent of polymorphonuclear leukocytes may be encountered in uncomplicated bronchiolitis and should not in themselves be regarded as evidence of bacterial causation or superinfection in the infant who is not too ill to be followed expectantly. Infants with associated pneumonia or otitis media and those too ill to be followed expectantly may be given ampicillin, 100 mg. per kilogram per day parenterally in four divided doses, until bacteriologic information is available for deciding on more precise therapy.

Cardiac failure is difficult to rule out in the infant with a rapid pulse and liver enlarged to palpation, but decompensation of a normal heart need not be feared. When a cardiac abnormality is suspected or known to exist and the severity of illness calls for all supportive measures available, digitalization must be on empirical grounds, since the high intrathoracic pressure secondary to expiratory obstruction of the bronchioles renders heart size and peripheral venous pressure unreliable as indicators of cardiac function.

Although use of corticosteroids has been advocated, the balance of existing evidence indicates that they are neither helpful nor harmful. The severely ill infant who does not respond to these supportive measures will require close monitoring of blood gases. This may be greatly facilitated by the cannulation of a peripheral artery such as the radial artery. Muscular exhaustion, respiratory effort that does not produce appreciable air exchange, arterial pO_2 values below 40 mm. Hg and pCO_2 values above 60 mm. Hg and rising point to respiratory failure and the need for further intervention. This requires endotracheal intubation or tracheostomy to provide for suctioning of the lower airway and institution of assisted ventilation. The details of care required at this level are best achieved by experienced personnel in an infant intensive care unit and are beyond the scope of this discussion.

Disorders of the Lungs and Pleura

REYNALDO D. PAGTAKHAN, M.D., *and*
VICTOR CHERNICK, M.D.

The pathophysiology of most pulmonary disorders involves a maldistribution of air and blood within the lungs and an increase in the work of breathing. The cause may be increased pulmonary secretions (pneumonia, cystic fibrosis), increased bronchial smooth muscle tone (asthma), edematous bronchial mucosa (bronchiolitis), extrinsic compression of the lung (pneumothorax, pleural effusion) or actual destruction of lung parenchyma (neoplasm). All disorders of lungs and pleurae may be classified according to whether there is a defect in normal expansion or distensibility of the lung (restrictive disease) or obstruction to air flow through the respiratory passages (obstructive disease) (Tables 1 and 2). Both restrictive and obstructive disease may cause inefficient gas transfer in the lung. Inefficient gas transfer may also occur as a primary disorder, such as a diffusion defect or insufficient alveolar ventilation secondary to altered respiratory control (Table 3). With severe diffuse disease the work of breathing may become so excessive that respiratory failure ensues.

The basic aim of therapy is to decrease the work of breathing and to ensure that inspired air is distributed properly to all portions of the lung so that adequate gas exchange may take place between alveolar air and the pulmonary capillary blood. Treatment of the majority of pulmonary disorders involves efforts to ensure a patent airway and expanded pulmonary parenchyma, control of parenchymal infection and surgery (Table 4).

Adequate tracheobronchial hygiene includes the use of bronchodilators, such as isoproterenol or epinephrine, which decrease smooth muscle tone and increase bronchial diameter. Bronchodilation results in a decrease in the work of respiration and aids in the removal of pulmonary secretions. Bronchodilators may be administered directly into the lung with either a nebulizer or an intermittent positive pressure machine. Recently, the intravenous use of isoproterenol (0.1 to 1.5 microgram per kilogram per minute) has been advocated in patients with status asthmaticus.

TABLE 1. Some Causes of Obstructive Respiratory Disease

SITE OF DISTURBANCE	SPECIFIC DISEASE CONDITIONS	
	Newborn	*Infancy and Childhood*
A. Upper airway		
1. Anomalies	Choanal atresia, Pierre Robin syndrome, laryngeal web, vocal cord paralysis, tracheomalacia, vascular ring	Tracheal stenosis, vascular ring, laryngotracheomalacia
2. Aspiration	Meconium, mucus, vomitus	Foreign body, vomitus
3. Infection		Laryngotracheitis, diphtheria, epiglottitis
4. Tumors	Hemangioma, cystic hygroma, teratoma	Papilloma, hemangioma, lymphangioma
5. Allergic or reflex	Laryngospasm from local irritation (intubation) or tetany	Laryngospasm from local irritation (aspiration, intubation, drowning) or tetany, allergy
B. Lower airway		
1. Anomalies	Bronchostenosis, bronchomalacia, lobar emphysema, aberrant vessels	Bronchostenosis, lobar emphysema, aberrant vessels
2. Aspiration	Amniotic content, tracheoesophageal fistula, pharyngeal incoordination	Foreign body, vomitus, drowning
3. Infection	Pneumonia, pertussis	Bronchiolitis, pneumonia, tuberculosis (endobronchial, hilar adenopathy), cystic fibrosis
4. Tumors		Bronchogenic cyst, teratoma, atrial myxoma
5. Allergic or reflex		Bronchospasm (allergic or secondary to inhalation of noxious gases)

TABLE 2. Some Causes of Restrictive Respiratory Disease

SITE OF DISTURBANCE	SPECIFIC DISEASE CONDITIONS	
	Newborn	*Infancy and Childhood*
A. Parenchymal		
1. Anomalies	Agenesis, hypoplasia, lobar emphysema, congenital cyst, pulmonary sequestration	Hypoplasia, congenital cyst, pulmonary sequestration
2. Atelectasis	Hyaline membrane disease	Thick secretions (postoperative)
3. Infection	Pneumonia	Pneumonia, cystic fibrosis, bronchiectasis, pleural effusion, pneumatocele
4. Alveolar rupture	Pneumothorax	Pneumothorax
5. Others	Pulmonary hemorrhage, pulmonary edema, Wilson-Mikity syndrome	Pulmonary edema, lobectomy, chemical pneumonitis
B. Chest wall		
1. Muscular	Diaphragmatic hernia, eventration	Amyotonia congenita, poliomyelitis, diaphragmatic hernia, eventration, muscular dystrophy
2. Skeletal malformations	Hemivertebrae, absent ribs, thoracic dystrophy	Kyphoscoliosis, hemivertebrae, absent ribs
3. Others	Abdominal distentions	Obesity, flail chest

TABLE 3. Some Causes of Inefficient Gas Transfer

SITE OF DISTURBANCE	SPECIFIC DISEASE CONDITIONS
A. Pulmonary diffusion defect	
1. Increased diffusion path between alveoli and capillaries	Pulmonary edema, pulmonary fibrosis, collagen disorders, *Pneumocystis carinii*, sarcoidosis
2. Decreased alveolocapillary surface area	Pulmonary embolism, sarcoidosis, pulmonary hypertension, mitral stenosis, fibrosing alveolitis
3. Inadequate erythrocytes and hemoglobin	Anemia, hemorrhage
B. Respiratory center depression	
1. Increased cerebrospinal fluid pressure	Cerebral trauma, intracranial tumors, meningitis, encephalitis
2. Excess central nervous system depressant drugs	Maternal oversedation, overdosage with barbiturates or morphine
3. Excessive chemical changes in arterial blood	Severe asphyxia (hypercapnia, hypoxemia)
4. Toxic	Tetanus

TABLE 4. Principles of Treatment of Lung Disorders

A. Prevention
  1. Disodium cromoglycate (Intal)
  2. Hyposensitization

B. Supportive therapy to enhance removal of secretions and decrease work of breathing
  1. Bronchodilators
     Adrenergic drugs (subcutaneous, oral, intravenous, nebulizer, intermittent positive pressure breathing)
     Aminophylline (intravenous, oral)
  2. Reduction of sputum viscosity
     Water (adequate systemic fluids)
     Pancreatic deoxyribonuclease (Dornavac)
     N-acetylcysteine (10 per cent Mucomyst)
     Appropriate antibiotics (aerosol, systemic)
  3. Gravity
     Postural drainage and chest "cupping"
  4. Deep breathing and cough (avoid cough-depressing drugs)
  5. Aspiration
     Tracheal suction
     Thoracentesis
     Bronchoscopy
     Lung lavage
  6. Tracheostomy

C. Treatment of primary disease
  Surgery
  Antibiotics
  Bronchodilators
  Digitalis

D. Emergency treatment
  Ensure patent airway (suction, intubation, bronchoscopy, tracheostomy)
  Oxygen
  Assisted ventilation
  B and C above

Although adrenergic drugs decrease bronchial smooth muscle tone, other actions depend on the type of drug used and are important when deciding on the optimal agent for use in inhalation therapy. Beta-adrenergic drugs, such as isoproterenol, increase myocardial contractility and are peripheral vasodilators. Thus, isoproterenol is not the best agent for conditions in which airway diameter is compromised by edematous and inflamed mucous membranes, but has more favorable cardiovascular effects than the alpha-adrenergic drugs. Isoproterenol is the agent of choice for the relief of bronchospasm. Recently, two drugs have been studied which are more specific β_2 agonists and are reported to act specifically on bronchial smooth muscle—orciprenaline and salbutanol.

Primarily alpha-adrenergic drugs, such as epinephrine or ephedrine, increase cardiac rate and are peripheral vasoconstrictors. The judicious use of epinephrine or ephedrine to shrink mucous membranes (e.g., in bronchiolitis, sinobronchitis) appears to be more effective in decreasing airway resistance. Aqueous Adrenalin, 1:1000 given subcutaneously (0.01 ml. per kilogram up to a dose of 0.5 ml.), is usually effective in asthma. Aminophylline given intravenously (12 mg. per kilogram per day in three or four divided doses), is very effective, but may be dangerous when higher doses are given. Rectal administration of aminophylline is not advised because absorption via this route is unpredictable.

Adequate drainage of pulmonary secretions requires that the viscosity of sputum be minimized. The best way to do this is to ensure adequate hydration of the patient with either oral or intravenous fluids. The use of maximal humidity in the inspired air also prevents drying of secretions. Iodides and expectorants have been shown to be less effective than adequate hydration except when used in very high doses. Two enzymes have been used extensively to decrease sputum viscosity, deoxyribonuclease (Dornavac) and *N*-acetylcysteine (Mucomyst). They are effective in decreasing viscosity in vitro, but the efficacy of these drugs in vivo has been questioned.

The force of gravity is used to promote drainage from the lungs, and adequate physiotherapy with postural drainage and chest percussion to loosen secretions is widely used and recommended. Elevation of the foot of the bed 12 to 18 inches is important for promoting drainage throughout the night, particularly in children with bronchiectasis. This procedure may alleviate the hacking night cough of children with postnasal drip.

Spontaneous coughing clears the large airway of mucus, and cough-depressing drugs must be avoided. Frequent nasotracheal suction clears the larger airways of mucus, promotes coughing and enhances the movement of mucus from the smaller airways. When secretions are an overwhelming problem, bronchoscopy should be considered and may be effective when other measures have failed. Tracheal catheterization and tracheobronchial lavage have recently been advocated to help in the removal of secretions. Tracheostomy may be necessary when secretions become overwhelming or if prolonged artificial ventilation is required. Vigorous supportive therapy in conjunction with specific drug therapy constitutes the basis for management of most disorders of the lung. There are situations, such as congenital anomalies, tumors, bronchiectasis or pneumothorax, which may require surgical intervention.

Emergency therapy is required when ventilatory failure is present, that is, when the patient is incapable of maintaining reasonable arterial blood oxygen or carbon dioxide tensions. The tracheobronchial tree must be cleared of secretions as well as possible by oropharyngeal or endotracheal suction. Bronchoscopy may be necessary for more effective aspiration of secretions. Oropharyngeal or endotracheal intubation is frequently necessary in the comatose child or in the patient with severe respiratory disease. Oxygen must be used as required to prevent cyanosis, thereby ensuring an adequate supply for metabolic activity even in the premature infant. Assisted ventilation, accomplished by the physician or by a variety of machines, is used when the patient is unable to maintain normal arterial blood gas tensions. Some pharmacologic agents which are useful during cardiorespiratory resuscitation are listed in Table 5.

Most pulmonary problems in the pediatric age group are managed using the principles outlined in Table 4. However, it must be pointed out that rigid scientific evaluation of many of the supportive procedures advocated for pulmonary diseases has not been carried out.

Specific prevention of pulmonary disorders is of course the primary aim of the physician. With allergic disease, such as asthma, some contend that hyposensitization is effective in preventing or decreasing the frequency of attacks. Disodium cromoglycate has been shown to be very effective in preventing attacks in some patients with asthma and has allowed a decreased use of corticosteroids.

NEONATAL ATELECTASIS

Failure to expand the lung at birth may be caused by immaturity; hyaline membrane disease; oversedation from maternal medications such as morphine; asphyxia; intracranial hemorrhage; aspiration of meconium or amniotic debris; delayed absorption of pulmonary fluid; pneumothorax; or congenital anomalies obstructing the airway, such as cysts, diaphragmatic hernia or tracheoesophageal fistula. Later in the neonatal period atelectasis is usually caused by pneumonia or aspiration of feedings secondary to pharyngeal incoordination.

Congenital anomalies may require emergency surgical therapy. Nalline (0.2 mg. per kilogram intravenously) is a specific morphine antagonist.* When aspiration of meconium or amniotic fluid debris is suspected in the delivery room, laryngoscopy and tracheal suction should be performed to remove as much of the aspirate as possible. Once appropriate cultures have been taken, aspiration and neonatal pneumonia are treated with penicillin intramuscularly (25,000 units per kilogram every 12 hours) and kanamycin (5 mg. per kilogram every 12 hours). Pharyngeal incoordination at birth is usually transient and is successfully treated by gavage feeding for several days.

Because the other causes of neonatal atelectasis cannot be treated directly, therapy is expectant and supportive. Oxygen is the most useful agent but must be used cautiously. In

* Naloxone (Narcan) is available in some countries and is believed to be superior to nalorphine (Nalline).

TABLE 5. Pharmacologic Agents Useful in Cardiorespiratory Emergencies

AGENTS*	STOCK SOLUTION *Quantity Supplied (ml.)*	*Concentration Per ml.*	INITIAL INTRAVENOUS DOSE *Per Kilogram*	*Maximum Dose*	*Remarks*
Levallorphan tartrate (Lorfan)†	1	1 mg.	0.01–0.02 mg.	1 mg.	May repeat q. 5 min. for 2 more doses. May cause respiratory depression
Sodium bicarbonate, 7.5%	50	0.9 mEq.	2–5 mEq.‡	45 mEq.	May repeat q. 10–15 min.
Tris-hydroxymethyl-aminomethane (THAM, 0.3 M)	1000	0.3 mEq.	2–5 mEq.	45 mEq.	May cause respiratory depression
Aminophylline	10	25 mg.	3–4 mg.		Place in drip chamber and give over 15–20 min. May repeat once after 30 min.
Epinephrine (Adrenalin, 1:1000)	1	1 mg.	0.01–0.04 mg.‡	0.5 mg.	May repeat q. 5 min.§
Isoproterenol hydrochloride (Isuprel, 1:5000)	1	0.2 mg.	0.0005–0.0015 mg.‡	0.04 mg.	Best given as a continuous infusion‡
Lidocaine, 2% (Xylocaine)**	5	20 mg.	0.5–2 mg.	100 mg.	May repeat q. 10–30 min.
Procainamide hydrochloride (Pronestyl)	10	100 mg.	4–8 mg.		Give over 5 min. with continuous ECG and BP monitoring. Repeat q. 5 min.
Calcium chloride, 10%	10	100 mg.	15–30 mg.‡	1 Gm.	Maximum is 2 ml. min.
Calcium gluconate, 10%	10	100 mg.	15–30 mg.‡	1 Gm.	Repeat q. 30–60 min. in infants and every 3–6 min. in older children
Mannitol, 20% (Osmitrol)‖	500	200 mg.	0.5–1.5 Gm.		Monitor heart rate. Give over 1–3 hour period
Urea, 30% (Urevert)	300	300 mg.	1.0–1.5 Gm.		Give over 30 min. period
Glucose, 50%	50	500 mg.	0.1–1.0 Gm.		

* Agents are listed by generic names; common trade name is in parenthesis.

† Manufacturer's precaution: Lorfan is for use in treatment of significant narcotic-induced respiratory depression. Lorfan is *ineffective* against respiratory depression due to barbiturates, anesthetics and other non-narcotic agents or *pathologic* causes, and may increase respiratory depression in these instances.

‡ May also be given by intracardiac route.

§ A solution with a concentration of 0.002 to 0.004 mg. per ml. is used for continuous infusion. Adjust rate according to patient's response.

** Manufacturer's precaution: Experience with lidocaine (Xylocaine) in children is limited.

‖ Manufacturer's precaution: Use of mannitol in pediatric patients has not been studied comprehensively.

the premature infant, concentrations higher than 40 per cent should be used only as long as necessary to combat cyanosis because of the danger of retrolental fibroplasia. When possible, arterial pO_2 should be closely monitored by using the umbilical, temporal or radial artery as a sampling site. Moreover, high concentrations of inspired oxygen may directly damage the lungs. The maintenance of a "neutral" body temperature (anterior abdominal skin temperature of 97.5° F.) is important because metabolic demands for oxygen are lowest at this temperature.

Frequent samples of arterialized capillary blood for pH, pCO_2 and bicarbonate provide data regarding overall alveolar ventilation and acid-base balance. Metabolic acidosis may require bicarbonate therapy; assisted ventilation is required for severe respiratory failure.

PNEUMOTHORAX

Pneumothorax and pneumomediastinum are more common in the newborn period than at any other time in childhood, occurring in 1 to 2 per cent of live births. The most common cause is iatrogenic, secondary to overzealous resuscitative efforts by the physician. However, spontaneous pneumothorax is found in 0.05 to 1 per cent of live births and is associated with aspiration of meconium, mucus or blood at the time of delivery in the vigorous term or postmature infant. Lubchenco reported a high incidence of spontaneous pneumothorax in premature infants and found that the lower the birth weight, the later the onset. She postulated that aspiration of feedings was the most likely cause. The only other conditions commonly associated with a pneumothorax in childhood are pneumatocele or lung cyst following staphylococcal pneumonia and asthma.

The essential first steps in management are, of course, to suspect the condition clinically and to confirm the diagnosis radiologically.

In the absence of continued air leak, asymptomatic and mildly symptomatic patients with a small pneumothorax will respond to conservative therapy consisting of close observation in an incubator with adequate humidity, warmth and oxygen. Frequent small feedings are advisable to prevent gastric dilatation, which may further compromise ventilation, and to minimize crying, which could worsen the pneumothorax or contribute to further gastric dilatation. In such patients the pneumothorax will clear in 24 to 48 hours and no further treatment will be required.

It has been shown that breathing 100 per cent oxygen will hasten the resorption of any loculated air, including pneumothorax, and this therapy has been used in full-term infants who have only mild respiratory distress or pneumomediastinum in the absence of pneumothorax. Experiments in rabbits have shown a six-fold increase in the rate of absorption of a pneumothorax during 100 per cent oxygen breathing. This therapy is contraindicated in the preterm infant because of the risk of retrolental fibroplasia. Obviously it is of no value when there is a continued air leak into the pleural space.

Close observation and a frequent check of vital signs are mandatory. Any sudden change, characterized by increased tachypnea, retractions and cyanosis, may indicate the development of a tension pneumothorax (defined as a pneumothorax with a pressure above atmospheric pressure). An increase in pressure within the thorax will impede venous return to the heart (so-called air block) and must be relieved immediately. A 50-ml syringe with a three-way stopcock, and an 18-gauge needle should always be available. In order to relieve the pressure within the thorax, the infant should be propped up, the needle inserted into the pleural space through the second intercostal space in the midclavicular line and the air aspirated. We recommend that needle aspiration only be done in an emergency situation, since there is a hazard of producing a lung tear with the sharp edge of the needle. Rarely a pneumomediastinum will interfere with venous return to the heart and aspiration of the mediastinal space via the suprasternal notch may be required.

It must be emphasized that conservative therapy should be considered only in asymptomatic or mildly symptomatic patients. In more severely affected infants the safest procedure is the insertion of a chest tube (tube thoracostomy) in the second intercostal space in the midclavicular line using a trochar and cannula. Underwater drainage is mandatory in order to prevent air from being sucked into the chest during inspiration. In the presence of continued air leak, suction should be applied at −10 to −15 cm. H_2O. The suction may be discontinued when air stops bubbling from the chest; it is rarely required for more than 24 hours. The tube may be removed 24 hours after air leak ceases, following radiologic evidence of complete expansion of the lung.

CONGENITAL LOBAR EMPHYSEMA

Acute respiratory distress at birth may be caused by overdistention of one or more lobes of the lung, usually the right upper or right middle lobe. More commonly this condition presents as progressive respiratory distress over the first month or two of life.

The cause is usually obscure, but emphysema may be secondary to expiratory airway obstruction caused by absence of cartilage, bronchomalacia, enlarged mucosal folds, extrinsic vascular or lymph node compression, bronchial distortion from an anterior mediastinal lung hernia or retained secretions. Often the surgical specimen is not helpful in supplying a cause, so that a primary alveolar disease has been suggested by some authors. About 10 per cent of patients have associated congenital heart disease. Chest film shows a large hyperlucent area containing vague lung and bronchovascular markings, compression of adjacent lobes and a shift of the mediastinum into the opposite hemithorax. Rarely a mucus plug may be removed at bronchoscopy; however, thoracotomy must not be delayed when respiratory distress is severe. Lobectomy is the treatment of choice.

ABNORMAL PULMONARY VESSELS

The most common anomalies of the pulmonary circulation are pulmonary sequestration, accessory lobe, arteriovenous fistula and anomalous pulmonary venous return.

Pulmonary sequestration (intralobar) refers to a mass of embryonic, cystic pulmonary tissue that is surrounded by visceral pleura and is not in communication with the airway. The mass is supplied by one or more large vessels from the thoracic or abdominal aorta, and venous drainage is usually into a pulmonary vein. Sixty per cent occur on the left side, usually in the lower lobe. Associated anomalies are rare. Pulmonary sequestration may be asymptomatic, but more commonly symptoms arise from infection through a fistula between the sequestration and the airway or digestive tract. Accessory lobes (extralobar sequestration) can occur anywhere from the thoracic inlet to the upper abdomen. However, 90 per cent are found in the left side and characteristically lie between the diaphragm and the left lower lobe outside the visceral pleura. The mass is supplied by small systemic arteries with venous drainage into the azygous system. They are usually asymptomatic, but, rarely, communication with the trachea, bronchi, esophagus, stomach or small bowel gives rise to symptoms. Associated pleuroperitoneal hernias are common. Infection should be treated with appropriate antibiotics, and the sequestration should be surgically excised.

Pulmonary arteriovenous fistula is a cavernous communication between the pulmonary artery and vein, producing a right-to-left shunt, and resulting in a decrease in arterial oxygen tension. Large shunts may result in cyanosis, polycythemia, dyspnea, clubbing of fingers and toes, hemoptysis or high output cardiac failure. Half the patients have generalized telangiectasis, often of the familial Osler-Weber-Rendu variety. The fistula is usually hilar or subpleural and contains numerous communications between the artery and vein. It occurs in the lower lobe in 60 per cent of cases; it is single in 65 per cent and unilateral in 75 per cent of cases.

Without treatment there are serious complications, including sudden exsanguination from a hemothorax or hemoptysis, subacute bacterial endocarditis and septicemia and brain abscess, and embolism or thrombosis secondary to the polycythemia. Thus, surgical treatment is recommended, and excisional therapy should be attempted with localized disease. Unfortunately, the removal of one lesion may be followed by the appearance of another lesion which may be ipsilateral or contralateral. Accordingly, Bosher *et al.* feel that maximum preservation of functioning lung tissue is important and have described a technique of local excision in a bloodless field in preference to segmental resection or lobectomy. When excision is impractical, in order to reduce the size of the shunt, ligation and division of as many individual arterial and venous branches as possible may be done under tourniquet control of the ipsilateral pulmonary artery.

LUNG CYSTS

True congenital lung cysts are rare and often difficult to distinguish from acquired cysts. A congenital cause is obvious only when cysts are found in the stillborn or newborn infant, because even the histologic finding of a ciliated columnar epithelial lining is not certain proof of a congenital origin. There are two types of congenital lung cysts: bronchogenic and pulmonary.

The majority of bronchogenic cysts are paratracheal, carinal, hilar or paraesophageal. Therapy is surgical excision.

A more common location for congenital cysts of the lungs is in the lung periphery and probably represents a disorder of bronchial growth that occurred at a later stage in fetal life than did the more central bronchogenic cysts. Needle aspiration of the tension cyst may be required as an emergency procedure. Treatment is surgical excision or resection.

Congenital cystic adenomatoid malformation of the lung is a rare variant of congenital pulmonary cysts, usually affecting premature infants with anasarca and hydramnios. Treatment is surgical excision.

The Wilson-Mikity syndrome, or pulmonary dysmaturity, is found in premature infants. The chief feature clinically is the persistent cyanosis requiring increased inspired oxygen concentrations, usually in the range of 25 to 35 per cent. Treatment is symptomatic. This condition should not be confused with bronchopulmonary dysplasia, which is caused by oxygen toxicity.

Acquired postpneumonic lung cysts or pneumatoceles are more common than congenital cysts and are found in about 10 per cent of patients with *Staphylococcus aureus* pneumonia, particularly in the first six months of life. Occasionally pneumatoceles follow pneumococcal, *Escherichia coli* or streptococcal pneumonia. The vast majority regress completely and should therefore be followed for several months before surgery is considered. Occasionally a pneumatocele will become infected, contain pus and require drainage or excision.

ASPIRATION PNEUMONIA

The aspiration of foreign substances into

the tracheobronchial tree will result in variable severity of clinical illness depending on the nature and the amount of the substance aspirated. The nature of the aspirated material in the newborn and early infancy period differs from that in the older child.

Neonatal Aspiration Pneumonia. In the neonatal period, aspiration pneumonias are usually due to the inhalation of amniotic fluid debris, including meconium or substances introduced into the respiratory tract through congenital abnormalities. Premature infants often regurgitate and aspirate feedings.

Treatment of *meconium aspiration* should begin in the delivery room. Usually the infants show signs of asphyxia and require resuscitation. Debris should be aspirated from the mouth and pharynx quickly and suction of the large airways performed via an endotracheal tube. In massive aspiration, 1 ml. of sterile saline should be injected into the endotracheal tube followed by further suction in an attempt to remove more debris. Further therapy is supportive. Metabolic acidosis is common and should be treated with sodium bicarbonate (see Table 4). Humidified warmed oxygen must be supplied in an appropriate concentration to correct arterial hypoxemia. Since meconium provides an ideal culture medium for *E. coli,* most authorities use prophylactic antibiotics. Although steroids have been advocated by some, there is no evidence of their efficacy in this condition. In addition, the use of steroids in the face of a possible bacterial infection may be hazardous. The aspiration may be so massive that respiratory failure ensues, requiring emergency artificial ventilation. Prospects for survival following massive meconium aspiration are poor.

Treatment of *tracheoesophageal fistula* will not be considered in detail here. The child must not be given oral feedings once the diagnosis has been established. He should be given intravenous fluids and other supportive therapy. Surgery is performed once the child is in optimal condition.

Aspiration of glucose water or milk may occur during the first few feedings in full-term infants and is a common complication in premature infants. Therapy, once again, is supportive. The role of steroids has not been proven unless acid gastric juice has been aspirated. In this situation, prednisone, 1 mg. per kilogram per day given in three divided doses, should be used. There is good evidence that sterile water is far less damaging to the lungs than is 5 per cent glucose water or saline, and perhaps first feedings should be sterile water.

Lipoid Pneumonia. Lipoid pneumonia may follow the inhalation of oily or fatty substances, such as cod liver oil, mineral oil, oily nose drops, castor oil and milk.

The optimal treatment is prevention. Educational programs in the community should point out the dangers of using these various substances. Once aspirated, the offending preparation should be withheld or used with the greatest care in order to prevent further reaction.

There is no specific therapy for lipoid pneumonia, although the use of steroids has been suggested. To date, no controlled studies of treatment with steroids have been reported.

Supportive therapy for this chronic condition is aimed at preventing intercurrent infections.

Hydrocarbon Aspiration Pneumonia. The ingestion of a hydrocarbon (e.g., gasoline, kerosene, furniture polish, lighter and cleaning fluids and certain insect sprays) is usually accompanied by its inhalation, thereby causing chemical pneumonitis. Treatment starts as soon as ingestion of hydrocarbon is detected. Usually some of the substance has already been inhaled, and immediate effort is made to prevent further aspiration.

Lavage is contraindicated unless large amounts of the substance have been ingested or the child is vomiting repeatedly. When performed, it should be done with the utmost care, because it may be associated with further aspiration and worsening of the pulmonary symptoms.

The child should be given saline cathartics. Mineral oil and olive oil have also been given to prevent absorption, although some researchers feel that mineral oil promotes rather than prevents absorption.

Of the children who ingest hydrocarbons, approximately 40 per cent develop significant pulmonary signs and symptoms. These children should receive humidified oxygen if the pulmonary reaction is so severe that dyspnea occurs. In patients with severe dyspnea, intermittent positive pressure therapy may be helpful. Bronchodilators, such as epinephrine 1:100 or isoproterenol 1:200, may be given with the nebulization, or, at times, epinephrine, 1:1000 (0.2 ml.), may be injected intramuscularly. Parenteral fluids should be given. If a secondary infection occurs, antibiotics are indicated.

In severely affected patients, many authorities recommend the use of corticosteroids to reduce spasm and inflammation of the bronchial tree. Prednisone may be given, 1 mg. per kilogram daily, divided into three doses. However, the efficacy of steroids has not been established.

MIDDLE LOBE SYNDROME

Brock has pointed out that the right middle lobe is particularly vulnerable to atelectasis because the right middle lobe bronchus is short, of small caliber and branches from the right main bronchus at an acute angle. Furthermore, the bronchus is surrounded by a cuff of lymph nodes which drains the upper and lower lobes, so that it is particularly subject to extrinsic compression by enlargement of these nodes.

Graham et al., in 1948, were the first to coin the term "middle lobe syndrome" to describe 12 adult patients who presented with an acute or insidious onset of hemoptysis and recurrent episodes of pulmonary infection. All had irreversible atelectasis and fibrosis of the right middle lobe due to chronic nonspecific lymphadenitis of the lobar lymph nodes. More recently many authors have extended the term "middle lobe syndrome" to apply to acute reversible atelectasis of the right middle lobe secondary to extrinsic compression by lymph nodes from any cause (tuberculosis, measles, pertussis, pneumonia, nonspecific).

Clinically, the adult and childhood diseases are similar, with the exception that hemoptysis is rare in the child. Treatment of right middle lobe atelectasis consists of vigorous supportive therapy and appropriate antibiotics (Table 4). If atelectasis persists at the end of four to six weeks, bronchoscopy and bronchography are advised. Bronchostenosis or bronchiectasis in the right middle lobe or nonfilling of the bronchus after selective injection warrants a middle lobectomy. In contrast, a normal bronchogram (except for the collapse) indicates less severe parenchymal disease and warrants further medical management. Lobectomy may be considered when atelectasis persists for 12 to 18 months despite vigorous medical management, including bronchoscopy. However, we have followed patients with atelectasis for longer periods of time and have documented reexpansion of the lobe.

BRONCHIECTASIS

Bronchiectasis is a condition in which there is chronic dilatation of one or more bronchi in varying form, degree and distribution. Cylindrical (fusiform, tubular) bronchiectasis is characterized by minimal and uniform dilatation of the larger bronchi. Irregular dilatation of the bronchi ending in a bulbous, distorted termination at about the fourth bronchial division is termed varicose bronchiectasis. When the dilatation increases progressively toward the periphery and ends in a cystic space, the type is known as saccular (cystic, globular).

The prevalence of bronchiectasis in childhood is most likely related to the smaller size of the airways and the greater tendency to obstruction by mucosal edema, secretions or enlarged lymph nodes. The sequence of events is one of obstruction, retention of secretions with a concomitant increase in intraluminal pressure, followed by infection which impairs bronchial muscle tone. Since the transluminal pressure is increased, bronchial dilatation occurs. With severe infection there is destruction of the elastic lamina, bronchial muscle and cartilage, so that when destruction is complete, the dilatation becomes cystic in nature. Destruction of the bronchi may be focal in nature. Histologically, however, the disease is usually more widespread than the bronchogram indicates.

Drainage of secretions from the lungs and vigorous control of infection are the mainstay of medical therapy. Postural drainage with chest pummeling should be performed several times daily. Continuous postural drainage of the affected area at night is likewise important. Since bronchiectasis frequently involves the lower lobes, the Trendelenburg or jack-knife position is commonly used to promote drainage during sleep. A member of the household should be taught chest physiotherapy, so that adequate treatment can be maintained. Moreover, continuous supervision by the physiotherapist is necessary to ensure that postural drainage is being properly carried out.

Bronchodilators, such as isoproterenol and epinephrine, relieve bronchospasm and thereby promote drainage. Drainage is further facilitated by thinning out the secretions. The most effective means of decreasing the viscosity of the sputum is to maintain an adequate oral intake of fluid. Bronchoscopy is indicated for the removal of extremely viscid secretions, or endobronchial granulation tissue.

During periods of acute infection, antibiotic therapy is guided by the results of the sputum culture. In patients who suffer from repeated episodes of acute infection, prophylactic antibiotics have been suggested on the basis of the clinical impression that they produce improvement. There has been no scientific documentation of the efficacy of prophylactic antibiotic in bronchiectasis. Favorable response to medical management is characterized by change in the character of sputum, the reduction of sputum volume and the relief of constitutional symptoms. Since the efficacy of medical management is unrelated to the degree of bronchiectasis, all patients should have a trial of conservative therapy. Medical management is a lifelong therapy and requires close supervision.

Surgical management must be considered under the following circumstances: (1) Failure of an adequate trial of conservative therapy, in which case resection of the most involved area may be done. (2) Recurrent, life-threatening hemoptysis. (3) Persistent symptoms with the bronchiectatic lesion localized to one segment or lobe. Another consideration for surgical resection may be the availability of health care facilities. Thus, surgical resection of a localized lesion may make it possible for an Eskimo or Indian child to return to his natural family and cultural environment sooner than if the child is required to remain in the vicinity of a large health care facility for medical management. It must be emphasized that surgical management should not be contemplated prior to careful observation and evaluation of the individual child and until an adequate course of medical management has been attempted.

Bronchiectasis should be a preventable disorder in children if close attention is paid to proper reaeration of lung tissue following pneumonia and if infection is promptly controlled by appropriate antibiotics. Foreign bodies should be removed promptly and postural drainage of the chest should be instituted to enhance removal of secretions. Similarly, the prevention of atelectasis in postoperative patients by deep breathing and coughing, along with the prompt control of infection, has virtually eradicated bronchiectasis as a complication of surgery.

ATELECTASIS

In older children, collapse or imperfect expansion of a lobe or lobes of the lung occurs usually secondary to bronchial or bronchiolar obstruction (obstructive type), but may also occur in the absence of demonstrable mechanical obstruction of the airways (nonobstructive type). Roentgenograms of the chest in both lateral and posteroanterior views are the most valuable diagnostic tools; however, differentiation between the two types is difficult. Clinical information is the most useful method of differentiating obstructive and nonobstructive atelectasis.

Irrespective of type, a segment that remains atelectatic is predisposed to insufficient drainage of secretions, infection and bronchial wall damage. Direct endotracheal suction may be necessary to facilitate drainage of secretions. Acute collapse of a significant portion of the lung can severely impair alveolar ventilation, thereby resulting in respiratory acidosis and hypoxemia.

In most respects, management of obstructive and nonobstructive atelectasis does not differ. The basic principles of therapy lie in removing obstruction or, when no obstruction is present, in assisting lung expansion by mechanical means. Thus, a foreign body must be removed promptly by bronchoscopy and infection must be controlled with appropriate antibiotics. Drainage of secretions and airway patency must be promoted with deep breathing and coughing, postural positioning and bronchodilators. Some have suggested the use of tube breathing, which increases dead space about three times normal and thereby stimulates deep respiration.

No categorical statement can be made regarding the length of time a lobe or segment should remain collapsed before surgery is planned. We have seen collapsed lungs reexpand after four years of intensive medical management.

EMPHYSEMA AND HYPERAERATION

Emphysema refers to a structural change in the lung and involves disruption of alveolar walls, resulting in the formation of multiple cystic spaces within the lung. The cysts may be centrilobular or panacinar. In some adults with emphysema there is an associated deficiency of circulating alpha-l-antitrypsin, and an autosomal recessive inheritance has been demonstrated. Alpha-l-antitrypsin–deficiency causing emphysema in childhood is extremely rare and more commonly has been associated with cirrhosis. Congenital lobar emphysema has been discussed earlier in this chapter.

In contrast, alveolar overdistention and hyperaeration on the chest film is commonly seen. The disorder can occur spontaneously in an otherwise normal lobe (or lobes) as a compensatory mechanism for loss of lung volume in adjacent areas (e.g., from atelectasis, agenesis, pneumonectomy). It may have an iatrogenic cause (e.g., injudicious positive pressure resuscitation) or may occur as a complication of, or in association with, ball-valve obstruction of the airways, anomalies of the great vessels or by a variety of bronchial and parenchymal disorders (e.g., congenital, aspiration, bronchospasm, bronchial edema, cystic fibrosis, retained secretions, tumors, right aortic arch with ventricular septal defect).

The timing and type of therapy depend on

the degree of respiratory difficulty resulting from compression of the normally functioning lung by the overdistended lobe or segment. Therapy varies according to the nature of the obstructing and nonobstructing mechanisms. Thus, when the patient is asymptomatic and the overaeration is limited to a lobe or portion of the lungs, as in agenesis or following lobectomy, no treatment is indicated. The presence of an adjacent lobar atelectasis requires specific therapy. Measures which reexpand the collapsed segments allow for return to normal of the overdistended segments. Treatment of localized overdistention, such as occurs secondary to bronchial obstruction caused by abnormal vessels, requires interruption of the obstructing vascular channels. Congenital lobar emphysema causing respiratory difficulty in a child requires immediate surgery. When a foreign body is suspected, direct bronchoscopic aspiration must be done.

The most common cause of overdistention and hyperaeration of the lung in childhood occurs with generalized expiratory airway obstruction disease, such as asthma or bronchiolitis. Therapy is directed at the underlying cause and includes adequate hydration and bronchodilators, physiotherapy and treatment of infection.

PULMONARY HEMOSIDEROSIS

Abnormal accumulation of hemosiderin in the lungs can occur as a primary lung disorder or secondary to cardiac or systemic vascular disease. Primary pulmonary hemosiderosis is the type more commonly encountered during childhood. Clinically, the patient suffers from recurrent episodes of respiratory distress, hemoptysis or hematemesis, pulmonary infiltrates and iron deficiency anemia. Roentgenograms of the chest usually reveal multiple fine densities with a patchy distribution which tends to change with time. Prussian-blue staining of a sputum specimen or of gastric or bronchial washings sediment may demonstrate hemosiderin-laden macrophages. Needle biopsy of the lung provides the most accurate method of diagnosis.

Since the fundamental cause of recurrent alveolar hemorrhages is unknown and the natural clinical history of the disorder is variable, therapy has mainly been empirical. In general, the prognosis is poor. During an episode of acute bleeding, the patient is maintained on intravenous fluids and nothing is given by mouth for 24 to 48 hours. Whole-blood transfusion is indicated to combat shock or severe anemia. Oxygen is given, sometimes by intermittent positive pressure machine, which in itself may hasten the cessation of bleeding. ACTH (adrenocorticotropic hormone), 10 to 25 units, or hydrocortisone in the dose of 4 mg. per kilogram per day is given intravenously for the first day or two. Later, when oral feeding can be started, usually two days after the onset of the acute episode, prednisone in the dose of 2 mg. per kilogram per day is administered by mouth. It must be emphasized that the minimum suppressive dose is given and this must be continued for at least three months. The dose may have to be increased or restarted if relapse occurs. Although steroids are advised, scientific proof of their value is lacking.

Since relapse remains a continuing danger, long-term follow-up is mandatory. Allergy to milk and milk products has been suggested by some as a cause of this condition and removal of milk from the diet has been used in some patients. However, the efficacy of this mode of therapy has not been proven. At best, it has found usefulness only in small infants.

Persistence of pulmonary symptoms or roentgenographic abnormalities may warrant use of the iron-chelating drug deferoxamine. The drug may be given intramuscularly, 25 mg. per kilogram per day divided in doses given every 8 hours. It is essential that urinary iron excretion be followed daily to gauge the effect of this therapy. Urinary iron excretion greater than 3 to 4 mg. per 100 Gm. of deferoxamine given, or 8 to 10 mg. per day, indicates removal of excessively accumulated iron.

Management of pulmonary hemosiderosis secondary to or associated with cardiac or renal dysfunction is basically the same. In addition, the primary cause must be treated. Thus, in the presence of congestive heart failure, digoxin and other anticongestive measures must be given.

PULMONARY EMBOLISM AND INFARCTION

Management of this disorder in infants and children, in whom the condition is exceedingly rare, is essentially based on the prevention of vascular stasis. Thus, severe dehydration must be avoided and treated promptly in diarrheal disease, cyanotic congenital heart disease, bacterial endocarditis and longstanding nutritional deficiencies. Emboli usually arise from the deep femoral and pelvic veins and are usually encountered following surgery. Fat emboli are most likely to be derived from compound fractures. Although the mortality is high, recovery is not necessarily related to the degree of parenchymal infarction. Morphine in the dose of 0.15 mg. per kilogram is given to allay fear and anxiety. The child must be placed in an oxygen tent for the relief of dyspnea and cyanosis. Although the administration of streptokinase and heparin has been associated with favorable results in adults, experience with these drugs in the pediatric patient is limited.

PULMONARY EDEMA

The child who develops pulmonary edema is usually very pale and cyanotic. Whether the onset is gradual or abrupt, respiratory distress is progressive and cough is productive of frothy, pink sputum. Cold sweats, audible wheezes, bubbling rales, tachycardia and an anxious appearance are evident. These clinical manifestations reflect the excessive accumulations of serous or serosanguinous fluid which has escaped from the pulmonary capillaries into the alveoli, bronchioles and bronchi.

Fundamentally, edema fluid accumulates in the lungs whenever pulmonary capillary transudation exceeds fluid clearance by the airways or lymphatic channels. A variety of causes can induce this disturbance. Thus, factors which increase resistance to the outflow of blood from the lungs (e.g., obstruction in the left side of the heart as in mitral stenosis), or factors which suddenly increase venous return (e.g., rapid or excessive intravenous infusion of fluids or blood), or both (e.g., adrenalin overdose), may result in a rapid extravasation of fluid into lung units due to the elevation of capillary hydrostatic pressure above that of the colloid osmotic pressure. The hydrostatic-osmotic pressure relationship may also be disturbed by a reduction in the osmotic pressure, as in acute nephritis or whenever serum protein concentration is acutely lowered (e.g., dilutional hypoproteinemia secondary to rapid intravenous infusion of fluids). Transudation of fluid may also result from capillary dilatation or increased permeability of capillary walls due to infections (e.g., pneumonia), asphyxia or chemical irritants (e.g., inhalation of chlorine gas, acid fumes, hydrocarbon and smoke). Interference with lymphatic drainage (e.g., congestive heart failure) or severe airway obstruction (e.g., severe bronchospasm) may also elicit or aggravate pulmonary edema by retarding or obstructing clearance of lung fluid from the terminal lung units.

Pulmonary edema results in a decrease in the lung compliance and a fall in vital capacity. The resistance to air flow is increased, and the work of breathing becomes exceedingly hard. Hypoxemia ensues and may be very severe because of venous-admixture-like perfusion. On the other hand, arterial carbon dioxide tension is usually below normal because of the hyperventilation induced by hypoxemia.

The therapeutic goals are two-fold: (1) relief of the functional disturbances and (2) reduction of capillary transudation by maintaining the hydrostatic-osmotic pressure relationship or facilitation of lymphatic or airway drainage. Inhalation of 100 per cent humidified oxygen delivered by mask and bag is started immediately, while aspiration of airway secretions, establishment of an intravenous route and monitoring of cardiovascular status and blood gas tensions are underway. Bubbling of oxygen through 50 per cent ethyl alcohol has been advised by some in order to disrupt the foamy secretions. Morphine decreases peripheral and pulmonary vascular resistance, allays anxiety and reduces the tachypnea. It is given in doses of 0.1 to 0.2 mg. per kilogram, and must be administered cautiously to patients with chronic lung disease. Venous return may also be reduced by placing the patient in a semirecumbent position. Tourniquets or blood pressure cuffs (inflated to a pressure between diastolic and systolic), applied to three extremities and rotated every 15 minutes, also lower blood return to the right side of the heart. Aminophylline decreases bronchospasm and increases cardiac output. It is given intravenously in doses of 3 to 4 mg. per kilogram over a 20- to 30-minute period. Unless dramatic improvement in oxygenation occurs, oxygen delivery has to be assisted by intermittent positive pressure ventilation (IPPV). IPPV also tends to reduce venous return.

Further therapeutic measures are aimed at controlling the primary disease process which precipitated the pulmonary edema. Rapid parenteral digitalization is indicated in the presence of congestive heart failure. Digoxin, 0.05 mg. per kilogram, is given in 24 hours; one-half of the total dose is given immediately; 25 per cent of the total dose is given 8 hours later and 25 per cent is given 16 hours later. Daily maintenance dosage is 20 per cent of the total digitalizing dose and is given in two divided doses. It is essential that electrocardiographic tracings be done before digitalization and that further dosage be guided by both clinical and electrocardiographic data. Ethacrynic acid* (1.0 mg.

* Manufacturer's precaution: Until further experience with ethacrynic acid is accumulated, therapy with oral and parenteral forms is contraindicated in infants.

per kilogram) or furosemide† (1.0 mg. per kilogram) will promote a prompt diuresis. Diuretic therapy has also been useful as an adjunct in the therapy of hypertension. More severe hypertension is best controlled by reserpine (0.07 mg. per kilogram per day) and/or hydralazine (0.15 mg. per kilogram per day). In the twin transfusion syndrome of the newborn or in a situation where lung edema results from excessive administration of parenteral fluids, phlebotomy can be lifesaving. In the former situation, removal of about 10 per cent of the blood volume is indicated. In the situation where the blood volume is expanded by an increase in plasma volume alone, exchange transfusion is indicated.

Pulmonary edema induced by epinephrine overdose has been reported to respond to phenoxybenzamine and chlorpromazine,‡ which are alpha-adrenergic antagonists. Phenoxybenzamine (1 to 3 mg. per kilogram) or chlorpromazine (0.5 to 1 mg. per kilogram) is given intravenously, and the dose is titrated according to the blood pressure response. Postoperative lung edema which occurs following a right pulmonary artery and ascending aorta anastomosis may require reoperation to decrease the size of the shunt or possible vascular obstruction. Massive doses of steroids (e.g., hydrocortisone, 5 to 8 mg. per kilogram every 8 hours for 72 hours) have been found useful in the resolution of pulmonary edema secondary to irritants (e.g., smoke inhalation).

PLEURAL DISEASE

The pleural cavity, normally only a potential space, may accumulate fluid or gas or both. Pleural effusion and pneumothorax constitute the most common disorders of the pleurae. Pneumothorax has already been discussed in an earlier section.

Pleural effusion is usually secondary to an underlying disease process located outside the pleurae. Whatever the initiating cause, there results an imbalance between extravasation of fluids from the pulmonary capillaries and reabsorption by venules and lymphatics in the pleural layers. Pleural transudation can occur as a consequence of an imbalance in the capillary hydrostatic-osmotic pressure relationship (e.g., congestive heart failure, vena caval obstruction, hypoproteinemia). Under these circumstances, the pleural fluid is a transudate (protein content less than 3 per cent; specific gravity less than 1.015; few cells, chiefly lymphocytes) and is termed hydrothorax (noninflammatory reaction).

In contrast, pleural transudation resulting from actual damage of the capillary walls or from interference with lymph drainage has been induced by an inflammatory or a neoplastic process. Early in the inflammatory process, fluid accumulation is minimal and chest pain dominates the symptomatology. Later, serous exudate accumulates. When the fluid becomes purulent (empyema) the patient is septic and chest pain is usually minimal.

Accumulation of blood in the pleural cavity (hemothorax) may occur secondary to (1) a penetrating injury of the chest wall with tearing of intercostal arteries; (2) spontaneous rupture of a subpleural bleb, tearing of a pleural adhesion or rupture of an aortic aneurysm; and (3) certain hemorrhagic disorders. Another form of noninflammatory intrapleural fluid accumulation is that of chylothorax. Leakage of chyle from the thoracic duct or its tributaries into the pleural space may result from (1) obstruction of the thoracic duct and its branches or of the left subclavian vein (e.g., mediastinal lymphadenopathy, neoplasm); (2) trauma to the chest wall (penetrating or nonpenetrating wound, accidental injury during thoracic surgery); or (3) a rare spontaneous occurrence in newborn infants. The chyle usually first accumulates in the mediastinum before rupturing into the pleural cavity. The milky white, opalescent fluid is diagnostic but is not present in the newborn infant before milk feeding has been started.

Significant accumulation of pleural fluid is associated with a reduced vital capacity and mismatching of ventilation and perfusion in the lung. The rate and amount of fluid accumulation determines the severity of the functional disturbance and, thus, the therapeutic approach.

Therapy is aimed at controlling the primary disease process and is supplemented by general supportive measures. Therefore, in the presence of respiratory distress, high concentrations of oxygen are given and evacuation of fluid is performed to relieve the restriction of lung expansion. Thoracentesis, in addition to being a therapeutic procedure, also helps in arriving at a more definitive diagnosis. The fluid obtained is stained for bacteria and cell morphology, examined for protein content and specific gravity and sent for culture.

Usually in the group of conditions causing hydrothorax, the pleurae are basically healthy and absorption of pleural effusion is very rapid

† Manufacturer's precaution: Furosemide should not be given to children until further experience is accumulated.

‡ Manufacturer's precaution: Chlorpromazine is not recommended for children under six months of age except when lifesaving.

once the initiating disorder is brought under control. Diuretics (e.g., furosemide, 1 mg. per kilogram intravenously) hasten the resolution of effusion and may be added to digitalization in the presence of congestive heart failure. When the cause is an intrathoracic obstruction (e.g., hilar adenopathy, neoplasm), the appropriate medical or surgical measures are instituted.

Other noninflammatory conditions require special management. Thus, hemothorax usually requires blood transfusion, tetanus toxoid or antitoxin if trauma has played a role, or a surgical procedure to ligate the bleeders. Fibrinolytic enzymes (e.g., pancreatic dornase) instilled into the pleural cavity is performed when clots have formed. Chest pain is relieved by analgesics. In chylothorax, repeated thoracentesis may be necessary and a safer procedure is closed drainage. Since protein loss may be significant, replacement must be given. If the leakage continues, surgical exploration may be considered.

An equally vigorous approach is required when the physician is confronted with an underlying inflammatory disease process. Appropriate antibiotics must be given in high doses. In the early stage when pain dominates the clinical picture and intrapleural fluid accumulation is minimal (dry or fibrinous pleurisy), analgesics (e.g., acetylsalicylic acid or codeine) are indicated. As the effusion becomes serofibrinous or purulent and increases in quantity, chest pain abates but dyspnea may ensue because of restriction of breathing. Thoracentesis is done and may have to be repeated if reaccumulation occurs. Since repeated thoracentesis may be traumatic to a child, continuous closed drainage connected to an underwater seal with or without suction is preferred. Drainage is continued until the lung has reexpanded and fluid has ceased to accumulate. When the foregoing measures fail to obliterate an empyema cavity, open thoracotomy with pleural resection is performed.

TUMORS OF THE CHEST

Less than 2 per cent of all malignant neoplasms occur in the childhood age group. In Bodian's series only 0.4 per cent of malignant tumors of childhood involved the respiratory tract. It is necessary, however, to add to this figure those neoplasms affecting the chest and its contents which, although histologically benign, may present life-threatening problems.

Once a chest tumor is suspected, a variety of diagnostic procedures is available to establish the anatomic site and the nature of the lesion. The plan of treatment can be decided once this investigation is complete.

Benign tumors involving the chest include hamartomas of the lung, which can usually be treated by local surgical removal, although lobectomy is sometimes indicated. Bronchial adenoma, papilloma and angioma present diagnostic difficulties because they simulate asthma, and the patient may be treated for this condition unnecessarily. Direct laryngoscopy and bronchoscopy are usually required for diagnosis and are necessary for local treatment of coagulation or local removal. Occasionally, more radical surgery is required. Jackson's dictum that "all is not asthma that wheezes" should always be kept in mind by the physician dealing with obstructive respiratory disease.

Many tumors of the chest cage are benign, although removal or biopsy may be necessary to prove this point. This category includes fibromas, chondromas and osteoid osteomas. Finally, a large thymic shadow in a fat healthy infant should not be accepted as the explanation for chest symptoms; the cause should be looked for elsewhere in the chest. In case of doubt when dealing with a radiologic shadow in the region of the thymus, angiography may be of assistance.

Primary malignant tumors of the chest are rare. Diagnosis is usually dependent on local exploration or biopsy.

Metastatic malignancy is rather more common. Wilms' tumor, neuroblastoma, retinoblastoma, leukemia, Hodgkin's disease, lymphoma and bone tumors may involve the lungs.

The treatment of a malignant tumor of the chest is determined by many factors and involves consideration of surgery, chemotherapy and irradiation. One or more of these approaches may be indicated, and decisions must be made on an individual basis for each patient.

Surgical removal of solitary metastatic tumors of the lung has resulted in prolonged survival and apparent cure in many cases. Thomford and Clagett list the criteria for selection of patients as follows: (1) Good risk for surgical intervention. (2) Primary lesion controlled. (3) No evidence of metastasis elsewhere in body. (4) Roentgenologic evidence of unilateral pulmonary involvement.

Chemotherapy used alone or in sequence with surgery or irradiation has met with varied success. The selection of the appropriate chemotherapeutic agent for a primary or secondary tumor of the chest in childhood is made primarily on the basis of the nature of the tumor. Thus, secondary lesions of Wilms' tumor and neuroblastoma, as well as thoracic involvement with lymphosarcoma and leukemia, are usually treated in a manner similar to treatment of these diseases when found elsewhere in the body. There are, however, a few specific instances in which tumors of the chest require therapy not frequently used elsewhere. Thus, recurrent malignant effusions (particularly due to lymphoma) which are nonresponsive to systemic therapy may respond to the intrapleural administration of nitrogen mustard. The total dose varies from 0.1 to 0.4 mg. per kilogram of body weight, depending on the patient's hematologic status. Systemic myelodepressive chemotherapy should not be given when intrapleural mustard is used because of the danger of an additive systemic effect. Mediastinal lymphomas at times may cause airway obstruction necessitating emergency therapy. At this time, therapy with nitrogen mustard and steroids is advisable to quickly reduce the tumor mass and diminish the associated edema.

In tumors involving the mediastinum, a superior vena caval syndrome may develop. Under these conditions, cytotoxic agents (such as nitrogen mustard) must not be given into the veins of the upper limb because of the danger of local tissue necrosis.

The irradiation of the lungs in childhood has to be considered as a palliative measure for inoperable pulmonary metastases of Wilms' tumors. When the lungs are directly exposed to the irradiation, some degree of radiation pneumonitis always occurs, but irreversible changes are related to the dose, the volume of tissue exposed and the rate at which therapy is given. The dose also has to be adjusted to the patient's age. If a thoracic bath treatment is given for pulmonary metastasis, the entire pleural surface and both lungs are irradiated through anteroposterior fields; the dose suggested up to the age of six years is 1200 to 1500 rads in three to four weeks measured as a central dose. After 10 to 12 years the full adult dose will be tolerated, but even then it is advisable to limit the dose to 2000 rads in four to five weeks. When a smaller volume of lung is irradiated, a relatively increased dose can be given accordingly. At the Children's Medical Center in Boston, Farber and his colleagues advise a dose of 1200 rads in 10 treatments over two weeks, in combination with actinomycin D in the treatment of metastatic Wilms' tumor.

These remarks would apply in general also to the treatment of multiple lung metastases of other radiosensitive tumors, such as neuroblastoma or Ewing's tumor, but the thoracic bath technique is by no means advocated as a routine measure.

If in Hodgkin's disease the mediastinum is being irradiated as the primary area of involvement or as the neighboring gland site being treated in continuity with the primary site, the lung parenchyma outside the treatment field should be protected from exposure to the beam of radiation.

References

General

Avery, M. E.: *The Lung and Its Disorders in the Newborn Infant.* Philadelphia, W. B. Saunders Company, 1968.

Cherniack, R. M., Cherniack, L., and Naimark, A.: *Respiration in Health and Disease,* 2nd ed., Philadelphia, W. B. Saunders Company, 1972.

Kendig, E. L., Jr. (ed.): *Disorders of the Respiratory Tract in Children.* Volume I: *Pulmonary Disorders in Children.* Philadelphia, W. B. Saunders Company, 1972.

Mellins, R. B., Chernick, V., Doershuk, C. F., Downes, J. J., Sinclair, J. C., and Waring, W. W.: Respiratory Care in Infants and Children. *Am. Rev. Resp. Dis.,* 105:461, 1972.

Schaffer, A. J., and Avery, M. E.: *Diseases of the Newborn,* 2nd ed. Philadelphia, W. B. Saunders Company, 1971.

Pneumothorax

Chernick, V., and Avery, M. E.: Spontaneous Alveolar Rupture at Birth. *Pediatrics,* 32:816, 1963.

Chernick, V., and Reed, M.: Pneumothorax and Chylothorax in the Newborn Period. *J. Pediat.,* 76:624, 1970.

Lubchenco, L. O.: Recognition of Spontaneous Pneumothorax in Premature Infants. *Pediatrics,* 24:996, 1969.

Macklin, C. C.: Transport of Air Along Sheathes of Pulmonic Blood Vessels from Alveoli to Mediastinum. *Arch. Intern. Med.,* 64:913, 1939.

Congenital Lobar Emphysema

Fischer, H. W., Lucido, J. L., and Lynxwiler, C. P.: Lobar Emphysema. *J.A.M.A.,* 160:340, 1958.

Mercer, R. D., Hawk, W. A., and Darakjian, G.: Massive Lobar Emphysema in Infants: Diagnosis and Treatment. *Cleveland Clin. Quart.,* 28:270, 1961.

Anomalies of Pulmonary Circulation

Bosher, L. H., Jr., Blake, D. A., and Byrd, B. R.: An Analysis of the Pathologic Anatomy of Pulmonary Arteriovenous Aneurysms. *Surgery,* 45:91, 1959.

Ellis, F. H., McGoon, D. C., and Kincaid, O. W.: Congenital Vascular Malformations of the Lungs. *Med. Clin. N. Am.,* 48:1069, 1964.

Pryce, D. M., Sellors, T. H., and Blair, L. G.: Intralobar Sequestration of Lung Associated with an Abnormal Pulmonary Artery. *Brit. J. Surg.,* 35:18, 1947.

Lung Cyst

Baghdassarian, O., Avery, M. E., and Neuhauser, E. B. D.: A Form of Pulmonary Insufficiency in Premature Infants. Pulmonary Dysmaturity. *Am. J. Roentgen.,* 89:1020, 1963.

Caffey, J.: On the Natural Regression of Pulmonary Cysts During Early Infancy. *Pediatrics,* 11:48, 1953.

Chin, K. Y., and Tang, M. Y.: Congenital Adenomatoid Malformation of One Lobe of a Lung with General Anasarca. *Arch. Path.*, 48:311, 1949.

Crawford, T. J., and Cahill, J. L.: The Surgical Treatment of Pulmonary Cystic Disorders in Infancy and Childhood. *J. Pediat. Surg.*, 6:251, 1971.

Kwittken, J., and Reimer, L.: Congenital Cystic Adenomatoid Malformation of the Lung. *Pediatrics*, 30:759, 1962.

Opsahl, T., and Berman, E. J.: Bronchogenic Mediastinal Cysts in Infants. Case Report and Review of the Literature. *Pediatrics*, 30:372, 1962.

Wilson, M. G., and Mikity, V. G.: A New Form of Respiratory Disease in Premature Infants. *Am. J. Dis. Child.*, 99:489, 1960.

Middle Lobe Syndrome

Billig, D. M., and Darling, D. B.: Middle Lobe Atelectasis in Children. *Am. J. Dis. Child.*, 123:96, 1972.

Brock, R. C.: *The Anatomy of the Bronchial Tree.* London, Oxford Medical Publications, 1946.

Dees, S. C., and Spock, A.: Right Middle Lobe Syndrome in Children. *J.A.M.A.*, 197:8, 1966.

Graham, E. A., Burford, T. H., and Mayer, J. H.: Middle Lobe Syndrome. *Postgrad. Med.*, 4:29, 1948.

Bronchiectasis and Atelectasis

Chernick, V., and Macpherson, R. I.: Respiratory Syncytial and Adenovirus Infection of the Lower Respiratory Tract in Infancy. *Clin. Notes Resp. Dis.*, 10:3, 1971.

Chernick, V., and Macpherson, R. I.: Bronchiectasis; in V. Kelly (ed.): *Brenneman's Practice of Pediatrics.* New York, Harper & Row, Publishers, 1972, Chap. 70.

Field, C. E.: Bronchiectasis: Third Report on a Follow-up Study of Medical and Surgical Cases from Childhood. *Arch. Dis. Child.*, 44:551, 1969.

Hyperaeration

Guenter, C. A., Welch, M. H., and Hammarsten, J. F.: Alpha-1-Antitrypsin Deficiency and Pulmonary Emphysema. *Ann. Rev. Med.*, 22:283, 1971.

Mittman, C.: Summary of Symposium on Pulmonary Emphysema and Proteolysis. *Am. Rev. Resp. Dis.*, 105:430, 1972.

Talamo, R. C., Levison, H., Lynch, M. J., Hercz, A., Hyslop, N. E., and Bain, H. W.: Symptomatic Pulmonary Emphysema in Childhood Associated with Hereditary Alpha-1-Antitrypsin and Elastase Inhibitor Deficiency. *J. Pediat.*, 79:20, 1971.

Pulmonary Hemosiderosis

Zinkham, W. H. Idiopathic Pulmonary Hemosiderosis; in V. Kelly (ed.): *Brenneman's Practice of Pediatrics.* New York, Harper & Row, Publishers, 1972, Chap. 81.

Pulmonary Edema

Ersoz, N., and Finestone, S. C.: Adrenaline-induced Pulmonary Oedema and Its Treatment. *Brit. J. Anaesth.*, 43:709, 1971.

Lloyd, E. L., and MacRae, W. R.: Respiratory Tract Damage in Burns: Case Reports and Review of the Literature. *Brit. J. Anaesth.*, 43:365, 1971.

Salem, M. R., Masud, K. Z., Tatooles, C. J., and Yanes, H. O.: Unilateral Pulmonary Oedema Following Aorta to Right Pulmonary Artery Anastomosis (Waterston's Operation). *Brit. J. Anaesth.*, 43:701, 1971.

Pleural Disorders

Bechamps, G. J., Lynn, H. B., and Wenzl, J. E.: Empyema in Children: Review of Mayo Clinic Experience. *Mayo Clin. Proc.*, 45:43, 1970.

Turner, J. A. P.: Staphylococcal Pneumonia: A Contemporary Rarity. *Clin. Pediat.*, 11:69, 1972.

Wolfe, W. G., Spock, A., and Bradford, W. D.: Pleural Fluid in Infants and Children. *Am. Rev. Resp. Dis.*, 98:1027, 1968.

Tumors of the Chest

Bodian, M.: Aspects of Cancer in Childhood; in D. Gairdner (ed.): *Recent Advances in Paediatrics*, 3rd ed. Boston, Little Brown and Company, 1965, pp. 266–293.

D'Angio, M., and Evans, E.: The Superior Mediastinal Syndrome in Children with Cancer. *Am. J. Roentgen.*, 93:537, 1965.

Koop, C. E., and Hernandez, J. R.: Neuroblastoma—Experience with 100 Cases in Children. *Surgery*, 56:726, 1964.

Russel, H.: Actinomycin D in Wilms' Tumor—Treatment of Lung Metastases. *Arch. Dis. Child.*, 40: 200, 1965.

Thomford, W., and Clagett, O. T.: The Surgical Treatment of Metastatic Tumors in the Lungs. *J. Thoracic Cardiovasc. Surg.*, 49:357, 1965.

5

Cardiovascular System

Congestive Heart Failure

BURTON W. FINK, M.D., *and*
ARTHUR J. MOSS, M.D.

The approach to treatment of the patient with signs and symptoms of congestive heart failure is shown in Table 1. It is mandatory that the correct cause of failure be established since the treatment varies with the cause.

Digitalis. In general, digoxin (Lanoxin) is the digitalis preparation most commonly used. This preparation has the advantage of multiple routes of administration, rapid action and rapid excretion. The dosage is weight- and age-related (see Table 2). The route of administration and the interval between doses is determined by the severity of failure (see Table 3).

If the patient is in early congestive failure and not vomiting, the oral route can be used. The intramuscular or intravenous route should be used in all other patients. If digoxin is administered orally or intramuscularly, one-half the estimated total dose is given initially, followed by two additional doses of one-fourth the total estimated dose at 6- to 8-hour intervals. Since the average digitalizing dose is an empirical calculation each patient must be titrated according to his response. When the desired response is achieved, a maintenance dose of one-fourth to one-third the total digitalizing dose is given in two divided doses at approximately 12-hour intervals. The drug effect should be monitored by pulse rate and electrocardiographic rhythm strips. It must be stressed, however, that no specific observation indicates when a patient is adequately digitalized.

DIGITALIS TOXICITY. When digitalis is given in excess, the patient may develop arrhythmias (particularly extrasystoles and heart block), vomiting, occasionally diarrhea and, rarely, accentuation of heart failure. The treatment of choice for digitalis toxicity is cessation of the drug and, when severe, administration of potassium chloride. This can be given orally (1 Gm. every 8 hours). It also can be administered intravenously as 40 mEq. in 500 ml. of 5 per cent glucose and water, given as a slow infusion with constant electrocardiographic monitoring. The total intravenous dose should not exceed 0.5 mEq. per kilogram per 24 hours. In life-threatening situations, peritoneal dialysis may be necessary.

Diuretics. Diuretics are used as an adjunct to digitalis (see Table 4). The major drugs are the mercurials, the thiazides, ethacrynic acid and furosemide.

Other Drugs. If pulmonary edema is present, morphine sulfate, 0.1 to 0.2 mg. per kilogram, is recommended.

Supportive Care. In addition to drug therapy, the patient may require oxygen, a semirecumbent position and, in some cases, a low sodium diet. Table 5 shows the relative sodium and potassium content of the most commonly available types of milk used for infants.

TABLE 1. Treatment of Congestive Heart Failure

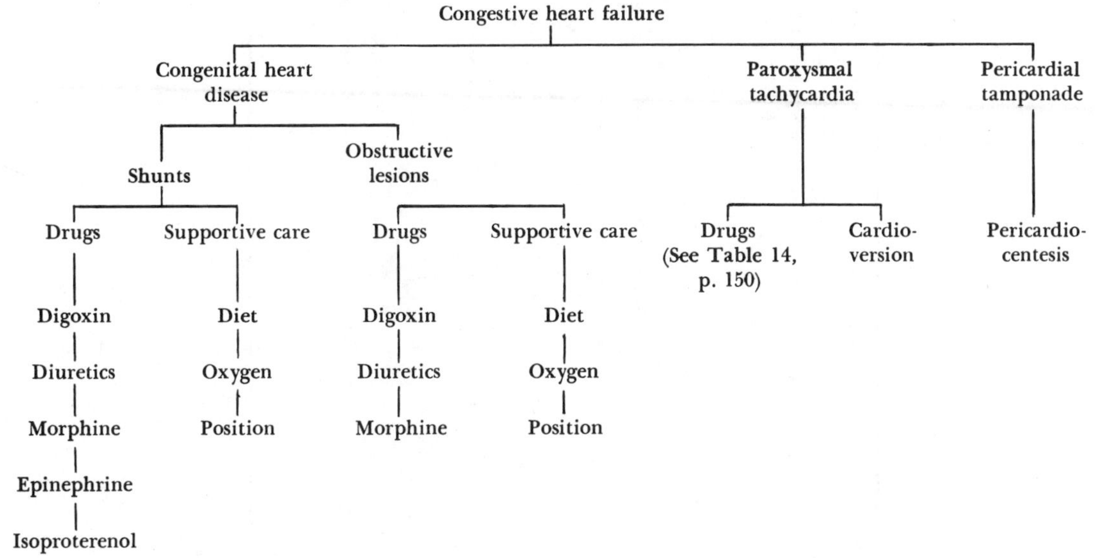

TABLE 2. Digoxin (Lanoxin)

HOW SUPPLIED	AGE	ESTIMATED TOTAL DIGITALIZING DOSE (*Oral or Intramuscular*)*	MAINTENANCE PROPORTION OF TOTAL DIGITALIZING DOSE
Elixir: 0.05 mg./ml. Tablets: (scored) 0.25 and 0.5 mg.; (unscored) 0.125 mg.	Premature infant (< 2500 Gm.)	0.04 mg./kg.	¼ to ⅓ in two divided doses per 24 hours
	Newborn infant (1 to 14 days)	0.05 mg./kg.	¼ to ⅓ in two divided doses per 24 hours
Ampules: 0.1 and 0.25 mg./ml.	Infant (14 days to 2 years)	0.06 to 0.075 mg./kg.	¼ to ⅓ in two divided doses per 24 hours
	Child (> 2 years)	0.03 to 0.05 mg./kg. (maximal total dose of 1.5 mg.)	¼ to ⅓ in two divided doses per 24 hours

* For intravenous administration, use 75 per cent of the dose shown.

TABLE 3. Characteristics of Digoxin (Lanoxin) Related to Route of Administration

ROUTE OF ADMINISTRATION	ONSET OF ACTION	PEAK ACTION	EXCRETION
Oral	1 to 2 hours	4 to 8 hours	4 to 7 days
Intramuscular	15 to 60 minutes	2 to 5 hours	4 to 7 days
Intravenous	5 to 30 minutes	2 to 5 hours	4 to 7 days

TABLE 4. Diuretics

DRUG	MODE OF ACTION	DOSAGE AND ROUTE	ONSET OF ACTION	HOW SUPPLIED	PRECAUTIONS
Meralluride (Mercuhydrin)	Inhibits tubular reabsorption	Newborn: 0.1 ml. intramuscularly Infant: 0.25 ml. intramuscularly Child 1 to 5 years: 0.5 ml. intramuscularly Child > 5 years: 1 to 1.5 ml. intramuscularly	2 to 3 hours	Ampules: 2 ml.	Requires adequate chloride levels
Chlorothiazide (Diuril)	Inhibits tubular reabsorption	20 to 40 mg./kg./day in two doses orally	1 to 2 hours	Syrup: 250 mg./5 ml. Tablets: 250 and 500 mg.	Use supplemental potassium
Hydrochlorothiazide (HydroDiuril)	Inhibits tubular reabsorption	2.0 to 3.5 mg./kg./day in two doses orally	1 to 2 hours	Tablets: 25 and 50 mg.	Use supplemental potassium
Spironolactone (Aldactone-A)	Aldosterone antagonist	1.5 to 3.0 mg./kg./day in two or three doses orally	1 to 2 hours	Tablets: 250 mg.	Causes potassium retention
Acetazolamide (Diamox)	Carbonic anhydrase inhibitor	5.0 mg./kg./day in one dose orally	1 to 2 hours	Tablets: 250 mg.	—
Ethacrynic acid*	Blocks sodium reabsorption	0.4 to 1.0 mg./kg./dose intravenously 10 to 20 mg./kg./day in four doses orally	10 to 20 minutes 1 hour	Vials: 50 mg. Tablets: 50 mg.	—
Furosemide† (Lasix)	Blocks sodium reabsorption	1 mg./kg./dose orally, intramuscularly or intravenously	1 to 2 hours orally 10 to 20 minutes intramuscularly 5 minutes intravenously	Tablets: 40 mg. Ampules: 10 mg./ml.	—

* Manufacturer's precaution: Infant dose of ethacrynic acid has not been established.
† Manufacturer's precaution: Until more experience is obtained, furosemide should not be given to children.

TABLE 5. Sodium and Potassium Content of Various Types of Milk

TYPE	SODIUM (*mEq./liter*)	POTASSIUM (*mEq./liter*)
Breast	7	14
SMA	7	14
PM 60/40	7	14
Similac	11	23
Enfamil	11	18
Isomil	13	18
Similac with iron	13	27
Soyolac	14	23
Mullsoy	16	40
Sobee	22	33
Homogenized	25	36
Skim	25	36

Congenital Heart Disease

BURTON W. FINK, M.D., *and*
ARTHUR J. MOSS, M.D.

The operative management of congenital cardiac defects varies somewhat from institution to institution depending on the facilities and personnel available. There has been a recent trend to perform definitive surgery in the first year of life. This is particularly true for transposition of the great arteries, tetralogy of Fallot and ventricular septal defect. Such an approach requires not only a skilled and experienced surgeon and cardiologist but also equally competent anesthesiologists, nurses and other supportive personnel. The recommendations that follow represent the current prevailing practice in most centers. With increasing experience, the trend to earlier surgery may well become the treatment of choice.

TETRALOGY OF FALLOT

The treatment of patients with tetralogy of Fallot (Table 1) is contingent upon a precise diagnosis. Since it may easily be confused with other entities, it is the general feeling that cardiac catheterization is indicated when cyanosis is present, regardless of the age of the patient. This usually provides an accurate diagnosis.

Hypoxic Episodes. These episodes, usually seen in infants, can be confused with seizures from noncardiac causes and are life-threatening. Treatment consists of oxygen, the knee-chest position and morphine sulfate (0.1 to 0.2 mg. per kilogram). Sodium bicarbonate injected intravenously (2 to 3 mEq. per kilogram) may be helpful. Isoproterenol is contraindicated.

Anemia. The patient with tetralogy of Fallot is subject to an iron deficiency anemia, which may be masked by the relatively normal hemoglobin levels. The administration of iron

TABLE 1. Treatment of Tetralogy of Fallot

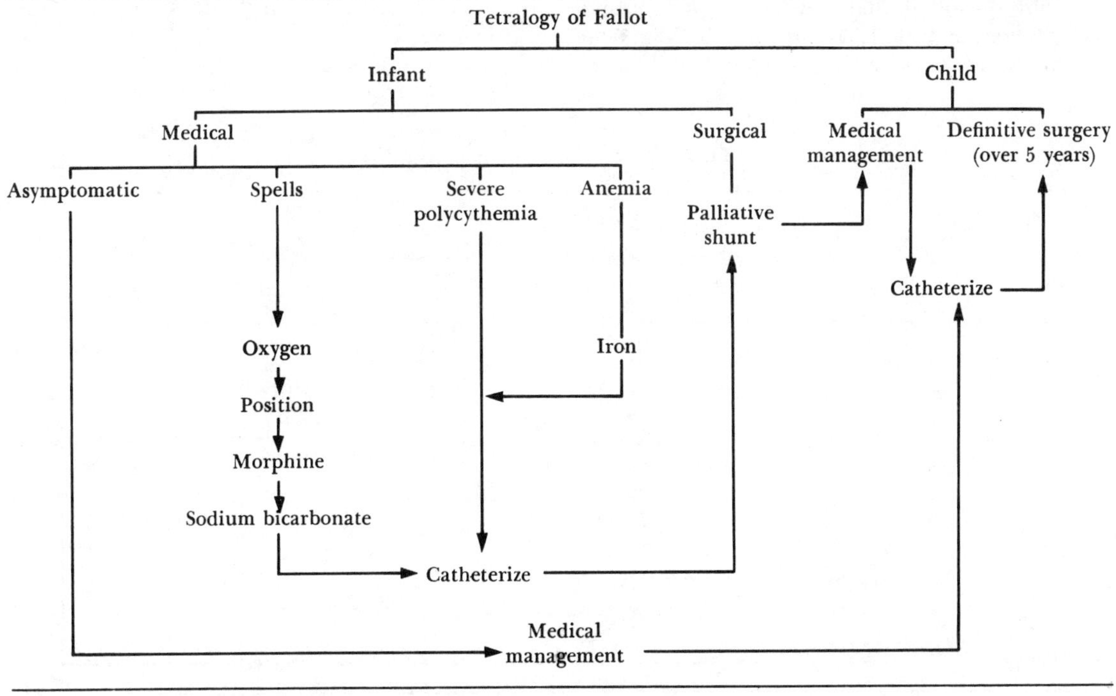

(6 mg. per kilogram daily, orally in three divided doses) will give more oxygen-carrying capacity to the patient but will increase the degree of cyanosis as the hemoglobin levels are elevated. Iron therapy probably should be discontinued if the hematocrit reaches 65 per cent or greater.

Surgical Management. Hypoxic episodes, or polycythemia with a hematocrit of 65 per cent or more, are indications for operative intervention. If the patient has not yet reached an age of five years, or a weight of 25 pounds, palliative surgery is indicated. The Potts procedure is an anastomosis between the left pulmonary artery and the descending aorta. The Blalock-Taussig procedure is an anastomosis between a subclavian artery and a main branch of the pulmonary artery. The Waterston procedure is an anastomosis between the ascending aorta and the right pulmonary artery. Each is designed to increase blood flow to the lungs. The Waterston procedure is currently in favor because of the relative ease of accomplishment and of correction at the time of definitive repair. The palliative procedure permits the patient to reach a satisfactory age for definitive repair (approximately five years) with reasonable growth and development.

In the asymptomatic patient, palliation is not necessary, and surgical intervention may be delayed until definitive repair can be accomplished. This consists of relief of the right ventricular obstruction and closure of the ventricular septal defect.

PULMONARY STENOSIS

The classic patient with valvular pulmonary stenosis is usually asymptomatic. When he reaches four to five years of age, and if the electrocardiogram shows right ventricular hypertrophy of a degree which suggests the need for operative intervention, heart catheterization should be performed (Table 2). If the pressure in the right ventricle exceeds 75 mm. of mercury at rest, surgical correction is indicated. Direct visualization of the valve, using open heart surgical techniques, permits repair of the valve in a way which reduces the chances of severe postoperative pulmonary insufficiency.

The infant with overwhelming pulmonary valvular obstruction (malignant pulmonary stenosis) however, is totally different. He develops cyanosis with heart failure and requires emergency cardiac catheterization. In this situation preparations must be made for immediate surgical relief. A Brock valvulotomy is the procedure of choice because of the relative speed with which it can be accomplished. The patient with malignant pulmonary stenosis is in jeopardy of his life during the catheterization and in the immediate preoperative period, until the valve is opened.

TRANSPOSITION OF THE GREAT ARTERIES

This lesion presents one of the true emergencies to the physician caring for patients with congenital heart disease (Table 3). The indications for catheterization are the presence of cyanosis or heart failure. One must be prepared to do a balloon septostomy at the initial catheterization.

Medical Management. Prior to catheterization it is advisable to determine the degree of metabolic acidosis and to correct it with sodium bicarbonate (2 to 3 mEq. per kilogram intravenously). Hypoxic episodes may occur and these should be treated with oxygen and

TABLE 2. Treatment of Pulmonary Stenosis

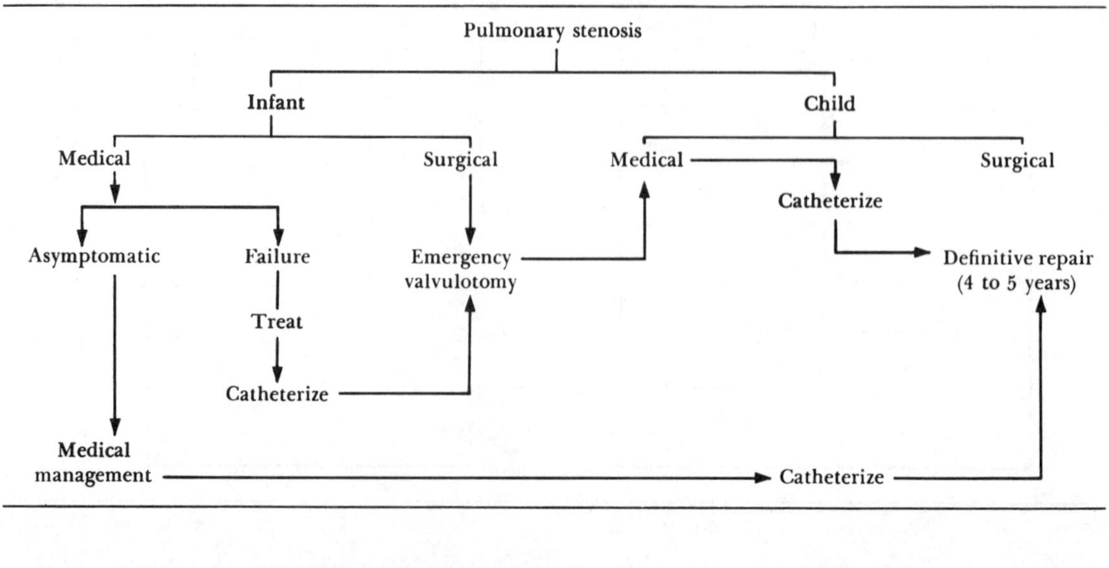

TABLE 3. Treatment of Transposition of the Great Arteries

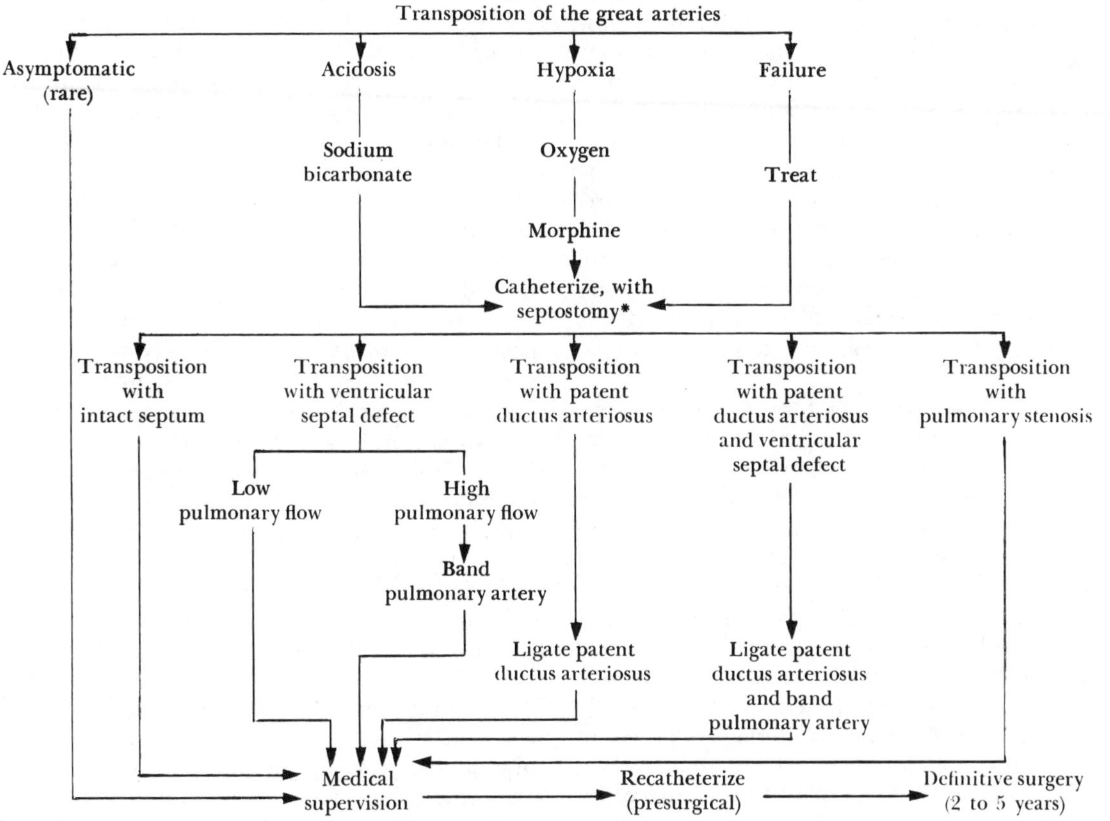

* If septostomy is not satisfactory, a septectomy should be performed.

morphine (0.1 to 0.2 mg. per kilogram). If the patient is in congestive heart failure, decongestive measures should be instituted.

Surgical Management. Although balloon septostomy is a palliative procedure performed in the catheterization laboratory by a cardiologist, it can be considered surgical treatment. As noted in Table 3, it is the treatment of choice in all patients with transposition of the great arteries, with or without coexisting congenital defects. When successful, this procedure immediately increases systemic oxygen saturation. When no additional abnormalities are present, the patient can be followed medically with repeat catheterization when indicated.

Total correction is best carried out at about two to five years of age. Currently, the Mustard procedure or some modification of it is the treatment of choice. Essentially this rebuilds the atrial chambers. A piece of pericardium is placed in such a way that it directs the superior and inferior caval flow to the mitral valve (from where it will ultimately enter the lungs) and directs the pulmonary venous return to the tricuspid valve (from where it will ultimately enter the systemic circuit).

If the patient has a coexisting ventricular septal defect, there is risk of pulmonary hypertension, and serial catheterizations are indicated. If increased pulmonary vascular resistance is suspected, banding of the pulmonary artery is recommended at an early age. Ultimate surgery involves removal of the band, correction of the ventricular septal defect and rebuilding of the atrium as described.

The patient with an associated patent ductus arteriosus also may develop pulmonary hypertension and require ligation of the ductus after creation of an atrial communication. The patient with a ventricular septal defect and pulmonary stenosis is deeply cyanotic but has a protected vascular bed and can usually be followed medically after a successful balloon septostomy. Repeat catheterization and definitive surgery at about the age of two to five years are recommended.

ATRIAL SEPTAL DEFECT

A patient with a secundum type of atrial septal defect is usually asymptomatic through childhood. He should be permitted unrestricted activity. When he reaches the age of four to five years, cardiac catheterization is indicated to confirm the diagnosis and to determine its physiologic significance. If the pulmonary flow is greater than 1.5 times the systemic flow, surgical correction is indicated. The lesion is usually repaired by direct suture, but if it is large, a prosthetic patch may be required.

A very rare infant will decompensate; he should be treated for congestive heart failure. Cardiac catheterization should be performed to confirm the diagnosis. Because of an increased risk of open heart surgery during infancy, medical management is preferred. If this is unsuccessful, however, the lesion should be repaired.

The patient with an ostium primum type of defect (which includes a cleft in the mitral valve) presents more frequently with congestive heart failure and requires earlier supportive care and perhaps earlier operation. The surgical repair is the same except that the cleft in the mitral valve is also repaired.

Table 4 indicates that the care of patients with secundum and primum defects is basically the same. This is true, except that patients with primum defects may present earlier and be more seriously ill. Some cardiologists prefer to delay operative intervention in the case of primum defects because of technical difficulties encountered in the repair of the mitral valve.

TRUNCUS ARTERIOSUS

The majority of patients with this lesion have increased pulmonary blood flow (types I, II and III) and experience early congestive heart failure requiring treatment as suggested elsewhere in the text. If they can be supported medically until they reach the age of about four years, surgery can be considered (Table 5). An aortic homograft, with the anterior leaflet of the mitral valve still connected, can be implanted in the wall of the right ventricle. The mitral valve leaflet is used to close the ventricular septal defect, thereby creating an intact right ventricle, with the aortic valve serving as the pulmonary valve. The pulmonary arteries are disconnected from the aorta and anastomosed to the graft (Rastelli procedure). Some surgeons currently use prosthetic material instead of homografts.

No surgical procedure is available at this time for the patient who has decreased pulmonary blood flow because of absent pulmonary arteries (type IV).

SINGLE VENTRICLE

The patient with a single ventricle may have early and devastating episodes of congestive heart failure with or without infection. Heart failure should be treated as outlined elsewhere in the text. Some patients survive until four or five years of age at which time, if the atrioventricular valves have supporting structures that insert within their own potential ventricular chamber, it may be possible to place a prosthetic patch within the ventricular chamber, thereby creating two separate ventricles. This requires extracorporeal circulation. Most

TABLE 4. Treatment of Atrial Septal Defect

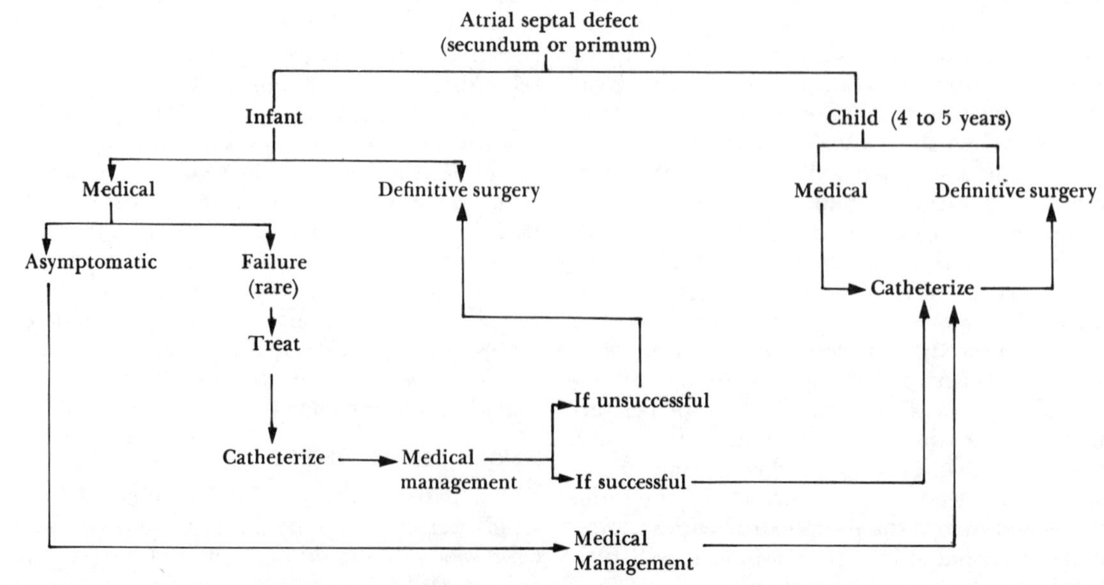

TABLE 5. Treatment of Truncus Arteriosus

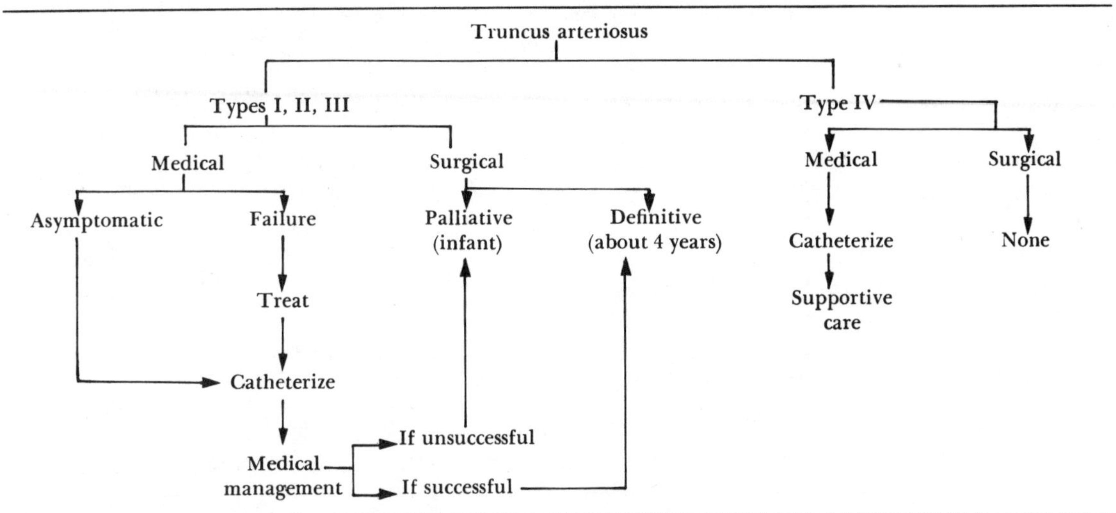

patients with single ventricle, however, do not have favorable intraventricular anatomy and prove to be inoperable.

ENDOCARDIAL FIBROELASTOSIS

The patient with this lesion usually presents in congestive heart failure during early infancy, which is treated. An occasional infant will respond satisfactorily and can be followed with medical supervision. The more usual course, however, is one of repeated episodes of congestive heart failure, each being more difficult to treat, with the patient ultimately expiring. No surgical procedure is available for this entity.

TUMORS

When a neoplasm obstructs the flow through a chamber, symptoms can be expected. Diagnosis can be accomplished with cardiac catheterization and appropriate angiographic techniques. Surgical removal is recommended.

When a neoplasm occurs within the myocardium, signs of cardiomegaly and congestive failure may result. Cardiac catheterization and angiocardiography may be necessary to establish the diagnosis. Surgical treatment is generally unsuccessful.

DOUBLE OUTLET RIGHT VENTRICLE

This entity is also known as origin of both great vessels from the right ventricle. This lesion can occur with pulmonary stenosis, in which case it resembles tetralogy of Fallot, and its care is similar to that of tetralogy of Fallot. It may also occur without pulmonary stenosis, in which case it resembles ventricular septal defect, and its management is similar to that of ventricular septal defect.

Cardiac catheterization is required in both instances to establish the diagnosis. Treatment is directed toward the correction of the intercardiac lesions, with redirection of flow through the two great vessels so that the right ventricular outflow is purely to the lungs and the left ventricular outflow purely to the aorta. Extracorporeal circulation is required.

PULMONARY ARTERIOVENOUS FISTULA

If the lesion is single, the affected portion of the lung should be removed and cure can be expected. If the lesion is multiple, a decision will have to be made as to the advisability of multiple resections.

SINUS OF VALSALVA ANEURYSM

This congenital anomaly may be asymptomatic and confused with a patent ductus arteriosus or, if ruptured, may present with devastating heart failure. If it is compensated, or if congestive failure cannot be controlled, surgical correction with extracorporeal circulation is indicated. Long-term medical management is not successful.

ANOMALOUS PULMONARY VENOUS CONNECTION

The significance of partial anomalous pulmonary venous connection is determined by the size of the left-to-right shunt. This information may be obtained at cardiac catheterization. Indications for catheterization are cardiomegaly, right ventricular hypertrophy in the electro-

TABLE 6. Treatment of Partial Anomalous Pulmonary Venous Connection

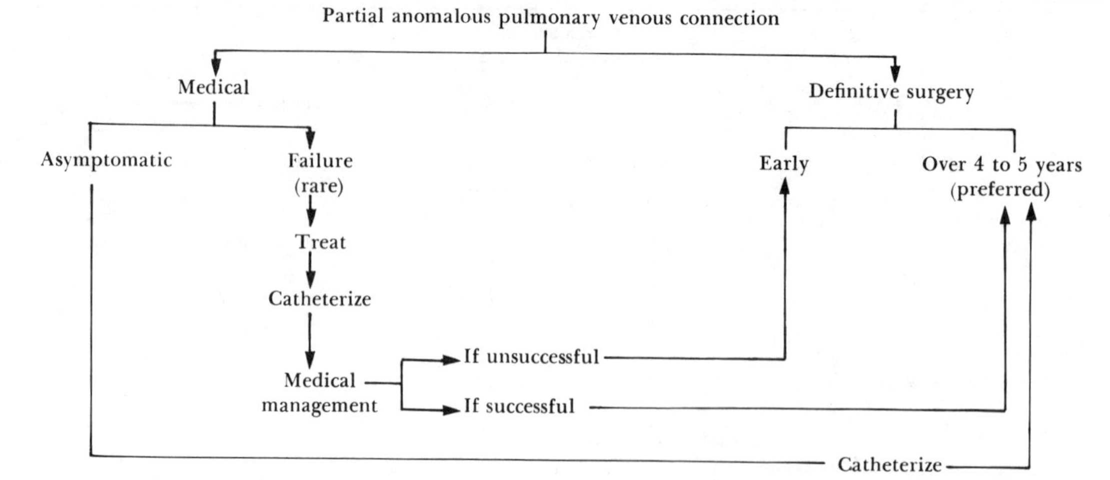

cardiogram, or clinical findings suggesting the presence of a significant shunt.

Patients with single anomalous veins are usually asymptomatic and need not be operated upon. Patients with partial anomalous connection may be indistinguishable from patients with atrial septal defect and require cardiac catheterization for differentiation. If pulmonary flow exceeds 1.5 times systemic flow, surgical correction is recommended. This is best done at age four to five years, using extracorporeal circulation. (See Table 6.)

When all veins drain anomalously, difficulty in early infancy can be forecast. The clinical condition may require early and urgent cardiac catheterization. If there is no obstruction to the veins, surgical correction with extracorporeal circulation can be attempted. If there is obstruction to the veins, marked pulmonary edema results, and this must be treated. Following that, surgical correction with extracorporeal circulation should be attempted. The mortality rate of this procedure is extremely high. Surgery is designed to reinstate the continuity of the pulmonary venous drainage to the left atrium and repair of the associated atrial septal defect. (See Table 7.)

PATENT DUCTUS ARTERIOSUS

The patient with patent ductus arteriosus may present with congestive heart failure during early infancy, or he may be asymptomatic.

If congestive failure ensues, adequate treatment must be accomplished. When it is compensated, cardiac catheterization is usually performed to confirm the diagnosis. Then, a

TABLE 7. Treatment of Total Anomalous Pulmonary Venous Connection

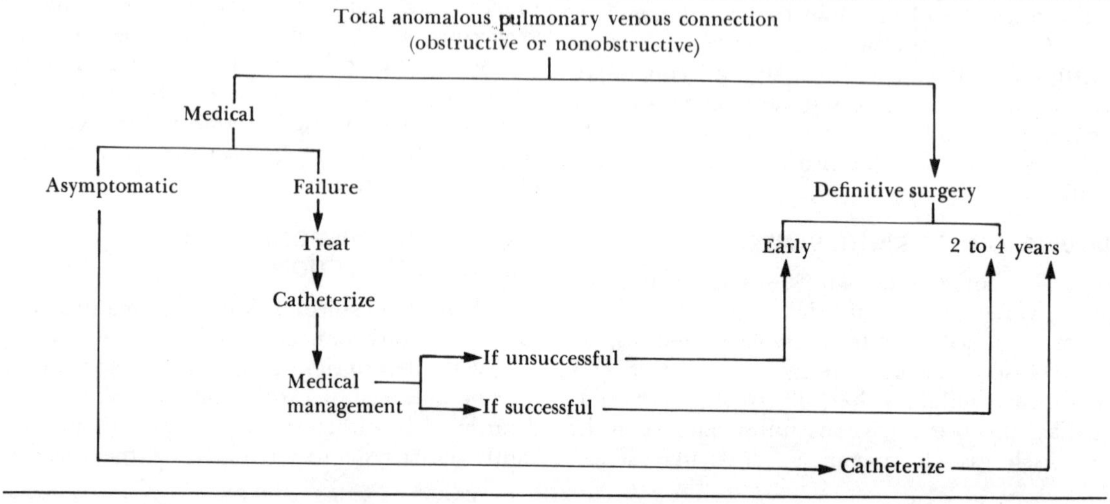

decision must be made as to whether the patient should be followed clinically or subjected to early surgical repair of the ductus as indicated in Table 8.

If the infant is asymptomatic, he can be followed clinically until the optimal age of two to five years is reached, and then surgical ligation or division of the ductus performed. Until this is accomplished, prophylactic antibiotics should be administered, particularly for dental extractions and oral surgery. The American Heart Association recommendations for this are as follow: Procaine penicillin, 600,000 units, with 600,000 units of crystalline penicillin, is given intramuscularly 1 or 2 hours before the procedure. This is followed by procaine penicillin, 600,000 units intramuscularly each day for two days. If absolute reliability is guaranteed, oral penicillin can be substituted, using 200,000 units of penicillin V (as a potassium salt) or 400,000 units of penicillin G, given four times the day of the procedure. An extra dose should be given 1 hour before the procedure. This should be followed by orally administered penicillin, four times each day for the next two days. If a patient is allergic to penicillin, erythromycin in the dosage of 40 mg. per kilogram per day in three or four doses, to a maximum of 1 Gm. per day, should be substituted.

AORTOPULMONARY SEPTAL DEFECTS

These lesions should be repaired using extracorporeal circulation. Although early operation is sometimes necessary, the lesion is optimally repaired when the patient reaches the age of four or five years. Differentiation from a patent ductus arteriosus is made by cardiac catheterization and angiocardiography.

ENDOCARDIAL CUSHION DEFECTS

The treatment of ostium primum defect (partial endocardial cushion defect) is covered in the section on atrial septal defect. Patients with the intermediate or total form usually present early in infancy in severe congestive heart failure, which is treated by the usual method. If failure is unremitting, banding of the pulmonary artery may be attempted. However, this is less successful than in the patient with a simple ventricular septal defect, because the increase in right ventricular pressure, secondary to the band, may be transmitted directly to the right atrium, placing the patient in intractable heart failure.

Some patients with the intermediate form, and a rare patient with the total form, can be maintained medically with attention being paid to the need for digitalis and the treatment of intercurrent infections. Correction of these defects may be attempted using extracorporeal circulation, but results thus far are discouraging. If the patient has advanced pulmonary vascular disease, and a high pulmonary vascular resistance, surgery is contraindicated. (See Table 9.)

COARCTATION OF THE AORTA

The infant with coarctation of the aorta may be asymptomatic or present with heart failure, which must be treated. If the diagnosis is in question, cardiac catheterization is indicated. If the diagnosis is clear, this may not be necessary. The optimal age for surgery is four to eight years. If the heart failure cannot be controlled medically, earlier surgical correction is indicated. The earlier surgery is required, the greater is the risk. In addition, the smaller

TABLE 8. Treatment of Patent Ductus Arteriosus

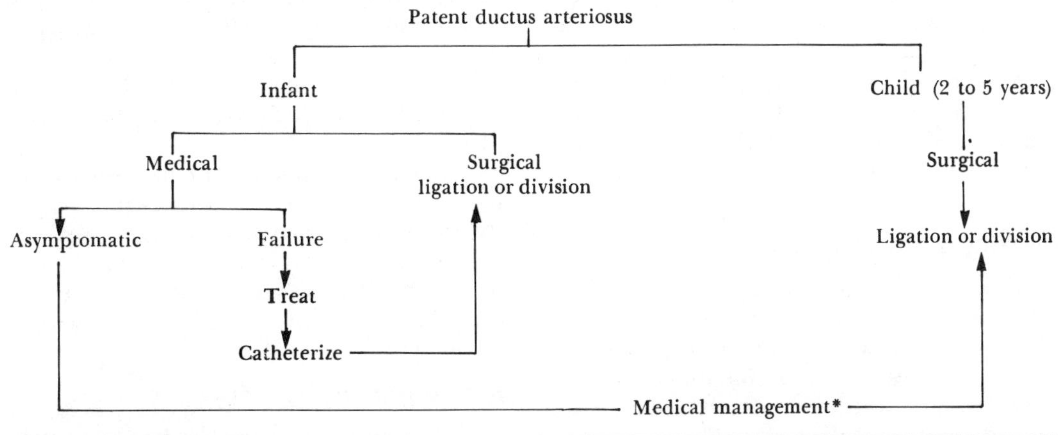

* Use prophylactic antibiotics until surgery is performed.

TABLE 9. Treatment of Endocardial Cushion Defect

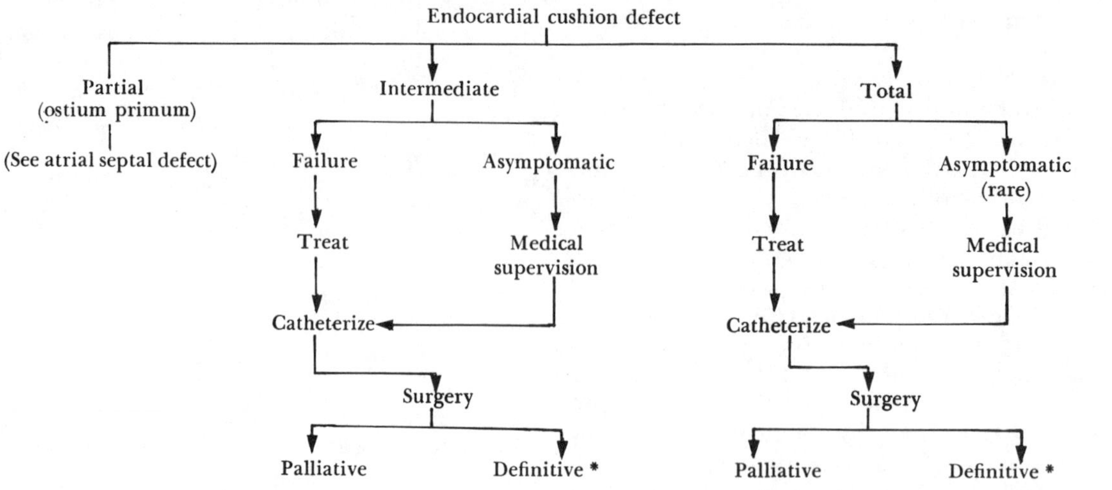

* Results discouraging.

the infant at the time of surgery, the higher the incidence of re-stenosis of the aorta. Normal physical activity is permitted until surgery is performed.

An important postoperative complication is the appearance of abdominal pain associated with paradoxical hypertension (mesenteric arteritis). This syndrome should be treated with a hypotensive agent, such as reserpine, 0.07 mg. per kilogram intramuscularly every 12 to 24 hours. Hydralazine hydrochloride (Apresoline) 0.15 mg. per kilogram every 12 to 24 hours, is often given with the reserpine.

Special attention should be given to the patient with the preductal type of coarctation of the aorta, with or without a hypoplastic aortic arch. These infants frequently have severe additional cardiac anomalies, are more seriously ill and require immediate diagnosis and early operation.

In the rare patient who has a complete interruption of the aortic arch, an attempt can be made to surgically bridge the interruption but the results are poor. If there are coexisting areas of abdominal coarctation, these can be repaired with either direct anastomosis or bypass grafts. (See Table 10.)

VENTRICULAR SEPTAL DEFECT

The infant with ventricular septal defect may present with congestive heart failure in early infancy, in which case the usual anticongestive measures should be instituted. Once it is compensated, cardiac catheterization is indicated to confirm the diagnosis. The patient then can be followed medically with attention to intercurrent infections and regulation of digitalis. However, if heart failure is intractable, surgery in infancy must be considered. This consists of either palliative banding of the pulmonary artery or definitive repair of the lesion.

Some patients with heart failure can be managed medically and maintained in a state of satisfactory compensation. In these, repeat catheterization is indicated in six to nine months.

In the patient with a small ventricular septal defect (asymptomatic and without cardiomegaly), cardiac catheterization and operation are not necessary. If the patient is symptomatic, and has cardiomegaly, cardiac catheterization should be performed prior to operation. If the pulmonary flow is 1.5 times the systemic flow, or greater, surgical correction using extracorporeal circulation is indicated. The optimal age for elective repair is four to five years. If the lesion is small, it can be closed with direct suturing, but if the lesion is large, a prosthetic patch may have to be sutured in place.

When pulmonary vascular resistance approaches or exceeds systemic vascular resistance, the shunt becomes balanced or reversed (Eisenmenger's complex) and operation is contraindicated. Prophylactic antibiotics are used as described for patent ductus arteriosus. (See Table 11.)

EISENMENGER'S COMPLEX

This entity is defined here as a ventricular septal defect, with pulmonary hypertension and

TABLE 10. Treatment of Coarctation of the Aorta

```
                        Coarctation of the aorta
                      (with or without other lesions)

        Infant                                                  Child
                                                             (4 to 8 years)

  Asymptomatic      Failure                                      Surgery

Medical management   Treat  ──────►  If unsuccessful ─┐
                      │                                │
                      If                               │
                   successful                          │
                      │                         Possible
                      │                      catheterization
                      │                                │
                   Possible                            │
                 catheterization                       ▼
                      │                          Early surgery
                      └────────────────────────────────────────────►
```

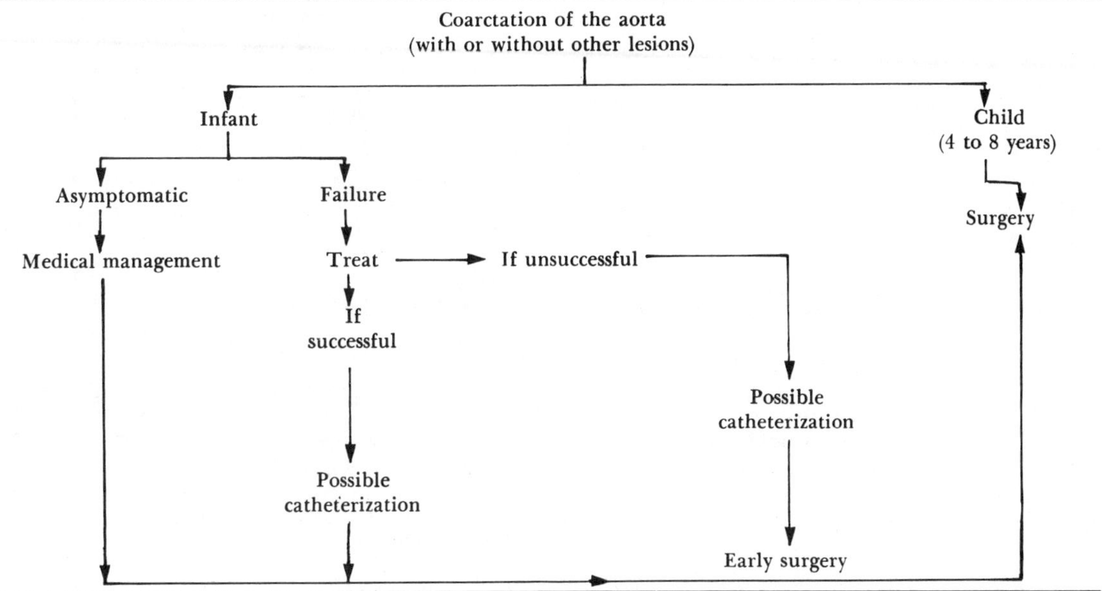

an increase in pulmonary vascular resistance to the point at which the dominant shunt through the defect becomes right to left. There is no satisfactory medical treatment available to these patients. Therapy is directed toward the treatment of intercurrent infections and, when present, polycythemia, syncope, dyspnea and chest pain. There is no definitive surgical treatment available since closure of the ventricular septal defect eliminates the escape valve and carries a 100 per cent mortality rate.

LEFT VENTRICULAR OBSTRUCTION

Patients with left ventricular obstruction may present either symptomatically or asymptomatically in infancy, early childhood or late childhood.

If congestive heart failure occurs early in life, aggressive treatment is indicated. The response to decongestive therapy may be poor. Early catheterization is indicated to determine the specific location and extent of the obstruction. If severe obstruction is present, surgery may be required using extracorporeal circulation. If the patient can be maintained medically in a good state of compensation, operation should be delayed as long as possible.

The child usually is asymptomatic. Barring symptoms of precordial pain, syncopal episodes or dyspnea, medical supervision at six-month to yearly intervals is indicated. Changes in the electrocardiogram suggesting left ven-

tricular hypertrophy or symptoms as already described warrant cardiac catheterization to determine the severity of the obstruction.

The exact time for surgical correction of congenital aortic stenosis and, in fact, the criteria are not completely agreed upon. It is accepted that syncopal episodes, precordial pain or electrocardiographic changes warrant cardiac catheterization. It is also clear that there need not be close correlation between electrocardiographic changes and severity of obstruction. It is generally agreed that if the systolic gradient across the aortic valve exceeds 75 mm. of mercury, surgery is indicated. It is also generally agreed that if the gradient is below 50 mm. of mercury, operation is not indicated. There is difference of opinion as to whether surgery should be done when the gradient is between these two values.

If the obstruction is a discrete subvalvular ring, a satisfactory result can usually be expected. If the valve is stenosed, and can be incised with a minimal degree of residual insufficiency, this is preferred to replacement of the valve. If, however, the valve is severely obstructed and irreparable, the valve replacement may be necessary. If a prosthetic device is inserted, continuous postoperative anticoagulation is probably indicated. The issue of anticoagulation in such instances is not completely settled. Extracorporeal circulation is required in all instances. (See Table 12.)

TABLE 11. Treatment of Ventricular Septal Defect

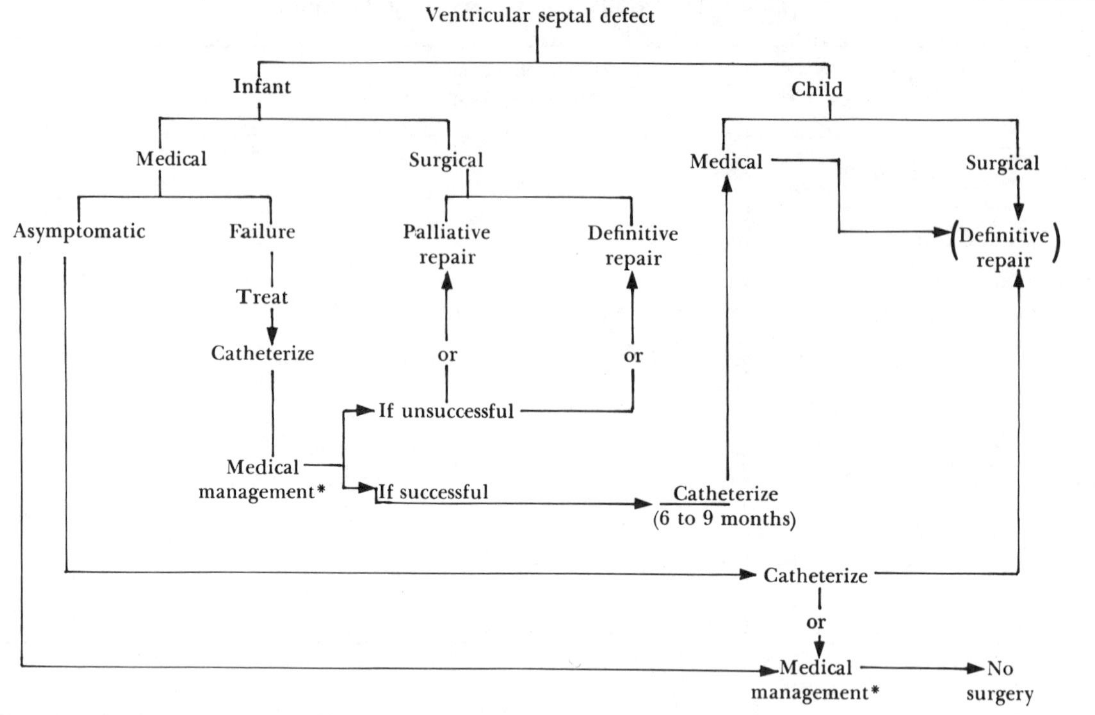

* Use prophylactic antibiotics until surgery is performed.

AORTIC ATRESIA (Hypoplastic Left Heart Syndrome)

The infant with aortic atresia presents in the early days of life with overwhelming congestive heart failure. No satisfactory treatment currently is available for this entity. Death occurs shortly after the onset of symptoms.

ANOMALIES OF THE AORTIC ARCH

If symptoms of esophageal or tracheal compression are present, and if a congenital anomaly of the development of the aortic arch system is suspected, chest roentgenograms following a barium swallow should be taken. Definitive diagnosis is made by aortography. The angiographic procedure performed in several planes permits adequate assessment of the vascular pathology. Surgery can then be accomplished with resection of the offending vessel, thereby relieving the compression and symptoms.

CONGENITAL ANOMALIES OF THE MITRAL AND TRICUSPID VALVES

Mitral Atresia. This lesion is usually seen in conjunction with the hypoplastic left heart syndrome. Early and overwhelming congestive heart failure is the presenting complaint. Medical management does not sustain life, and no surgical correction is available at present.

Mitral Stenosis. When congenital mitral stenosis is seen as an independent lesion, early symptoms can be expected. These often respond poorly to medical management and may require early surgery. The valves are often not reparable, and if replacement is necessary, the surgical results are far from satisfactory. If successful, one can anticipate the need for repeated valve replacement with growth.

Mitral Insufficiency. Isolated mitral insufficiency is uncommon. This lesion usually occurs in association with an ostium primum defect or other forms of endocardial cushion defect. If the patient develops heart failure which is refractory to medical management, surgical intervention is necessary. Operation consists of plication or valvular replacement. Continuous anticoagulant therapy is generally employed if a prosthetic valve is used.

Tricuspid Atresia. The patient with this entity typically has diminished blood flow to the lungs, and therapy must be directed to improving this situation and preventing hypoxic episodes. Systemic artery to pulmonary artery shunts and superior vena cava to pulmonary artery anastomoses (the Glenn operation) are the procedures of choice. The hypoxic episodes can be treated with oxygen and morphine sulfate, 0.1 to 0.2 mg. per kilogram intramuscularly. Frequently the communication between

TABLE 12. Treatment of Left Ventricular Obstruction

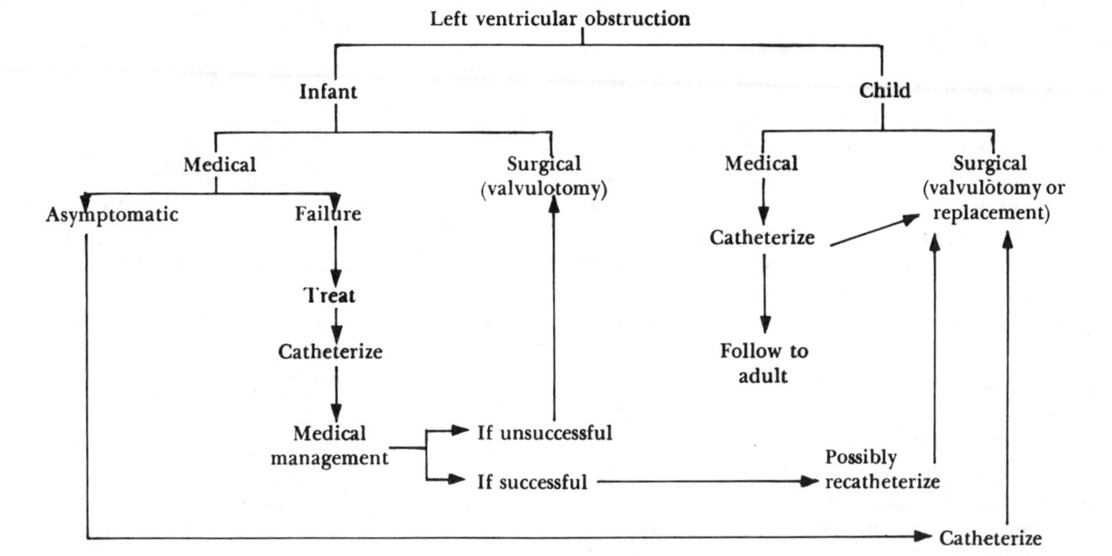

the right atrium and the left atrium is inadequate and requires enlargement. This can be accomplished either by balloon septostomy during the initial catheterization or by an atrial septectomy at the time of operative palliation.

The presence of cyanosis with or without electrocardiographic findings and hypoxic episodes warrants cardiac catheterization early in life.

Tricuspid Stenosis. Tricuspid stenosis is almost always seen with other lesions. Treatment is dependent on the coexisting disorders.

Ebstein's Anomaly. The patient with this anomaly may present early in infancy overwhelmingly ill, in either acute congestive heart failure or with an arrhythmia. Either disorder must be treated by the usual methods. Cardiac catheterization is necessary for diagnosis. If response to medical supervision is satisfactory, this can be continued indefinitely. However, if the patient does not respond satisfactorily to medical treatment, surgical intervention is required. Operations currently available are the Glenn procedure (anastomosis of the superior vena cava to the pulmonary artery) and valvular replacement. (See Table 13.)

Tricuspid Insufficiency. Although congenital tricuspid insufficiency may be an iso-

TABLE 13. Treatment of Ebstein's Anomaly

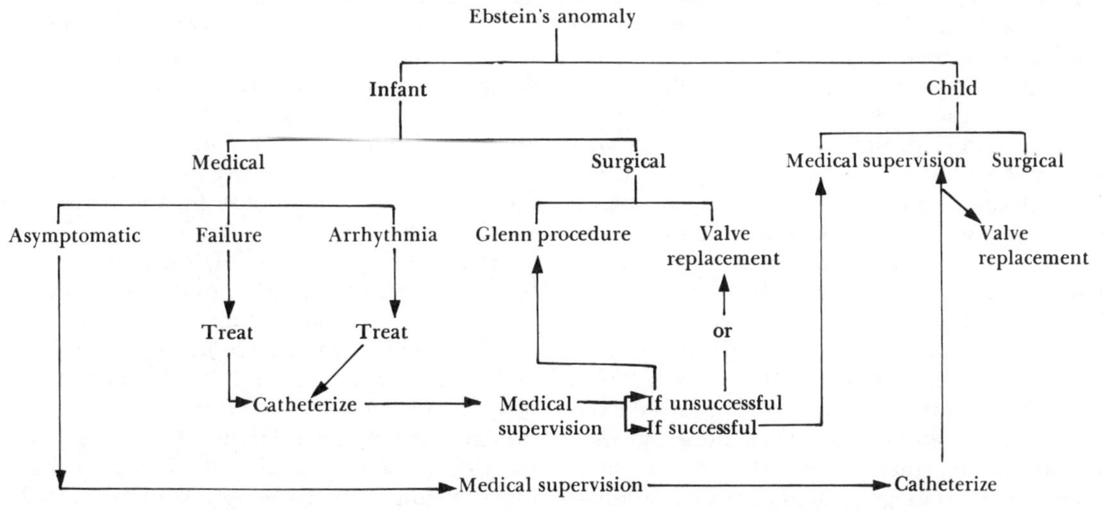

lated lesion, it is almost always seen with other anomalies. Its treatment is dependent upon the coexisting lesions.

CORONARY ARTERY ANOMALIES

Anomalous Origin of the Left Coronary Artery from the Pulmonary Artery. Ever since it was discovered that the major flow of blood in this anomaly may be from the aorta through the anomalous vessel into the pulmonary artery, two methods of approach to treatment have been suggested: One is simple ligation of the coronary artery at the insertion into the pulmonary artery; the other is creation of a bypass graft from the aorta to the anomalous coronary artery. Each is best accomplished beyond the age of three months. It is mandatory, however, that heart catheterization (with appropriate angiographic techniques) be performed prior to operation.

Origin of the Right Coronary Artery from the Pulmonary Artery. This lesion is usually asymptomatic and does not require surgery.

Coronary Arteriovenous Fistula. This entity may be confused with a patent ductus arteriosus and requires cardiac catheterization for definition. If it is present, and if a small coronary artery is involved, simple ligation is the treatment of choice. If a major branch is involved, coronary reconstruction may be required.

TABLE 14. Drugs Used for Treatment of Supraventricular Tachycardia

DRUG	DOSAGE
Digoxin (Lanoxin)	See text
Quinidine	6 mg./kg. every 3 to 5 hours five times a day intramuscularly
Procainamide (Pronestyl)	15 mg./kg. every 6 hours orally; 6 mg./kg. every 6 hours intramuscularly
Lidocaine (Xylocaine)	1 mg./kg. intravenously*
Neostigmine† (Prostigmin)	0.05 to 0.5 mg. subcutaneously as a single dose
Phenylephrine hydrochloride (Neo-Synephrine 1%)	0.1 mg. increasing by 0.1 mg. every 30 minutes up to 0.5 mg. intravenously
Metaraminol (Aramine)	50 mg./100 ml. 5% dextrose by intravenous drip
Norepinephrine (Levophed)	4 ml./1000 ml. 5% dextrose by intravenous drip
Propranolol (Inderal)	0.1 mg./kg. intravenously

* Manufacturer's precaution: Experience with lidocaine in children is limited.

† The administration of neostigmine (Prostigmin) for treatment of supraventricular tachycardia is not listed in the manufacturer's package insert indications. However, this use of neostigmine has worked well in our experience.

CARDIAC ARRHYTHMIAS

Abnormal rhythms of sinus origin do not require therapy. Extrasystoles of atrial or nodal origin also do not require treatment. Ventricular extrasystoles that are unifocal in origin or infrequent in occurrence, or which disappear with exercise, do not require treatment. If they are from multiple foci, consecutive, or increase with exercise, their cause should be investigated.

Treatment of supraventricular tachycardia should be considered in terms of whether the onset is in infancy or in older childhood. In infancy the usual methods of vagal stimulation —carotid sinus pressure, vomiting or eyeball pressure—are usually ineffective. Digoxin is the drug of choice. The intravenous or intramuscular route should be used, depending upon the severity of the situation. Other drugs which have a vagotonic effect can be used and are listed in Table 14.

Cardioversion can be used initially to convert the arrhythmia. If digitalis has been given prior to cardioversion, great care must be exercised in the use of countershock since ventricular fibrillation due to digitalis toxicity may occur. Low wattage should be used initially with gradual increase in the strength of shock, depending upon the response of the patient. The amount of initial wattage depends upon the size of the patient and varies from 10 to 50 wattseconds. Once converted, the patient is maintained on digoxin for six months. If a second episode occurs, and conversion to sinus rhythm is successful, digoxin is continued for one to two years.

In the older child, the methods of conversion are the same as in the infant but in a dosage range appropriate for age. There is a greater tendency for repeated episodes in this group of children, and maintenance digoxin is usually given for one to two years. With recurrent episodes, propranolol in the dosage of 10 to 50 mg. per day can be given in addition to, or sometimes instead of, digoxin, particularly when the Wolff-Parkinson-White syndrome is the cause of the arrhythmia.

First and second degree heart block usually do not require treatment. If the first degree block is due to administration of digoxin, caution in further use needs to be exercised, but the drug is not discontinued. Complete heart block requires treatment if syncopal episodes or heart failure occurs. Isoproterenol can be tried in the dose of 5 to 20 mg. every 3 to 4 hours sublingually. If this is ineffective in preventing the symptoms, implantation of a permanent pacemaker is indicated.

PERICARDITIS

It is essential that the cause of pericarditis be determined before treatment is instituted. Therapy is directed mainly to the primary cause. If signs of tamponade occur, pericardiocentesis is indicated. However, pericardiocentesis may also be indicated to establish a definitive diagnosis. In the case of constrictive pericarditis, pericardiectomy is required. Pericarditis may occur with myocarditis.

MYOCARDITIS

Treatment for myocarditis is directed toward the primary cause of the disease as well as its secondary effects. If congestive heart failure or arrhythmias occur, they should be treated in the usual manner.

Hypertension

SOL LONDE, M.D., ALAN ROBSON, M.D., *and* DAVID GOLDRING, M.D.

The establishment of blood pressure standards for normal children of different ages and of both sexes has emphasized that blood pressure readings considered normotensive for an adult may represent significant hypertension in the younger child. Although severe chronic hypertension is not a common problem in the pediatric population, children with systolic and diastolic blood pressures consistently above the 95th percentile for their age are not infrequently seen. Moreover, hypertensive encephalopathy is seen in the pediatric age group, frequently occurring at lower blood pressures than in adult patients.

Blood pressure should be measured with the patient at rest and accustomed to his surroundings, and with the correct size of blood pressure cuff as recommended by the American Heart Association. Anxiety or agitation may result in falsely elevated values for blood pressure, as may the use of too small a cuff. Too large a cuff may result in erroneously low values.

If hypertension represents a medical emergency, treatment should be instituted immediately. However, whenever possible, investigations into the cause should be completed before starting therapy, since some drugs interfere with the interpretation of diagnostic tests, and since the primary drug of choice for the treatment of acute and chronic hypertension is different. In addition, it should also be determined whether there may be an underlying, surgically treatable cause for the elevated blood pressure, such as coarctation of the aorta, renal artery stenosis, unilateral renal disease, primary aldosteronism, pheochromocytoma and, less frequently, Wilms' tumor or neuroblastoma.

Severe hypertension (systolic values above 170 mm. Hg or diastolic values above 100 mm. Hg) usually requires early treatment. The need for treatment in patients with more moderate elevations of blood pressure is determined by several factors, including the patient's age, the underlying cause of the hypertension and whether hypertension is persistent or intermittent. For example, we are more inclined to treat a patient with moderately elevated blood pressure due to acute glomerulonephritis than a child of the same age with the same degree of hypertension appearing after genitourinary tract surgery, since hypertension in the latter situation is usually transient.

ACUTE HYPERTENSION

The drugs most frequently used in the treatment of acute hypertension in the pediatric age group are hydralazine and reserpine given either alone or in combination. Hydralazine lowers blood pressure without reducing renal blood flow and is of special value in patients with compromised renal function. When given alone, a starting oral dose of 0.75 mg. per kilogram per day can be given in four to six divided and equally spaced doses. If there is no response, the dose can be progressively increased to a maximum of 3.5 mg. per kilogram per day. If the patient is nauseated, the drug can be given intramuscularly in an equivalent dose. The onset of action may be delayed even when the drug is given intravenously, but effects are usually seen within 1 to 2 hours after oral administration and within 10 to 80 minutes when it is given parenterally. The response lasts 4 to 6 hours. Side effects occur infrequently. Headaches, which respond to antihistamines, and flushing may be seen but rarely present a major problem.

Reserpine acts up to 24 hours with a maximum effect 2 to 6 hours after ingestion. A response can be seen within an hour after intramuscular injection. The starting dose of up to 0.07 mg. per kilogram (not to exceed a maximum initial dose of 2 mg.) is usually repeated at 12-hour intervals. Depression may result from reserpine administration in older children but is rarely seen in younger children. Nasal congestion, sedation and bradycardia are more troublesome. Reserpine should not be administered to patients who are to undergo surgery, to patients with a pheochromocytoma, if catecholamine levels are to be determined, or in conjunction with guanethidine or methyldopa or with any cough mixtures or decongestants that contain sympathomimetic amines.

The use of hydralazine and reserpine together is often effective when one of the drugs alone has failed to produce an adequate response. When using this combination, reserpine is given in usual dosage at 12-hour intervals, and hydralazine is given initially in a reduced dosage of 0.15 mg. per kilogram per dose, as needed at up to 4-hour intervals to regulate spikes of hypertension. If a greater response is required, we have given larger doses of hydralazine than this without encountering any difficulties. Side effects from this combination are encountered less frequently than when reserpine is given alone.

Emergency Situations. If a patient does not respond adequately or sufficiently rapidly to the administration of reserpine and hydralazine, we have had good response to the use of the ganglionic blocking agent pentolinium tartrate given subcutaneously. Some patients, especially those with renal insufficiency, are particularly sensitive to this drug, and to avoid hypotension the standard preparation of pentolinium tartrate (10 mg. per ml.) should be diluted with sterile normal saline to 1 mg. per ml. in a tuberculin syringe. An initial dose of 0.1 ml. of the diluted solution is injected subcutaneously in a peripheral part of an arm with a blood pressure cuff in place proximal to the site of injection. If there is no response, subsequent doses are doubled progressively and are given at 10- to 20-minute intervals until adequate control is obtained. The onset of action of this drug is rapid, often within minutes, and constant monitoring of blood pressure is necessary. If response is too great, the blood pressure cuff is temporarily inflated to reduce venous return and thus lower the rate of absorption of the drug. When the correct dose has been determined, it can be repeated as needed at up to 4-hour intervals.

Intravenous methyldopa can also be effective in rapidly lowering the blood pressure. The initial dose is 2 to 4 mg. per kilogram. If there is no initial response, subsequent doses can be doubled or quadrupled and given at 4- to 6-hour intervals. Side effects include bradycardia, sinus arrhythmia and drowsiness.

Intravenous sodium nitroprusside may lower blood pressure in patients with intractable severe hypertension. It has to be prepared in the hospital pharmacy. We have followed Loggie's* regimen of giving the drug as a constant infusion. The initial dose, 0.004 microgram per kilogram per minute, is increased until a satisfactory response is obtained with a dose of approximately 1 microgram per kilogram per minute. Higher doses have been used in adults.

Diazoxide (Schering Corporation), originally developed as a diuretic and later used to treat hypoglycemia, has been found to lower blood pressure in patients with intractable hypertension. It should be given intravenously as a rapidly administered, single injection in a dose of up to 10 mg. per kilogram.† It acts rapidly and its effects last approximately 24 hours. It is important to give a large dose (5 mg. per kilogram) initially, since resistance may develop if smaller, more frequent doses are given. Hyperglycemia has not been a problem in the patients we have treated.

CHRONIC HYPERTENSION

When designing a long-term regimen for treating chronic hypertension, it is important to make it simple, using only a single drug whenever possible. Many parents willingly purchase a sphygmomanometer and quickly learn to measure blood pressure accurately, ensuring good control of blood pressure in the home and reducing the frequency of visits to the physician's office. Since short-term benefits of therapy may not be readily apparent to parents, it is very important to discuss with the family the reasons for therapy and possible side effects. By taking such simple measures, the therapeutic regimen is more likely to be followed correctly.

Especially in the patient with chronic hypertension, too-rapid correction of hypertension may result in hypotensive symptoms, even though blood pressure values may still be above normal. In such circumstances the dose of hypotensive drugs should be temporarily reduced. When the blood pressure has increased moderately, therapy can be reinstituted with an appropriate reduction in dose. Optimum treatment should probably aim at the eventual reduction of blood pressure to normal values.

---

* Loggie, J.: Hypertension in Children and Adolescents. II Drug Therapy. *J. Pediat.*, 74:640, 1969.

† Manufacturer's precaution: The safety of the intravenous use of diazoxide in children has not yet been established.

Long-term treatment with oral hydralazine (up to 200 mg. per day; a lupus-like syndrome may develop when larger doses are given for several months) or reserpine (up to 2 mg. per day‡) may be effective in treating chronic hypertension, but we prefer the use of other drugs such as oral methyldopa. The usual starting dose of methyldopa (10 mg. per kilogram per day) is given in three divided doses. If there is no response, the dosage can be increased as high as 60 mg. per kilogram per day. In small children, administration of the drug may be difficult, since only 250-mg. tablets are available. Drowsiness or an acquired hemolytic anemia may result, but side effects are rare with the drug. Methyldopa should not be used in conjunction with reserpine because of their incompatibility; in addition, it interferes with the diagnostic tests for pheochromocytoma.

Successful long-term control of chronic hypertension has been achieved with guanethidine and requires only a single daily dose given in the morning. The initial dose approximates 0.2 mg. per kilogram per day. We usually start with either 5 or 10 mg. per day, depending on the size of the child, and have usually observed a response with daily dose of 25 mg. per day or less. The drug has little effect when the patient is in the supine position; thus, patients should sleep with several pillows or with the head of the bed elevated on blocks. Blood pressure should be monitored in the supine and upright position as well as after exercise. Postural hypotension usually observed early in the morning is the main side effect and can be averted by instructing the patient to get out of bed slowly, sitting for a few seconds before attempting to stand. Mild diarrhea is an occasional complication. The drug is incompatible with reserpine and is ineffective if given with the antidepressants imipramine and desipramine.

We do not use diuretics alone to treat hypertension. The hypotensive effects of the drugs already discussed can be potentiated by the use of either a low salt diet or diuretics. Chlorthalidone, because of its longer action, is given as a single morning dose of 2 mg. per kilogram. Dietary salt restriction may potentiate the hypotensive effects of the diuretics, but severe salt restriction is rarely needed and is not well tolerated by patients. The diuretics mentioned may be relatively ineffective in the presence of marked renal insufficiency and can be replaced by furosemide§ given in a single daily dose of approximately 0.5 mg. per kilogram. Each of the diuretics results in negative potassium balance, and furosemide is a potent saluretic and kaliuretic agent which should not be used in patients with normal renal function.

Used alone, spironolactone, an aldosterone inhibitor, may have a mild hypotensive effect. We have restricted its use (2 mg. per kilogram per day) to patients with evidence of secondary aldosteronism, and it may be useful to decrease the hypokalemia associated with the use of diuretics.

Recent evidence suggests that the combination of hydralazine, propranolol and a diuretic is very effective in the control of moderate or severe hypertension. Although there is still limited experience with this regimen to date, it appears to produce no major side effects.

SPECIAL SITUATIONS

The hypertension seen in patients taking high doses of *steroids* may be prevented by the patient's strict adherence to a 1-Gm. salt diet, or can usually be controlled by oral hydralazine. Diuretics may be needed to control edema in some of these patients, but they should be avoided whenever possible since they potentiate the hypokalemic effect of the steroids.

Therapy is rarely required for the hypertension seen with *coarctation of the aorta,* although treatment of the postoperative hypertension which can persist for 10 to 14 days may reduce the incidence of complications, such as abdominal arteritis or mesenteric artery thrombosis. Hydralazine and reserpine are the drugs of choice in this situation, as they are in the treatment of hypertension secondary to *raised intracranial pressure.* In acute oliguric *renal failure,* severe fluid overload may make patients refractory to conventional hypotensive therapy, and dialysis with fluid removal is then required to control the hypertension. In patients on chronic dialysis, blood pressure appears to be directly related to salt intake. Rigid control of dietary salt or more frequent dialysis is required if such patients develop hypertension.

Although the hypertension associated with *pheochromocytoma* has been treated preoperatively with both phentolamine and phenoxybenzamine, recent data suggests that better re-

‡ Note: Reserpine 2 mg. per day is greater than the dosage recommended by the manufacturer. The manufacturer states: Initial dose is 0.5 mg. daily for one to two weeks. Maintenance dose is 0.1 to 0.25 mg. daily. Higher doses should be used cautiously because serious mental depression and other side effects may be increased considerably.

§ Manufacturer's precaution: Furosemide should not be given to children until further experience is accumulated.

sults are obtained by the use of phenoxybenzamine (1 to 2 mg. per kilogram) alone, given every 12 hours. The dosage should be adjusted by measuring blood pressure in both the supine and the upright positions, and the drug should be continued for 7 to 10 days prior to surgery.

There is now evidence that *essential hypertension* may begin in the pediatric age group and may well be the most frequent type of hypertension encountered by the pediatrician in practice. Usually of mild degree, and frequently associated with a positive family history of hypertension and with obesity, the natural history of hypertension in these asymptomatic patients is not yet known, nor has the role of hypotensive therapy in these patients been determined.

Hypotension

SOL LONDE, M.D., ALAN ROBSON, M.D., *and* DAVID GOLDRING, M.D.

Hypotension cannot be defined in terms of absolute systolic and diastolic pressures, especially in infants and children whose blood pressure changes with age. Perhaps it is best to consider hypotension as a sudden drop in blood pressure which results in failure of cellular function on the basis of inadequate perfusion.

Hypotension is encountered as an acute life-threatening emergency in infants and children who suffer any of a number of catastrophic events listed in Table 1. Effective therapy requires an understanding of the specific fundamental disorder, of basic cardiovascular, renal and pulmonary dynamics, of fluid and electrolyte balance and of antibiotic usage. It is beyond the scope of this discussion to describe in detail the pathogenesis of the derangements in body functions, and so the major physiologic responses to these severe disturbances are listed in Table 1. Also, some of the general principles of therapeutic management are listed in the table and will be mentioned briefly here. It should be stressed that hypotension is usually one of a number of very serious disturbances in body function in these emergency states, and treatment should be directed not only toward the correction of hypotension but more importantly and primarily toward correction of the specific underlying cause.

Monitoring. The ultrasonic Doppler technique has made it possible to measure and monitor blood pressure in small children and premature infants. Blood pressure as well as other vital body functions should be continually assessed. Thus, central venous pressure, heart rate and rhythm, temperature, body weight, fluid intake and output, pO_2, pCO_2, pH, cardiac output, serum osmolality, serum electrolytes, urine, hemoglobin, hematocrit, platelets, white blood cells and clotting mechanism must be monitored, and bacterial cultures (blood, spinal fluid, tracheal fluid and so forth) should be obtained as necessary.

Transport of Patient. When the critically ill child is some distance from the medical center, it is imperative to institute emergency therapeutic measures (fluids, digitalization, antibiotics and so forth), before transporting him. A well-equipped ambulance with trained personnel should be used, and the physicians at the medical center should be alerted. At the hospital, the appropriate emergency therapeutic regimen should be implemented with dispatch in an intensive care unit if one is to avert cardiac arrest, which may occur in any of the emergencies listed in Table 1.

Fluid Replacement. Initial extracellular fluid replacement is vital in most of these emergencies because of diminished blood volume, dehydration and anhydremia. When fluids are administered, it must be remembered that insensible water loss and water loss due to high fever are proportionately greater in the young and that renal function is immature during the first weeks of life. Thus, the turnover of water, sodium and potassium is greater in infancy and water requirement is about 150 to 200 ml. per kilogram per 24 hours. The volume of the initial parenteral infusion of Ringer's lactate or 0.9 per cent saline has to be adjusted for each patient depending on the estimation of the degree of dehydration, anhydremia and hypovolemia. In congestive heart failure the volume of fluid given has to be less because of the hypervolemia, and should therefore be 50 to 100 ml. per kilogram in 24 hours. The diminished cardiac output and hypotension due to exsanguinating severe hemorrhage can be promptly helped by the immediate administration of Ringer's lactate or 0.9 per cent saline (20 to 30 ml. per kilogram of body weight in 10 to 15 minutes). This should be followed as soon as possible by transfusion with whole blood of 20 ml. per kilogram body weight given over a period of 20 to 60 minutes. The rapidity of administration and the amount of blood given is governed by the status of the patient and the estimate of blood loss. In barbiturate intoxication, 10 per cent glucose in Ringer's or 0.9 per cent saline may be given initially to

TABLE 1. Causes of and Therapy for Hypotension

	PHYSIOLOGIC DERANGEMENT					THERAPY††					
Condition†	*Blood Volume*	*Hypoxemia*	*Respiratory Distress*	*Renal Function*	*Blood (B) or Plasma (P)*	*Respiratory Assistance: Endotracheal Tube (ET) or Tracheostomy (T)*	*Digoxin*	*Diuretics*	*Morphine Sulfate*	*Iso-proterenol*	*Antibiotics*
1. Diarrhea and/or vomiting	↓	+*	+*	↓	B** or P**	ET**	0	0	0	+**	+**
2. Endotoxic shock	↓*	+	+	↓	B** or P**	ET	+**	+**	0	+	+
3. Acute, severe blood loss‡	↓	+*	+*	↓*	B	ET**	0	0	0	+**	0
4. Severe burn	↓	+*	+*	↓*	B and P	T**	+**	+**	+**	+**	+
5. Congestive heart failure	↑*	+	+	↓	0	ET**	+	+	+	+	+**
6. Untoward drug reactions											
a. Anaphylactic shock	↓*	+	+	↓*	B** or P**	ET	0	0	0	0	0
b. Barbiturate intoxication	↓	+*	+*	↓*	0	ET**	0	+**	0	+**	0
c. Imipramine intoxication§	?	+*	+*	↓*	0	ET**	0	0	0	0	0
7. Acute adrenal insufficiency	↓	+	+	+*	0	ET**	0	0	0	0	0

†† *Oxygen therapy* should be used for all of the listed conditions. *Fluids* are indicated in all of the disorders. In patients with congestive heart failure due to congenital heart defects, cautious administration of fluids in reduced amounts is indicated, especially in the postoperative period (see text, under Fluid Replacement).

† *Tachycardia* and *hypotension* are observed in all of these conditions. The *cardiac output* is down in all, and in 6(c) it may be depressed.

** May be needed.

* May be present.

‡ After 24 to 48 hours, the blood volume may be increased.

§ Hypotension is postural. Discontinuation of drug and institution of bedrest have been effective.

induce diuresis, and in acute adrenal insufficiency, 5 per cent glucose in 0.9 per cent saline should be used.

The metabolic acidosis in diarrhea or endotoxic shock is treated with sodium bicarbonate. The amount needed is calculated as follows: desired bicarbonate level (20 to 25 mEq. per liter), minus the patient's actual bicarbonate level, times 0.6, times kilogram body weight is equal to the mEq. of bicarbonate to be given. In congestive heart failure, one-fourth to one-half of this amount should be given over a 6- to 8-hour period to reduce the possibility of hypernatremia, water retention and alkalosis. It should be noted that the full dose of bicarbonate may not be needed because the high serum lactic acid (anaerobic metabolism) causing the acidosis may be quickly metabolized as heart function improves.

Respiratory Assistance. The infant or child with a severe burn, especially if it involves the face and neck, may need a tracheostomy for more effective respiratory assistance. This is also true of the occasional infant or child during the immediate postoperative period after extensive open heart surgery for congenital cardiac malformations. Since such patients are usually weak, a volume-limited ventilator should be used because the infant or child may have a superimposed pulmonary infection and an increased or changing lung compliance. Patients in severe congestive heart failure, endotoxic shock, imipramine or barbiturate intoxication may be tided over the critical period with an endotracheal tube.

Adrenergic Drugs. In conditions such as acute congestive heart failure and endotoxic shock, improvement in cardiovascular hemodynamics may be achieved by isoproterenol, a beta-adrenergic stimulating agent which dilates the arterioles (thus reducing vascular resistance) and improves cardiac output. In addition, the patient is benefited by the drug's positive inotropic and chronotropic properties. The drug also reduces airway resistance and pulmonary vascular pressure. Isoproterenol should be given at a rate of 0.2 microgram per kilogram per minute and the blood pressure should be monitored.

Epinephrine hydrochloride is indicated as immediate treatment for anaphylaxis; 0.2 to 0.5 ml. of a 1:1000 solution should be given parenterally and repeated in 15 to 20 minutes, if necessary.

Levarterenol bitartrate is indicated in anaphylactic shock and in acute adrenal insufficiency. This drug is given intravenously as 1 ml. of a 0.2 per cent solution in 250 ml. of diluent at 2 micrograms per square meter per minute and should be titrated using constantly monitored blood pressure as a guide.

Steroids. Massive doses of dexamethasone (5 mg. per kilogram of body weight) or its equivalent have been recommended as an adjunct to treatment of endotoxic shock, but the use of this drug is still controversial.

Immediate administration of hydrocortisone is indicated for acute adrenal insufficiency. The recommended dose for immediate intravenous use is 25 mg. for infants and 50 mg. for children. This same dose can then be given as an infusion every 4 hours until the patient is stable. The patient should also be given desoxycorticosterone acetate intramuscularly (1 mg. for an infant and 2 to 4 mg. for a child).

Other Measures (Table 1). Digoxin should be given intravenously or intramuscularly (0.03 mg. per kilogram of body weight) as a total digitalizing dose. Some have recommended higher doses, but we feel that this increases the risk of toxic reactions. One-half of this dose is given at once, one-fourth in 3 to 6 hours, and one-fourth during the next 3 to 6 hours. The amount of digoxin may be increased to 0.1 mg. per kilogram of body weight as a total digitalizing dose if necessary, depending on the response of the individual patient.

Morphine sulfate is strongly recommended for the restless, agitated infant in acute congestive heart failure (0.1 to 0.2 mg. per kilogram of body weight). In an effort to suppress sodium resorption by the kidney and thus decrease edema, a diuretic agent is indicated and ethacrynic acid* has been found very effective. The dose is 1 mg. per kilogram of body weight intravenously, and this may be repeated in 12 hours.

The above discussion touched briefly on the more important causes of hypotension and their management. The salvage rate will depend on the ability of the physician to make an accurate diagnosis with dispatch and on the institution of immediate appropriate therapy in a well-staffed and well-equipped intensive care unit.

Peripheral Vascular Disease

WARREN G. GUNTHEROTH, M.D., *and*
D. EUGENE STRANDNESS, JR., M.D.

Peripheral vascular disorders of whatever cause will present with similar findings on initial inspection: obstructed veins will result in

* Manufacturer's precaution: Infant dose of ethacrynic acid has not been established.

markedly reduced arterial flow, and the results of arterial spasm may be identical to those of permanent arterial obstruction at the time of onset. Therapy, however, varies from minimal medical treatment to amputation, requiring a thoughtful approach to diagnosis as well as to selection of treatment.

PERIPHERAL ARTERIES: VASOACTIVE DISORDERS

Raynaud's Disease. Raynaud's phenomenon is a vasospastic disorder with a characteristic sequence of pallor, cyanosis and rubor. Criteria for the diagnosis of Raynaud's disease are excitation of the vasospastic disorder by cold or emotion, bilaterality, absence of gangrene and absence of an underlying primary disease.

Therapy should be conditioned by the generally favorable prognosis of Raynaud's disease. Surgical sympathectomy is rarely, if ever, indicated in the primary disorder. If the symptoms are bothersome, selection of a warm, dry climate is helpful but not mandatory. Clothing selection should be directed toward conserving body heat rather than just covering the affected extremities; our studies show that cold applied directly to the affected extremity is less likely to produce vasospasm than is general body cooling. The clothing should not be tight-fitting; hard-finish, tightly woven material is essential to block wind, and bulky woolen clothing is necessary for insulation against cold. In girls, particularly adolescents, increased muscular activity is probably beneficial in reducing suspectibility to cold.

Medications have not been successful in eliminating Raynaud's phenomenon in our patients, but they have reduced the severity and frequency of episodes in every instance. Although several similar drugs may be equally effective, we have used tolazoline (Priscoline), a direct-acting agent that substantially increases flow in vasospastic vessels without generalized flushing or hypotension. The beginning dose is 0.5 mg. per kilogram four times a day. (Adult dosage is begun at 25 mg. four times a day and may be increased to 50 mg. six times a day.) The major precaution in the use of tolazoline is in patients with gastritis or ulcers, since the medication stimulates gastric secretions. In addition to tolazoline, reserpine has been useful in small doses, 0.1 to 0.25 mg. daily by mouth.

Therapy is rarely required for two related disorders, acrocyanosis and livedo reticularis, except for cosmetic reasons.

Erythromelalgia. Although the number of cases of erythromelalgia is smaller than that of Raynaud's disease, the symptoms are so much more debilitating that therapy must be considered briefly. Erythromelalgia presents as a peripheral hyperreactivity to heat, the counterpart to reaction to cold in Raynaud's disease. The hot, swollen and tender hands and feet are extraordinarily unpleasant, and have led to suicide in a young adult in our hospital. Therapy should be directed toward physical factors as well as medicinal factors. Cooling of the body in general, as well as cool soaks to the affected extremities, brings some degree of relief. Ephedrine has been effective in some instances, 0.5 mg. per kilogram every 4 to 6 hours (average adult dose, 25 mg.). To avoid the excitability effect of ephedrine, we usually add a tranquilizer or sedative. Aspirin is definitely worth trying on a regular basis (every 4 hours), not only for its analgesic effects but also because there are indications that endogenous bradykinin may be involved and aspirin is almost specific as a blocker. Other authorities have suggested that erythromelalgia is a form of "peripheral migraine," and that release of serotonin is responsible. Accordingly, they have suggested antiserotonin medications, such as methysergide. However, cyproheptadine is a safer antiserotonin preparation. The adult dose is 4 mg. three times daily, increased as necessary up to eight times daily. For children, an average dose is 0.08 mg. per kilogram. A curious side effect of the drug is stimulation of appetite, in addition to drowsiness, both of which may be desirable in some instances.

Causalgia. Although a deep wound with injury to a major nerve trunk leading to "major causalgia" is easily diagnosed, forms of minor causalgia often elude prompt and effective treatment by masquerading as primary vascular disorders. Unilateral vascular disorders, particularly when associated with exquisite tenderness, swelling and abnormal perspiration, should suggest post-traumatic sympathetic dystrophy, a form of minor causalgia. The vascular disorder is most often vasospastic, but we have successfully treated a boy with sympathetic dystrophy resembling unilateral erythromelalgia. Therapy is the same regardless of the vascular disorder: paravertebral sympathetic blockade with injections of 1 per cent lidocaine. If the diagnosis is correct, subjective relief is striking and will last for several hours. Permanent improvement will depend on vigorous physical therapy, beginning at once under the effect of the block, continuing for days or weeks and usually requiring additional injections at intervals. It is imperative to interrupt the cycle of pain, disuse osteoporosis and so forth, and exercise of the affected limb is the essential part of the therapy. The main function of sympathetic blockade is to permit relatively painless exercise of the limb. Sympathectomy is rarely, if ever, indicated in the treatment.

PERIPHERAL ARTERIES: OBSTRUCTIVE DISORDERS

Trauma. The immediate goal of therapy for traumatic interruption of arterial flow is to prevent loss of tissue and limb. Continuity of the arteries must be restored, spasm relieved, intraluminal clots removed and prevented and tissue edema managed so that the arterial lumen is not compromised. None of these aspects of care may be neglected without jeopardizing the future growth of the limb and its function without claudication.

Restoration of adequate circulating blood volume is of primary importance, not only for the preservation of life but also to permit intelligent judgment of the state of the local circulation. Although actual gangrene is rare in children, a nonoperative approach to vascular injury prolonged beyond 6 to 8 hours may lead to subsequent weakness and atrophy. Thus, the ultimate function of the limb should govern the acute management, and early intervention by a skilled surgeon may be truly conservative. If the diagnosis of spasm is entertained, the period of nonintervention should be relatively brief, and the assumption tested by nonsurgical sympathetic block. Arteriography may be helpful in locating the site and extent of obstruction, but the use of a transcutaneous Doppler flowmeter is less traumatic and may be repeated at will.

Proper surgical technique will include scrupulous debridement; end-to-end anastomosis if adequate vessel length is available to avoid tension, and autogenous vein graft replacement otherwise; complete removal of distal clots; relief of arterial spasm; and fasciotomy to control complications of edema and hematoma.

Congenital Stenosis. Peripheral arterial stenosis rarely produces any definite signs or symptoms when it is congenital, reflecting the remarkable ability of youthful tissues to develop collateral circulation.

Arteritis. Inflammatory disease of arteries may occur locally or as part of a widespread disorder (see discussion of polyarteritis, p. 380). The latter is rare, although the former may be more common than recognized. When smaller arteries are involved, a muscle biopsy is the only means of certain diagnosis. The most effective treatment is identification and removal of sensitizing drugs, infection or toxin and, in severe generalized arteritis, the use of steroids. Major vessel arteritis due to local irritation, such as the thoracic outlet syndrome, may require resection of the first rib and arterial thrombectomy.

PERIPHERAL ARTERIES: FISTULAS

Trauma. It is quite possible that the most frequent cause of this disorder in the pediatric age group is needle puncture of the femoral vein by physicians. The treatment is obviously surgical after the diagnosis is established, with proper caution that closure of the fistulous connection does not compromise the arterial lumen.

Congenital. The need for treatment and the probability of success vary according to whether the fistulas are multiple or single, whether they are large vessel or small and whether the vital organs are involved directly or by virtue of inseparable involvement of the arterial supply of that organ. There is no satisfactory therapy for multiple, small fistulas, but large vessel fistulas, if well localized, may be satisfactorily divided or removed if there is adequate circulation to vital tissues peripheral to the fistula.

PERIPHERAL VEINS: THROMBOPHLEBITIS

Thrombophlebitis is rarely a pediatric problem, but its occurrence is attended by considerable risk to life if treatment is not prompt and effective. The aggressiveness required in the therapeutic approach depends on the extent of the thrombophlebitis, whether it is progressing in spite of medical therapy and whether pulmonary embolism has occurred.

Massive deep thrombophlebitis (phlegmasia cerulea dolens) involves the entire limb with massive edema, severe pain and cyanosis. The presence and quality of the distal pulse depend on the general status of the patient, particularly the blood volume and pressure, the degree of arterial spasm and the degree of edema at the site of the pulse. The value of thrombectomy is controversial but should be considered if the diagnosis is established within 24 hours of the onset of symptoms. The location of the thrombus in the deep venous system before surgery and the success of thrombectomy should be determined by either contrast phlebography or Doppler ultrasonic flow mapping. Venous ligation or plication (usually at the level of the inferior vena cava) should be considered in patients who develop pulmonary emboli while on adequate anticoagulant therapy.

Less massive thrombophlebitis is termed phlegmasia alba dolens or "milk leg," because of the pale, swollen appearance of the extremity. The treatment is conservative for this condition and consists primarily of anticoagulation. Initial heparinization is 150 to 200 U.S.P. units per kilogram intravenously, the dose subsequently adjusted according to the Lee-White clotting time at 4-hour intervals. The clotting time should be 20 to 30 minutes prior to the next dose. Heparin is continued until the circulatory status of the limb is satisfactory and oral sodium warfarin is begun. Heparin may be discontinued when the prothrombin time is twice the normal control (20 to 30 per cent on the Quick scale). The initial dose may be calculated on the basis of 1 mg. per kilogram and adjusted according to daily prothrombin levels until a stable dosage has been determined. Total duration of warfarin therapy should be at least six weeks. The patient should be kept at bed rest until tenderness has subsided, with the legs elevated to 20 degrees. Elastic bandages are applied from the feet to the upper thigh, and tailored support hose are mandatory before ambulation is begun.

If pulmonary embolism occurs, or if there is progression of the thrombophlebitis on adequate heparin therapy, plication of the inferior vena cava should be considered.

SMALL VESSEL DISORDERS

Frostbite. Rapid rewarming with moderately warm water (40 to 42° C.) should be promptly initiated if the extremity is still frozen or cold. However, for those situations in which the physician may be consulted by radio or telephone, and the patient is still remote from hospitalization, rewarming should not be undertaken unless all danger of refreezing is eliminated. The duration of rewarming required will depend on the depth to which the tissue is frozen; and if there is through and through freezing, rewarming of the deeper layers may require over an hour. The subsequent care is one of fastidious hygiene of the injured extremity for a lengthy period; extirpation or amputation should be delayed, since surprising recovery is characteristic of frostbite injuries. Daily care should include gentle cleansing, avoidance of pressure or even light contact, bed rest and analgesics until the acute inflammation has subsided. After that stage, physical therapy is essential to restore gradually full range of motion; whirlpool baths may aid in this.

Purpuric Disorders. Small vessel thrombosis may occur with a normal platelet count (nonthrombocytopenic purpura) or with a low platelet count (thrombocytopenic purpura). The treatment varies according to the underlying disorder. The most dramatic forms of purpura are those that are progressive, causing a consumptive coagulopathy. Treatment, therefore, is anticoagulation with heparin.

References

Guntheroth, W. G., et al.: Raynaud's Disease in Children. *Circulation,* 36:724, 1967.

Guntheroth, W. G., et al.: Post-traumatic Sympathetic Dystrophy. Dissociation of Pain and Vasomotor Changes. *Am. J. Dis. Child.,* 121:511, 1971.

Strandness, D. E., Jr.: *Collateral Circulation in Clinical Surgery.* Philadelphia, W. B. Saunders Company, 1969.

Winsor, T., and Hyman, C.: *A Primer of Peripheral Vascular Diseases.* Philadelphia, Lea & Febiger, 1965.

Purpura Fulminans

E. RICHARD STIEHM, M.D.

Purpura fulminans (postinfectious gangrene) is a disorder of unknown cause, characterized by the abrupt appearance of massive purpuric areas of the skin with bleeding and necrosis. In most cases, there has been a preceding infectious disorder, such as mild viral respiratory infection, chickenpox or streptococcal infection, suggesting that this disorder may be a hypersensitivity reaction. There are significant morbidity (loss of soft tissue, amputation) and mortality rates. Frequently there is confusion with the cutaneous manifestations of meningococcemia. In about half of the cases, there are the typical abnormalities of intravascular coagulation (thrombocytopenia, hypofibrinogenemia, prolonged prothrombin, thrombin and partial thromboplastin times, low factors II, V and VIII and elevated levels of serum fibrin split products). Examination of the affected skin reveals vasculitis and thrombosis.

Treatment. Baseline coagulation studies should be done. If there is laboratory evidence of intravascular coagulation, heparin therapy (100 to 150 units per kilogram of body weight every 4 hours intravenously) should be started immediately and continued until coagulation tests are normal and the skin lesions are improving (see Disseminated Intravascular Coagulation).

If the tissue damage is extensive, with or without evidence of intravascular coagulation, low molecular weight dextran (Dextran 40,

10 per cent solution in 5 per cent dextrose) is recommended to increase capillary blood flow and diminish stasis. The dose is 10 ml. (1 Gm.) per kilogram infused over 2 to 4 hours. It is given every 12 hours for the first one or two days, and then every 24 hours until adequate healing is underway.

Corticosteroids have been used in many cases but their benefit is in doubt. Hydrocortisone, 10 to 20 mg. per kilogram per day intravenously, or prednisone, 2 mg. per kilogram per day orally, is recommended. Prompt supportive treatment of shock, infection and anemia is indicated. If bleeding occurs as a result of depletion of coagulation factors, fresh blood, fresh or fresh frozen plasma or fibrinogen should be given after heparinization. Hyperbaric oxygenation has been used successfully in a single case. The involved skin areas should be treated locally like a burn; plastic surgery often is required.

Complications of treatment include rare hypersensitivity reactions to dextran (minimized by the use of Dextran 40 rather than Dextran 70), hepatitis from blood products and circulatory overload.

References

Allen, D. M.: Heparin Therapy of Purpura Fulminans. *Pediatrics*, 38:211, 1966.

Hattersley, P. G.: Purpura Fulminans. Complete Recovery with Intravenously Administered Heparin. *Am. J. Dis. Child.*, 120:467, 1970.

Hjort, P. F., Rapaport, S. I., and Jorgensen, L.: Purpura Fulminans. Report of a Case Successfully Treated with Heparin and Hydrocortisone. Review of 50 Cases from the Literature. *Scand. J. Haemat.*, 1:169, 1964.

Smith, H.: Purpura Fulminans Complicating Varicella. Recovery with Low Molecular Weight Dextran and Steroids. *Med. J. Australia,* 2:685, 1967.

Waddell, W. B., et al.: Purpura Gangrenosa Treated with Hyperbaric Oxygenation. *J.A.M.A.*, 191:971, 1965.

Disseminated Intravascular Coagulation

E. RICHARD STIEHM, M.D.

Disseminated intravascular coagulation refers to the activation of the coagulation mechanism within the circulation. This has two severe effects: (1) coagulation factors are consumed so rapidly that an acquired bleeding disorder develops, characterized by hypofibrinogenemia or afibrinogenemia (defibrination), thrombocytopenia and low levels of factors II, V and VIII, and (2) fibrin thrombi are deposited in the vasculature, causing tissue damage to organs such as the skin, kidney, gastrointestinal tract and brain.

Disseminated intravascular coagulation is common in a great number of disorders; however, it is rarely accompanied by life-threatening bleeding or tissue damage. Severe disseminated intravascular coagulation with defibrination may occur in pediatric patients with a variety of disorders, including bacterial sepsis (notably meningococcemia), certain viral, fungal and rickettsial infections, hemolytic transfusion reactions, hemangiomas, snakebites, malignancies (neuroblastoma, leukemia), hemolytic-uremic syndrome and purpura fulminans. Disseminated intravascular coagulation with defibrination occurs in newborns following traumatic deliveries or abruptio placentae, or those with a macerated twin. Tissue damage is especially severe in purpura fulminans, meningococcemia and snakebite.

Diagnosis of disseminated intravascular coagulation is readily made by specific coagulation assays; often these are unavailable in an emergency. Laboratory tests of value are prolongation of the thrombin, prothrombin and activated partial thromboplastin times, low levels of factors I (fibrinogen), II, V, VIII and platelets, and elevated levels of fibrin split products in the serum (as a result of secondary fibrinolysis of deposited fibrin). For most clinical situations, hypofibrinogenemia (fibrinogen less than 150 mg. per 100 ml.), thrombocytopenia (platelets less than 100,000 per cubic millimeter), prolongation of the thrombin time and elevated levels of fibrin split products are the most characteristic laboratory abnormalities. Additional coagulation studies should be done whenever possible and repeated on a serial basis. Afibrinogenemia can be rapidly diagnosed at the bedside by failure of immediate clot formation after addition of topical thrombin to recently drawn blood. Afibrinogenemia as a result of primary fibrinolysis (lysis of circulating fibrinogen), a rarity in adults, has not been described in children.

Treatment. Treatment of severe disseminated intravascular coagulation is initially aimed at removing the stimulus for coagulation. This is accomplished by prompt treatment of the underlying disease, such as use of antibiotics for infections, chemotherapy for malignancies and surgery or radiation for hemangiomas. In many instances no further treatment is necessary. The decision to use anticoagulants to prevent further fibrin deposition is dependent on the likelihood of continuing intravascular coagulation and the degree of tissue damage already present. Thus, anticoagulation is not usually indicated in the treatment of septic shock, despite evidence of disseminated intravascular coagulation, since adequate antibiotic therapy should halt the process. Further, in the newborn period and in the hemolytic-uremic syndrome, active intravascular coagulation may have stopped by the time the bleeding or tissue damage is recognized. However, if the cause of the disseminated intravascular coagulation is such that the process cannot be interrupted (e.g., in purpura fulminans or a viral disease) or if there is a grave risk of loss of soft tissue or extremities with additional thrombosis, heparin therapy should be instituted.

Heparin is the drug of choice because of its rapid action, potent anticoagulating activity and ease of neutralization. Oral anticoagulants are not recommended because of their slow onset of action. Baseline coagulation studies should minimally include a fibrinogen level, a platelet count, a thrombin time and an activated partial thromboplastin time. Samples of blood for fibrin split products and specific coagulation assays should also be obtained if the laboratory can perform them. Heparin is given rapidly intravenously in a dose of 100 to 150 U.S.P. units per kilogram of body weight and repeated at 4-hour intervals. Blood for repeat coagulation studies should be obtained prior to the next dose. The partial thromboplastin time should be kept between 60 and 70 seconds by adjusting the heparin dose.

An increase in platelets, fibrinogen and consumable clotting factors indicates successful interruption of the intravascular coagulation. Heparin is continued until control of the underlying disease is achieved and intravascular coagulation has ceased. Heparin is then discontinued for 8 hours and repeat coagulation studies are performed. If these remain in the normal range, it may be assumed that the process is over.

Excessive heparinization can be reversed with protamine (1 mg. for 100 units of heparin) given intravenously. Give one-half the calculated dose intravenously slowly and recheck the partial thromboplastin time; if it remains prolonged, administer the remainder of the dose. Heparin should not be used in the presence of central nervous system bleeding or long-standing azotemia.

For bleeding with disseminated intravascular coagulation, coagulation factors are replaced by administering fresh whole blood (10 to 20 ml. per kilogram), fresh or fresh frozen plasma (10 to 20 ml. per kilogram) or fibrinogen (100 mg. per kilogram). There is a risk in using replacement therapy in ongoing intravascular coagulation until heparinization has been accomplished, since fibrin deposition may be accelerated by supplying additional fibrinogen.

Exchange transfusion with fresh blood has been used successfully in a few patients with disseminated intravascular coagulation. Low molecular weight dextran may be of value in the treatment of excessive tissue destruction (see Purpura Fulminans). The value of fibrinolytic agents such as urokinase has not been established. Complications of treatment include bleeding with overheparinization, transfusion hepatitis and circulatory overload.

References

Abildgaard, C. F.: Recognition and Treatment of Intravascular Coagulation. *J. Pediat.*, 74:163, 1969.

Corrigan, J. J., Jr., Ray, W. L., and May, N.: Changes in the Blood Coagulation System Associated with Septicemia. *New England J. Med.*, 279:851, 1968.

Gross, S., and Melhorn, D. K.: Exchange Transfusion with Citrated Whole Blood for Disseminated Intravascular Coagulation. *J. Pediat.*, 78:415, 1971.

Hathaway, W. E., Mull, M. M., and Pechet, G. S.: Disseminated Intravascular Coagulation in the Newborn. *Pediatrics*, 43:233, 1969.

Hathaway, W. E.: Care of the Critically Ill Child: The Problem of Disseminated Intravascular Coagulation. *Pediatrics*, 46:767, 1970.

McKay, D. G.: *Disseminated Intravascular Coagulation: An Intermediary Mechanism of Disease.* New York, Hoeber Medical Division, Harper & Row, Publishers, 1965.

Stuart, R. K., and Michel, A.: Monitoring Heparin Therapy with Activated Partial Thromboplastin Time. *Canad. M. A. J.*, 104:385, 1971.

Rheumatic Fever*

BENEDICT F. MASSELL, M.D.

There are three main aspects of the management of rheumatic fever patients: (1) treatment of acute (active) rheumatic fever, (2) prevention of group A streptococcal infections of the upper respiratory tract and (3) treatment of possible streptococcal infections if these should occur in spite of preventive measures.

ACUTE (ACTIVE) RHEUMATIC FEVER

The objectives of treatment during the acute stage of rheumatic fever are to relieve symptoms, to save lives of patients who are extremely ill and to prevent or minimize resid-

* The studies on which this article is based were supported by the Barney Siegal Research Fund and P. H. S. grants 150 from the Maternal and Child Health Service and HE-04957 from the National Heart Institute.

ual heart disease. Present-day therapy involves chiefly the use of drugs—particularly penicillin or other antistreptococcal agents, and aspirin, adrenocortical steroids or other anti-inflammatory drugs. Strict bed rest, which at one time was considered to be of therapeutic importance, is necessary only in the presence of severe joint symptoms, chorea or severe carditis with congestive heart failure. The use of penicillin and other antistreptococcal agents, which are of great indirect value in therapy, are discussed in the last two main sections of this article. The application of diuretics and digitalis, which may be needed as supplementary treatment in patients with congestive heart failure, is discussed elsewhere.

Anti-inflammatory Drugs: Selection of Aspirin or Prednisone. The two most commonly used anti-inflammatory (antirheumatic) drugs are aspirin and prednisone (an adrenocortical steroid). They are used to suppress joint symptoms, fever and other systemic manifestations of inflammation, and to suppress inflammation of cardiac tissues (active carditis). Prednisone is much more potent than aspirin as an anti-inflammatory agent, but it is also more likely to produce undesirable or even serious side effects. Selection of either aspirin or prednisone depends on the presence or absence of significant murmurs when the patient is first seen, the severity of cardiac involvement in patients who are found to have significant murmurs and the time elapsed from onset of rheumatic fever to when the physician first sees the patient.

From the point of view of therapy, patients with rheumatic fever can be divided into three groups: patients without significant murmurs, patients with congestive heart failure or pericarditis in addition to significant murmurs and patients with significant murmurs but without congestive heart failure and pericarditis.

Patients Without Significant Murmurs. On the whole, these patients have an excellent prognosis, provided they do not have a recurrence of rheumatic fever. Therefore, aspirin, which will readily control fever and joint symptoms, is the drug of choice for patients in this category. However, these patients should be kept under close medical supervision, especially during the first few weeks of their illness, in order to be sure that the cardiac findings are not changing. If significant murmurs should develop during aspirin therapy, a change to prednisone treatment may be indicated.

Patients with Congestive Heart Failure or Pericarditis. The presence of either or both of these manifestations during acute rheumatic fever is practically always a sign of severe carditis with a potentially high mortality. All such patients also have significant murmurs and nearly all have considerable cardiac enlargement. In this group, prednisone is usually life-saving and is definitely the antirheumatic drug of choice.

Patients with Significant Murmurs in the Absence of Congestive Heart Failure and Pericarditis. For these patients, who constitute a middle group with regard to prognosis, the immediate threat to life is slight; the chief risk is the development of permanent valvular damage.

Significant murmurs characteristic of valvular involvement during acute rheumatic fever sometimes lessen in intensity and even disappear completely either by the time the acute attack has subsided or during the next several years—provided recurrences of rheumatic fever can be avoided. In general, prognosis with regard to loss of murmurs is better for patients without cardiomegaly than for patients with enlarged hearts, better for patients without aortic diastolic murmurs than for patients with such murmurs and better for patients with slight (grade 2) apical systolic murmurs than for patients with systolic murmurs of moderate (grade 3) or loud (grade 4) intensity.

Even when the foregoing factors are taken into consideration, treatment of acute rheumatic fever with prednisone results in a lower incidence of residual signs of rheumatic heart disease than when aspirin is used. Furthermore, when significant murmurs persist, the degree of residual heart damage is less in prednisone-treated patients than in aspirin-treated patients. The earlier in the acute attack that therapy is started, the greater the difference in favorable results. Therefore, except when there is a high risk of serious steroid side effects, we generally select prednisone rather than aspirin for patients in this third category—especially when treatment can be started within three weeks after the onset of rheumatic fever. When more than three weeks has elapsed from onset of acute rheumatic fever, fibrotic changes and possibly other changes have developed in the heart valves and other cardiac tissues and cannot be influenced by anti-inflammatory drugs.

Dosage Schedules of Aspirin and Prednisone. The objective of therapy in rheumatic fever is to administer antirheumatic drugs for a sufficient length of time to cover the duration of most self-limited attacks of the disease and to administer the drugs in sufficient dosage to obtain a maximum degree of suppression of the rheumatic inflammatory process without producing serious toxic effects. Since most initial attacks of rheumatic fever subside within 9 to 12 weeks, we have selected 9 to 12 weeks as the period of treatment with both aspirin and prednisone.

When aspirin is used, the total daily dosage is calculated on the basis of 90 mg. per kilogram (2/3 grain per pound) of body weight, and this total daily amount is given by mouth in four divided doses approximately every 6 hours, preferably with milk or other food. If the clinical response (especially the response of fever and joint symptoms) is not adequate, the daily dose can be increased to 100 mg. per kilogram (3/4 grain per pound) or even to slightly larger amounts. However, daily amounts approaching 130 mg. per kilogram (1 grain per pound) often are toxic. Treatment at the initial dosage level is continued for a total of 7 to 10 weeks, and then the daily amount is gradually decreased over an additional two weeks. If the dosage is not tapered toward the end of treatment, abrupt discontinuation may be followed by fever and other "rebound" manifestations.

When prednisone (5-mg. tablets) is used, a highly suppressive dose for most rheumatic fever patients is 12 tablets (60 mg.) a day given by mouth in four divided doses every 6 hours. For children weighing less than 40 pounds, the daily amount is reduced by about one-third. In patients who are extremely ill with severe carditis (especially when there is a combination of congestive heart failure and pericarditis), we sometimes begin with 100 mg. a day. The initial dosage level is continued for three weeks, and then the daily amount is reduced very gradually over the remaining six to nine weeks of the treatment period.

Rebounds, manifested chiefly by fever and elevation of the sedimentation rate, sometimes occur toward the end of the treatment period or shortly after prednisone has been discontinued. However, these rebounds are usually mild and self-limited and do not require additional therapy.

Alternate-day prednisone (or other steroids) administration is not suitable for the treatment of acute rheumatic fever.

Toxic Effects of Aspirin and Precautionary Measures. An anaphylactic type of reaction (asthma or angioneurotic edema) to very small amounts of aspirin can occur in individuals who have an idiosyncrasy for the drug. However, this kind of reaction is rare and can be avoided by reviewing the history of possible previous reactions before beginning therapy.

Abdominal distress, nausea and vomiting are sometimes due to local irritation of the gastrointestinal tract, but these symptoms are generally mild or absent when the recommended dose of aspirin is used and especially when the aspirin is given with food. If such symptoms are present and persist, they may be prevented by supplementing each dose of aspirin with an antacid.

Tinnitus, with possibly some impairment of hearing, may occur when aspirin treatment is begun. This symptom often will disappear even when therapy is continued. If it persists, however, a decrease in aspirin dosage may be required.

Systemic toxicity, recognized by the presence of hyperpnea, usually does not occur with the recommended dose. However, because hyperpnea is a potentially serious sign and because it can be readily detected by inspection, patients being given aspirin for rheumatic fever should be kept under reasonably close medical supervision. The development of definite hyperpnea is an indication for decreasing the dose of aspirin.

Gastrointestinal hemorrhage (usually recognized by the presence of black stools) can be severe, but fortunately this is an uncommon complication of aspirin therapy – especially when aspirin is given with food.

Keeping serum salicylate levels between 20 and 30 mg. per 100 ml. may be helpful in regulating aspirin dosage and in avoiding serious toxic reactions—but determining salicylate serum levels should not and cannot replace examination of the patient and evaluation of his clinical response.

Side Effects of Prednisone and Precautionary Measures. A number of so-called side effects have been reported in patients with a variety of conditions being treated with prednisone and other adrenocortical steroids. These side effects include hormonal effects that alter the patient's appearance and adverse reactions that are potentially serious.

The adverse—and potentially serious—reactions include adrenal insufficiency, sodium and fluid retention, excess potassium excretion, hyperglycemia and glycosuria, elevation of blood pressure, psychoses, convulsions, myopathy of leg muscles, osteoporosis with compression fractures of the spine, peptic ulcer with perforation or gastrointestinal bleeding and the development and spread of bacterial and viral infections.

Although these potentially serious effects are very infrequent when prednisone is selected as the adrenocortical steroid and when the recommended treatment schedule is used, it is important that all patients receiving prednisone therapy be kept under close medical supervision and that the physician be prepared to alter the course of therapy if dangerous reactions develop.

Administration of prednisone suppresses the normal physiologic activity of the patient's adrenal cortex, but the steroid being given prevents the patient from having symptoms of adrenal insufficiency. Serious adrenal insufficiency can develop, however, if prednisone therapy is discontinued abruptly. Hence, if discontinuation of therapy is indicated, it is advisable to taper the dose over a period of three to four weeks, or to reduce the dose rapidly to 3 tablets (15 mg.) per day and then reduce the daily amount very slowly over three to four weeks before stopping all therapy.

Although sodium and fluid retention is usually not a problem with prednisone (in contrast to some of the other adrenocortical steroids), it is worthwhile to prescribe a low sodium diet until steroid dosage reaches low levels.

Development of myopathy of the leg muscles can be detected at an early stage by allowing patients mild physical activity out of bed as soon as their fever and joint pain have responded to therapy. In addition, the "chair test" can be used periodically. With this test the patient is asked to step up on a chair of appropriate height for the child's size. Normally, the chair test is performed with ease. Difficulty in the child's getting up on the chair may be a sign of weakness of the leg muscles. In my experience, advanced myopathy develops only when patients are kept on a regimen of strict bed rest, during which muscle weakness can occur without being apparent until it has become severe.

In children receiving adrenocortical steroids (including prednisone), probably one of the greatest risks is the development and spread of infection. Fortunately, most bacterial infections can be controlled with antibiotic therapy and most viral infections do not become overwhelming. The one exception is chickenpox (varicella). Although this disease is usually mild in children, during steroid therapy it may become extremely extensive and sometimes rapidly fatal. Because of the potential seriousness of chickenpox, the following precautions should be kept in mind for children who do not have a history of previous definite chickenpox:

1. Most important, every effort should be made to avoid the patient's exposure to other children in hospital in-patient departments and in the waiting rooms of hospital clinics and physicians' offices. If it is impossible to prevent such exposure, the use of prednisone (or other adrenocortical steroids) may need to be abandoned unless the risk of severe carditis seems to outweigh the risk of chickenpox.

2. If the patient is inadvertently exposed to chickenpox, every effort should be made to administer within three days either zoster immune globulin (5 ml. intramuscularly) or zoster immune plasma (1 ml. per pound of body weight up to a maximum of 80 ml. by slow intravenous infusion). These materials, made from the blood of adults about one month after recovery from herpes zoster, apparently will prevent or lessen the severity of chickenpox, but both are in short supply and difficult to obtain. The Center for Disease Control of the Public Health Service in Atlanta, Georgia, is presently preparing zoster immune globulin and has set up distribution centers in most major cities of the United States.

3. The possible prophylactic capacity of pooled gamma globulin (available commercially or from local health departments) should be kept in mind even though the value of this material has not yet been established. Pooled gamma globulin can be used in one or both of two ways. The first involves the intramuscular injection of 5 ml. every month for about four months, beginning about one week after the start of prednisone therapy. This regimen possibly will prevent or ameliorate a number of other viral diseases in addition to chickenpox. The second method involves the intramuscular injection of extremely large amounts of pooled gamma globulin as soon as possible after exposure to chickenpox. We have given 1 ml. of pooled gamma globulin per pound of body weight up to as much as 80 ml. in divided doses over a period of two to four days. (Note: The dose of 1 ml. of gamma globulin per pound of body weight exceeds the manufacturer's recommended rate. The total dose of 80 ml. of gamma globulin exceeds that recommended by the manufacturer.)

4. The possible therapeutic value of cytosine arabinoside (cytarabine) should be seriously considered in the event that chickenpox actually develops. The use of this material (an antiviral compound) is still experimental; information about its therapeutic and prophylactic status can be obtained from centers doing cancer research.

Hormonal effects that alter appearance are common during large-dose steroid therapy (including prednisone therapy). Varying degrees of weight gain, "mooning" of the face and abdominal fullness occur in practically all patients. A "buffalo hump," striae of the skin and hirsutism occur in about two-thirds of the patients, and acne develops in about one-third. Striae are more common in patients between 10 and 16 years of age and also more common in females than in males.

Although the hormonal effects that alter appearance are often disturbing to patients and their parents, it is reassuring to know that, with the exception of striae, all of them will disappear again within a few months after prednisone has been discontinued. Striae usually lose their discoloration slowly and become less noticeable after one or two years, but some residual faint scars may continue for several years or even indefinitely. In general, the more severe and extensive the striae are during therapy, the more noticeable the residual scars are likely to be.

When striae are extensive, they often involve the skin over the upper arms and over the inner aspect of the legs as far down as the knees, and residual scars in these areas may be disconcerting to patients, especially female patients. This fact must be given consideration in the selection of aspirin or prednisone for the treatment of adolescent females, in whom striae occur most often. Nevertheless, when the use of prednisone is decidedly preferable with regard to the course of carditis, the risk of this hormonal effect must be ignored.

PREVENTION OF STREPTOCOCCAL INFECTION

In the preantibiotic era, intercurrent group A streptococcal respiratory infections were common among patients convalescing from rheumatic fever. These infections often caused rheumatic recrudescences, which in turn prolonged the attacks and frequently resulted in an increase in the incidence and severity of heart damage. Thus, the daily or continuous administration of penicillin or other antistreptococcal drugs, by preventing streptococcal infections and rheumatic fever recrudescences, is indirectly of great therapeutic value. The control of group A streptococcal infection undoubtedly plays a major role in making rheumatic fever run a self-limited course.

Duration of Prophylaxis. The administration of penicillin or other antistreptococcal drugs in prophylactic dosage should be started as soon as the diagnosis of rheumatic fever has been established, and should be continued following recovery at least until adult life is reached. Since the risk of rheumatic fever recurrences decreases with increasing age in adults, and since the risk also decreases as the number of years from a previous attack increases, it is reasonably safe to discontinue prophylaxis in adults who show no residual signs of rheumatic heart disease. However, since patients with rheumatic heart damage are particularly vulnerable to recurrences and since such recurrences may cause further heart damage, even a slight risk is too much for patients with rheumatic heart disease. Therefore lifetime prophylaxis is recommended if signs of residual rheumatic heart disease are present by the time adulthood is reached.

Prophylactic Regimens. Any of the following prophylactic regimens may be used to reduce the risk of group A streptococcal infection:

INTRAMUSCULAR BENZATHINE PENICILLIN G (BICILLIN). The dose is 1.2 million units (in 2 ml.) every four weeks. This regimen provides the best available protection against group A streptococcal infections. However, if the interval between injections is extended beyond four weeks, the degree of protection rapidly decreases. The disadvantage of this method is that it involves a greater risk of anaphylactic or other allergic reactions than does penicillin given by mouth. Furthermore, the injections are painful, and in some patients the pain may be quite severe and may last for as long as one or two days.

PENICILLIN BY MOUTH. Either buffered penicillin G or potassium penicillin V (phenoxymethyl penicillin) may be given in a dose of 125 mg. (200,000 units) three times every day. Buffered penicillin G has the advantage of being relatively inexpensive, but it does not give quite as high blood levels as penicillin V and it preferably should be given on an empty stomach. Penicillin by mouth, even three times daily, does not afford as much protection against group A streptococcal infections as does intramuscular benzathine penicillin. This difference may be explained in part by the fact that patients for whom oral penicillin has been prescribed may sometimes forget to take their medication.

Although penicillin by mouth has never led to the development of penicillin-resistant group A streptococci, there is evidence that it has induced penicillin-resistance in other organisms which are normally in the mouth flora —including bacteria in the gingival tissues. If such resistant bacteria should enter the blood stream and cause bacterial endocarditis, it is conceivable that treatment of this complication might be more difficult than if the mouth organisms had not become penicillin-resistant.

A related but probably more important effect of prophylactic penicillin by mouth is the increase in the throat flora of penicillinase-producing staphylococci and the induction of increased amounts of penicillinase by these staphylococci. The presence of penicillinase in the tissues of the throat may destroy the relatively small amounts of penicillin that are given for prophylaxis. This may be one of the explanations for instances in which group A streptococcal infections occur in spite of prescribed penicillin prophylaxis.

The foregoing effects of penicillin given by mouth presumably are related to the temporary presence of a high local concentration of penicillin on the surface of the tissues of the mouth and throat, a condition that does not develop when prophylactic penicillin is given in the form of injectable benzathine penicillin. This high local concentration of penicillin probably could be prevented to a great extent by having the patient drink a whole glass of water with each dose of penicillin and swirl the water around the mouth before swallowing.

SULFADIAZINE, ERYTHROMYCIN AND CLINDAMYCIN BY MOUTH. In patients who may be allergic to penicillin, any one of these drugs can be given by mouth for prophylaxis against group A streptococcal infections and recurrences of rheumatic fever. The use of these drugs in place of penicillin by mouth would also have the advantage of not producing penicillin-resistant mouth organisms and not inducing penicillinase by staphylococci.

Sulfadiazine has the advantage of being relatively inexpensive, but it has the disadvantage of being only bacteriostatic (rather than bactericidal) for group A streptococci. The usual prophylactic dose of sulfadiazine is 0.5 Gm. twice daily, and that of erythromycin is 250 mg. twice daily.*

Clindamycin (Cleocin), though still classified as investigational for use in prophylaxis, has been found by us to be effective for the prevention of group A streptococcal infections in a dose of 75 mg. two or three times daily. It is effective when given with food, and when so given, it only rarely causes digestive symptoms.

TREATMENT OF POSSIBLE STREPTOCOCCAL INFECTIONS

Although the daily or continuous administration of penicillin or other antistreptococcal drugs reduces the incidence of group A streptococcal infections, such prophylaxis is not always effective. When streptococcal infections occur in spite of prophylaxis, these infections may be subclinical (without symptoms) or clinical. Whether clinical or subclinical, the infections may cause an antibody response and under these circumstances they may cause recurrences of rheumatic fever. A major difficulty in the recognition of these infections is the fact that throat cultures, which ordinarily are useful in diagnosis, may be masked by the prophylactic regimen and thus may be falsely negative.

Subclinical streptococcal infections are almost impossible to recognize until there has been a rise in antistreptolysin O titer or other streptococcal antibody, by which time it is too late to prevent rheumatic fever recurrences. Even if very frequent throat cultures were taken periodically (a program that is not especially practical), the masking effect of prophylaxis would often interfere with the detection of group A streptococci.

Prophylaxis may also mask throat cultures in clinical group A streptococcal infections, but an evaluation of symptoms and the response to a therapeutic trial will usually allow for adequate treatment of these infections and the prevention of rheumatic fever recurrences.

The most common symptoms of group A streptococcal infections are a definite sore throat (usually pain on swallowing) plus definite fever (usually 101° F. or higher in children). Definite fever alone (i.e., without sore throat) sometimes is also a manifestation of streptococcal infection. On the other hand, most head colds (coryza), respiratory illnesses with predominant cough and sore throat without fever usually are not due to group A streptococcal infection.

On the basis of the foregoing, our policy for management of rheumatic fever patients receiving daily or continuous prophylaxis is as follows:

1. Whenever there is an illness characterized by a combination of sore throat and definite fever, or by definite temperature elevation to 101° F. or higher without sore throat, prompt treatment is started with penicillin or other antistreptococcal drugs—even if a throat culture is also obtained just before therapy is started.

2. Definite response of fever and other symptoms within one to two days is an indication to continue therapy for a full 10 to 14 days —even if a throat culture taken before treatment is reported to be negative for beta-hemolytic streptococci.

3. Failure of fever to respond to large amounts of penicillin or other reliable antistreptococcal drugs constitutes strong evidence against a streptococcal cause and is an indication to reduce dosage to a prophylactic level.

Dosage Schedules for Treatment. BENZATHINE PENICILLIN G. A dose of 1.2 million

* Manufacturer's precaution: Sulfadiazine should not be used in infants under two months of age.

units injected intramuscularly provides therapeutic levels for 10 days or longer. One such injection is usually considered adequate, but supplementary penicillin by mouth will ensure effectiveness. Intramuscular benzathine penicillin G should be considered for children for whom oral medication had been prescribed for prophylaxis. When symptoms of a possible streptococcal infection develop in children who are already being given periodic intramuscular injections of benzathine penicillin G for prophylaxis, an additional injection of this preparation can be given with or without supplementary penicillin by mouth.

PENICILLIN BY MOUTH. Large amounts of penicillin by mouth can be used alone or as a supplement to intramuscular benzathine penicillin G. For this purpose, buffered penicillin G or potassium penicillin V can be given in a dose of 375 mg. to 500 mg. (600,000 to 800,000 units) four times daily.

ERYTHROMYCIN AND CLINDAMYCIN. One of these two antibiotics should be used in patients who may be allergic to penicillin. *Sulfadiazine* (or other sulfonamides), which may be useful for prophylaxis, *should not be used for treatment* of suspected streptococcal infections. The sulfonamides are bacteriostatic rather than bactericidal and may not eradicate group A streptococci from the deep tissues of the upper respiratory tract. The therapeutic dose of erythromycin is usually 250 mg. four times daily. The therapeutic dose of clindamycin (Cleocin) is 150 mg. to 300 mg. four times daily, preferably with food.

The Problem of Persistent Positive Throat Cultures. Although penicillin given for prophylaxis may mask group A streptococcal infections and result in falsely negative throat cultures, a somewhat different situation is sometimes encountered in which throat cultures are persistently positive for group A streptococci. Such positive cultures may be detected during the administration of daily or continuous penicillin for prophylaxis or following one or more 10-day courses of penicillin given for the treatment of group A streptococcal infection.

Although there may be a number of possible mechanisms to explain this situation, one cause that we have demonstrated involves the inactivation of penicillin by the presence of penicillinase-producing staphylococci in the throat flora. Whatever the mechanism may actually be, we have found that a combination of penicillin and erythromycin, each given by mouth in therapeutic dosage for 10 days, will often eradicate group A streptococci that could not be removed from the upper respiratory tract by large amounts of oral or intramuscular penicillin alone. One possible explanation for this apparent synergistic effect of the two antibiotics is that erythromycin suppresses the penicillinase-producing staphylococci and thus prevents inactivation of penicillin—at least during the 10-day course of treatment. During this period, the normally bactericidal action of penicillin becomes effective.

Although studies have not yet been done with a combination of clindamycin and penicillin, it is likely that this combination could also be used in instances of persistent positive throat cultures for group A streptococci.

6

Digestive Tract

Abnormalities, Injuries and Diseases of the Oral Region

ROBERT A. VICKERS, D.D.S., *and*
ROBERT J. GORLIN, D.D.S.

The pediatrician may be called upon to render emergency dental and oral treatment. Prompt, intelligent disposition of these conditions is often a significant factor in the maintenance of a healthy and esthetically pleasing dental apparatus throughout the patient's life. In addition, a fundamental knowledge of other alterations of oral cavity constitutes, in the very least, a basis for sound patient management for a host of general health problems.

ACUTE TRAUMA OF DENTAL AND ORAL TISSUES

Hemorrhage

Oral hemorrhage in children usually results from acute trauma. Rarely, unusual bleeding may follow minor oral surgical procedures, such as tooth extraction. All wounds are managed by examination and debridement of necrotic tissue and foreign material. Primary closure or application of folded sterile gauze pressure dressings for 15 to 40 minutes is usually sufficient. The mouth should not be rinsed, since clots are easily dislodged from their moist environment. Absorbable gelatin sponge (Gelfoam) cut to size and saturated with thrombin, or warm, moistened tea bags have also been used for persistent bleeding.

If bleeding continues, an oral surgeon should be consulted. Appropriate tests should be done to exclude the possibility of blood dyscrasia and other complicating factors.

Tooth Fracture

If a tooth receives a severe, sharp blow, fracture often occurs. This fracture may be visible and involve the clinical crown of the tooth; or it may be invisible and involve the invested or root portion but be evident on a dental radiogram. In either instance dental consultation should be immediate. It should be emphasized that the physician should recommend that the child see the family dentist or pedodontist within the shortest possible time.

Fractures of the crowns of teeth are treated by covering surfaces with a protective, crown-shaped plastic or metallic cap. The cap is secured in position by a sedative dressing, such as a mixture of zinc oxide and eugenol, which minimizes pulpal hyperemia and protects against irritation by thermal and chemical factors. If fracture of the tooth crown involves the pulp portion, treatment is either pulp removal with sealing (ideally), pulpotomy (slightly less successful) or extraction.

Root fractures, though rare in primary teeth, are immobilized in situ by supportive wire ligation of affected and neighboring teeth. Extraction may be deemed necessary in some cases.

It is worth emphasizing that early dentition performs a valuable space-maintaining function for the subsequent permanent dentition. Early loss of primary teeth adversely affects the development of a properly aligned permanent dentition.

Tooth Displacement or Loss; Replantation

Intrusion or forceful impaction of primary maxillary incisors is common during the first three years of life. The entire clinical crown may become embedded in bone and soft tissue.

Primary attention should be given to treatment of the soft tissues. No attempt should be made to reposition the teeth after the accident. A dental radiogram should be made to detect fracture of the root or alveolar process. It is almost never possible to predict with accuracy whether injury has occurred to the underlying permanent successor. Intruded teeth usually re-erupt within one month after injury. Over half of the teeth will be retained; the rest undergo either pulpal necrosis or inflammatory resorption.

Displaced, but not intruded, permanent but *not* primary, teeth are repositioned. If the teeth are severely loosened, the prognosis is poor, especially if the roots are completely formed and the teeth are permanent ones.

Replantation of an avulsed permanent tooth is usually unsuccessful, since it will probably undergo subsequent resorption. Replantation is, however, still recommended, since the tooth is occasionally retained and will serve as a space maintainer. The tooth is gently cleansed, care being taken not to remove adherent periodontal ligament. The tooth is then placed in a mild antiseptic solution and the child referred to a dentist or pedodontist for root canal filling of the tooth, replantation and splint construction for immobilization.

It is desirable to examine carefully patients with oral trauma to exclude an associated fracture of the jaw or facial bones. There is considerable value in the use of a panographic dental x-ray machine for this purpose.

Oral Electric Burns

Occasionally a child, usually between one and two years of age, suffers flash burns of the lips, tongue and other oral structures when sucking on the free end of a live electric extension cord or, more rarely, when biting through an electric wire. The commissural areas of the lips are especially involved.

Therapy consists of tetanus immunization, parenteral tube feeding when indicated and blood transfusions for patients hemorrhaging from labial arteries. Severe bleeding from the labial arteries may be delayed for over a week, and it is important to be aware of this complication. Usually only minimal immediate local care is needed for the burn wound. Although a few authors have suggested early resection and skin grafting, the majority advocate conservative treatment, allowing spontaneous healing followed by reconstructive procedures, since microstomia or webbing is a frequent result.

Oral Self-Mutilation

Occasionally a physician or dentist is called upon to see a child who had an unexplained denudation of the roots of one or more teeth. This may be due to self-mutilation with the fingernail, but at times an instrument such as a bobby pin has been used. Such a child may be emotionally disturbed. Severe cheekbiting is often done by these children. Psychiatric referral may be indicated.

FACIAL TRAUMA

A maximal effort must be made to avoid interference with subsequent growth and development in the surgical care and handling of both hard and soft tissues in the child. Fractures of the facial structures should, where necessary, be corrected by closed reduction and immobilization. If open reduction is required, such surgery should be minimal. Insertion of wires and pins must be avoided whenever possible, since they may interfere with bone development.

Fractures of the facial bones are often difficult to diagnose radiographically in the child because of the delicate multicontoured nature of bones comprising the facial skeleton. A panoramic radiogram may be of greater help. Injuries are often unrecognized at the time of injury, and only with subsequent distorted growth and development can prior injury be determined. This is especially the case with nasal skeleton fractures.

Uncorrected, displaced fractures of the maxilla can lead to flattening of the mid-face and are best treated by closed reduction through elevation of fragmented bones attached to and adjoining the soft tissues. If effective reduction cannot be accomplished, implants may be utilized subsequently to restore continuity. Refracture and repositioning of fragments is a formidable procedure and should only be done following cessation of the rapid growth phase.

Mandibular fractures are best corrected by realignment and immobilization utilizing interdental wiring. This technique is the least traumatic and does not interfere with bone development. A correct dental occlusion is the key to successful realignment.

Fracture of the mandibular condyle or injury to the temporomandibular joint may rarely be complicated by ankylosis or mandibular hypoplasia.

DISORDERS OF TOOTH GROWTH AND DEVELOPMENT

In general, if possible the first dental examination should be carried out before the second birthday.

Nursing Bottle Syndrome

The pediatrician should advise the parents concerning the hazard of nocturnal bottle feeding with either milk or sugar-sweetened solutions. Owing to decreased salivary flow, oral clearance is reduced and rapid, massive dental destruction is possible.

Congenitally Missing and Conical Crowned Teeth

In about 4 per cent of persons, one or more permanent teeth, other than third molars, fail to develop. The teeth most commonly absent are maxillary lateral incisors and maxillary and mandibular second premolars. Space maintenance may be required, and dental consultation should always be suggested.

There may be complete (anodontia) or partial (hypodontia) lack of tooth formation in X-linked recessive hypohidrotic ectodermal dysplasia. The teeth that are present often have conical crowns. The female heterozygote not uncommonly also has deficient or conical crowns. Pronounced deficiency of teeth and conical crown form may also be seen in incontinentia pigmenti. Full or partial dentures may be constructed by a pedodontist when the child is three years of age or younger, but preferably this should be carried out at school age. With continued growth of jaws, new prostheses should be constructed.

Amelogenesis Imperfecta and Similar Conditions

Amelogenesis imperfecta and similar conditions are related either to failure of proper deposition of the enamel matrix or to inadequate calcification of this matrix. There are numerous separate entities under the general term amelogenesis imperfecta. The most common form of amelogenesis imperfecta is inherited as an autosomal dominant trait and affects both primary and secondary dentitions. Other forms have other types of inheritance patterns and clinical manifestations. Commonly there is an associated anterior open bite which must be corrected orthodontically.

Early coverage of the posterior teeth by stainless steel crowns and of the anterior teeth by acrylic or porcelain jackets may be indicated, since the enamel is thin and crumbles, leaving the tooth crowns devoid of enamel covering and prone to dental decay. A recently employed effective technique is acid etching of the enamel, which is then covered by a resin which adheres to the treated enamel to restore normal contour.

Dentinogenesis Imperfecta

Dentinogenesis imperfecta occurs most often (about 1 in 9000 births) as an isolated entity, but it also may be seen in association with osteogenesis imperfecta. In either instance the condition is inherited as an autosomal dominant trait. The teeth have an opalescent, bluish-gray or brown color. The enamel is rapidly worn off, and crowns or full dentures are not uncommonly indicated after the resultant attrition. Crowns and prosthetic appliances are recommended early for maintenance of vertical dimension of the jaws and face.

INTRINSICALLY STAINED AND HYPOPLASTIC TEETH

Hemolytic Conditions

Dental changes following hemolytic disease in the newborn are manifested as yellow-green stained enamel and dentin and hypoplasia of enamel of the cusp tips of deciduous dentition. Permanent teeth are not affected. Treatment consists of the dental restoration of hypoplastic teeth.

Tetracyclines

Yellow-gray, bright yellow, gray-brown or darker discoloration of teeth which may or may not be accompanied by hypoplasia of the enamel has been traced to tetracycline therapy during the period of tooth formation. Tetracyclines have caused tooth defects in children when administered to mothers in the last trimester of pregnancy and to mothers nursing infants, as well as when administered to the child. Some researchers have found that the effects are dosage-dependent, while other workers have failed to establish such dependence. Individual susceptibility to tetracyclines varies, which probably accounts for these different results. Tetracyclines used during periods of tooth formation at levels exceeding 75 mg. per kilogram nearly always cause enamel hypoplasia.

As many as 35 per cent of children in a pediatric medical practice have been noted to demonstrate such changes. Comprehensive studies on the frequency of permanent tooth staining have yet to appear. Diagnostically, a yellow to yellow-brown fluorescence is noted under ultraviolet light, peaking at 340 to 370 millimicrons. Although no treatment is necessary, severe hypoplasia may require dental restoration of teeth. Jacket crowns or acid etching and resin application may be desirable in case of severe staining.

Other Disorders of Tooth Calcification

In addition to the previously mentioned causes, many systemic conditions may interfere with matrix formation and calcification. These include rickets, hypoparathyroidism and various disorders accompanied by high fever.

Disorders in Tooth Eruption

Primary teeth erupt prematurely about once in 3000 live births. They may be present at birth (natal teeth) or may erupt within the first month (neonatal teeth). This disorder may be inherited as an autosomal dominant trait or be associated with a syndrome such as pachyonychia congenita, Ellis–van Creveld syndrome or oculomandibulodyscephaly. If the teeth are loose or interfere with nursing (see Riga–Fede disease), they should be gently extracted.

The most common disturbance in the eruption of teeth is caused by premature loss or extraction of neglected permanent or primary teeth. Loss of a first permanent molar without subsequent space maintenance may result in serious malocclusion. Early, premature loss of a primary tooth impairs mastication and may result in improper eruption or impaction of the permanent tooth. When teeth are lost prematurely, therefore, construction of a space maintainer by the dentist is necessary.

CYSTS

Epstein's Pearls or Bohn's Nodules

This condition is characterized by small keratin cysts most frequently on the alveolar ridge or midline of the palate in the infant. Clinically, they appear as small multiple white blebs which burst spontaneously.

Odontogenic Cysts

Numerous varieties of cysts of the jaws originating from epithelial remnants of the embryologic tooth-forming structures may be encountered. Frequently asymptomatic and detected by routine dental x-rays, they may manifest symptoms such as facial or bony swelling. Surgical removal by curettage is the treatment of choice. Multiple cysts of the jaws may be observed as part of the multiple nevoid basal cell carcinoma syndrome.

Fissural or Nonodontogenic Cysts

Cysts of the jaws and neighboring soft tissues originating from embryologic epithelium not associated with tooth-forming structures are also observed. Because many of these cysts are found in areas where fusion of embryologic processes occurs they may also be termed fissural. Individual examples have been delineated, such as thyroglossal duct cyst, median anterior palatal cyst, branchial cleft cyst, nasolabial cyst and globulomaxillary cyst.

DEFORMITIES OF THE FACE, JAWS AND MOUTH

Torus Mandibularis

This condition is represented by single or multiple, unilateral or bilateral, bony growths on the lingual aspect of the mandible in the region of the premolars. It is rarely found in young children but develops slowly and manifests itself at puberty or later. By adulthood, as much as 10 per cent of the population shows this condition. The growth is of no significance unless it interferes with dental prosthesis. Treatment if indicated consists of surgical removal.

Torus Palatinus

This entity is characterized by a nodular or lobular bony growth in the midline of the hard palate. Like its mandibular counterpart, it is rare in infants and is usually not evident until puberty. In the adult population it is noted in 25 per cent of females and 15 per cent cent of males. Treatment if indicated consists of surgical removal.

Micrognathia

Diminished size of the jaw may result from many causes, such as trauma, radiation, various developmental disorders and childhood rheumatoid arthritis. It may be unilateral or bilateral. Chin implants (plastic or cartilage grafts) have proved effective.

Prognathism

Enlargement or anterior placement of the lower jaw may be absolute or relative and is often a hereditary trait. After the jaws have ceased to grow (usually at 16 or 17 years), the patient is referred to an orthodontist and oral or maxillofacial surgeon for correction. Many successful surgical techniques are available.

Malocclusion

Various types of disturbed development of the face and jaws may result in malocclusion.

Underdevelopment of the maxilla or of the mandible (micrognathia) or overdevelopment of the mandible may require special surgical procedures after puberty. Incompatibility of tooth size and jaw size may result in spacing, crowding or irregularity of teeth. Prolonged retention of primary teeth may result in delayed eruption of permanent teeth. Neglected primary or permanent teeth may be lost prematurely. Early consultation with an orthodontist is indicated to resolve problems associated with malocclusion.

Thumb-Sucking

Thumb-sucking is certainly a common phenomenon during the first two years and should be considered normal, although some children never exhibit this habit. Whether this habit, if prolonged, will produce an effect upon the dentition probably depends upon several factors, including the frequency and duration of the habit and the amount and direction of pressure exerted. Most children stop thumb-sucking before the age of five years. If the habit is continued for more than four years, some may develop malocclusion.

Corrective appliances should be used *only* when the child has expressed a desire to rid himself of the habit! Patient and parental cooperation is essential for the success of corrective appliances. These may be constructed by the dentist, orthodontist or pedodontist and should not be painful or interfere with occlusion. They should be used *only* as a reminder!

Abnormal Labial Frenum

Spacing between permanent central incisors is physiologically normal, and eruption with distal inclination is expected in younger children. This is usually corrected as the lateral incisors erupt approximately a year later and the canines erupt three or four years later. Only when the frenum forms a wide band with lingual attachment to the palatine papilla and when the palatine papilla blanches when intermittent tension is placed on the frenum, or when gingival recession occurs, should surgical intervention be considered.

Fistulas of Lateral Soft Palate

Rare congenital anomalies, the fistulas may be unilateral or bilateral. Not uncommonly they are associated with agenesis of the palatine tonsils. Surgical closure may be necessary to prevent food from being forced into the nasopharynx.

Hemifacial Hypertrophy

This refers to unilateral hypertrophy of facial and oral structures of hypertrophy combined with enlargement of an extremity or even half the body. The asymmetry is almost always present at birth, although it may become accentuated at puberty. The hair is coarse and of a different shade on the involved side. About 15 per cent of these patients are mentally retarded. Embryonal tumors may be associated. Plastic surgery may be necessary for cosmetic reasons.

Idiopathic Masseteric Hypertrophy

This condition is seen in about 1 per cent of the population; it is possibly twice as common in males and often bilateral. It is rare before puberty. No treatment is necessary, but familiarity with the condition is necessary to rule out parotid gland pathology.

Progressive Hemifacial Atrophy

Romberg's syndrome consists of slowly progressive atrophy of essentially half the face accompanied most often by contralateral jacksonian epilepsy, trigeminal neuralgia and changes in the eyes and hair. In about 7 per cent of patients there is associated atrophy of half the body. Surgical or cosmetic correction may be elected.

Oral-Facial-Digital Syndrome I

This bizarre syndrome is X-linked dominant and lethal in the male. It is characterized by asymmetric cleft palate, bifid, trifid or tetrafid tongue and various digital anomalies. The tongue is often repaired, largely for cosmetic reasons.

Cleft Lip and Cleft Palate

Clefts of the primary and/or secondary palates are included among the more common congenital anomalies. A vast amount of data has been gathered about facial clefts, only a small portion of which can be presented here.

Clinically, there is great variability in the degree of cleft formation. The minimal degrees of involvement include such anomalies as bifid uvula, linear lip indentations or so-called intrauterine healed clefts, and submucous cleft of the soft palate. A cleft may involve only the upper lip or may extend to involve the nostril and the hard and soft palates. Isolated palatal clefts may be limited to the uvula (bifid uvula), or they may be more extensive, cleaving the soft palate or both the soft and hard palates.

Cleft lip–cleft palate makes up about 50 per cent of the cases, with cleft lip and isolated cleft palate each being about 25 per cent, irrespective of race.

Cleft lip with or without cleft palate would appear to occur in about 1 (range, 0.6 to 1.3) per 1000 Caucasian births. The incidence appears to be increasing, probably due to declining postnatal mortality, decreasing operative mortality, steadily improving operative results and attendant increase in marriage and childbearing.

The prevalence is higher in Orientals (about 1.7 per 1000 births) and lower among Negroes (approximately 1 per 2500 births).

Isolated cleft lip may be unilateral or bilateral (approximately 20 per cent). When unilateral, the cleft is more common on the left side (about 70 per cent), although no more extensive. Lips are somewhat more frequently cleft bilaterally (approximately 25 per cent) when combined with cleft palate. Cleft lip–cleft palate is more common in men. About 85 per cent of bilateral cleft lips and 70 per cent of unilateral cleft lips are associated with cleft palate.

Cleft lip is not always complete (i.e., extending into the nostril). In about 10 per cent of cases, the cleft is associated with skin bridges or Simonart's bands.

Isolated cleft palate appears to be separate from cleft lip with or without cleft palate. It has been demonstrated that siblings of patients with cleft lip with or without cleft palate have an increased frequency of the same anomaly but not of isolated cleft palate, and vice versa.

Children with isolated cleft palate not uncommonly (about 30 per cent) have associated congenital anomalies.

The incidence of isolated cleft palate among Caucasians and Negroes would appear to be between 1 per 2000 births and 1 per 2500 births, respectively. It may be somewhat more common among Orientals. It is more common in females. Breakdown of cleft palate according to extent clearly indicates that whereas a 2:1 female predilection exists for complete clefts of the hard and soft palates, the ratio approaches 1:1 for clefts of the soft palate or uvula only.

Cleft uvula appears to be an incomplete form of cleft palate. The incidence of cleft uvula is about 1 per 80 Caucasian individuals.

The frequency of cleft uvula among various Amerindian groups is quite high, ranging from 1 per 9 to 1 per 14 individuals. In Negroes it is extremely rare (1 per 300).

Treatment of cleft lip/palate is complex and involves several disciplines. Most persons would agree that the best treatment is provided by the "team approach," where the team might consist of a maxillofacial surgeon, otolaryngologist, pedodontist, orthodontist, prosthodontist, speech pathologist, human geneticist, psychologist and social worker. The considerable overlap of interest and concern of this clinical problem relating structure, function and well-being of the patient demands the diagnostic and treatment skills of all these professions for an extended period of time.

The development of adequate speech and language skills is an important concern. Speech and language are behaviors which are learned primarily through audition. Since there is a relatively high incidence of ear pathology and consequent hearing loss (primarily conductive) in the young cleft palate population, early identification and treatment is important to ensure optimal hearing function during the speech and language developmental years.

Early closure of the palatal cleft provides a more optimal mechanism with which to produce speech. Surgical closure of the secondary palate can be performed with a variety of techniques. The primary goal of surgery is to achieve a complete closure of the hard and soft palate and provide a soft palate which has good length and mobility.

Attainment of good length and mobility of the soft palate becomes important in the processes of deglutition and speech. For both functions, velopharyngeal closure, or the ability to seal off the nasal cavity from the oral cavity, is required. Although velopharyngeal closure for speech and certain nonspeech activities, such as deglutition and blowing, is sphincteric in nature, involving movements of palatal and pharyngeal structures, the soft palate is considered the prime mover in accomplishing closure.

If velopharyngeal closure is not achieved following the initial surgical procedures, food and liquids may be directed into the nasopharynx during deglutition. Similarly, speech may be characterized by excessive air escapage through the nose accompanying consonants which require intraoral pressure for their production, and excessive nasal resonance perceived as hypernasality.

Although the primary technique to evaluate the adequacy of the velopharyngeal closure mechanism for speech is the speech product itself, other techniques involve direct oral-pharyngeal-nasal observations, radiography and air pressure–air flow instrumentation.

Secondary procedures to correct the velopharyngeal inadequacy for speech may be indicated. Such procedures may include a surgical pharyngeal flap, prosthodontic speech appliances (speech bulb or palatal lift) or a pharyngeal implant. Because treatment choice depends on a number of surgico-dento-speech considerations and because the inadequacy of velopharyngeal mechanism for speech may be due to several anatomic and physiologic variations, complete diagnosis and evaluation is required by all members of the cleft palate team.

In some persons with cleft lip/palate, velopharyngeal closure may be achieved with the aid of tonsillar and adenoidal tissue. Decision as to the complete removal of these tissues in this population should be made with caution, as persistent hypernasality and audible nasal air emission may result.

It should be pointed out that velopharyngeal inadequacy for speech is not unique to persons with cleft lip/palate but may occur in a number of other congenital anomalies and syndromes involving the craniofacial complex.

If the cleft only involves the primary palate, following the initial surgical repair the relationship between structure and speech is less clear, although the presence of a number of deviant dental conditions, oronasal fistulas or dental appliances may be hazards to good speech production. Appropriate referral for, and proper timing of, speech therapy may be indicated.

Dental specialty observations and treatment for the patient with cleft lip/palate are important as they relate to occlusion, appearance, adequate oral functions (mastication, deglutition, speech) and good oral hygiene. The status of the dentition can make an important difference in treatment choice.

Cleft palate teams are currently broadening their interest to include diagnostic and treatment services for a variety of developmental anomalies of the face, jaws and mouth, some of which are presented in this section.

Lateral Facial Cleft

Lateral facial cleft (macrostomia; transverse or horizontal facial cleft; cleft cheek) is caused by failure of penetration of mesoderm between the embryonic maxillary and mandibular processes. The cleft may be unilateral or bilateral, partial or, rarely, complete, extending from the angle of the mouth toward the ear. In many cases, the cleft extends above or below the tragus.

It appears to be more common in males and, when unilateral, occurs more often on the left side. It may be an isolated phenomenon, but more frequently it is associated with other malformations. There does not appear to be a genetic basis for this anomaly.

Lateral facial cleft may be found with the first and second branchial arch syndrome (hemifacial microsomia – i.e., hypoplasia of the ascending ramus and condyle of the mandible, ear tags, and microtia), oculoauriculovertebral dysplasia (essentially hemifacial microsomia with epibulbar dermoids and hemivertebrae) and, rarely, mandibulofacial dysostosis.

Oblique Facial Cleft

Oblique facial cleft is extremely rare and is variable in appearance. Most commonly it is associated with cleft lip and extends to the inner canthus of the eye. In some cases, the cleft runs lateral to and does not involve the ala of the nose, passing near the outer canthus into the temporal region. It may be superficial but more often separates the underlying bone. When the cleft reaches the orbital margin, the eyelid may be uncovered. It has been stated to represent failure of mesodermal penetrance between the maxillary, median nasal and lateral nasal processes. Only rarely, however, does the oblique facial cleft follow the epithelial grooves, and other explanation should be sought.

The cleft may be unilateral or bilateral. The oblique cleft is nearly always associated with cleft lip, cleft palate or lateral facial cleft. There does not appear to be any evidence of a genetic role.

Double Lip

Rarely one notes a transverse replication or prolapse of maxillary labial tissue. This may occur alone or in combination with blepharochalasis and nontoxic thyroid enlargement (Ascher's syndrome). Simple surgical excision of the excess mucosa is usually necessary for cosmetic reasons.

Commissural Lip Pits

This developmental condition, probably genetic, may occur bilaterally or unilaterally and is characterized by pits 1 to 4 mm. deep at the angles of the mouth. They occur in about 12 per cent of the population and about 25 per cent of these are bilateral. No treatment is necessary.

Lower Lip Pits

Inherited as an autosomal dominant trait and sometimes associated with cleft lip or cleft palate, these pits (at times only one is present) are located on the vermilion of the lower lip on either side of the midline. At times they are situated on a snoutlike process. Surgical excision is usually necessary for cosmetic reasons or because of the annoying secretion of saliva from the orifices.

GINGIVAL AND PERIODONTAL DISORDERS

Severe gingivitis is uncommon in children, though a mild, reversible form is seen in about 40 per cent of children 6 to 11 years of age.

Eruption Gingivitis

A mild, temporary gingivitis may be seen during deciduous tooth eruption which abates after tooth emergence. Treatment is rarely indicated. Eruption of the permanent teeth is often accompanied by a mild gingivitis, possibly related to the fact that the surrounding gingiva receives little, if any, protection from the tooth during early eruption, the gingiva becoming inflamed by continued irritative, abrasive action of food. No treatment is required other than institution of improved oral hygiene.

Marginal Gingivitis

Inflammation of the marginal gingiva in children is usually associated with poor oral hygiene and, at times, the presence of an abnormal occlusion. Treatment consists of correcting tooth-brushing technique and removing plaque and food debris.

Necrotizing Ulcerative Gingivitis (Vincent's Infection)

This condition is extremely rare in children, occurring far more commonly in young adults. It is infectious but not contagious. (Most cases of so-called Vincent's infection in children are actually acute herpetic gingivostomatitis.) The condition seems to be associated with lowered resistance and invasion of the oral tissues by organisms normally present in the mouth, principally *Borrelia vincentii* and fusiform bacilli. The interproximal gingival papillae are destroyed, and a pseudomembrane covers the marginal gingiva. The gingivae bleed easily and are painful, and not uncommonly there is malaise, fever, loss of appetite and a fetid odor.

The disease is treated by débridement, subgingival curettage and dilute (3 per cent) hydrogen peroxide mouthwashes. In addition, if the process is accompanied by systemic symptoms such as fever, oral administration of penicillin V is indicated, 25,000 to 50,000 units per kilogram per 24 hours divided into four doses. Ordinarily the process, if treated, subsides within 48 hours. It is important that dental consultation be recommended, for the usual sequelae of acute infection may lead to chronic disease of supporting or periodontal structures.

Oral Candidosis (Thrush)

Treatment of oral candidiasis is limited to infants with visible lesions, particularly when these affect food intake. One course of nystatin (Mycostatin) is usually sufficient for treatment. This consists of dropping 1 ml. (100,000 units) of the suspension in the mouth, swabbing the involved areas and repeating four times daily until about three days after the lesions have cleared.

If treatment has been given properly the first time, recurrence of oral candidosis should make one suspect an underlying problem, such as a rare case of thymic aplasia. In older infants and children, oral candidosis is usually a complication of antibiotic therapy. Less frequently it might result from other forms of therapy, such as with antimetabolites or an antihistaminic regimen. Recurrent oral candidosis, occasionally combined with skin involvement, should make one suspect a hormonal defect, malignancy or immunologic disorder, particularly one associated with defective cellular immune mechanisms. Therapy with nystatin in children with associated underlying conditions is usually only temporarily effective.

Herpes Simplex

Distinction should be made between primary and secondary (recurrent) disease. In the former, herpetic gingivostomatitis and inoculation herpes simplex are the most common manifestations. Recurrent lesions occur in various locations, there being a predilection for transitional zones from skin to mucosa. The primary infection occurs in early life, although clinical disease is produced in less than 1 per cent of patients. Regardless of whether the primary infection is clinical or subclinical, recurrent herpetic lesions develop later in many persons, being precipitated by many different factors. Not all individuals suffer from recurrent herpes simplex. It has been estimated that from 70 to 90 per cent of the population are carriers of the virus after 14 years of age.

Primary Herpetic Gingivostomatitis. Primary herpetic gingivostomatitis usually occurs between 1 and 5 years of age. Rarely is it observed in adults. The acute vesicular lesions last from five to seven days and are accompanied by high fever, dehydration, malaise and nausea. Initially, the gingiva becomes swollen, with associated salivation, fetor oris, dysphagia and painful lymphadenopathy. The oral mucous membranes, especially those of the gingiva and tongue are sites of round to oval, sharply demarcated, disseminated vesicles or erosions which are 2 to 4 mm. in size, painful, covered by a yellowish pseudomembrane and surrounded by a red margin. The intact vesicle rarely lasts for more than 24 hours. After about 10 to 14 days, the primary infection subsides without scar formation. Treatment consists of dietary supplements and the preservation of electrolyte balance in severe anorexial dysphagia.

Secondary (Recurrent) Herpes Simplex. The most common form of herpetic infection, secondary herpes simplex, possibly affects 50 per cent of the adult population. After a prodromal period of 24 to 48 hours, marked by a burning sensation in the region of the forming lesions, the eruption appears. This consists of groups of small clear vesicles that soon become transformed into pustules or crusted confluent erosions. The usual oral location is the lip-skin junction. Recurrences generally occur at the same sites.

A variety of stimuli may precipitate recurrent herpes simplex. These include fever, sunlight, food allergy, mechanical trauma and possibly even psychosomatic factors.

Subjective complaints extend from mild itching or burning to severe pain, in addition to the cosmetic inconveniences involved. After 4 to 10 days, the crusted lesions heal without scarring.

Secondary herpes simplex may very rarely involve the oral cavity proper, where, in contrast to primary gingivostomatitis, it affects only circumscribed areas such as the hard palate and gingiva.

The most effective treatment is decapitation of the vesicles as soon as they form, painting the base with a 5 per cent solution of neutral red dye and then exposing the lesions to a bright light for 10 minutes. This procedure is repeated twice a day for two days. In many cases this reduces the duration of the lesions from 10 to 14 days to two to four days.

Recurrent Aphthous Stomatitis

Recurrent aphthous stomatitis (aphthae, canker sores) is a disorder that affects about 20 per cent of the population. The disorder is of unknown etiology although various agents, such as trauma, psychosomatic factors, food allergy, autoimmune factors and L form of alpha-hemolytic streptococci, have been blamed. None, however, has met with general agreement. Herpes simplex has been ruled out as a causative agent in the majority of instances.

The patient is often aware of a burning sensation in the affected mucosa during the prodromal stage. The mucosa becomes focally erythematous and necrotic, with formation of single or multiple, round to oval ulcerations usually 2 to 10 mm. in diameter. About 10 per cent are larger than 1 cm. The ulcer is covered by a grayish white fibrinous exudate and surrounded by a bright red halo. It usually persists for one or two weeks and heals without scarring. Nearly any oral site may be involved, but the labial, buccal and lingual mucosa is affected most often. Many patients experience a half-dozen recurrences per year. Females may be affected somewhat more often than males.

Treatment consists of giving relief in the form of Orabase covering or 5 per cent topical Xylocaine ointment until the lesions resolve. Duration is usually 5 to 10 days.

Hand-Foot-and-Mouth Disease

Hand-foot-and-mouth disease is a vesicular disorder affecting both skin and mucosa; it is caused by several Coxsackie viruses, principally group A, type 16. Several epidemics have occurred, predominantly affecting children in Canada, the United States and England. In some cases, group A Coxsackie viruses, types 5 and 10, have been isolated. The epidemics have occurred most often during the warm summer months.

Those affected are usually children under 10 years of age, principally those one to five years old, although adults may be affected. After an incubation period of between two and six days, the cutaneous lesions appear. Although there may be as many as 100, usually there are no more than 20 to 30 flaccid superficial vesicles located on the borders of the palms and soles and ventral surfaces and sides of the fingers and toes. The lesions first appear as red papules, 2 to 10 mm. in diameter, which change within a day or two to flaccid gray vesicles that resolve within one to two weeks.

The oral lesions, often 5 to 10 in number, usually appear as painful aphthae 2 mm. or less in diameter, the vesicular phase being very short-lived. They can involve any area of the mouth, but the lips and buccal mucosa principally are affected. The pharynx rarely is involved. Healing occurs within 5 to 10 days. Cervical adenitis may occur but is not marked.

Constitutional symptoms are not severe. There are mild malaise and anorexia, and the temperature usually is below 100° F.

In most cases the clinical picture is so clear as to exclude nearly all other conditions. Inoculation of suckling mice with the vesicle fluid and tissue culture should be employed for diagnosis. Treatment is not necessary, since the lesions seldom last more than a few days and are not markedly painful.

Herpangina

Herpangina, is an acute infectious syndrome of childhood occurring in children up to six years of age; it is only rarely found in older children. It belongs to disorders caused by the Coxsackie viruses and, at times, the echo viruses.

After an incubation period of two to nine days (average, four days), the disease begins with acute symptoms accompanied by high fever, vomiting, headache, pain in the extremities, conjunctivitis, dysphagia and other symptoms that resemble those of appendicitis or early poliomyelitis or meningitis. The clinical findings in the oral cavity significantly aid diagnosis. On the soft palate, uvula and fauces are found several (3 to 10) small reddish vesicles on an erythematous base. They are usually symmetric and develop with the acute symptoms. After rupture, superficial aphthous lesions form and last from four to six days. The fever diminishes rapidly but, at times, a regional lymphadenitis persists.

The location of the vesiculoaphthous lesions is quite characteristic, but similar efflorescences may occur in the pharynx and, rarely, in the anterior part of the mouth. The suggestive name "herpangina" should not cause confusion with primary herpetic gingivostomatitis, since in most cases herpes simplex does not involve the tonsils and their surroundings. Moreover, herpetic gingivostomatitis is characterized by longer duration and more severe pain and halitosis.

Probably herpangina is not produced by Coxsackie viruses alone but simultaneously by other viruses as well: group A Coxsackie viruses, types 7, 9 and 16, group B Coxsackie viruses, types 1, 2, 3, 4 and 5 and ECHO viruses 9 and 17. Without doubt, only a small percentage of all cases of herpangina are recognized, since the infection often takes a nonspecific or abortive course.

Treatment is not necessary since the disorder resolves rapidly. Topical viscous Xylocaine ointment may be of aid in lessening the pain and dysphagia.

Puberty Gingivitis

A rather characteristic marginal gingivitis occurs at puberty. It is usually limited to the anterior part of the mouth, the interproximal papillae becoming bulbous. Therapy consists of improved oral hygiene only.

Gingival Fibromatosis

This generalized enlargement of the gingiva is often genetic, being inherited as an autosomal dominant characteristic. The gingivae seem to enlarge until the permanent teeth are covered by a hard, firm, painless gingiva, which may displace the teeth. There are several varieties, some with associated systemic abnormalities.

Therapy consists of surgical removal of the hyperplastic tissue. Recurrence within a year is not uncommon, and repeated gingivectomies may be required. Special precautions during the postoperative phases and scrupulous oral hygiene lessen the likelihood and the rapidity of recurrence.

Dilantin Gingival Enlargement

A generalized, painless hyperplasia of the gingiva is associated with prolonged therapeutic use of Dilantin sodium. In some patients the gingiva may actually cover the teeth. The degree of hyperplasia appears to be most closely related to oral hygiene: the poorer the hygiene, the more pronounced the enlargement. Gingival surgery may be indicated in severe hyperplasia. Excellent oral care retards regrowth. Vigorous tooth-brushing and gingival massage, either manual or with an electric toothbrush, are indicated.

Premature Periodontal Destruction

Inflammation of supporting structures of teeth, such as gingivae, bone and periodontal ligament, is so rare in children that the clinician is alert to its frequently systemic implications. It is seen in more than 90 per cent of children with *Down's syndrome* (trisomy 21). Not uncommonly in these children there is loss of the mandibular incisors because of alveolar bone loss. Scrupulous oral care must be given to children with this condition. Early loss of anterior deciduous teeth – the permanent dentition is almost always spared – is seen in *hypophosphatasia* due to lack of cementum.

Severe periodontal destruction occurs about both deciduous and permanent teeth in the *Papillon–Lefevre syndrome.* This is a rare autosomal recessive condition associated with infantile palmar and plantar hyperkeratosis. Periodontal therapy has been of no avail. Early periodontal destruction is also seen in many *neutropenias* and in *acatalasemia. Histiocytosis X* is frequently associated with periodontal destruction and early, individual tooth loss, especially in the molar areas of the primary teeth. Surgical curettage, radiation and, recently, chemotherapy have been used. Most important, children with *leukemia* frequently present with oral signs resembling periodontitis. This may take the form of engorged, edematous gingival tissue or periodontitis. The gingivae rapidly become necrotic, with associated exfoliation of teeth. Good oral hygiene in these children is extremely important.

TONGUE

Geographic Tongue

This condition is noted in 1 to 6 per cent of the population and in most cases is asymptomatic. The dorsum of the tongue shows characteristic smooth, shiny erythematous areas which are slightly depressed below the surrounding normal papillae. These patches disappear and reappear in different areas and at different times throughout the person's life. There appears to be no treatment for this condition except to allay the parents' fear that the child may have a serious disorder.

Scrotal Tongue

Often misdiagnosed as fissured tongue, this condition is characterized by tongue papillae divided into groups and clumps by small fissures which may not be apparent until the tongue is folded. There seems to be a linear progression in the prevalence of this entity with age, being seen in 1 per cent of infants, in approximately 2.5 per cent of children and in 4 per cent of young adults. Scrotal tongue may also be part of the Melkersson–Rosenthal syndrome and is also found frequently in mongolism. The condition does not adversely affect the patient, and no treatment is recommended.

Fissured Tongue

As much as 10 per cent of the population manifests at least two midline fissures. In addition it is not uncommon to note fissures parallel to or at right angles to the central grooves. A severe form, occurring in 1 to 1000 births, is often part of a continuum of lingual clefts and is treated accordingly. No treatment is required for the mild, more common form.

Bifid Tongue

Bifid tongue occurs either as an isolated finding or in association with median clefts of the lower lip and mandible or with the orofacial digital syndrome. In this latter condition the tongue may even be trifid or tetrafid. This condition is noted in approximately 1 in 10,000 births. In most cases the tongue is divided only at the tip. No treatment is indicated for minor clefts, whereas a straight-line closure is recommended for more severe cases.

Congenital Macroglossia

Enlarged tongue may be relative or absolute. Most cases are due to lymphangioma or other angiomatous malformations. Cystic hygroma may be present. The tongue surface often is irregular or papillary with 1- to 3-mm. blister type nodules. Radiation therapy has generally proved unbeneficial. Most successful treatment is a combination of sclerosing agents and corrective surgery.

The tongue may also be enlarged in type 2 glycogen storage disease or in the macroglossia-omphalocele syndrome. Both conditions are inherited as autosomal recessive traits. Differential diagnosis of macroglossia should also include neurofibromatosis.

Median Rhomboid Glossitis

This entity is not truly a glossitis. It has been considered to be caused by embryonal failure of the tuberculum impar to submerge, that is, to be covered by the lateral lingual tubercles. Nevertheless, it is innocuous. Its incidence is about 1 in 400 persons with a 3 to 1 male predilection. Classically, it is characterized by a smooth to nodular, elevated or depressed area void of papillae, located just anterior to the circumvallate papillae on the dorsum of the tongue. No treatment is required.

Aglossia or Microglossia

A rare congenital anomaly, this condition is often associated with adactylia. There is usually a grooved anterior alveolar process. Speech is not as disturbed as might be expected. No therapy is possible.

Lingual Thyroid

This condition has been explained as a partial or complete embryologic failure of the thyroid gland to descend from the foramen cecum to its normal position in the neck. It is characterized by multiple nodules of thyroid tissue on the dorsum of the tongue in the area of the foramen cecum or within the body of the tongue. In rare cases all the thyroid tissue remains on or in the tongue. The condition is seen in possibly 10 per cent of the male and female population, and the amount of ectopic tissue varies from a few acini to nodules 1 cm. in diameter. No treatment is required for small, discrete lesions. Larger lesions which may by position become traumatized should be removed surgically. However, no lingual thyroid tissue should be removed until the presence of thyroid tissue elsewhere is ascertained.

Black Hairy Tongue

This entity is characterized by an elongation of the filiform papillae and concurrent growth of a black pigment-producing fungus. The development of black hairy tongue is most often associated with antibiotic therapy. The condition is harmless and usually disappears spontaneously. Although treatment is not necessary, frequent application of 20 per cent aqueous caprylate or of 0.25 per cent triamcinolone acetonide in an adhesive base is effective. In addition, the patient should brush the dorsum of the tongue two or three times daily.

Ankyloglossia

This condition has been arbitrarily defined as the inability to elevate the tongue tip above a line extending through the commissures of the lip when the mouth is open because of a congenitally short lingual frenum. No treatment is required in mild forms because the defect rarely interferes with speech. In extremely severe forms the frenum should be clipped in infancy.

Riga-Fede Disease

In cases of natal or neonatal teeth, the tongue is drawn over the incisal edges during the sucking reflex and an ulcer develops on the ventral tip. Removal of the teeth may be necessary if smoothing of the edges does not eliminate the condition.

WHITE LESIONS OF THE ORAL MUCOSA

Lichen Planus, Hyperkeratosis and Leukoplakia

Although these conditions merit consideration in differential diagnosis in the adult, they are almost never seen in children. Benign intraepithelial dyskeratosis, white spongy nevus and hereditary dyskeratoses are examples of hereditary white lesions of oral mucosa.

Burns

Aspirin, various toothache drops and other chemicals held in a restricted area of the oral mucosa cauterize and whiten the tissue. If the etiologic agent is removed, the lesion heals.

SALIVARY GLAND DISORDERS

Sialolithiasis

Salivary calculus may be deposited in the salivary gland, or, more commonly, the excretory ducts. This may result in blockage with resultant pain and swelling. It is rare in children. The submandibular gland is most often affected. There is usually a history of intermittent, transient, painful swelling that may be more pronounced during eating. It may be associated with an acute suppurative process. Chronic obstructive conditions may lead to glandular atrophy. Probing, radiographic and sialographic studies should be done to locate the sialolith. If deposits cannot be readily removed by gentle probing or massage, surgical removal is necessary. Supportive therapy includes antibiotics, analgesics and salivary stimulation.

Sialadenitis and Other Conditions

Sialadenitis with inflammation and swelling may result from bacterial and viral infections. Appropriate antibiotics are indicated. *Xerostomia* and *ptyalism* may be related to oral and systemic infections. Malformations, cysts and other conditions may also yield chronic sialadenitis. *Neoplasms* should always be kept in mind when considering the salivary glands. Juvenile hemangioendothelioma of the parotid gland and mucoepidermoid carcinoma (or tumors) are the most common salivary tumors of children. Treatment is surgical.

Retention Cysts (Mucocele)

Mucous retention cysts result from rupture of a duct of a minor salivary gland, allowing the mucus to spill out into the connective tissue where it is treated as a foreign substance by the body. The mucocele occurs most often on the mucosal surface of the lower lip. It may also appear on the buccal mucosa, oral floor or ventral surface of the tip of the tongue (cyst of Blandin-Nuhn). Treatment consists of complete excision of the mucocele and the offending group of minor salivary glands and duct. Incision and drainage yield temporary improvement only.

NEOPLASMS

Numerous types of benign and malignant neoplasms may occur early in life. Two of the more fascinating benign ones seen in infancy are the *melanotic anlage tumors* of neural crest origin and the *congenital epulis,* which is a granular cell myoblastoma.

Congenital Epulis of the Newborn

This benign tumor is present at birth, usually pedunculated and located on the maxillary or mandibular gingiva, usually in the anterior region. It is limited almost exclusively to female infants. Histologically, it is similar to a granular cell myoblastoma but without associated pseudoepitheliomatous hyperplasia. Treatment is simple surgical excision.

Pigmented Anlage Tumor of Neural Crest Origin

This benign tumor usually occurs in the anterior maxillary gingiva of infants less than six months of age. It may grow rapidly and is usually deeply pigmented. Surgical excision is necessary. Even though it is benign, postsurgical recurrence is noted in about 10 per cent of cases.

Malignant Tumors

The prognosis of malignant neoplasms in children is generally grave. Because of frequent lymphadenopathy in childhood, symptoms of neoplasia may be ignored. Thorough oral examinations, including manual palpation of soft and hard tissues, and cooperation of dentist, pediatrician and pathologist are essential in diagnosis, treatment and post-treatment management.

THE HANDICAPPED CHILD

In handling the dental problems of children handicapped by cerebral palsy, mental retardation, hemophilia, phobias, severe cardiac problems and many other handicaps, special procedures are indicated. In some instances patient cooperation can be elicited by special care or by use of sedatives or tranquilizing drugs, making routine dental care possible in the dental office. In many cases dental treatment in the hospital with general anesthesia is preferable.

References

Finn, S. B.: *Clinical Pedodontics.* 3rd ed. Philadelphia, W. B. Saunders Company, 1967.

Gorlin, R. J., and Goldman, H. M. (eds.): *Thoma's Oral Pathology.* St. Louis, The C. V. Mosby Co., 1970.

Gorlin, R. J., and Pindborg, J. J.: *Syndromes of the Head and Neck.* New York, The McGraw-Hill Book Co., 1964.

Kutscher, A. H., et al.: *Pharmacotherapeutics of Oral Disease.* New York, The McGraw-Hill Book Co., 1964.

Witkop, C. J., and Wolf, R. O.: Hypoplasia and Intrinsic Staining of Enamel Following Tetracycline Therapy. *J.A.M.A.,* 185:1008, 1963.

Salivary Gland Tumors

WALTER P. WORK, M.D.

Primary tumors of the major salivary glands occur less frequently in children than in adults. The parotid is more frequently involved than the submandibular gland. These structures may also be the site of metastases from distant primary malignancies, or be involved by encroachment from adjacent or constitutional neoplasia.

Surgery is often the treatment of choice as in the adult. Radiation therapy used alone or in combination with surgery can be efficacious. However, few young patients are treated with x-ray therapy because of the inherent dangers encountered even with high energy radiation. Full tumor dosage can retard growth of bony and soft tissue structures about the head and neck and, as a result, radiation deformities may be apparent in later years. Likewise, these large doses of radiation may later subject the child to development of new neoplasms about the head and neck. Smaller doses of radiation therapy may be feasible in lymphoma lesions of the parotid and adjacent lymph nodes.

Chemotherapy has not been used effectively in pediatric patients with primary, recurrent or metastatic disease.

Hemangiomas. This tumor is the most frequently diagnosed tumor of the parotid gland in the infant. Rapid growth may be evident during the first few weeks of life. However, it is usually satisfactory to observe the patient for evidence of spontaneous involution, which usually occurs by three years of age. If involution does not occur, surgery may be indicated. In this instance the facial nerve is preserved.

Lymphangiomas. Lymphangiomas involve the major salivary glands by encroachment and less frequently as a primary localized lesion. Thus, adjacent areas of involvement may be the upper part of the neck, face, floor of the mouth, tongue and pharynx. Rapid growth, infection, airway obstruction and hemorrhage within the lymphangioma are indications for surgery. In most instances the facial nerve is preserved and excision is subtotal, even though the submandibular and parotid glands are included in the dissection. Recurrence is minimized by the placement of an iodoform pack in the substance of the tongue, floor of the mouth and upper part of the neck at the conclusion of excision. This pack is removed gradually over 10 or so days. Tracheostomy is performed in selected patients as part of the treatment.

Benign Mixed Tumors. These tumors occur in the older child and teenager. They appear as primary lesions, most frequently in the parotid gland as a slowly enlarging, painless noninflammatory mass. Total removal of tumor, including a generous portion of normal gland, is essential with preservation of the facial nerve at the first surgery. Benign mixed tumors in the submandibular gland in these age groups are rare. However, when they do occur, surgical excision is the treatment of choice.

Although recurrence rate of this benign tumor is high, particularly if the initial surgery is inadequate, malignant degeneration is infrequent. Benign recurrent disease must be surgically excised (total parotidectomy) with preservation of the facial nerve.

Mucoepidermoid Tumors. As in the adult, the biologic behavior of this ductal tumor is difficult to predict from permanent microscopic tissue examination. Attempts to make these predictions from frozen section only compound the difficulties. Hence, the surgeon must cooperate fully with the pathologist in treatment even to the point of wound closure and the performance of definitive surgery at a later date only after diagnosis is confirmed by microscopic examination of permanent tissue sections.

Surgery is the treatment of choice in any instance. In our hands, radiation therapy has not proved efficacious either as an initial method of therapy or later in combination with surgery. Surgery is the treatment of choice for recurrent lesions, also.

Undifferentiated Malignant Tumors. Undifferentiated malignant tumors are second in occurrence only to the mucoepidermoid tumor in children. If this tumor is suspected by the physician, incisional biopsy may be indicated. Since this tumor is characterized by rapid invasion of adjacent tissues and spreading by lymph channels, it is not unusual for the physician to note advanced disease at first examination of the patient. There may be an infiltrating, nonmovable mass with facial nerve dysfunction and cervical lymph node involvement. Radiation therapy may be the treatment of choice directed at arrest of the disease or palliation for the patient. Even patients selected for radical surgical excision carry a poor prognosis.

Adenocystic Adenocarcinomas (Cylindromas). This malignancy rarely occurs as primary disease in major salivary glands of the child. Therefore, as contrasted with the adult, the clinical behavior of this tumor in younger patients is little understood. However, using guidelines established in adults, treatment should consist of a combination of surgery and radiation therapy.

Squamous Cell Carcinomas. This also is a rare malignant tumor of major salivary gland origin in the child. Surgical excision probably should be the treatment of choice initially. In certain patients, radiation therapy may be used in combination with surgery.

Recurrent Bacterial Parotitis

EDWARD J. O'CONNELL, M.D.

Recurrent bacterial parotitis is a very uncommon condition. Involvement may be unilateral or bilateral. This condition can occur from the newborn period to adulthood; the peak incidence in childhood is from age 5 to 10 years. Although extensively investigated, the precise cause and pathogenesis remain unknown. Recurrent parotitis has been associated with allergic factors, various degrees of obstruction of Stensen's duct and ductal dilatation (sialectasis). Most improve spontaneously during older adolescence.

Management of the acute episode is directed at providing symptomatic relief, reestablishing salivary flow and giving specific antibiotic therapy. The usual symptomatic measures suffice, including administering aspirin for analgesia and applying heat to the gland. To achieve salivary flow, the gland should be milked periodically. Parents are instructed to do this. Some of the purulent material expressed from Stensen's duct should be cultured. Usually, typical oral flora are grown: *Streptococcus viridans, Staphylococcus aureus,* pneumococci and occasionally beta-hemolytic streptococci. Antibiotics have not been proven effective, but until further data are available their use seems appropriate. Ampicillin, 50 to 100 mg. per kilogram body weight orally every 6 hours, to a maximum dose of 500 mg. every 6 hours, should be given for 10 days. If the patient is penicillin-sensitive, erythromycin, 30 to 50 mg. per kilogram body weight every 6 hours, to a maximum dose of 500 mg. every 6 hours, may be given for 10 days. Most episodes last four to six days.

When the acute process has resolved, methods of prevention should be attempted. These are, however, not predictably effective. Patients should be advised to chew gum in an attempt to achieve salivary flow. Periodic massage of the gland is also suggested. Approximately 20 per cent of patients have fewer recurrences while on long-term antihistamine therapy such as diphenhydramine hydrochloride, 3 to 5 mg. per kilogram body weight three times a day, to a maximum dose of 300 mg. in 24 hours.

If recurrences continue, a sialogram should be performed to demonstrate the appearance of the duct structure, which may be normal, obstructed in some fashion or dilated (sialectasis). Many patients improve after this procedure.

Other forms of therapy, such as continuous antibiotics, autogenous vaccine, steroids and radiation, have no role in the treatment of recurrent bacterial parotitis. Because improvement is usually spontaneous, surgery is seldom indicated.

Thyroglossal Duct Cysts and Branchial Cysts and Fistulas

WERNER D. CHASIN, M.D.

THYROGLOSSAL DUCT CYSTS

Thyroglossal duct cysts arise from the normal thyroglossal duct of the embryo when this fails to become obliterated. They should be removed because they may become infected, they may break to the surface forming a permanent thyroglossal duct fistula and they are cosmetically conspicuous. Removal is seldom urgent, except when the cysts become infected or when they cause choking sensations.

The treatment of choice is total removal of the cyst or fistulous tract, including the stalk, which usually runs through or near the body of the hyoid bone up through the floor of the mouth and the root of the tongue to the foramen cecum of the tongue. Incision and drainage of the cyst is indicated only to treat an acute infection; it is not curative in eliminating the lesion. Through a horizontal skin incision, the cyst is dissected free and the stalk followed up to the hyoid bone. The central 1.5 cm. of the bone is removed, and the stalk is followed and cored out of the floor of the pharynx and root of the tongue up to the foramen cecum. The muscles of the tongue and the pharyngeal floor are closed with absorbable sutures, the subcutaneous tissues of the neck and the skin are sutured and the wound is drained with a soft rubber dam. Postoperative discomfort is mild, and the child may be discharged in four to six days. Thyroglossal duct fistulas are treated in identical fashion, with the additional removal of an ellipse of skin surrounding the caudal cervical opening of the sinus tract.

BRANCHIAL CYSTS AND FISTULAS

Branchial clefts and fistulas are congenital anomalies of the neck, which probably result from incomplete fusion of the branchial arches of the embryo. These anomalies include the following varieties: (1) branchial cyst, which is located in the side of the neck usually anterior and deep to the upper half of the sternomastoid muscle, and which may have no communication with either the pharynx or the skin of the neck, (2) branchial sinus, which is a tract buried in the deep structures of the neck, and which communicates at one end either with the pharynx or with the cervical skin, (3) branchial fistula, which is an epithelial-lined tract that courses from the pharynx through the structures of the neck to open on the skin of the side of the neck, (4) preauricular sinus, which opens on the skin in front of the upper half of the ear or in the auricle or external auditory canal and (5) the rare cervicoaural fistula, which is a tract running from the external auditory canal through the soft tissues of the neck, opening onto the cervical skin behind the angle of the mandible.

The treatment of choice for all the varieties of branchial cysts, sinuses and fistulas is complete excision during the first operation. In many cases the surgery may be quite complex, because these lesions may be located deep in the neck in intimate relationship with the carotid vessels, related nerves and walls of the pharynx. Even the innocent-appearing tiny preauricular sinus may require for its complete excision deep dissection in the parotid and periauricular areas, because it may branch extensively beneath the skin over the parotid gland and may communicate with the eustachian tube. Complete excision of these anomalies is usually successful. Incomplete removal, because of the surgeon's failure to follow the deep extensions of these tracts, invites recurrence of the lesions and necessitates secondary operations, which are usually more difficult because of postsurgical and postinflammatory scarring.

Disorders of the Esophagus

LAWRENCE K. PICKETT

ESOPHAGEAL ATRESIA WITH TRACHEOESOPHAGEAL FISTULA

The infant with respiratory difficulty due to excessive mucus should have immediate anteroposterior and lateral x-rays. An air esophagogram on either or both views may be suggestive or diagnostic of esophageal obstruction. Air in the abdominal viscera is evidence of a tracheoesophageal fistula.

The diagnosis of esophageal atresia can be confirmed by attempting to introduce a plastic feeding tube into the esophagus through the nose. If an obstruction is met, the tube is strapped in place and under careful fluoroscopic control and with the baby held upright, a small amount of contrast material, usually

Hypaque, is introduced into the tube to form a meniscus at the bottom of the pouch. The level of the upper esophageal pouch can be noted. Films of the entire chest and abdomen are obtained to demonstrate air in the intestine to confirm the presence of tracheoesophageal fistula, and also to investigate the possibility of intestinal obstruction distal to the stomach.

Once the type of esophageal atresia has been determined, a tube or plastic sump drainage tube is again placed, ideally under fluoroscopic control, at the bottom of the pouch, strapped securely and placed on constant suction. This aspirates the saliva and prevents tracheal obstruction from overflow of saliva. The infant is elevated at an angle of 45 degrees. Any severe dehydration is then rapidly corrected. During hydration, the infant should be taken to an operating room where a gastrostomy is carried out under local anesthesia. This prevents further reflux of gastric contents into the lungs and allows for decompression of the intestinal tract. While hydration is being completed, the aspiration pneumonia is treated with antibiotics, preferably penicillin and kanamycin given in appropriate dosage. After the gastrostomy has been completed, the child is kept in cold steam and is elevated at an angle of about 45 degrees so there will not be esophageal reflux. The gastrostomy tube, preferably number 16 or 18 French, should be kept on simple drainage to keep the gastrointestinal tract decompressed.

During this period of observation, other congenital anomalies, such as congenital heart disease or renal anomalies, can be investigated. In the full-term infant, once a maximum state of hydration and control of infection have been obtained, and if there are no obvious complicating anomalies of other systems, definitive surgical correction is undertaken. The exact method of repair is determined by the anatomy and type of fistula. In the most common type—that is, esophageal atresia with tracheoesophageal fistula from the main stem bronchus or bifurcation of the trachea—we now employ the end-to-side anastomosis, with simple ligation of the tracheoesophageal fistula with number 0 silk; and then careful end-to-side, one-layer anastomosis, tying the knots on the inside between the end of the upper pouch and the side of the distal esophagus. This anastomosis permits maximum blood supply to the distal esophagus. The discrepancy between the two esophageal segments is overcome by dissection of the upper esophageal segment where the blood supply is intramural and will not be compromised by extensive dissection. The approach is extrapleural with resection of the segment of the fourth rib in a posterolateral approach. Following completion of the anastomosis, the retropleural space is drained with a number 12 catheter put on suction in order to keep the dead space from being occupied by serum or blood which will compress the lung. If the pleura has been entered, an intrapleural catheter is occasionally necessary for expansion of the lung for the first 24 to 48 hours. Following the operation the child is kept elevated at a 45 degree angle because of cardioesophageal incompetence. Feeding is instituted through the gastrostomy tube 24 to 48 hours after the operation, depending on the age of the patient and the evident gastrointestinal function.

In the case of premature infants, simple ligation and division of the tracheoesophageal fistula by the retropleural approach is carried out under local anesthesia after gastrostomy and hydration of the child. The upper pouch is kept on sump suction until adequate size is obtained, generally 2500 Gm. Secondary repair of the esophagus is then carried out with an end-to-end anastomosis via a transpleural approach. This is then drained retropleurally with a chest catheter left in place for five days in case of an esophageal anastomotic leak.

Types of esophageal atresia other than those commonly encountered are treated according to the anatomy. Type I is esophageal atresia without tracheoesophageal fistula. Type III occurs when the upper pouch is at the thoracic inlet and may be treated by dilatation of the upper pouch; the upper pouch is elongated with mercury bougies until a primary anastomosis can be done. If dilatation is unsuccessful, marsupialization of the upper esophageal pouch is necessary and colonic replacement may be accomplished after 12 to 18 months of age.

Common to all types of esophageal atresia repair is the necessary care in postoperative feeding due to cardioesophageal incompetence. The gastrostomy tube must always be left open so that vomiting or regurgitation can take place up the tube in case of overfeeding or lower intestinal obstruction. Careful hydration is always essential. Antibiotic coverage with penicillin and kanamycin in the immediate postoperative phase is generally indicated.

ESOPHAGEAL STENOSIS AND STRICTURE

Esophageal Stenosis. Occasionally, instead of esophageal atresia, one may encounter esophageal stenosis. The position of the stenotic area can be demonstrated by the contrast material at the diagnostic evaluation, as noted in the discussion of esophageal atresia. Mild stenosis can be treated by antegrade esophageal dilatation by esophagoscopy and the placing of a filiform catheter and filiform follower dilator through the area. Most severe strictures should be treated by the establishment of a gastrostomy for feeding purposes, and by retrograde Tucker dilatations with graduated dilators brought through the stenotic area from below. If the esophageal stenosis is resistant to dilatation, a direct operative approach is needed. The details of the operative technique will vary depending on the site of the stricture, whether it is mucosal or whether it involves the full thickness of the esophageal wall. Details must vary with the anatomy encountered.

Inflammatory Esophageal Stricture. Esophageal stricture has been caused by reflux esophagitis associated with a hiatus hernia. It often responds to conservative treatment with antacids, frequent feedings and antispasmodics. Only in the most extreme conditions must operative intervention be undertaken. The operative correction of such strictures is discussed later under hiatus hernia.

CHEMICAL BURNS OF THE ESOPHAGUS

Inflammatory stricture of the esophagus secondary to chemical burns is treated in various ways, depending on the extent of the burn and the nature of the agent. When a caustic burn of the esophagus is suspected, the child is admitted to the hospital, placed on nothing by mouth, given ampicillin in the customary dosage for his age and started on steroid therapy or prednisone, 1 mg. per kilogram body weight per day. Between 24 and 48 hours after admission, the child is taken to the operating room where an esophagoscopy is done under general anesthesia to determine the extent of the esophageal burn. If no burn is found, therapy is discontinued and the patient discharged. If there is circumferential burn of the esophagus, no further attempt at esophagoscopy is made and the child is returned to the ward and continued on the steroid and chemotherapy for two weeks. At the end of this time, evaluation of the esophagus by esophagogram is made. Depending on symptomatology, the diet progresses from clear fluids to nourishing fluids to a soft diet. If no stricture is evident on x-ray, a second cautious esophagoscopy is carried out to determine the extent of healing. If the lesion seems to be resolving, steroids are tapered over a one-week period, ampicillin is discontinued and the child is sent home. If there is a stricture present or if there is diminution in the lumen of the esophagus, gentle bougienage or dilatation is carried out using the mercury-filled bougies. If the stricture is prolonged and extends through more than one-third of the esophagus, a gastrostomy is done for feeding and for purposes of retrograde esophageal dilatation on whatever schedule is necessary to keep the esophagus functional. It is generally not necessary to dilate these strictures more than once every three weeks, but repeated dilatations can be done depending on the needs of the patient. Since instituting steroid therapy, we have encountered very few resistant strictures that have needed dilatation. If, however, the lesion is persistent and continues to be symptomatic after six dilatations, esophageal resection and/or colonic replacement should be undertaken. In this instance the multiple anesthetics for dilatation and the danger of perforation at each dilatation are greater than for the single operation for esophageal replacement. On the other hand, if the stricture will respond to dilatation, the scarred esophagus and possibly competent cardioesophageal junction are far preferable to colonic interposition. With the use of steroids and antibiotics, stricture formation has become a rarity.

CHALASIA AND ACHALASIA

Chalasia is a condition characterized by cardioesophageal relaxation: there is inappropriate cardioesophageal function and consequent reflux. After the baby is fed there is immediate reflux into the esophagus, causing vomiting, the symptoms mimicking those of pyloric stenosis. Once the diagnosis of chalasia is made, whether or not an associated hiatus hernia is diagnosed, the child should be elevated 45 degrees in a so-called esophageal chair after feeding, and he should receive thickened feedings with antispasmodics for a period of four to six weeks. The condition is generally self-terminating and self-correcting and rarely leads to surgical problems.

Achalasia or cardiospasm may be confused with esophageal hiatus hernia and a resultant stricture secondary to peptic esophagitis. It may be due to intrinsic disease in the wall of the esophagus with attendant cardioesophageal stenosis. Most of these patients respond to dilatations done in antegrade fashion by passing a filiform through the esophagoscope and through the narrowed area to the stomach. Gentle dilatations with filiform follower dilators are done to an appropriate size; generally, on the first dilatation a number 22 to 24 is used, rapidly progressing with subsequent dilatations up to a number 30 to 32. Most cases of achalasia in infants will respond to dilatation and will not require surgical intervention.

Achalasia in older children is a rare occurrence. The literature indicates that a modified Heller procedure with an esophageal myotomy is a proper form of therapy. A longitudinal incision is made through the fiber muscular layers of the stomach and esophagus down to the mucous membrane. The mucous membrane is not penetrated. Suitable separation of the esophagus provides relief from the obstruction.

HIATUS HERNIA

Enthusiasm for surgery for hiatus hernia varies tremendously, depending on the geographic location of the surgeon. My belief is that this is a totally reversible abnormality which can in most cases be treated conservatively with the same therapy as is used for chalasia. Frequent feedings, antacids, 5 ml. of Gelusil given between feedings, maintenance of an upright position after feedings and antispasmodics, such as 10 to 15 drops of Donnatal, will result in reversal of most cases of extensive evident hiatus hernia or so-called congenital short esophagus.

If the condition is not discovered early in infancy but only after peptic esophagitis and stricture have resulted, operative intervention should be undertaken. The type of operation varies, depending on the amount of stricture and obstruction of the esophagus. Proper repair of the esophageal hiatus with reconstruction of the intra-abdominal esophagus, and often some form of fixation of the stomach intra-abdominally to the lower side of the diaphragm, is essential in completing the repair. Again, the details may roughly be described as the Allison operation, but how it is carried out depends on the anatomy of the situation. It should once more be noted that most cases of hiatus hernia respond to conservative therapy. It is only the rare instance that will require operative intervention.

Vomiting

GERALD W. FRIEDLAND, M.D., *and*
PHILIP SUNSHINE, M.D.

Vomiting occurs in many normal infants and children and in about 60 per cent of normal newborns. It may also be the principal manifestation of relatively benign conditions, such as motion sickness or an acute emotional upset. But, in both infants and young children, it may be an important early sign of obstruction or inflammation anywhere in the gastrointestinal tract from the mouth to anus; of inflammatory lesions of almost any organ system; of numerous metabolic disturbances; of increased intracranial pressure; of adverse effects of medications; or of poisoning. In many instances the vomiting will subside when the primary causative agent has been treated, or when medications, which can irritate the stomach if administered orally, are given by the rectal or intramuscular route.

The purpose of this section is to discuss the management of vomiting with emphasis on those conditions in which the *prime symptom* is vomiting.

RECURRENT VOMITING IN HEALTHY BABIES

When the normal infant sucks, he swallows not only milk but also a considerable quantity of air. Some of this air finds its way into the intestine. Fortunately, a simple method exists for eliminating most of the swallowed air—the burp. During burping, about 5 to 10 ml. of milk are usually lost with the air. When greater quantities, in the range of one-third to one-half the intake, are vomited after almost each feeding, the infant merits careful observation.

If the infant is otherwise healthy, simple measures should be attempted initially. During the first few days of life, gastric irritation from ingestion of irritating meconium, blood or amniotic fluid can be eliminated by simple gastric lavage. Feeding is then commenced after 12 to 24 hours, beginning with small quantities (½ to 1 ounce) of dilute formula (10 to 12 calories per ounce), which is gradually increased in quantity and strength.

The majority of cases of persistent vomiting in otherwise healthy babies can be successfully dealt with by the practicing pediatrician or general practitioner in a logical manner. The means of delivery of the feeding, the type of feeding or the burping process may be at fault. Poor delivery in breast fed infants can be due to retraction of the nipple; in bottle fed infants, an inadequate hole in the nipple is a common cause. Vigorous sucking of the hungry infant in both instances results in the swallowing of inordinate quantities of air. The hole in the nipple of the feeding bottle can be enlarged by plunging a red-hot needle into it. It should be sufficiently large to permit the total feeding to be administered in no more than 20 minutes.

Changes in the formula will sometimes

alleviate the vomiting. If the formula is too dilute, the infant may need to consume an excess quantity to satisfy his needs, and may vomit the excess. Conversely, too great a concentration may be irritating and lead to vomiting.

How the mother burps the infant may be important. The infant should be burped both before and after feeding, and for a period of about 20 minutes thereafter the infant should be kept in a sitting position. Infant seats can effectively maintain the infant upright and relieve the parent of much of the tedium of this task. When the infant is placed in a crib, the prone position is preferable to the supine. Both in the upright and prone position, air in the upper part of the stomach, rather than food, is regurgitated, and the likelihood of pulmonary aspiration is reduced. In these positions, gravity aids gastric emptying.

When the simple measures outlined fail to remedy the vomiting, and if the infant does not thrive, loses weight or has blood-streaked vomitus, more detailed investigation is required so that specific therapy can be instituted.

Infants who have an allergy to milk or other foods may present with vomiting or diarrhea or both. The therapy for these infants is discussed under the section entitled Allergy.

Any neonate whose vomitus contains bile must be suspected of having an intestinal obstruction or sepsis, and should be worked up accordingly. Bile-stained vomitus indicates disease until proved otherwise.

VOMITING IN PREMATURE INFANTS

Premature infants (particularly tiny babies, weighing 1200 Gm. or less) frequently suffer from two feeding difficulties: first, aspiration of food due to incoordination of sucking, swallowing and breathing; and, second, gastroesophageal reflux after feeding due to immaturity of the lower esophageal sphincter mechanism. Although reflux can lead to vomiting, more frequently in tiny infants (weighing 1200 Gm. or less), refluxed gastric contents are expelled no further than the pharynx and back of the mouth. Unlike the mature infant, the presence of regurgitated food in the premature infant's pharynx and esophagus does not initiate deglutition or secondary esophageal peristalsis. A pool of regurgitated food may lie in the back of the mouth and pharynx, and spill over into the larynx with resultant aspiration.

The deglutition difficulties necessitate gavage feedings, either intermittent or via an indwelling catheter, depending on the nursing staff's preferences. Pooling of regurgitated food at the back of the mouth and pharynx poses a major nursing problem because nurses will not detect its presence unless they open and inspect the infant's mouth. Nurses caring for a premature infant must, therefore, place the infant right-side-down in a semi-Fowler position after feeding. The nurses must also open the infant's mouth at frequent intervals and inspect both mouth and posterior pharynx for the presence of regurgitated milk.

VOMITING IN INFANTS WHO ARE SMALL FOR GESTATIONAL AGE

For some totally unexplained reason, infants who are small for gestational age tend to vomit more often than do normal-sized infants. Because many infants who are small for gestational age develop hypoglycemia, feedings of 5 to 10 per cent dextrose (depending on the infant's maturity) are commenced within 1 to 2 hours after delivery. Since these infants often vomit intermittently during the first 12 to 24 hours of life, oral feedings of dextrose may not be sufficient or appropriate to prevent hypoglycemia, and glucose must be administered intravenously.

GENERAL PRINCIPLES IN THE MANAGEMENT OF VOMITING OF INFANTS AND CHILDREN

Certain general principles of management apply to many types of vomiting. When vomiting is copious, oral feedings should be stopped for several hours. Thereafter, infants should receive clear liquids (½ teaspoon of table salt and 1 tablespoon of sugar per quart of water) in small feedings, followed by half-strength and then full-strength formula when such are tolerated. Older children tolerate carbonated drinks, such as ginger ale and cola, as well. Sweetened tea and dilute bouillon are also satisfactory. Dry crackers and toast can then be introduced, followed by a bland and then a normal diet as vomiting subsides. More severe fluid and electrolyte losses require immediate intravenous replacement in the hospital, as outlined under Fluid Therapy in Pediatrics.

A further problem associated with vomiting is pulmonary aspiration. Sometimes such episodes of aspiration lead to cardiorespiratory arrest, which requires resuscitation. In all mechanical obstructions, preoperative nasogastric suctioning is necessary, and this should be continued in the postoperative period until evidence of obstruction and ileus no longer exists. Other vomiting infants are best nursed in the prone or prone-Trendelenburg position, which minimizes the tendency to pulmonary aspiration. When vomiting is due to primary or secondary chalasia or hiatal hernia, the infant should be maintained in the upright position, as will be discussed later.

DRUG THERAPY

In order to understand the drug therapy of vomiting, it is necessary to appreciate how various stimuli affect the vomiting center and where antiemetic drugs act to inhibit these stimuli. The vomiting center lies in the dorsal portion of the lateral reticular formation. Drugs and toxins do not act directly on the vomiting center; instead, they exert their influence on the chemoreceptor trigger zone, an area in the medulla oblongata through which emetic impulses are conveyed to the vomiting center. Impulses derived from the labyrinths, for example, those generated in children susceptible to motion sickness, may pass through the 8th nerve and cerebellum and stimulate the trigger zone. Some impulses bypass the chemoreceptor trigger zone and act directly on the vomiting center. Included in this category are impulses originating in the nerve endings of the gastrointestinal tract and mediated through the vagus and sympathetic nerves, as well as those arising from psychologic factors and obnoxious sights and smells.

None of the antiemetic drugs acts directly on the vomiting center. They exert their influence either on the chemoreceptor trigger zone or on the labyrinths. As a result, they are most effective when used to counteract impulses passing through the chemoreceptor trigger zone or arising from the labyrinths.

Before describing the antiemetic drugs which may be used, it is important to emphasize that in most cases, vomiting will cease when the causative disease process and fever are relieved. Antiemetic drugs contribute little, if anything, to the management of vomiting in these circumstances. They also possess unpleasant side effects. Certain specific indications exist for the use of antiemetic drugs, and they can be helpful if correctly used.

Phenothiazine Derivatives. Certain phenothiazine derivatives act as potent antiemetic agents. But some children receiving phenothiazine derivatives develop extrapyramidal side effects, which, although temporary, are unpleasant. Moreover, these side effects are particularly liable to occur in precisely those children most in need of an antiemetic agent; namely, the acutely ill child and the child who is dehydrated from the vomiting and diarrhea of gastroenteritis. Indeed, adequate urinary output must be established before phenothiazine derivatives are administered. Phenothiazine derivatives may also mask important developing signs and symptoms when the diagnosis is uncertain. Despite these objections, phenothiazine derivatives are widely prescribed for control of vomiting in children. If the physician elects to use them, he should do so only if the child is closely supervised and adequately hydrated.

Of the phenothiazine derivatives available, prochlorperazine (Compazine) is the most effective. It should not be used for children under 20 pounds or under two 2 years of age. Since part or most of the drug will be lost by vomiting if it is administered orally, rectal administration is recommended. Dosage schedules are as follows: for children weighing 20 to 29 pounds, 2½ mg. once or twice a day, not to exceed 7½ mg. per day; 30 to 39 pounds, 2½ mg. two to three times per day, not to exceed 10 mg. per day; 40 to 85 pounds, 2½ mg. three times a day or 5 mg. two times a day, not to exceed 15 mg. per day. Suppositories for children are available in 2½-mg. and 5-mg. dosages. It is advisable to prescribe the 2.5-mg. dosage as 2½ mg. because it may be confused with the 25-mg. suppository available for adults. Promethazine hydrochloride (Phenergan) is also effective in the treatment of vomiting in infants and children, especially when it is secondary to gastroenteritis. The dosage varies from 12.5 to 25 mg. intramuscularly, depending on the age and size of the child.

Nonphenothiazine Antiemetic Drugs. Several nonphenothiazine derivatives are used for the treatment of vomiting in children. Included in this category are trimethobenzamide (Tigan),* which shares the piperazine side chain of prochlorperazine, and diphenidol (Vontrol).† Although these drugs produce less sedation and are considered slightly safer than prochlorperazine, they are proportionately less efficacious and generally more expensive. Prochlorperazine remains the standard drug for use in children.

Certain drugs, although not usually considered antiemetics, possess this pharmacologic action in a limited number of specific conditions. For example dimenhydrinate (Dramamine) is effective in controlling the vomiting of motion sickness and benign paroxysmal vertigo. For therapeutic or prophylactic use, children 8 to 12 years of age can be given 25 to

---

* Manufacturer's precaution: Injectable form of trimethobenzamide (Tigan) is not recommended in children.

† Manufacturer's precaution: Oral form of diphenidol (Vontrol) is not recommended for children under 25 pounds or six months of age. Subcutaneous or intravenous administration is not recommended for children of any age.

50 mg. orally or rectally three times daily. Children under six years of age may be given 6.25 mg. three times daily. The dosage may be further increased until drowsiness and atropine-like symptoms occur.‡

RECURRENT VOMITING ASSOCIATED WITH ABDOMINAL MIGRAINE OR ABDOMINAL EPILEPSY

Phenobarbital, 7.5 to 15 mg. twice a day, will usually prevent electroencephalographically-proved occult abdominal epilepsy. Dilantin, although effective, frequently produces undesirable side effects. Some side effects, although purely cosmetic (for example, hirsutism, gingival hyperplasia and measles-like rashes), may cause psychologic upset, especially in girls, and the child may refuse to take the drug. Serious side effects occur much less frequently. The use of Dilantin suspension is not recommended; poor suspending qualities invariably result in nonuniformity of dosage, too little medication being present in the upper part of the bottle and too much in the lower part.

Attacks of vomiting due to migraine will respond to treatment with ergotamine tartrate. Younger children are given one-half of a Cafergot suppository (1 mg. ergotamine tartrate, plus 50 mg. caffeine) rectally early in an attack. This can be repeated half an hour later if necessary. Older children will respond to 1 to 2 mg. ergotamine tartrate (½ to 1 tablet Ergomar) sublingually, repeated half an hour later if necessary (maximum dose, 4 mg.).

RECURRENT ACETONEMIC VOMITING

Recurrent acetonemic vomiting is a condition characterized by vomiting, of variable duration, in an infant or child in whom symptoms and signs indicating disease of a specific organ or system are absent. The diagnosis can only be suggested when thorough investigation fails to reveal organic disease.

Treatment is symptomatic. For mild to moderate cases, administration of antispasmodics and antacids will relieve symptoms during an attack. Dicyclomine hydrochloride (Bentyl) is an effective antispasmodic which produces few atropine-like side effects. Infants are given half a teaspoon (5 mg.) of the syrup three or four times daily; this can be increased to 10 mg. (1 teaspoon of the syrup or 1 tablet) in older children. Rarely, in susceptible children, marked atropine-like side effects occur, necessitating reduction in dosage or cessation of therapy. A combination of aluminum hydroxide and magnesium hydroxide prevents constipation induced by aluminum hydroxide. Infants and young children can be given 2 to 4 ml. with each feeding. Older children are given 1 teaspoon every 2 hours. If vomiting is severe, the child may become rapidly dehydrated and develop ketosis. Dehydration, acidosis and electrolyte disturbances require correction with the appropriate parenteral replacement. Phenothiazine derivatives have proven extremely useful in controlling vomiting in this condition.

Long periods without food seem to precipitate relapses and ketosis. This can be prevented by giving a regular midnight snack.

Formerly, this condition was believed to cease spontaneously at puberty. Recent investigations, however, have shown that this is not the case.

RECURRENT VOMITING DUE TO HYPERAMMONEMIA

Infants or children who have "recurrent acetonemic vomiting," or who are diagnosed as having abdominal epilepsy or migraine, may have hyperammonemia. Measurement of the concentration of ammonia in blood should be performed about ½ to 1 hour postprandially; if hyperammonemia is found, the cause of this abnormality must be defined. Most commonly a defect in urea biosynthesis is encountered, especially ornithine transcarbamylase (OTC) deficiency. This defect is found almost exclusively in females. If OTC deficiency occurs in males, it usually results in death in the neonatal period. Appropriate dietary therapy consisting of a low protein intake (1.0 to 1.2 Gm. per kilogram) should be instituted in order to prevent hyperammonemia, but at the same time the protein intake should be adequate to ensure appropriate growth.

HIATAL HERNIA

Hiatal hernia is a common cause of persistent vomiting. It can present in a number of different ways, especially in infants and children; persistent vomiting, hematemesis, failure to thrive, iron deficiency anemia and respiratory infections are commonly associated with hiatal hernia, but more exotic presentations include Sandifer's syndrome, the rumination syndrome, protein-losing enteropathy and finger clubbing.

Sandifer's syndrome involves torsion spasms of the head and neck and, occasionally,

‡ Note: The dosage of dimenhydrinate for children under six years of age has not been established by the manufacturer. The dosage listed here is that recommended by A. M. Chutorian, in *Current Pediatric Therapy*, 4th ed., 1970.

also of the upper part of the torso; the limbs are almost never involved. The *rumination syndrome* occurs when a child regurgitates food, and then rechews and reswallows it; sometimes some of the food dribbles out of the mouth. The child's head is usually extended, with the mouth open, and the tongue makes sucking motions just before regurgitation. Both Sandifer's syndrome and the rumination syndrome involve abnormal movements and are associated with hiatal hernia; they may therefore be somehow related. The rumination syndrome is sometimes thought to be psychogenic, but this is doubtful.

Persistent vomiting in infants has also been ascribed to relaxation or dysfunction of the lower esophageal sphincter (the vestibule); in other words, chalasia. *Primary chalasia* is due to a maturation defect and occurs in premature or very young infants. *Secondary chalasia,* which is probably caused by depression of the function of the vagal nuclei, occurs in infants who have lesions of the central nervous system, acute pyelonephritis, uremia and other systemic illnesses. Most cases diagnosed as "chalasia" are, in fact, due to small hiatal herniae.

Treatment of hiatal hernia in infants and children may be either medical or surgical. Medical therapy consists of small feedings, thickened formula and around-the-clock maintenance of an upright position. Simple elevation of the head of the crib is not sufficient. Antacids and parasympathomimetic drugs are of unproved value. Medical therapy should be continued for at least two months. Surgery is required when symptoms do not respond to medical therapy or if severe esophagitis with stricture develops.

A large variety of operative procedures are now available for repair of neonatal hiatal hernia. Each procedure has strong advocates, but any operation that maintains the vestibule in its normal anatomic position will usually succeed. About 25 per cent of patients undergoing surgery will have recurrence of symptoms.

OTHER GASTROINTESTINAL DISORDERS ASSOCIATED WITH RECURRENT VOMITING

Many congenital anomalies can present with episodes of persistent vomiting. Although vomiting usually manifests itself at birth, or soon after, it may not appear until the child is older; sometimes not even until adulthood. Some of the more common anomalies responsible for recurrent vomiting include Ladd's bands, malrotation, congenital defects in the mesentery, duodenal diaphragm, annular pancreas, duplications and Meckel's diverticulum. Some of these conditions can be associated with severe, crampy abdominal pain at the time of vomiting, particularly Ladd's bands and malrotation. If a barium examination of the intestine is not performed when the symptoms are most evident, the examination may appear normal and the patient might erroneously be thought to have psychogenic vomiting. The treatment for these congenital anomalies is the appropriate surgical procedure.

The treatment of pylorospasm and duodenal ulcers is discussed elsewhere in this volume.

Constipation

DAVID R. FLEISHER, M.D.

Persons who pass firm, highly segmented stools a few times a week or less, with dyschezia, are often referred to as being constipated. They do not develop fecal retention or soiling. This stool pattern results from a tendency to exaggerated nonpropulsive contraction of the distal colon and sigmoid. Patients with this type of constipation range in years from early infancy to old age. Firm, segmented stools are evidence of a normal variant of colon function, not a pathologic process. Treatment is usually not indicated. Stool softeners, oral mineral oil or bran may be helpful in cases of secondary anal irritation or fissure. Cathartics and enemas should be avoided because they are unnecessary and intensify the existing tendency to colon spasm.

Constipation is a term also applied to a quite different process—chronic functional fecal retention. This is a progressive disorder, not a physiologic variant of normal. It does not involve hypercontractility of the autonomically innervated smooth muscle of the distal colon and sigmoid, but rather the somatically innervated striated muscle of the pelvic floor. This kind of constipation affects children from nursery school age to early teens. It often causes incapacity and occasionally may cause extrinsic obstruction of the lower urinary tract.

Management of chronic functional fecal retention is based on the concept that normal development of control over defecation has been interrupted or that previously acquired competence has been lost. It may occur when family life is disturbed by conditions that create an atmosphere of bitterness or uncertainty, e.g., intense marital discord. The genesis of the syndrome may be traceable to very early infancy. Parents may become concerned because they may see their baby straining to pass stool, because he has missed a day or because the doctor was concerned by the presence of blood in his stool during the newborn nursery stay. They may fear that absence of a bowel movement for a day or so will lead to intestinal obstruction, that his system will be "poisoned" or that internal rupture will occur. Intervention is in the form of enemas or suppositories. When discomfort recurs, experience leads to quicker incrimination of intestinal malfunction. Intrarectal manipulations are again tried. The idea becomes established that the baby needs special help, that without it he could not pass stools adequately. Gradually, help in the form of rectal intervention may become routine. Instead of the toddler's gradually acquiring self-control in response to his parents' expectations, he is manipulated from without. His recalcitrance increases. His bowel movements become an increasingly distressful, central issue of family concern. The motivation for learning self-control gives way to a feeling of being assaulted. His parents have taken over the responsibility for regulation of his bowels. He becomes further removed from approaching the task. The child responds to the fecal urge by automatically tightening his muscles. As retained feces accumulate, enemas, suppositories and laxatives become less effective and are met with more resistance.

Eventually, the clinical picture becomes fullblown: large fecal masses are palpable in the abdomen. After a week or two of retention the patient develops abdominal cramps. His appetite wanes. He becomes less playful. He makes visible efforts to prevent leakage as the fecal urge becomes more frequent. Then, "diarrhea" episodes occur, during which the patient has involuntary soilage and may run to the toilet many times. Several days of distress may then culminate in the very difficult passage of a gigantic stool. The child is exhausted. Soilage and discomfort stop temporarily. Fecal retention resumes and the cycle is repeated. Other children are unable to pass sizable stools for many weeks at a time. They are chronically uncomfortable and soil continuously.

As the syndrome becomes well established, the school-age child becomes overwhelmed by his loss of control. Then, characteristic attitudes of an almost dissociative nature develop. He seems to be indifferent to the problem and may vigorously deny that he has a problem. At the same time, he gives a history of not being able to feel the fecal urge. Instead of placing his soiled underwear in an appropriate place, he may secrete it in bizarre locations.

Parents and older children cannot feel empathy with the child when he soils. They have no recollection of the difficulties they experienced as toddlers during their own process of acquiring control. Perceptual-motor skills, once mastered, seem simple and automatic. The child's soiling, refusal to use the toilet and apparent nonchalance cause great vexation. Of all the indiscretions and accidents that might befall a school-age child, fecal soiling is the one that evokes the most intense deprecation from peers and parents and is the most damaging to self-esteem. This constitutes a vicious cycle.

Management. The pediatrician should learn the fears and misconceptions harbored by the parents and by the child so that he may allay them. Attitudes concerning defecation are often influenced by information of a folklore nature. Fecal retention does not produce a toxic state or headaches. Retention of stool for a week or more may produce discomfort, but not disease. Passing stools frequently or regularly is not healthier than passing them infrequently or sporadically. Normal stooling patterns in healthy persons vary widely.

A course of anal dilatation will usually produce more harm than benefit. If children with ectopic anus or imperforate anus and rectoperineal fistula are excluded, congenital anal stenosis is extremely rare. The narrowness of the anal canal is determined by the vigor with which the patient tightens his levator ani muscles during digital examination. The diagnosis of anal stenosis is untenable in patients who have passed stools of normal caliber.

Functional disorders of elimination do not conform to the pneumococcal pneumonia model of disease. There is no specific medication that can be applied to the patient who then recovers by the passive process allowing it time to work. The malfunction develops because distress either prevents a child from developing this normal skill or causes him to lose it. The child is "cured" when he becomes able to grapple with and overcome the emotional and physical distress he feels when he experiences the fecal urge and tries to pass stool. He regains control primarily as a result of his own efforts. In their work together, the pediatrician and the parents attempt to discover which measures are helpful to their child and which measures hinder him in his efforts.

Certain skills are mastered by a person only if he is left alone. Socially appropriate elimination is such a skill. One of the principal goals of management is allowing a child autonomy. To achieve this, the parents must be able to stop direct intervention into the child's rectum as well as coercive ministrations to induce defecation. Parents must allow the child complete responsibility for his own bowel movements. The issue should cease being a focus of exaggerated family concern.

These changes in attitude are difficult. It is acutely distressing for a parent to watch his child in discomfort, knowing that emptying the rectum will offer temporary relief. However, the parent must be helped to understand that intervention of this sort will make the child's assuming control of the problem more remote.

It is appropriate for the pediatrician to perform diagnostic procedures to rule out Hirschsprung's disease, other obstructive lesions, sensorimotor defects of the pelvic floor and abdominal musculature, hypothyroidism and hypercalcemic states. He must clarify the concept that the essential defect is not inherent in the feces but rather in the child's difficulties in organizing the process by which it is passed. He should clarify the pathogenesis of symptoms, such as cramps, overflow soiling and retentive posturing. He should effectively reassure the parents that although there may be great discomfort, there is little danger in refraining from active intervention. The pediatrician must be accessible to and supportive of the parents when they find it too difficult and are about to resort to rectal intervention. An immediate office visit can be very reassuring during times of crisis. Parents are helped by learning that their problem is not unique—that other families have experienced the same disorder and have overcome it.

The pediatrician should develop a rapport with the child and, by private conversations, help him acknowledge the existence of his problem and reassure him of his ability to overcome it. As the child's attitudes mature, he will begin to feel primarily responsible for overcoming his problem. In the majority of cases, retention is not a long-term condition. Avoidance of rectal intervention, helping the parents to allow the child to be in control, administration of stool softeners or lubricants and supportive follow-up care usually suffice.

In many cases, intense emotional difficulties are apparent on first contact and symptoms began after a long period of trouble-free defecation, thereby making aganglionosis unlikely. The disorder of defecation is just one of several major areas of difficulty in the child's life. It may be preferable in such cases to defer an "organic" work-up and have the patient evaluated by a competent child psychiatrist. If no improvement occurs despite progress in the emotional area, the pediatrician still has the option of pursuing a thorough evaluation of the structure and function of the child's colorectum and pelvic floor. The advantage of this approach is that it will not cause harm, it may lead to resolution of the symptoms as well as to progress in helping the child and family in a much broader context and it avoids the expense and stress of diagnostic studies.

However, *the prerequisites for effective psychiatric referral* should be met: (1) The parents appreciate their child's emotional distress; lecturing parents who are not yet able to recognize the presence of emotional distress in their child usually results in dissatisfaction with the pediatrician and loss of rapport. (2) The parents view referral to a mental health facility as a potentially useful step. Many parents are quite unwilling to seek professional help even though they recognize and are worried by the emotional distress they see in their child. (3) A competent child psychiatrist or other appropriate mental health facility must be available in the family's locality. (4) The referral is economically feasible. (5) The pediatrician remains responsible for the diagnosis and treatment of the child's organic symptoms; he does not refer the patient to a psychiatrist to cure a physical symptom such as fecal retention. Patients resent such referrals, since they may infer that the physical symptom is "all in the head" and not taken seriously by the physician. Patients are more likely to accept a psychiatric referral for the purpose of alleviating acknowledged emotional distress.

If the physical symptom subsides as the patient improves emotionally, the physician's job of diagnosing and treating the retentive fecal soiling is made much easier. "Transferring" a patient with physical symptoms to the sole care of a psychiatrist is irresponsible, and unfair to both psychiatrist and patient; it would be analogous to transferring a toddler with suspected intussusception to the sole care of a radiologist.

In prolonged, difficult cases, it is sometimes helpful to hospitalize the child for a week or more to allow him freedom by temporarily lifting the burden of responsibility from his parents and observing what happens. His passing a bowel movement by himself is very reassuring to his parents, who have doubted his ability to do this. If he experiences discomfort, it is reassuring to the parents to observe that he survives it without damage and without outside intervention. Barium studies can be performed to ascertain the absence of aganglionosis and other obstructions. A series of enemas and laxatives may be necessary prior to and following barium enema to prevent barium impaction.

Care and time should be taken to involve the child as a cooperating participant in the diagnosis rather than allowing him to be a victim of tests. Frequent conversations with the parents, including separate discussions with each parent, are useful in strengthening rapport and appreciating the sources of parental distress. At the end of the hospitalization, considerable data have been collected from diagnostic tests and observations of feelings and behavior. A conference with both parents is useful so that the material can be reviewed, future management planned and a basis for supportive follow-up established.

Mineral oil given orally is useful, provided rectal leakage does not intensify the family's distress. The notion that any medication cures fecal retention should be avoided, since it obscures the fact that the cure is achieved primarily by the child's own efforts.

A fairly common error is mistaking nonretentive fecal soiling for overflow soiling secondary to fecal retention. Mineral oil in these instances only worsens a most distressing symptom.

Prognosis. Some children quickly recover after the condition is clarified and coercion is stopped. They may experience relapses during periods of emotional stress but past experience in overcoming fecal retention usually makes recovery from a new episode much easier.

Other patients take much longer to improve. In many instances, emotional difficulties within the family are of such magnitude that it is impossible for the parents to adopt more facilitative attitudes or for the child to cope effectively with his problem. In such cases, the pediatrician's function is to support the parents in their avoidance of coercive intervention and to help them become aware that emotional difficulties exist and that their child's lack of improvement is symptomatic of these difficulties. Many parents can be helped toward the realization that psychologic evaluation may be useful.

References

Anthony, E. J.: An Experimental Approach to the Psychopathology of Childhood; Encopresis. *Brit. J. Med. Psychol.*, 30:146, 1957.

Bellman, M.: Studies on Encopresis. *Acta Pediat. Scand.*, Suppl. 170, 1966.

Mendeloff, A. I.: Defecation; in C. F. Code (ed.): *Handbook of Physiology*. Baltimore, Williams & Wilkins Co., 1967–1968, Section 6, Vol. IV.

Chronic Nonspecific Diarrhea Syndrome

Irritable Colon of Childhood

MURRAY DAVIDSON, M.D.

Despite continued separation of an ever-increasing number of distinct disease entities associated with diarrhea, there remains a considerable number of children who have nonspecific persistent or recurrent diarrhea. The condition occurs especially among children between one and three years of age. In this group, diarrhea is characterized by recurrent episodes of loose bowel movements, varying in number from 3 to 10 per day (usually five or less) and containing mucus but no blood, which worsen during periods of emotional or physical stress (e.g., respiratory infections or teething). The presence in the stool of grossly visible, undigested vegetable fibers, together with extracellular starch granules upon microscopic examination, sometimes leads to the mistaken impression that it is a form of malabsorption; hence the loosely (and incorrectly) applied pseudonyms of starch intolerance or mild celiac disease. The children gain weight and develop normally. It is our belief that this condition is not a disease state but instead is a juvenile form of functional hyperreactivity of the distal colon to stress. When present in adults, this condition is referred to as irritable colon, spastic colon or mucous colitis.

The initial therapeutic approach to this condition is its proper diagnosis. Before initiating treatment, the physician must be satisfied that he has ruled out the two principal differential diagnostic possibilities: a malabsorptive condition or a chronic low-grade infection. Malabsorption should be suspected whenever the onset of diarrhea can be traced to the neonatal period rather than to the usual time of onset of irritable colon at between six months and one year of age, whenever it continues beyond four years of age or whenever the youngster presents with small size and weight. Cystic fibrosis of the pancreas is the malabsorptive condition with which the syndrome of irritable colon of childhood may most frequently be confused. Whenever the disease is even remotely suspected, sweat electrolyte examination must be performed. We have also observed patients with congenital disaccharidase deficiencies whose condition was mistaken for this syndrome on rare occasions. If these diseases are suspected, they should be ruled out by examinations of fresh stools for pH and for reducing substances, and by appropriate disaccharide tolerance tests. When infection is suspected, appropriate bacteriologic studies are indicated.

Once one is convinced that neither malabsorption nor infection is the cause of the symptoms, the main factor in treatment is a reassuring discussion with the parents. It is useful to point out that proper management consists of attention to the entire child, not simply to the manner or frequency with which he manages to rid himself of excreta. The normal physical development of most of these children should be emphasized to help parents realize that the symptoms do not reflect a disease state and that malabsorption for nutriments is not occurring.

Although we have demonstrated excessive water loss in the stools, it is not of sufficient magnitude that dehydration or electrolyte imbalance ensues. The problem is not related to kinds of foods ingested and requires no special dietary management. Adherence to the restrictive, high protein, low fat and simple sugar regimens often recommended imposes unnecessary emotional burdens on child and mother and tends to be confusing if symptoms recur despite strict adherence to the prescribed regimen. A limited diet may even predispose to perpetuation of symptoms. On a number of occasions we have observed prompt and complete remission of an episode, for reasons not entirely clear, with no change other than introduction of a full diet.

Since patients virtually always come from families in which some other members, parents or siblings, are also affected by functional bowel complaints, acceptance of the explanation is frequently made easier. Once reassured that the prognosis is excellent and that the symptoms will wax and wane without regard to food intake, parents are often relieved and content with little else in the way of management. It is our belief that prescription of drugs might minimize the therapeutic advantages gained from frank discussion and reassurance that the condition is not a "disease," and we therefore rarely prescribe them.

Absorbent antidiarrheal agents, such as kaolin, with or without added pectins, and antispasmodics appear to be of little value. For the most part, except as indicated for any associated respiratory infection, antibiotics are also without benefit. Certain agents have been found empirically to be helpful, but their effectiveness is not predictable in all instances. Methylcellulose preparations, presumably through their hydrophilic properties, may occasionally impart cohesiveness to a watery stool. Most available preparations are not suitable for use in children because of their unappetizing granularity. Tablets, e.g., Cellothyl, may be crushed and given in small amounts of diluent twice daily. These drugs may also be administered as wafers, which can be taken twice daily instead of cookies, covered with jam or jelly. Toxicity is so low that it is not an important consideration.

In some cases, administration of sulfisoxazole (Gantrisin), 0.1 to 0.2 Gm. per kilogram per day, has been reported to be of value.* Approximately 30 to 50 per cent of all patients respond dramatically to 150 to 950 mg. of diiodohydroxyquin (Diodoquin) daily, divided into two or three doses. Other antimicrobials generally do not have the same effect. Both of these agents have been widely prescribed as relatively safe for long periods of administration. This is not entirely true. Reactions to sulfa, either skin rashes or more serious agranulocytosis, have been reported with sulfisoxazole. Diiodohydroxyquin is believed to be largely insoluble and nonabsorbable. However, the infrequent instances of dermatitis and anal diiodohydroxyquin are probably due to a form of iodism that results from absorption either of the unchanged drug or of iodine that has been dissociated from the organic nucleus in the intestinal lumen. Diiodohydroxyquin has also been observed rarely to lead to serious eye involvement; retinal changes and lenticular opacities have been reported.

Avoidance of chilled fluids is suggested, because laboratory studies indicate that in these children, and in others with diarrheal tendencies, sudden introduction of cold material into the stomach may stimulate colonic propulsion and the urge to defecate.

References

Cohlan, S. Q.: Chronic Non-Specific Diarrhea in Infants and Children Treated with Diiodohydroxyquinoline. *Pediatrics,* 18:424, 1956.

Davidson, M., and Bauer, C. H.: The Value of Microscopic Examination of the Stool for Extracellular Starch in the Diagnosis of Starch Intolerance. *Pediatrics,* 21:65, 1958.

Davidson, M., and Wasserman, R.: The Irritable Colon of Childhood (Chronic Nonspecific Diarrhea). *J. Pediat.,* 69:1027, 1966.

---

* Manufacturer's precaution: Systemic sulfonamides are contraindicated in infants under two months of age.

Intractable Diarrhea

MURRAY DAVIDSON, M.D.

Precise delineation of the point at which acute infantile diarrhea should be viewed as intractable varies with the author. In this section, the definition, modified from Avery, includes diarrhea in infants under six months of age, longer than two weeks in duration and severe enough to lead to dehydration. These infants require hospital treatment with parenteral fluid administration, and it is understood that they have negative cultures for specific infections, such as salmonella, shigella and pathogenic *E. coli,* and for ova or parasites.

The management of intractable diarrhea touches on four major problems: (1) maintenance of an anabolic nutritional state, (2) correction and avoidance of fluid and electrolyte deficits, (3) effecting cessation of the diarrheal process itself and (4) definition of the possible underlying diagnosis. The relative importance and degree of emphasis applied to each of these four points vary with the particular expert who discusses the topic. In this discussion, each topic will be dealt with separately, to indicate some of the rationales for this author's point of view and, where appropriate, to point out alternate attitudes.

Nutritional State. It is generally agreed that children with diarrhea require adequate nutrition to recover from their disease. What is not agreed upon by many authors is whether the caloric and protein needs of the infant should be met by oral feeding or by another route. Among authors who choose oral feedings, there is disagreement about the length of time the patient should initially be starved after admission to the hospital. As early as 1924, Park expressed the view that one should disregard the stools and think more of assimilation of food by the child. Studies by Chung and coworkers in 1948 showed that although oral feeding was associated with increased stool losses in patients with infantile diarrhea, the quantities of nitrogen, fat and electrolytes which were absorbed also increased. They also suggested that the overall duration of the diarrhea was not adversely influenced by oral feedings.

The literature provides abundant evidence that protein is adequately absorbed even among infants with prolonged periods of diarrhea. Similarly, unless there is a disturbance in disaccharidase activity, carbohydrates are well tolerated. On the other hand, if patients with intractable or persistent diarrhea are not fed adequate calories and protein and begin to suffer signs of malnutrition, there is a prompt diminution in serum amino acid levels and blood sugar, with a concomitant decrease in the tissue turnover rate of rapidly metabolizing organs, including the liver, the pancreas and the intestinal mucosa. Decrease in synthetic rates of these organs, with resultant diminished elaboration of digestive secretions, impedes further protein, carbohydrate and fat digestion and assimilation in severely malnourished children.

From a practical point of view, prevention of this self-perpetuating catabolic state should begin in the early stages, and we therefore adopt a uniform attitude concerning oral feedings for all infants in the early acute phase of diarrhea and dehydration. Starvation for an initial period of 12 to 24 hours may diminish continuing losses and lead to quicker homeostatic readjustment during rehydration therapy. Initial restriction of oral feedings is additionally useful for the child who enters the hospital with acute gastroenteritis and who may also be vomiting. However, following this initial starvation period, oral clear fluids are introduced for one to two feedings. If the feedings are tolerated, the patient is ready for milk. Some authors advocate avoidance of cow's milk for a few days after treatment for acute diarrhea because of the reported tendency to absorption of whole proteins with development of antibodies in this state, or because of the difficulties that might result from secondary lactase insufficiency. However, for the vast majority of infants it makes little difference what feeding one chooses. We prefer boiled skim milk diluted with equal quantities of water for the first 24 hours of oral therapy. Boiling denatures the protein. Dilution lowers the lactose load to levels easily tolerated by virtually all infants whose diarrhea has persisted for less than 48 hours. Following this period, boiled skim milk is given at full strength for the next 24 hours, after which the infant is ready for reintroduction of his normal formula, or of whole milk and bland nonfatty solid foods if these have previously been taken. We follow this refeeding regimen whether diarrhea recurs or not. Of course, for the purposes of this section it is assumed that diarrhea should have recurred and should have been present for at least two weeks in an infant whose subsequent course entitled him to be included among those with *intractable diarrhea.*

Certain rules must be followed with this refeeding regimen. Continual parenteral fluid therapy in accordance with the discussion that follows is mandatory. Feedings are given at 3- to 4-hour intervals in relatively normal volumes for the age of the infant. Small hourly feedings should be avoided, since these induce the gastrocolic reflex and simply lead to increased numbers of stools.

Even if lactase insufficiency had not been a problem at the outset of therapy, it might develop at a later point. In this event, feedings should be changed from cow's milk to either a predigested formula, meat base preparation or soy bean formula. None of these mixtures contain lactose and they should therefore be tolerated. Some authors suggest, on the basis of limited evidence, that acute infantile diarrhea may lead not only to disaccharidase (i.e., digestive) insufficiency, but also to a transport defect for monosaccharides. In this case, a carbohydrate-free formula would appear to be indicated, but there is real danger in the feeding of caloric mixtures free of carbohydrates to infants with diarrhea. Physiologically, water and electrolytes are passively absorbed (solvent drag) only as a result of carbohydrate absorption in the upper small intestine. Outpouring of large volumes of fluid into the upper intestine, associated with diarrheal conditions in which toxic material increases the normal secretory process of the upper intestine, has clearly been demonstrated to be corrected by oral administration of a solution of an actively transported sugar (glucose). Such improvement in direction of net fluid losses in the upper intestine decreases fecal losses. Thus, the presence of isotonic amounts of sugar in an oral feeding mixture is not only useful for its caloric value and protein-sparing action but also serves to help compensate for losses of fluid and electrolytes and to reverse the process which perpetuates diarrhea. Omission of this material from the mixtures used in feeding is contraindicated.

If adequate amounts of calories and protein are provided by mouth in infants with intractable diarrhea, it is not necessary that these infants be coincidentally or alternately treated with parenteral alimentation. Despite increasing popularity for this treatment, we have rarely found it necessary in infants with diarrhea in whom adequate oral feedings were instituted early in the course of management. Small babies with intractable diarrhea are among the most difficult patients to manage with intravenous feedings. Such complications as infection, hyper- and hypoglycemia, ketoacidosis and mechanical difficulties, with need for regular and frequent replacement of the lifeline occur most often in this age group, especially among those with infectious or diarrheal conditions.

Fluid and Electrolyte Homeostasis. The most important corollary to the oral maintenance of the nutritional and caloric needs in infants with intractable diarrhea is to appreciate that such feedings produce variable effects on fluid and electrolyte homeostasis. Oral feedings may in some patients increase losses by aggravating the diarrhea or, conversely, they may be retained by other patients and thus compensate for losses. It is therefore extremely important to adopt a consistent policy that total reliance for maintenance of fluid and electrolyte balance should be by the parenteral route and that fluid and electrolyte homeostasis be totally separated from nutritional considerations.

Three types of fluid are commonly employed in hydration therapy: (1) Colloid preparations are primarily used for blood volume expansion and include whole blood, plasma, dextran, 5 per cent albumin or a hypertonic combination of electrolytes and glucose. In addition, plasma and blood may be used to supply proteins and immune substances. (2) Solutions designed for repair of fluid and electrolyte deficits usually contain about 60 mEq. of sodium and 15 mEq. of potassium with the balancing 75 mEq. of anions distributed in an approximately 3 to 1 ratio of chloride to bicarbonate or lactate. (3) Solutions primarily intended to meet the maintenance needs of an infant should contain no more than a total of 45 to 50 mEq. of cations, fairly evenly distributed between sodium and potassium, and an equal amount of anions distributed in a 3 to 1 ratio of chloride to lactate. A number of available commercial "maintenance" solutions fit this description and may in addition contain small amounts of calcium, magnesium and other cations and anions.

Successful continuing oral feeding of an infant with *intractable* diarrhea rests on institution of a consistently adequate regimen of parenteral fluids in the earliest *acute* phases of disease. This includes combined ongoing maintenance and replacement therapy. Once repletion of initial fluid and electrolyte losses has been made, the infant is begun on appropriate amounts of maintenance fluid for each 24-hour period. The amounts used are 150 ml. per kilogram for infants in the age range we are discussing, i.e., birth to six months of age. It is our practice to divide these into three equal 8-hour aliquots. In addition, a crude estimate of 20 to 25 ml. water loss for each stool passed is made for continuing diarrhea in infants in this age group. The infant is checked every half hour for bowel movements and these are charted by the nurse. At the end of each 8-hour work period, appropriate amounts, i.e., 20 to 25 ml. per loose stool, of *replacement* fluid is added to the next 8-hour aliquot of the daily *maintenance* fluid. In this way, fluid and electrolyte homeostasis is maintained and any deleterious effects of oral feedings on fluid and electrolyte losses are not allowed to get out of hand.

It is obviously important that patients be examined regularly for signs of distention and possible pooling of material in their gastrointestinal tracts. Children are weighed daily and laboratory data from serum samples are used as additional guides for refinement of this clinical "on the spot" type of ongoing hydration therapy.

Parenteral maintenance and replacement therapy is utilized simultaneously with oral feedings until replacement requirements fall below 100 ml. per day, i.e., less than four stools daily, in the face of adequate oral intake. At this point it is safe to discontinue intravenous therapy on a trial basis, which usually remains permanent.

Clearing of Diarrhea. In most instances this persistent, combined oral-parenteral pattern of therapy may be rewarded by gradual cessation of a diarrheal process whose previous intractability goes unexplained. The infants are usually in good nutritional state at this point, since they have not been exposed to excessive periods of starvation or to periods of rapid shifts in electrolyte and fluid homeostasis.

However, rather than simply hope for spontaneous remission, the physician must be alert to possible perpetuation of diarrhea by secondary changes which have become superimposed on the original causes. In the face of the persistent diarrhea, fresh stool specimens must be examined at least once daily for pH and reducing substances. For these tests, one must be certain to utilize a liquid part of the stool, or to suspend more formed stool in distilled water to solubilize hydrogen ions. As discussed under the section on feeding, lactase insufficiency may develop later, even if not a problem at the outset.

Regular and repeated examinations of stool specimens for overgrowth of particular organisms, such as enteropathogenic *E. coli* or staphylococci must also be performed. Although examination for enteropathogenic *E. coli* should be performed if typing for these organisms is available, a five- to seven-day oral trial of neomycin is indicated in any patient in whom acute diarrhea has persisted, especially if shifts in normal colonic flora are considered because antibiotics had been given at the outset of treatment. We have also observed a number of such patients who, not having responded to neomycin, improved with lactobacillus therapy. It is our routine to follow an unsuccessful period of neomycin therapy with approximately one week of thrice-daily feedings of lactobacilli, either as dry cultures or in yogurt and buttermilk, in this group. It is not necessary to be concerned about lactase insufficiency when using yogurt or buttermilk, since the lactase in these preparations has been fermented to small-chain acids in the process of preparation of these cultured milk products. One must be certain, however, to cease administration of antibiotics during this period for maximal effectiveness.

Investigation and Additional Treatment. Although many authors stress that the persistence of infantile diarrhea must be investigated rapidly, it is our own feeling that many infants are overexposed to diagnostic procedures which tend to weaken them and make their resistance to the diarrheal process less effective. If one reviews the literature on the subject, there is clearly little need to carry out exhaustive (and thereby exhausting) studies in these children, since among the many autopsies reported, findings were nonspecific. We prefer to proceed slowly with diagnostic procedures and to permit infants adequate opportunity for maintenance of normal nutrition and fluid balance with slow recovery from the process.

A simple and systematic approach is taken to uncover the underlying diagnoses, which must be considered for corrective therapy. When there is repeated abdominal distention, blood in the stool, explosive stools or vomiting, an obstructive or secondarily acquired inflammatory lesion of the lower colon should be suspected. Specific diagnoses in these categories include Hirschsprung's disease, stenotic lesions of the lower colon and enterocolitis. Plain films of the abdomen will usually suggest these diagnoses. If confirmed by barium enema, early performance of a colostomy proximal to the site of the disease is imperative if the intractable diarrhea is to improve.

Regular urine examinations for infection are necessary. Congenital obstructive lesions of the urinary tract with progressive renal insufficiency may be associated with intractable diarrhea in the young infant. If suspected, intravenous pyelography usually points to the diagnosis.

In children with central nervous system lesions, such as subdural hematoma, intractable diarrhea may be present, usually associated with persistent vomiting and failure to thrive. Other conditions which must be considered are endocrine lesions such as adrenogenital syndrome, hyperthyroidism or catecholamine-secreting tumors. Patients with immunoglobulin insufficiency and colonic floral changes, or those with cystic fibrosis, might present initially with intractable diarrhea in infancy.

The important diagnostic point to be stressed is that more often than not, the diarrheal process proves to be nonspecific in origin. The rapid and complete work-up stressed by many authors may prove harmful to a sick infant and may thus impede recovery. Judicious and well-spaced simple diagnostic tests, e.g., cultures, specimens of blood not requiring too great a volume, urine collections and/or an iontophoretic sweat collection, may be carried out without undue stress to the infant and with considerable reliability to rule a specific diagnosis in or out.

References

Avery, G. B., Villavicencio, O., Lilly, J. R., and Randolph, J. G.: Intractable Diarrhea in Early Infancy. *Pediatrics,* 41:712–721, 1968.

Carpenter, C. C. J.: Cholera Enterotoxin—Recent Investigation Yields Insights into Transport Processes. *Am. J. Med.,* 50:1–7, 1971.

Chung, A. W., and Holt, L. E., Jr.: Place of Oral Feeding in Diarrhea. *Pediatrics,* 5:421, 1950.

Hyman, C. J., Reiter, J., Rodnan, J., and Drash, A. L.: Parenteral and Oral Alimentation in the Treatment of the Nonspecific Protracted Diarrheal Syndrome of Infancy. *Pediatrics,* 78:17–29, 1971.

Pierce, N. F., Sack, R. B., Mitra, R. C., Bamwell, J. G., Brigham, K. L., Fedson, D. S., and Mondal, A.: Replacement of Water and Electrolyte Losses in Cholera by an Oral Glucose-Electrolyte Solution. *Ann. Int. Med.,* 70:1173–1181, 1969.

Preoperative and Postoperative Care of Patients Undergoing Gastrointestinal Surgery

STEPHEN L. GANS, M.D.

Preoperative Care. General preparation for gastrointestinal surgery in all instances includes correction of any depletions, such as fluids and electrolytes, whole blood or blood components, vitamins and nutritives where possible. Needless to say, this is proper for all surgical and most nonsurgical conditions, and these subjects are dealt with in greater detail elsewhere in this book.

Preparation of the bowel itself depends on the site of the lesion (proximal or distal) and the presence or absence of an acute inflammatory process or obstruction. In the patient undergoing gastric or upper intestinal surgery and who is without inflammation or obstruction, simply withholding feedings for 12 hours (in the neonate, 4 hours) is adequate; a nasogastric tube is placed in the stomach before induction of anesthesia.

When acute inflammation is present, peristalsis is diminished or has ceased and fluid and air collect in the bowel, much the same as in the presence of a true mechanical obstruction. Under these circumstances the bowel should be decompressed by passing a nasogastric tube into the stomach as soon as the condition is known. This is best accomplished by using as large a tube, well lubricated and with *several* holes cut near its end, as will pass through the nares a measured distance into the stomach. The tube should be connected to intermittent suction and should be irrigated every 2 hours with a measured amount of normal saline (10 ml. in the neonate, more in the older child) to ensure its patency, and its position adjusted if the irrigating fluid is not returned. A tube that is not working is more harmful than no tube at all. It should *not* be plugged while the patient is being transported for x-rays or to the operating room. Small infant feeding tubes are not adequate for gastric decompression.

Before *elective* lower intestinal surgery the patient should be placed on a liquid or low residue diet for three to four days and bowel sterilization should be considered. The best results have been obtained with a combination of mechanical cleansing with warm normal saline enemas twice each day and a 72-hour program of chemical treatment. Although several medications and regimens have been found to be adequate, the most efficient in our hands has been oral kanamycin and nystatin in cherry or orange syrup according to the following dosage schedule:

Under 1 year	kanamycin	250 mg.
	nystatin	50,000 units
1–2 years	kanamycin	350 mg.
	nystatin	75,000 units
2–3 years	kanamycin	400 mg.
	nystatin	100,000 units
4–5 years	kanamycin	500 mg.
	nystatin	200,000 units
6–8 years	kanamycin	1000 mg.
	nystatin	500,000 units

One dose is given every 2 hours for four doses, then every 6 hours for the remainder of the 72-hour period before surgery. When a colostomy is present, a 1 per cent solution of kanamycin should be instilled into the distal loop, and per rectum after each enema; in Hirschsprung's disease without colostomy, each enema should be followed with such an instillation during the preparatory period. Supplemental vitamin K should be used if this regimen is prolonged for any reason.

A rare complication of this method is the development of a staphylococcal enterocolitis, and a more hypothetical complication is an increased incidence of tumor growth at the anastomotic site where bowel malignancies are resected. However, when properly chosen according to sound surgical principles, the method can be used to good advantage.

In *emergency* situations involving lower intestinal surgery, such preparation is not feasible. Moreover, in the newborn the gastrointestinal tract is relatively sterile and there is no need for preoperative bowel sterilization. In the older neonate or infant this problem must be met by choice and method of surgical procedure and by postoperative care.

When an indwelling bladder catheter is a necessary adjunct to the surgical procedure, this is best introduced in the operating room where sterile conditions are more secure.

Postoperative Care. Only aspects of postoperative care pertaining to the gastrointestinal tract will be discussed here; other features of general supportive treatment are covered elsewhere.

We strongly recommend that all tubes, drains and postoperative enemas be managed under the direction of a member of the operating team who knows the details of the operation and who is in a position to assess the condition of the bowel and security of any suture line.

The first basic need is effective decompression of the stomach and intestines until normal peristalsis is present and an anastomosis is patent. The use of a nasogastric tube in the manner described under Preoperative Preparation is satisfactory in most instances of short duration. Suction or gravity drainage should continue until good peristalsis is audible and flatus is passed or, when there is an anastomosis, at least three days. When long-term decompression is anticipated and critical, gastrostomy should be considered at the time of surgery. This procedure and its management are discussed elsewhere.

Feedings may be started when decompression is discontinued. Progress is made from clear liquids to low residue diet to full diet for age as quickly as is tolerated by the patient.

In the absence of mechanical or neostomal obstruction, failure of the gastrointestinal tract to move gas along in normal fashion after 72 postoperative hours suggests *adynamic ileus*. Treatment consists in prolongation of decompression by the previously described methods, attention to possible deficiences in fluids, electrolytes and vitamins, the free use of oxygen (within safe limits) and patience.

Finally, in catastrophic problems involving the bowel, when it will not function properly over a considerable period of time, much benefit can be derived by the use of total intravenous nutrition while permitting the intestines to recover.

Differences of opinion exist as to either the value or possible complications from the *routine* use of antibiotics following gastrointestinal surgery. Believing that the greatest harm comes from going to either extreme, we suggest the following. Cultures should be made at surgery from free peritoneal fluid and from any open intestinal lumen. Antibiotics should not be used routinely for most gastric and upper intestinal surgery, but should be more commonly considered for lower bowel surgery. When suppuration is present in the peritoneum, when excessive contamination complicates the procedure, when questionably viable bowel remains in the peritoneal cavity or when a suture line is considered to be insecure, antibiotics should be used. In the neonate, we prefer the penicillin and kanamycin combination, in the higher dosage range. In older patients, ampicillin is a good initial choice. Adjustments should be made according to the results of cultures.

Ileostomy. Ileostomy is most commonly used in the treatment of ulcerative colitis, but it also occasionally used in the neonate with meconium ileus, atresia of the ileum or Hirschsprung's disease involving the entire colon.

When used for meconium ileus, a loop ileostomy is made and a spur-crushing clamp is applied at the time of surgery. The proximal loop empties the intestinal tract. The distal loop is irrigated every 12 hours with a solution of Viokase powder, ½ teaspoonful in 30 ml. of saline, until the lower bowel is cleared of inspissated meconium. Sometimes it is necessary to irrigate the proximal loop and also the rectum in order to accomplish this purpose. A small plastic collecting bag is glued to the skin around the ileostomy at the time of surgery. This not only assists in measuring the output, which at times is quite copious, but also protects the surrounding skin from the irritating effects of ileostomy discharge. In a few days the spur between the proximal and distal loops becomes necrotic and the spur crushing clamp comes out. Now the contents of the proximal loop can pass into the distal loop. This can be assisted by blocking the opening in the skin with a close-fitting plastic cap, which directs the intestinal juices along. Often the ileostomy will then shrink considerably and even close spontaneously in time. If it does not, it should be closed surgically. If the losses from the ileostomy are great despite the open communication of loops and the plastic cap, surgical closure should be carried out without further delay.

Ideally, ileal atresia is treated by a primary anastomosis. However, in some cases the dilated proximal bowel end and the worm-like distal end are brought out as a double-barreled ileostomy. The spur-crushing clamp and the plastic bag are applied at the time of surgery. The distal loop and the rectum can be irrigated with normal saline until open throughout. When the spur is crushed out, a communication exists as previously described and the same anatomic, mechanical and clinical principles prevail as in the foregoing paragraph.

Ileostomy, either temporary or permanent, has a very important place in the treatment of ulcerative colitis. The parents must understand its implications, and when possible a simple explanation should be given to the child.

The ileum is brought out about 1 inch beyond the skin, and an eversion stoma is made by suturing its edges to the subcuticular fascia. This spout is enclosed immediately by an adhesive plastic bag with a hole cut in it to fit the stoma, and the bag is glued to the skin. The child is encouraged to lie on his right side, so that intestinal contents will fall away from the abdominal wall and into the bag.

In the postoperative period copious spillage from the ileostomy may pose a problem in fluid management. Replacement therapy is aided by measurement and analysis of the discharge as well as frequent checks of the blood chemistries. In a few days, the ileostomy discharge becomes thicker in consistency and the amount of fluid loss diminishes rapidly. Paregoric or Kaopectate, given every 3 or 4 hours in doses appropriate for age, will assist in reducing loss from intestinal output.

Postoperative bags are reapplied every other day following surgery. They may be cemented to the skin directly or attached to the skin with double-sided Marlen adhesive discs. In 10 days to 2 weeks after operation, the ileostomy should be settled sufficiently to permit careful measurement for a permanent bag. Some of the appliances are made of rubber, some of plastic and some of neoprene or allied compounds. Instructions for use are supplied by the manufacturers. The important thing to remember is that no one type is suitable for all patients. Finding a suitable pouch may be a matter of trial and error.

When removing the pouch, cement solvent should be used to prevent the irritative trauma to the skin which occurs if the bag is pulled off. Gum karaya powder is then dusted on the skin and the excess blown away after two minutes, or a gum karaya washer is applied. The pouch is then glued to the skin with a thin layer of cement. If properly selected and applied, it will adhere to the abdomen for a period of at least 24 hours without any damage to the skin or stoma and will be accident-proof during that time. Needless to say, the appliance should be most carefully cleansed before reapplication.

Skin irritation is an ever-present threat and occurs in varying degrees of severity. There are many ways to cope with this problem, but all of them depend on the degree of meticulousness with which the patient is treated. The two causes most frequently observed are contact with feces and improper handling of the cement or solvent. Poor appliance fitting may be responsible for the former. Should any portion of the skin present a red, wet surface, dust gum karaya powder on it and blow away the residue. The cement can be applied right over the powdered area. Karaya gum washers will prevent many of the skin problems that arise. Finding the best cement is a trial-and-error procedure. It is advisable to make a patch test 24 hours before a new cement or solvent is used.

Persistent raw areas or shallow ulcers present a more difficult problem, because an appliance will not adhere properly to this kind of skin. Meticulous cleansing and drying and the use of aluminum hydroxide gel in combination with karaya may be helpful. A neglected ileostomy may be a torturous thing. Sometimes it is necessary to place the patient in the prone position on a Bradford frame so that all discharges from the intestine flow directly into a pan underneath until healing is accomplished.

Persistent odors can be satisfactorily eliminated by using Derifil, a highly purified and potent chlorophyll derivative, one to six tablets a day placed in the bag, or Nilodor drops as directed. If the odor problem is coupled with excessive gas, activated charcoal taken by mouth or placed in the bag is helpful.

Although most children with ileostomies can eat a normal diet, some may experience difficulties with certain foods. In general, low residue diets are tolerated the best: lean meats, liver, hard boiled eggs, cottage cheese, rice, gelatin, simple sugars, cooked cereals, orange juice, clear soups and some cooked vegetables. It is advisable to avoid or use great care with the following: cabbage, turnips, corn on the cob or whole kernel corn, onions, nuts, raisins, coconut, berries with seeds, highly spiced or seasoned foods and large amounts of candy or sweets, especially chocolate.

Complications are better avoided than treated. Fistulas are usually the result of faulty application or fitting of the bag. Most strictures occur at skin level and respond to gentle daily dilatation with the finger. Minor degrees of prolapse or herniation may be controlled by the wearing of an elastic girdle over the appliance. More severe strictures, prolapse or herniation may require surgical revision. Obstruction may be due to edema or may result from eating large amounts of high residue foods. Irrigation with warm normal saline using a soft rubber bulb syringe or Foley catheter will bring relief.

Accustoming a child to the presence of an ileostomy and its care is a task of patience and forbearance. However, in most instances children respond in a manner that most adults would do well to emulate. Local ileostomy clubs are a source of great technical aid and psychologic encouragement.

Colostomy. Colostomy is used as a temporary bowel-decompressing or stool-diverting arrangement in infants or children with aganglionic megacolon, ectopic or imperforate anus or other anorectal anomalies, atresia or stenosis of the colon or severe injuries to the anus or lower bowel. There are many different types of colostomy, and the site and type will depend on the location and nature of the lesion being treated as well as on the definitive or reconstructive procedures planned for the future.

Postoperative Care. Many surgeons recommend a waiting period of 24 or more hours before opening the colostomy, but we have had no complications, particularly in the newborn with relatively sterile stool, as a result of making this opening immediately at the time of surgery. A plastic bag with a hole cut in its double-faced adhesive backing is worked over the colostomy and glued to the abdominal wall. This is kept in place until it starts filling with stool. Gas can be permitted to escape by pricking the bag with a pin. This transparent bag permits one to measure fluid or blood loss and to observe viability of the colostomy and onset of function without having to change dressings. It also seals fecal drainage from a nearby incision and helps prevent skin irritation.

The plastic bag may be discarded and replaced every day or when full. When the incision is healed and the stools are becoming formed, the plastic bag can be replaced by a strip of petrolatum gauze over the bowel ends and covered with an ordinary diaper. Some parents prefer to use adherent plastic bags more or less permanently, as with an ileostomy. Others simply handle the colostomy as an abdominal "anus," by using the usual cleansing and diapering techniques.

Care of Bowel and Stoma. Satisfactory results are brought about by widely differing methods. In many infants, no special handling is necessary, particularly if the colostomy is to be present for a short time only. In others, the skin quickly becomes irritated or breaks down unless meticulous care is given. This can be controlled through diet, irrigations or local skin therapy, singly or in combination. Constipating or low residue diets, depending on age, assisted by paregoric or Kaopectate where necessary, will prevent constant soiling with its resulting irritation. Irrigation of the bowel thoroughly once daily or every other day, combined with the above-mentioned diet, may result in no intervening spontaneous stools, thus allowing the skin to heal. The best local therapy is cleanliness. Acid soaps and a very dilute vinegar solution are better than alkaline soaps and tap water. Zinc oxide ointment should be applied for minor irritation; antimonilial (Vioform), antibacterial (neomycin) or anti-inflammatory (hydrocortisone) preparations should be used when indicated.

Occasionally the skin becomes inflamed because of bag adhesives or adhesive solvents, or by traumatic adhesive bag removal. Under such circumstances this method should be discarded, or at least the cement or solvent changed after adequate skin tests elsewhere on the body.

Tincture of benzoin painted over the area regularly will toughen the skin. A drying lotion (calamine) will help relieve itching. Bleeding from the stoma or mucocutaneous junction is common and can be easily controlled by applying a layer of petrolatum over the bleeding surface. More serious bleeding may require cauterization or electrocoagulation.

Stricture usually occurs at the skin level.

This is not ordinarily a problem in the infant with soft stools and a temporary colostomy. In others, gentle daily dilatations will open the aperture to a satisfactory size. If it does not, surgical removal of a circle of skin and resuture of the mucosal margins are easily accomplished maneuvers.

Pylorospasm

HARRY MEDOVY, M.D.

Pylorospasm is to a large extent a diagnosis of exclusion. The description by Ellis appears to be the most acceptable: "Pylorospasm is a term applied to a group of hypertonic infants showing infrequent explosive vomiting without visible gastric peristalsis and in whom no pyloric tumour is palpable." One might add that a gastric x-ray series fails to show evidence of significant pyloric obstruction. Spence classes pylorospasm with "neuromuscular disorders of organ function" and compares it with congenital laryngeal stridor, colonic dysfunction of the spastic constipation type and adynamic ileus of the newborn. Symptoms are often present from birth and rarely persist beyond the sixth month.

Since infants suspected of this disorder rarely come to surgery, and gradual recovery is the rule, the pathophysiology can only be surmised. Whether these cases are in fact atypical or mild examples of pyloric stenosis, or whether they represent a disorder of neuromuscular function is not known.

General Treatment. Once other causes of vomiting in this age group are excluded by history, examination and, if necessary, radiologic study, the parents should be reassured about the self-limited nature of the problem. All the details of the infant's feeding should be reviewed, including quality and quantity of feedings, frequency, prefeeding and postfeeding positioning and maternal attitudes.

The following points should be stressed in maternal counseling: (1) a quiet environment; (2) in bottle fed babies a nipple with an opening large enough to ensure that the feeding can be completed without undue effort and in a reasonably short time; (3) the baby held as for breast feeding with interruptions of the feeding at least once for burping, and then positioning in the crib on the right side with the head of the crib elevated.

Frequent weighing should be discouraged on the basis that weight gain is likely to be irregular in any event; a poor weight gain one week may be followed by a substantial gain the following week. Frequent checking of the weight by the mother may only add to her anxiety. The baby should be re-fed if a considerable portion of a feeding is vomited within half an hour of receiving it.

Drug Treatment. Sedation of the infant and the use of anticholinergic drugs are often indicated. Used in proper dosage with careful attention to signs of toxicity (drowsiness, flushing, rapid pulse, high fever), they minimize vomiting and ensure reasonable rest for infant and mother. If signs of toxicity appear, one or two doses should be omitted, and then treatment restarted.

Phenobarbital, 8 mg., is given before the first, last, and mid-day feedings in the form of the elixir phenobarbital. The dose or the timing may be altered to ensure a restful but not oversedated infant.

The addition of anticholinergic drugs, which inactivate acetylcholine, thus blocking transmission of impulses from the parasympathetic nerve to the end-organ, is thought to give more satisfactory results. The trend has been to use products made of a combination of phenobarbital with methscopolamine (Donnatal Elixir), 1 to 1.5 ml., or methscopolamine and butabarbital (Restropin Pediatric Drops), 1½ drops per pound of body weight before each feeding (20 drops from a calibrated dropper equals 1 ml.). The recommended dose is given before each feeding and may need to be increased or decreased in any particular infant under one year of age, depending on the amount of sedation produced by the phenobarbital, which is included in this product.

Prognosis. The prognosis for recovery is excellent, and recurrence is unusual once the symptoms are controlled. Treatment may need to be maintained for two to four weeks, occasional cases giving trouble as late as six months of age.

Pyloric Stenosis

HARRY MEDOVY, M.D., *and*
COLIN C. FERGUSON, M.D.

The treatment of choice is surgery, and the accepted procedure is the Fredet-Ramstedt operation. Under optimal conditions (early diagnosis, adequate preoperative and postoperative care, experienced surgeon and anesthetist, good nursing) morbidity is minimal and the mortality rate less than 1 per cent.

It should be borne in mind that when such satisfactory conditions are not available, the morbidity and mortality rates may be considerable. If cases of pyloric stenosis are encountered only occasionally, and experienced surgeons and anesthetists are not available, the infant should be transported without delay to the nearest pediatric center.

Preoperative Therapy. Persistent vomiting in infancy results in loss of hydrogen and chloride ions, exchange of hydrogen ion for potassium at the cellular level, and loss of potassium in the urine. All but the milder cases of hypokalemic alkalosis are accompanied by dehydration. The infant with pyloric stenosis therefore requires replacement of water, sodium, chloride and potassium. In all but the mildest cases with no dehydration, hemoglobin and hematocrit levels, routine urinalysis, serum sodium, potassium and chloride concentrations, carbon dioxide content and blood urea nitrogen should be determined.

Cases of pyloric stenosis may be placed in one of three groups, based on clinical evaluation and assisted, when indicated, by laboratory studies. In group 1 (mild) disease, there is no significant dehydration and electrolytes are normal. This group includes most cases of pyloric stenosis. These patients should be operated on within 24 hours of admission. These infants usually tolerate glucose and saline feedings by mouth and are fed until 8 hours before operation. If the infant vomits, oral feeding is stopped and replaced by intravenous administration of maintenance fluids (1500 ml. per square meter or 100 ml. per kilogram per 24 hours), using a solution containing one part normal saline (25 to 50 mEq. of sodium, 40 to 60 mEq. of chloride), three parts 5 per cent glucose and water, and potassium (20 mEq.) per liter.

In group 2 (moderately severe) disease, there is mild dehydration (less than 10 per cent of body weight) with normal electrolytes or mild metabolic alkalosis (carbon dioxide content less than 35 mEq. per liter). These infants are given nothing by mouth. Maintenance plus deficit fluids are given intravenously for 24 hours before operation. A suitable solution contains one part normal saline (50 to 60 mEq. of sodium, 50 to 70 mEq. of chloride), two parts 5 per cent glucose and water, and potassium chloride (20 to 30 mEq.) per liter.

In group 3 (severe) disease, severe dehydration (greater than 10 per cent of body weight) and metabolic alkalosis (carbon dioxide content greater than 35 mEq. per liter) are present. These infants are given nothing by mouth. Maintenance plus deficit fluids are given intravenously for 24 to 48 hours before operation. A suitable replacement solution contains one part normal saline (75 mEq. of sodium, 90 to 100 mEq. of chloride) one part 5 per cent glucose in water, and potassium chloride (30 to 40 mEq.) per liter. As a general rule it is not necessary to achieve normality in electrolyte levels before operation, but at least 50 per cent of the estimated fluid deficit should be replaced. When alkalosis appears to be resistant to correction within 24 hours using the foregoing regimen, additional potassium should be added to the solution, bringing the maximal potassium content up to 40 mEq. per liter. When shock and circulatory collapse are prominent features, whole blood or plasma (20 ml. per kilogram) is indicated at the start of treatment.

In all cases, once a diagnosis is made, a Levin tube is inserted and the stomach emptied of its contents. The tube is left in place and nothing is given by mouth before operation.

Surgery in pyloric stenosis is not an emergency, but it should be carried out as soon as the patient is hydrated, in electrolyte balance and ready to tolerate the procedure. To avoid possible aspiration of retained gastric contents, the stomach must be emptied before induction of anesthesia. During induction and the operation, it is important to maintain the infant's body temperature. This is satisfactorily accomplished by wrapping the extremities and by placing a warm-water mattress under the baby.

Postoperatively, a Levin tube is left in place and aspirated manually each hour with a 10-ml. syringe or connected to continuous suction. At 3 to 5 hours, the Levin tube is removed and glucose feedings are started. A longer period of suction (8 to 24 hours) may be required in conditions resulting in excessive postoperative pyloric edema. These include incision of duodenal mucosa during pylorotomy, excessive duodenal and bowel trauma during operation, pylorotomy on the infant aged seven weeks or older, and resolving gastritis in the severe group.

The initial feeding is 1 ounce of glucose, and this is increased by 5 ml. at each 3-hour feeding. If three or four glucose feedings are well-tolerated, the infant is given half-strength formula every 3 hours. About 24 hours postoperatively, or when the 2- or 2½-ounce feeding is reached, the infant is started on his usual formula.

If a feeding is vomited, the infant is fed 3 hours later with a similar amount of glucose. If two successive feedings are vomited, a Levin tube is passed, and the stomach lavaged with 30 ml. of normal saline solution. If vomiting continues despite this measure, the infant is given a further 4 hours of nothing by mouth and intermittent gastric suction; then feedings are reinstituted. Maintenance intravenous fluids are given for 12 to 18 hours postoperatively.

Once the infant is retaining his usual formula, he should be discharged as soon as possible. This is usually the second postoperative day for infants with ready access to the hospital, and the fourth or fifth postoperative day for infants referred from more distant areas.

The breast fed baby with pyloric stenosis should be put back on breast feeding as soon as the first two or three glucose feedings have been given postoperatively. If preferred, the mother's breast milk may be expressed and the first few postoperative feedings given by bottle.

Peptic Ulcer

THEODORE C. JEWETT, Jr., M.D.

Peptic ulcer, a frequently encountered problem in adults, is being recognized with increasing frequency in children. However, the typical clinical syndrome in the adult is usually not seen in the child until early adolescence. From birth until seven or eight years of age, the child with peptic ulcer usually presents as an acute surgical emergency because of complications. In the child beyond eight years of age, the adult pattern of the disease begins to appear.

The treatment of peptic ulcer in children is best managed in relation to the age of the patient rather than the artificial division of medical or surgical considerations. Most peptic ulcer disease has both medical and surgical implications, and teamwork is important for a successful result.

ULCER IN CHILDREN UNDER EIGHT YEARS OF AGE

Almost all infants and children under eight years of age with peptic ulcer disease present as an acute surgical emergency. Many have a primary medical illness. The surgical complications in this age group are hemorrhage or perforation and, at times, a combination of both. The pediatrician's major role in this emergency is prompt recognition of the disaster and immediate surgical consultation. The pediatrician's continued assistance is most valuable to the surgeon in the management of this problem, particularly if the ulcer is secondary to a medical disease.

Upper gastrointestinal tract hemorrhage in the newborn is most often thought to be due to hypoprothrombinemia or ingested maternal blood. These patients invariably cease bleeding spontaneously, and the exact cause may remain obscure. However, a few cases are due to acute gastroduodenal ulcerations, and these may exsanguinate or progress to perforation if the pediatrician is not alert to this possibility. The mortality rate from these complications in this age group approaches 100 per cent if surgical correction is not instituted early.

Once free intraperitoneal air is seen radiographically, laparotomy is indicated, particularly in the infant whose peritoneal defenses are poorly equipped to localize a free perforation.

Massive bleeding is best treated by meticulous blood replacement and continuous observation by the pediatrician and surgeon. If the hemorrhage does not diminish within 24 hours or if the blood loss exceeds replacement, surgical control is necessary.

Radiologic confirmation of a suspected bleeding ulcer in the young infant is usually not helpful, because these ulcers are shallow and often are not seen by barium meal study. This study should be done, however, if the patient's condition permits, if only to rule out other causes of upper gastrointestinal tract bleeding in this age group.

Surgical intervention in these patients should be directed toward only the acute complication. Perforations are most often on the anterior wall and should be closed with a single transverse layer of silk sutures and reinforced with an omental patch. Bleeding ulcers are best treated by duodenotomy or gastrotomy with suture ligation of the bleeding vessel.

ULCER IN CHILDREN OVER EIGHT YEARS OF AGE

Patients over eight years of age with peptic ulcer disease present less frequently as acute surgical emergencies. Most are diagnosed following an upper gastrointestinal roentgen study for chronic abdominal pain. Response to medical therapy results in a high incidence of healing of the ulcer.

Chronicity, bleeding, perforation or obstruction may occur in this age group as a complication of peptic ulcer. Occasionally, these complications may be secondary to a more serious illness. We have seen complicated ulcer in this age group with unsuspected brain tumor and non-beta cell adenoma of the pancreas (Zollinger-Ellison syndrome).

The management of peptic ulcer in the child parallels the accepted treatment in adults. The keystone of ulcer therapy is neutralization of the hydrochloric acid. Diet and antacids are important.

During the early stages of treatment, a bland diet should be used, preferably as small, frequent feedings. Once the acute symptoms have subsided, a regular diet devoid of spices may be given. Antacids are used to buffer the hydrochloric acid every 1 or 2 hours between meals, and at night, every few hours for pain if necessary. Aluminum hydroxide may cause constipation; however, this can be controlled by using a preparation containing magnesium, such as Maalox. Skimmed milk may be substituted at times for the antacids; however, regular milk should be avoided because of its high fat content. Coffee, tea and cola derivatives must be restricted.

Anticholinergics and sedatives are seldom necessary in the treatment of ulcer in children. The anticholinergic drugs are poorly effective in controlling hydrochloric acid secretion when given orally unless the doses given are so large that they cause unpleasant side effects. Sedation for the child with peptic ulcer is usually unnecessary but may be a valuable adjunct for the agitated patient.

The physician treating a child with ulcer disease should strive to strengthen the doctor-patient relationship. Time should be taken to explain to the parents and child the relationship of anger, hostility and stress to the production of ulcer. Possible discord at home or at school should be investigated and, if present, corrected. The physician's role as educator and advisor in ulcer disease often is the most important phase of treatment. Medical therapy as outlined should be continued for six to eight weeks. Treatment should be reinstituted whenever symptoms suggestive of ulcer recur.

Surgical consultation should be promptly sought when the complications of ulcer (bleeding, perforation, intractability or obstruction) appear. Of these, upper gastrointestinal tract hemorrhage is the most common. Immediate treatment should be directed toward replacement of blood volume and control of hydrochloric acid secretion. A central venous catheter is useful both to serve as a reliable, fast conduit for blood replacement and to measure central venous pressure. Nasogastric suction is used to remove all hydrochloric acid and, if necessary, to lavage the stomach with chilled saline. If hemorrhage lessens, a constant drip of milk or aluminum hydroxide is started through the nasogastric tube. If bleeding continues uncontrolled, surgical intervention is necessary. Simple duodenotomy with suture ligation of the bleeding vessel, rather than subtotal gastrectomy, is recommended in children.

Perforation, the second most common complication, usually presents as an acute abdominal catastrophe with few prodromal symptoms of ulcer. The nature of the perforation is often not discovered until the abdomen is opened. Surgical closure of the perforated duodenal ulcer should be done transversely with omentum placed over the closure. Postoperative nasogastric decompression is necessary until normal peristalsis returns. Supportive therapy is necessary with antibiotics, plasma derivatives or blood.

Intractability, obstruction and recurrent bleeding or recurrent perforation require surgical control of the production of hydrochloric acid. Surgical procedures available vary from vagotomy and pyloroplasty to subtotal gastrectomy. It is strongly recommended that vagotomy and pyloroplasty be the operation of choice. This offers a high degree of success in checking the production of hydrochloric acid without subjecting the child to the possible complications of retarded growth and development, "dumping syndrome" or malabsorption problems. If this simple procedure fails, subtotal gastrectomy may be done.

Gastritis

LAWRENCE K. PICKETT, M.D.

Acute gastritis may be defined as an acute inflammation of the mucosa of the stomach, histologically nonspecific and resulting in excessive gastric secretion and vomiting, or gastric hemorrhage.

Types of Gastritis. Gastritis may be the result of infection of enteric origin, usually viral, but occasionally associated with the exanthems of childhood or bacterial infection. Another more diffuse type is that associated with excessive steroid dosage, stress, central nervous system disorders or burns.

Treatment and Prognosis. Treatment of gastritis involves putting the stomach at rest to decrease gastric secretions. In severe cases, this is done with a nasogastric tube; in the milder cases restriction of oral intake is sufficient. Most of the viral disorders are self-terminating. Bacterial disease may be treated more specifically with antibiotic therapy, depending on the organism. The gastritis associated with the exanthems is self-limiting and usually mild. In the case of hemorrhagic gastritis associated with steroids, stress, central nervous system disorders or burns, the treatment is more complex. Keeping the stomach at rest by using a nasogastric tube on suction with frequent irrigations is important to decrease gastric acidity as well as to determine the extent of the bleeding and to measure blood loss. Frequent irrigations with chilled saline seem to decrease the amount of bleeding but rarely can be considered definitive therapy. The use of antacids, as frequently employed, is without a physiologic basis, since the gastric secretions in the various forms of stress or steroid ulcerations are not increased. In addition to gastric decompression, treatment of the source—i.e., supportive therapy for the burns, operative intervention or supportive therapy for the central nervous system disorder and, in the case of steroids, discontinuance of the medication—is as important in the treatment of the hemorrhagic gastritis as any specific form of therapy. If the diagnosis is confirmed by x-ray and/or gastroscopy and if there is no evident single bleeding point, such as a duodenal ulcer or varices, surgical intervention is most often disappointing in treatment of the hemorrhage. Vagotomy and pyloroplasty have been advocated but have not been found to be as useful as removal of the source of stress or supportive therapy until the underlying condition is corrected.

Another form of gastritis is that caused by the ingestion of corrosives. It should be treated immediately by acid or alkali instillation, depending on the nature of the corrosive. Despite the risks of perforation, a nasogastric tube should be placed and kept on suction so that the stomach is kept at rest, thus decreasing gastric secretions. When corrosives reach the stomach in sufficient quantities to cause gastritis, there is a high incidence of gastric perforation. Those in whom gastritis is suspected should be closely observed, and with any development of peritoneal signs surgical intervention with plication or excision of the ulcerated area should be undertaken. The use of the nasogastric tube in the case of corrosive gastritis may be impossible or unwise in view of the associated oral and esophageal burns. If gastric atony or acute retention is noted, laparotomy with gastrostomy may be lifesaving, anticipating gastric perforation.

Malformations and Malrotations of the Stomach and Intestine

LAWRENCE K. PICKETT, M.D.

DIAPHRAGMATIC HERNIA

Once the diagnosis of diaphragmatic hernia is suspected, a nasogastric tube should be inserted to evacuate air from the stomach and to ensure that additional air is not introduced into the intestine to cause an increasing space-occupying lesion and further respiratory embarrassment. The child should be placed in a high-oxygen environment with humidity. If assisted respirations are necessary with intubation, great care should be taken in the amount of pressure exerted. Positive-pressure assistance may cause rupture of the hypoplastic lung associated with diaphragmatic hernia, and may result in fatal pneumothorax. The patient should be elevated at a 40-degree angle and preparation for operation made immediately. Correction of the acidosis associated with hypoxia may be undertaken during preparation for operation, but no delay in operative intervention should be allowed despite the inevitable blood-gas disturbance associated with underventilation.

An appropriate dosage of atropine should be used prior to surgery, the amount depending on the size of the child. In view of the marked respiratory embarrassment and consequent poor gas exchange, it may not be possible to accomplish surgical anesthesia. The space-occupying lesion in one side of the chest causes a shift of content toward the mediastinum and seriously impairs gas exchange in the contralateral lung. As in assisted respiration in the preoperative phase, the anesthetist must be most cautious with the amount of positive pressure anesthesia used during the operation, since overexpanding a hypoplastic lung can cause serious irreparable damage.

An incision in the upper part of the abdomen is made transversely or in a paramedian fashion, depending on the surgeon's preference. A catheter should be introduced into the chest through the diaphragmatic defect to allow the vacuum to be equalized; the intestines are then removed as rapidly as possible from the chest. This allows expansion of the contralateral lung, and anesthesia can then be introduced by the anesthetist in the emergency situation. After the viscera have been liberated from the chest, a careful search should be made for a sac which, if missed, will cause the formation of a cyst—a space-occupying lesion in the postoperative period that will interfere with expansion of the lung. The diaphragm is repaired with the remnants in whatever manner is suitable. A two-layer closure with a single layer of mattress sutures, reinforced by interrupted 3–0 silk sutures, is adequate. No attempt should be made by the anesthetist to expand the lung, since it is often unexpanded, immature or hypoplastic and requires time for its normal development. A gradual resorption of air from the pleural cavity over a period of a week to

10 days following operation gradually expands the lung, with an attendent shift to the mediastinum; this process is far superior to indwelling catheters, suction or positive pressure.

During surgery, the viscera should be inspected for associated anomalies. The viscera that have migrated into a diaphragmatic hernia have an associated malrotation which should be corrected. Any bands across the duodenum should be carefully lysed. The viscera should be replaced in the abdominal cavity and, when possible, layer closure is carried out. When layer closure will interfere with diaphragmatic excursion and cause severe intra-abdominal pressure that will restrict aeration, only the skin is closed, and the resultant ventral hernia is closed at a later date.

Immediately postoperatively the stomach should remain decompressed, by means of nasogastric suction or via a gastrostomy that was performed before abdominal closure, until gastrointestinal motility has been reestablished. A gastrostomy should be used in most newborn infants with diaphragmatic hernia, and in some older children. The primary postoperative problems are respiratory. The gastrostomy frees the upper airway of the semiobstructive and irritating tube and offers not only decompression but also an avenue of early alimentation for the seriously ill infant. The gastrostomy is performed in the conventional manner of Stamm. Blood gases should be carefully measured, and acidosis resulting from the hypoxia should be corrected. Volume-controlled respirator assistance may be necessary to correct respiratory acidosis, which is extremely common particularly in newborn infants. When the blood gases are corrected and the baby is making respiratory efforts on his own, assisted respirations can continue. Respiratory assist should be discontinued as soon as possible so that the endotracheal tube can be removed to prevent damage to the larynx and trachea. The baby should remain elevated about 40 degrees from the prone position, in a high-humidity and controlled-oxygen environment. Also, in the postoperative period, glucose determinations should be followed closely, since hypoglycemia may complicate hypoxia and cause central nervous system damage, particularly in the neonate.

In those infants who require surgical correction in the first 24 hours of life, there remains a high mortality rate despite all the precautions mentioned above. Early diagnosis, careful monitoring of the blood gases and attention to the intricate details of pulmonary assistance are essential if the neonatal mortality rate is to be lowered. Older children present fewer problems than the neonate, and should be able to be corrected with a low mortality rate.

OMPHALOCELE AND GASTROSCHISIS

Omphalocele or congenital hernia into the umbilical cord may present as a small, easily reducible protrusion; closure is accomplished with a primary abdominal wall repair and without respiratory embarrassment.

In the larger lesions with a larger abdominal defect where the viscera cannot be returned to the abdominal cavity without severe respiratory embarrassment and difficulty with abdominal wall repair, the abdominal wall can be reconstituted with commercially available Silastic-covered Teflon mesh. This can be sutured to the edge of the rectus muscle and brought together with sufficient tension so that the skin can be closed over it. In serial steps immediately after the first few postoperative days, segments of this Silastic sheeting can be removed, reconstituting the abdominal wall in three or four stages; in this manner, complete abdominal repair is accomplished in three to four weeks postoperatively. Because of the use of foreign material, the infant should be protected by antibiotic therapy—penicillin or kanamycin in appropriate doses—until all the foreign material has been removed.

In *gastroschisis,* which is a defect lateral to the umbilicus with the cord intact, the bowel is quite often matted, covered with a heavy layer of fibrin with encased, trapped amniotic fluid. A similar situation may exist with a ruptured omphalocele. When it is ruptured in utero, this bowel should be carefully inspected to find areas of atresia or malformation secondary to constriction. The amniotic fluid should be liberated and the viscera returned to the abdomen, using the Silastic sheeting procedure described above. The sheeting may be removed as the edema disappears from the bowel, reconstituting the abdominal wall in two to three weeks postoperatively.

With all abdominal wall closures for omphalocele or gastroschisis, the anesthetist should not use relaxing drugs, since too tight a closure can be accomplished, with subsequent respiratory embarrassment. Postoperatively, attention should be paid to possible hypoglycemia, since this is frequently associated with umbilical defects and may lead to disastrous central nervous system damage.

MECKEL'S DIVERTICULUM

The majority of Meckel's diverticula are found as incidental findings during surgery for another cause. If the surgical manipulation involved in the primary cause for operation does not contraindicate it, the Meckel's diverticulum should be excised at the time of operation. Should, however, the primary procedure contraindicate prolonging the procedure or opening the intestine, the diverticulum should be operated on electively at a later date. Surgical excision may be accomplished either by oblique division of the diverticulum at its base, with subsequent two-layer closure; however, should there be palpable evidence of gastric mucosa extending down into the lumen of the intestine, sleeve resection with end-to-end ileoileostomy should be carried out. I prefer an open anastomosis with a two-layer closure, the outer layer being 5–0 nonabsorbable material and the inner layer being 5–0 chromic catgut. In the small child, interrupted sutures should be used throughout to prevent stenosis.

When Meckel's diverticulum is the primary finding at operation and has been involved in inflammation or bleeding, care should be taken in simple excision to make sure that inflammatory reaction or ulceration does not impair the viability of the adjacent bowel or its healing potential. Generally, when there is marked inflammation around the Meckel's diverticulum, a segmental resection of the ileum is indicated, performed in an open manner as indicated above.

When the Meckel's diverticulum is the lead point of an intussusception and is found during the reduction of the intussusception, the condition of the patient will dictate whether primary resection should be carried out, or whether complete reduction should be accomplished and resection carried out at a later date. In no case should primary resection be done if the patient's condition is precarious or if the bowel is so damaged that it will compromise healing after an anastomosis. In most cases, primary resection can be carried out, but edema of the bowel wall and the question of viability of the bowel will dictate the proper procedure.

Supportive care after the resection is obviously indicated, along with fluid and electrolyte as well as blood replacement, if there has been blood loss, until restoration of intestinal function. Nasogastric suction is usually adequate for decompression. Antibiotics are rarely indicated unless there has been peritoneal contamination at the time of anastomosis or secondary to perforation. If there has been contamination, broad-spectrum coverage of both gram-negative and gram-positive organisms should be provided, usually with penicillin and kanamycin in the customary dosage for the weight of the patient.

Omphalomesenteric Remnants. Since Meckel's diverticulum is the most frequent form of omphalomesenteric duct remnant of the embryonal human, it represents the major problem in imperfect embryology of the gut. It may, however, exist as patent omphalomesenteric duct with discharge of intestinal contents through the umbilicus, which is noted shortly after birth. If fecal material is present at the umbilicus, x-rays and other injection studies are rarely indicated, since total excision of the omphalomesenteric duct should be carried out in a manner similar to the operation for Meckel's diverticulum. There is some urgency to the operation, since ileal prolapse and fluid and electrolyte loss may accompany the patent omphalomesenteric duct. Immediate surgery will prevent complications arising from these sources.

The persistence of other omphalomesenteric remnants may result in an umbilical polyp or granuloma which does not respond to cauterization and the usual measures employed. Careful probing should be carried out at the time of operation to make sure there is no communication with the intestinal tract. When there is an umbilical polyp or cyst, or other evidence of omphalomesenteric duct remnant, the peritoneum should be opened in the midline to be sure that the remainder of the omphalomesenteric duct is not in existence. Occasionally there will be a band from the umbilicus to the position of the Meckel's diverticulum, creating a potential for volvulus. Obviously, such a band should be divided. Simple excision of the umbilical remnant of the omphalomesenteric duct should be carried out with the preservation of the umbilicus.

INTESTINAL OBSTRUCTION

Intestinal obstruction is generally heralded by colicky abdominal pain; vomiting, which progresses to bile-stained vomitus; abdominal distention and cessation of bowel movements. All of the above may occur in varying degrees, depending on the nature of the obstruction (complete or incomplete) and the level of the obstruction.

Once the diagnosis has been made by the presence of bile-stained vomitus, the general appearance and condition of the child should be ascertained. In the newborn infant the level of obstruction can generally be determined by a prone and upright film of the abdomen, depending on the number of gas-filled loops. Occasionally a barium enema is needed to demonstrate patency of the large bowel or malrotation with possible duodenal bands and/or volvulus.

In the older child, one is aided by the progression of symptoms, the x-ray appearance and the physical examination of the abdomen. Tenderness and peritoneal irritation are easier to elicit in the older child than in the newborn; these warn of impending perforation or catastrophe due to impaired bowel viability. After the diagnosis has been established, restoration of fluid and electrolyte depletion should take top priority. There are only two circumstances in which careful fluid and electrolyte balance should be done precipitously: when there is evidence of vascular impairment of the gut wall, or when there is a closed loop obstruction. In either case, the losses may be greater than can be restored and valuable time and viability of the bowel wall may be lost with the delay. So-called crash hydration should be accomplished. In cases of suspected midgut volvulus, intussusception or closed loop obstruction, hydration should be instituted and continued during the operation and postoperatively. Hydration should be carried out with a hypotonic solution until voiding takes place, and sodium and potassium should be added according to losses measured in the serum. Whole blood can be used to combat shock if the viability of the bowel wall is in question. Full correction of losses should be accomplished only rarely, in view of continued loss into the "third space." When hydration is underway and some urine flow is established, operation should proceed with all urgency.

The primary principle in managing duodenal obstruction is that most forms should be treated with duodenojejunostomy rather than by a direct attack on the stenotic area. High forms of intestinal obstruction, in the jejunum or upper ileum, are best treated with direct end-to-end anastomosis. Lower forms of obstruction, where there is marked size discrepancy between the distal and proximal bowel, may be treated by exteriorization resection of a Mikulicz-type if viability is in question. When segments of the small bowel are missing and atresia is found, all attempts to preserve the terminal ileum should be made. Success in treatment of the short gut syndrome is more frequently encountered when the terminal ileum can be salvaged.

Obstruction Due to Malrotation and Volvulus—A True Emergency. Midgut volvulus will generally occur in a clockwise direction, requiring derotation in a counterclockwise direction. Once viability of the bowel has been ascertained and bands of the duodenum lysed, one should be particularly certain that there is no intrinsic obstruction of the duodenum and no extrinsic bands. A proper treatment for malrotation is the so-called Ladd's procedure, with freeing of all the attachments of the colon, leaving the cecum and colon on the left side of the abdomen, with the duodenum descending on the right side of the abdomen freed of bands and obstruction. Any attempts to fix the bowel in any certain position leads to localized volvulus and obstruction rather than to prevention of recurrent midgut volvulus.

Obstruction Due to Aganglionic Megacolon. Though this subject is treated in detail elsewhere, the newborn with aganglionic megacolon presents a tremendous challenge. Thirty per cent of the children with this condition will manifest their problem by diarrhea rather than by obstipation. Barium enema will reveal anatomic continuity and give some hint as to the presence of aganglionic megacolon. A well-defined aganglionic segment may be hard to demonstrate by x-ray. This may be confirmed in the newborn period only by rectal biopsy. Once the diagnosis has been made, colostomy should be performed at the transition zone under frozen section control, with definitive resection being done when the child reaches a sufficient weight of 20 to 25 pounds. The definitive resection can be done electively at an optimum time rather than during a time of depletion in the newborn period.

Duplications of the Stomach and Intestine. Duplications of the stomach and small intestine generally manifest themselves by intestinal obstruction but may also be noted because of bleeding or the presence of an abdominal mass. Each duplication must be treated on its own specific indications; no general rules can be set down for management.

Generally, the duplication will share a wall with the normal intestine and require intestinal resection with an end-to-end anastomosis. The extent of the duplication should be outlined as completely as possible with barium studies before operation. The varieties of duplication in continuity, such as a total hindgut duplication, are treated as the situation indicates, with resection of one or the other segments of the bowel, the remaining segment being the one that is more functional or more easily reconstructed.

CONCLUSION

Only the highlights of treatment of malformations of the stomach and intestines have been dealt with here. Details can be found in suitable surgical texts. The important principles of careful hydration before operation, of restoration of fluid and electrolyte losses and of meticulous attention to surgical technique are of the utmost importance. Proper anesthetic support, realization that delays can be fatal in the case of impaired blood supply, and hour-to-hour observations in the postoperative period are essential to success.

Gastrointestinal Foreign Bodies

J. ALEX HALLER, JR., M.D.

Gastrointestinal foreign bodies are usually a problem in children six months to three years of age. During this time the child becomes increasingly mobile and inquisitive and yet has insufficient insight to avoid ingestion of dangerous foreign bodies. As a general rule, any object which can be swallowed to the stomach will pass through the intestinal tract without subsequent difficulty. The exception to this statement are the sharp foreign bodies which may become imbedded in the mucosa and carry a potential for perforation. Thus, our only concern with smooth or round foreign bodies is whether they proceed through the esophagus or not. The most common point at which foreign bodies become lodged is at the cricopharyngeal area of the upper esophagus. Not infrequently, children who have swallowed foreign bodies to this level have recurring episodes of attempted vomiting, and may have associated respiratory distress if edema develops and encompasses the surrounding epiglottal tissues. If the object is radiopaque, the diagnosis is easily made with a routine chest x-ray. In our own experience, esophagoscopy to remove such foreign bodies should be carried out only after endotracheal anesthesia has been established. This is increasingly important in the younger child, because his tracheal airway may be compromised by endoscopic manipulation in the upper esophagus. Under light, general anesthesia, administered through an endotracheal tube, the esophagoscope can be slipped into the upper part of the esophagus and the offending foreign body grasped with an appropriate forceps and removed.

If the rounded object, such as a penny or marble, reaches the stomach, intelligent neglect is in order. These patients can be followed as outpatients, with occasional x-rays if the object is radiopaque. These objects should pass in the stool within two to five days. In rare instances, in which the foreign body remains lodged in the stomach or in some other portion of the gastrointestinal tract for longer than two weeks, we have recommended laparotomy and operative removal.

If the foreign body is sharp, such as an opened safety pin or an object with sharp points which passes into the stomach, we have been more cautious and admitted these patients to the hospital in order to have them under observation during the period of passage of the foreign body. Almost all such objects will pass without difficulty in the stool in two to five days. Daily x-rays are taken, and if the object fails to move significantly for a day or two, this is taken as an indication that it has become imbedded in the mucosa and perforation is impending. Such objects are therefore surgically removed. Other evidences of potential perforation, such as fever, tachycardia and vomiting, are also indications for exploration. Fortunately, most foreign bodies, both sharp and smooth, pass without difficulty through the intestinal tract in a short period of time, and under appropriate observation, the child is best managed without operative intervention.

Intussusception

J. ALEX HALLER, JR., M.D.

Intussusception is a disease process of the intestine in which telescoping of a proximal segment of the intestine (the intussusceptum) into the lumen of the distal intestine (the intussuscipiens) occurs. This invagination may reduce spontaneously but generally persists and results in mechanical intestinal obstruction with evidences of partial to complete blockage of the terminal ileum and colon. Approximately two-thirds of the patients are seen within the first year of life, usually between the fifth and ninth months. In other parts of the world this condition may occur at a later time, and has also been reported in adults. In the vast majority of infants with intussusception, no definite pathologic abnormality in the bowel wall or mucosa is found. Since intussusception occurs in well-nourished infants and at a time when many are changing their dietary intake, nutritional changes have been implicated in the etiology. In a small percentage of cases a specific abnormality may be present in the wall, such as polyp, Meckel's diverticulum or hypertrophied lymphoid patch. Large lymph nodes have been implicated, but whether they actually represent cause or effect is not known. A viral gastroenteritis not infrequently is associated with intussusception, suggesting that there may be a causal relationship with possible hypertrophy of the Peyer's patches in the terminal ileal segment.

The large majority of intussusceptions begin at the ileocecal valve and extend for variable distances into the colon, occasionally presenting through the anus as a dramatic form of prolapse. When telescoping begins, there is increased peristaltic activity which drives the intussusceptum further downstream. As the mesentery with its contained blood vessels is pulled with the telescoping bowel, there first occurs obstruction to venous drainage accompanied by lymphatic obstruction. This results in increasing edema and incarceration of the intussusceptum. If this persists, there may be arterial obstruction as well, leading to ischemic necrosis and perforation. The progressive edema with the outpouring of goblet cell mucus and some blood results in the mucoid, reddish stools which are referred to as currant jelly stools. The end stage of this process is obviously ischemic gangrene of the bowel wall and, ultimately, perforation and septicemia.

The usual clinical presentation of a child with intussusception is suggestive of intestinal obstruction. Typically it occurs in a well-nourished child of approximately six months of age who has intermittent episodes of cramping abdominal pain, identifiable by the child's doubling up and crying out in pain, with 30- to 45-minute periods of quiet and relaxation inbetween. These symptoms subside often and recur after a short interval. After a few hours, the colicky pain may be associated with the mucoid stool with reddish discoloration. If the condition persists until impending ischemic necrosis occurs, the child may become apathetic and pallid and show evidence of increasing dehydration and the onset of septicemia.

The positive physical signs of this condition are largely those of lower intestinal obstruction. The abdomen is usually tightly distended with some tenderness to palpation but without spasm, unless perforation has occurred. In approximately 90 per cent of the cases a soft, doughy, sausage-shaped mass is palpable in the right lower quadrant and can usually be moved about. The precise diagnosis is established by a carefully performed barium enema which, at the same time, is often therapeutic.

The two forms of therapy currently used in the United States consist of (1) hydrostatic pressure reduction, and (2) operative reduction. On our service at Johns Hopkins, we prefer the nonoperative technique of hydrostatic pressure reduction, since it avoids general anesthesia and laparotomy in more than 70 per cent of the patients in our experience. Critics of this technique are concerned that nonviable bowel might be reduced by barium enema management. Both experimental and clinical experience contradicts this concern, provided the barium column is carefully controlled at a height less than 3 feet 6 inches. Another objection is that the diagnosis may be uncertain and that one cannot be sure of complete reduction when intussusception is present. If the barium column refluxes freely into the small intestine after reduction of the colonic intussusception, the reduction is usually complete. While it is true that specific causes, such as polyps, will not be corrected by this nonoperative treatment, the occurrence of polyps is so rare in young infants that it is statistically insignificant. In older children and adults, barium enema reduction should be considered the first stage in management and an elective operative procedure subsequently carried out because of the high incidence of specific etiology.

Barium enema, along with the associated hydrostatic pressure phenomena, is not a substitute for operative intervention, but it is the diagnostic procedure which may be followed by successful reduction. If the nonmanipulative barium enema fails to reduce the intussusception or if there is any question concerning the completeness of reduction, the patient is taken directly to the operating room for the standard operative procedure.

In practice, when the diagnosis of intussusception is considered, the patient is tentatively scheduled for operation, intravenous fluids are begun, nasogastric suction is instituted and the patient is taken to the x-ray department for the barium enema, where the surgeon and the radiologist, and perhaps the pediatrician, are in attendance. The enema catheter is connected to an overhead reservoir of thin barium, which is measured at a height of no more than 3 feet 6 inches above the patient. Under fluoroscopic control, the barium is permitted to run into the rectum without manipulation. The barium column usually progresses rapidly to the point of the intusssusception, where the round head of the advancing barium column suddenly becomes concave, forming the so-called C sign of intussusception. As the hydrostatic pressure increases, the column of barium widens, the meniscus opens and the intussusceptum is displaced more proximally. This is repeated until the intussusceptum is reduced. If during the course of the procedure no progress occurs in reduction for 15 to 30 minutes, the attempted enema reduction is abandoned and the patient is taken to the operating room for surgical reduction.

The operative technique is usually performed through a right lower quadrant muscle-splitting incision. The intussusception can usually be reduced by manual progressive compression of the bowel distal to the intussusception. If it is easily reduced, there should be little question about viability. If reduction is not readily accomplished, resection should be performed. The present trend is toward direct resection and primary end-to-end anastomosis.

The operative mortality in most hospitals is higher than the very low barium enema mortality, lending further emphasis to the advisability of hydrostatic reduction as a first step in overall management. Recurrence of the condition following reduction is rare. When it occurs, it nearly always reflects the presence of a specific intestinal lesion.

References

Benson, C. C., et al.: *Pediatric Surgery*. Vol. 2. Chicago, The Year Book Medical Publishers, 1962.

Gross, R. E., and Ware, P. F.: Intussusception in Childhood: Experience from 610 Cases. *New England J. Med.*, 239:645, 1948.

Haller, J. Alex, Jr.: *Principles of Surgery*. New York, McGraw-Hill Book Company, 1969, pp. 1387–1389.

Power, D'A.: The Hunterian Lectures on the Pathology and Surgery of Intussusception, *Brit. Med. J.*, 1:381, 453, 514, 1897.

Ravitch, M. M., and McCune, R. M., Jr.: Reduction of Intussusception by Barium Enema: A Clinical and Experimental Study. *Ann. Surg.*, 128:904, 1948.

Ravitch, M. M., and McCune, R. M., Jr.: Reduction of Intussusception by Hydrostatic Pressure: An Experimental Study. *Bull. Johns Hopkins Hosp.*, 82:550, 1948.

Ravitch, M. M.: Intussusception in Infancy and Childhood. An Analysis of 77 Cases Treated by Barium Enema. *New England J. Med.*, 259:1058, 1958.

Snyder, W. H., Jr., Kraus, A. R., and Chaffin, L.: Intussusception in Infants and Children: Report of 143 Consecutive Cases. *Ann. Surg.* 130:200, 1949.

Hirschsprung's Disease

ORVAR SWENSON, M.D.

Hirschsprung's disease, or congenital megacolon, is a rare entity which has always attracted a great deal of attention among clinicians. A possible reason is the similarity between symptoms and signs of this condition and those of severe habit constipation. The practicing physician and pediatrician are always alert to the possibility of a case of Hirschsprung's disease because much can be done for these children therapeutically.

Hirschsprung's disease is difficult to diagnose because of its rarity—the average physician probably sees no more than one case in a lifetime. Because of the limitations of space, only the salient features can be mentioned here. In neonates these are vomiting (often with bile-stained vomitus), abdominal distention and obstipation. In older children the features are constipation (present from birth) and bouts of severe abdominal distention, but never is there fecal soiling and no or minimal feces are found in the rectum on rectal examination.

Once the diagnosis has been made, one may perform either a primary resection of the aganglionic segment or a colostomy. In children over 10 months of age who are in good condition, primary resection is advisable. In children in poor condition and in infants, a colostomy is preferred. The position of the colostomy is determined by biopsy, and it is placed at the junction of the normal and the aganglionic colon. We have found it a good practice to wait until a patient weighs 20 to 30 pounds before performing a definitive operation with resection of the colostomy and the aganglionic segment with a pull-through type of anastomosis.

We have not found it necessary to prepare the colon with a course of antibiotics to reduce the bacterial count of the intestinal content. Such a program was tested but discontinued because of an increased rate of enterocolitis postoperatively. Since most of our patients have a colostomy, the only preparation necessary is to make sure that blood is available for transfusion. The operations are performed with a two team set-up. The abdominal operation consists of resecting the bowel beyond the colostomy, or, in a patient who does not have a colostomy, beyond the point where the ganglion cells end. This can be determined only by biopsies since visual observation can be misleading.

The dissection is most difficult in the depth of the pelvis, since one must prevent damage to the neural elements deep in the pelvis. By keeping the dissection on the bowel wall, no structures in the pelvis are damaged. The dissection must be carried down to a point where one can see the mucocutaneous margin with ease when the distal colonic segment is prolapsed. It is essential that the proximal bowel prolapsed through has adequate length and excellent blood supply so that when the anastomosis is made, there is no tension on the suture and prompt healing occurs.

The resection of the distal segment should be low enough to include a large part of the internal sphincter posteriorly. It is best to make this an oblique anastomosis with the anterior portion of the rectal wall 2 to 3 cm. in length. We have found that by resecting a part of the internal sphincter, the incidence of postoperative enterocolitis is significantly reduced.

The treatment of patients with total aganglionosis is exactly the same as that just described, except that instead of a colostomy, an ileostomy is made. The ileum is brought down to the anal canal in a manner identical to that described for partial aganglionosis of the colon.

These patients have frequent bowel movements for several months after surgery, but gradually this subsides. One boy whom we have followed for 20 years has two bowel movements a day. The incidence of complications with this procedure is acceptable. The mortality rate is less than 2 per cent. The results are excellent and 98 per cent of patients are essentially normal. Follow-ups for as long as 20 years now show maintenance of excellent results.

Recently the technique of resection has been modified, particularly in Europe. In the United States, authorities have advocated a so-called segmental resection in which a considerable part of the aganglionic segment is left in place. We have seen a number of patients who have undergone this type of operation; although they have been helped for two, three or four years, they tend to have a recurrence of symptoms severe enough to require further therapy. Consequently, it is felt that the segmental resection is inadequate. From a theoretical standpoint, this can be postulated because only a part of the aganglionic segment is removed. Certainly, if the concept of the pathology and physiology of this disease is correct—and extensive experience has proved this to be the case—inadequate resection of the diseased bowel would result in a recurrence of symptoms of the disease, as we have seen in a number of patients.

More recently, another way of bringing normal bowel down to the perineum has been suggested. This technique entails leaving the rectum in place. Because a large part of the diseased bowel is left in place, it is predicted that the long-term results of this operation will not be satisfactory.

Because we have been able to achieve excellent results in 98 per cent of patients by resection of the aganglionic segment with reapproximation of the colon, it would seem unwise to experiment with techniques that are likely to give poor results. Not one in a series of 284 patients has had urinary incontinence. Fecal incontinence may be present postoperatively for three to four months in 1 or 2 per cent of our patients, but never has it extended beyond this period. Ninety-eight per cent are continent immediately after operation, and remain so. In a group of older male patients, there has been no disturbance of ejaculation.

Ulcerative Colitis and Regional Enteritis

MARCEL PATTERSON, M.D.

The recent literature has many articles about granulomatous colitis or Crohn's disease, as distinguished from idiopathic ulcerative colitis. These distinctions are based on clinical and pathologic findings, but from the standpoint of therapeutics the goals are the same: to quell diarrhea, to restore nutrition and to control systemic symptoms and local complications as they arise. Treatment in either condition is empirical and pragmatic and, of necessity, will continue to be until we have a clearer idea of the etiology and pathogenesis of these diseases.

The problems mount in the young; often they have total colon involvement when first seen, and these particular patients respond more poorly to treatment. Furthermore, they run a higher risk of developing cancer the longer they live, although it is said that the risk with Crohn's colitis is less. The disabling effects of this chronic illness on physical and mental growth, coupled with the undesirable effects of prolonged corticosteroid therapy, make careful assessment of our therapeutic efforts imperative. Permanent ileostomy looms as a formidable disability, but with the alternative of chronic invalidism or early death, it can be tolerated.

One hopes for a really new and exciting therapeutic breakthrough with these diseases, and occasionally one does see dramatic and gratifying responses with present treatment. But because of the prognosis, the importance of an accurate diagnosis cannot be overemphasized.

Therapeutic modalities available to the physician are diet, nutritional aids, drugs for controlling pain and diarrhea, corticosteroids, immunosuppressive agents and antibacterial agents. None seems quite as potent as the physician himself. These patients and their families require much support and sympathetic understanding. Some thought needs to be given to career goals, since the chronicity and relapsing course of this illness require goals that are realistic in terms of talents and strength.

During acute exacerbations, particularly with febrile episodes, bed rest is advisable. If the patient's condition permits daily activities, relief from required physical education and permission to leave school rooms on demand should be arranged. Nothing can be more emotionally shattering to a teenager than public fecal soilage.

DIET AND NUTRITIONAL AIDS

Maintaining nutrition requires ingenuity. Foods should be offered that appeal to the taste with minimal restrictions. Large amounts of fats, as well as high-residue foods, such as leafy vegetables or fruits, tend to aggravate diarrhea; in general, a low residue, fat-restricted diet is better tolerated, with emphasis on protein foods. Too many diet restrictions can aggravate malnutrition. At the beginning, I restrict milk and milk products. Some patients tolerate milk poorly and in some it may play a role in the pathogenesis of these diseases. Commonly, Negroes, Indians and Orientals are lactase-deficient and large amounts of milk aggravate diarrhea and flatulence. If milk and its products offend, a period of restriction of two to three weeks should decrease symptoms. Reintroducing milk and noting the effect on diarrhea and abdominal symptoms may give further support to the idea of intolerance. Since milk provides much of the essential nutrient calcium, it should not be discarded casually.

The diet by choice or restriction may be inadequate in vitamins, and a daily multivitamin supplement is advisable, although nothing suggests that vitamins are directly important in this illness. Hypoprothrombinemia may develop when broad-spectrum antibiotics are used or when bile salt absorption is poor. In this case, parenteral vitamin K may be useful.

Anemia accompanies inflammatory bowel disease, and iron may not help if infection is prominent. Iron stores should be measured and replaced where deficient. If oral iron is poorly tolerated, parenteral therapy should be considered. Terminal ileal disease may impair B_{12} absorption, as well as absorption of bile salts. In this case, parenteral administration of B_{12} may be needed to improve the anemia.

Electrolytes need careful monitoring, particularly when diarrhea and vomiting are prominent or corticosteroids are used. Deficits should be corrected as they arise. Oral potassium supplements may be needed, although they are capable of producing diarrhea.

In the very ill child, restricting all foods may be necessary. Two recent developments, elemental diets and hyperalimentation, make it easier to do this. The so-called elemental (space) diets, i.e., Vivonex or W. T. Low Residue Food, consist of monosaccharides, amino acids, vitamins and minerals. Though not particularly palatable, they can be infused through a fine plastic tube placed in the upper duodenum. Absorbed in the first few feet of the small bowel, this diet maintains nutrition with a minimium of stimulation of gastrointestinal secretions and without residue to stimulate the colon. The place of these diets in the treatment of colitis and enteritis has not been fully explored, but this approach seems reasonable and less hazardous than intravenous hyperalimentation.

ANTIDIARRHEAL AGENTS

Diphenoxylate hydrochloride (Lomotil), as a tablet or liquid, is well tolerated and effective in controlling diarrhea for many patients. The usual dose after age 12 is two tablets four times a day; under 12 to age eight the dose is 1 teaspoon or 1 tablet five times a day; for children five to eight, 1 teaspoon four times a day is recommended.

Traditionally, the narcotic drugs codeine (15 to 30 mg.), paregoric (4 ml.) and tincture of opium (10 drops) have been used for diarrhea. Their potential for addiction makes their use worrisome, but there are occasions when Lomotil does not control symptoms and tolerance seems to develop. By alternating these agents with Lomotil, they may be used safely for short periods and be effective. Dosage need not be rigid but should be regulated to control symptoms; some patients will not require these drugs more than once or twice a day. Toxic megacolon is a calculated risk with their use.

The use of bland hydrophilic mucilloids (Metamucil, Konsyl) may thicken stool and prevent soilage. The usual dose is 1 heaping teaspoon at bedtime or twice a day. They should be avoided when strictures are present, and sometimes they aggravate more than help.

Synthetic anticholinergics are disappointing in these diseases. Their action on colon motility is questionable, and they can produce ileus and sometimes precipitate obstruction. Their ability to check diarrhea or control pain is not impressive. On occasion, I prescribe Elixir of Donnatal or a similar barbiturate-belladonna alkaloid mixture, but in small doses (½ teaspoon three times a day and on retiring) and primarily for its sedative effect. Occasionally, the minor tranquilizing drugs have been helpful.

ANTI-INFLAMMATORY–IMMUNOSUPPRESSIVE AGENTS

Corticosteroids can control symptoms. In general, if the rectum is involved with disease it is well to start with topical steroids since they have less systemic effects, can slow diarrhea and may reverse proctoscopic findings.

The extent of the disease dictates the choice of topical therapy: for diseases limited to the rectum or rectosigmoid, steroid suppositories, usually inserted on arising and at bedtime can be tried. Two such preparations available are Wyanoids HC (15 mg. hydrocortisone) and Anusol-HC (10 mg. hydrocortisone).

Where the colon is more extensively involved, 50 mg. of hydrocortisone sodium succinate (Solu-Cortef), dissolved in a small bottle of saline (250 ml.) connected to tubing usually used for parenteral feedings and attached to a rectal catheter, can be given as an enema. Patients can be taught to regulate the flow and insert the solution to allow retention and avoid expulsion. This therapy has the disadvantage that the water-soluble steroids are unstable and must be prepared daily. If this is tolerated, the dose can be increased to 100 mg. hydrocortisone and the diluent increased to bathe the entire colon.

There are several enema preparations commercially available, such as plastic squeeze bottles with 100 mg. of hydrocortisone (Cortenema) or methyl prednisolone powder, 40 mg. per bottle (Medrol EnPak), packaged with a plastic container to suspend the powder in water and tubing for enema insertion. Prescribed at bedtime, one hopes that the material will be retained overnight. These preparations are suspensions and need to be well shaken before use, since the drug tends to settle out. Also, preparations forcefully squeezed into the rectum often act as enemas and are promptly expelled. Lately, hydrocortisone acetate (90 mg.) mixed with a foaming agent (Cortifoam) has been introduced to improve retention.

If topical steroids help, they do so promptly. Within a few days, tenesmus subsides, stools decrease and proctoscopy shows a lessening of inflammation. Some patients retain fluid but usually undesirable side effects are not a problem. The biggest difficulty with topical therapy has been that some youngsters resist the insertion of materials into their rectums and others refuse to try it. If their use evokes strong emotional reaction, this method of treatment should be discarded.

How long should one continue topical therapy? A lack of response in four to five days usually means no response will occur, but if symptoms abate no one is sure when treatment should be stopped. I arbitrarily set two weeks to change daily treatments to every second or third day, and by the third or fourth week I stop treatments. If symptoms recur, treatments are resumed on a daily basis. Some patients have continued treatment with topical preparations for months on a two- or three-times-a-week basis; others use this therapy for a few days to control mild exacerbations.

Certain generalizations can be made about topical steroid treatment: it is expensive, it tends to be less effective with repeated exacerbations and for some it does not help; in a few patients, symptoms are aggravated. The extent or type of colon disease or small bowel involvement should not deter its being tried if there is any evidence of rectal disease. Some patients' symptoms are helped even when x-ray and proctoscopic changes are not modified. Furthermore, topical steroids combined with systemic steroids may be more effective. They should be tried in combination even though either agent alone has failed.

Systemic steroids should be used when more conservative methods fail and should be maintained at as small a dose as possible for the control of symptoms. Steroids do retard growth and can produce side effects as undesirable as the illness under treatment.

When the decision is made to use systemic steroids, the initial dose should be large, i.e., prednisone, 40 to 60 mg. per day with a plan to taper the dose as soon as symptoms are controlled. If no response is obtained within a week, little is gained by pushing the dose upward; rather one should switch to adrenocorticotropic hormone (ACTH, 40 to 60 units daily) given either intravenously or intramuscularly. ACTH sometimes produces dramatic effects when oral or systemic prednisone or hydrocortisone in a comparable or larger dose has failed. As symptoms improve, the dose is tapered 5 to 10 units every second or third day, and the symptom response is observed. As the ACTH dose is tapered, oral prednisone is begun (20 to 30 mg. daily) with the eventual goal being to maintain the patient on the smallest oral dose of prednisone that will control symptoms. This is usually between 5 to 15 mg. daily. Once steroids are started they will need to be continued; relapses can be expected within a few days to weeks if they are stopped abruptly. Prolonged use of a small dose is usually well tolerated. The steroid dose must be dictated by the response. If exacerbations occur, increasing the dose 5 to 10 mg. per day may control symptoms and tapering can be started again on a slower schedule. Alternate-day or intermittent dosage schedules have been suggested to reduce complications but are not as effective as daily medications.

Those individuals whose symptoms are not controlled with steroids or who can only be controlled by doses that produce severe side effects should be considered for azathioprine treatment. Azathioprine (Imuran), 1 mg. per kilogram per day, combined with steroids may make it possible to use a tolerable dose of steroid while avoiding the usual azathioprine dose of 2 to 5 mg. per kilogram per day.* Therapeutic responses are more gradual and not as dramatic as with corticosteroids. The toxicity of azathioprine demands careful observation of blood, kidney and liver function. Anorexia, nausea and epigastric discomfort occur frequently. At the moment, many investigators are studying the place of immunosuppressive therapy in inflammatory bowel disease and a clearer picture of its value should be appearing shortly.

ANTIBACTERIAL AGENTS

Antibiotics have been most useful in controlling secondary infections, i.e., perirectal abscess or intra-abdominal sepsis but have not been helpful in uncomplicated ulcerative colitis or Crohn's disease. On many occasions when given for another problem such as a respiratory infection, they seem to exacerbate colitis symptoms. They should be used with clear indications.

The mode of action of salicylazosulfapyridine (Azulfidine) a diazo compound of salicylic acid and sulfapyridine, in inflammatory bowel disease is not known. It is only partially absorbed. Although its effectiveness in producing remission of ulcerative colitis has been documented by controlled clinical trials, it has been less well studied in Crohn's disease. Small dose maintenance therapy appears to reduce relapses.

The usual dose is 2 Gm. (one 500-mg. tablet four times a day) in adults and 40 mg. per kilogram in children, divided in three to six doses over a 24-hour period. A large initial dose is recommended: 4 to 8 Gm. to 12 Gm. (24 tablets) in adults and 75 to 150 mg. per kilogram for children in six to eight divided doses over a 24-hour period. In some patients, the larger dose must be maintained to control symptoms. The tablets are large and sometimes not well accepted by children. Anorexia, nausea and vomiting are common with large doses, but these symptoms may be eliminated by using the enteric-coated tablet or by reducing the dose.

Other adverse reactions are not rare and include rash, fever, headache, muscle pains and blood dyscrasias, such as agranulocytosis, thrombocytopenia, leukopenia, methemoglobinemia and hemolytic anemia, particularly in patients with glucose-6-phosphate dehydrogenase deficiency. The urine may turn orange-yellow if alkaline, and similar discolorations of the skin have been reported.

Obviously this drug must be given under careful supervision and patients watched for clinical signs of fever, sore throat, pallor, purpura or jaundice. Complete blood counts should be done at least weekly when therapy is begun. If the drug can be tolerated early, late difficulties with administration over several months are rare.

Other sulfonamides have been tried in colitis, particularly Sulfathalidine, but the reported results have not been encouraging.

SURGERY

Bowel perforation demands prompt colectomy. Such leaks can occur quite insidiously in patients receiving large doses of steroids and should be carefully watched for. Other complications, such as hemorrhage, toxic megacolon and obstruction, which do not respond promptly to treatment will require a colectomy. The difficult decision comes in defining intractability. It would be helpful if there were firm criteria, but there are not; one factor that must be eliminated in decision making is our own frustrations at inadequate therapeutic measures that only partially control this disease. Rather, we must assess the disability and risk of further medical treatment against colectomy and ileostomy. Total colon involvement, severe perirectal disease, intra-abdominal abscesses, growth failure and other serious complications, such as iritis or arthritis, not controlled after a reasonable trial with medical treatment are indications for surgery. Furthermore, if prolonged and heroic doses of corticosteroids are required with all the dismal and inevitable side effects, this seems an unreasonable price to pay for the control of this illness.

Crohn's disease treated surgically has a high incidence of recurrence and further surgery can produce nutritional invalids from inadequate bowel. Once the diagnosis is firmly established, further surgery should be delayed as long as possible.

In conclusion, surgery in ulcerative colitis and regional enteritis requires considerable

* Manufacturer's precaution: Imuran is investigational for this use.

skill. An ileostomy poorly constructed will make life intolerable. Therefore, when the decision is made to choose surgery, the very best and experienced surgeon available should be consulted.

References

Dyer, N. H.: Medical Management of Crohn's Disease. *Clinics in Gastroenterology,* 1:449–467, 1972.

Kirsner, J. B.: Ulcerative Colitis 1970—Recent Developments. *Scand. J. Gastroent.,* Suppl. 6, 63–91, 1970.

Jewell, D. P., and Truelove, S. C.: Azathioprine in Ulcerative Colitis: An Interim Report on a Controlled Therapeutic Trial. *Brit. Med. J.,* 1:709–712, 1972.

Patterson, M., Castiglioni, L., and Sampson, L.: Chronic Ulcerative Colitis Beginning in Children and Teenagers—A Review of 43 Patients. *Am. J. Dig. Dis.,* 16:289–297, 1971.

Peritonitis

ERIC W. FONKALSRUD, M.D.

Children with bacterial peritonitis, regardless of cause, usually experience hypovolemia and are best treated prior to surgery by expeditious infusion of irradiated plasma, 10 to 20 ml. per kilogram of body weight, and buffered Ringer's lactate solution or 5 per cent dextrose in half-normal saline. A central venous pressure catheter may supplement frequent recording of pulse and urinary output to determine the volume of fluid replacement necessary before the operation should be undertaken.

Aqueous penicillin (20,000 to 50,000 units per kilogram of body weight) is administered intravenously every 8 hours, and kanamycin (7.5 mg. per kilogram) is given intramuscularly every 12 hours. Fever is lowered with rectal aspirin or by a cooling mattress. A nasogastric tube is inserted routinely.

Patients with suspected ruptured appendix are placed in the semiFowler position and given analgesics intravenously (morphine sulfate, 1 mg. per 5 kilograms body weight). After 1 to 2 hours of fluid replacement and antibiotic therapy, operation is performed on patients with intestinal perforation or other inflammatory conditions that require prompt surgical management.

Intraoperative irrigation of the peritoneal cavity with saline solution has been used with diffuse peritonitis. This has not been employed when a walled-off abscess is drained. Peritoneal irrigation with dilute kanamycin solution has not found wide use in pediatric patients. Peritoneal cultures and smears should be obtained at operation and appropriate changes made in the antibiotic regimen when the organism and sensitivity are identified. The most common organisms cultured from the peritoneal cavity in children are *Escherichia coli, Staphylococcus aureus* and Pseudomonas. External drainage is used in most children with peritonitis; a rubber drain is used, with the central wick brought through the wound.

A prolonged period of postoperative ileus is to be expected, and vigilant management of fluid, electrolyte and nitrogen losses is imperative. Plasma has been effective in supplementing daily requirements of maintenance fluids. Antibiotics are continued until the patient has been afebrile for 48 hours. Subphrenic and pelvic abscesses are not uncommon and may require surgical drainage if not relieved by antibiotics. Intestinal obstruction due to adhesions may develop weeks or months after peritonitis, and females have been reported to have a decrease in fertility.

Lymphatic Obstruction of the Gastrointestinal Tract

PETER R. HOLT, M.D.

Intestinal lymphatic obstruction can be caused by congenital or acquired intrinsic diseases of the small intestine and by extraintestinal obstruction to lymphatic flow from the bowel. The therapy differs if the principal manifestation is chylous ascites or exudative enteropathy.

Considerable lymphatic obstruction may occur in celiac disease, regional enteritis, Whipple's disease, intestinal and mesenteric involvement with lymphoma and tuberculosis; the therapy is that of the primary disease. Extraintestinal obstruction to lymph flow in constrictive pericarditis is treated by pericardectomy. Localized obstruction by a single lymph cyst or tumor or peritoneal band is treated by abdominal exploration and surgical excision if this can be achieved without damage to the intestinal vasculature. When intestinal lymphangiectasia is localized or a large lymphatico-intestinal fistula is demonstrated, resection of involved bowel is indicated.

In severely sick patients, particularly after repeated paracenteses, replacement of fluid and electrolytes is imperative and intravenous plasma or albumin may be necessary. When tetany occurs, supplemental calcium or magnesium is needed. The diet should contain less than 100 mg. per kilogram of long chain fat daily (preferably in the form of linoleic acid to avoid essential fatty acid deficiency). To increase caloric intake, fat can be administered in the form of medium chain triglycerides. These are available as a powder (Portagen) containing 18 per cent protein, 22 per cent fat and 460 calories per 100 Gm., and can be diluted to make a formula for infants providing 20 calories per fluid ounce. This formula is nutritionally balanced and may be used as the sole source of food. The administration of Portagen has resulted in gastrointestinal distress or diarrhea in some patients. Most commonly this has been due to intolerance of the high lactose load present in the formula. Low lactose preparations of medium chain triglyceride combined with caseinate or hydrolyzed protein (Pregestimil) are now available direct from Mead Johnson Company for patients who do not tolerate Portagen.

Protein supplements in the form of mixed amino acids can be given, and parenteral fat-soluble vitamins are needed if significant steatorrhea is present. Supplemental oral iron preparations are often necessary. Lymphopenia and hypogammaglobulinemia are frequent, and recurrent infections need specific antibiotic therapy and occasionally parenteral gamma globulin. If tense ascites is troublesome, small paracenteses for relief are indicated, but special attention to sterility is essential because of the threat of infection. Recurrent paracenteses should be avoided because considerable loss of fluid, electrolytes and nutrients will follow. The potent diuretics show promise in treating chylous ascites and chronic peripheral edema but have not yet been approved for use in infants. Such a diuretic is furosemide* (Lasix) or ethacrynic acid† (Edecrin), 1 mg. per kilogram starting dose, orally or systemically, usually twice daily to a maximum of three times daily. These diuretics may be used indefinitely if the level of serum potassium is checked carefully.

If these measures fail, lymphaticovenous anastomosis of a dilated abdominal lymphatic vessel to the reflected saphenous vein just below a valve has been successfully employed. Peritoneal-venous anastomoses have been used for the therapy of chronic chylous ascites.

* Manufacturer's precaution: Furosemide should not be given to children until further experience is accumulated.

† Manufacturer's precaution: Infant dose of ethacrynic acid has not been established.

Cirrhosis and Tumors of the Liver

HARVEY L. SHARP, M.D.

CIRRHOSIS

A more definitive diagnosis than cirrhosis is essential for the optimal therapeutic approach to this aspect of hepatic disease. Identification of the inciting agent or process allows an attack on the primary problem rather than on the secondary manifestations. The supportive approach alone eventuates in a downhill struggle. Certain inherited disorders can be managed effectively by either diet or drugs. Also crucial is the early identification of inherited disorders in siblings to prevent any severe manifestations of the disease process.

The overall nutritional balance of the child with cirrhosis is generally dictated by the number of functioning hepatocytes. Special diets are not particularly helpful in children with cirrhosis, although the child should be encouraged to eat frequently and include foods with protein until signs of hepatic encephalopathy develop. Once ascites becomes significant, the sodium should be reduced in the diet.

One must familiarize parents with the signs and symptoms of potential fatal complications due to infection, hemorrhage and drugs. Such signs as fever, excessive thirst, black stools, lethargy or inappropriate behavior should signal the parents to contact their physician for early evaluation.

Ascites. A cautious conservative approach must be taken in the management of ascites, because electrolyte and fluid imbalance can easily precipitate hepatic coma, especially following metabolic alkalosis. Therefore, the diuretic management of ascites in liver disease requires more careful monitoring than does ascites in renal disease.

When mild ascites appears, salt restriction should be tried. Sometimes, surprisingly, long symptom-free intervals can be obtained by the administration of salt-poor albumin to ascitic children when the serum albumin level is below 2.5 Gm. per 100 ml. One aims for a serum albumin level of 3.0 Gm. per 100 ml. with the administration of 1 Gm. per kilogram of albumin per day (or 12.5 Gm. a day in the younger child and 25 Gm. in older children).

The first diuretic to be tried with progressive ascites is spironolactone (Aldactone), 3 mg. per kilogram per day, because usually there is no significant potassium loss. The dosage can be progressively increased to as high as 10 mg. per kilogram per day. The urine should be monitored for sodium-potassium ratios. When this urinary electrolyte ratio is greater than one, it is useless to pursue higher Aldactone doses to mobilize the ascites fluid. If no response from Aldactone is obtained, chlorothiazide (Diuril) is started at 10 mg. per kilogram per day and gradually increased to 40 mg. per kilogram if needed. Electrolytes must be closely monitored. Potassium replacement is essential to prevent metabolic alkalosis. Paracentesis with adequate intravenous colloid replacement is reserved for patients in severe respiratory embarrassment with nonresponsive ascites.

Comfort may be obtained in refractory cases by severe limitation of fluid intake, similar to the treatment of inappropriate antidiuretic hormone secretion. The fluid intake should equal the urine output plus 300 ml. per square meter. Another regimen in end stage liver disease is Lasix,* 60 mg. per square meter per day in two divided doses, and Aldactone, 62.5 mg. per square meter per day in four doses. Losses of more than a kilogram a day can precipitate fluid shifts dangerous to the well-being of the child.

Infection. A fever in a child with cirrhosis should elicit a careful evaluation for the following serious infectious complications: pneumonia, sepsis, meningitis and peritonitis. The most common causative organisms have been pneumococci, with *E. coli* and beta streptococci the less likely causes. A child with ascites who presents with abdominal pain and fever should be tapped with an intracath in the midline below the umbilicus. If the patient has had previous surgery or peritonitis, a surgeon should assist by providing a more direct look via an incision small enough to avoid intestinal puncture. Since these patients are prone to repeated septic episodes with pneumococci, I feel it is advantageous to administer prophylactic penicillin after the first episode. Immunization by pneumococcal polysaccharide may be a more scientific and safer approach to prophylaxis in the future.

Coagulation and Hemorrhage. Splenectomy should not be done for thrombocytopenia. The platelet count never gets low enough to cause serious hemorrhage. Nosebleeds are quite common in these patients but rarely cause significant bleeding. One of the parameters for hemorrhage and adequate blood replacement is the child's thirst and its alleviation by colloid replacement. As soon as the child reaches the hospital, an adequate line for blood infusion should be inserted. Transfusions with fresh blood are preferable, after colloid has been given to stabilize the blood pressure and initiate urine output. Twenty-five milligrams of vitamin K should be given slowly intravenously. Vital signs and urine output should be monitored closely. If evidence of persistent gastrointestinal bleeding is present, a soft lavage tube should be passed and the stomach aspirated and washed with iced saline. After bleeding has stopped, 250 to 500 mg. of neomycin may be administered through the tube four times a day. Two and one-half per cent neomycin enemas should be given to clear the blood from the bowel and alter the colonic bacteria to decrease the ammonia load to the liver.

Fortunately, gastrointestinal bleeding tends to be milder in children than in adults and usually can be conservatively managed. If blood loss persists or replacement is difficult, vasopressin† may be administered slowly intravenously over 10 to 20 minutes in doses of 10 to 20 units in 25 ml. of saline to temporarily reduce portal venous pressure. This dose can be repeated at 2- to 4- hour intervals if effective. Rarely is it necessary to insert a Sengstaken-Blakemore balloon tube, but pediatric sizes are available. Emergency surgery for exsanguinating bleeding from gastritis, ulcer or esophageal varices (unresponsive to the measures above) has not been necessary in the last 12 years.

Drugs. The drug most dangerous, besides diuretics, to the cirrhotic patient is aspirin, because of its propensity to initiate gastrointestinal bleeding. Thus, all parents must be told to use Tylenol for acute fever or pain. Anabolic steroids may improve nutrition and give some relief from pruritus, but one must accept the risk of (1) cholestasis and (2) peliosis hepatitis. Any drug may not be metabolized normally, but narcotics, long-acting sulfonamides, tetracyclines, Ilosone, Dilantin, phenothiazines and oxyphenisatin laxatives should be avoided. Halothane should not be used as an anesthetic agent, particularly if the patient has had a febrile reaction with previous exposure.

Hepatic Coma. Coma is usually the result of end stage liver disease, but certain other factors can precipitate coma. These include infection, electrolyte and fluid imbalance from

* Manufacturer's precaution: Lasix (furosemide) should not be given to children until further experience is accumulated.

† Manufacturer's precaution: Vasopressin has not been approved for intravenous use.

diuretics, surgery and hemorrhage. Diuretics should be stopped and the appropriate fluid regimens instituted. After hypovolemia has been corrected, fluid is limited to 1000 ml. per square meter. Protein should be restricted and gradually increased to 1 Gm. per kilogram when tolerated. Local antibiotics are given rectally and orally as summarized in the previous paragraph. Blood glucose levels and electrolytes are monitored closely, with appropriate correction in the intravenous fluids containing customarily between 5 and 10 per cent glucose. Huge replacements with potassium chloride are often necessary, limited only by decreasing urinary output associated with a rise in the blood creatinine.

TUMORS OF THE LIVER

Primary malignant and benign tumors of the liver require a surgical approach provided that only one lobe is involved and that no metastatic foci are present. Adequate catheters for rapid blood replacement are necessary prior to any resection attempt. Chemotherapy and radiation are only palliative. A benign adenoma or hamartoma is a joy to find at laparotomy.

In contrast, more clinical judgment is required for the management of infantile hepatic hemangioendothelioma, because the correct therapeutic approach is unknown. These lesions eventually regress spontaneously, similar to skin hemangiomas. Hence, if heart failure is not a severe problem, these children can be safely watched. Usually the lesion diffusely involves the liver and lobectomy is therefore not feasible. The severity of the heart failure dictates how aggressive the therapeutic approach should be. Radiation, three small doses of 150 rads, may be enough to tide the infant over until the lesions spontaneously regress. Recently, prednisone, 40 mg. every other day with gradual weaning over several weeks, has been reported to be beneficial. Otherwise, ligation of the hepatic artery has been reported to be successful. Cavernous hemangioma of the liver presents in the newborn with shock from vascular rupture. After a diagnostic abdominal tap, immediate surgery is the only hope for this rare disorder.

Aggressive therapy has been successful in metastatic Wilms' tumor. The most beneficial treatment thas been the use of actinomycin D plus radiation. One must be aware that the initial postoperative radiation to the right kidney bed may cause a focal hepatic lesion in the field, simulating a metastatic lesion. Metastasis has also responded to vincristine.‡ Even wedge resection of isolated metastatic lesions has resulted in cures.

Neuroblastoma with early hepatic involvement for some strange reason has a fairly good prognosis. Unfortunately, late metastatic involvement may only be palliated by vincristine‡ and Cytoxan (cyclophosphamide).

Portal Hypertension

SHEILA SHERLOCK, M.D.

Portal hypertension is nearly always due to obstruction to blood flow in the portal venous system. It can be divided into two main categories: presinusoidal, and sinusoidal or postsinusoidal. In the presinusoidal type of portal hypertension, the obstruction is in the main portal vein or in the portal vein radicles in the portal tracts. In the sinusoidal or postsinusoidal form of disease, the obstruction is at the level of the sinusoids, the central hepatic vein or in the main hepatic vein. This is the more prominent form in the cirrhoses. It is important to make the distinction. In the presinusoidal type of portal hypertension, hepatocellular function is intact, whereas in the second form, it is defective and liver cell failure is liable to be precipitated by hemorrhage.

In childhood the presinusoidal (extrahepatic) portal vein occlusion is more frequent. In the neonatal period, obstruction of the portal vein is usually secondary to umbilical sepsis. The infection spreads along the umbilical vein to the left branch of the portal vein and hence to the main portal vein. The portal vein may be obstructed by an abscess at the hilus of the liver following other neonatal infections. It may also follow an exchange transfusion through the umbilical vein.

In later childhood, infection is equally important, and conditions causing liver abscess, such as osteomyelitis and pylephlebitis following an appendix abscess or even a clinically missed appendicitis, must be included. Congenital anomalies of the portal venous system are exceedingly rare.

Congenital hepatic fibrosis is a rare form of intrahepatic presinusoidal portal hypertension. It is due to deficiency of terminal branches

‡ Manufacturer's precaution: Vincristine sulfate is investigational for radiation-resistant medulloblastomas. It is recommended only for treatment of acute leukemia in childhood.

of the portal vein in the densely fibrotic portal zones of the liver. It is readily confused with cirrhosis.

Cirrhosis can be due to previous neonatal hepatitis, viral hepatitis, Wilson's disease, galactosemia, tyrosinosis or other metabolic liver disease or active chronic ("lupoid") hepatitis, and in many instances it is cryptogenetic. Postsinusoidal portal hypertension can follow toxic involvement of the central hepatic veins due to Senecio (Ragwort). Rarer causes of postsinusoidal portal hypertension in childhood include congenital valves and webs in the hepatic veins and vena cava and constrictive pericarditis.

Diagnosis and Investigation. Treatment depends upon accurate localization of the site of obstruction and, if possible, knowledge of the cause.

A careful history should be taken of pyrexia and sepsis in the neonatal period, neonatal jaundice and viral hepatitis. A family history of conditions such as Wilson's disease or galactosemia should be noted.

Special examinations should include slit lamp examination for the presence of Kayser-Fleischer rings, the stigmas of cirrhosis, particularly vascular spiders, jaundice, firm hepatomegaly, edema and ascites. The features of portal hypertension include splenomegaly and dilated epigastric abdominal wall veins, the flow being upward.

Special Investigations. Serum biochemical tests include determination of the serum bilirubin, transaminase and gamma globulin levels, all of which tend to be increased in cirrhosis in young people. Too much attention should not be paid to the serum alkaline phosphatase value, which exceeds adult values in normal infants and children. The hemoglobin and, if possible, the serum iron level should be estimated and a blood film studied as an index of gastrointestinal hemorrhage. The leukocyte and the platelet count may be depressed secondary to enlargement of the spleen. A barium series is performed to confirm esophageal and gastric varices.

Delay in diagnosis is usually due to failure to perform liver biopsy and splenic venography. In children these may be done under general anesthesia on the same occasion. The intrasplenic pressure is estimated at the same time, and this is used as a baseline for further serial determinations. It is also useful to confirm that portal hypertension is present. The splenic pressure may be normal if the portal-systemic collateral circulation is sufficiently great. If the spleen has already been removed, selective celiac or mesenteric angiography via the femoral artery may be done. The portal circulation is followed by exposing serial films, and the portal vein and portal-systemic collaterals are visualized in the venous phase of the angiogram.

There may be doubt whether to perform these special and rather complicated investigations in an apparently otherwise well child who has splenomegaly. They are virtually without risk and should be undertaken without delay once portal hypertension is diagnosed, even before hemorrhage has taken place. Knowledge of the anatomy of the portal system and the cause of the portal hypertension allows management to be rational and enables any surgical procedure to be tailored to the actual state of the portal system.

Management Before and Between Hemorrhages. Apart from any treatment necessary for underlying cirrhosis, the child should be allowed to lead as normal a life as possible. He should attend ordinary school, and provided the spleen is not too large, games and physical education may be allowed. Particularly vigorous sports, such as football, must be forbidden. The child should not be allowed to become overly tired. The school principal should be informed of the situation, and the parents should not press the child to be overly competitive in either work or play.

Note should be taken of fecal color and the parents told to report if it becomes black. Hemoglobin estimations should be done if the child appears anemic or passes black stools. Oral iron treatment is given as required. The cirrhotic child requires occasional estimations of the prothrombin time, and intramuscular vitamin K_1 (5 mg.) may be useful from time to time.

Hemorrhage commonly follows an upper respiratory tract infection, and these should be avoided if possible and all necessary inoculations given. If infection develops, it should be taken seriously and broad-spectrum antibiotics given from the start. Drugs containing acetylsalicylic acid must be avoided.

Undue attention should not be paid to the platelet and leukocyte counts. Although both may be low, the effects on the patient are not definite. Multiple infections are unusual. Low values should not indicate splenectomy.

Management of Hemorrhage. If the diagnosis is in doubt and the technique has not been performed previously, an emergency percutaneous splenic venogram must be done.

If the patient is cirrhotic, hepatic precoma and coma may be precipitated by the hemorrhage. This should be anticipated by giving no protein by mouth, keeping the bowels moving freely, giving an enema if necessary and prescribing oral neomycin, 15 mg. per kilogram four times a day for three days. All types of sedation should be avoided. If the child has extrahepatic portal venous obstruction and normal hepatic function, there is virtually no danger of the development of hepatic precoma. The precoma regimen is therefore unnecessary, and sedation can be given as required. It is unusual for these patients to bleed before the age of three years.

Blood transfusion is usually necessary. In patients with extrahepatic portal obstruction, hemorrhages are likely to be multiple over years. The greatest possible care must be taken to preserve peripheral veins for further transfusions and to give absolutely compatible blood.

If liver cell function is adequate, the bleeding usually ceases spontaneously. If liver cell function is deficient and if the bleeding continues, I prefer to use vasopressin (Pitressin) intravenously, although this route is not recommended by the manufacturer. This drug lowers portal venous pressure by constriction of the splanchnic arterial bed, causing an increase in resistance to the inflow of blood to the gut. It controls hemorrhage from esophageal varices by lowering portal venous pressure. A large dose, 1 unit per 3 kilograms of body weight is given well diluted in 5 per cent dextrose intravenously in 10 minutes. Mean arterial pressure increases transiently, and portal pressure decreases for three-quarters to one hour.

The stomach is aspirated every 30 minutes through a gastric tube, and control of hemorrhage is shown by the disappearance of blood from the aspirate and by serial pulse and blood pressure readings. Abdominal colicky discomfort and evacuation of the bowels, together with facial pallor, are usual during the infusion. If these are absent, it may be questioned whether the vasopressin is pharmacologically active. Inert material is the most common cause of failure. Regular vasopressin injections may be repeated in 4 hours if bleeding recurs, but efficacy decreases with continual use. The ultimate failure of vasopressin to control terminal hemorrhage reflects hepatocellular failure rather than improper method of treatment.

The value of vasopressin is its simplicity of use. In an emergency it can even be used in the home. Special nursing and medical care are not essential. The short duration is obviously unsatisfactory, and the side effects are unpleasant even if short-lived. However, this dosage is necessary to achieve an adequate reduction in portal pressure.

If vasopressin fails to produce the desired effect, the Sengstaken trilumen esophageal compression tube is used. A special small-sized tube is available for pediatric use. A rubber tube is inflated in the esophagus at a pressure of 20 to 30 mm. Hg, slightly greater than that expected in the portal vein. Another balloon, to be filled with weak radiopaque solution, is in the fundus of the stomach. The third lumen communicates with the stomach. The tube is passed relatively easily if the pharynx is well anesthetized. When the tube is in position, traction has to be exerted and this causes difficulty. Too little traction means that the gastric balloon falls back into the stomach. Too much traction causes discomfort, with retching, and potentiates gastroesophageal ulceration.

The compression tubes are very successful in controlling bleeding from esophageal varices. They do, however, have many complications. They should not be left inflated longer than 24 hours. Their use should be part of a plan of management culminating either in surgery or in withdrawal of the tube and conservative treatment if the patient's condition is too poor. Complications include obstruction of the pharynx with consequent asphyxia, aspiration pneumonia and ulceration of pharynx, esophagus and fundus of the stomach. The tube is not well tolerated by the patient. Skilled nursing is required for supervision of the patient while the tube is in position.

Emergency surgery is rarely necessary. If bleeding does not cease or if it recurs and active intervention becomes essential, the best surgical method is probably transthoracic, transesophageal direct ligation of the bleeding varices. In patients having normal liver function, and in whom the splenic venogram has shown a portal or splenic vein of adequate caliber, a portacaval or splenorenal shunt may be performed. Emergency shunt surgery has a high mortality rate if the patient has cirrhosis, and if possible should be avoided in these circumstances.

Elective Surgery. Prophylactic surgery is not indicated. The patient must have bled from varices before operation can be considered. The choice of procedure depends largely upon the state of the portal venous system as revealed by splenic venography or selective splanchnic angiography. If the portal vein is patent and of adequate caliber, end-to-side portacaval anastomosis is the most satisfactory procedure. In experienced hands this operation carries a low mortality rate of less than 5 per cent. Because of vein size, the operation can rarely be undertaken before the age of 10 years. It carries a small risk of shunt encephalopathy. In children this is particularly small, and in the presence of a normal liver, e.g., obstruction to the portal vein at the hilus of the liver, the chances are almost nonexistent. In the presence of cirrhosis, the possibility varies with the degree of underlying damage to the liver. The operation should not be performed in the presence of jaundice, ascites or a past history of hepatic coma.

Splenorenal anastomosis may be considered in portal venous occlusion if the splenic vein is of adequate size. It is less efficient than a portacaval anastomosis, because the shunt is small and often occludes. The danger of post-shunt encephalopathy, however, is very small.

Superior mesenteric vein–inferior vena caval shunt is used to treat portal hypertension in patients who have occlusion of the portal and splenic veins, making neither available for anastomosis. The vena cava is transected just proximal to the junction of the two iliac veins, and the distal segment is ligated. The proximal segment is then anastomosed to the side of the intact superior mesenteric vein. Technically it may not be easy. Failures may be due to superior mesenteric vein thrombosis, and the mortality rate is about 16 per cent. Ligature of the inferior vena cava is inevitable. Nevertheless, this operation, provided it is done by an experienced surgeon, provides a better chance of improvement in patients with extrahepatic portal venous obstruction than do the various local attacks on esophageal or other varices.

Direct attacks on the varices and on various dangerous collaterals are numerous and rarely of long-lasting benefit. They include splenectomy, transection of the esophagus, partial and total gastrectomy and partial esophagectomy. In general, they are not to be recommended. Patients with extrahepatic portal venous obstruction rarely die of exsanguinating hemorrhage. Conservative management usually helps them over the acute episode. Bleeding becomes more infrequent as time allows for the opening of collateral vessels to the renal and lumbar veins. Ultimately, portal pressure may decrease. This possibility may be lessened with repeated operations and removal or transection of such benign collaterals. The operative and postoperative mortality rate of the local operations on varices in a cirrhotic patient with borderline liver function is high, and the ultimate benefit doubtful.

Reference

Sherlock, S.: *Diseases of the Liver and Biliary System.* 4th ed., revised. Philadelphia, F. A. Davis Co., 1971, p. 199.

Chronic Aggressive Hepatitis

HARVEY L. SHARP, M.D.

Currently, the only proved use of immunosuppressive therapy is in chronic aggressive hepatitis or liver transplantation. Chronic aggressive hepatitis may present in a variety of ways, such as (1) nonresolving hepatitis, (2) recurrent hepatitis, (3) indolent hepatosplenomegaly or (4) a mass in the abdomen. All affected patients have elevated hepatic cellular enzymes. Many have evidence of other "autoimmune" disease processes, such as thyroiditis, ulcerative colitis or diabetes, or simulate lupus erythematosus (LE) without kidney involvement. Weakly positive or suspicious LE clot tests, the presence of tart cells and other positive tests for immune phenomena are often found. When evidence for an "autoimmune" disease is not present, Wilson's disease must be ruled out. Serum gamma globulin levels are often strikingly elevated as high as 4 to 8 Gm. per 100 ml. Australia antigen has not been found in our patients.

A liver biopsy is important for ultimate prognosis, but an open liver biopsy should not be undertaken in a severely ill child. Coagulation studies sometimes prohibit even attempting a closed percutaneous needle biopsy. In these circumstances, an abnormal LE clot test, gamma globulin levels above 5 Gm. per 100 ml. or evidence of a circulating anticoagulant is sufficient evidence to initiate therapy.

The following pathologic changes are usually found in liver biopsy specimens: Aggressive inflammation, including many plasma cells, with piecemeal necrosis altering the hepatocytes along the limiting plate, are the most important and prominent pathologic changes found in the portal areas. In contrast, the liver biopsy of chronic persistent hepatitis contains only chronic inflammation without invasion of the limiting plate and little evidence of portal fibrosis. No immunosuppressive therapy is necessary for this second entity and the outlook for the patient is good. A lack of significant inflammation in the liver prior to any therapeutic endeavor also indicates that medication will be of little benefit. On the other hand, if the biopsy is obtained after 10 days of steroid therapy, the plasma cells may have vanished. The amount of necrosis, inflammation, fibrosis, cirrhosis and regenerative nodules varies with the individual patient. The long-term prognosis is poorer in those patients with marked cirrhosis and regenerative nodules on the initial biopsy and lack of evidence of an immune phenomenon by laboratory testing. Obviously, massive necrosis is a poor immediate sign for even initial recovery.

Treatment is initiated with prednisone at 40 mg. per square meter per day. This dose is continued until liver function tests show marked improvement. If no improvement is seen in one week, the dose is increased to 60 mg. per square meter per day. When it is clear that the patient is improving, the steroids are switched to every other day at double the original dose. High-dose steroid therapy continues until liver function studies return completely to normal. Then the every-other-day prednisone dose is gradually tapered, but liver function tests are constantly monitored with each change. It is customary to find that patients require around 25 mg. of prednisone every other day to avoid exacerbation of their disease as evidenced by liver enzyme elevation.

Six-mercaptopurine (6MP) may be helpful in several circumstances. (1) We tend to use it in conjunction with prednisone because of the psychologic effects in teenage girls secondary to hypercortisonism. In these instances we have accepted the risk of using two immunosuppressive drugs, believing we can decrease the prednisone dose sooner and thus maintain the patients on 6MP alone. This regimen has not always been successful; therefore, both drugs are sometimes required to maintain normal liver function. (2) We add 6MP when the patient is not responding well to the prednisone. This has been successful on occasion but the need to do this is a poor prognostic sign. (3) Rapid mortality in two four-year-old girls treated with prednisone has prompted me to use 6MP alone in similar instances, with satisfactory results. (4) An early relapse after discontinuation of medication may respond nicely to 6MP alone. The dose of 6MP is always less than 1 mg. per kilogram per day. Higher doses have been associated with evidence of liver toxicity or very severe white blood cell depression.

Low doses of immunosuppressive therapy are continued for two to four years. Exacerbations after discontinuation of medication usually occur within six months of withdrawal. After one year off medication the outlook is good. The immediate response to high-dose prednisone is usually rapid in contrast to the response to 6MP, which may require four to six weeks before improvement is seen. Gamma globulin levels rapidly decrease to normal with prednisone, whereas the levels decrease less rapidly with 6MP. When splenomegaly does not rapidly resolve with prednisone, severe cirrhosis is already present; this is a poor long-term prognostic sign. The leukopenia seen with 6MP is usually prevented by prednisone. The side effects of hypercortisonism, including obesity, osteoporosis and increased susceptibility to infection, are even more apparent in patients with liver disease. We particularly watch for evidence of a gastrointestinal ulcer and add antacids on a 2-hour schedule as soon as any signs appear. Initially, we monitor electrolytes and frequently find that we need to add supplemental liquid potassium chloride to prevent metabolic alkalosis even when the patient is not receiving diuretics. Eyes are closely observed for cataracts by slit lamp examination. The 6MP dosage is decreased when peripheral white counts drop to the 3000 to 4000 range, and it is stopped at counts under 3000. Another reason for temporarily stopping the 6MP arises when herpes simplex infections occur. A minor side effect of 6MP is thinning of the hair. Patients are warned of the possible teratogenic effects of 6MP and are counseled to avoid becoming pregnant. Neither drug should be started for 7 to 10 days after an open liver biopsy in order to allow time for adequate wound healing.

The therapeutic objective is to suppress the active destruction of hepatocytes by inflammation in order to prevent further necrosis and collapse which result in cirrhosis. Liver function tests are monitored, and completely normal studies are an indication of adequate therapy. The results of this aggressive therapeutic approach were last summarized in 1968, and the details can be found in the reference following this article. Subsequently, the series has continued to expand, but we have not had any further deaths in our long-term follow-up studies.

Reference

Page, A. R., Good, R. A., and Pollara, B.: Long-term Results of Therapy in Patients with Chronic Liver Disease Associated with Hypergamma Globulinemia. *Am. J. Med.*, 47:765, 1969.

Congenital Abnormalities of the Gallbladder and Bile Ducts

HARVEY L. SHARP, M.D.

Obstructive jaundice during infancy may be associated with several entities, including severe hemolytic anemia, infections (generalized septicemia, urinary tract infection, syphilis, toxoplasmosis, rubella and cytomegalic inclusion disease), galactosemia, cystic fibrosis and alpha-l-antitrypsin deficiency.

The most common disease of the biliary system, extrahepatic biliary atresia, is fatal unless bile can physiologically leave the liver. Therefore, every effort must be made to reinstitute bile drainage as quickly as possible.

The rose bengal ^{131}I clearance method assures a preoperative diagnosis of complete obstruction and obviates unnecessary surgery on infants with intrinsic nonoperative problems. This procedure requires careful performance, following an accurate intravenous injection, to measure the total amount of isotope cleared in a two-day collection of stools uncontaminated by urine. A percutaneous liver biopsy, although not diagnostic, can be complementary if bile duct proliferation, particularly pseudoductular formation, is found. At present, other tests related to liver function have been nondiagnostic.

Management. SURGERY. Although significant coagulation abnormalities are rarely seen early in the disease, prothrombin time, partial thromboplastin time and platelet count should be determined. An abnormality in the first two values may usually be corrected by administering 5 to 10 mg. of vitamin K. At laparotomy a liver biopsy is performed. Cholangiography is attempted through the gallbladder, if present, with only a small amount of dye injected through a tightly secured polyethylene tube. This study visualizes the common duct when present. A simple surgical procedure cures the patient if a distal obstruction is found. Unfortunately, this is not the usual location of the atresia. When the hepatic radicles are not visualized, the dye injection is repeated with gentle occlusion of the distal part of the common duct. If no patent system is found after thorough investigation of the extrahepatic biliary tree, the porta hepatis should be explored. This proposed undertaking is derived from postmortem evidence of biliary-lined cystic structures bulging from the porta hepatis. Because such structures communicate with intrahepatic bile ducts, this is a potentially drainable area. This difficult dissection requires experience, because during initial exploration these structures can be mistaken for lymphatics. Simple needle insertion into this region is misleading because the bile is too thick to be aspirated.

Any infant presenting with a mass extrinsic to the liver, who may also have abdominal pain, intermittent jaundice or significant vomiting, has either a choledochal cyst or an anomaly of the cystic duct resulting in an enlarged gallbladder. In addition, all infants in whom jaundice persists for six months ought to have a laparotomy.

If no abnormality of the extrahepatic system is found, external drainage of the gallbladder is provided. The number of bile ducts per portal area in the liver biopsy needs to be determined. Clearing of jaundice following drainage of gallbladder bile indicates that such patients may respond to the resin cholestyramine.

CHOLESTYRAMINE. Cholestyramine (Questran) is an oral resin medication which exchanges its chloride ion for bile acids excreted into the duodenum. The bile-acid binder is available to alleviate pruritus in patients who have patency of the biliary system. In addition, liver function (except for alkaline phosphatase) and liver size return toward normal if the levels of serum bile acids are decreased to the normal range. Beginning dosage is 2 Gm. four times a day mixed in a suitable vehicle, such as orange juice, applesauce or milk formula. The dosage is increased until normal values for serum bile acids are obtained. We have given as much as 16 Gm. a day to infants and 36 Gm. to older children, in contrast to the dosage of 4 to 12 Gm. used to control pruritus in adults. The original resin had a peculiar taste, but with continual improvement it is now fairly palatable. Adults have taken as much as 28 Gm. a day to lower the cholesterol level under study conditions. [The manufacturer recommends a usual dose of 12 Gm. per day (maximum of 24 Gm.) for adults and for children over six years of age. The manufacturer also stipulates that the dosage for children under six years has not been established.]

Some patients, particularly those whose livers contain less than one bile duct per portal triad, may benefit from this therapy. The following possible side effects have been noted: An interference with the absorption of fat-soluble vitamins can be prophylactically prevented by the administration of water-soluble vitamins (10,000 units of vitamin A, 800 to 1600 units of vitamin D, vitamin K as 2.5 mg. a day by mouth or 10 mg. a week intramuscularly and vitamin E as 100 units of Aquasol E). Metabolic acidosis may develop infrequently because of the absorption of the chloride ion, but it responds readily to sodium bicarbonate. Calcification or stones within the biliary tree have been reported in two adults with liver disease. Iron deficiency anemia may develop with long-term high-dose administration. We find minimal problems in getting our patients to take this resin, because the relief from pruritus provided by this medication compensates for any unpalatability, and the improvement in liver function and weight gain gives continual encouragement. Perhaps when it is introduced in the first year of life, there may be less taste discretion by the infants. In children with xanthomas, a diet low in cholesterol with two-thirds of the fat in unsaturated form has been helpful in addition to the cholestyramine.

MEDIUM CHAIN TRIGLYCERIDES. Improvement in the nutritional status in biliary diseases can be achieved in two-thirds of patients by the ingestion of medium chain triglycerides (Portagen), which are transported by the portal vein to the liver for rapid utilization. This form of fat is reasonably well absorbed even in the absence of pancreatic lipase or bile salts. A decrease in stool volume within 10 days and a gain in weight within the first month of administration are noted. This nutritional gain cannot be accounted for by improvement in the disease process. Those who do not gain weight usually have evidence of quite severe liver dysfunction. The liquid formula, a complete dietary supplement, is started at 8 ounces on the first day, increased by 8 ounces for each of the next two days and then maintained at 24 to 28 ounces a day. A slow dietary initiation avoids the cramping or diarrhea secondary to the higher osmolar load. The sodium content of Portagen is 370 mg. per quart, based on reconstitution at 20 calories per fluid ounce. A change in diet may be necessary when ascites develops if the patient does not respond readily to diuretics.

Recently, Pregestimil (AD3200) has become available from the same company (Mead Johnson). In addition to the medium chain triglycerides, it contains carbohydrates in the form of dextrose, and protein in the form of casein enzymatically hydrolyzed and charcoal-treated to reduce allergenicity. These alterations may prove to be more beneficial nutritionally. We have found it helpful for the increasing number of newborns, now being seen in the intensive care units, with the combination of short gastrointestinal tracts, hyperalimentation lines and obstructive jaundice.

PHENOBARBITAL. For years phenobarbital has been known to have a marked choluretic action in rats, but the basic mechanism is unknown and not related to alteration of bile salts in the rodent. Recently, phenobarbital has been shown to increase bile flow in children with intrahepatic obstructive jaundice but patent bile duct systems. These children have abnormal bile salt metabolism which is altered by this medication. We have used phenobarbital in the following circumstances: (1) in patients who fail to respond to cholestyramine, (2) in patients with minimal bile salt secretion from the liver, and (3) in newborn infants with obstructive jaundice in combination with short gut difficulties. The beginning dose is 3 mg. per kilogram per day, which can be gradually increased every two weeks up to 5 to 6 mg. per kilogram per day. Some can tolerate even higher doses. The clinical responses have not been as dramatic as we have seen following the administration of cholestyramine, but phenobarbital has benefited certain patients. It is poorly tolerated in children with long-term cirrhosis. They become quite irritable or drowsy owing to the higher phenobarbital plasma levels. Other side effects include suppression of immunity and bone changes with long-term administration. Its effect on other drugs used in patients with liver disease has not been evaluated in the clinical situation.

References

Sharp, H. L., Carey, J. B., Jr., White, J. G., and Krivit, W.: Cholestyramine Therapy in Patient with a Paucity of Intrahepatic Bile Ducts. *J. Pediat.*, 71:723, 1967.

Sharp, H. L., Krivit, W., and Lowman, J. T.: The Diagnosis of Complete Extrahepatic Obstruction by Rose Bengal ^{131}I. *J. Pediat.*, 70:46, 1967.

Sharp, H. L., and Mirkin, B. L.: Effect of Phenobarbital on Hyperbilirubinemia, Bile Acid Metabolism, and Microsomal Enzyme Activity in Chronic Intrahepatic Cholestasis of Childhood. *J. Pediat.*, 81:116, 1972.

Diseases of the Pancreas

ERIC W. FONKALSRUD, M.D.

PANCREATITIS

Although pancreatitis is an uncommon disease in children, it does occur with sufficient frequency to warrant consideration in the differential diagnosis of abdominal pain and vomiting. Pancreatitis in children rarely is caused by peptic ulcer or choledocholithiasis as is characteristic in adults. The signs and symptoms in children are similar to those observed in adults, frequently the manifestations of an acute surgical abdomen. Several types of pancreatitis have been recognized in children (Fonkalsrud et al.).

Pancreatitis Associated with Steroid Therapy

Pancreatitis develops occasionally in children with collagen vascular diseases, nephrosis or other conditions that have been treated with steroids or immunosuppressive drugs such as azathioprine. The mechanism by which steroids induce pancreatitis is unclear, although it is believed that the underlying disease may be a predisposing factor. It is also unclear whether steroids should be discontinued for the duration of the pancreatitis in such patients, although immunosuppressive therapy should be terminated. Laparotomy in these acutely ill patients should be avoided. Hyperamylasemia helps to distinguish this condition from acute appendicitis.

Obstructive Pancreatitis

Pancreatic obstruction in the child usually is due to congenital malformation of the ducts and rarely to common bile duct obstruction. Choledochal cysts, stenosis or hypoplasia of the common bile duct, stenosis of the duct of Santorini or ampulla of Vater and annular pancreas may cause pancreatitis. Treatment of this form of pancreatitis should be directed toward operative relief of the obstruction by choledochointestinal or cholecystointestinal anastomosis, sphincterotomy or duodenojejunostomy.

The worm *Ascaris lumbricoides* has produced pancreatitis in children by mechanical blockage of the pancreatic ducts. Antihelmintic drugs, such as piperazine syrup (3 Gm. daily for two days for children weighing from 25 to 45 kilograms), may prevent recurrence but rarely relieves the acute obstruction in the pancreatic or common bile ducts. Operative removal of the parasite usually is required.

Choledocholithiasis is extremely uncommon in young children and is seen only rarely in adolescents. Cholecystectomy and choledocholithotomy usually are followed by resolution of the pancreatitis. Pancreatitis also has been observed in children with acalculous cholecystitis, presumably as a consequence of the closely situated inflammatory process.

Post-Traumatic Pancreatitis

Blunt and penetrating abdominal injuries may be followed by acute pancreatitis in children. If the duct is unobstructed and drainage is satisfactory, formidable pancreatitis usually does not develop in the traumatized pancreas. Because post-traumatic pancreatic pseudocysts in children usually are very thin-walled, enteric anastomosis is technically very difficult or unfeasible.

Pancreatitis Due to Systemic Infection

Pancreatitis caused by mumps is not uncommon, and the diagnosis usually can be based on clinical signs, such as abdominal pain and nausea. Rest usually is all that is required for these patients; they rarely need hospitalization.

Generalized sepsis, such as that which follows a ruptured appendix, has produced hemorrhagic pancreatitis. Major hemorrhage may ensue because of intravascular coagulopathy and frequently is fatal.

Hereditary Pancreatitis

This unusual form of recurrent pancreatitis is believed to be caused by multiple areas of duct stenosis and usually produces symptoms before the age of five. Operative drainage of the pancreatic duct by means of a Puestow procedure or lateral pancreaticojejunostomy should be performed early to prevent lithiasis, diabetes, steatorrhea and pseudocysts.

Idiopathic Pancreatitis

In many children, pancreatitis occurs in the absence of obvious causative factors. The mortality rate in this group of patients is high, regardless of therapy.

Management. Replenishment of body fluids and blood is of primary importance and may be guided by variations in the central venous pressure and blood electrolytes. Volumes greater than 3000 ml. per square meter of body surface area per day may be necessary. Normal saline or Ringer's lactate solution should be given initially, with irradiated plasma (10 to 20 ml. per kilogram of body weight per 24 hours) to compensate for pooling of fluids in the abdomen. When urinary flow becomes adequate, a solution containing 5 per cent dextrose and half-normal saline plus 20 to 40 mEq. (1.5 to 3 Gm.) per liter of potassium chloride should be used. When acute fluid losses have been corrected, the daily fluid requirement may be calculated on the basis of 1500 ml. per square meter of body surface area per 24 hours plus replacement of nasogastric drainage, using 5 per cent dextrose and half-normal saline plus 20 to 30 mEq. of potassium chloride per liter. Albumin (25 to 50 Gm.) or plasma (10 ml. per kilogram of body weight) should be given daily in divided doses.

Aspiration of abdominal fluid may help to alleviate respiratory distress if the diaphragm is elevated. Calcium gluconate (10 per cent), in a dose of 40 to 100 ml. per day, should be added to the intravenous fluids if hypocalcemia is present. When there are bowel sounds and flatus is passed, clear liquids may be started and the diet gradually progressed to solids with high carbohydrate and low fat content. Gastric stimulants, such as tea and coffee, should be avoided.

Hormonal stimulation of the pancreas by secretin should be reduced, and gastric and pancreatic function should be depressed with nasogastric suction and anticholinergic drugs, such as atropine sulfate, 0.01 mg. per kilogram of body weight, administered subcutaneously every 4 to 6 hours, but not to exceed 0.4 mg. per dose. A smaller dose should be used if excessive dryness of the mouth, flushing of the skin, dilatation of the pupils or hyperpyrexia occurs. Propantheline bromide may be given intramuscularly in four equal doses totaling 1.5 mg. per kilogram per 24 hours, although atropine is preferred during the first two to four days of therapy.

Pain and sphincter spasm may be relieved or prevented by the intramuscular administration of meperidine hydrochloride, 1 to 1.5 mg. per kilogram of body weight every 4 to 6 hours. Morphine is contraindicated.

Broad-spectrum antibiotics usually are recommended once the diagnosis of acute pancreatitis is established, particularly if duct obstruction is the cause.

Surgical drainage of the peritoneal cavity with large sump catheters may be of great benefit to patients with acute hemorrhagic pancreatitis.

ANNULAR PANCREAS

Complete annular pancreas frequently occurs in association with duodenal atresia and causes obstruction high in the intestine of the newborn, with bilious emesis and minimal abdominal distention. The diagnosis may be established by the characteristic "double bubble" appearance on abdominal roentgenograms. A number 10 short rubber nasogastric tube should be inserted and attached to low intermittent suction. If the infant is less than 48 hours old, minimal preoperative hydration usually is necessary. After typing and crossmatching for blood, and administration of phytonadione (vitamin K), 1 mg. intramuscularly, surgical correction should be undertaken. A side-to-side duodenoduodenostomy (two-layer anastomosis) is performed to relieve the obstruction. The pancreas should not be divided. Biliary obstruction rarely occurs in these patients. A Stamm tube gastrostomy with a number 16 rubber mushroom catheter is recommended.

In infants who have been vomiting, serum electrolyte determinations should be performed, and appropriate electrolyte solutions should be administered prior to operation. Approximately one-third of these infants are mongoloid.

In patients with incomplete annular pancreas or with complete annular pancreas but incomplete duodenal obstruction, obstructive symptoms may not be seen for months or even years. Upper gastrointestinal contrast roentgenograms are essential to establish the diagnosis. Duodenoduodenostomy is recommended for these patients and usually is attended with low risk.

HYPOGLYCEMIA

Hypoglycemia in infants and children usually requires a carefully planned investigation to determine the cause. Surgical treatment has been particularly beneficial in children with functioning islet cell adenomas and idiopathic hypoglycemia, presumably due to islet cell hyperplasia. Medical or surgical treatment must be instituted before irreparable brain damage occurs.

The functioning islet cell adenoma is one of the few completely curable causes of hypoglycemia in childhood. Functioning islet cell carcinoma is uncommon in the pediatric age group.

The diagnosis may be strongly suspected on the basis of a positive Whipple's triad: (1) spontaneous hypoglycemia accompanied by central nervous system or vasomotor system symptoms, (2) repeated fasting blood sugar determinations below 50 mg. per 100 ml. and (3) relief of symptoms by oral or intravenous administration of glucose. The most valuable laboratory aid is the frequent determination of the blood sugar level after various periods of fasting or exercise.

When the presence of an islet cell adenoma is confirmed or even suspected, laparotomy should be performed. If one or more discrete adenomas are found, they may be removed generally by simple enucleation or local wedge resection. If an adenoma cannot be visualized or palpated after extensive mobilization of the pancreas, pancreaticoduodenal resection with removal of the head of the pancreas is more likely to yield the adenoma than is blind resection of the body and tail of the gland. Although two-thirds of islet cell adenomas occur in the body and tail of the gland, these lesions usually are more readily exposed than are adenomas concealed in the head and uncinate process. An intravenous solution containing 10 per cent dextrose is administered during the operation as the gland is manipulated. The blood sugar level in most patients is elevated to 200 or 300 mg. per 100 ml. during the postoperative period, gradually returning to normal values three to five days later. Small amounts of regular zinc insulin may be given during this period.

In children with idiopathic severe hypoglycemia, which usually appears within the first two years of life, serious consideration should be given to performing a blind distal 75 per cent pancreatectomy. If islet cell hyperplasia is present in the tissue removed, a favorable result and good prognosis usually may be anticipated.

PANCREATIC NEOPLASMS

Ulcerogenic tumors of the pancreas (Zollinger-Ellison syndrome) have been reported in children under 15 years of age; they are familial in many instances. These tumors may be suspected when peptic ulcers are in unusual locations, when the 12-hour gastric secretory volume and free acidity are unusually high, and when peptic ulceration recurs despite good medical or surgical management. Diarrhea is an important symptom and may occur without ulceration.

Total gastrectomy as the initial definitive ulcer procedure has yielded the best survival rate; this should be combined with resection of the tumor (if feasible) short of total pancreatectomy. Since 61 per cent of these patients have malignant tumors, 44 per cent of which have metastasized when first diagnosed, gastrectomy and pancreatectomy may not be possible. Since these malignancies may be slow growing, wide resection, combined with radiotherapy to control the peptic ulcer and the tumor, may be rewarding.

Carcinoma of the pancreas is uncommon in infants and children. Most of these tumors are nonfunctioning islet cell tumors and begin in the head of the gland. Longterm survival has been reported in several children following pancreaticoduodenectomy. When extensive resection of the pancreas is performed, insulin and pancreatic exocrine supplements must be given. Cotazym, 1 to 3 tablets after each meal, has been most successful in our experience. Weight and growth generally can be maintained by a high carbohydrate, high protein, low fat diet. Initially, frequent feedings may be necessary to minimize the symptoms of the "dumping syndrome."

PANCREATIC TRAUMA

Traumatic disruption of the pancreas is not uncommon after blunt abdominal injuries in children and, if unrecognized, may be fatal. Repeated serum amylase determinations and frequent examinations of the patient should lead to the diagnosis. Depending upon its severity, pancreatic injury is usually followed by tachycardia, hypotension, abdominal pain and signs of peritonitis, ileus and hyperamylasemia.

If pancreatic or other intra-abdominal injury is suspected, laparotomy should be performed promptly. Injuries of the tail of the gland usually are best treated by resection of that portion, with careful ligation of the distal duct and closure of the gland. Injuries in the midportion or head of the gland frequently may be repaired by careful closing of duct lacerations and stenting with a Silastic tube brought through the ampulla and into the duodenum.

Pancreaticointestinal anastomosis with an isolated intestinal segment may be successful for more extensive injuries, although the likelihood of pancreatic leak is great. Total pancreatectomy and duodenectomy rarely are necessary after abdominal trauma. If the head of the gland is severely injured, the tail of the pancreas should be salvaged, if possible, and attached to an isolated intestinal segment.

PANCREATIC CYSTS

Pancreatic pseudocysts may develop after pancreatic injury and usually are manifested by abdominal distention, the presence of a mass, nausea, emesis and hyperamylasemia. Upper gastrointestinal contrast roentgenograms help to establish the diagnosis. Such cysts in children, in contrast to adults, are not easily drained into the intestinal tract. The cyst wall generally is very thin and may not hold sutures. If the pancreatic duct is unobstructed, such cysts generally close with external tube drainage over a period of one to three months. If the duct is obstructed, reconstruction of the duct or pancreatic drainage into the intestine may be necessary.

True pancreatic cysts in childhood are very uncommon, and malignant cysts have not been reported in this age group. True cysts may be associated with ductal obstruction, and radiographic examination of the duct should precede resection of the cyst.

References

Fonkalsrud, E. W., Henney, R. P., Riemenschneider, T. A., and Barker, W. F.: Management of Pancreatitis in Infants and Children. *Amer. J. Surg.*, 116:198, 1968.

Cystic Fibrosis

PAUL A. DI SANT'AGNESE, M.D.

For a proper approach to the treatment of cystic fibrosis it is essential that the generalized nature of the disease be understood as well as the pathogenesis of most complications (pulmonary, pancreatic, hepatic and intestinal). These are secondary to obstruction of organ passages by "mucous secretions" which have an abnormal physicochemical behavior due to an as-yet-unknown inherited error of metabolism. In addition, the potential threat posed especially in hot weather by the abnormally high sweat electrolyte levels should be appreciated. It is clear, therefore, that until the basic defect in cystic fibrosis is uncovered, a rational, effective and lasting treatment cannot be devised. At present, therapy is mainly palliative, aimed at combating, slowing or preventing some of the secondary or tertiary complications of this disease.

Although early diagnosis and treatment and aggressive therapy during serious pulmonary complications are effective in prolonging the life of patients, the natural variation in the severity of cystic fibrosis is an important factor in determining the outcome.

GENERAL CARE

Quality of Life and Activity. The leading of as normal a life as possible by the patient should be the ultimate goal. Activities (school, competitive sports and so forth) should be restricted only as indicated by the patient's tolerance. If the patient is a child, he should be encouraged to attend school; if he is an adolescent or a young adult, he should continue his studies or obtain a job and work within the limits of his capacities. It has been clearly shown that regardless of physical condition or severity of illness, patients who withdraw from their surroundings and who are excessively dependent on their mothers do much worse than those who maintain contacts with the outside world.

Immunizations. Routine immunizations against diphtheria, tetanus, pertussis and poliomyelitis should be performed at appropriate ages. Booster doses should be given when indicated. Live virus measles vaccine is mandatory in all susceptible patients if their condition permits, since complications following rubeola may be serious or even fatal. Influenza vaccine is recommended especially in patients with pulmonary involvement, even if minimal. A bout of influenza may initiate serious pulmonary disease or cause a severe relapse when pulmonary disease is already present.

Principles of Treatment. A multidisciplinary approach to the manifold problems presented by the patient with cystic fibrosis and his family is needed. The role of the physician should be complemented by that of the social worker, the physical therapist and, at times, the psychiatrist. The parents must clearly understand all of the therapeutic measures to be carried out at home so that they can cooperate to the fullest extent, and the genetic aspects of this disease should be available to the family.

The following principles of treatment should be kept in mind: (1) Therapy should be individualized. (2) Active therapy of the pulmonary involvement deserves the major emphasis, since the lung disease dominates the clinical picture and usually determines the fate of the patient. (3) The effects of pancreatic deficiency are less important to the ultimate outcome, although proper attention should be paid to maintenance of good nutrition, including avoidance of vitamin deficiencies. Dietary measures are needed only when pancreatic deficiency is present. (4) Additional salt is required by all patients in hot weather (unless contraindicated by cor pulmonale) regardless of the pancreatic status, especially if the patient is exercising in the open air or if air conditioning is not available in the home.

PULMONARY INVOLVEMENT

Treatment of the pulmonary involvement is based on the following: (1) the evacuation of mucopurulent secretions by physical methods and at times by use of aerosol solutions, and (2) the appropriate and timely use of antimicrobial agents to combat infections. Both modes of therapy are essential to therapeutic success.

Physical Therapy. It is generally agreed that physical therapy to relieve bronchial obstruction due to accumulated secretions is needed on a continued basis by patients with even minimal pulmonary involvement. It has been proposed that physical therapy methods be used prophylactically in patients who have no clinical or roentgenographic evidence of pulmonary involvement. We do not subscribe in general to this philosophy.

Both the patient and the therapist should be comfortable during drainage. Any type of clothing worn by the subject should be loosened or removed and there should be a supply of disposable tissues conveniently at hand along with a container for expectorated secretions. The patient is placed on a firm padded board or table that can be inclined to the proper angles for drainage of the middle lobe, lingula and the basal sections of both lower lobes. Infants are best positioned on a pillow over the extended legs of the therapist. Frequency, duration of treatment and positions to be used should be individually prescribed on the basis of careful segmental auscultation of the chest and a review of the chest x-ray.

After positioning the patient, clapping, cupping, deep breathing, assisted coughing, thoracic squeezing and vibration are used. Mechanical vibrators are less effective than hand vibration; however, in the case of the young adult living away from home, or where assistance with postural drainage is not available, mechanical devices may be useful.

Aerosol Therapy. One should distinguish between interrupted inhalational therapy usually done in conjunction with postural drainage, and mist tent therapy. The object in both cases is to hydrate bronchial secretions and to assist their evacuation by physical therapy methods. To penetrate to the smaller bronchial subdivisions, aerosol particles must be 0.5 to 5 microns in size. Hand operated nebulizers do not deliver particles of adequate size. A small nebulizer, such as that used in the treatment of asthma, is sufficient for interrupted aerosol therapy, but for continuous nebulization in a "mist tent" a large capacity nebulizer is needed. Compressed air can be used as a propellant with the aid of an appropriate pump. Frequently used are ultrasonic nebulizers, which produce a very thick mist with particles of small diameter, and which are quiet. Solutions generally recommended contain 10 per cent propylene glycol in distilled water.

Our recommended schedule for *interrupted nebulization* consists of three steps: *Step 1:* Postural drainage for 5 to 10 minutes, to be done at least twice a day in the morning and evening and, if necessary, at mid-day. *Step 2:* Nebulization with the solution described for 10 to 15 minutes (following Step 1, this permits the moisture particles to penetrate further along the bronchial tree). *Step 3:* Following nebulization, repeat the postural drainage for 15 to 20 minutes.

In contrast to the universal acceptance of physical therapy methods, *mist tent therapy* is quite controversial. If it is employed, a large capacity nebulizer with a compressor, or an ultrasonic nebulizer should be used with the same solution that was mentioned previously. According to the severity of the disease, the patient can be in a mist tent for 24 hours a day or just for the night and naps. We have the impression that this type of treatment is variably effective and should be tried, if needed. It is quite helpful in some patients and of limited value in others. We tend to use mist tent therapy in a patient hospitalized for acute relapse of his pulmonary disease, in conjunction with all of the other physical therapy and antibiotic treatments, but we are very selective in choosing patients to use the tent at home during the sleeping hours. It may become quite hot inside the tent; during the summer, air conditioning of the room is helpful. It should be mentioned that some people in this country and many in England do not use mist tent therapy regularly or at all and have overall results which are not incomparable with the ones claimed by those who do. Mist tent therapy also has been advocated as a prophylactic treatment to prevent the onset of pulmonary involvement. This has not found general acceptance and we ourselves do not subscribe to this theory. Among other considerations is the question of making therapeutic cripples of patients who conceivably may go on for many years before the onset of pulmonary involvement despite the lack of any kind of prophylactic treatment. Prophylactic treatment of this kind is certainly detrimental to the quality of life and to making the patient feel as much as possible similar to his normal peers.

Whether interrupted nebulization or mist tent therapy is used, clean equipment in good working order is essential to successful treatment and to avoidance of complications. Daily or at least weekly thorough cleaning of inhalation therapy equipment decreases the chances of significant contamination.

Expectorants are useful at times: e.g., saturated solution of potassium iodide (S. S. K. I.), 0.25 to 0.5 ml. in two to four doses a day. Syrup of hydriodic and/or Organidin also have been used. Excessive or prolonged use of iodides in patients with cystic fibrosis has led to goiters and hypothyroidism. *Antihistamines* are generally to be avoided because of their drying effect on secretions. *Bronchodilators* are generally not too effective and it has been shown repeatedly that the majority of patients with cystic fibrosis do not have bronchial spasm. However, if bronchial spasm is present, especially if the patient has bronchial asthma in addition to cystic fibrosis, bronchodilators can be incorporated in the aerosol solutions. Isoproterenol (0.05 to 0.5 ml. of a 1:200 solution of Isuprel) or phenylephrine (2 to 3 ml. of 1/8 per cent solution) can be added to each intermittent aerosol treatment. *Mucolytics* are usually not very effective and can be irritating if their use is prolonged. *N*-acetyl-cysteine (Mucomyst) in a 5 to 20 per cent solution, can be tried during interrupted nebulization. *Buffered* L-*arginine* has been reported to improve pulmonary function, but we have no experience with this agent. *Enzyme preparations* (trypsin, hyaluronidase and so forth) are irritating and have not been beneficial. *Steroids* generally have not been useful and should not play a part in the routine management of patients with cystic fibrosis. However, under special circumstances when extreme bronchial spasm is present, especially in infants, these agents can be tried for short courses (hydrocortisone, 5 to 10 mg. per kilogram daily intravenously, or prednisone, 1 mg. per kilogram per day orally) in addition to all the other types of therapy that are used. Aminophylline by intravenous administration also has been used in recommended doses (see p. 131) in acute bronchospasm.

Antibiotic Therapy. Therapeutic courses of intensive antibiotic therapy are indicated during acute exacerbation of the pulmonary disease and in an attempt to halt progressive deterioration.

The choice of the antibiotic agent should be based whenever possible upon in vitro susceptibility tests of the bacterial pathogens isolated by culture from the respiratory tract. However, if the situation is so acute that it is not possible to wait one to three days for the bacteriologic reports, we start patients on one of the broad-spectrum antibiotics, usually chloramphenicol,* which is in general the most effective. If we suspect the presence of pseudomonas based on the greenish color of the sputum, parenteral gentamicin and even carbenicillin may be added.

The routes of administration selected (e.g., parenteral, oral, inhalation, or all three simultaneously) depend on the severity and acuteness of the disease and on the antibiotic agent to be used. As in all antibiotic therapy these agents should be given for a long enough period and in sufficient doses to be effective. A therapeutic course of antibiotic therapy, therefore, is usually not less than seven days and may extend to 15 days or even longer if necessary, and full recommended therapeutic doses of the agent(s) of choice should be given. Because of the possibility of parenteral administration of antibiotic agents plus the need for good physical therapy and other types of supportive treatment (e.g., oxygen therapy), hospitalization is recommended during most of the periods of intensive antibiotic therapy.

A fairly wide variety of antibiotic agents is available. The respiratory flora of patients with cystic fibrosis usually consists primarily of *Staphylococcus aureus hemolyticus* and/or *Pseudomonas aeruginosa* if they have received antibiotic therapy on previous frequent occasions. Other organisms, such as *H. influenzae,* Proteus and *E. coli,* are less common. Therefore, an anti-staphylococcal agent alone, or in combination with a drug effective against pseudomonas, is commonly used. This is true even if *Staphylococcus aureus* is not present in the sputum or nasopharyngeal culture, on the assumption that this is the organism responsible for the basic infection in the pulmonary involvement of cystic fibrosis. If the staphylococcus is resistant to penicillin G, the penicillinase-resistant semisynthetic penicillins and the cephalosporins are usually selected, the dosage depending on the route of administration as well as on the age of the patient.

As antipseudomonas drugs, gentamicin (5 mg. per kilogram per 24 hours intramuscularly or intravenously, with a range of 3 to 5 mg. in three divided doses) and carbenicillin (400 mg. per kilogram per day in six divided doses by intravenous administration), usually with the addition of probenecid‡ (250 mg. orally four times a day) have been effective. The combination of gentamicin and carbenicillin is usually considered synergistic, and both can be used together in life-threatening situations.

Among the broad-spectrum antibiotics, chloramphenicol has been the most effective agent, but because of the risks of bone marrow suppression and optic neuritis (the latter especially after prolonged administration), its use should be avoided whenever equally efficacious antibiotics are available. If used, it should be given for only a short time (one to four weeks), parents should be forewarned to seek immediate medical advice if diminution of visual acuity occurs, and blood counts should be obtained at least once a week.

If possible, an antibiotic with fewer side effects should be used. If the child is below the age of eight years, one of the penicillins in combination with ampicillin should be used; the latter, of course, is useful also against *Hemophilus influenzae* and *Proteus mirabilis.*

* Manufacturer's precaution: Chloramphenicol is not recommended for intravenous or intramuscular pediatric use. Chloramphenicol sodium succinate has been approved for intravenous pediatric use.

‡ Manufacturer's precaution: Probenecid is not recommended for children under two years of age.

If the patient is above the age of eight years, one of the tetracyclines is usually preferred.

Erythromycin, colistin, streptomycin and kanamycin have been widely used in the past with varying success; however, they have been supplanted by the newer antibiotic agents, especially in view of the potential toxicity of the latter two.

Aerosol Antibiotic Therapy. This is regarded as a form of topical treatment and only as an adjunct to systemic administration. Published studies have shown that aerosol antibiotic therapy can be effective, especially when the same antibiotic is used as is given by the oral or parenteral route. It has been our custom to add some of these agents during periods of intensive antibiotic therapy in the hospital when drugs are given by the oral or parenteral route. Penicillin G (100,000 units per ml. four times a day), nafcillin‖ (100 to 250 mg. per ml. four times a day), ampicillin (125 to 250 mg. per ml. four times a day), and gentamicin (5 to 10 mg. per ml. four times a day) have been used. In our hands, neither neomycin, polymyxin B or colistin have proven useful when administered in this manner.

Continued Antibiotic Therapy. In our experience and that of most others, some severely ill patients cannot be controlled effectively without antibiotic therapy for long periods of time (months or even years). We prefer to use one of the oral antistaphylococcal agents or one of the tetracyclines (always only if the child is older than eight years) and administer this agent in the smallest dose sufficient to prevent reappearance of symptoms as determined by trial and error. We do not favor rotation of antibiotics. Long-term administration of antibiotics in small dosage is treatment and not true prophylactic administration, which we feel is not indicated. The principal argument against this method of therapy is the risk of increased resistance of strains of *Staphylococcus aureus* to antibiotics and the colonization with *Pseudomonas aeruginosa* and other resistant bacteria. This is true, but at times one's hand is forced by the constant recurrence of symptoms and the menace of a rapidly progressive pulmonary disease if no treatment is given.

Surgical and Other Treatment. *Pulmonary surgery* is rarely indicated because of the generalized nature of the lung involvement in most patients. However, approximately 2 per cent of patients with cystic fibrosis have a pulmonary disease sufficiently localized so that resection can be attempted. Lobectomy of one or more lobes of the same lung, or even total pneumonectomy, has been performed with at least temporary success. Spread to the previously unaffected lung parenchyma after resection of a severely affected lobe, however, is a possible hazard.

Tracheostomy before surgery, in order to permit adequate evacuation of secretions and, if necessary, assisted ventilation during the postoperative period, has been used to advantage. The importance of a surgeon experienced in surgery on patients with cystic fibrosis cannot be emphasized enough. The necessity for vigorous and aggressive supportive treatment (physical therapy, electrolyte balance and antibiotics both against staphylococcus and pseudomonas) in the postoperative period, with the fullest cooperation between surgical and medical teams, is mandatory.

When surgical procedures are performed on patients with pulmonary involvement, care must be employed in the selection of *preanesthetic* and *anesthetic agents.* When possible, local anesthesia is preferable to general anesthesia; preanesthetic agents that increase the viscosity of secretions or cause drying of pulmonary secretions should be avoided if possible; anesthetic agents that produce a minimum of bronchial irritation should be used. Morphine, codeine and other drugs that depress the cough reflex or that cause excessive sedation are contraindicated as either pre- or postoperative medication.

Bronchoscopy for drainage has been used with some success by skilled operators; in general, because of the risks involved in the procedure, it should be attempted only in selected cases.

Repeated small episodes of hemoptysis are not uncommon in patients with severe pulmonary involvement, especially in the older age group; they are of poor prognostic significance but need no special treatment provided the prothrombin time is normal. *Massive hemoptysis,* however, is an unusual and serious complication that has been seen with increasing frequency in the older age group in recent times. There may be a sudden, massive, fatal exsanguinating hemorrhage. More often there is clinical or laboratory evidence of blood loss and at times hemorrhage sufficiently great to require transfusion. An attempt should be made to localize the bleeding site. Intravenous injection of fluorescein during bronchoscopy with a fiber optic bronchoscope has yielded some results. Simple bronchoscopy can be attempted, and if the patient bleeds profusely during the

‖ Manufacturer's precaution: Intravenous use of nafcillin in neonates and children is investigational.

procedure, localization may be possible. If the bleeding is copious and repeated and if localization is certain, resection of the affected lobe or even total pneumonectomy can be attempted. However, on several occasions lobectomies have been performed and later it was found that the bleeding site had not been removed.

Pneumothorax, often repeated and at times bilateral, has also been seen with increasing frequency in recent years, especially in older patients. It is of poor prognostic significance and poses a problem in treatment. At the moment we have adopted the following system: If the pneumothorax is unilateral and not more than 15 per cent, hospitalization and observation are indicated; if it is more than 15 per cent or bilateral, closed thoracotomy with tube insertion is performed. In general, after three attacks of recurring pneumothorax, repeated instillation of a sclerosing agent is tried (Atabrine, 100 mg. in 10 ml. or more distilled water four times a day). This induces a slow pleural reaction with fever and leukocytosis and frequently good results. Alternatively, if the patient's condition permits, open thoracotomy with resection of blebs and pleural scarification or pleural stripping has been performed with success. Vigorous physical therapy or deep tracheal suction is needed during the first postoperative days to avoid the accumulation of intrabronchial secretions resulting from splinting of the operated hemithorax due to pain, despite the danger of pneumothorax occurring on the other side.

Tracheostomy and nasotracheal intubations in very ill patients in order to permit mechanical ventilation with a respirator has in general been unsuccessful, and there is agreement that it should be avoided except for selected cases. Usually it has prolonged life for a period measured in days or weeks, and it is very difficult to wean the patient from the mechanical respirator. The hazards of both tracheostomy and endotracheal intubation have decreased somewhat since the introduction of Silastic and polyvinyl tubes.

Assisted ventilation, as previously stated under tracheostomy, has not been very effective and should be reserved for selected cases. *Intermittent positive pressure breathing* (IPPB) machines in general should be used only in the hospital and with due care because of the danger of inducing a pneumothorax.

Permanent tracheostomy to facilitate suction of secretions usually is not done but has been performed with some success in occasional older patients.

Pulmonary lavage with a total volume of saline of many liters should be performed only by an expert operator; while mandatory in other conditions (e.g., alveolar proteinosis), it is of limited use in patients with cystic fibrosis because of technical difficulties (size of the equipment needed and so forth). It should be reserved for older patients who have previously had fairly good pulmonary function and pCO_2 values of more than 50 to 60 mm. Hg, but who develop an episode of persistent bronchial obstruction. *Tracheobronchial lavage* without complete filling of the lavaged lung is questionably effective, and there is no objective proof that this procedure helps the patient. If very small volumes of liquid are used, any possible benefit gained is outweighed by the risks of bronchoscopy. However, the recent introduction of the fiber-optic bronchoscope offers hope for the simplification of these procedures. *Deep tracheal aspiration* is often effective and should be used in severely ill patients; however, it is necessarily limited to older individuals who cooperate with the procedure. It is generally agreed that normal saline is a better solution for all types of lavage than is *N*-acetyl-cysteine (Mucomyst), which may cause severe irritation of the tracheobronchial mucosa and bronchial spasm.

Digitalis for cor pulmonale is useful because it can improve cardiac contractility and slow the heart rate to physiologic levels. While cor pulmonale is notoriously difficult to diagnose, it can be assumed that any patient with a pO_2 of less than 50 mm. Hg or a pCO_2 greater than 45 mm. Hg has cor pulmonale. However, the dangers of administration of digitalis to anoxic patients should be kept in mind. Many pediatric cardiologists feel that once digitalization is started it should be maintained for the lifetime of the patient. *Diuretics* are important adjuncts to the treatment of cor pulmonale and in general diuretic agents such as the thiazides, furosemide (Lasix) ** or ethacrynic acid (Edecrin)†† in recommended dosage are used. Of course, the usual precautions should be used to avoid potassium depletion. In general, only short courses of diuretic treatment are needed in patients with cystic fibrosis, usually one day to one week, but at times in very severely ill patients continued diuretic therapy may be necessary.

** Although the manufacturer cautions against the use of furosemide in children until further experience is accumulated, I have used it quite extensively in older patients with cystic fibrosis.

†† Manufacturer's precaution: Infant dose of ethacrynic acid has not been established.

Oxygen therapy should be ideally correlated with measurements of O_2 content of the blood. If the blood pH is low, this will enhance the dissociation of oxygen and hemoglobin and necessitate higher oxygen tensions for achieving the same levels of saturation. As little oxygen concentration as is needed to improve the oxygenation of the blood should be used: 28 per cent to 40 per cent. In general, concentrations of oxygen of more than 50 per cent for more than a few hours should be considered hazardous (CO_2 narcosis, tissue damage and so forth). Despite the dangers of oxygen therapy, it has been shown that the degree of pulmonary hypertension correlates with the severity of hypoxia.

GASTROINTESTINAL TRACT COMPLICATIONS

Pancreatic Deficiency. More than 85 per cent of patients with cystic fibrosis have pancreatic deficiency and consequent maldigestion and malabsorption with abnormal stools, steatorrhea and azotorrhea and potentially liposoluble vitamin deficiencies. The pancreatic achylia is readily compensated by a diet of high caloric, high protein and moderate fat content in conjunction with administration of pancreatic extracts. It is the general experience that infants and small children with this disease have much more of a need for *dietary measures,* whereas these appear to become less necessary with advancing age. However, individual variations are found in the need for dietary measures at all ages, and the patient's appetite and character of the stools should be a guide to the dietary intake. It is generally agreed that the nutritional state is more closely correlated with the severity of the pulmonary infection than with pancreatic function. Recent longitudinal studies of older patients with cystic fibrosis have shown virtually no correlation between dietary restriction and a number of parameters, such as degree of steatorrhea, azotorrhea, eventual growth achieved, state of nutrition, severity of the pulmonary disease and other manifestations of the disorder.

Commercially available powdered high protein milk preparations can be used to advantage in the first few weeks of life; subsequently, skim milk is advised until later childhood, when homogenized milk can be given if the patients tolerate it. Soybean milk preparations do not provide adequate protein and should not be given to infants with cystic fibrosis, since hypoproteinemic edema has been seen under such circumstances. *Liposoluble vitamin supplements* in water-miscible preparations should be provided every day in double the usual recommended dose. If hypoprothrombinemia due to vitamin K deficiency is present, administration of vitamin K_1 (phytonadione, 1 to 2 mg. intramuscularly) is indicated. However, occasionally if there is an extensive and long-standing cirrhosis of the liver, the response to vitamin K administration may not be adequate. *Pancreatic extracts* improve intestinal absorption and the nature of the stools and are usually needed with each meal. Many commercial products are available: we have usually used either Cotazym or Viokase. Dosage depends on the preparation selected and, in particular, on the patient's clinical response. Constipation and anorexia may result if the dose of pancreatic extracts is excessive. Colace (50-mg. capsules twice a day) has been found effective under these circumstances.

Medium chain triglycerides are absorbed better than other longer chain fats and have been used as dietary supplements. This can be done by the use of appropriate formulas containing medium chain triglycerides (Portagen) or the medium chain triglyceride oil used for cooking.

Anabolic steroids have been useful in increasing appetite and promoting weight gain, but only short repeated courses are recommended in order to avoid side effects. Claims that they have improved the respiratory disease have not been substantiated.

Lactase Deficiency. Lactase deficiency has been described in some patients with cystic fibrosis. In most cases it does not give rise to any clinical symptoms and its significance is uncertain, but in others there are persistently loose stools and abdominal cramps despite the institution of dietary restrictions for pancreatic deficiency. In these instances, after the proper diagnostic evaluation, it is necessary to limit the dietary lactose intake.

Treatment of Obstructive Complications. A number of obstructive complications of the gastrointestinal tract may be present at various ages; treatment is usually surgical. The most frequent is *meconium ileus,* which is present in 5 to 10 per cent of all cystic fibrosis patients and which accounts for a very significant proportion of all intestinal obstruction of newborn infants. Details of the operative procedures are to be found in the literature. It is important to keep in mind that one-half of all cases of meconium ileus are complicated by either volvulus or atresia. Gastrografin enemas have been introduced recently and in many instances have been effective in avoiding surgical intervention if the meconium ileus is not complicated. In many clinics, patients with meconium ileus and meconium peritonitis (not to be confused with ileus, but at times associated with it) are put on prophylactic antibiotic therapy (usually ampicillin and kanamycin) for a few days. It is our strong recommendation that if a diagnosis of cystic fibrosis cannot be immediately established in a newborn who is suspected of having this disease because of intestinal obstruction, he should be treated with a high protein formula and pancreatic replacement therapy until the age of three or four weeks when a reliable sweat test can be obtained easily. If the patient then is shown not to have cystic fibrosis, nothing will have been lost; much will have been gained if the patient turns out to have this disorder. Needless to say, vigorous antibiotic and other therapy is given if there is any evidence of the onset of pulmonary involvement.

Regardless of age, however, all patients with cystic fibrosis are subject to intestinal obstructive complications. These result from solid or semisolid content where the fecal stream is normally liquid, which is due to the abnormal character of the fecal contents. *Fecal masses* are usually in the cecum, 3 to 5 cm. in diameter, hard, mobile and nontender. Although firmly adherent to the mucosa and giving rise to abdominal pain when extruded, they are usually passed spontaneously and no treatment is necessary. Constipation should be avoided; dioctyl sodium sulfosuccinate (Colace 50 mg. twice a day), a temporary moderate increase in dietary fat intake and a concomitant decrease in pancreatic enzyme therapy have been helpful in this respect. *Volvulus, meconium ileus equivalent* (intestinal obstruction) and *intussusception* are not infrequently encountered in older patients with cystic fibrosis. The latter two complications often result in incomplete obstruction. Intussusception may respond to reduction by barium enema and partial obstruction may respond to repeated high colonic enemas. Mucomyst orally (5 ml. of a 10 per cent solution four times a day) has been used with satisfactory results. If not, surgical intervention is needed and many times it is possible to reduce the intussusception or to break up the fecal mass causing the obstruction without intestinal resection. Time is of the essence in instituting treatment, because if adhesions have already formed in the case of intussusception, surgery will be inevitable.

Cystic fibrosis is by far the most common cause in this country of *rectal prolapse,* especially in infants and young children. It is estimated that as many as 15 to 20 per cent of all patients with cystic fibrosis may have this complication. Although the pathogenesis is uncertain, the rectal prolapse responds so well to medical and dietary treatment that surgical intervention is rarely if ever needed.

Focal biliary cirrhosis is frequently found in the liver at autopsy, and recent evidence indicates that as many as 20 to 30 per cent of patients may have some abnormality of their liver function tests. However, even in *widespread multilobular biliary cirrhosis,* which occurs in only 2 to 3 per cent of patients, large areas of liver parenchyma remain normal because of the focal nature of the disease, and therefore hepatic function remains adequate. Treatment is nonspecific, especially in view of the fact that a high protein diet is followed by most patients with this disease. If hematemesis or melena occurs as a consequence of *portal hypertension,* they should be treated as they would be in any other patient, including the eventual performance of shunting procedures. Surgeons usually prefer not to perform shunting operations in a child who is still growing rapidly because of the small size of the vessels and the change in their caliber due to age.

There is no unanimous consent as to the treatment for *obstructive neonatal jaundice* in cystic fibrosis. Only seven cases have been reported so far and they all seem to be due to the presence of inspissated bile causing extrahepatic obstruction. While surgical intervention may be necessary in some cases, a more conservative approach is frequently successful.

ABNORMAL SALT LOSS

Massive salt depletion through sweating in hot weather may present a real medical emergency. The administration of saline solution intravenously is urgently needed in such instances to reconstitute the extracellular fluid volume and to avoid cardiovascular collapse; as much as 10 ml. of isotonic saline solution per kilogram within 15 minutes may have to be given, followed by appropriate fluid replacement therapy. Additional sodium chloride (2 to 4 Gm. per day) should be taken orally by all patients in hot weather, regardless of their pancreatic status, provided cor pulmonale does not contraindicate it.

OTHER COMPLICATIONS

Moderate to severe oral *glucose intolerance* is not uncommon in older patients with cystic fibrosis and may lead to *glycosuria.* This should not be confused with the genetic diabetes mellitus, none of whose characteristic complications and postmortem findings is present. It is probably due to anatomic disorganization of the islands of Langerhans by the fibrotic process. Dietary restriction and at times oral antidiabetic agents are sufficient, but some patients require the addition of insulin. *Genetic diabetes mellitus* may in some instances occur coincidentally with cystic fibrosis, and its treatment should follow the same lines as in any other patients with this condition, keeping in mind the additional problems and dietary restrictions indicated in the presence of pancreatic achylia and consequent malabsorption.

Ten to 15 per cent of patients with cystic fibrosis have recurrent *nasal polyps* which may require polypectomy.

SOCIAL, PSYCHOLOGIC AND PSYCHIATRIC CONSIDERATIONS

Cystic fibrosis is not only a medical problem but a social one as well, owing to the devastating emotional and financial stresses on the family. There is need for a compassionate, helpful, understanding attitude on the part of the physician and, when needed, support and assistance by a psychologist and psychiatrist. Every effort must be made to prevent the patient from dominating the family emotionally and to allay the guilt feeling and consequent overconcern or hostility of the parents, which are apt to develop in relation to an inherited, severe and progressive disease. The support of a medical social worker familiar with the problems of this disorder is desirable to allay the family's emotional response as well as to help them utilize community resources to the fullest extent.

Adolescents and young adults with cystic fibrosis grow up with an unusual number of stresses related to their physical appearance, conflicts in their upbringing and increased awareness of the future. Recent studies have shown that generally the father needs to be encouraged to become more involved with the patient and that, conversely, the mother needs to be helped to allow the patient greater independence and responsibility. Both parents and patients need to be aware of the benefits of an environment with free communication about cystic fibrosis.

The role of the physician is very important in helping the parents to allow the patient to develop normally emotionally; to listen to the patient's concerns; and to lead group discussions of parents and, at times, of older patients in terms of offering practical and concrete ways to deal with daily concerns (e.g., handling separation, going to college, seeking employment and reorienting their goals more realistically). Both male and female patients who marry need special counseling both before and after marriage to deal with common fears and frustrations. Specific concerns about sterility or adoption need to be discussed and then discussed again after the patient has had time to digest the facts. Finally, the physician should encourage the patient to continue school or work if at all possible. Those who have had to stop, for whatever reason, have become lonely and depressed, and have had low self-esteem.

References

di Sant'Agnese, P. A.: The Pancreas: in W. E. Nelson, V. C. Vaughan and R. J. McKay (eds.): *Textbook of Pediatrics*. 9th ed. Philadelphia, W. B. Saunders Company, 1969, pp. 854–869.

Guide to Diagnosis and Management of Cystic Fibrosis, 2nd ed., 1971. National Cystic Fibrosis Research Foundation, 3379 Peachtree Road, N.E., Atlanta, Ga. 30326.

Huang, N. N. (ed.): *Guide to Drug Therapy in Patients with Cystic Fibrosis*, 1972. National Cystic Fibrosis Research Foundation, 3379 Peachtree Road, N.E., Atlanta, Ga. 30326.

Malabsorption Syndrome and Intestinal Disaccharidase Deficiencies

FIMA LIFSHITZ, M.D.

In recent years the malabsorption syndrome in children and infants has been more easily recognized. The malabsorption syndrome is characterized by failure to thrive, weight loss and passage of abnormal stools. Malabsorption from any cause decreases the total caloric intake and malnutrition often ensues. Malabsorption can lead to malnutrition in any age group and socioeconomic bracket.

A precise diagnosis of the pathophysiologic alterations associated with the malabsorption syndrome is essential for rational treatment. Table 1 lists some of the most frequent diseases and disorders that form part of the malabsorption syndrome, classified according to the pathophysiologic mechanisms.

GENERAL PRINCIPLES OF THERAPY

Basic medical principles should be applied in the management of disorders causing malabsorption syndrome and malnutrition in the pediatric age group. In severely ill patients emergency fluid therapy given intravenously should be employed to restore blood volume and correct acid-base and electrolyte abnormalities. The general principles of parenteral fluid therapy should be followed. However, patients with the malabsorption syndrome are particu-

TABLE 1. Disorders Composing the Malabsorption Syndrome

DISORDERS WITHIN INTESTINAL LUMEN	DISORDERS OF INTESTINAL MUCOSAL CELL TRANSPORT
Inadequate Digestion	*Nonspecific (Generalized Malabsorption)*
Pancreatic exocrine insufficiency (single or multiple)	Celiac disease
Acid hypersecretion	Tropical sprue
Gastric resection	Skin diseases
Altered bile salt metabolism	Radiation
Short gut syndrome	Drugs
Intestinal stasis syndrome	Mucosal infiltration (parasites, bacteria, neoplasm, amyloid)
	Circulatory disturbances (ischemia, congestive heart failure)
	Specific (Selective Malabsorption)
	A-beta-lipoproteinemia
	Specific amino acid transport defects
	Specific vitamin and mineral malabsorptions
	Disaccharidase deficiencies
	Monosaccharide transport defects

DISORDERS OF INTESTINAL LYMPHATIC TRANSPORT	DISORDERS CAUSED BY MULTIPLE FACTORS	UNCLASSIFIED
Primary lymphatic disease	Malnutrition	Hypogammaglobulinemias
Whipple's disease	Bacterial overgrowth	Endocrinopathies
Secondary disturbed circulation	Protein-losing enteropathy	Ganglioneuroma
	Carbohydrate intolerance in diarrheal disease	Bovine protein hypersensitivity
	Hard water intake	

larly prone to have any of several of the following complications: acidosis, hypoproteinemia, hypopotassemia, hypocalcemia and hypomagnesemia. Therefore, one must be careful when supplying intravenous potassium, alkaline solutions or serum albumin, since any of these may precipitate tetany and convulsions or even cardiac arrest due to latent hypocalcemia. In some patients who are severely dehydrated or in shock, whole blood or plasma transfusions may be lifesaving. Fasting should be kept to a minimum to avoid the perpetuation of the diarrheal process and starvation. Once the dehydration and the electrolyte imbalance are corrected, oral intake should be initiated.

With the development of intravenous hyperalimentation, total prolonged parenteral nutrition has become practical. This technique is of importance in treating some patients who have disorders of the gastrointestinal tract and malabsorption syndrome. Indications for its use are short bowel syndrome, particularly following massive intestinal resection, intestinal tract fistulas and certain inflammatory processes of the gastrointestinal tract. This type of therapy may be the optimal method for adequate feeding to allow these patients to recover or to improve their nutritional status before and after surgery. In addition, intravenous hyperalimentation may be employed in patients whose nutrient requirements cannot be met by the gastrointestinal tract alone. However, this technique should not be used when more rational, specific treatment is available. There are several severe complications that are frequently found in patients receiving intravenous hyperalimentation at any medical center and even under the best of circumstances. Examples are sepsis and hyperosmolar-hyperglycemic dehydration.

SPECIFIC GUIDELINES OF THERAPY

Disorders Within the Intestinal Lumen: Inadequate Digestion

Pancreatic Exocrine Insufficiency. Inadequate digestion from pancreatic insufficiency may be treated by the oral administration of pancreatic enzymes. Patients with pancreatic exocrine insufficiency of any sort as well as those with specific processes, such as cystic fibrosis, trypsinogen deficiency, enterokinase deficiency and lipase deficiency, are candidates for replacement therapy. There are several products available for pancreatic replacement. Cotazym (300-mg. capsules) has lipolytic activity; each capsule may digest 17 Gm. of dietary fat. Viokase (powder, 1.5 Gm. per teaspoon, or 325-mg. tablets) has good lipase activity and protein hydrolysis. It is cheaper than other products. All of these products have an unpleasant odor and taste. Generally, the extract is fed at the beginning of the meals to ensure intake. The powder must be added to the food just prior to its administration in order to minimize its decomposition in vitro; for the same reason it is not wise to combine it with warm foods. The required dosage of these preparations varies from patient to patient. Adequate replacement is judged by the character and the decrease in the frequency of the stools. Infants usually require 1/4 to 1/2 teaspoon with each feeding; children from 5 to 10 years of age require two to four tablets per meal. Since lipase is inactivated by a pH of less than 4.5, it may be helpful to administer these preparations with sodium bicarbonate (0.2 Gm. per kilogram per day). Overdosage of pancreatic extracts induces constipation. Patients with pancreatic exocrine insufficiency and bone marrow failure may require additional blood transfusions and corticosteroid therapy. In all instances the diet should be supplemented with medium chain triglycerides (see below, Dietary Therapy).

Acid Hypersecretion. Marked acid hypersecretion associated with Zollinger-Ellison syndrome is preferably managed by resection of the tumor; however, since an isolated obvious tumor is rare, total gastrectomy is preferred by most surgeons. Some patients with malabsorption after gastrectomy have bacterial overgrowth in the afferent loop, which may be temporarily reduced with oral broad-spectrum antimicrobial drugs (see below). Conversion of the Billroth II to a Billroth I anastomosis, if possible, is advisable in these cases.

Altered Bile Salt Metabolism. DECREASED SYNTHESIS. When decreased conjugated bile salts cause steatorrhea, replacement therapy may be feasible. Congenital or acquired bile salt deficiency might be treated by conjugated bile salt preparations; i.e., Decholin Tablets, 0.25 to 0.75 Gm. three times a day. The dose should be gradually increased to this level because of the possibility that diarrhea might be induced.

EXCESSIVE LOSS. When bile salts are lost, loss of fat in the stools occurs. If hepatic synthesis is capable of keeping the bile salt pool at nearly normal levels, fat digestion and absorption is only moderately impaired, with slight to moderate loss of fat in the stools. This kind of diarrhea and malabsorption can be alleviated by feedings of cholestyramine (a bile-salt binding resin). However, if hepatic synthesis of bile salt is not capable of maintaining the bile salt pool, maldigestion and malabsorption of long chain triglycerides occur with severe excretion of fat in the stools. This kind of diarrhea and malabsorption cannot be controlled by adsorption of bile salt alone but by a combination of adsorption of bile salts with cholestyramine and substitution of medium chain triglycerides for long chain fats in the diet. Cholestyramine resin (U. S. P.)* (Cuemid Powder, Questran, 2 to 4 Gm. four times a day) may be given mixed in orange juice or milk formula. It should be kept in mind that this preparation interferes with the absorption of vitamins A, D and K and other nutrients and may produce hyperchloremic acidosis. Malabsorption of fat might be worsened by cholestyramine if the dose exceeds 12 Gm. a day. Cholestyramine might be useful in patients with ileal resection, biliary fistula or ileal bypass.

ALTERED METABOLISM. When bile salt metabolism is altered by bacterial overgrowth resulting in deconjugation of bile salts, cholestyramine is not effective. In these instances the therapy should be directed toward controlling bacterial overgrowth (see later).

Short Bowel Syndrome. Extensive bowel resection might cause a malabsorption syndrome. These patients have significant increases in total gastric acidity and rate of acid production. Hypersecretion may be limited to the postoperative period or persist for months. In the presence of gastric hypersecretion, pancreatic and intestinal enzymes may be inactivated owing to lowering of intraluminal pH with resultant azotorrhea and steatorrhea. Vagotomy and pyloroplasty or gastroenterostomy should not be considered as a primary therapy in such patients because hypersecretion is usually self-limited and the decreasing gastric emptying time following surgery may worsen steatorrhea. To combat excessive duodenal acidity, effective antacid should be used in adequate dosages; i.e., sodium bicarbonate, 0.2 Gm. per kilogram per day, or magnesium-aluminum hydroxide (Maalox, tablets or oral suspension). Feedings may be initiated with a dilute glucose electrolyte solution. If the infant has frequent watery bowel movements while taking this solution, it is unlikely that he will be successfully fed by mouth. The use of parenteral hyperalimentation in this type of patient should be considered. However, if dilute glucose and electrolytes are tolerated, frequent feedings of small amounts of formula may be offered. It is advisable to begin feedings with a simple hyposmolar formula containing low concentrations of glucose, protein hydrolysate and medium chain triglycerides. Full caloric supply should not be attempted by mouth until diarrhea has subsided. Intravenous

---

* Manufacturer's precaution: Dosage of cholestyramine resin (Questran) for children under six years of age has not been established.

hyperalimentation can be employed to meet the calorie requirements. After this diet is tolerated, it may be changed to an isomolar formula with 5 per cent glucose, which provides a full caloric supply and, later, to a more complex formula which contains disaccharides and even lactose as a source of carbohydrate. Medium chain triglycerides should be continued in the diet. In patients with smaller resections limited to the ileum, cholestyramine treatment might be helpful. Should bacterial overgrowth occur, antibiotic treatment is indicated. Malabsorption of water-soluble vitamins usually does not occur except for folic acid and vitamin B_{12}.

Disorders of Intestinal Mucosal Cell Transport: Nonspecific (Generalized Malabsorption)

Gluten-Induced Enteropathy (Celiac Disease). Most cases of celiac disease (childhood and adult) respond to elimination of gluten from the diet. This regimen must be lifelong. It is of utmost importance that the dietary exclusion of gluten and its components be as strict as possible. Frequently, neither the physician nor the patient is alert to the possibility that gluten is present in commercial preparations in the form of "fillers" or "additives." Such factors are frequently involved in the "failure of gluten-free diets."

Most investigators agree that the improvement in patients with celiac disease is related to the degree to which gluten is eliminated from the diet. Improvement can be observed clinically by reduction in diarrhea and steatorrhea, by weight gain and by loss of abdominal distention. These symptoms are usually alleviated in a few days. At the same time tests of intestinal absorption show a progressive return to normal. When a series of jejunal mucosa biopsies are performed, it is possible to demonstrate a marked improvement in the mucosal structure, with the villi often showing an almost normal appearance; however, such a pronounced degree of improvement may take several months.

If gluten is readministered to a patient with celiac disease who has been on a gluten-free diet, a variable response may be observed. In some, a return of symptoms may be induced almost immediately or in a matter of days; in others the malabsorption might be delayed, with symptoms being either mild or subtle. However, when objective observations are made, changes may be observed quite early. Biochemical documentation of increased fecal fat excretion and of changes in the proximal jejunal mucosa as early as one day after administrating gluten can be documented.

In most published reports, good response to the use of a gluten-free diet has been observed in almost all patients with celiac disease. When dietary treatment fails, at least three factors should be considered: The dietary restriction may have been inadequate, the patient may have an intestinal villous atrophy due to a disorder other than celiac disease or there may be other complicating features.

One should be reluctant to consider dietary therapy a failure unless the patient has been hospitalized and the response to treatment has been observed under the close supervision of the physician and the dietitian. As pointed out above, there are several possible errors in the diagnosis of celiac disease. The mucosal lesion with a flat villous surface, although characteristic of this entity, is not specific for this disease. Patients with agammaglobulinemia, enterocolitis, granulomatous disease and carcinoma of the duodenum, and even secondary generalized malnutrition might show severe atrophy of the intestinal mucosa not related to celiac disease. These patients fail to respond to gluten-free diets. A group of patients, with severe malabsorption, extensive atrophy of the jejunal mucosa and few or no Paneth cells, who failed to respond to gluten-free diets has also been described. A "true" failure of gluten-free diet in celiacs also occurs. Initially the response to gluten withdrawal may be limited by the secondary malnutrition and pancreatic insufficiency. Subsequently the superimposition of a malignant process such as lymphoma may account for failure to respond to a gluten-free diet.

Oats were originally considered to be deleterious to the patient with celiac disease, but recent observations have not supported this belief. Oats might be included in the diet of these patients without observing adverse effects clinically, biochemically or morphologically.

Before the use of gluten-free diets, corticosteroids were used to treat celiac disease and led to a reasonable degree of clinical improvement. However, usually this does not correct the steatorrhea to the extent observed after dietary therapy, and the mucosal biopsy tends to remain abnormal. In patients who are treated initially with steroids and in whom a response is achieved, gluten restriction almost always results in further improvement. Patients with Paneth cell deficiency respond to steroids.

Elimination of milk from the diet has enhanced the degree of clinical improvement in patients with celiac disease. The possibility that they may have lactose intolerance secondary to mucosal atrophy with secondary lactase deficiency should be kept in mind. Lactose-free diets, however, are usually not necessary in the treatment of these patients. The demonstration of low disaccharidase activity in a single upper small intestinal mucosal biopsy specimen or a diminished rise in blood sugar levels after an oral dose of specific sugar may indicate some alterations in the handling of sugars in this region of the gut, but if not accompanied by diarrhea of the type seen in carbohydrate-intolerant patients, i.e., excretion of carbohydrates and acid stools, it does not necessarily indicate a defective handling of sugar by the small intestine as a whole. Confusion seems to exist between the presence of disaccharide intolerance in a patient, and disaccharidase deficiencies in a biopsy specimen. Only occasionally patients with celiac disease have been found to show symptoms of sugar intolerance. If the stools are liquid and acid and contain carbohydrates, then it might be necessary to institute a lactose-free or even a lactose- and sucrose-free diet initially, in addition to the gluten-free diet. The symptoms of sugar intolerance are found to disappear within 48 hours and weight gain begins immediately in infants in whom the symptoms are due to celiac disease with associated carbohydrate intolerance. As soon as the pH of the stool returns to normal and carbohydrate excretion ceases, gradual introduction of carbohydrates into the diet should be initiated. Even in patients with marked carbohydrate intolerance, lactose might be given in the diet within the first month of recovery.

Tropical Sprue. Tropical sprue responds dramatically to administration of broad-spectrum antimicrobial drugs (tetracycline,† 50 mg. per kilogram per day for two weeks). Recovery is hastened by the concomitant administration of vitamin B_{12} (20 micrograms intramuscularly daily for one week) and folic acid (15 mg. orally daily for two weeks, followed by 5 mg. daily for four to five months).

Other Alterations. The malabsorption due to diffuse regional enteritis may be alleviated somewhat by the administration of steroids, provided the patient does not have bacterial overgrowth due to chronic obstruction or to fistula. Diffuse nongranulomatous ileojejunitis may improve temporarily with the administration of prednisone (2 mg. per kilogram a day).

In patients with *Giardia lamblia* infection, there may be a response to quinacrine therapy (8 mg. per kilogram per day for five days; maximum 300 mg. per day), or the response to metronidazole (Flagyl, 250 to 750 mg. per day according to age for 10 days)‡ is highly successful. In smaller children, 10 to 20 mg. per kilogram per day is used. A second treatment might be administered after one week of rest if *G. lamblia* persists.

Disorders of Intestinal Mucosal Cell Transport: Specific (Selective Malabsorption)

A-Beta-Lipoproteinemia. There is no known specific treatment of patients with A-beta-lipoproteinemia. However, the malabsorption can be improved by the administration of medium chain triglycerides.

Specific Amino Acid Transport Defects. In patients with specific amino acid transport defects, dietary treatment might also be offered. A low protein diet may be given to patients with conditions such as familial protein intolerance, or a specific amino acid can be eliminated from the diet, such as in methionine malabsorption. The reverse might also be necessary; a high protein diet is required to stimulate absorption of protein in patients with Hartnup disease.

Specific Vitamin and Mineral Malabsorptions. Patients with selective malabsorption of vitamin B_{12} respond well to parenteral administration of this vitamin given monthly (see later, Nonspecific Replacement Therapy). Also, patients with congenital malabsorption of folic acid respond to the administration of this vitamin (see later, Nonspecific Replacement Therapy). Selective deficiencies of mineral absorption, such as familial hypomagnesemia, have also been recognized. Treatment is magnesium supplementation given parenterally during the acute stage and later as an oral supplement. In patients with familial chloride diarrhea there is a defect in chloride absorption. Treatment with potassium chloride, 2 to 14 mEq. per kilogram per day, to maintain normal serum electrolytes and pH will allow improvement and gradual compensation of the growth retardation.

Disaccharidase Deficiencies. Human intestinal disaccharidase activity is accounted for by a mixture of at least five alpha-glucosidases, all of which have maltase activity, some of them

† Manufacturer's note: The use of tetracyclines during tooth development (last half of pregnancy, infancy and children to eight years of age) may cause permanent discoloration of teeth. This adverse reaction is more common during long-term use of the drug but has been observed following repeated short-term courses.

‡ Manufacturer's precaution: Metronidazole (Flagyl) is considered investigational for this use.

having in addition sucrase and/or isomaltase activity; and the beta-glucosidases, which have the lactase activity. There might be a specific enzyme deficiency as a congenital defect, or there might be secondary multiple enzyme deficiencies as acquired defects. In any instance disaccharidase deficiencies impair the digestion of dietary disaccharides and carbohydrate intolerance occurs, with diarrhea, acid stools and excretion of carbohydrates.

The treatment of disaccharidase deficiencies must be directed toward correcting the carbohydrate intolerance and the diarrheal disease. All the clinical symptoms will improve when the specific carbohydrate is eliminated from the diet. The dietary treatment of carbohydrate intolerance in diarrheal disease is described below. This type of therapy should be instituted as soon as the diagnosis of carbohydrate intolerance is made. During the acute stage of the illness of any specific disaccharidase defect there might be associated disaccharidase deficiencies secondary to the diarrheal course. Therefore, elimination of all the carbohydrates that are not tolerated is indicated. However, after recovery, only the specific incriminating disaccharides need be eliminated from the diet. In patients with alpha-glucosidase deficiencies there is usually an intolerance to sucrose and isomaltose. Maltose is usually well tolerated; however, there have been a few patients described who have maltase deficiency and who are unable to tolerate maltose as well. On the other hand, in patients with lactase deficiency, lactose will have to be eliminated from the diet and the other disaccharides might be included since they are usually absorbed normally. In these congenital forms of the disease a prolonged adherence to the dietary regimen is necessary. The disaccharide should be sufficiently restricted from the diet to keep the patient symptom-free and growing at a normal rate. In all instances of congenital disaccharidase deficiencies a gradual increased tolerance of the specific carbohydrates might be observed. The patients may eventually tolerate an ordinary diet, but with certain limitations throughout life in regard to their specific intolerance. Even patients with lactase deficiency can consume some milk without any problem. On the other hand, in patients with lactose intolerance and lactosuria, lactose should be eliminated from the diet as well. However, these patients require a very strict adherence to the lactose-free diets for a limited time only. Once the acute stage is over, a normal diet might be tolerated.

An isolated intestinal lactase deficiency, and/or a decreased blood sugar rise after lactose oral loads, is often found in large segments of the population. These findings may indicate the presence of some alterations in the handling of lactose. However, if not accompanied by clinical lactose intolerance, this sugar need not be eliminated from the diet. Multiple disaccharidase deficiencies are usually found in association with other alterations and in many instances of the malabsorption syndrome as secondary acquired alterations. However, only patients who have clinical evidence of carbohydrate intolerance need be treated. Disaccharidase deficiencies diagnosed in a biopsy specimen need not be treated.

Premature infants have a relative lactase deficiency that results in a diminished capacity to digest and absorb lactose. They usually do not have diarrhea while on milk formula feedings. However, they may develop metabolic acidosis, with a drop in blood pH and serum CO_2, when fed lactose. These patients may be treated by lactose-free formulas during the first three weeks of life.

Monosaccharide Transport Defects. Infants with congenital glucose-galactose malabsorption cannot be kept free from symptoms unless they are fed a diet containing fructose as the only carbohydrate. However, gradually they might be offered some solid or semisolid food items with low starch content. Between two to three years of age these patients may tolerate ordinary children's food, but with certain limitations in regard to milk- and starch-containing foods (bread, potatoes and cereals). They can usually consume one glass of milk, two or three sandwiches and two small potatoes daily without major trouble. These diet restrictions then have to be followed for the rest of their lives. Whenever diarrhea is induced there must be a reduction of the various carbohydrates that are being fed. On the other hand, if no gastrointestinal symptoms occur, the patient may have an intake of these nutrients to provide for normal growth and development.

Patients with the acquired form of monosaccharide malabsorption do not tolerate any carbohydrates, including monosaccharides such as fructose. These alterations usually follow an acquired episode of gastroenteritis and are accompanied by inflammation and bacterial overgrowth of the upper segments of the small intestine with positive duodenal cultures. The culture of the duodenal fluid in the upper segments usually yields bacteria in concentrations above 10^7 per ml. The treatment consists of carbohydrate-free formulas during the acute stage of the illness. During this period utmost care should be exercised to provide glucose parenterally to avoid hypoglycemia. Specific antibiotic therapy to reduce the duodenal infection is indicated and may allow a more rapid recovery. After the diarrhea improves, feedings of small concentration of glucose by mouth should be initiated at a concentration of 1 per cent. Gradual increments in the concentration of glucose from 1 to 5 per cent may follow as long as this solution is tolerated. The intravenous administration of glucose is gradually reduced when carbohydrate intake by mouth is at a 3 per cent level. After a 5 per cent glucose intake is tolerated, disaccharide might be introduced in the diet, starting with maltose, and following with isomaltose, sucrose and finally lactose, as described in the section on carbohydrate intolerance in infants with diarrhea. Should glucose malabsorption persist after a period free from diarrhea, an attempt should be made to diagnose and treat persistent duodenal infection or other alterations.

Abnormalities of Intestinal Lymphatic Transport

Abnormalities of intestinal lymphatic transport associated with malabsorption may be effectively managed in some cases. For example, in *congenital lymphangiectasia* the protein loss, which is moderate, will be reduced considerably by the administration of a medium chain triglyceride or a low fat diet. *Whipple's disease,* caused by an unknown microorganism visible on electron microscopy, responds dramatically and, it appears, permanently to continuous administration of tetracycline or other broad-spectrum antimicrobials. Withdrawal of therapy is almost always associated with a recurrence of the disease in a period of weeks to months. The mild malabsorption which results from *constrictive pericarditis* is corrected by pericardiolysis.

Abnormalities Caused by Multiple Factors

Malnutrition. In human and in experimental protein and protein-calorie malnutrition, the small intestinal mucosa retains its morphologic and functional integrity longer than other tissues. However, eventually intestinal mucosal atrophy ensues and malabsorption syndrome occurs as a part of primary protein malnutrition. Exocrine pancreatic insufficiency contributes in part to the malabsorption syndrome of patients with protein deprivation and, ordinarily, its dysfunction precedes that of the bowel. It is important to know whether malabsorption in many instances is primary or secondary to severe malnutrition.

Bacterial Overgrowth. The presence of bacterial overgrowth in the upper segments of the small bowel is important in the genesis of malabsorption. Under normal circumstances the duodenal fluid is sterile. Heavy overgrowth of bacteria is defined as a concentration of more than 10^6 organisms per ml. of intestinal fluid. The elimination of the bacteria from the upper segments of the small intestine may result in improvement of the malabsorption.

Excision of a fistula or resection of blind loops due to multiple stricture might be curative. When corrective surgery is not possible, oral administration of specific antimicrobials should be given after appropriate cultures are obtained. These preparations might be rotated on a schedule as indicated by bacterial and antibiotic sensitivity studies. The culture of intestinal fluid by transintestinal tubes may be very helpful. Chronic stasis in the small intestine with bacterial overgrowth in scleroderma and diabetic neuropathy requires continuous administration of broad-spectrum antimicrobials.

Protein-Losing Enteropathy. In any patient with protein-losing enteropathy, an extensive search must be made of the cardiovascular system and the gastrointestinal tract for a treatable lesion. Multiple causes might be associated with protein-losing enteropathy, and they all require specific treatment in each instance.

Carbohydrate Intolerance in Diarrheal Disease. In severe diarrheal disease of infancy, carbohydrate intolerance usually occurs. Any child with diarrhea who excretes carbohydrates in the stools (more than 0.25 per cent reducing substances and 1+ glucose) and who has acid feces (pH of less than 6) has carbohydrate intolerance. Using these criteria, this complication occurs in up to 77 per cent of infants with severe diarrhea during the acute stage of the illness. In the treatment of diarrheal disease of infancy the selection of the appropriate formula mixture to initiate feedings once dehydration and electrolyte imbalance are corrected is most important. A brief period of 6 to 24 hours of fasting and then a gradual build-up of nutrients is indicated for the start of treatment. Although oral fluids are initiated, it is important to continue the intravenous infusion of electrolyte solutions to maintain vascular volume and renal function and to replace stool losses. During the acute stage of the illness oral feedings may be initiated with a dilute electrolyte mixture containing glucose (to make the solution isotonic) to ensure that the patient tolerates oral fluids and that vomiting is no longer a problem.

However, milk or other infant feeding preparations can be given soon afterwards. Patients fed with carbohydrates which are tolerated possibly may be given a full caloric intake without increased stool losses of water and electrolytes. However, there might be other disturbances of the intestine, in addition to those of carbohydrate absorption, which dictate careful resumption of milk feedings. The amount of intake is gradually increased up to 150 ml. per kilogram of body weight as the infant recovers from the illness sufficiently to develop a good appetite. As soon as excessive stool losses are no longer a problem, intravenous infusion should be stopped.

Since lactose intolerance is a frequent occurrence in severe diarrheal disease, the administration of a feeding preparation containing carbohydrates other than lactose as a source of calories is recommended. Infants with a short diarrheal course of less than one week's duration usually tolerate other disaccharides and may therefore be given a lactose-free disaccharide-containing diet. Those patients who have had a prolonged diarrheal course usually have a generalized disaccharide intolerance and should therefore be treated with a disaccharide-free, glucose-containing formula. These diets are now commercially available and they may be routinely employed as a starting formula for all infants hospitalized for severe diarrhea, provided that glucose is not given in a concentration above 5 per cent.

The use of carbohydrate-free formulas should be reserved for those patients who continue to have diarrhea and glucose intolerance. Carbohydrate-free feedings are not without danger; hypoglycemia might ensue as a severe complication during the acute stage or after recovery. Utmost care should be exercised to provide parenteral glucose to those infants throughout the time they are not fed carbohydrates. Fructose-containing formulas should be reserved for treatment of infants with specific congenital glucose-galactose malabsorption. In diarrheal disease of infancy there is infection and inflammation of the small intestine; the permeability of the intestinal mucosa is therefore altered, with markedly decreased transport of fructose.

The capacity to tolerate carbohydrates is rapidly recovered after the diarrhea ceases. An increased number of sugars and more complex carbohydrates may be given to the patient soon afterward. As soon as glucose is tolerated, maltose is introduced, followed by isomaltose, sucrose and finally lactose. This can be done by feedings of Dextri-Maltose as a source of carbohydrates in the carbohydrate-free formula. Subsequently, the diet is expanded with cereal and starches, table sugar and, finally, regular milk formula. Even patients with severe forms of carbohydrate intolerance tolerate lactose within four months of the acute stage of the illness. An attempt should be made to diagnose other abnormalities if carbohydrate intolerance persists.

Hard Water Feedings. In infants the hardness of the water might be a factor in inducing malabsorption. This should be suspected when the patient repeatedly improves after admission to the hospital and deteriorates when he is fed at home. Water is considered hard when it contains 100 to 200 parts per million of minerals. The treatment is to substitute the water supply and prepare infant formula with soft water, containing less than 50 parts per million of minerals.

Unclassified

Immune-Deficiency Disorders. Replacement therapy with intramuscular gamma globulin injections has occasionally controlled steatorrhea in some of these patients. However, in others it has persisted. It has been pointed out that gamma globulin concentrates used for replacement therapy contain predominantly gamma globulin fraction, which does not replace deficient gamma A and M globulins. Many patients with hypogammaglobulinemia have suffered from enteric infection, particularly *Giardia lamblia.* Eradication of this parasite from the intestine has controlled diarrhea and steatorrhea on several occasions. In these patients, antibiotic therapy may also be effective even without the presence of specific pathogens. Occasionally, fresh plasma transfusions have been lifesaving and may control steatorrhea and diarrhea.

Endocrinopathies. Frequently the presenting diagnosis of a patient with hypoparathyroidism is malabsorption syndrome. A patient with malabsorption syndrome who has an elevated serum phosphate level should be suspected of having hypoparathyroidism; specific vitamin D therapy should be instituted. Dihydrotachysterol (Hytakerol, 0.25 mg. per ml. or 0.125-mg. capsules in doses varying from 0.5 mg. to 2 mg. per day by mouth is sufficient to control this disease. A normal serum calcium may be maintained and urinary calcium excretion should be kept at less than 100 mg. per day. In other instances there may be hypothyroidism, and replacement therapy with thyroid hormone should be given [thyroid (U. S. P.) doses vary from 1 to 3 grains, depending upon age].

It has been emphasized in recent literature that steatorrhea in a diabetic may be associated with pancreatic insufficiency, celiac disease or diabetic neuropathy. Severe visceroneuropathy is more common in the young, poorly controlled diabetic. Gastrointestinal symptoms are often intermittent and usually respond to improved diabetic control.

DIETARY THERAPY

In general, the diet should be selected after the specific diagnosis has been established. The diet should provide an adequate amount of calories to allow normal weight increments and catch-up growth. Emphasis should be given to treating the patient rather than the stools. Increasing stool losses might be associated with an increased food intake. However, the increased proportion of nutrients being absorbed might be sufficient to improve the nutritional status of the patient.

Medium Chain Triglycerides. An increasing body of evidence suggests that the administration of medium chain triglycerides as the predominant source of fat in the diet is of benefit to patients with malabsorption, particularly to those with short gut syndrome, regional enteritis, inadequate digestion due to exocrine pancreatic insufficiency, A-beta-lipoproteinemia and abnormalities of intestine lymphatic transport of fat. Medium chain triglyceride preparations might also be considered for patients with severe malabsorption of any sort as a supplement to the diet when there is severe malnutrition, in addition to other modes of therapy during the initial phase of treatment or as the only treatment in specific entities. The rationale for the use of this agent is that medium chain triglycerides are more easily hydrolyzed than are long chain triglycerides, requiring little conjugated bile salts or pancreatic enzymes. In addition, medium chain fatty acids are more readily taken up and transported by the mucosal cells. Finally, they find their way into the portal vein, not requiring incorporation into chylomicrons and entrance to the lymphatics to complete their absorption. Medium chain triglycerides are available as oil, or as powder (Portagen), which can be dissolved to make a liquid formula, and as the medium chain triglyceride used in food preparations. The side effects include high blood levels of medium chain fatty acids, specifically in patients with impaired hepatic function. Therefore, in patients with liver disease caution must be exercised to avoid coma. Additionally, medium chain triglyceride therapy can induce diabetic ketoacidosis in susceptible individuals. The administration of medium chain triglycerides may induce gastrointestinal symptoms and diarrhea; therefore, the dose should gradually be built up.

Gluten-Free Diet. For details of the gluten content of foodstuffs, specific tables should be consulted.* In general, any food containing wheat, wheat flour, rye, barley or malt should be eliminated from the diet. Careful efforts should be made to avoid foods that frequently contain concealed "gluten," including meatloafs, canned meat dishes, frankfurters, cold cuts, beer and ale, commercial salad dressings and some commercial ice creams, food prepared with bread, and cracker crumbs. Other foods are allowed. Rice, soy, potatoes or cornmeal flour may be used as "breading" or in preparations of stuffing or gravies.

Source and Concentration of Carbohydrate, Protein and Fat, and Osmolar Load of Commercial Products Frequently Used in Infant Feedings. The amount, the type and the number of nutrients in each of the formulas vary. It is important to know the basic differences in each of these preparations to understand the therapeutic effects and to plan specific dietary intakes. A frequent error is the diagnosis of "milk allergy," with excellent response and improvement after the formula is changed to one with a different protein source. However, often the carbohydrate source is also changed and the improvement of these patients might be related to the simultaneous lactose elimination. We now know that the majority of these infants have lactose intolerance, not milk protein allergy. In addition to the source and concentrations of the various nutrients, it is important to consider the osmotic load that the formulas provide. Hyperosmolar formulas may induce diarrhea and malabsorption, even though they are an adequate source of carbohydrate, protein and fat. Table 2 summarizes data on the source and concentration of these nutrients as well as the osmolar loads of the most frequently employed commercial products in infant feedings at a normal dilution (20 calories per ounce).

Other sources of carbohydrates in food as well as in medications should be considered. The carbohydrate content of food may be found in specific tables.† The common carbohydrates in fruits are fructose, glucose, sucrose and starch; in vegetables, sucrose and starch; in mature dry

* See *Current Pediatric Therapy 5*, pp. 11–18.

† See Cornblath, M., and Schwartz, R. (eds.): Disorders of Carbohydrate Metabolism in Infancy. Philadelphia, W. B. Saunders Company, 1966, pp. 281–284.

TABLE 2. Analysis of Commercial Products Used in Infant Feeding

FORMULA	CARBOHYDRATE (Gm./100 ml.)		PROTEIN (Gm./100 ml.)		FAT (Gm./100 ml.)		OSMOLALITY (mMol./liter)
Bremil	lactose	7.0	skim milk	1.5	peanut, coconut and corn oil	3.7	307
Enfamil	lactose	7.0	skim milk	1.5	soy, corn and coconut oils	3.7	293
Similac	lactose	7.0	skim milk	1.8	coconut, soy and corn oils	3.6	293
Similac (PM 60/40)	lactose	7.6	electrodialyzed whey, skim milk	1.6	corn and coconut oils	3.5	427
SMA	lactose	7.2	skim milk, electrodialyzed whey	1.5	oleo, coconut, oleic (safflower) and soybean oils	3.6	300
Lonalac	lactose	4.8	casein	3.4	coconut oil	3.5	259
Mull-Soy	sucrose	5.2	soy flour	3.1	soy oil	3.6	236
Neo-Mull-Soy	sucrose	6.4	soy protein isolate	1.8	soy oil	3.5	253
ProSobee	sucrose, corn syrup solids	6.8	soy protein isolate	2.5	soy oil	3.4	252
Soyalac	sucrose, dextrins-maltose-dextrose	6.7	soybean solids	2.2	soybean oil	3.8	203
Isomil	sucrose, corn syrup solids, corn starch	6.8	soy protein isolate	2.0	corn and coconut oils	3.6	200
Meat Base Formula	sucrose, modified tapioca starch	4.2	beef hearts	2.9	sesame oil	3.3	147
Lofenalac	corn syrup solids, arrowroot starch, sucrose	8.7	Specially processed hydrolyzed casein	0.4	corn oil	2.7	362
Nutramigen	sucrose, tapioca starch	8.6	enzymically hydrolyzed casein	2.2	corn oil	2.6	468
Portagen	corn syrup solids, sucrose	7.8	sodium caseinate	2.4	fractionated coconut oil, corn oil (trace)	3.3	346
Probana	banana powder, dextrose	7.9	whole milk curd, nonfat dry milk, enzymically hydrolyzed casein	4.2	butterfat, corn oil	2.2	653
Pregestimil	dextrose, tapioca starch	8.8	enzymically hydrolyzed casein	2.2	fractionated coconut oil, corn oil (trace)	2.8	715
Cho-Free*	Formula base does not contain carbohydrate	0.02	soy protein isolate	1.9	soy oil	3.4	113

* Cho-free does not provide 20 calories per ounce unless carbohydrate is added. The manufacturers recommend the addition of dextrose, 6 tablespoons per 26 fluid ounces, to make the solution isocaloric. However, this provides a 12 per cent carbohydrate solution with an excessive osmolar load of approximately 773 mMol. per liter. In a 5 per cent glucose concentration the osmolar load is approximately 391 mMol. per liter. The specific amounts of each carbohydrate in formulas containing several sugars may be obtained from the manufacturer.

Carbohydrate-free formulas should not be administered without providing parenteral glucose, since hypoglycemia might be induced.

legumes, sucrose and starch; in cereal and cereal products, starch and small amounts of sucrose; and in spices and condiments, starch. Syrups and other sweets usually contain glucose, maltose and polysaccharide dextrins. Honey contains fructose and glucose. Milk and milk products are the major sources of lactose. Milk of any sort contains lactose in concentrations varying from 3.8 per cent in yogurt to 7 per cent in human milk. Goat's milk contains 4.7 per cent lactose.

NONSPECIFIC REPLACEMENT THERAPY

In patients with malabsorption syndrome of any cause there may be associated vitamin and mineral deficiencies. Specific treatment should be given after the diagnosis is made. The possibility of vitamin A, B, E, D and K deficiency should be considered. Vitamin B_{12} and folic acid deficits may also be present. Severe potassium and magnesium deficiency is often encountered. Iron deficiency and anemia are frequent. The treatment of specific alterations is as follows:

Vitamin A. 10,000 to 20,000 units daily of a water-soluble preparation.

Vitamin B_6. 2.5 mg. per day. If convulsion of unknown cause occurs, give up to 5 to 10 mg. per day.

Vitamin B_{12}. Treatment of pernicious anemia must be individualized. In general, 1000 to 5000 micrograms provide a hematologic response. This dose can be given as 100 micrograms per day for two or more weeks. Maintenance therapy is 2 micrograms per day or a single injection every month or every other month.

Folic Acid. Treat anemia with 5 to 10 mg. daily for seven days. Parenteral administration (1 mg. per day for four to five days) is required if there is diarrhea or difficulties in giving the medication by mouth. Maintenance therapy with 5 to 10 mg. daily may be required.

Vitamin K. 2 to 5 mg. daily, orally or parenterally, to correct the prothrombin time.

Vitamin E. 15 mg. of tocopherol daily until normal levels are restored.

Iron. The dosage of oral ferrous sulfate should be calculated on the basis of the elemental iron content of the preparation used. These range from 25 mg. per ml. for the concentrates given in drop form (Fer-In-Sol iron drops), to 8 to 10 mg. per ml. for the elixir and syrup given by teaspoon (Fer-In-Sol elixir). The recommended dosage of these preparations is 6 to 8 mg. per kilogram per day, given in three or four divided doses. Iron dextran parenteral preparations may be given when malabsorption obviates the use of an oral preparation during the acute stage of illness. The dose should be calculated according to the following formula: weight in kilograms $\times$ (13.5 — patient's hemoglobin in Gm. per 100 ml.) $\times$ 2.5 = milligrams of iron needed. The total dose can be given in divided portions at daily intervals during the acute stage. This dose will not replace iron stores. This can later be achieved by the oral route if malabsorption improves.

Vitamin D. Vitamin D deficiency with or without hypocalcemia responds to a single oral dose of 600,000 units. This may be given in one dose or divided in four doses over a 24-hour period. There is no advantage to giving vitamin D_2 parenterally, even if there is severe intestinal malabsorption. It is wise to mix vitamin D with medium chain triglyceride oil. The usual vitamin D_2 preparation is diluted with propylene glycol and provides 400 to 800 units per ml. Careful attention should be paid to not giving this medication, since giving this high a dose would produce propylene glycol toxicity.

Calcium. CALCIUM GLUCONATE. Hypocalcemic tetany frequently occurs in patients with malabsorption and must be treated during the acute stage with intravenous calcium: calcium gluconate (9 per cent calcium, 100 mg. per ml. vials), 20 mg. per kilogram per dose, not exceeding 2 Gm. Inject slowly and stop if bradycardia occurs. Do not give intramuscularly or subcutaneously. Calcium supplements might be given by mouth as well; however, a positive response should follow the large dose of vitamin D administration. If hypocalcemia persists, magnesium deficiency must be considered.

CALCIUM CHLORIDE. Calcium chloride (27 per cent calcium) dosage in infants is 1 to 2 Gm. per day by mouth, and in children 2 to 4 Gm. per day by mouth. Give in milk, not exceeding a 5 per cent concentration.

CALCIUM LACTATE. Calcium lactate (13 per cent calcium) dosage is 0.5 Gm. per kilogram per day by mouth in divided dosages.

CALCIUM GLUCONATE. Calcium gluconate (9 per cent calcium) dosage is 0.5 Gm. per kilogram per day. Infants should receive 3 to 6 Gm. per day, and children 6 to 10 Gm. per day by mouth, not exceeding a 10 per cent concentration.

NEO-CALGLUCON SYRUP. 4 ml. of Neo-Calglucon Syrup (calcium gluconogalactogluconate) is equivalent to 1 Gm. of calcium gluconate (90 mg. calcium).

Magnesium. Hypomagnesemia is treated with magnesium given parenterally, either intravenously or intramuscularly, 3 mEq. per kilogram per day, with a maximum of 60 mEq. per day. Intravenous magnesium is given by slow drip with blood pressure and cardiac monitoring.

MAGNESIUM SULFATE. Magnesium sulfate [$MgSO_4 \bullet 7H_2O$ (U. S. P.) 50 per cent solution] provides 4 mEq. magnesium per ml. for intravenous or intramuscular administration.

MAGNESIUM CHLORIDE. 4 Gm. of magnesium chloride ($Mg \bullet Cl_2 \bullet 6H_2O$) provides 40 mEq.

MAGNESIUM CITRATE. 6 Gm. of magnesium citrate ($MgHC6H_5O_7 \bullet 5H_2O$) provides 40 mEq.

Any of these magnesium salts added to water to 100 ml. makes a solution which provides 0.8 mEq. of magnesium per ml. for oral intake, at a dose of 2 to 3 mEq. per kilogram per day. The dose should be built up gradually to avoid diarrhea.

DIAGNOSIS BY TRIAL OF THERAPY

The diagnosis of the malabsorption syndrome is occasionally substantiated by a therapeutic trial. Examples are as follows: clinical and biochemical response to a gluten-free diet (celiac disease); to withdrawal of lactose or other specific carbohydrates (lactose intolerance, disaccharide or monosaccharide intolerance and/or disaccharidase deficiencies); to elimination of specific bovine milk protein (allergy); to a course of broad-spectrum antibiotics (Whipple's disease, bacterial overgrowth); to therapy with specific hormones (hypothyroid, hypoparathyroid, diabetes); or to a therapeutic trial of antiparasitics (*Giardia lamblia* infestation). Response to pancreatic extracts in pancreatic insufficiency is also often an aid in the diagnosis. Response to adrenal steroids is rather nonspecific. In addition, the exact diagnosis of specific disease entities may have to await the improvement of malnutrition and the secondary digestive and absorptive alterations. However, the response to therapy should never be employed instead of a diagnostic work-up.

Disorders of the Anus and Rectum

STEPHEN L. GANS, M.D.

ECTOPIC OR IMPERFORATE ANUS; ANORECTAL STENOSIS

For purposes of management, these congenital anomalies are divided into three categories. In the first group are those in which meconium is demonstrated in a tract on the perineum or in which there is a thin layer covering the end of the bowel. These should have an immediate definitive corrective operation. In the second group are those in which meconium is freely discharged on the perineum or in the vaginal fourchette. Operation can be postponed for about three months. The orifice is kept open by dilations when necessary, and impaction is prevented by dietary regulation and occasional enemas. In these two groups the prognosis is excellent and there are few complications. The third group consists of those cases in which the terminal end of bowel communicates with the urinary tract or vagina, or ends blindly at some distance from the peritoneum. Preliminary colostomy is done and definitive correction is postponed for a period of three to six months, or longer when indicated.

Congenital or postoperative stenoses are both treated initially by progressive dilatation with well-lubricated dilators, and later with the finger. Rarely, it is necessary to cut a thick fibrous ring before dilatation can be carried out.

RECTAL PROLAPSE

Mild degrees of prolapse usually recede spontaneously. Treatment of constipation or diarrhea, if present, will assist in this process. More severe degrees of prolapse may need manual replacement. This can be done by gentle insertion of a finger, covered with a finger cot and well lubricated, into the lumen of the protruding mass and pushing it back into place, in the manner of performing a rectal examination. If the prolapse comes out between bowel movements, it is sometimes helpful after reduction to strap the buttocks together with adhesive tape.

By using the foregoing methods of assistance, almost all cases are self-limiting and the condition will improve and disappear with the growth of the child. In the unusual circumstances in which this does not occur, more radical methods of treatment may become necessary. Injections of sclerosing solutions into the submucous or retrorectal areas at regular or irregular intervals have not been consistently satisfactory. Surgical procedures are rarely indicated and range from packing gauze between the rectum and presacral fascia, to various types of resections and rectosigmoidopexies.

ANAL FISSURE, CRYPTITIS AND PAPILLITIS

Almost all of these conditions respond to conservative measures, and surgery is reserved for the complications of longstanding or untreated cases. Hard bulky stools are changed by dietary measures and the use of stool softeners and mineral oil. Initially, large doses of dioctyl sodium sulfosuccinate (Colace) in milk or fruit juice, 20 mg. three or four times daily, are used in infants and small children, and this can be reduced as the effects are noted. Mineral oil, 5 ml. or more morning and night, is a helpful lubricant. Anal spasm is reduced by frequent warm baths (three or four a day) and the use of soothing suppositories with hydrocortisone (Desitin HC or A and D HC) after each bath and each bowel movement. Anesthetic suppositories or ointments are of little value and may sensitize the anus and surrounding skin. This regimen should be continued for at least two weeks, although symptoms may subside in a few days.

If conservative measures fail, the infant should be hospitalized and undergo proctoscopy under general anesthesia. If an anal ulcer or chronic indurated fissure is present, it should be excised. Deep crypts can be incised. If none of these complications is present, simple dilatation of the anal sphincters under anesthesia will greatly assist in bringing about improvement along with continuation of the previously described medical measures.

Prolonged untreated cryptitis or fissure may result in other complications, namely, anorectal abscess and fistula in ano.

ANORECTAL ABSCESS

Before fluctuation is evident, resolution may occur with frequent warm baths or packs (four or five times daily) and the use of antibiotics. Failure to improve in 24 to 48 hours, and the presence of fluctuation, are indications for incision and drainage under a general anesthesia. Postoperatively, warm baths are continued and the area is kept clean by frequent washing with a bland antibacterial soap, such as povidone-iodine (Betadine Surgical Scrub Skin Cleaner) to avoid seeding of nearby irritated areas. Many will heal completely and permanently, but attention should be directed to bowel habits to prevent a recurrence. A number will go on to the next phase or complication, fistula in ano.

FISTULA IN ANO

A number of these conditions will heal and disappear with only warm baths and local cleanliness, as well as attention to bowel habits (see Anal Fissures). If resolution does not occur in four weeks, the infant should be hospitalized for surgical treatment, i.e. fistulotomy, or fistulectomy. The wound is allowed to close spontaneously, with warm baths and local cleanliness as the only postoperative treatment.

HEMORRHOIDS

Hemorrhoids are rarely a primary problem in infants and children. Warm baths and attention to bowel habits will usually obtain satisfactory results, unless the distended veins are due to another primary cause such as portal hypertension or intra-abdominal tumor. Rarely, hemorrhoidectomy is indicated because of recurrent pain, ulceration and bleeding that does not respond to the above-mentioned treatment.

TRAUMA

Damage to the anus or rectum may occur from impalement by falling or sitting on sharp or elongated objects. Injuries occasionally occur by the use of rectal thermometers, enemas, anoscopes or anal dilators. The wound may be extraperitoneal or intraperitoneal and may result in hemorrhage or inflammation (intraperitoneal or perirectal). Roentgenographic examination of the abdomen for possible pneumoperitoneum will assist in determining the type of treatment.

When intraperitoneal perforation has occurred, immediate operation is indicated, with closure of the perforation and proximal colostomy. For lower lesions, careful inspection of the anus, digital examination, and anoscopy under general anesthesia may be necessary to delineate the wound. Lesser wounds may be treated by irrigation with normal saline solution, debridement and loose primary suture. More extensive and complicated wounds may need a diverting colostomy and drainage of the extrarectal areas. Perirectal or anal abscesses or fistulas may complicate this injury.

FOREIGN BODIES

Foreign bodies will almost all pass in 24 to 48 hours. If they do not, or if a larger foreign body is impacted, general anesthesia will be necessary. The sphincters may be dilated or even cut in order to remove the large impacted foreign body, and smaller incarcerated objects may be removed through an anoscope. Enemas are contraindicated, but mineral oil may be helpful, given orally.

PRURITUS ANI

The causes of this condition may be coarse or moist underclothing, uncleanliness, pinworms, anal fissure or fistula in ano. The treatment is to correct any of these causes. Hydrocortisone ointment may be helpful while awaiting results of treatment.

7

Blood

Anemias of Iron Deficiency, Blood Loss, Renal Disease and Chronic Infection

JAMES A. WOLFF, M.D.

ANEMIA OF IRON DEFICIENCY

One of the most frequently encountered errors in the therapy of pediatric hematologic disorders is the indiscriminate use of iron medication. As a result, many infants and children with diseases such as heterozygous thalassemia or mild hereditary spherocytosis are given oral iron preparations periodically by a succession of physicians. This therapy is ineffective and in some cases deleterious. Therefore careful history-taking and physical examination and appropriate diagnostic procedures must be carried out before embarking on treatment with iron. Moreover, treatment of iron deficiency consists not only in the replenishment of deficient body stores of iron but also in the elucidation of the cause of this deficit. Except in infants and young children, nutritional iron deficiency anemia is uncommon in most areas of the United States today. In older children, chronic blood loss is of more importance. Therefore, even when a history of inadequate dietary intake of iron is obtained, search for possible blood loss from the intestinal tract by means of examinations of at least three stools for occult blood is essential.

For subjects in whom the diagnosis of iron deficiency anemia presumably has been established, oral rather than parenteral iron therapy is almost always indicated. Both ferrous and ferric forms of iron compounds are available for the treatment of iron deficit anemia. Since iron is absorbed in the ferrous state and since ferrous iron preparations are as well tolerated in pediatric patients as are ferric compounds, treatment with a simple ferrous compound, ferrous sulfate, is the drug of choice. Adjuvants to increase iron absorption are not necessary, despite the recommendations of many pharmaceutical concerns.

The dosage of iron required should be calculated on a weight basis. Five mg. of elemental iron per kilogram of body weight daily in three divided doses will produce a maximal response. It has been shown that absorption of iron may be somewhat better when it is given between meals, although an adequate response may be obtained if given with food in the occasional patient who does not tolerate therapy on an empty stomach. A reticulocyte count should be performed one week after start of treatment, at which time a significant rise should be found if an appropriate response has occurred. The hemoglobin level will be restored to normal usually within four weeks. At this time, body stores of iron still will be deficient. Therefore, further treatment, for at least two months, is necessary.

Parenteral therapy is required rarely. The primary indication is in those subjects who are likely not to receive the medication as prescribed, because of ignorance, indifference or misunderstanding on the part of parents or guardians. Very rarely, parenteral iron may be required because of gastrointestinal intolerance to oral iron or because of underlying disorders leading to malabsorption of the medicinal compound. For such subjects, an iron dextran compound (Imferon) can be given intramuscularly. This material contains 50 mg. of elemental iron per ml. In order to prevent local irritation, it should be given deeply into the muscle, with a Z type of injection. To calculate in milligrams of elemental iron the total amount of parenteral iron required, the following formula may be used:

$$\frac{\text{Desired hemoglobin} - \text{current hemoglobin}}{100} \times \text{Blood volume (ml.)} \times 3.4 \times 1.5$$

Transfusions are indicated rarely in the treatment of iron deficiency anemia. Immediate restoration of the hemoglobin to normal may be required when an acute surgical emergency intervenes, when the anemia is complicated by severe infection or heart failure or when the hemoglobin level is below 3 Gm. per 100 ml. In such instances, packed red cell transfusions are more suitable than administration of whole blood. A maximum of 15 ml. per kilogram of body weight should be given at one time, slowly, at a rate not to exceed 40 ml. per hour. If heart failure is present or expected, 5 to 7 ml. of packed cells per kilogram of body weight should not be exceeded for the first transfusion.

The use of prophylactic iron therapy in infancy has been the subject of much discussion before and since the recommendation in 1971 of the Committee on Nutrition of the American Academy of Pediatrics* that all infants receive an iron-fortified formula for the first 12 months of life. Prior to 1971, medicinal iron fortification of the diet during the first year of life had been used primarily for premature infants. The proponents of prophylactic iron administration to all infants have marshaled strong evidence for this practice. It is certain that iron-fortified milk for the first year is desirable for infants in areas of the country where the usual infant diet is for various reasons inadequate, or for infants in a deprived socioeconomic environment. For other full-term infants, the necessity for iron-fortified formula throughout the first year of life is more questionable. Available iron-fortified formulas contain 12 mg. of elemental iron in each 13 ounces of concentrated formula for reconstitution, which will provide sufficient prophylactic supplemental iron for both premature and full-term infants.

BLOOD LOSS ANEMIA

Anemias resulting from acute blood loss are normocytic and normochromic. When hemorrhage has been sufficient to become life-threatening or to produce considerable morbidity, transfusion of blood is indicated. When the bleeding has been less severe but has resulted in some degree of anemia, it is preferable to administer oral iron medication in order to replenish the hemoglobin iron lost as a result of hemorrhage. In those instances of blood loss anemia for which transfusion is considered necessary, whole blood is preferable to packed cells, in order to restore the plasma volume as well as lost red cells and hemoglobin. For the usual hemorrhage requiring whole blood transfusion, 20 ml. per kilogram of body weight may be given, ordinarily not to exceed the volume obtained from 500 ml. of whole blood at a single transfusion, unless bleeding continues. With continuous bleeding, larger amounts may be necessary. If an abnormal bleeding problem is present, use of corrective factors may be helpful, as discussed elsewhere.

Chronic blood loss results in iron deficiency anemia. Transfusions are rarely required in this type of iron deficit anemia. The indications and types and volumes of transfusions mentioned in the previous section, Anemia of Iron Deficiency, are applicable. Considerations concerning iron therapy, already noted, are also relevant to chronic blood loss anemia.

ANEMIA OF RENAL DISEASE

The anemia of chronic renal disease with uremia is primarily the result of inadequate erythropoietic response in the presence of low-grade hemolysis as a consequence of both intracorpuscular and extracorpuscular factors. When the anemia is severe, transfusions of packed red cells should be given. We do not give transfusions to children with otherwise uncomplicated chronic renal disease whose hemoglobin level remains above 7 Gm. per 100 ml. If hypertension is a complication of the renal problem or if the child has evidence of heart failure, smaller volumes of sedimented red cells than advised in the previous section on Anemia of Iron Deficiency should be used.

Epistaxis is a common complication of chronic renal disease, and gastrointestinal hemorrhage may also be seen. This bleeding diathesis is presumably the result of an abnormality of platelet function. As a result, superimposed iron deficiency secondary to blood loss may aggravate the already existing anemia. In such instances, administration of oral iron in the form of ferrous sulfate should be given in a dose of 5 mg. per kilogram of body weight per day in three divided doses.

Superimposed megaloblastic anemia as a result of dietary deficiency resulting in low serum folate levels has been reported in children with chronic renal disease. This has been very uncommon in our experience. If megaloblastic blood production is documented, ad-

* Committee on Nutrition: Iron Fortified Formulas. *Pediatrics,* 47:786, 1971.

ministration of folic acid, 5 mg. by mouth daily, will produce a partial correction of the anemia.

In acute glomerulonephritis, with or without azotemia, a low-grade anemia frequently occurs as a result of hemodilution because of increased plasma volume. No therapy is indicated for the anemia since spontaneous correction will occur as the basic process subsides.

ANEMIA OF CHRONIC INFECTION

The anemias associated with chronic infection result primarily from inadequate erythropoiesis because of inadequate iron utilization. Despite adequate iron stores, impaired release of iron by the reticuloendothelial system results from chronic infection. Essential to the treatment of the anemia is an attempt to eliminate the infection. Unless the nature of the underlying disease process is determined with subsequent eradication of the infecting organism, correction of the anemia cannot be accomplished. Persistence of severe anemia may require the use of periodic blood transfusions. The hemoglobin level at which transfusion is indicated will vary from subject to subject. Unless other complications are present which would dictate transfusion at a higher level of hemoglobin, such as a necessity for surgical intervention, we do not advise transfusion unless the hemoglobin is less than 7 Gm. per 100 ml. In the anemia of chronic infection, packed red cell rather than whole blood transfusions are used.

Aplastic and Hypoplastic Anemia

ROBERT C. NEERHOUT, M.D.

APLASTIC ANEMIA

Aplastic anemia is a disorder characterized by pancytopenia of the peripheral blood in association with marked reduction of normal marrow hematopoietic elements (red cell, granulocyte and platelet precursors). Bone marrow aspiration followed by biopsy confirmation is mandatory to rule out maturation arrest or neoplastic replacement as the cause. Although cases of presumed aplastic anemia with normocellular or even hypercellular bone marrow have been described, their inclusion in this group must be accepted with some skepticism.

Cases may be divided into congenital and acquired forms. The congenital form is most frequently associated with a variety of other congenital anomalies (as in Fanconi anemia), but familial forms without associated anomalies have been reported. Acquired forms of the disease are largely associated with exposure to any one of a large variety of hematopoietic toxins, most notably chloramphenicol, nonbarbiturate anticonvulsants, organic solvents and pesticides. Current information on compounds implicated in the cause of aplastic anemia can be obtained from the Bureau of Drugs of the Food and Drug Administration. Any suspected compounds should be reported to this agency. An exhaustive search for possible hematopoietic toxins is indicated since the prognosis of cases where a toxin is identified and removed may be better than that in cases where no toxin is identified (and repeated exposure may therefore continue). Acquired aplastic anemia has also been noted following infectious diseases, most notably infectious hepatitis.

The mortality from aplastic anemia is mainly related to overwhelming infection (secondary to neutropenia) or bleeding (secondary to thrombocytopenia). This is particularly true in the acquired forms of the disease where the onset may be more acute and the pancytopenia more severe than in the congenital forms. The overall mortality rate, even with intensive therapy, is generally 50 per cent (or higher) and death may occur within the first weeks or months of the disease. It is difficult to predict which cases will have a fulminant course, but this is most likely to be seen in acquired disease with severe pancytopenia and a markedly acellular marrow. An aggressive approach to this form of disease with possible bone marrow transplant must be given stronger consideration as this technique becomes increasingly available.

Good supportive care remains the most important therapeutic objective aimed at tiding the patient over the aplastic phase to allow the marrow a chance to recover. Maintenance of an adequate hemoglobin level above 5 to 6 Gm. per 100 ml. can be easily attained by packed cell transfusions. The use of a few selected compatible donors for all transfusions reduces the possibility of hepatitis and transfusion reactions. Complete blood typing, including minor blood groups in addition to ABO and Rh(D), prior to any transfusion provides useful information in selecting the best donors. This is particularly helpful if hemolytic transfusion reactions begin to occur after multiple transfusions. If pyrogenic transfusion reactions develop, they may be minimized by saline washing of the donor red cells prior to administration. In patients surviving several years with continued transfusion requirements, the frequency of transfusion must be carefully considered to minimize, if possible, the development of hemosiderosis.

Replacement transfusion of platelets to control hemorrhage can be quite beneficial if used judiciously. Platelets harvested at room temperature and administered within a few hours have proven effective in elevating the platelet count and controlling hemorrhage early in the course of the disease. The use of one platelet pack (i.e., the platelets harvested from one unit of whole blood) per 10 pounds body weight will usually attain hemostatic levels. After repeated platelet transfusions, antiplatelet antibodies will develop which decrease the effectiveness of this mode of therapy. This problem can be reduced if techniques for selecting histocompatible donors (HL-A identical, identical twin) are available. Because of these difficulties, the use of "prophylactic" platelet transfusions in an attempt to maintain a minimal acceptable platelet count is not recommended. Platelet transfusion should be utilized vigorously at the first sign of a significant bleeding episode but not for minor problems such as skin petechiae or purpura. All thrombocytopenic patients should carefully avoid the ingestion of any drug known to interfere with platelet function, most notably aspirin and antihistamines. Potential platelet donors should be screened for recent ingestion of such compounds since their platelets may be hemostatically ineffective.

Attempts to control granulocytopenia by transfusion have proven largely unsuccessful because of low cell yield and shortened cell survival. The use of buffy coat preparations from normal donors presents technical problems which make this procedure unfeasible. Utilization of patients with chronic granulocytic leukemia who have white cell counts in excess of 200,000 per cubic mm. may be considered if such a donor can be located. Here again, the short survival of such transfused cells makes this approach relatively ineffective. The development of automated cell separators and closed bag leukocyte collection systems should increase the availability of granulocyte replacement therapy in the near future.

Because of the lack of adequate granulocyte replacement, infection must be primarily approached from the viewpoint of prevention and antibiotic therapy. A major source of severe infection is from "within" the patient himself; i.e., from the normal flora of the skin and gastrointestinal tract. Consequently, strict isolation procedures are of limited value, but exposure to people with known infection, particularly respiratory, should be avoided. Procedures which break the normal skin barrier (e.g., finger punctures for blood counts, venipuncture, intravenous therapy) should be performed with scrupulous aseptic technique. Such sites should also be carefully examined for subsequent infection and treated vigorously. Prolonged intravenous therapy with indwelling catheters should be avoided. The use of chronic nasal packing to control epistaxis should be approached with caution as the incidence of secondary sinusitis appears to be high. Febrile episodes, particularly when associated with chills or other systemic signs, should be treated with broad bactericidal antibiotic coverage after cultures of blood, urine, throat and so forth have been obtained. Febrile episodes should not be treated with aspirin but with nonsalicylate antipyretics such as acetaminophen.

Specific drug therapy aimed at improving the hematologic status remains a controversial issue. Despite occasional reports to the contrary, corticosteroid drugs probably have little direct effect on marrow recovery. Consequently, the prolonged use of corticosteroids as a single drug for this purpose is not indicated. As with most thrombocytopenic states, corticosteroids may have an ameliorating effect on associated bleeding problems, presumably through improved platelet-vascular interaction or "vascular tone." Prednisone in doses of 1 to 1.5 mg. per kilogram per day can be used during episodes of clinical bleeding and may diminish the need for platelet transfusions at these times. Corticosteroid therapy alone should not be relied upon for controlling severe bleeding where platelet transfusion is more beneficial. The prolonged administration of corticosteroids to improve hemostasis must be considered with caution because of the increased susceptibility to infection associated with their immunosuppressive properties.

The use of androgen compounds as a form of myelostimulatory therapy in childhood aplastic anemia can now be viewed from the vantage point of nearly 15 years of therapeutic trial. Unfortunately, no truly controlled studies with this form of therapy have been carried out and the actual therapeutic potential of androgen therapy remains in question. Most studies aimed at elucidating the mode of action of androgen have been performed in adults with a variety of causes for bone marrow failure and thus may not be directly applicable to children. These studies do show, however, that the more generalized and severe the marrow depression, the less likely a response to androgen therapy will occur. Recent reports of patients treated with androgen therapy show mortality figures in the range of 70 per cent or greater. Such results may indicate that only the more severe forms of the disease are currently being referred to medical centers for therapy. This observation must be tempered by the fact that earlier series with improved mortality figures generally included patients who had survived prolonged periods prior to being treated and thus did not represent the more fulminant form of the disease.

A variety of androgenic compounds have been used, but the most convenient forms are sublingual methyltestosterone* (1 to 2 mg. per kilogram per day) or oral oxymetholone† (3 to 6 mg. per kilogram per day). The latter drug is generally preferred because it has less virilizing side effects. If oral therapy cannot be tolerated, parenteral testosterone propionate‡ (1 to 2 mg. per kilogram per day) may be utilized, but this adds the possible complication of bleeding into injection sites. In children, androgen therapy has generally been combined with corticosteroids administered in low dosage (0.5 mg. per kilogram per day to a maximum of 20 mg. per day). This combination of corticosteroid with androgen may offset the anabolic effects of androgen administered as well as provide some hemostatic function. Since no studies have been carried out in children to evaluate the relative effectiveness of androgen plus corticosteroid therapy compared with androgen therapy alone, the use of the traditional combination therapy is generally recommended. Evidence from uncontrolled studies suggests that corticosteroids add nothing to the myelostimulatory effect of androgen and, consequently, their dosage should be kept to a minimum and the drug discontinued if infection or other side effects become a significant problem. Alteration of liver function tests have been noted in as many as 80 per cent of patients on androgen therapy. Evidence of increasing hepatocellular damage requires discontinuation of therapy.

Response to androgen therapy is slow with little hematopoietic change noted for many weeks or even months. Although the majority of patients responding to therapy show evidence of improvement by six months, reports of patients responding only after 1 to 1½ years of therapy make the definition of an adequate clinical trial difficult. Initial signs of response include lessening of transfusion requirements coupled with an increase in reticulocytes. Hematologic recovery in association with androgen therapy is most complete in the red cell line with less optimal return of granulocytes and platelets. The primarily red cell response is in keeping with the observation that the action of androgen is mediated through its effect on erythropoietin. The desultory response to androgen makes it of limited value in the acute fulminant form of the disease where the mortality within the first weeks or months is so high. Since the response is slow, however, early institution of therapy is indicated with the hope that good supportive care will tide the patient over this acute phase.

In patients with acquired aplastic anemia, androgen therapy can usually be tapered off and discontinued when a satisfactory hemoglobin level (10 to 11 Gm. per 100 ml.) has been attained. Persistent granulocytopenia or thrombocytopenia is not an indication for continued therapy when an adequate red cell response is reached. Patients with congenital aplastic anemia will relapse if the drug is stopped and chronic therapy is required to support erythropoiesis. Recent experience suggests that these patients often become refractory after prolonged treatment and become aplastic again despite continued therapy at increased dosage.

A truly effective form of therapy for severe aplastic states with marked marrow hypocellularity remains to be found. Vigorous supportive care is of critical importance to these patients. Myelostimulatory therapy with androgen would have to be classified as "the best we have to offer" at this time. Whether such therapy actually reverses an otherwise progressively downhill course or merely accentuates an otherwise spontaneous reversal has yet to be proven. Although still an experimental form of therapy, bone marrow transplantation would appear to offer the most potential hope to those patients with rapidly progressive acquired disease. Early referral to centers capable of critically evaluating such patients for transplantation is, in my opinion, indicated.

HYPOPLASTIC ANEMIA (ERYTHROID HYPOPLASIA, PURE RED CELL APLASIA)

The term hypoplastic anemia is reserved for patients demonstrating a selective diminution of marrow erythroid precursors without significant involvement of granulocytic or megakaryocytic cell lines.

Congenital forms of the disease typically present by the first four to six months of life and are not associated with other major anomalies (Diamond-Blackfan syndrome). Recent reports have stressed the association of hypoplastic

---

* Note: Methyltestosterone is considered investigational for this use, since approval has not been officially stated in the package insert.

† Note: Oxymetholone is considered investigational for this use, since approval has not been officially stated in the package insert.

‡ Note: Testosterone propionate is considered investigational for this use, since approval has not been officially stated in the package insert.

anemia with a variety of congenital anomalies, particularly triphalangeal thumbs. Although less common, this latter group should be stressed to avoid classification of these patients with those having the more severe pancytopenic state associated with radial limb abnormalities (Fanconi anemia).

Treatment is aimed at supporting hemoglobin levels with transfusions while attempting to stimulate erythropoiesis with corticosteroids. Since granulocytopenia and thrombocytopenia are not part of this disease, infection and bleeding are not noted. Consequently, the prognosis is much more favorable than that of aplastic anemia. Prednisone in a dose range from 15 to 30 mg. per day will elicit a response in the majority of patients. Response is indicated by a reticulocytosis within one to two weeks after initiating therapy. If no response is noted, higher doses of prednisone should be attempted for a period of a few weeks before considering a patient to be a therapeutic failure. Occasional patients have responded to the addition of androgen compounds (as described under Aplastic Anemia) when they have not responded to corticosteroid alone. Because of the side effects and toxicity of androgen, this should be used only after an adequate trial of corticosteroid. Prolonged drug therapy in an unresponsive patient is not indicated. When a therapeutic response is attained and the hemoglobin level has reached 10 to 11 Gm. per 100 ml., the corticosteroid medication should be shifted to an alternate-day schedule and then gradually reduced in small increments every month until a minimal dose is reached which is capable of sustaining the hemoglobin level.

Corticosteroid therapy should be initiated as soon as the diagnosis is made. Experience has shown that the younger the child, the more likely a good response will be seen. This may be purely an age-related phenomenon, but it also appears to be related to the degree of hemosiderosis found in patients who have received multiple blood transfusions prior to corticosteroid therapy. Occasional spontaneous remissions have occurred even after many years in this disease and this possibility should be kept in mind when evaluating long-term therapy.

Transient forms of erythroid hypoplasia have been noted in children and may initially be difficult to distinguish from the congenital form. Age is an important differential point, since the congenital form typically presents before six months of age while the transient forms may occur at any age. Prolonged but self-limited erythroid hypoplasia in infants has been noted as a complication of hemolytic disease of the newborn. The cause is often more obscure in the older child with erythroblastopenia, although it is frequently associated with an infectious disease. Any child presenting with such a picture should be carefully evaluated for the possibility of an underlying hemolytic anemia with shortened red cell survival time. Exposure to hematotoxic drugs or chemicals must also be considered. Since this process is generally self-limited, only supportive care in the form of packed cell transfusions is necessary and corticosteroid therapy is not indicated. In areas of nutritional deprivation, a form of acquired pure red cell aplasia which responds to riboflavin has been noted in children with marasmus.

References

Bloom, G. E.: Disorders of Bone Marrow Production *Pediat. Clin. N. Am.*, 19:983, 1972.

Diamond, L. K., and Shahidi, N. T.: Treatment of Aplastic Anemia in Children. *Seminars Hemat.*, 4:278, 1967.

Grumet, F. C., and Yankee, R. A.: Long Term Platelet Support of Patients with Aplastic Anemia. *Ann. Int. Med.*, 73:1, 1970.

Heyn, R. M., Ertel, I. J., and Tubergen, D. G.: Course of Acquired Aplastic Anemia in Children Treated with Supportive Care. *J.A.M.A.*, 208:1372, 1969.

Killander, A., Lundmark, K–M, and Sjölin, S.: Idiopathic Aplastic Anaemia in Children. Results of Androgen Therapy. *Acta Paediat. Scand.*, 58:10, 1969.

Li, F. P., Alter, B. P., and Nathan D. G.: The Mortality of Acquired Aplastic Anemia in Children. *Blood*, 40:153, 1972.

Lovric, V. A.: Anaemia and Temporary Erythroblastopenia in Children. A Syndrome. *Aust. Ann. Med.*, 1:34, 1970.

Sanchez-Medal, L., Gomez-Leal, A., Duarte, L., and Rico, M.G.: Anabolic Androgenic Steroids in the Treatment of Acquired Aplastic Anemia. *Blood*, 34:283, 1969.

Santos, G. W.: Application of Marrow Grafts in Human Disease. *Am. J. Path.*, 65:653, 1971.

Sjölin, S., and Wranne, L.: Treatment of Congenital Hypoplastic Anaemia with Prednisone. *Scand. J. Haemat.* 7:63, 1970.

Megaloblastic Anemia

JAMES A. WOLFF, M.D.

Megaloblastic anemias in the pediatric age group are relatively uncommon. They are almost always the result of a congenital or acquired deficiency of folic acid or of vitamin B_{12}, secondary to dietary causes, a result of interference with absorption or caused by drugs which block the action of folic acid.

Folic acid deficiency in infancy is seen primarily following infections in those infants who have been fed milk low in folic acid, such as goat's milk, or who are premature. Intestinal malabsorption due to conditions such as celiac disease also may lead to deficiency of this vitamin. Methotrexate, a folic acid antagonist, and the anticonvulsant diphenylhydantoin are the drugs which most commonly lead to megaloblastic anemia as a result of interference with activity or absorption of folic acid. Increased demand for folic acid, as in thalassemia or sickle cell anemia, may lead to superimposed megaloblastic anemia.

Vitamin B_{12} deficiency causes megaloblastic anemia less commonly than does folic acid deficiency in the pediatric age group. Juvenile pernicious anemia due to deficiency of intrinsic factor is rare. One type, seen in infants or young children, is due to a congenital absence of secretion of intrinsic factor. It is not associated with gastric atrophy or humoral antibodies. The second type, occasionally seen in older children, is similar to pernicious anemia of adults. Congenital specific malabsorption of vitamin B_{12} has also been described. Other uncommon causes are due to interference with activity or absorption of vitamin B_{12}, such as anomalies of the small intestine or regional enteritis, respectively.

The treatment of megaloblastic anemia should be conditioned by the consideration that large doses of vitamin B_{12} may cause hematologic response in folate-deficient patients and that large doses of folic acid may produce a hematologic response but not prevent neurologic relapse in juvenile pernicious anemia. Therefore, even when the nature of the deficiency is reasonably certain, large therapeutic doses of either agent should be avoided. The necessity for extremely rapid response in infants and children is rarely required, as it may be in the older severely anemic patient.

The folic acid–deficient subject may be treated adequately with daily doses of 0.5 to 1 mg. by mouth. Since commercial preparations contain 1 mg. per tablet or per teaspoon, a dose of 1 mg. orally daily is usually prescribed. Parenteral treatment is required for severe intestinal diseases, in subjects with congenital or acquired anomalies of the small intestine or for very rare cases of congenital folic acid malabsorption. Folinic acid, in doses of 3 mg. daily intramuscularly, should be used to treat folic acid antagonist (Methotrexate, Daraprim)–induced megaloblastic anemia. Treatment or elimination of the underlying disorder or cause which has produced the megaloblastic change must accompany specific therapy, if possible. For example, celiac disease will necessitate a gluten-free diet, or goat's milk-induced folate deficiency requires dietary alteration. Although treatment with folic acid may be terminated after several weeks if the hemoglobin level has been restored to normal, careful observation is required for at least six months to ascertain that relapse will not occur.

Megaloblastic anemia due to vitamin B_{12} deficiency requires parenteral treatment. In cases of intrinsic factor deficiency, congenital specific malabsorption of vitamin B_{12} or uncorrectable small intestinal lesions, lifelong treatment with vitamin B_{12} is necessary. Small doses, 10 micrograms daily intramuscularly, may be given until hematologic response, as indicated by adequate reticulocytosis and rise in hemoglobin, has occurred. Thereafter, 250 micrograms intramuscularly should be given monthly. Although nervous system complications are seen very rarely in juvenile pernicious anemia, if they do occur there is no evidence that the neuropathy requires more vitamin B_{12} than the hematologic abnormality.

Hemolytic Anemia

EUGENE KAPLAN, M.D.

The treatment of symptomatic hemolytic anemia associated with extrinsic disorders, such as burns, infections, malignancies and microangiopathies, is essentially that of the primary disturbance. Immunohemolytic anemias in childhood are usually mild and self-limited and require no treatment. Supportive packed red cell transfusion may be used when acute hemolytic anemias result in hemoglobin concentrations below 8 Gm. per 100 ml. Occasionally, warm antibody autoimmune hemolytic anemia in children is more persistent and will require a course of oral prednisone, 2 mg. per kilogram per day, for several weeks or until a satisfactory response is obtained.

Elective splenectomy is indicated for all children with congenital spherocytic hemolytic anemia. This is best delayed until after the fourth year of life to minimize the hazard of postsplenectomy sepsis. In the immediate postoperative years these children should receive appropriate antibiotics at the onset of recognized bacterial infections. Severe recurrent anemia in the first year of life may require transfusions at intervals of one to three months. Acute episodes of erythroblastopenic crisis in later years are supported by packed red cell transfusion during the brief period until return of marrow erythropoietic activity.

The treatment of congenital nonspherocytic hemolytic anemia associated with specific erythrocyte enzyme defects includes supportive transfusions for severe anemia and consideration of an elective splenectomy in older children whose severe anemia is persistent. The benefit of splenectomy is far less predictable than it is in children with congenital spherocytosis. Episodic attacks of anemia in drug- or chemical-induced hemolytic disturbance associated with G6PD-deficient erythrocytes may require supportive red cell transfusion, but with care to select a blood donor not affected by a similar inherited red cell defect.

In some newborn infants with congenital hemolytic anemia, either spherocytic or nonspherocytic, severe hyperbilirubinemia may require replacement transfusion to prevent kernicterus.

Thalassemia

HOWARD A. PEARSON, M.D.

There is no curative therapy for thalassemia. Therefore, therapeutic measures may be supportive, symptomatic or directed at managing the disease and forestalling and treating its complications.

THALASSEMIA MAJOR (COOLEY'S ANEMIA)

This severe anemia results from homozygosity for thalassemia. It is usually a severe refractory anemia, accompanied by marked hypertrophy of erythropoietic tissue at medullary and extramedullary sites.

Transfusion. These children usually must receive transfusion of normal red cells at frequent intervals.

Recently a more aggressive transfusion regimen has been adopted in which the hemoglobin level is not permitted to fall below 9.5 Gm. per 100 ml. Patients maintained at these higher levels experience fewer clinical symptoms and probably do not develop cosmetic problems as severe as do those who are permitted to become more anemic. The vigorous transfusion program appears to be effective palliation for what is still a chronic and ultimately fatal disease.

Blood transfusion should be carefully performed. The blood should be freshly drawn, group-specific and type-specific, and checked for compatibility by the indirect globulin cross-matching technique. Use of packed or sedimented cells is preferred. Ten to 15 ml. per kilogram of packed cells can be safely given as a single transfusion; in older patients, 1 unit of packed cells (250 ml.) is given for each 20 kilograms of body weight. This volume can be expeditiously infused in about 2 hours. When larger amounts of blood are necessary, divided transfusions should be given in successive days.

Allergic and febrile episodes frequently occur in these patients, even in the absence of a hemolytic type of transfusion reaction. Pretransfusion administration of 25 to 50 mg. of diphenhydramine (Benadryl)* and aspirin may minimize these reactions when given orally.

Splenectomy. Splenectomy is indicated for relief of mechanical symptoms resulting from massive enlargement of this organ and for hypersplenism (which may bring about thrombocytopenia, leukopenia and increased transfusion requirements). These hematologic abnormalities improve after splenectomy, but otherwise the operation does not change the course of the disease.

Following splenectomy, as many as 30 per cent of these patients develop fulminating sepsis, which is due primarily to pneumococci. Splenectomy should be delayed as long as possible, and therapy with oral penicillin, 200,000 units per day, has been advocated for a year or two afterward.

Folic Acid Deficiency. Occasionally a superimposed folic acid deficiency may develop, and oral folic acid in a dose of 5 mg. per day for two to three weeks is recommended. There is no evidence that administration of folic acid or any other hematinic substance has any long-term beneficial effect. Any form of medicinal iron is strictly contraindicated.

Gallbladder Disease. Many patients develop pigmentary gallstones. Cholecystectomy is indicated when episodes of biliary colic or obstructive jaundice occur, and the gallbladder should be examined at splenectomy and removed if stones are present.

Complications of Iron Overload. Patients with thalassemia major usually succumb in the second decade of life from the effects of chronic anemia, hypoxia and tissue iron overload. The iron overload derives from blood transfusion and from increased absorption of dietary iron. Cardiac complications are particularly serious, and intractable congestive heart failure is a frequent terminal complication. Therapy requires maintenance of the hemoglobin above 10 Gm. per 100 ml., digitalis, salt restriction and diuretics.

At present, there is no effective way to treat iron overload. Chelating agents which mobilize tissue iron and facilitate its urinary excretion have been used experimentally in thalassemia major and include deferoxamine

* Manufacturer's precaution: Diphenhydramine (Benadryl) is not for use in premature or newborn infants.

(Desferal) and diethylenetriamine pentaacetate (DTPA). The consensus is that the small amount of iron removed even by vigorous chelation therapy does not justify regular use of these agents with their attendant toxic side effects, although investigation in chelation therapy is continuing.

THALASSEMIA MINOR

Hemoglobin levels average 2 to 3 Gm. per 100 ml. below normal. This condition is commonly mistaken for iron deficiency anemia. Iron therapy is not only ineffective but indeed potentially detrimental.

Patients with the thalassemia trait should be reassured that their mild anemia is nonprogressive. They should be given genetic counseling and advised that the trait is frequent in persons of Greek and Italian backgrounds, and that if they marry a similarly affected person, a proportion of their children may have thalassemia major. Parents who have had a child with thalassemia major should be made aware of the average 25 per cent chance of repetition in subsequent pregnancies.

Hemolytic Reaction to Transfusion Of Incompatible Blood

HARRY J. SACKS, M.D.

The management of a hemolytic reaction involves immediate treatment of hypotension with fluids and volume expanders, and immediate diuresis with hyperosmotic mannitol, urine alkalinization and steroids. Complications of mannitol are avoided by attention to its contraindications.

Clinical use of 20 per cent mannitol for diuresis has not been studied comprehensively in the pediatric patient. However, its successful use for reversible oliguria in adults makes it a logical choice for trial in similar problems in the pediatric age group.

The most important hazards of this regimen are heart failure and water intoxication. These can be avoided if the following contraindications to the use of 20 per cent mannitol are observed: (1) anuria or worsening oliguria in spite of one or two doses of 20 per cent mannitol, (2) severe dehydration, (3) severe pulmonary congestion, frank edema or heart failure, (4) active intracranial bleeding except during craniotomy, (5) oliguria known to be due to advanced chronic renal disease.

Finally, although not strictly a part of treatment, this situation always serves to present the following questions: (1) Was the patient being observed during the transfusion? (2) Did the laboratory, ward and identification procedure meet the minimal standards as given in the AABB Technical Methods and Procedures Manual, the modern standard of reference for technical and administrative procedure in blood banking? (3) Were the therapeutic materials and a written protocol immediately at hand when the reaction occurred?

General Treatment. 1. Two issues are at stake: the diagnosis and the mode of treatment. In practical terms one must be guided by the immediate clinical findings and later be persuaded by the results of the time-consuming laboratory tests as to the true state of affairs. Therefore because *time is critical,* when the clinical signs of hemolytic reaction are characteristic or even questionably so, the following regimen should be immediately instituted. For small children and infants appropriate reduction in amounts is indicated, with particular care required in dehydrated infants.

2. The transfusion must be stopped instantly by nurse or doctor; because the vein must be kept cannulated, 5 per cent mannitol* in water (or whatever intravenous solution was used to start the transfusion) is connected via new intravenous tubing into the needle and allowed to barely flow. If possible, connect a three-way stopcock into the needle to facilitate future blood samplings or for parenteral therapy. The residual donor blood is promptly sent to the laboratory along with the blood samples for study.

3. Interrupt the infusion long enough to withdraw a 5-ml. and up to a 30-ml. sample of blood. Discard the former and place some of the latter into EDTA anticoagulant, some into a prothrombin time anticoagulant and another portion into clean, dry tubes for appropriate tests. (*Do not squirt the blood into the tubes because this produces hemolysis.*)

4. The nurse or doctor must verify the identity of the patient and donor bottle.

5. Using a dose of 0.3 Gm. per kilogram of 20 per cent mannitol containing 45 mEq. per square meter of sodium acetate, infuse in 5 to 10 minutes up to a maximum of 20 Gm. of the mannitol and up to 90 mEq. of sodium acetate.

6. Following this, infuse 5 per cent mannitol in water containing 45 mEq. sodium acetate per liter and titrate its infusion rate so that it is the same as the urine flow.

7. Using a dose of 2 mg. per kilogram,

* Manufacturer's precaution: Use of mannitol in pediatric patients has not been studied comprehensively.

inject up to 200 mg. of prednisolone sodium succinate into the tubing.

8. Attempt a urine collection at this time to note its color. If it is not grossly bloody, send it to the laboratory for occult blood and routine urinalysis. Initiate monitoring of hourly output, specific gravity and pH. If the patient cannot void, catheterization must be resorted to because the urine output is essential as a guide to immediate diagnosis, fluid intake and renal function.

9. If the subsequent 3-hour output does not attain 60 to 100 ml. per hour in the child weighing more than 20 kilograms [and a proportionately smaller amount in the small child (40 ml. per hour per square meter) or infant (10 ml. per hour per square meter)], the 20 per cent mannitol dose should be repeated—providing that the previously listed contraindications still do not apply. If oliguria persists after two such doses, treatment for irreversible renal failure must be considered.

10. Once diuresis has been induced, continue an intake to allow a urine output as previously outlined for the next 48 hours. This at first is accomplished by intravenous therapy with attention to needed electrolyte requirements, and gradually switched to oral intake if possible. Urine pH should be maintained above 7.4, and blood pH should be monitored to avoid alkalosis.

11. Steroid therapy, prednisone orally in a dose of 0.5 mg. per kilogram per day up to a maximum of 40 mg. per day, is continued for 24 to 48 hours.

12. If the laboratory results refute the possibility of a hemolytic reaction, this regimen can be terminated at any point.

Specific Additional Procedures. 1. If hypotension threatens or is present, one must use albumin or other volume expanders or pharmacologic agents as the case may be. If it is not certain that the hypotension is due to volume depletion, a central venous catheter should be promptly passed to provide a means of monitoring right atrial pressure as fluids are infused.

2. Under virtually no circumstances should blood or red cells be used until the diagnosis has been clarified and the available blood units rechecked.

3. Anemia which results in the oxygen-want syndrome can usually be treated with oxygen until the laboratory can resolve the issue. As soon as compatibility is achieved, whole blood or packed cells can be used as indicated; but even then danger may be present unless a thoroughly sophisticated serologic work-up is carried out. Whole blood or red cells should be withheld until such study is carried out, unless the severity of oxygen lack necessitates a calculated risk.

4. Coagulation defects resulting in severe hemorrhage are best treated with fresh frozen plasma even before their nature can be elucidated but after blood samples have been collected for study. Thrombocytopenia below 50,000 per cubic millimeter, if associated with prolonged bleeding time, will have been treated by the steroid dose and later by platelet or fresh blood transfusion if necessary. Finally, if signs of a hemorrhagic diathesis become intractable, the possibility of disseminated intravascular coagulation must be considered and appropriate therapy instituted.

5. Pain and pyrogenic and allergic symptoms are treated symptomatically.

Hemolytic Disease of the Newborn

(Erythroblastosis Fetalis)

JOHN N. LUKENS, M.D.

Current therapeutic approaches are effective in salvaging approximately 50 per cent of those fetuses and neonates who are otherwise doomed to die from erythroblastosis fetalis. Since the severity of disease is determined by prenatal rather than by postnatal events, it is of paramount importance that the efforts of the obstetrician and pediatrician be closely integrated. Identification of the fetus which will benefit from antenatal transfusion and prediction of the postnatal implications of concurrent prematurity and hemolytic disease are important team functions. If facilities for meeting the anticipated needs of the fetus and infant are not immediately available to the team, early consultation with a perinatal treatment center should be sought.

In the discussion which follows, management of hemolytic disease of the newborn is considered against the framework of chronologic milestones. Prenatal management entails detection of maternal sensitization by means of the indirect antiglobulin (Coombs) test, quantitation of fetal hemolysis by serial analysis of amniotic fluid and, finally, plotting the course of therapy with respect to fetal transfusion and timing of delivery. Postnatal management is designed to correct significant anemia and to maintain the serum bilirubin concentration below those levels which are associated with bilirubin encephalopathy.

PRENATAL MANAGEMENT

Detection of Fetal Hemolytic Disease. A provisional diagnosis of fetal erythroblastosis is made if the mother's serum contains antibodies directed against RH(D)-positive red blood cells. Blood typing is done on all women at the time of the first prenatal visit. If the mother's blood type is Rh(D)-negative, an indirect antiglobulin (Coombs) test is done at 12 to 16 weeks', at 28 to 32 weeks' and again at 36 weeks' gestation. If no antibody is detected by the 36th week, one may conclude that the fetus is not affected and the pregnancy may be permitted to continue to term. On the other hand, an antiglobulin test which is positive in a titer greater than 1:32 at any time during pregnancy constitutes presumptive evidence for fetal hemolytic disease. Subsequent monitoring of the fetus is achieved by analysis of amniotic fluid.

The mother's history with respect to previous pregnancies and blood transfusions, and knowledge of the father's blood type and zygosity with respect to Rh (D) are helpful in assessing the relative risk of fetal disease. If the mother has had an affected infant by a previous pregnancy and if the father is presumed to be homozygous for the Rh (D) factor, the magnitude of fetal disease can be expected to be at least as great as that observed in the previous infant. The pregnant woman who has given birth to an affected infant is best followed with serial amniocenteses.

Assessment of Severity of Fetal Disease. The hemoglobin concentration of cord blood at birth varies inversely with the concentration of bilirubin in amniotic fluid. Hence, measurement of the amniotic fluid bilirubin concentration provides a valuable means for quantitating fetal anemia.

Amniocentesis is indicated if the indirect Coombs antibody titer is greater than 1:34 or if the mother has delivered a previously affected infant. In the first sensitized pregnancy, the initial amniocentesis is done at 28 to 29 weeks' gestation. Earlier examination of the amniotic fluid is indicated if the maternal antibody titer is unusually high (greater than 1:128). The timing of the first amniocentesis for women who have delivered an affected infant is determined by the severity of disease in the previous offspring. In general, the initial amniocentesis is done approximately 10 weeks prior to the gestational age of the previously affected infant at the time of delivery. (If the former infant was born with severe disease at 34 to 37 weeks' gestation, the first amniocentesis is performed at 24 to 27 weeks.) Amniocenteses are repeated at intervals of one to three weeks. The frequency of amniotic fluid examinations is dictated by the magnitude and by the trend of bile pigment concentration.

By convention, bilirubin concentration in amniotic fluid is determined indirectly as the increase in optical density at 450 millimicrons above the projected slope of the spectrophotometric curve of amniotic fluid (ΔO.D. 450). As the amniotic fluid volume increases with advancing gestation, the concentration of bile pigments contributing to the ΔO.D. 450 decreases. Hence, interpretation of the spectrophotometric analysis of amniotic fluid is possible only with an accurate assessment of gestational age. Quantitation of the severity of fetal hemolytic disease is based on two observations: the magnitude of the ΔO.D. 450 (relative to gestational age) and the *trend* of ΔO.D. 450 readings on serial specimens. A graph, constructed by Liley from data culled from several hundred pregnancies, permits interpretation of both variables.* The graph, which relates ΔO.D. 450 to gestational age, defines three zones of severity of fetal disease. A ΔO.D. 450 reading which falls in zone 1 identifies a fetus who, if affected, has only mild disease. A reading falling in zone 2 signifies intermediate disease and one falling in zone 3 portends severe disease or impending death from erythroblastosis fetalis. Further, a high reading which rises or remains flat with advancing gestation is associated with prenatal or neonatal death, whereas a falling ΔO.D. 450 suggests a favorable prognosis for fetal survival.

Management of Fetal Disease. Amniocentesis provides a window through which the natural course of fetal disease is viewed. On the basis of data derived from amniocenteses, prenatal management is charted with respect to fetal blood transfusion and the timing of delivery.

If the prognosis for fetal survival is good, pregnancy is allowed to continue to the 38th week of gestation. Termination of pregnancy at 38 weeks imposes little risk of neonatal respiratory distress, decreases the duration of fetal exposure to maternal antibodies and permits delivery of the infant at a time when the immediate availability of obstetric, pediatric and blood bank personnel is assured. If the prognosis for fetal survival is poor (a flat or rising ΔO.D. 450 in high zone 2 or in zone 3) and if the gestational age of the fetus is 34 weeks or greater, prompt induction of labor is indicated. Termination of pregnancy prior to 34 weeks' gestation is interdicted by the insurmountable problems of immaturity. Severe disease in the

---

* Liley, A. W.: *Amer. J. Obstet. Gynec.*, 86:485, 1963.

previable fetus is treated with intrauterine transfusion.

Intrauterine transfusion is indicated if the amniocentesis data portend fetal death prior to the 34th week of gestation. For technical reasons, intrauterine transfusion is generally not attempted prior to the 28th week of gestation. Established fetal hydrops (diagnosed by the injection of a radiopaque dye into the amniotic cavity) is rarely reversed by intrauterine transfusion. For this reason, the diagnosis of hydrops is considered a contraindication for fetal transfusion.

The experience and skill of the obstetric team undertaking intrauterine transfusion are of utmost importance for the success of the procedure. Consequently, it is appropriate that this operation be restricted to those centers which have demonstrated expertise with the technique. Fresh, group O Rh (D)-negative blood, cross matched with the mother's serum, is used for the transfusion. Fifty to 75 ml. of washed, lightly packed red blood cells are infused into the fetal peritoneal cavity through a needle passed through the mother's anterior abdominal wall. Following an intrauterine transfusion, amniocenteses are of no value in monitoring fetal disease. The intrauterine transfusion is repeated one to two weeks after the first procedure and thereafter at three- to four-week intervals until the pregnancy is terminated.

POSTNATAL MANAGEMENT

If the pediatric team is to anticipate effectively the immediate needs of the newly born infant, it is essential that they be conversant with the milestones of prenatal surveillance and management. Fresh whole blood, cross matched with maternal serum, should be available at the time of birth if the severity of disease necessitates interruption of pregnancy prior to 38 weeks' gestation.

Management at Birth. Decisions regarding the immediate care of the neonate are based on the appearance of the infant at birth and on laboratory analysis of cord blood. Pallor, purpura, hepatosplenomegaly, edema and/or ascites signify severe involvement; together, these physical findings constitute indication for prompt exchange transfusion. If the infant is not distressed at birth, the decision for proceeding with an exchange transfusion is postponed until the results of cord blood studies are available. Cord blood is collected to determine hemoglobin concentration, packed cell volume (hematocrit), reticulocyte count, blood type, direct antiglobulin (Coombs) test and bilirubin (direct and indirect) concentration. The diagnosis of isoimmune hemolytic disease is confirmed by the demonstration of fetomaternal Rh (D) incompatibility and a positive direct antiglobulin reaction.

Indications for Exchange Transfusion. The cornerstone of therapy for erythroblastosis fetalis is exchange transfusion. This crude but effective procedure permits removal of red blood cells vulnerable to premature destruction, effects prompt correction of anemia, facilitates relief of congestive heart failure and achieves a reduction of serum and tissue bilirubin. Exchange transfusion is performed in order to (1) ameliorate heart failure, (2) correct significant or progressive anemia and (3) maintain the serum bilirubin below those levels which are associated with brain injury:

1. An exchange transfusion is performed at birth if congestive heart failure or frank hydrops fetalis is apparent. By creating a volume deficit of 10 to 20 ml. and by increasing the hemoglobin concentration, hypervolemia is corrected and the venous pressure is reduced.

2. In the absence of signs of cardiac decompensation, an exchange transfusion is conducted if the venous hemoglobin concentration is less than 12 Gm. per 100 ml. at birth or at any time during the first 24 hours. If untreated, infants who are anemic at birth experience a progressive decrease in hemoglobin concentration and potentially severe hyperbilirubinemia.

3. Reduction of serum bilirubin by exchange transfusion should be accomplished if (a) the serum indirect bilirubin is 20 mg. per ml. or greater at any time during the first week of life, (b) the clinical manifestations of early (and reversible) bilirubin encephalopathy are detected or (c) the rate of rise in serum bilirubin suggests that a peak level of 20 mg. per 100 ml. will be exceeded.

Unfortunately, there is no reliable level of serum bilirubin below which bilirubin encephalopathy does not occur. As a result, it is important that the bilirubin level at which exchange transfusion is done not be rigidly defined. The decision to proceed with an exchange transfusion should be based not only on the level of indirect-reacting bilirubin but also on the presence or absence of those factors known to predispose to kernicterus: asphyxia, acidosis, hypothermia, hypoglycemia, hypoproteinemia, extreme prematurity, sepsis and exposure to certain drugs (sulfonamides, salicylates, heparin, caffeine). These factors, alone or in combination, predispose to kernicterus at levels of unconjugated bilirubin below 20 mg. per 100 ml. Consequently, exchange transfusion is performed in the sick neonate whose serum bilirubin is less than 20 mg. per 100 ml. if he demonstrates the early signs of kernicterus: lethargy, hypotonia, poor suck, weak cry, hypothermia. Finally, because bilirubin levels during the first day of life have predictive value with respect to the subsequent magnitude of bilirubinemia, an exchange transfusion is indicated if the indirect bilirubin is in excess of 5 mg. per 100 ml. at birth, 9 mg. per 100 ml. at 6 hours, 12 mg. per 100 ml. at 12 hours, or 15 mg. per 100 ml. at 24 hours of age.

If an exchange transfusion is not performed at birth, the infant's hemoglobin and serum indirect bilirubin are measured again at 4 and 8 hours of age, and thereafter at 12- to 24-hour intervals. More frequent observations are made as the criteria for exchange transfusion are approached.

Conduct of Exchange Transfusions. The procedure requires an operator familiar with the technique and with its potential complications, an assistant, appropriate hardware and mechanisms for monitoring the infant's body temperature and for warming donor blood. Instructions for performing the procedure are presented in detail in a previous edition.† The present discussion is restricted to recommendations regarding the selection of donor blood, the choice of anticoagulant and the use of albumin.

Donor Blood. Type O Rh (D)-negative blood is used for the exchange transfusion. Blood of the infant's ABO type may be given if there is no fetomaternal ABO incompatibility. It is important that donor red cells be cross matched with both maternal and infant sera. For this reason, a sample of the mother's blood must accompany the infant who is transferred to another institution for the procedure.

Anticoagulant. Infant tolerance of donor blood is determined to a large extent by the anticoagulant into which the blood is collected. Judicious selection of the appropriate blood requires knowledge of the relative advantages and potential toxicities of blood bank anticoagulants.

Acid-citrate-dextrose (ACD) blood has a number of disadvantages, especially for the sick neonate and for the small premature infant. Infusion of ACD blood is attended by a proclivity to acidosis, hypocalcemia, hypoglycemia and tissue hypoxia. For reasons which are not clear, severe erythroblastosis is often associated with islet cell hyperplasia and hyperinsulinemia. The vulnerability of the infant to hypoglycemia is augmented by anticoagulants rich in dextrose. The glucose load evokes an exaggerated insulin response. Hyperinsulinemia, in turn, is followed by hypoglycemia. As a result, apnea and/or seizures due to hypoglycemia may be observed 1 to 3 hours following an exchange transfusion with ACD blood. Further, the 2, 3-diphosphoglycerate (2, 3-DPG) content of red blood cells stored in ACD declines rapidly. As the concentration of 2, 3-DPG decreases, the oxygen affinity of hemoglobin increases. Red blood cells deficient in 2,3-DPG contribute little to tissue oxygenation.

Citrate-phosphate-dextrose (CPD) blood imposes slightly less of an acid load and functions normally with respect to oxygen dissociation. The oxygen affinity and 2,3-DPG content of red cells stored in CPD remain unchanged over five days. CPD blood contains about two-thirds as much dextrose as ACD blood. Delayed hypoglycemia may be observed.

The use of heparin as an anticoagulant circumvents the problems of acidosis, hypocalcemia and hypoglycemia. Since heparinized blood must be used shortly after collection, its 2,3-DPG content is unaltered. Unfortunately, heparinized blood must be discarded if not used within 24 to 48 hours of its collection.

For small premature and sick term infants, heparinized blood is preferred. CPD blood is used for the mature neonate who is not severely compromised. If ACD or CPD blood is used for an exchange transfusion, the infant's blood glucose is checked with Dextrostix 1 to 2 hours after completion of the procedure. Low levels of glucose are confirmed by quantitative analysis. Symptomatic or chemical hypoglycemia is corrected with an infusion of a 10 per cent dextrose solution.

Albumin. An infusion of albumin prior to the exchange transfusion induces a prompt shift of unconjugated bilirubin from extravascular sites to plasma and thereby facilitates removal of approximately 40 per cent more bilirubin. When an exchange transfusion is done for hyperbilirubinemia, 25 per cent salt-poor human albumin (1 Gm. per kilogram) is given 1 to 2 hours prior to the procedure. Albumin priming is contraindicated in the infant with severe anemia of congestive heart failure.

Adjuvant Measures. Phototherapy has not been shown to decrease the need for exchange transfusion in infants with erythroblastosis fetalis due to Rh (D) incompatibility. With brisk hemolysis, the rate of bilirubin production exceeds the capacity of light to effect decomposition. Since the relationship between serum bilirubin concentration and observed icterus is altered by phototherapy, it is imperative that

† Bowman, J. M., in Gellis, S. S., and Kagan, B. M. (eds.): *Current Pediatric Therapy 5*. Philadelphia, W. B. Saunders Company, 1971, p. 262.

the serum bilirubin be monitored closely if phototherapy is used.

Phenobarbital administration has been suggested on theoretical grounds because of its capacity to accelerate bilirubin conjugation. The equivocal results observed in a limited number of infants studied under controlled conditions preclude acceptance of phenobarbital as an adjuvant to therapy at this time.

Late Anemia. Whether or not the infant with erythroblastosis fetalis is subjected to an exchange transfusion, a progressive decrease in hemoglobin concentration during the first six weeks of life is expected, This "late" anemia develops because the erythroid marrow fails to increase the production of red blood cells in response to continuing hemolysis. The hemoglobin concentration is checked at weekly intervals during the first six weeks. A transfusion of sedimented red cells is given if the hemoglobin falls below 5 Gm. per 100 ml. An infusion of 2 ml. of red blood cells per kilogram body weight is followed by an increase in the hemoglobin concentration of 1 Gm. per 100 ml. Because maternal antibodies persist in the infant's circulation through the second month of life, Rh (D) -negative red blood cells, compatible with both maternal and infant sera, are used.

Erythroblastosis due to ABO Incompatibility. Erythroblastosis fetalis due to fetomaternal A or B incompatibility differs from that duc to RH (D) incompatibility in several respects. A prenatal diagnosis of erythroblastosis due to ABO incompatibility cannot be made with confidence. Since fetal distress due to A or B incompatibility does not occur, no antenatal therapeutic efforts are necessary. The affected infant is born at term with little or no anemia. Hyperbilirubinemia is the sole expression of the disorder requiring therapeutic intervention.

The diagnosis of erythroblastosis fetalis due to ABO incompatibility rests on the demonstration of appropriate fetomaternal incompatibility and on consistent clinical and hematologic features. Ninety per cent of the mothers of affected infants have group 0 red blood cells. The infant's blood type is group A or, less frequently, group B. Although the direct antiglobulin test may be weakly positive at birth, it is usually negative by 24 hours of age. Currently available techniques for the detection of "immune" anti-A and anti-B are of little or no diagnostic or prognostic value. Severe anemia, reticulocytosis and normoblastosis are not observed. The most impressive feature of the peripheral blood smear is prominent spherocytosis.

The indications for exchange transfusion based on hyperbilirubinemia are the same as those outlined for infants with Rh (D) isoimmune hemolytic disease. For exchange transfusion, group O Rh (D)-specific, low titer blood is used. Once again, donor red blood cells must be compatible with both maternal and infant sera.

Because bilirubin generation is considerably less than with Rh (D) incompatibility, phototherapy may circumvent the need for exchange transfusion in some infants. When exposed to lights within 72 hours of birth, infants with ABO hemolytic disease experience lower mean peak bilirubin levels and require approximately 50 per cent fewer exchange transfusions. Nevertheless, the early institution of phototherapy provides no guarantee against the need for exchange transfusion. Phototherapy should not be used if the indications for exchange transfusion already prevail. Once phototherapy is instituted, the serum bilirubin must be monitored compulsively lest unwittingly the infant be denied a necessary exchange transfusion.

PREVENTION

The administration of anti-Rh (D) gamma globulin to unsensitized mothers following the birth of Rh (D) -positive infants has proved highly effective in preventing maternal sensitization. Protection may be sustained through two or more pregnancies.

Prevention of primary Rh (D) immunization is achieved by the intramuscular injection of 1 ml. (equivalent to 300 micrograms of anti-Rh[D]) of Rhogam (Ortho Diagnostics, Raritan, New Jersey) within 72 hours of delivery. This material is given only if the mother's blood type is RH(D)-negative and if her indirect antiglobulin (Coombs) test is negative. If these prerequisites are met, immunoprophylaxis is indicated: (1) following delivery of an Rh (D)-positive infant, (2) following a spontaneous or therapeutic abortion and (3) following the inadvertent transfusion of Rh (D)-positive red blood cells. In the latter situation, the amount of Rhogam given is determined by the volume of incompatible blood infused. One ml. (300 micrograms) of Rhogam inactivates 10 ml. of incompatible whole blood.

Sickle Cell Disease

ROLAND B. SCOTT, M.D.

Rational therapy of sickle cell disease is based upon recognition that this syndrome is divisible into a number of clinical types of variable occurrence and morbidity. Moreover, the course of the disease is usually characterized by periods of remission and exacerbation (crises). The approach to treatment is generally based upon the nature of the crisis and the presence of complications.

CRISES

For clinical and therapeutic purposes, the crises may be classified as follows:

1. Thrombotic, infarctive, symptomatic, vasoocclusive or pain crisis—pain in the area of erythrostasis with little or no change in hemoglobin, reticulocytes, bone marrow or other laboratory findings in the blood. Fever, if present, is often lowgrade.

2. Aplastic, hypoplastic or aregenerative—pain, rapid and severe decrease in hemoglobin and reticulocytes with hypoplastic bone marrow. Viral infections have been frequently associated with this type.

3. Hemolytic, hyperhemolytic—pain, fever, increased rate of red cell destruction, drop in hemoglobin and red blood cell levels, increase in reticulocytes, as a rule, and hyperplastic bone marrow.

4. Sequestration—rather sudden and massive collection of large amounts of erythrostasis in visceral organs, especially the spleen. This may be associated with debilitation, weakness or shock and a decrease in red cells and hemoglobin in the peripheral blood.

5. Mixed, such as thrombotic-hemolytic variety.

Treatment. A crisis may occur without demonstrable precipitating causes, but in childhood, intercurrent infections are often associated with exacerbations of the syndrome.

Thrombotic crises are the most frequently observed variety. They vary considerably in frequency, duration and intensity. Mild forms characterized mainly by pain and lassitude can often be treated satisfactorily in the home by measures that include bed rest, water taken orally and anodynes or analgesics. The water by mouth (120 ml. per kilogram per 24 hours) is administered in aliquots at hourly intervals. After 24 to 48 hours, broth and other clear fluids are added. Anodynes or analgesics include acetylsalicylic acid (aspirin, Empirin), 65 mg. per kilogram per 24 hours, divided into four or more doses, acetaminophen (Tempra, Tylenol) in single doses of 60 mg. for infants under one year of age, 60 to 120 mg. for children one to four years, 120 to 240 mg. for children four to eight years and 240 mg. for children eight to 12 years, propoxyphene hydrochloride (Darvon),* 3 mg. per kilogram per 24 hours divided into four to six doses orally, and papaverine in dosages of 6 mg. per kilogram per 24 hours divided into four doses and administered either intramuscularly or orally.

My associates and I have employed indomethacin (Indocin)† with salutary effect in the treatment of thrombotic type of crises characterized by pain, fever, tenderness and local soft tissue swelling, particularly involving the extremities. Several patients exhibited partial or complete immobilization when joints were involved. The dosage used was 1 mg. per kilogram of body weight, administered orally every 6 to 8 hours until symptoms and signs abated. The drug was then tapered and discontinued as the crisis was controlled. We observed no adverse side effects when the agent was used in this type of short-term program. Hospitalization may be necessary, however, if symptoms such as pain, dehydration and vomiting become refractory to treatment at home.

Hemolytic and aplastic crises may vary in intensity, but they are likely to be of sufficient severity to warrant hospitalization for special measures, such as intravenous therapy. Oxygen is indicated for severe anemia and shock, especially as an emergency measure while the patient is being prepared for blood transfusions or for complications such as pneumonia and respiratory distress. As a rule, oxygen should not be given beyond the emergency period because prolonged use can cause suppression of erythropoiesis. Certain clinicians have reported on the use of hyperbaric oxygen in selected patients in crisis. However, the results have not been uniformly salutary. Antibiotics are of greatest usefulness in the treatment of specific complications, such as septicemia, meningitis, pneumonia and osteomyelitis.

ACTH and the adrenal corticosteroids have limited usefulness in the treatment of crises. Steroids are favored over ACTH mainly because of their greater convenience in treating both ambulatory and hospitalized patients. The agents currently used include prednisone (Meticorten), methylprednisolone (Medrol) and triimcinolone (Aristocort). They are used generally for two classes of patients:

1. Hospitalized children treated for severe crises (aplastic or hemolytic) may be benefited

---

* Manufacturer's precaution: The safety of propoxyphene hydrochloride (Darvon) in children has not been established.

† Manufacturer's precaution: Indomethacin (Indocin) is contraindicated in children 14 years of age and under.

if the drug is used as an adjunctive agent with transfusions and other measures for the control of shock, debility and anorexia. (Most of these patients are also receiving antibiotics for associated infections and have had blood cultures taken at the time of admission.) A five-year-old child would receive about 4 or 5 mg. of one of the previously mentioned steroids three or four times during the first 24 hours. This dosage is given for a few days and then tapered and discontinued.

2. Ambulatory patients who do not require hospitalization may be benefited by intermittent or short-term steroid therapy. This plan has been used in the treatment of the hand-foot syndrome, which is observed most frequently in infants and small children who exhibit painful swelling of the hands and feet, including the fingers and toes. This syndrome is often associated with a thrombotic-like crisis with only slight changes in the characteristic blood cell counts usually exhibited by these children.

Some of these patients can be satisfactorily managed on an ambulatory basis by the oral administration of a steroid (methylprednisolone or triamcinolone, 2 to 4 mg. as a single dose repeated at 4- to 6-hour intervals during a 24-hour period). Staggered doses of an oral antibiotic medication may be included in the regimen for associated infections. The steroid is continued only long enough to relieve local pain and swelling, and then the dosage is tapered and the drug discontinued. Mothers usually report observable improvement in a few days, and medication can usually be discontinued after about two weeks. Occasionally, symptoms return and a second course of therapy is required. Patients vary in their response to the drug, and the physician may find it necessary to adjust the dosage schedule in an effort to ascertain the minimal effective dosage. Parents should be fully informed of the nature of the medication and advised to protect these children against unnecessary exposure to chickenpox. These children should have the benefit of x-ray examination of the involved parts in order to exclude the possibility of osteomyelitis (salmonella).

TRANSFUSIONS. Blood transfusions are used less frequently than formerly. It is generally recognized that as long as these children are comfortable and able to carry out their normal daily activities, such as playing, eating and school attendance, no special measures need be directed toward changing the status of their hemoglobin, erythrocyte and leukocyte levels (which tend to stabilize at mean values of 7.7 Gm. per 100 ml., 2.6 million per cubic millimeter and 16,000 per cubic millimeter, respectively). The unwarranted use of blood transfusions in this disease unnecessarily exposes the patient to a number of hazards, including hemolytic reactions, bone marrow suppression, homologous serum hepatitis and hemosiderosis. This agent should be reserved for strict indications. In general, it is the policy of our clinic to reserve blood transfusions in these patients for the following conditions: (1) severe crisis associated with debility, excruciating pain and anemia (less than 5 Gm. of hemoglobin), (2) formidable complications, such as pneumonia, meningitis, septicemia or osteomyelitis, (3) elective or emergency surgical operations and (4) when other measures have failed to control the crises.

Whole blood transfusions are definitely indicated in aplastic, sequestration and hemolytic crises when the hemoglobin level is falling at an alarming rate. In this situation a hemoglobin value less than 4 or 5 Gm. is hazardous and should be supported by whole blood.

Small transfusions of packed cells (6 to 10 ml. per kilogram of body weight administered daily until the hemoglobin level reaches about 10 Gm.) are often useful in situations in which one must use caution to avoid overloading the circulation, as in pneumonia and cardiomegaly.

Some clinics have used partial exchange transfusions prophylactically at intervals of six to eight weeks in an effort to maintain 15 to 30 per cent of normal donor cells in the patient's circulation at all times as a preventive measure against frequent crises. This program, which has been used chiefly in adults, does not materially change the status of the anemia or other hematologic values; however, by their presence normal cells decrease the absolute number of sickle cells and thus reduce blood viscosity. This method of therapy has many obvious hazards and limitations and in pediatric practice is applicable only to the occasional selected patient whose crises are severe and frequent and cannot be managed satisfactorily by less formidable measures.

OTHER FLUIDS. In 1955 Barreras Areu reported the successful treatment of 12 children with active disease by the use of sodium citrate and sodium lactate solutions administered orally and intravenously. He observed an increase in the erythrocyte counts without the use of blood transfusion. In 1958 Greenberg and Kass reported that four of six crises in patients with sickle cell disease responded promptly by relief of pain after the intravenous administration of large amounts of sodium bicarbonate (3.3 mEq. per kilogram of body weight per hour). In both studies the investigators attributed their results to the inhibition of the sickling phenomenon by an increase in the plasma pH. My colleagues and I have tried alkali therapy of this type, but we find it to be no more effective than nonelectrolyte-containing solutions (glucose and dextran) in the control of crises. The safe use of electrolyte fluids, moreover, requires periodic examination of the patient's blood (carbon dioxide–combining power or pH) to avoid severe degrees of alkalosis.

In 1971 the salutary effect of orally administered sodium citrate for crises was reported. The dosage was 60 ml. of a 10 per cent solution diluted to 400 ml. every 2 hours for the first 24 hours. The case series was small and the double-blind method of evaluation was not used.

In 1964 Schwartz and McElfresh conducted a double-blind study on the comparative therapeutic effect of intravenous infusion of sodium bicarbonate (3.3 mEq. per kilogram per hour) versus infusions of comparable quantities of sodium chloride used as a control for the relief of painful crises. They observed that once the crisis was present, alkalization of the blood was no more effective than saline in achieving relief.

My associates and I have observed the disappearance of pain and other symptoms of crises in children with sickle cell anemia after the intravenous administration of 6 per cent dextran in 5 per cent fructose in a dosage of approximately 25 ml. per kilogram of body weight given at the rate of 3 ml. per minute. In six of nine cases especially studied, we observed an increase in the total mass of hemoglobin (without blood transfusion). This finding, with other evidence, suggests that the effectiveness of various fluids (electrolytes as well as dextrose, plasma, dextran, and similar fluids) is nonspecific and is derived primarily from their ability to mobilize stagnant or trapped cells in organ depots and to return them to circulation in the peripheral blood vessels.

Recently, urea in invert sugar has been advocated for the control of sickle cell crises. This mode of therapy (intravenous and oral) is still in the experimental stage and conclusive evaluation remains to be achieved. The cyanates (sodium and potassium) are currently under experimental evaluation for the treatment of sickle cell anemia.

Surgical Procedures. Elective surgical operations for the removal of diseased tonsils and adenoids, for the repair of hernias, for dental extractions and for other reasons should be carried out during a quiescent stage of the disease. Blood transfusions should be given as necessary to bring the hemoglobin level to at least 10 Gm. before the child is subjected to general anesthesia and surgery.

Older children with this disease sometimes have gallstones (calcium bilirubinate) and may require cholecystectomy. Abdominal pain in children with sickle cell anemia may simulate appendicitis, cholecystitis, salpingitis, ileus and other intra-abdominal diseases. Sickle cell anemia should be considered in the differential diagnosis of all Negro patients with acute abdominal pain.

Splenectomy has been performed for selected cases of sickle cell anemia by some investigators. In general, their criteria for the operation include frequent hemolytic crises, persistent splenomegaly and clinical and laboratory evidence of hypersplenism. My colleagues and I have observed few cases that have satisfied these composite criteria for splenectomy. The procedure is not curative and not without hazards, but it is of value in carefully selected patients in whom extracorpuscular hemolytic factors can be clearly demonstrated. Splenectomy should be considered when splenomegaly is associated with pancytopenia or with severe recurrent episodes of sequestration crises.

Emergency splenectomy is, of course, indicated for splenic rupture, which rarely occurs after exposure to low barometric pressure and anoxia during high altitude airplane flights.

Other Therapeutic Agents. Many drugs, including acetazolamide (Diamox), anticoagulants (Dicumarol and heparin), cobalt, Priscoline, magnesium sulfate and phenothiazines (Promazine), were used in the past by various investigators. These particular drugs are not recommended because they are ineffective in preventing or aborting the symptoms of crises. Moreover, some of them have serious toxic side effects.

Occasionally it may be necessary to prescribe codeine alone or in combination with Empirin for severe pain in children. The repeated use of narcotics (codeine, Demerol, morphine) should be avoided, however, because of the danger of addiction.

In general, iron-containing medication should not be given as a therapeutic measure to patients with sickle cell anemia. Because of the shortened survival time and excessive hemolysis of erythrocytes in this disease, serum iron is usually increased and tissue hemosiderosis is a characteristic finding. Moreover, iron is not effective in relieving the anemia. On the other hand, children with the sickle cell trait on occasion (usually for dietary reasons) do exhibit iron deficiency anemia, for which advice about diet and a hematinic may be indicated.

In North America, patients with sickle cell anemia require, as a rule, only such vitamin supplements as would be needed by any growing child. Megaloblastic anemia with deficiencies involving folic acid and vitamin B_{12} has been described as a complication of sickle cell anemia in Africa and some sections of the West Indies.

My colleagues and I have observed biochemical evidence of folic acid deficiency in patients with sickle cell anemia who were clinically asymptomatic (except for laboratory demonstration of anemia). We have not observed any significant relief of clinical symptoms in children with thrombotic pain or aplastic crises after folic acid medication.

In a study involving three small children with aplastic crises, Pearson and Cobb were also unable to find convincing evidence that the symptoms were due to folic acid deficiency. Pierce and Rath, however, reported hematologic response after oral folic acid supplementation (1 mg. daily) in two adult patients. In the present state of our knowledge, the significance of biochemical abnormality of folic acid metabolism in sickle cell anemia is uncertain, and specific administration of folic acid would not seem to be necessary in North American children with sickle cell anemia.

Some workers administer polytherapeutic mixtures (antimalarials, vitamins, antibiotics or long-acting sulfonamides) for prophylaxis in some developing countries in which malaria, malnutrition and severe infections have a significant effect upon the morbidity and mortality rates of children with sickle cell disease.

Testosterone has been reported to halt or prevent crises in some subjects. Unfortunately, this therapy leads to premature appearance of secondary sex characteristics in prepubescent children.

COMPLICATIONS

Many complications have been described in sickle cell anemia, including congestive heart failure, hematuria, aseptic necrosis of bone, osteomyelitis (especially due to salmonella), leg ulcers, priapism, chorioretinitis and amblyopia, pneumonia and pulmonary infarction, nephrosis, frostbite and cerebrovascular accidents. Only a few of these conditions will be discussed briefly here.

Pneumonia. This is a frequent complication in children with sickle cell anemia. In addition to antibiotic therapy, oxygen and small transfusions (6 to 10 ml. per kilogram of body weight) of packed red cells are administered daily until the hemoglobin level reaches 12 Gm.

Priapism. Fortunately, this complication does not occur frequently in children. Treatment, in general, is conservative. Many remedies and modes of therapy have been used by various clinicians. If compresses and analgesics fail to relieve the pain and congestion, needle aspirations of the corpora cavernosa appear to yield the most satisfactory results.

Aseptic Necrosis of Bone. This complication may seriously impair function, particularly when the bones of the weight-bearing extremities are involved. Involvement of the femoral neck and head may produce radiographic changes that are difficult to distinguish from the classic Legg-Calvé-Perthes disease. The condition is best managed by conservative (nonoperative) orthopedic procedures.

Hematuria. Intermittent hematuria may occur in homozygous sickle cell anemia, sickle cell trait and the sickle cell variant hemoglobinopathies. It is apparently less frequently observed in children than in adults. Conservative measures are recommended because the bleeding stops spontaneously in most patients.

Immergut and Stevenson found epsilon amino caproic acid to be useful in the control of this type of hematuria in three Negro adult patients. One of these received 1000 mg. four times daily for two weeks. The agent presumably acts by inhibition of the fibrinolytic activity of urokinase present in normal urine.

The intravenous infusion of distilled water and urinary alkalinization are reported to arrest hematuria in adult patients.

Leg Ulcers. Leg ulcers as complications of sickle cell anemia are less frequently observed in children than in adults. This condition tends to become chronic and intractable to treatment. The most effective method of therapy appears to be a regimen that requires control of local infection, bed rest, transfusions of whole blood to maintain the hemoglobin level around 11 to 12 Gm. and the application of Unna's boot.

It has been reported that zinc sulfate (220 mg. given three times daily) caused the healing of leg ulcers in adult patients three times faster than in a placebo-treated group.

Heart Failure. Myocardial weakness and dilatation may result from chronic anoxia and severe anemia. The administration of oxygen (50 per cent concentration) in a tent and the judicious use of small transfusions of packed erythrocytes (6 ml. per kilogram of body weight) often result in considerable decrease in heart size. Congestive heart failure is an indication for digitalization. Digoxin is satisfactory for oral or parenteral administration. The oral digitalizing dose (tablet or liquid) is 0.06 to 0.10 mg. per kilogram of body weight for infants less than two years and 0.04 to 0.09 mg. per kilogram for children more than two years old. Half of the calculated dose is given initially, and the remainder is taken in equal parts at 6- to 8-hour intervals. The daily maintenance doses may be calculated at one-fourth the digitalizing dose. They are given in two divided doses 8 to 12 hours after full digitalization. If the emergency requires parenteral use of the drug, the dosage can be calculated at two-thirds the oral dose.

Salmonella Infections. Hematogenous osteomyelitis is a rare complication of salmonellosis in normal patients; however, children with sickle cell anemia appear to have a predisposition to this type of infection. Management entails sensitivity studies of the microorganism's response to several antibiotics and the selection of the appropriate agent or combination of drugs. During the treatment of these infections it is advisable to use not only in vitro sensitivity studies but also in vivo determinations of the ability of the patient's own serum to inhibit growth of microorganisms in serial dilutions of 1:100.

Chloramphenicol, 50 to 100 mg. per kilogram per 24 hours in divided doses orally (or chloramphenicol sodium succinate by continuous intravenous infusion), and tetracyclines‡ (Terramycin), in dosage of 25 to 50 mg. per kilogram per 24 hours in four oral doses, are often effective.

In some cases of salmonella osteomyelitis, streptomycin (20 to 40 mg. per kilogram per 24 hours divided into two or three intramuscular doses), along with a tetracycline or chloramphenicol with crystalline penicillin G (25,000 to 50,000 units per kilogram per 24 hours divided into four to six doses) has proved to be an effective therapeutic combination. Ampicillin also has been used for the treatment of salmonella osteomyelitis. Dosages of 150 to 200 mg. per kilogram per day after an initial dose of 50 mg. per kilogram intravenously have been recommended. The antibiotics should be continued until the patient is completely asymptomatic clinically and until blood cultures are negative and roentgenograms demonstrate healing in the case of osteomyelitis. Surgical drainage and curettage may be necessary.

‡ Manufacturer's note: The use of tetracyclines during tooth development (last half of pregnancy, infancy and childhood to age eight years) may cause permanent discoloration of teeth. This adverse reaction is more common during long-term use of the drugs but has been observed following repeated short-term courses.

MANAGEMENT DURING PERIODS OF REMISSION

In the periods between crises, opportunity should be taken to determine and record the physical and hematologic status of the patient. This is also a good time to carry out elective procedures, such as dental care and tonsillectomy. During the winter and spring months, when respiratory infections are more frequent, it may be helpful to place the young child on prophylactic antibiotic therapy because intercurrent infections are the chief precipitating factors in exacerbations (crises). Moreover, pneumonia and meningitis caused by pneumococcal organisms are statistically more common in these patients. Unfortunately, effective drugs and vaccines are not generally available for the viruses that commonly infect the respiratory tract. The regimen of prophylactic medication is reserved mainly, but not exclusively, for children of preschool age.

Lehmann and coworkers recommend sodium bicarbonate in preventing crises and acidosis rather than in affecting sickle cells once the crisis has developed. Their dosage is between 500 and 1000 mg. per kilogram of body weight per day divided into 6- or 8-hour doses. The aim is to keep the urine sufficiently alkaline to give a blue reaction with litmus paper. The bicarbonate dosage is increased as soon as the urine becomes acidic. It is claimed that this prophylaxis against crises can be carried out indefinitely, provided kidney function is normal. A regimen of this kind must be reserved for carefully selected patients and families.

Because of the chronicity and intractability of the disorder, it is important to provide the parent (and older child) with general guidance and education about the nature of the illness. A booklet has been found helpful in achieving this plan.§

VARIANT FORMS

Sickle cell–hemoglobin C disease and sickle cell–thalassemia are the two most commonly encountered variant forms in my experience. As a rule, these syndromes are not as severe clinically as ordinary homozygous sickle cell anemia. The usual clinical types of crises also occur in these variant forms of the disease and are

§ Scott, Roland B., and Kessler, Althea D.: *Sickle Cell Anemia and Your Child.* Published by the Center for Sickle Cell Anemia, Howard University, College of Medicine, Washington, D. C. 20001.

treated as described for ordinary sickle cell anemia. Because of the mildness of the anemia, transfusions of whole blood are rarely indicated in sickle cell–hemoglobin C disease.

Polycythemia

J. LAWRENCE NAIMAN, M.D.

Since polycythemia rubra vera (increased numbers of red cells, white cells and platelets) is extremely rare in childhood, the terms polycythemia and erythrocytosis may be considered synonymous. Polycythemia is generally secondary to some underlying disorder and is usually asymptomatic. Its occurrence should therefore be regarded more as a challenge to diagnosis than as a signal for therapy.

NEONATAL POLYCYTHEMIA

In a plethoric newborn with high capillary hemoglobin concentration or hematocrit, the diagnosis of polycythemia should not be accepted unless verified with venous blood (hemoglobin over 22 Gr. per 100 ml. or hematocrit over 65 ml. per 100 ml.). In most infants there are no symptoms other than plethora, and phlebotomy is not indicated. Such infants should be observed closely, however, and watched for certain complications:

1. *Hyperviscosity* may cause respiratory distress, cyanosis and twitching, which suggest impaired circulation in the lungs or brain. Cerebral thrombi may lead to residual brain damage.

2. *Increased red cell breakdown* may cause hyperbilirubinemia.

3. *Metabolic abnormalities* such as hypocalcemia or hypoglycemia may contribute to twitching and irritability.

The presence of any of the above symptoms is an indication for efforts to reduce the red cell volume. This is best carried out by partial exchange transfusion with fresh frozen plasma, using the same equipment and technique as in conventional exchange transfusion. Pre-exchange blood samples should be obtained from the umbilical vein for determination of hemoglobin, hematocrit, glucose, calcium and bilirubin, and for special studies to rule out maternal-fetal transfusion (fetal hemoglobin concentration, serum IgM and mixed red cell agglutination test). The infant's blood is removed in aliquots of 10 ml. and replaced with an equal volume of group-specific fresh frozen plasma, aiming at a final venous hematocrit of 60 ml. per 100 ml. or less. A simple formula to estimate the required volume of exchange is as follows:

$$\text{Volume of exchange (ml.)} = \frac{100 \times \text{weight (kg.)} \times (\text{observed Hct.} - \text{desired Hct.})}{\text{observed Hct.}}$$

The presence of hypoglycemia or hypocalcemia requires appropriate correction with intravenous hypertonic glucose or calcium.

When the polycythemia results from a twin-to-twin transfusion, the anemic donor (usually the sicker of the two) deserves priority and may require prompt blood transfusion. If the anemia is severe and accompanied by signs of shock, group O Rh-negative whole blood (20 ml. per kilogram) should be given rapidly through an umbilical venous catheter. Otherwise, simple transfusion with appropriately cross matched packed red cells may be given to raise the infant's hemoglobin to 13 to 14 Gr. per 100 ml.

POLYCYTHEMIA BEYOND THE NEWBORN PERIOD

Primary Polycythemia. An isolated increase in the concentration of red cells in the absence of an underlying cause (see below) is termed primary erythrocytosis. It may be familial and, since it is usually asymptomatic, treatment is not necessary.

Secondary Polycythemia. DUE TO HYPOXIA. Most commonly this occurs in children with cyanotic congenital heart disease and represents a beneficial adaptive response. However, when the hematocrit exceeds approximately 75 per cent, the increased blood viscosity results in reduced systemic blood flow and a net worsening of the hypoxia. Symptoms such as headache, fatigability and irritability may be relieved by efforts to reduce the hematocrit to about 60 per cent. This may be accomplished either by repeated phlebotomy alone, or phlebotomy coupled with infusion of an equal volume of fresh frozen plasma (erythropheresis). The latter method, although slightly more tedious, is recommended because it avoids any acute changes in total blood volume which may lead to hypotension and cerebrovascular accidents. Exchange volumes of 7 to 8 ml. per kilogram are repeated once or twice weekly until the desired hematocrit is reached, and then at less frequent intervals as determined by the patient's hematocrit and symptoms. A convenient system for carrying out the erythropheresis can be constructed from a Venotube Twin Site* (Abbott Venotube 30, Catalogue

* Abbott Laboratories, North Chicago, Illinois 60064.

No. 4522) connected to a number 14 or 16 needle inserted in the child's vein under local anesthesia. A large syringe (30 to 50 ml., depending on the size of the child) is attached to the female end of the Venotube. After each syringeful of blood is removed, an equal volume of plasma may be infused through one side arm. The other side arm may be used for irrigation of the system with heparinized saline.

Erythropheresis is also recommended to correct the hemostatic defects of such patients prior to cardiac surgery. A rapid reduction of hematocrit may be achieved by phlebotomies of 5 ml. per kilogram, replacing with equal volumes of plasma and repeated daily until a hematocrit of about 60 per cent is reached. Postperfusion bleeding may be further reduced by transfusion of fresh frozen plasma (10 ml. per kilogram) and platelet concentrates (1 unit per 5 kilograms) after the patient is taken off the heart pump.

Hypoxia from chronic pulmonary disease is usually not accompanied by polycythemia severe enough to cause symptoms. If the hematocrit should exceed 75 per cent, a trial of phlebotomies is worthwhile to see whether there is any improvement in dyspnea or exercise tolerance.

DUE TO INAPPROPRIATE INCREASE IN ERYTHROPOIETIN SECRETION. This type of polycythemia may occur with renal tumors or cysts, hydronephrosis and tumors of the adrenal, liver and cerebellum. Identification and correction of the underlying disorder will eliminate the polycythemia.

DUE TO AN ABNORMAL HEMOGLOBIN WITH INCREASED OXYGEN AFFINITY (E.G., HEMOGLOBINS CHESAPEAKE, RANIER). The degree of polycythemia in such individuals is generally not great enough to require treatment.

Leukopenia, Neutropenia and Agranulocytosis

JOHN N. LUKENS, M.D.

The term *leukopenia* designates an absolute decrease in the number of circulating white blood cells. Minor variations in numbers of peripheral blood leukocytes are observed in normal children of different ages. For practical purposes, however, leukopenia may be defined as a state characterized by fewer than 4000 white blood cells per cubic mm. of blood, irrespective of age. Leukopenia most frequently results from a decrease in the number of neutrophils (*neutropenia*). An absolute neutrophil count (calculated as the product of the total white blood cell count and the percentage of neutrophils in the differential leukocyte count) of less than 1500 per cubic mm. constitutes neutropenia. Less frequently, leukopenia is due to an absolute lymphopenia or to concurrent neutropenia and lymphopenia. Leukopenia and neutropenia are commonly associated with varying degrees of anemia and thrombocytopenia. The term *agranulocytosis* is used to designate a state characterized by severe neutropenia and normal numbers of circulating red blood cells and platelets. Technically, agranulocytosis implies an absolute deficiency of eosinophils, basophils and monocytes as well as neutrophils. By convention, however, the term is used to mean severe, isolated neutropenia.

Recognition of lymphopenia serves to direct attention to specific diagnostic possibilities. On the other hand, lymphopenia rarely lends itself to therapeutic manipulation. In contrast, neutropenia is attended by a predictable risk of life-threatening infection. Scrupulous attention to management of the patient is of utmost importance if infectious complications are to be prevented or effectively treated. Consequently, the following discussion is confined to the therapeutic implications of neutropenia.

The causes of neutropenia are legion. An understanding of the pathogenesis of neutropenia and an appreciation for its anticipated severity and duration are basic to rational management of the patient. Prior to embarking on a therapeutic program, it is important to review in detail the child's exposure to drugs; to identify associated hepatic, pancreatic or splenic disease; and to examine peripheral blood and bone marrow with respect to cellular morphology and maturation. In addition, evaluation of family members, screening of serum for atypical antibodies, cultures of body fluids and leukokinetic studies may be necessary.

MANAGEMENT OF THE NEUTROPENIC CHILD

The treatment of neutropenia is dictated by the projected course of the patient with respect to infectious complications, by the magnitude of neutropenia and by the presence of associated disease. Because variations in numbers of blood neutrophils do not necessarily reflect events in the tissue pool of neutrophils, it is appropriate that treatment be based on patient needs rather than on an arbitrary level of blood neutrophils. Despite severe neutropenia, some children experience little or no increase in the frequency or severity of infectious illnesses. These children have normal numbers of neutrophil precursors in the bone marrow and an abundance of mature neutrophils in nasal and conjunctival exudates. One may conclude that sufficient numbers of neutrophils may be mobilized in response to physiologic stimuli. Aggressive therapeutic intervention is unwarranted. Other children, whose neutropenia is of comparable magnitude, are subject to recurrent, protracted, devastating infections. For them, intensive supportive measures may be lifesaving. In general, host response to infection is not impaired until the absolute neutrophil count falls below 1000 per cubic mm. Patients with neutrophil counts between 500 and 1000 per cubic mm. are subject to a slight but significant increase in infectious complications. Neutrophil counts of less than 500 per cubic mm. are associated with an impressive proclivity for severe infections. At any level of granulocytes, the frequency of infectious episodes is greater if there is concurrent systemic disease. The neutropenic patient with leukemia is more vulnerable to infection during relapse than during periods of remission.

Specific Therapy. Regrettably, the majority of neutropenic states do not lend themselves to correction by therapeutic measures currently available. In the absence of a primary disease requiring myelosuppressive therapy, it is of utmost importance to protect the patient from exposure to drugs, chemicals and physical agents which have the potential to injure bone marrow. Drugs which have been implicated in the pathogenesis of neutropenia include the sulfonamides and their derivatives, anticonvulsants, aminopyrine, phenothiazines, tranquilizers and antithyroid agents. Withdrawal of the neutropenic patient from all drugs may have important diagnostic as well as therapeutic significance. If drug therapy is indicated for an associated or intercurrent illness, it is recommended that the recognized side effects of candidate drugs be carefully scrutinized for evidence of blood or bone marrow toxicity.

Although controlled data are lacking, anabolic steroids are widely acknowledged to improve bone marrow function in children and adults with aplastic anemia. Since remissions in this condition are characterized by an increase in blood leukocytes as well as erythrocytes, androgens have been advocated for patients with isolated neutropenia as well. Unfortunately, the published experience with androgens in neutropenic states is anecdotal and unconvincing. A therapeutic course of androgen should be undertaken only with an understanding of the experimental nature of the trial and an appreciation for the hepatic toxicity of the drug. Oxymetholone* is given in a dose of 2 to 5 mg. per kilogram body weight per day for a minimum of three months.

Splenomegaly from any cause is commonly associated with sequestration of peripheral blood cells. If the rate of sequestration exceeds the regenerative capacity of the bone marrow, pancytopenia ensues. Although children with splenomegaly and splenic sequestration are regularly neutropenic, the neutropenia is rarely of sufficient magnitude to precipitate infectious complications. Asymptomatic neutropenia in the child with splenomegaly is best managed by careful observation and suppression of surgical enthusiasm. The child with recurrent or progressive infections and splenic neutropenia poses a most difficult therapeutic problem. Splenectomy in children is not to be undertaken lightly, since splenic extirpation early in life imposes a risk of life-threatening pneumococcal sepsis. This risk is greater for children with primary disorders of bone marrow function or immune responsiveness. The sole reliable diagnostic criterion for splenic neutropenia is the correction of neutropenia by splenectomy. Consequently, the therapeutic utility of the procedure cannot be predicted with confidence. Splenectomy should be considered only if the bone marrow is rich with neutrophil precursors. In the presence of bone marrow hypoplasia, splenectomy serves only to potentiate the infectious complications of neutropenia.

Pharmacologic doses of corticosteroids induce an increase in circulating neutrophils in hematologically normal individuals. The neutrophilia is due in part to a shift of marrow granulocytes to the circulating compartment and in part to a decrease in the egress of neutrophils from blood to tissues. The use of corticosteroids as primary therapy for neutropenia is to be condemned. Not only do steroids have the potential for masking bacterial infections, they further compromise the patient whose ability to mobilize a tissue inflammatory response is already impaired.

Management of Infectious Complications. The ultimate concern for all neutropenic patients is infection. As a result, the major thrust of patient management entails implementation of preventive measures and diligent attention to each febrile episode.

Preventive Measures. The patient or parent is instructed in the essentials of good

* Note: Oxymetholone is considered investigational for this use, since approval has not been officially stated in the package insert.

personal hygiene. Aggressive perirectal abscesses frequently result from minor injury to the perianal area. Consequently, the use of rectal suppositories and rectal thermometers is avoided. A stool softener (Colace, 50 to 100 mg. daily) is given in order to prevent anal fissures. Isolation precautions are not generally exercised, since the greatest threat to the patient is imposed by his own enteric flora rather than by environmental microorganisms. The prophylactic administration of antibiotics is contraindicated. Their use provides no protection against systemic infections, ensures the emergence of resistant organisms and creates an environment favorable for the growth of *Candida albicans.*

Programs designed to reduce exposure of the patient to both exogenous and endogenous microbial flora are presently under investigation in a number of centers. These programs necessitate isolation of the patient in specially designed units which filter room air. Patient sterilization is achieved by the topical application of antiseptic and antibiotic agents, by the provision of sterile food and by the oral administration of nonabsorbable antibiotics (vancomycin, gentamicin, and Mycostatin). This approach has been used primarily to protect leukemic patients who are undergoing intensive treatment with myelosuppressive agents. Combined gut sterilization and barrier isolation decrease the risk of infections in severely neutropenic subjects. Nevertheless, for leukemic patients, there is no benefit with respect to remission rates or duration of survival. The role of this experimental approach in the protection of neutropenic patients remains to be determined.

Management of Suspected or Documented Infection. Infection is suspected whenever fever occurs. This policy applies to patients whose primary disease may produce fever, as well as to patients with isolated neutropenia. Recognition of infection in the neutropenic patient is difficult. Often, infection is not betrayed by characteristic signs and symptoms: febrile responses are atypical, exudates are scanty and nonpurulent and the blood leukocyte response is minimal or absent. Invasive organisms are not confined to the site of initial colonization and, as a result, septicemia occurs without signs of localized infection. If early control of disseminated infection is to be achieved, each febrile episode must be carefully evaluated, appropriate cultures must be obtained and prompt institution of antibiotics must be effected.

The selection of antibiotics is based on knowledge of the types of infections most commonly experienced by neutropenic patients. Bactericidal agents are used in preference to bacteriostatic drugs. The responsible organisms are ubiquitous microbes of low pathogenicity: *Pseudomonas aeruginosa, Escherichia coli, Staphylococcus aureus, Aerobacter aerogenes, Klebsiella pneumoniae* and other members of the enteric flora. Once cultures are obtained, a therapeutic course of cephalothin and gentamicin is begun. Cephalothin is administrated in a dose of 200 mg. per kilogram per 24 hours. The drug is given by intravenous push at 2- to 3-hour intervals. Gentamicin is infused intravenously at 8-hour intervals in a total daily dose of 5 mg. per kilogram body weight. If skin lesions suggestive of pseudomonas septicemia are observed (ecthyma gangrenosum) or if pseudomonas is recovered by culture, both carbenicillin and gentamicin are given. Carbenicillin is infused intravenously at 4-hour intervals in a dose of 400 mg. per kilogram per 24 hours. Carbenicillin and gentamicin should not be mixed in the same bottle.

Antibiotics are continued until the infecting microorganism is identified and its sensitivities are characterized. Thereafter, the therapeutic program is tailored to selectively suppress the isolated pathogen. If no organism is recovered from cultures of body fluids, decisions regarding the duration of antibiotic administration are based largely on the patient's temperature chart. If fever resolves within 48 hours of the initiation of treatment, the drugs are continued for at least 7 to 10 days. On the other hand, if no defervescence is observed, one may conclude that the antibiotic combination is of no value. In this situation, the drugs are discontinued after a total of 3 to 4 days. The risk of superinfection with resistant organisms interdicts the long-term administration of antibiotics.

Granulocyte transfusions may be of benefit in the treatment of established infection in selected neutropenic patients. Since many prospective recipients of leukocyte infusions have been sensitized to leukocyte antigens by prior transfusions of whole blood or platelets, random donors cannot be used with profit. Leukocyte transfusions are used with success when efforts are made to select donors with HL-A compatible leukocytes, when transfusions are initiated early in the course of the infectious illness and when transfusions are repeated daily until the infection is eradicated or until bone marrow function is restored. Unfortunately, plasmapheresis procurement techniques are expensive and demanding of donors and professional personnel alike. As a result, leukocyte infusions remain an experimental approach to the treatment of established infections.

Acute Leukemia

DONALD P. PINKEL, M.D.

In the past, childhood leukemia has been considered to be a uniformly fatal disease. The goal of management has been prolongation of life in comfort by sequential or cyclic administration of antileukemic drugs and use of supportive measures. However, results of recent studies indicate that acute lymphocytic leukemia can no longer be considered an incurable disease and that palliation is no longer an acceptable approach to its treatment.

LYMPHOCYTIC LEUKEMIA

Total therapy of acute lymphocytic leukemia, utilizing a combination of several antileukemic agents and necessary supportive treatment, has resulted in a 17 per cent seven-year *leukemia-free* survival rate for children admitted for treatment studies at St. Jude Children's Research Hospital in 1962 to 1965. Patients admitted to the 1967 to 1968 study have a 51 per cent four-year *leukemia-free* survival rate.

The method of treating acute lymphocytic leukemia described here is based on 10 years of experience with total therapy. It is recommended for all childhood leukemia cases that are characterized by lymphocytes, lymphoblasts and stem cells. The treatment of acute and chronic myelocytic leukemia is discussed separately.

Drugs Used. *Prednisone* is a synthetic corticosteroid hormone that produces lysis of lymphoblasts and lymphocytes and inhibits proliferation of lymphoid tissue; it also exerts a nonspecific hemostatic effect in patients with thrombocytopenic bleeding. It causes protein deficiency with muscle atrophy by promoting gluconeogenesis, and it reduces resistance to infection. Less frequently it causes serious sodium retention and hypertension or precipitates hyperglycemia and ketosis. In the patient who is not taking food, its potassium-wasting effect can lead to hypochloremic alkalosis and hypokalemia.

Vincristine is a natural alkaloid that produces rapid destruction of lymphoblasts, stem cells and several other types of neoplastic cells. Its primary toxicity consists of peripheral neuropathy, both sensory and motor, with paresthesias, loss of deep tendon reflexes, extensor weakness and frank paresis. Abnormal erythropoiesis, immunosuppression, muscle wasting, constipation, ileus, convulsions, hypertension and hyponatremia due to inappropriate secretion of antidiuretic hormone also result from its administration. Paravenous injection leads to tissue necrosis.

Methotrexate is a synthetic antimetabolite of folic acid that causes inhibition of purine and pyrimidine synthesis, preventing synthesis of deoxyribonucleic acid (DNA). It produces mucosal ulceration, vomiting, abdominal cramps, diarrhea, alopecia, megaloblastic anemia, hepatic fibrosis and suppression of hematopoiesis. It decreases resistance to infection. Oral methotrexate is usually discontinued during treatment with intrathecal methotrexate.

Mercaptopurine is a synthetic antimetabolite of guanine that inhibits DNA synthesis. It causes vomiting, diarrhea, alopecia, mucosal ulceration, toxic hepatitis and suppression of hematopoiesis. It depresses immune response and lowers resistance to infection.

Cyclophosphamide is a synthetic alkylating agent that inhibits DNA synthesis. It produces vomiting, alopecia, toxic hemorrhagic cystitis, mucosal ulceration and suppression of hematopoiesis and immunity. Prolonged administration may cause fibrosis of the urinary bladder.

Definitions. *Complete remission* means that the patient is free of symptoms and signs attributable to leukemia, that the peripheral blood counts are normal except for drug-induced neutropenia or thrombocytopenia and that the bone marrow demonstrates active hematopoiesis and contains 5 per cent or less lymphoblasts and stem cells.

Relapse is the reappearance of leukemia as manifested by the appearance of more than 10 per cent lymphoblasts and stem cells in the marrow progressive to 40 per cent or more of these cells, or by the appearance of central nervous system leukemia, visceral infiltration or symptoms and signs attributable to leukemia.

Central nervous system leukemia is diagnosed when leukemic blast cells are found in the Wright-stained centrifugate of a sample of spinal fluid. When morphology is questionable, another sample is obtained in a week.

Evaluation of Patients. Complete and accurate evaluation of the patient is the first step in the treatment of leukemia. Often the patients have infections or harbor organisms such as *Pseudomonas aeruginosa* that are potentially pathogenic after chemotherapy is initiated. Malnutrition is a frequent problem that impedes successful chemotherapy and regeneration of normal hematopoiesis. Metabolic and electrolyte abnormalities are common, especially when the patient has extensive renal infiltration or has been under treatment with nephrotoxic antibiotics. Hemorrhage may be apparent or occult; it is usually due to thrombocytopenia rather than to other coagulation defects. Central nervous system leukemia is present in 5 per cent of patients at the time of diagnosis; it is usually asymptomatic at that time.

The following studies are carried out on all patients prior to therapy:

1. Complete history and physical examination; height, weight, head and chest measurements; dietary evaluation; initiation of Stuart Growth Grid and Nellhaus Head Circumference Chart.

2. Hemoglobin; white blood cell, differential, platelet and reticulocyte counts; bone marrow examination.

3. Lumbar puncture with examination of Wright-stained sediment for leukemic cells.

4. Electrocardiogram; intravenous pyelogram with a urinary bladder film after voiding; chest, sinus and skeletal roentgenograms.

5. Blood chemistries: urea nitrogen, uric acid, bilirubin, serum glutamic oxaloacetic transaminase, alkaline phosphatase, prothrombin time, proteins, sodium, potassium and chlorides.

6. Urinalysis.

7. Mouth, throat, rectal, blood, urine, spinal fluid and bone marrow cultures for bacteria and fungi; Gram-stained smears of any infected lesions and examination of urine sediment for bacteria and fungi.

8. Serologic tests: hepatitis-associated antigen; cytomegalovirus, varicella-zoster and toxoplasma antibody titers.

9. Tuberculin (PPD) skin test and other skin tests such as histoplasmin or coccidioidin in endemic areas.

10. Evaluation of cultural, ethnic and family background of child and parents.

Induction of Complete Remission. The purpose of the initial phase of treatment is to rapidly relieve the sick child of bleeding, infection and metabolic problems and to restore him to a happy, ambulatory state. A combination of antileukemic drugs is used that rapidly destroys leukemic tissue without interfering with hematopoietic regeneration and without causing nausea. Vincristine, 1.5 mg. per square meter, is injected intravenously once weekly, and prednisone, 40 mg. per square meter, is administered in two or three divided doses daily by mouth. After 28 days of this combination, the bone marrow is reexamined. If less than 5 per cent lymphoblasts and stem cells are present, the second phase is started. If not, vincristine and prednisone are continued for an additional week or two and marrow examination is repeated. If the marrow remains leukemic, the cell type diagnosis may be erroneous or this may be an unusual instance of refractory acute lymphocytic leukemia, in which case the patient should be referred to a center where experimental drugs such as L-asparaginase are available.

Fever usually indicates infection and after thorough examination and appropriate bacterial smears and cultures have been taken, full dosages of appropriate bactericidal antibiotics are administered *intravenously without delay.* If the child has been on penicillin, infection with *Staphylococcus aureus, Escherichia coli* or Klebsiella-Aerobacter is suspected. If he has received broad-spectrum antibiotics, Pseudomonas or Candida infection is suspected and the patient is treated accordingly pending cultures. *Prolonged antibiotic therapy is avoided.* Repeat smears and cultures are taken when fever persists or recurs following initial defervescence; antibiotics are changed as indicated. *Do not wait for an abscess or cellulitis to "point."* Inject 0.2 to 0.3 ml. of saline into the lesion, aspirate quickly and make a Gram-stained smear and cultures of the aspirate. Immediate determination by Gram-stained smear of whether the infecting organism is gram-positive or gram-negative may be lifesaving. Antibiotic sensitivity tests are performed by the Kirby-Bauer method on significant isolates, particularly gram-negative bacteria. In the interpretation of bacterial and fungal cultures, the physician in charge of the patient, not the laboratory technician, should determine what isolate is significant or not and what is a contaminant or not. Selection of isolates for antimicrobial sensitivity tests should also be directed by the physician.

The antibiotics used are penicillin G for *Streptococcus pyogenes* and *Streptococcus pneumoniae;* kanamycin for Klebsiella-Aerobacter, *E. coli* and Proteus species; oxacillin for *S. aureus;* streptomycin for *E. coli* and some Klebsiella-Aerobacter organisms; chloramphenicol* for Salmonella, *Hemophilus influenzae* and *E. coli;* gentamicin for *E. coli* and Enterobacter; gentamicin and carbenicillin in combination for Pseudomonas; Mycostatin orally every 3 hours for oral candidiasis; and amphotericin B or 5-flucytosine for systemic candidiasis. Dos-

* Manufacturer's precaution: Chloramphenicol is not recommended for intravenous or intramuscular pediatric use. Chloramphenicol sodium succinate has been approved for intravenous pediatric use.

ages larger than those conventionally recommended are used during the first two to three days of infection. For undiagnosed sepsis, intravenous cephalothin and gentamicin are often administered pending results of cultures.

Although widely discussed, the value of "life islands" and granulocyte transfusions from normal donors to control infection remains unsubstantiated. Minimization of hospital admissions and stays, handwashing by personnel and room isolation are important measures, however.

Metabolic problems, such as hyperuricemia, azotemia and hyperkalemia, often occur as leukemic tissue is catabolized during the first three to four days of chemotherapy, liberating toxic breakdown products of nucleic acids and proteins. The following precautions are taken:

1. Liquid intake and urinary output are measured and recorded; urine pH and specific gravity are checked three to four times a day at the bedside; urinalysis is obtained and blood urea nitrogen, potassium and uric acid values are measured daily for three days or until normal.

2. A liquid intake of 2000 to 3000 ml. per square meter per day is maintained. Potassium-containing multiple electrolyte solutions *are not given.* It must be remembered that potassium is liberated from catabolized leukemic cells; prednisone causes sodium retention and potassium excretion; excretion of xanthine compounds may cause sodium depletion; and renal tubular function may be abnormal because of leukemic infiltration, hyperuricemia, vincristine therapy or concurrent administration of nephrotoxic antibiotics. *Intravenous fluid and electrolyte therapy is tailored to the needs of the individual patient and monitored with blood chemistries.*

3. Allopurinol, 100 to 150 mg. per square meter every 12 hours orally, is started prior to chemotherapy and continued for three days or until the uric acid level is normal.

4. Sodium bicarbonate, 1 Gm. per square meter every 6 to 8 hours, is administered orally to maintain urine pH at 6.0 to 6.5. The intravenous route is used when necessary, employing a smaller dose of bicarbonate and accompanied by careful monitoring of blood pH and carbon dioxide.

Once the initial destruction of leukemic tissue is completed, usually within three to four days, these precautions can be terminated.

Fresh whole blood is used for anemia in order to avoid further reduction in circulating platelets. Platelet-rich plasma can be used for thrombocytopenic hemorrhage, but thrombocytopenia without bleeding requires no special treatment. While a bleeding tendency exists, deep venipunctures, intramuscular injections and instrumentation with catheters, tubes and laryngoscopes are avoided; clothing is kept loose.

Good nutrition is important for optimal tolerance of chemotherapy and regeneration of normal hematopoietic tissue. Soft drinks and "junk foods," such as cakes, cookies and potato chips, are avoided and emphasis is placed on adequate proteins, calories, vitamins and minerals, using supplementary preparations when indicated.

Central Nervous System Therapy. Past studies indicate that approximately one-half of children with acute lymphocytic leukemia develop central nervous system relapse while still in hematologic remission. This is apparently because of failure of antileukemic drugs to penetrate the meninges and cerebrospinal fluid in effective levels. The chance of relapse at this site increases with increasing duration of hematologic remission. The purpose of this treatment phase is to eliminate leukemic tissue in the central nervous system and thus to prevent central nervous system relapse from terminating complete remission.

As soon as bone marrow remission (less than 5 per cent lymphoblasts and stem cells) has been achieved, ^{60}Co teletherapy, in a total midplane tissue dose of 2000 to 2400 rads, is administered to the entire cranial vault through two opposing ports in approximately 15 treatments over a 2½- to 3-week period (Fig. 1). For children under one year of age, the dose is limited to 1500 rads.

Starting on the third day of radiotherapy, intrathecal methotrexate is administered. At lumbar puncture, cerebrospinal fluid, approximately 12 ml. per square meter, is removed from the patient and methotrexate, 12 mg. per square meter, is injected. The methotrexate solution consists of 1 mg. of methotrexate per ml. of physiologic saline solution. Several precautions are used to avoid adverse reactions to intrathecal methotrexate. The lumbar puncture must be atraumatic, spinal fluid is allowed to flow freely and is not aspirated and the saline diluent is free of preservatives. The methotrexate solution is kept no longer than 15 days at 4° C. and is filtered through a 0.22-micron millipore filter and brought to room temperature prior to administration. The solution is injected without aspiration over 15 to 30 seconds, and the stylet is reinserted before the needle is withdrawn. If the lumbar puncture is traumatic, repeat puncture and methotrexate

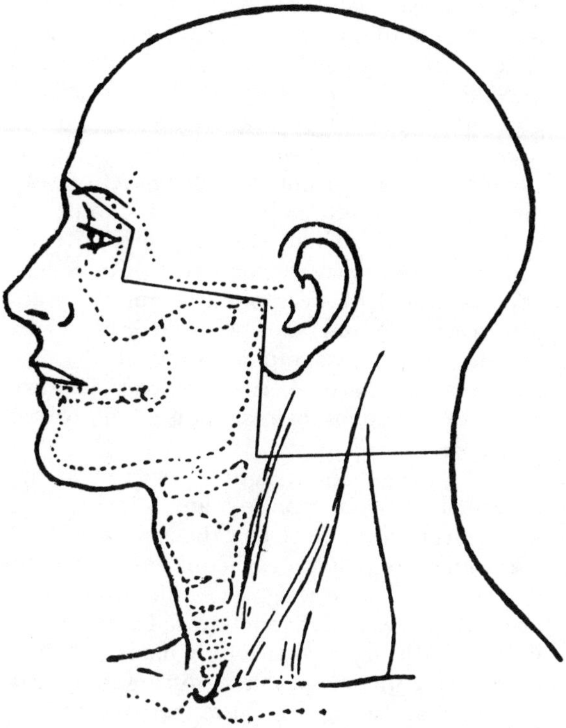

FIGURE 1. Cranial irradiation, 2400 r total midplane dose, is administered early during complete remission through two lateral portals as outlined above.

injection should be deferred for a day or two. Methotrexate is instilled into the subarachnoid space twice weekly during the course of radiotherapy for a total of five doses. Mild pleocytosis and protein elevation sometimes occur by the fourth or fifth dose. Leucovorin is *not* administered.

The parents and child are warned of alopecia and arrangements are made for a hairpiece, if indicated, before epilation. The hair regrows within three to four months but its color and texture are frequently different.

Concurrent systemic chemotherapy (see next section) is reduced if the white blood cell count drops below 2000 per cubic mm., but irradiation is not interrupted for leukopenia. Oral methotrexate is discontinued during the period when intrathecal methotrexate is being administered.

Continuation Therapy. This phase is initiated as soon as bone marrow remission is achieved and central nervous system therapy started. It is continued throughout central nervous system therapy and for the subsequent 2½ years. The purpose is to eliminate all residual leukemic cells, particularly those outside the central nervous system. Drugs that act by inhibition of DNA synthesis and that are tolerable and effective for long-term treatment are used.

The chemotherapy regimen consists of mercaptopurine, 50 mg. per square meter per day orally in one dose; methotrexate, 20 mg. per square meter once weekly; and cyclophosphamide, 200 mg. per square meter once weekly. The cyclophosphamide and methotrexate usually are given on the same day and can be given orally or intravenously.

These dosages are reduced or increased in order to maintain the white blood cell count between 2000 and 3500 per cubic mm. *This biologic parameter is the prime criterion for dosage.* If severe vomiting, diarrhea or mucosal ulceration develops, the drugs are interrupted and then resumed when symptoms and signs clear. Alopecia and sporadic vomiting are *not* indications for interrupting therapy. Cyclophosphamide-induced vomiting usually begins 4 to 6 hours after administration and continues for 24 hours; antiemetics are sometimes useful in preventing this.

Cyclophosphamide cystitis can be prevented usually by a liberal fluid intake started one day before the drug is taken and continued for two days afterward, and by the patient emptying his bladder frequently during the day and at least once during the night after receiving the medication.

Jaundice is an absolute indication for interrupting the drugs, but it is rarely due to them.

During continuation chemotherapy a white blood cell count is obtained weekly prior to methotrexate and cyclophosphamide administration. The hemoglobin level is measured and a blood smear evaluated once or twice monthly. At three-month intervals the bone marrow is reexamined, a lumbar puncture is performed and the spinal fluid sediment is examined for leukemic cells. At the same time the blood urea nitrogen, creatinine, bilirubin, alkaline phosphatase, serum glutamic oxaloacetic transaminase and prothrombin time are repeated and a routine urinalysis performed. Roentgenograms of the chest, estimation of bone age, a bromsulphalein clearance test and a creatinine clearance test are performed every six months. Roentgenographic study of the urinary bladder once or twice a year for evidence of cyclophosphamide-induced fibrosis is advisable.

The height and weight of each child are measured at least monthly and recorded on the Stuart Growth Grid, and the Nellhaus Head Circumference Chart is maintained. If the child's height and weight decline from their original percentile channel to a lower one, a thorough dietary evaluation is made. Malnutrition is a major problem during leukemia chemotherapy and predisposes the child to serious infection and excessive drug toxicity. Parents of leukemic children tend to cater to their children's dietary whims, substituting soft drinks, cookies and similar items for nutritious foods. In addition, the disruption of normal family routine by frequent trips to the physician, the depression of appetite by anxiety and the toxic effects of antileukemic drugs all interfere with nutrition. If growth impairment continues and physical evidence of undernutrition develops in spite of dietary counseling and supplements of proteins, vitamins and minerals, the dosages of antileukemic drugs are reduced until improved nutrition is established.

Sometimes asymptomatic infections during remission reduce drug tolerance and impair nutrition and growth. The patient should be carefully studied for chronic sinusitis or otitis if he is not doing well. Elimination of chronic infection is essential to optimal continuation chemotherapy.

Parents are warned to protect their children from contagious disease, particularly varicella-zoster infection. If exposure to varicella occurs in a child who has not had this disease previously as determined from his history and by a negative baseline antibody titer for varicella-zoster virus, chemotherapy is terminated for three weeks and zoster immune globulin† is administered. Varicella or disseminated herpes zoster infections are sometimes treated with 2 to 4 units of fresh white cell–rich plasma from donors convalescing from herpes zoster. The efficacy of this treatment is unproved. Two antiviral agents, cytosine arabinoside and idoxuridine, are reported to be effective in these patients, but their value has not been established by controlled studies and their side effects are hazardous.

Parents are advised to contact the physician when fever and other signs of infection occur. In the presence of serious infection, chemotherapy is interrupted and specific bactericidal antibiotic therapy is administered after appropriate smears and cultures for bacteria and fungi are taken. For hospitalized patients, antibiotics are given intravenously and in larger than conventional dosages. Because infection may progress very rapidly in these children, treatment is usually started without waiting for results of cultures. Again, immediate Gram-stained smears, indicating whether gram-positive cocci, gram-negative bacilli or fungi are the predominant organisms, are important.

Pneumonia due to *Pneumocystis carinii* is a leading hazard during combination chemotherapy and usually occurs independent of white blood cell count depression. The diagnosis is strongly suspected when the patient has fever, chest pain, mild to severe tachypnea, cough and flaring of the alae nasi, regardless of whether infiltration is seen on chest roentgenography. Pulmonary needle aspiration and staining of a smeared aspirate with methenamine silver nitrate (Gomori's method) reveals the diagnosis. Antileukemic chemotherapy is discontinued when the diagnosis is made or suspected. Pentamidine isethionate (obtained by telephoning the Parasitic Diseases Drug Service, National Disease Control Center, Atlanta, Georgia) is administered in a dosage of 150 mg. per square meter once daily intramuscularly for five days and then 100 mg. per square meter once daily for an additional five days along with supportive measures, such as oxygen and parenteral fluids. Side effects of pentamidine are azotemia, hypoglycemia and local tissue reaction at injection sites. The hypoglycemia can be avoided by using intravenous fluids containing 5 to 10 per cent glucose.

Other serious infections occurring during remissions are toxoplasmosis, viral hepatitis and encephalitis and cytomegalic inclusion disease.

Chronic subdural hematomas may occur in children with acute lymphocytic leukemia and are difficult to diagnose. They should be suspected in children with nonmeningeal central

† Not available commercially. Consult National Disease Control Center, Atlanta, Georgia.

nervous system symptoms such as convulsions, hemiplegia or coma.

Emotional support of the child and his family is an important part of therapy. The physician must "tune in" on each family and relate to it within its particular frame of reference. The family needs to feel that the physician is competent, concerned and candid. The older child should be told his diagnosis.

Hospitalization can be minimized if the patients are observed carefully in clinic and if their potential problems are anticipated and headed off. At this institution the majority of children with acute lymphocytic leukemia are not admitted to the hospital.

The question of when to stop chemotherapy in the child who has stayed in complete remission for a long while is unresolved. It is our current observation that most children who have received adequate "prophylactic" central nervous system irradiation and have remained in continuous complete remission for 2½ to 3 years continue in complete remission after termination of chemotherapy. We therefore recommend cessation of therapy after 2½ years of maximum tolerated combination chemotherapy and a course of cranial radiotherapy exceeding 2000 rads. After chemotherapy is stopped, an immunologic "rebound" is usually observed with bone marrow and peripheral blood lymphocytosis that can resemble early relapse. This usually subsides within a year.

Experimental techniques such as bone marrow transplantation and multiple injections of BCG vaccine have no established value in leukemia therapy at this time.

OTHER TYPES OF CHILDHOOD LEUKEMIA

Acute myelocytic leukemia is diagnosed only when there is clear differentiation of leukemic cells to myelocytes or typical Auer rods are present. Treatment of this form of leukemia is unsatisfactory and no standard therapy is worthy of recommendation. Referral to a research center engaged in development of new and better methods of treating this disease is preferable.

At present, we treat acute myelocytic leukemia in the following manner. To induce remission, we administer a combination of three drugs: mercaptopurine, 75 mg. per square meter per day orally for 28 to 42 days; vincristine, 1.5 mg. per square meter once a week intravenously for four to six weeks; 6-azauridine,‡ 15 Gm. per square meter per day intravenously for the first 10 days.

‡ Not available commercially; for experimental use only.

Precautions are similar to those taken for acute lymphocytic leukemia. Allopurinol is generally omitted, but if it is required because of hyperuricemia, the dosage of mercaptopurine is reduced to 37.5 mg. per square meter per day. The dosage of 6-azauridine occasionally must be decreased because of somnolence and diffuse slow wave dysrhythmia on electroencephalogram.

Prednisone, 40 mg. per square meter daily by mouth, may be used in short courses if thrombocytopenic bleeding is a problem. In contrast to acute lymphocytic leukemia, patients with acute myelocytic leukemia often have other coagulation defects.

After induction of remission the following combination is used for continuation chemotherapy: mercaptopurine, 75 mg. per square meter once a day orally, and cytosine arabinoside, 150 mg. per square meter once a week. The dosage is adjusted to biologic tolerance so that the white blood cell count remains between 2000 and 3500 per cubic mm. Severe vomiting, diarrhea or mucosal ulcerations may require temporary cessation or reduction of chemotherapy. Treatment is continued until relapse.

The toxic effects of cytosine arabinoside are similar to those of mercaptopurine: depression of hematopoiesis, mucosal ulcerations, vomiting, diarrhea, hepatic dysfunction and immunosuppression.

The investigational combinations of daunorubicin and cytosine arabinoside or of thioguanine and cytosine arabinoside have been recommended for acute myelocytic leukemia.

Acute monocytic leukemia is uncommon in children. It is diagnosed only when there is definite evidence of monocytic differentiation of the leukemic cells. Treatment is unsatisfactory and remissions are uncommon. The drug regimen described for acute myelocytic leukemia can be used.

Erythromyelocytic leukemia may have a longer course than acute myelocytic leukemia, but it is usually refractory to chemotherapy. The regimen for acute myelocytic leukemia can be used.

Chronic myelocytic leukemia, which must be differentiated from leukemoid reactions, is of two types in children. One resembles the adult type and demonstrates the Philadelphia chromosome (Ph^1). Treatment with busulfan usually leads to reduction in white blood cell count and organomegaly and relief of symptoms. Busulfan is administered in an initial dose of 2 mg. per day and increased *gradually* to 4 to 6 mg. per day depending on the white blood cell count response. When the white blood cell count drops to approximately 30,000 per cubic mm., the dose is reduced to 2 to 4 mg. daily and continued at a level sufficient to maintain the count at 5000 to 10,000 per cubic mm.

Intermittent administration of busulfan is reported to be as effective and less toxic than its continuous use. The toxic effects of busulfan include depression of normal hematopoiesis, skin pigmentation, amenorrhea, a wasting syndrome with features of Addison's disease and a pulmonary disease characterized by cough with progressive dyspnea.

The *juvenile non-Philadelphia chromosome (Ph^1 negative) type of chronic myelocytic leukemia* tends to occur in younger children. Unlike the adult type, the patient usually has thrombocytopenia and hemorrhage at the time of diagnosis and the disease is refractory to chemotherapy. Supportive measures, such as cautious transfusions of fresh whole blood and fresh platelets, may prolong life, and irradiation or chemotherapy may reduce white blood cell counts and splenomegaly.

We have observed two pairs of siblings with disease resembling the juvenile type of chronic myelocytic leukemia. Three children developed remissions after splenectomy; two remain in clinical and hematologic remission after six years.

WHO SHOULD TREAT CHILDREN WITH LEUKEMIA?

The physician in private practice sees few children with leukemia and cannot be expected to remain current with advances in treatment. Often he does not have the clinical laboratory, blood bank, pharmacy and nursing resources that are required for management of these patients. The time and energy that it takes to see a leukemic child through a severe infection, a metabolic crisis or a bleeding episode may be more than one can spare from a busy practice. For these reasons, referral to a university clinic or a cancer study center is frequently advocated.

On the other hand, many hematology units and cancer clinics have a pessimistic view of leukemia therapy and do not provide modern treatment for their leukemia patients. Often they fail to give the continuous comprehensive care these patients require. Different physicians see the children on each clinic visit and primary care is sometimes relegated to inexperienced house staff without adequate supervision.

Because of the complexity of childhood leukemia, each patient needs a personal physician who is acquainted with all fields of medicine: infectious disease, nutrition and metabolism as well as hematology and cancer chemotherapy. The physician must be willing to take consistent responsibility for the patient and to make the necessary services available to him as needed. Whether this "right physician" is a hospital-based specialist in a hematology or cancer center, or an internist, pediatrician or general practitioner in a community is of secondary importance.

In the mid-South the majority of children with leukemia are treated cooperatively by community-based physicians and a childhood cancer center. At the center each child is assigned to his own physician. Weekly supervision and home care are provided by the physician in the community. Initial and periodic evaluation, treatment plans, drugs and hospitalization are provided at the center by the staff physician assigned to the patient.

References

Aur, R. J. A., et al.: Central Nervous System Therapy and Combination Chemotherapy of Childhood Lymphocytic Leukemia. *Blood,* 37:272, 1971.

Aur, R. J. A., et al.: A Comparative Study of Central Nervous System Irradiation and Intensive Chemotherapy Early in Remission of Childhood Acute Lymphocytic Leukemia. *Cancer,* 29:381, 1972.

Borella, L., et al.: Immunological Rebound after Cessation of Long Term Chemotherapy in Acute Leukemia. *Blood,* 40:42, 1972.

Crowther, D., et al.: Combination Chemotherapy Using L-Asparaginase, Daunorubicin, and Cytosine Arabinoside in Adults with Acute Myelogenous Leukaemia. *Brit. Med. J.,* 4:513, 1970.

Galton, D. A. G.: Chemotherapy of Chronic Myelocytic Leukemia. *Seminars Hemat.,* 6:323, 1969.

Gee, T. S., et al.: Treatment of Adult Acute Leukemia with Arabinosylcytosine and Thioguanine. *Cancer,* 23:1019, 1969.

Holton, C. P., and Johnson, W. W.: Chronic Myelocytic Leukemia in Infant Siblings. *J. Pediat.,* 72:377, 1968.

Johnson, H. D., and Johnson, W. W.: *Pneumocystis carinii* Pneumonia in Children with Cancer. *J.A.M.A.,* 214:1067, 1970.

Simone, J.: Treatment of Children with Acute Lymphocytic Leukemia. *Advances Pediat.,* Vol. 19, 1972.

Simone, J., et al.: Fatalities During Remission of Childhood Leukemia. *Blood,* 39:759, 1972.

Walters, T., et al.: 6-Azauridine in Combination Chemotherapy of Childhood Acute Myelocytic Leukemia. *Cancer,* 29:1057, 1972.

Hemorrhagic Disorders

THOMAS F. NECHELES, M.D.

Bleeding episodes frequently present as medical emergencies and one is often tempted to jump in immediately with therapy. If the patient shows signs of cardiovascular decompensation or bleeding into a vital organ, this may be unavoidable, but there is always sufficient time to draw appropriate samples to establish a diagnosis. Emergency replacement therapy will depend on the type of bleeding encountered: hypovolemia with cardiovascular embarrassment requires the use of volume expanders and packed red cells, and bleeding into vital organs associated with petechiae may indicate the need for platelet-rich plasma and/or frozen plasma. Use of the latter may, however, be hazardous in the presence of disseminated intravascular coagulation (DIC) and contribute to the bleeding problem. Only rarely is there insufficient time to examine a smear of the peripheral blood to evaluate the number of platelets as well as the presence of fragmented red cells (schistocytes). Once the possibility of DIC has been eliminated, plasma products can be used as indicated. However, a definitive etiologic diagnosis is needed for specific therapy, for possible prophylactic treatment and for discussion of prognosis and genetic aspects with the patient and his family.

The hemostatic mechanism consists of three components: the plasma clotting factors, the platelets and the vascular system. Defects in each component can, in general, be either congenital or acquired. Many of the latter are secondary to other underlying disease processes and these must be treated, if possible, before the long-term integrity of the hemostatic system can be restored.

COAGULATION DISORDERS (DISORDERS IN THE PLASMA CLOTTING FACTORS)

Emergency Therapy. If one is faced with a bleeding patient with an abnormal prothrombin time (PT) and/or prolonged partial thromboplastin time (PTT) in the absence of significant thrombocytopenia or schistocytes on the peripheral blood smear, one can assume that one is dealing with a disorder of the plasma clotting factors and, in the absence of other information, infusion of fresh frozen plasma is the treatment of choice. The usual dose is 10 ml. per kilogram, which can be repeated every 8 to 24 hours as symptoms indicate. Usually the laboratory is able to establish a definitive diagnosis before a second infusion becomes necessary. Minor bleeding episodes, such as prolonged epistaxis or bleeding following dental extraction, can often be controlled by local measures and do not require plasma infusions. Pressure packs with thromboplastic agents such as Oxycel supplemented with a few drops of a concentrated solution of Adrenalin (1:100 strength) will often suffice. By avoiding the use of nonspecific plasma therapy, one can often establish an exact diagnosis in a much shorter time and allow the use of specific replacement therapy, if necessary, as well as alleviate the normal anxiety in the patient and his family.

Congenital Coagulation Disorders

Classical Hemophilia (Factor VIII Deficiency). Classical hemophilia is a congenital deficiency of factor VIII inherited as a sex-linked recessive trait. Patients with this disease are classified as mild, moderate or severe depending on the level of factor VIII present in the nonbleeding state (since factor VIII is consumed during bleeding episodes, levels taken at the time of acute episodes will not accurately reflect the level normally present in the patient). Patients with known factor VIII deficiency are best treated with concentrates containing high levels of factor VIII activity (Table 1); use of fresh-frozen plasma or fresh whole blood is at best only a second choice. Replacement therapy can be used as treatment of acute bleeding episodes, as short-term prophylaxis prior to surgery or dental procedures, or as long-term prophylaxis to prevent most, if not all, bleeding episodes.

Acute bleeding episodes can be of three types: rapid bleeding through a skin wound or into the gastrointestinal tract, bleeding into a closed space such as a joint or bleeding into soft tissues. All may be life-threatening under some circumstances and all require prompt attention. Our usual course is to give a rapid infusion of one of the factor VIII concentrates in a quantity calculated to be sufficient to elevate plasma levels to 75 per cent or more. We use the formula

$$\text{Expected level (in \% of normal)} = \frac{\text{AHF (antihemophilic factor) units administered}}{\text{Body weight (in kg.)} \times 0.4}$$

to calculate the initial loading dose and then, if the patient is in the hospital, repeat one-half of this dose every 12 hours. A simple slide-rule calculator is available from Hyland Laboratories for this calculation. If the patient is to be treated as an outpatient, as many patients with joint or soft tissue bleeding are, therapy is repeated at 24-hour intervals at the full dose. If bleeding is severe, as in the case of a gastrointestinal hemorrhage or the fracture of a major bone, the dose of factor VIII must be doubled and the interval between injections shortened to 8 hours. Therapy is monitored by factor VIII levels taken immediately prior to the injection of the next dose. However,

TABLE 1. Blood Products Useful in the Treatment of Bleeding Disorders

PREPARATION	MAJOR FACTOR(S)	VOLUME	USUAL REGIMES *Initial**	USUAL REGIMES *Maintenance**	HALF-LIFE OF MAJOR FACTOR(S)
Fresh-frozen plasma	All	200 ml.	10 ml./kg.	5 ml./kg./6 hr.	12–24 hr.
Cryoprecipitate	Factor VIII and fibrinogen	10 ml.	10 ml./5 kg.	10 ml./5 kg./12 hr.	12 hr.
Factor VIII concentrate (Hyland)	Factor VIII	7 ml.	25 units/kg.	12 units/kg./12 hr.	12 hr.
(Courtland)	Factor VIII	25 ml.	25 units/kg.	12 units/kg./12 hr.	12 hr.
Factor IX concentrate (Cutter)	Factor IX (II, VII, IX, X)	10 ml.	20 units/kg.	10 units/kg./24 hr.	24 hr.
(Hyland)	Factor IX (II, VII, IX, X)	30 ml.	20 units/kg.	10 units/kg./24 hr.	24 hr.
Fibrinogen—no longer recommended for clinical use					

* This suggested dose schedule should be modified by the clinical response of the patient and by the results of detailed laboratory studies.

since factor VIII determinations are rarely available when one needs them, a return of the partial thromboplastin time to within the normal range indicates a level of at least 25 to 30 per cent and is usually sufficient for monitoring purposes. In the case of bleeding into a joint or soft tissues, therapy for one to two days usually suffices; progress is evaluated by measurements taken at clearly marked points (we usually instruct the parent to mark, with a ballpoint pen, the point on the joint or extremity where measurements using a tape are made). Bleeding from a wound, into the gastrointestinal tract, or around the site of a fracture usually requires more prolonged therapy, which may range from seven to 10 days or more.

Short-term prophylactic therapy is used to prepare the patient for surgery or major dental work. Under these circumstances, the aim is to provide hemostatic levels during the period of risk, i.e., until primary wound healing occurs. The dosage required depends to some extent on the amount of bleeding encountered, but if preparation has been adequate, bleeding should be minimal. The usual course is to infuse sufficient concentrate immediately prior to surgery to raise the circulating level to 100 per cent (as calculated by the formula previously given) and repeat one-half the initial dose at 12-hour intervals. Close cooperation with the surgical staff is essential, especially to ensure that proper monitoring is carried out and that subtle signs of bleeding are not overlooked. Using this program, we have been able to carry out major surgery, including portacaval shunts and bowel resections, in patients with severe hemophilia.

Long-term prophylactic therapy is a relatively recent development in the treatment of hemophilia. Such therapy was not possible prior to the widespread introduction of the commercial concentrates, and was facilitated by the development of the concept of home therapy: parents or patients giving concentrate on a predetermined schedule. Initial fears of an increased incidence of sensitization have proved unfounded. The aim of most such programs is to maintain a minimum level of 10 per cent, a level sufficient to prevent most bleeding episodes. Therapy is individualized for each patient, but most programs prescribe 250 to 500 units of concentrate every two to three days. Such prophylactic therapy does not, of course, preclude the prompt administration of additional AHF for acute episodes. The selection of patients suitable for inclusion in such a program presents some problem. In general, this therapy is limited to those patients who are having recurring bleeding episodes and whose basal factor VIII level is below 1 per cent. Placing a patient on a prophylactic program does not relieve the physician of his supervisory responsibilities. It is hoped that there will be fewer visits for acute bleeding episodes, but initially at least the patient must be carefully monitored with repeated factor VIII levels to determine the optimal schedule for administration of the concentrate; moreover, once the patient is regulated, his physician must pay continued attention to the ancillary care of the hemophiliac (see below). Plasma factor VIII levels should be repeated at 6-month intervals to detect the possible appearance of inhibitors; the development of inhibitors precludes further prophylactic therapy and limits the use of factor VIII concentrates to emergency situations. Although it is possible to have the patient visit the physician at regular intervals to receive prophylactic infusions, for most patients a considerable advantage is gained if the patient or his family (or a visiting nurse) can administer the concentrate at home. This obviates the necessity for office or hospital visits with the attendant travel and waiting. Teaching the patient or his family may not be easy, but patience and understanding will overcome most normal fears. The help of a nurse-practitioner in this area may be invaluable.

The appearance of circulating inhibitors to factor VIII requires reevaluation of the proper management of the patient. Inhibitors appear in about 5 per cent of all patients with classified hemophilia and apparently are unrelated to the number of prior infusions. These inhibitors are probably antibodies specific to factor VIII activity and clinically are characterized by a reduced or absent response to otherwise adequate infusions of factor VIII concentrate. Once factor VIII inhibitors are present, prophylactic therapy is useless and may indeed be harmful since *any* infusion of factor VIII activity will call forth an amnestic response, i.e., cause a secondary rise in antibody (inhibitor) activity 7 to 10 days following the infusion.

In the patient with inhibitor, minor bleeding episodes are treated with local measures (ice packs, pressure dressing and so forth); the use of factor VIII is avoided. On the other hand, in life-threatening situations four courses are available: (1) Massive amounts of factor VIII concentrate may be infused, enough to "swamp" the inhibitor and provide therapeutic levels of factor VIII activity. (2) Porcine or bovine factor VIII, which has different antigenic determinants and thus *may* not be inactivated by the circulating inhibitor, may be used. (In vitro tests may give a hint but are not completely reliable for indicating the usefulness of either material; only a clinical trial gives definitive data.) Since these materials are derived from a different species, specific antibodies to each will eventually develop and so the use of each is a one-shot affair—useful in a single episode. (3) Antimetabolites (usually cyclophosphamide) may be given in a large dose (10 to 20 mg. per kilogram intravenously) at the time of the initial infusion in an attempt to prevent the amnestic response. (4) Plasmapheresis may be tried in an attempt to reduce the titer of circulating antibody. A combination of techniques (1) and (4) may be successful even in patients with a high titer of inhibitors, particularly if the newer cell separator centrifuges are available. A combination of these techniques—administration of antimetabolites with the initial dose of factor VIII, use of sufficient factor VIII concentrates to "swamp" the circulating inhibitor, plasmapheresis with administration of factor VIII concentrates to replace the volume removed and, if all else fails, the use of bovine or porcine factor VIII—should be sufficient to tide most hemophiliacs with inhibitors over even the most severe bleeding episodes. These procedures, however, require close cooperation between a clotting laboratory, the blood bank and the clinician.

Various ancillary measures have been proposed at one time or another in the therapy of hemophilia. Some of them, such as the use of peanut oil in the preventive therapy of bleeding episodes, have been thoroughly discredited. Others, such as the use of epsilon-aminocaproic acid to control clot breakdown and, thus, further utilization of circulating factor VIII, are of dubious value. Still others, such as the use of steroids (prednisone in a dose of 2 mg. per kilogram per day for five days) in hemarthrosis to suppress the inflammatory response and possibly impede the development of interarticular fibrosis, are probably of some value, but definitive proof is still lacking. Controlled studies in this area are difficult to carry out since well-defined endpoints are usually lacking.

All too often patients with hemophilia are treated in the emergency room as a series of disconnected acute episodes, and there is little or no long-term continuity of care. A patient with hemophilia has a chronic disease similar in many respects to diabetes mellitus. Long-term survival without major disability is now a practical goal but depends on close cooperation between a number of specialty services all attuned to the particular problems of this disease. Hemarthrosis frequently requires orthopedic consultation with the preparation of bivalve casts and possibly the use of sleeping splints to help correct contractures. Once the acute bleeding episode is past, the physical therapist is called in to begin exercises to the affected joints: first passive exercises to maintain or regain mobility and then active exercises to strengthen muscles around the affected joint. Continuous exercises are prescribed to maintain the stability of the joint and to prevent, as far as possible, further bleeding episodes. Preventive dental care is also essential, since extensive dental work almost invariably requires hospitalization and prophylactic concentrate therapy. Of particular importance is the avoidance, if possible, of intramuscular injections. This is especially true in dental care, where the use of local anesthesia (nerve blocks) is contraindicated, but also extends to the use of intramuscular antibiotics, intramuscular preoperative medications and so forth.

One should only give intramuscular injections if the site is suitable for direct application of pressure and if one is able to apply such pressure for at least 10 minutes. Thus, routine immunizations should be given with care and, in the severe hemophiliac, preferably at the time when factor VIII concentrates are being administered.

Attention to the social aspects of this problem is also important. The ultimate goal is to ensure that these boys will develop into healthy functional adults. Group therapy, as practiced on an informal basis by the National Hemophilia Foundation (25 W. 39th St., New York, New York 10018) and the regional and local chapters, is helpful, especially in reassuring the parents that other families can live with this problem. Social service follow-up is helpful in ensuring that families are aware of the resources available in the community for schools, transportation, vocational advice and training, and blood replacement, if necessary. The physician must also be prepared to spend considerable time with the growing boy explaining the disease, the therapy and the precautions which are necessary. The boy must be given the opportunity to ask questions and discuss his problems. The necessity for avoiding contact sports such as football and basketball should be pointed out and the reasons given. The physician can also advise on the use of items such as padded plastic head protectors, especially during the ages when the child is active but not yet old enough to understand the importance of avoiding head injuries. Close continuous cooperation between the physician, the patient and his family is necessary to achieve a happy and essentially normal childhood and adolescence.

A major cause of trouble in hemophilia is the use of drugs that interfere with platelet reactions and make the bleeding tendency more severe (Table 2). Percodan and Darvon compound, both of which contain aspirin, have been used for joint pain in hemophilia, with disastrous results. *No bleeder should receive any of the drugs listed in Table 2.*

von Willebrand's Disease. This is a congenital bleeding disorder affecting platelet aggregation and factor VIII synthesis. It is inherited as an autosomal dominant gene; thus, both boys and girls are affected. Clinical symptoms are usually mild and many affected individuals are diagnosed only through family studies. Bleeding problems are usually limited to epistaxis and bleeding following dental extractions, but occasionally major trauma or surgical procedures can be followed by excessive bleeding. Hemarthrosis is rare.

TABLE 2. Drugs Which Are Known to Interfere with Platelet Function

Aspirin (acetylsalicylic acid)
Glyceryl guaiacolate (found in many cough preparations)
Phenacetin
Butazolidine
Phenothiazides (especially Compazine, Thorazine, Sparine and Periactin)

The major cause of clinical problems in patients with von Willebrand's disease is epistaxis. Although the nosebleeds are usually mild, they often recur with sufficient frequency to lead to a severe iron deficiency anemia. Pressure and/or nasal packing is usually sufficient to stop the bleeding, but recurrence is common. Topical thrombin and/or the application of a few drops of concentrated Adrenalin (1:100) to the pack may be useful in stopping the bleeding. Occasionally, however, infusions are required. Fresh-frozen plasma or cryoprecipitate immediately augments the circulating factor VIII level and in addition serves as a precursor for endogenous factor VIII production. The usual initial dose is 10 ml. per kilogram of fresh-frozen plasma or 1 bag of cryoprecipitate per 10 kilograms. This dose is usually repeated at 24-hour intervals if necessary. Glycine-precipitated factor VIII concentrates (Hyland or Cutter) are not as useful in von Willebrand's disease, since their use does not lead to the secondary rise seen with the less purified preparations. Patients with von Willebrand's disease are prone to iron depletion because of repeated epistaxis and therefore should be placed on iron supplementation (ferrous sulfate, 6 mg. per kilogram per day, or as indicated).

Factor IX Deficiency (Christmas Disease). Factor IX deficiency has clinical features similar to mild to moderate classical hemophilia (factor VIII deficiency). Inherited as a sex-linked recessive characteristic, Christmas disease is one of the more common of the congenital bleeding disorders. Differentiation from classical hemophilia is important because concentrates useful in the therapy of the latter are of little or no value in the Christmas disease. Factor IX is present in refrigerated, fresh-frozen and lyophilized plasma. The initial dose of any of these plasma preparations is 10 ml. per kilogram, but because of the longer half-life of factor IX, the dose need only be repeated at 24-hour intervals. Concentrates of factor IX (plus factors II, VII and X) are now available (Konyne, Cutter Laboratories; Proplex, Hyland Laboratories) for the treatment of serious bleeding episodes or of preoperative prophylaxis. The use of these preparations may be associated with an increased risk of hepatitis, but this is a hazard common to many products prepared from pooled plasma, not unique to factor IX preparations, and the possible risk must be weighed against the potential benefit of the infusion. The dose of concentrate sufficient to achieve plasma levels of 50 per cent is roughly one vial (500 units) per 10 kilograms of body weight. This dose is repeated at 24-hour intervals until adequate hemostasis is achieved, usually in 48 to 72 hours. Long-term prophylactic therapy in patients with factor IX deficiency has not, in our experience, been found necessary but certainly is now feasible. The indications are similar to those in factor VIII deficiency.

Factor XI (Plasma Thromboplastin Antecedent) Deficiency. This is a rare autosomal dominant disorder which in its clinical symptomatology resembles mild to moderate hemophilia. No concentrates are currently available and bleeding manifestations are treated with infusions of fresh plasma. The biologic half-life of factor XI is 24 hours, so infusions are repeated at 24- to 36-hour intervals.

Factor I (Fibrinogen) Deficiency. Factor I deficiency is a rare autosomal recessive disorder comparable in clinical severity to mild hemophilia. Bleeding manifestations usually follow severe trauma, but epistaxis is also said to be common. Most episodes can be controlled with local measures, including pressure packs and the use of topical Adrenalin. Massive bleeding, bleeding into inaccessible sites or preoperative preparation for surgery requires infusions. Since fibrinogen is stable in bank blood, infusions of practically any form of plasma (fresh, fresh-frozen or lyophilized) will be adequate to provide hemostasis. Concentrates of human fibrinogen are also available but their use is not, at present, recommended because of a very high risk of hepatitis. Cryoprecipitate of Factor VIII is fibrinogen-rich and is the therapy of choice.

Factor II (Prothrombin) Deficiency. This is also a rare autosomal recessive bleeding disorder similar in terms of clinical severity to mild hemophilia. Prothrombin is present in fresh plasma, fresh frozen plasma or in bank blood which is less than 72 hours old; replacement therapy is therefore not difficult. It is also present in adequate amounts in factor IX concentrates (Konyne or Proplex), and these preparations can also be used. Since factor II has a half-life of 72 hours, infusion need not be repeated as frequently as in factor IX deficiency.

Factor XIII Deficiency. This is a rare autosomal recessive bleeding disorder in which the hemorrhagic manifestations may not become evident until 24 to 48 hours following formation of the initial clot. Patients having or suspected of having this deficiency must therefore be observed for three to four days following a bleeding episode or infusion therapy to ensure that the clot does not break down and bleeding resume. Most bleeding episodes can be managed with local measures; replacement therapy requires the use of fresh-frozen plasma given at 24- to 48-hour intervals. There is no concentrate presently available for the treatment of bleeding due to factor XIII deficiency.

Acquired Bleeding Disorders

Vitamin K Deficiency. Probably the most common acquired bleeding disorder is due to a deficiency of the factors (II, VII, IX and X) which are dependent on vitamin K for their synthesis. The underlying deficit may be nutritional, due to liver dysfunction, or secondary to medications. Nutritional defects include dietary deficiency, malabsorption or prolonged diarrhea. Liver dysfunction includes the immature liver of the newborn (especially of the premature infant), obstructive jaundice and parenchymal liver disease. Drugs may interfere with the action of vitamin K (such as the warfarin derivatives) or may interfere with its synthesis by the intestinal flora and its absorption (such as some antibiotics).

In those patients in whom the bleeding defect is due to a deficiency of vitamin K, correction of the prolonged prothrombin time can usually be achieved with a single intramuscular dose of vitamin K_1 (Mephyton); 1 to 2 mg. will usually begin to act within 4 to 6 hours. However, the prothrombin time will usually continue to be prolonged for 24 to 48 hours. The administration of vitamin K_1 even intravenously, therefore, cannot be depended upon to treat serious acute bleeding episodes but must be supplemented by the administration of the appropriate factors, either in the form of plasma or as the factor IX concentrates (Konyne or Proplex), which also contain adequate amounts of factors II, VII and X. A lack of response to low doses of parenteral vitamin K usually indicates some degree of liver impairment, and repeated doses, except in rare instances, do not lead to an improvement in the response and may indeed lead to hemolysis and jaundice in susceptible individuals. The frequent practice of administering repeated high doses of vitamin K to patients with bowel surgery or liver disease is unjustified. The treatment of bleeding in patients with liver disease is complicated by the multiple disorders which are frequently found. Not only is there a decrease in the vitamin K–dependent coagulation factors, but thrombocytopenia is frequently present (sometimes, but not always, due to hypersplenism) and vascular abnormalities (such as esophageal and gastric varices) are common. Disseminated intravascular coagulation (see p. 160) often complicates liver disease. Acute bleeding episodes are best treated with whole fresh blood, although fresh-frozen plasma plus packed red cells can be used when fresh blood is not available. The presence of profound thrombocytopenia (platelet counts of less than 25,000 per cubic mm.) mandates the use of platelet concentrates to control bleeding episodes.

Fibrinolysins. Circulating fibrinolysins are an extremely uncommon cause of bleeding in children. Those that do occur are usually associated with a malignancy, such as promyeloblastic leukemia, where breakdown of the malignant cell is thought to cause fibrinolytic activators. Extracorporeal perfusion during open heart surgery is also thought to produce some fibrinolytic activity, although this is usually minor. An abnormality of the euglobulolysis time associated with clinical signs of bleeding never justifies a trial of epsilon-aminocaproic acid (EACA or Amicar), since the fibrinolysis may be secondary to disseminated intravascular coagulation. If heparin therapy produces no improvement, EACA may be added. EACA should not be given to an unheparinized, bleeding patient. A loading dose of 70 mg. per kilogram body weight is followed by 15 mg. per kilogram every 8 hours until bleeding ceases. EACA should be used with caution in the face of urinary tract bleeding, since inhibition of the normal urinary fibrinolytic mechanisms may lead to acute urinary tract obstruction. It must be reiterated that clinically important circulating fibrinolysins are uncommon in pediatrics, and treatment with EACA is rarely indicated.

Inhibitors. Circulating inhibitors to one of the normal coagulating factors is usually secondary to repeated replacement therapy such as in factor VIII or factor IX deficiency, where roughly 5 per cent of all patients eventually develop this complication. The spontaneous occurrence of circulating inhibitors has also been observed in patients with systemic lupus erythematosus, rheumatoid arthritis and dermatitis herpetiformis. The inhibitor may be directed against any one of a number of the coagulation factors and is an IgG immunoglobulin. Treatment of bleeding due to the presence of a spontaneous inhibitor is similar to that outlined for therapy in the presence of factor VIII inhibitors (p. 283). Long-term therapy with immunosuppressive drugs appears to be more successful with spontaneous inhibitors than in treating the inhibitors found in hemophilias. There are, however, no controlled studies on the use of immunosuppressive drugs.

PLATELET DISORDERS

Idiopathic Thromboycytopenic Purpura (ITP). ITP is an acute, usually self-limited disease in childhood frequently following infections but just as frequently having no apparent antecedent illness. Acute thrombocytopenia is frequently associated with few or no symptoms and children appear to tolerate very low platelet counts for a prolonged period of time. Acute bleeding episodes, when they occur, can be catastrophic; prior to the advent of the use of corticosteroids and platelet concentrates, a significant number of children died of acute intracranial hemorrhage. It is usually possible to prevent this complication by judicious use of corticosteroid and platelet replacement therapy, but since most children with ITP never experience such bleeding episodes, the selection of patients for therapy is sometimes difficult. In general, however, children with platelet counts above 20,000 to 25,000 per cubic mm. do not have spontaneous bleeding manifestations, and counts above 50,000 per cubic mm. are sufficient to support normal hemostatic mechanisms even in the face of severe trauma, including surgery. Therapy can therefore safely be limited to those children with platelet counts below 20,000 per cubic mm. or in whom surgery cannot be deferred. The 20,000 to 25,000 platelet count is not an absolute level, and frequently children whose platelet count is much lower can go for prolonged periods without problems; retinal hemorrhages, retinal petechiae and petechiae in the posterior oropharynx, however, suggest increased susceptibility to central nervous system hemorrhage.

Acute bleeding episodes, such as severe gastrointestinal or genitourinary bleeding, or signs of impending bleeding, such as retinal petechiae and hemorrhages, are treated with platelet concentrates. Even though the recovery of transfused platelets may be poor and platelet survival is markedly reduced, a definite, albeit temporary, hemostatic effect is usually achieved. If sufficient numbers of platelets are given frequently enough, most bleeding episodes can be controlled. The quantity and frequency of transfusions depend on the effectiveness of the antibody, an activity for which we have no clinically useful in vitro test. One unit of platelet concentrate per 5 kilograms of body weight given every 12 hours is usually sufficient to control the hemorrhagic manifestations in acute ITP and is continued only as long as active bleeding continues. Children who have severe thrombocytopenia (platelet counts of less than 20,000 to 25,000 per cubic mm.) but who do not have clinical signs of a severe bleeding diathesis are usually treated with prednisone in a dose of 2 mg. per kilogram of body weight given once a day by mouth. There is no objective evidence that corticosteroid therapy either shortens the recovery phase or increases the effectiveness of the circulating platelets, but it appears that steroids reduce the bleeding tendency in thrombocytopenic children, perhaps by reducing capillary fragility. Prednisone therapy is usually continued until the platelet count rises to levels above 100,000 per cubic mm. The dose is then rapidly tapered and discontinued. A slight (25 per cent or less) transitory drop in the count is seen in some patients but rarely is sufficient to require resumption of steroid therapy.

Seventy-five per cent or more of all children with acute ITP recover in six months or less. The percentage is probably higher, but many children with acute ITP undoubtedly never come to the attention of the physician and recover spontaneously. That small group of children who fail to recover in six months can be divided into two groups: those who never respond to steroid therapy and those who have a profound drop in platelet count when steroid therapy is discontinued. The latter group usually responds when therapy is reinitiated. One again starts with a dose of 2 mg. per kilogram per day. When the platelet count again rises, the dose is tapered to a level which is just sufficient to maintain the count. This dose is maintained until the platelet count rises or problems (gastrointestinal symptoms, growth failure, hypertension and so forth) arise from continued steroid therapy. Most clinicians will wait for 6 to 18 months before considering splenectomy, but this decision must be tempered by the clinical condition of the patient. If the patient is stable and requires little or no therapy, the decision can be put off for two years or more; if, on the other hand, the child requires large doses of corticosteroids to maintain his platelet count in a range found necessary to avoid bleeding episodes, and particularly if this dose is associated with serious clinical side effects, splenectomy may have to be carried out before six months are up. Finally, in the rare child who fails to respond to steroid therapy and who has continued bleeding manifestations controlled only by the frequent administration of platelet concentrates, splenectomy may have to be carried out very early in the clinical course.

The majority of children with ITP who come to surgery respond to splenectomy. This is particularly true of those individuals who initially responded to corticosteroid therapy. Patients who fail to respond to surgery are usually considered candidates for immunosuppressive therapy, particularly with azathioprine (Imuran). Although occasional responses are seen, the results in general have been disappointing.

Thrombocytopenia in the Newborn. This may be due to the passive transfer of maternal antiplatelet antibody, to perinatal sepsis, to hemolytic disease of the newborn, to congenital leukemia or to congenital aplastic anemia. The most common cause appears to be perinatal sepsis, such as rubella, toxoplasmosis, cytomegalic virus, syphilis or neonatal bacterial infection. The decrease in platelet count is usually moderate and rarely results in hemorrhagic complications. Platelet concentrates can be used if bleeding problems occur, but primary therapy should be directed, when possible, to the underlying infection.

The thrombocytopenia frequently found associated with severe hemolytic disease of the newborn is usually thought to be due to sequestration of platelets within an enlarged spleen. Exchange transfusions, particularly with bank blood, may accentuate the drop in platelet count. Hemorrhagic manifestations are rare, but when they occur they may be treated with platelet concentrate transfusions. One should also attempt to use whole fresh blood whenever possible.

Neonatal thrombocytopenia due to the passive transfer of maternal antiplatelet antibody is probably rare but may occur in mothers who have, or who have a history of, ITP or systemic lupus erythematosus. Isoimmunization against antigens specific to platelets as well as to the more generally distributed HL-A antigens may also occur. Since the maternal IgG has a relatively long half-life in the fetal circulation, thrombocytopenia may persist up to four to six weeks. These infants present with skin and mucosal bleeding manifestations at, or shortly after, birth. Intracranial hemorrhages are more common in this age group than in the older child and are a leading cause of mortality in neonatal thrombocytopenia. Because of this hazard, treatment is aggressive: platelet concentrates are given if hemorrhagic manifestations are present and as soon as the diagnosis is established. One unit of platelets per 5 kilograms of body weight can be expected to elevate the platelet count to safe levels and can be repeated at 12- to 24-hour intervals until the bleeding manifestations are controlled. Prednisone in a dose of 2 mg. per kilogram may increase "vascular integrity" but is usually ineffective in the treatment of thrombocytopenia due to passively transferred antibody.

In rare instances, neonatal thrombocytopenia may also be the presenting sign of congenital aplastic anemia or congenital leukemia. The amegakaryocytic thrombocytopenia in congenital aplastic anemia may be present for a variable period of time before a decrease in granulocytes or red cells becomes evident. Both aplastic anemia and congenital leukemia are diagnosed by examination of the bone marrow. Basic therapy should be directed against the underlying disease, but the immediate management of bleeding manifestations usually requires the use of platelet concentrates.

Secondary Thrombocytopenia. There are a number of disease entities which can present with bleeding manifestations and thrombocytopenia. Some of these, such as sepsis, have already been mentioned. A few others deserve comment. Thrombocytopenia has been associated with the administration of several drugs, the most noteworthy of which is quinidine, although other drugs have at times been implicated. In at least some instances the drug plays the role of a haptene in an antigen-antibody reaction. Withdrawal of the drug results in a prompt increase in the platelet count; the use of platelet concentrates or corticosteroids is rarely necessary. Cyanotic congenital heart disease can also be associated with a mild thrombocytopenia but is usually not the cause of bleeding problems; the thrombopathy associated with this entity (see below) is probably of greater clinical significance.

Thrombocytopenia can also be caused by sequestration of platelets in a giant hemangioma. Interestingly enough, the platelet count may respond for a time to corticosteroid therapy. This is usually only of temporary benefit and if the thrombocytopenia is symptomatic, surgical resection or radiation of the hemangioma may become necessary.

Hypersplenism is still another cause of secondary thrombocytopenia; occasionally the degree of splenic sequestration may be sufficient in itself to indicate the need for splenectomy.

Finally, several congenital disorders may be associated with thrombocytopenia. Chief among these is the Wiskott-Aldrich syndrome, where the hemorrhagic manifestations may be the presenting clinical aspect. Although splenomegaly is frequently present, splenectomy is not indicated in this disorder. Bleeding manifestations are frequently episodic and appear to be alleviated by short courses of prednisone. Administration of platelet concentrates is indicated only for serious hemorrhages.

Platelet Concentrates. Platelet concentrates represent the most useful form of replacement therapy in the treatment of most forms of thrombocytopenia (with the thrombocytopenia of DIC a notable exception). Improvements in the techniques of collection and preservation have enhanced recovery and survival of transfused platelets. Storage at room temperature (25° C.) rather than at 4° C. allows platelet concentrates to be kept for several days rather than 8 to 12 hours as was formerly true; and, finally, the increasing use of component transfusion therapy, rather than the almost universal use of whole blood, has increased the availability of platelet concentrates. Because of the smaller volume, platelet concentrates are more useful in severe thrombocytopenia than is either fresh whole blood or platelet-rich plasma. The latter should be used only when the administration of either red cells or plasma protein components is also indicated.

One unit of platelet concentrate per 7 kilograms of body weight will raise the platelet count significantly in the absence of platelet antibodies or abnormal sequestration (such as in an enlarged spleen). The effective half-life of transfused platelets is about four days; thus, in the absence of bleeding, platelet transfusions can be spaced at about two- to four-day intervals.

The prophylactic use of platelet transfusions, except in the neonatal period, is unwise because of the eventual development of isosensitization. This is uncommon when 10 or less units of platelets (or fresh whole blood) have been administered, but the frequency of sensitization increases rapidly above this point. The use of HL-A compatible donors can be lifesaving in the thrombocytopenic patient who has become sensitized. Antigenic systems unique to platelets appear to be a less common cause for isoimmunization. In the patient who has become sensitized, as evidenced by poor platelet recovery following transfusion and shortened survival, in the absence of ITP or hypersplenism, the use of family donors may lead to an increase in the clinical benefit derived from platelet transfusions.

Functional Platelet Defects (Thrombopathy). The primary disorder in this group of syndromes is a defect in the aggregation of platelets defined as an in vitro defect in ADP-, ephedrine-, or collagen-induced aggregation. The platelet count is usually normal but the bleeding time is prolonged. The congenital forms of this syndrome (Glanzmann's hereditary thrombasthenia) are quite common. The patients have an increased susceptibility to bruising with a tendency to bleed excessively, with epistaxes and menorrhagia. These individuals usually require no therapy. The acquired form of platelet dysfunction is usually seen in association with cyanotic congenital heart disease, uremia and the use of certain drugs, where the platelet dysfunction appears to be more significant than the mild thrombocytopenia which may also be present. These patients do not appear to have serious hemorrhagic tendencies, and an increased incidence of prolonged epistaxis appears to be the major clinical manifestation of this syndrome. However, it appears prudent to correct the abnormality, as far as possible, prior to cardiac surgery. Prednisone (0.4 mg. per kilogram per day by mouth) given for three days prior to surgery usually improves the bleeding time but does not appear to affect the in vitro aggregation abnormalities.

VASCULAR DEFECTS

Congenital Defects

Hereditary disorders of the vascular component of the hemostatic system are quite uncommon. The best known of these is hereditary hemorrhagic telangiectasia, where multiple telangiectases scattered throughout the mucous membranes and gastrointestinal tract may lead to recurrent epistaxes and/or gastrointestinal hemorrhage. The bleeding is usually controllable by local measures, and transfusions are rarely indicated. However, the patients frequently become iron deficient and iron supplementation is often indicated.

In the Ehlers-Danlos syndrome, the tendency to bruise easily is due to a poor collagen substructure of the vascular bed. There is no effective treatment other than the avoidance of trauma.

A number of families have been described in whom multiple individuals have an increased tendency to bruise easily and the women frequently complain of menorrhagia. There is often a history of prolonged bleeding following dental extractions or surgery. The characteristic laboratory abnormality is a prolonged bleeding time. Plasma coagulation factor levels and in vitro tests of platelet function are normal. Treatment is, in general, unsatisfactory and the only recourse is the administration of whole blood if bleeding is excessive as judged by a marked fall (greater than 20 per cent) in hematocrit or by signs of decompensation of the cardiovascular system.

Acquired Defects

Scurvy in the past was a common cause for vascular purpura but is now quite infrequent in this country because of vitamin C supplementation of most commercial infant formulas. The major bleeding manifestations are hemorrhages into the skin following even the slightest trauma. In children, subperiosteal hemorrhages with bone tenderness are quite typical. Treatment consists of 50 mg. of ascorbic acid given four times a day for a week. Maintenance therapy (50 mg. per day) can then be continued for another three months.

Septic thrombi can be mistaken for petechiae but occur in the absence of thrombocytopenia or other bleeding manifestations and are usually slightly tender to palpation. The causative organism can frequently be cultured from the thrombus by careful aspiration. Treatment is directed against the underlying infection.

Anaphylactoid purpura (Henoch-Schönlein or allergic purpura) is thought to be a hypersensitivity reaction, related to acute nephritis, in which there is a diffuse acute inflammatory reaction around the capillaries and small arterioles. It is relatively common in children and should be distinguished from acute ITP, which it may resemble. In anaphylactoid purpura, however, the petechiae and ecchymoses are typically distributed over the buttocks, lower extremities and face, with few on the trunk, and the platelet count is normal. Scalp edema and joint involvement may be prominent. The uncomplicated case requires no therapy and recurrences are uncommon. There are two possible complications, however, which require therapy. The most common is colicky abdominal pain related to vasculitis and edema of the bowel wall. This may be accompanied by vomiting, diarrhea and gastrointestinal hemorrhage. In the occasional patient, the gastrointestinal involvement leads to intussusception and perforation, which requires surgical intervention. Because of this hazard, children in whom the abdominal symptoms are prominent are best treated with a short course of prednisone (2 mg. per kilogram per day by mouth), which is continued until there are no fresh skin lesions. Most children with allergic purpura show some degree of microscopic hematuria and proteinuria during the acute stages of the disease. In a majority of patients these abnormalities rapidly resolve and there is no evidence of residual renal damage. In about 5 to 10 per cent of cases, however, urinary abnormalities persist beyond six months and eventually evolve into a picture indistiguishable from chronic nephritis and end-stage renal disease. If this is recognized early enough, the use of immunosuppressive therapy (Imuran or cyclophosphamide) appears to be associated with subsidence of signs of active disease and stabilization of renal function. Because of the possibility of persistent renal involvement, children who have had an episode of anaphylactoid purpura should have a routine urinalysis at six and 12 months following the acute episode.

The Immunodeficiency Diseases

RICHARD A. GATTI, M.D., *and*
ROBERT A. GOOD, M.D., PH.D.

Immunodeficiency can be divided into two basic syndromes: B-cell deficiency syndrome (associated with deficits of humoral immunity) and T-cell deficiency syndrome (associated with deficits of cell-mediated immunity). (See Table 1.) Each syndrome is characterized by a distinct constellation of infection. Patients with various primary immunodeficiency diseases manifest parts of each syndrome, depending on the type and extent of their deficiencies. Treatment is based on careful diagnostic evaluation of these immunologic deficits in each patient.

B-cell deficiency syndrome is characterized by recurrent severe bacterial infections, such as pneumonitis, otitis media, pyoderma, meningitis and diarrhea, as well as by poor growth and eczema. Malabsorption, arthritis and an extremely severe form of hepatitis are also seen. Leukemia occurs in 5 to 10 per cent of these patients. Serum immunoglobulins are either present in very low levels or absent; isohemagglutinin titers are low; the Schick test remains positive after diphtheria-pertussis-tetanus immunization; antibody production following antigenic stimulation is very poor. Plasma cells are absent in bone marrow, lymph nodes and intestinal lamina propria.

Treatment of this syndrome centers on providing good pulmonary hygiene to minimize the progressive destruction of recurrent lung infections and on correcting the immunoglobulin deficits. Since only IgG (gamma globulin) is available commercially in the United States, treatment has been limited to correction of IgG levels, except in rare situations in which plasma infusions have been used to raise IgM, IgA and IgE levels. Because hepatitis is such a devastating disease in these patients, a "buddy" donor is found (usually a parent) and used repeatedly as the plasma donor. Plasma is taken from donors by plasmapheresis to minimize hemoglobin loss. The efficacy of plasma therapy in these patients remains unproved, although certain patients appear to have fewer and less severe clinical infections. In patients suffering from cell-mediated immune deficits as well, all blood products, including plasma, should be irradiated before being administered. In patients with isolated IgA deficiency, anti-IgA antibodies may be present. Such patients may suffer severe anaphylactoid reactions following transfusion with plasma or blood products containing IgA. If such a patient requires cellular transfusion, the cells should be washed carefully and administered as packed cells.

T-cell deficiency syndrome is characterized by recurrent severe viral and fungal infections. Candidiasis is seen in most patients with this syndrome. Vaccination with live viruses is contraindicated and has been fatal in a number of patients; BCG vaccination has led to similar consequences. These patients lack small lymphocytes in peripheral blood, lymph nodes and bone marrow and consequently have little or no capacity to manifest delayed hypersensitivity skin responses. In vitro lymphocyte responses to phytohemagglutinin, allogeneic cells and antigens are poor.

TABLE 1. Immunodeficiency Diseases

PRIMARY IMMUNODEFICIENCY DISEASE	TYPE OF DEFECT
Infantile X-linked agammaglobulinemia (Bruton)	Absence of B-cells
Thymic hypoplasia (pharyngeal pouch syndrome of DiGeorge)	Absence of T-cells
Severe combined immunodeficiency (Swiss)	Absence or abnormality of lymphoid stem cells
Common variable immunodeficiency (late onset)	Variable B-cell defects; T-cell deficiency
Immunodeficiency with Wiskott-Aldrich disease	B-cell synthesis of antibody to some polysaccharide antigens; T-cell dysfunction
Immunodeficiency with ataxia-telangiectasia	B-cell secretion of IgA; T-cell dysfunction
Selective IgA deficiency	B-cell secretion of IgA
Thymoma-agammaglobulinemia	B-cell deficiency; T-cell deficiency

Because such patients lack the ability to reject any homografts, transfused blood from a histo*in*compatible donor can produce a graft-versus-host reaction consisting of high fever, morbilliform rash, hepatosplenomegaly, bloody diarrhea, pancytopenia and death approximately 14 days after transfusion. If blood transfusion is inevitable in a patient with cell-mediated immune deficiency, well-oxygenated blood should receive at least 2000 R before being administered to the patient. This dose of irradiation may not be sufficient to halt proliferation of small lymphocytes in poorly oxygenated blood. The incidence of malignancy in patients with various forms of T-cell deficiency is approximately 10 per cent.

Patients with *stem cell deficiencies* fail to develop either B-cells or T-cells and thus manifest the signs and symptoms of both B-cell and T-cell deficiency syndromes.

Gamma Globulin Therapy. Maintenance of IgG levels above 300 mg. per 100 ml. greatly reduces the frequency of bacterial infections in patients with hypogammaglobulinemia. To approach this level, an initial loading dose of 1.5 ml. of the standard 16.5 per cent gamma globulin solution per kilogram of body weight is administered intramuscularly. This loading dose may be divided in half and the second aliquot given a few days after the first, since this quantity is painful to receive. Because the average half-life of gamma globulin is 24 to 30 days, a maintenance dose of 0.6 ml. per kilogram is administered every three to four weeks. The clinical response of the patient is the most useful guide to appropriate modification of this schedule. Measurement of serum gamma globulin levels before each dose during the first few months of therapy is also helpful in schedule and dosage adjustments.

PRECAUTIONS. Currently available commercial gamma globulin contains gamma globulin aggregates which may produce anaphylactoid shock if injected intravenously. Swiss investigators have emphasized the hypersusceptibility of hypogammaglobulinemic patients to gamma globulin aggregates. Reactions on this basis may occur even after intramuscular administration. These usually are mild but are severe in an occasional patient. Reactions may be characterized by gastrointestinal symptoms, joint pains, back pain, dyspnea and syncope shortly after injection. Aqueous epinephrine should be readily available whenever gamma globulin is administered. Occasionally, true allergic reactions to gamma globulin have occurred in hypogammaglobulinemic patients.

Complications. *Pneumocystis carinii* pneumonitis carries an ominous prognosis in patients with hypogammaglobulinemia. Its insidious onset, often accompanied by eosinophilia and characterized by the absence of rales on physical examination, makes early diagnosis very difficult. In very young patients with hypogammaglobulinemia and suspected pneumocystis pneumonia, we recommend starting therapy even if the organism cannot be found on smears of tracheal aspirate. We have used open lung biopsy in these small children with minimal addition to morbidity and with much advantage in establishing a diagnosis. Successful treatment has been accomplished with pentamidine isethionate, 4 mg. per kilogram per 24 hours intramuscularly over a two-week period.* A second and even third course of therapy may be necessary if signs and symptoms consistent with the disease reappear.

Antibiotic Treatment. Despite gamma globulin therapy, chronic sinopulmonary and ear infections are frequent. Long-term therapy with the tetracyclines in addition to specific antibiotic therapy seems to be of value in some patients. In general, treatment of acute bacterial infection in patients with humoral immune deficiency requires accurate bacteriologic diagnosis followed by intensive specific antibiotic therapy. As an aid to therapy while awaiting results of microbiologic cultures, the following list of the most frequent constellations of infection is given:

B-CELL DEFICIENCY
Pneumococcus
Hemophilus influenzae
Streptococcus
Pseudomonas aeruginosa
Meningococcus sp.
Hepatitis virus
Pneumocystis carinii

T-CELL DEFICIENCY
Candida albicans
Rubeola virus
Varicella
Vaccinia
Cytomegalovirus
Acid-fast bacteria
Histoplasmosis
Enteric pathogens
Pneumocystis carinii

Cellular Reconstitution. In patients with severe combined immunodeficiency, treatment with gamma globulin and antibiotics has not altered the ominous prognosis of death before one year of age. Bone marrow transplantation, on the other hand, has restored over a dozen

* Pentamidine isethionate is not commercially available. It must be obtained from the Parasitic Disease Drug Service, National Disease Control Center, Atlanta, Georgia.

infants with this disease to healthy, immunologically competent children. In most cases, a compatible bone marrow donor has been available among the siblings of the patient. Compatible histocompatibility matches can be expected in 25 per cent of siblings. Bone marrow transplants utilizing nonidentical donors, including parents of patients, have resulted in graft-versus-host reactions which, when coupled with sepsis, have been fatal in almost all cases. Further, life-threatening and even fatal graft-versus-host reactions have occasionally been observed with marrow from matched siblings when immunosuppressive agents, such as cyclophosphamide, have been used.

Bone marrow transplantation has also been efficacious in patients with Wiskott-Aldrich disease. Improvement, in one case, has been long-lasting. In another, improvement was transient. In both cases, marrow donors were HL-A identical siblings.

In patients with thymic hypoplasia (DiGeorge), transplantation of fetal thymus into the rectus abdominis muscle sheath has resulted in immunologic reconstitution. These infants lack both thymus and parathyroid glands and therefore suffer not only from a cell-mediated immune deficiency but also from neonatal hypocalcemic tetany. On the other hand, not all infants with this clinical syndrome are completely T-cell deficient. Some infants apparently have small remnants of thymic tissue and may manifest only a delayed maturation of the T-cell compartment.

WISKOTT-ALDRICH DISEASE

This syndrome consists of recurrent infections, thrombocytopenia and an eczematoid rash and is transmitted as a sex-linked recessive trait. These patients die from bleeding secondary to the thrombocytopenia, from overwhelming infection usually with pneumococcus organisms or from malignancy. One in 10 patients dies with malignancy, most often of a lymphoreticular form. Platelet transfusions are often life-saving for such patients. Steroids are of little avail in treating the thrombocytopenia and increase the danger of infection. Bone marrow transplantation has already been discussed above. Recently, clinical improvement and a transient reversal of skin anergy have been observed in several patients following administration of transfer factor extracted from lymphocytes of a donor sensitive to antigens to which the patient had been previously anergic. Anergy and eczema return after several months. This form of therapy has little if any noticeable effect on platelet levels.

CHRONIC GRANULOMATOUS DISEASE

This is an X-linked recessive disorder characterized by recurrent septic granulomatous lesions and a high mortality rate. The pathogenesis involves an inability of the neutrophils to kill ingested microorganisms. Once these organisms are inside the neutrophils, they are protected from the action of antibiotics. Antibiotic therapy is, thus, often ineffective or very slow in eradicating infection in these children. The most common sites for septic lesions include lung, skin, liver, lymph nodes and bones. The constellation of infection one sees in this disease includes:

- Staphylococcus
- Klebsiella sp.
- *Aerobacter aerogenes*
- *Serratia marcescens*
- *Candida albicans*
- Aspergillus
- Nocardia
- Other catalase-positive bacteria

These patients must be followed closely throughout their lives. Abscesses must be handled aggressively with incision and drainage, with extensive culturing of the exudate for bacterial and fungal organisms and with large doses of broad-spectrum antibiotics until specific microbiologic information is available to dictate more appropriate antibiotics. Since these children have normal capabilities for antibody formation, some of the newer antibacterial vaccines may prove useful in this situation. Gamma globulin therapy has been tried; however, convincing evidence for its effectiveness is lacking. Genetic counseling should be an important part of the total care since it is now possible in most families to recognize carriers as well as an occasional patient with the autosomal recessive form of the disease.

References

Bortin, M. M.: A Compendium of Reported Human Bone Marrow Transplants. *Transplantation,* 9:571, 1970.

Fudenberg, H. H., et al.: The Primary Immune Deficiencies. Report of a World Health Organization Committee. *Pediatrics,* 47:927, 1971.

Gatti, R. A., and Good, R. A.: The Immunological Deficiency Diseases. *Med. Clin. N. Am.,* 54:281, 1970.

Good, R. A., et al.: Fatal (Chronic) Granulomatous Disease of Childhood: A Hereditary Defect of Leukocyte Function. *Seminars Hemat.,* 5:215, 1968.

Holmes, B., et al.: Chronic Granulomatous Disease in Females. A Deficiency of Leukocyte Glutathione Peroxidase. *New England J. Med.,* 283:217, 1970.

Spitler, L. E., et al.: The Wiskott-Aldrich Syndrome. Results of Transfer Factor Therapy. *J. Clin. Invest.,* 51:3216, 1972.

8

Spleen and Lymphatic System

Management of Patient after Splenectomy

LOUIS K. DIAMOND, M.D.

The syndrome of overwhelming post-splenectomy infection (OPSI) deserves separate consideration inasmuch as its course, especially its speed of progression, is far different from that usually seen in individuals with intact spleens. (What is said here about the post-splenectomy syndrome applies equally well to congenital absence or to hypoplasia of the spleen, and to certain functional aplasias of the spleen, e.g., in some sickle-cell anemias.) Necessary are constant alertness to the danger of the occurrence of OPSI, early recognition of its onset and prompt specific treatment. The frightening speed of the spread of infection is characterized by a progression from a slight sore throat and malaise at onset to coma and death from bacteremia, septicemia and meningitis within 12 to 18 hours. The causative organism is most commonly the pneumococcus, less often *Hemophilus influenzae* and, rarely, the meningococcus. All of these organisms have a distinctive carbohydrate capsule and multiply very rapidly. Splenic function is therefore important as an in-line blood filter and as a processor of antibody production on first contact with one of these bacteria.

Management of OPSI is as follows:

1. When the average responsive child of about three years of age or older complains that he feels ill or develops a sore throat, a headache or nausea followed by vomiting, the parents should be impressed with the need to notify the physician promptly. Within the first hour or two from onset of symptoms, in conjunction with the physical examination, the nasopharynx and blood should be cultured for bacteria and, unless a diagnosis of some other illness seems likely, the patient should be started on antibiotic therapy. Ampicillin is the drug of choice because of its general effectiveness against the pneumococcus, as well as the influenza bacillus and the meningococcus. The dosage should be at the maximum level for the size of the patient, probably 250 mg. every 4 hours for the first 24 hours and then every 6 hours until recovery is evident. Intravenous administration is indicated when bacteremia or meningitis is likely, or confirmed, or if oral medication cannot be tolerated. If the causative organism is identified as the pneumococcus, aqueous penicillin may be used (see Pneumococcal Infections).

If the family physician is not able to see the patient within a few hours to assume full responsibility, it is advisable for the parents to be instructed to start ampicillin treatment to guard against the possibility of uncontrolled pneumococcal infection. Occasionally, if a viral infection is the cause of the illness, the patient may receive ampicillin unnecessarily for 48 hours; nevertheless, this is far preferable to failure to treat a pneumococcal invasion if it is actually occurring.

2. For the child under three years of age, or sometimes even an older child who cannot be trusted to complain or otherwise indicate when a sore throat or other early symptoms of an upper respiratory infection have their onset, it is safer to use prophylactic ampicillin medication routinely from the time of splenectomy. For prophylactic treatment, a schedule of 125 mg. of ampicillin twice daily should protect against infection with pneumococcus or the other organisms responsible for the syndrome under discussion. If sensitivity to ampicillin develops, one of the other antibiotics which combat these particular organisms should be used.

3. When a postsplenectomy patient develops signs of serious infection, such as high fever, chills, severe headache, stiff neck, drowsiness or coma, it is imperative that a diagnostic workup be performed promptly and treatment started simultaneously. In addition to the complete physical examination, a white blood count and differential should be obtained; swabs of the nasopharynx should be cultured for organisms, followed by cultures of the blood and spinal fluid. The spinal fluid should be smeared on a glass slide and examined immediately while routine analysis is being carried out. With pneumococcal meningitis, the spinal fluid may appear relatively clear yet contain many organisms which can be recognized easily by a Gram's stain. Treatment for suspected bacteremia and meningitis should be vigorous and comprehensive. Ampicillin should be administered intravenously in full dosage. For hypovolemia and dehydration from fever, sweating and vomiting, parenteral fluids containing glucose should be given intravenously. To combat possible adrenal hemorrhage (Waterhouse-Friderichsen syndrome), corticosteroids, blood, plasma or albumin infusion may be indicated.

A new approach to the much-desired protection against pneumococcal infection in the asplenic individual consists of the use of polyvalent pneumococcal vaccines for immunization. This should induce specific antibodies in about two weeks to two months after subcutaneous injection. Such immunization is best given at least one to two weeks before splenectomy to patients in whom the operation can be scheduled in advance, or as soon after splenectomy as possible if the operation has been done without such preliminary preparation. This protective immunization against the common types of pathogenic pneumococci should materially diminish the hazard of OPSI and improve the prognosis for the spleenless individual.

References

Diamond, L. K.: Splenectomy in Childhood and the Hazard of Overwhelming Infection. *Pediatrics*, 43: 886, 1969.

Eraklis, A. J., Kevy, S. V., Diamond, L. K., and Gross, R. E.: Hazard of Overwhelming Infection after Splenectomy in Childhood. *New England J. Med.*, 276:1225, 1967.

Haller, J. A., Jr., and Jones, E. L.: Effect of Splenectomy on Immunity and Resistance to Major Infections in Early Childhood: Clinical and Experimental Study. *Ann. Surg.*, 163:902, 1966.

Shinefield, H. R., Steinberg, C. R., and Kaye, D.: Effect of Splenectomy on the Susceptibility of Mice Inoculated with *Diplococcus pneumoniae*. *J. Exp. Med.*, 123:777, 1966.

Congestive Splenomegaly, Splenic Cytopenia and Trauma to the Spleen

THOMAS F. NECHELES, M.D.

The causes of splenomegaly are outlined in Table 1. Any one of these may, at one time or another, be associated with some degree of hypersplenism. When possible, therapy is directed at the underlying primary cause. Frequently, however, the primary disease is not amenable to treatment, and one must consider when and how to treat the hypersplenic syndrome. Mild to moderate degrees of hypersplenism or splenic sequestration are usually tolerated with no difficulty. It is only when the degree of splenic uptake exceeds the ability of the bone marrow to compensate that hypersplenism become a significant factor in the management of the patient.

Splenomegaly and, indeed, evidence of hypersplenism are therefore not in themselves sufficient indications for splenectomy. Indications usually include (1) incidental splenectomy secondary to vascular surgery in the portal system, (2) presence of symptomatic hypersplenism, (3) splenectomy following splenic trauma and (4) evidence of mechanical discomfort due to a massively enlarged organ. Malignancies involving the spleen are in themselves rarely indications for removal of the organ; surgery is indicated only when the tumor is truly localized to the spleen (such as an isolated hemangiosarcoma of the spleen) or when removal of the spleen is important in evaluation of the disease. Splenectomy is usually indicated in hereditary spherocytosis, even when the hemolytic process is well compensated, because the operation is usually "curative," with cessation of hyperhemolysis and the associated potential complications (hyperbilirubinemia with increased incidence of gallstones).

CONGESTIVE SPLENOMEGALY

Congestive splenomegaly is usually associated with increased pressure within the portal or splenic vasculature. This may be secondary to cardiovascular decompensation, in which case therapy is directed toward the systemic problem, or to vascular obstruction within the portal or splenic system. This obstruction may be intrahepatic, usually secondary to primary liver disease; extrahepatic (portal vein thrombosis or cavernous transformation of the portal vein); or in the splenic vein (splenic vein thrombosis). By far the most common is pri-

TABLE 1. Splenomegaly in Childhood

I. Primary
  A. Infection
    1. Viral
    2. Parasitic
    3. Bacterial
  B. Malignant
    1. Lymphoproliferative disease
      a. acute lymphocytic leukemia
      b. lymphoma, lymphosarcoma
    2. Hodgkin's disease
    3. Myeloproliferative disease
      a. acute myelocytic leukemia
      b. chronic granulocytic leukemia
    4. Reticuloendotheliosis
    5. Isolated tumors
  C. Storage disease
    1. Gaucher's
    2. Niemann-Pick
    3. Other rare forms
II. Secondary
  A. "Work Hypertrophy"
    1. Hereditary spherocytosis
    2. Red cell enzyme defects (glycolytic)
      a. pyruvate kinase deficiency
      b. other rare forms
    3. Hemoglobulinopathies
      a. sickle cell anemia (in first decade of life)
      b. HbC disease and variants
      c. thalassemia major and variants
    4. Erythroblastosis
    5. Iron deficiency
  B. Congestive Splenomegaly
    1. Secondary to circulatory overload
    2. Secondary to vascular obstruction
      a. portal vein obstruction
      b. splenic vein obstruction
    3. Secondary to hepatic disease
  C. Systemic autoimmune diseases
    1. Systemic lupus erythematosus
    2. Rheumatoid arthritis
    3. Other (acute immune hemolytic uremia and so forth)
III. Idiopathic

mary hepatic disease, although portal vein thrombosis is not uncommon in childhood and splenic vein thrombosis is occasionally seen in the newborn.

Symptomatology, therapy and prognosis vary somewhat with the location of the obstruction. Splenic vein obstruction is associated with isolated splenomegaly and causes no signs of liver dysfunction or portal hypertension; it is cured by simple splenectomy. In general, the prognosis is good.

Extrahepatic portal vein obstruction is associated with splenomegaly, signs of increased portal pressure, but no signs of hepatic dysfunction. The portal hypertension is reflected in an increased collateral circulation, the most significant of which is dilatation of the veins around the esophagogastric junction with the formation of submucosal varicosities. Hemorrhage from such varicosities can be triggered by practically any trauma, including coughing, vomiting or straining at stools. The bleeding may be slight, detectable only by stool guaiac tests, or it may be massive and even life-threatening. Fortunately, in the absence of preexisting severe anemia or cardiac disease, children rarely die of gastrointestinal hemorrhage. However, massive gastrointestinal bleeding is a medical emergency and the patient should immediately be admitted to the hospital, preferably to an intensive care unit where careful monitoring is available. The patient is placed on bed rest and given nothing by mouth. Circulatory collapse is prevented by transfusion of whole blood, packed red cells, plasma or plasma expanders, depending on what is available and the urgency of the situation. Transfusion therapy must be tempered by the observation that moderate hypotension is often associated with diminution or cessation of bleeding. The use of intravenous Pitressin* (20 units diluted in 20 ml. saline given over 10 to 15 minutes and repeated at 1- to 2-hour intervals) may also decrease the portal venous pressure. Local pressure may be applied at the esophagogastric junction by a Sengstaken-Blakemore tube, but this is rarely indicated in children and usually is quite unsatisfactory. Part of the difficulty is the lack of adequate cooperation on the part of the patient; even heavy sedation is insufficient to make the tube tolerable. Direct ligation of the bleeding varices is a temporary expedient used to stop massive bleeding episodes; its use is rarely indicated in children. Surgical procedures designed to reduce the portal pressure frequently provide long-term symptomatic relief, especially in patients with extrahepatic portal vein obstruction. The procedure should be delayed as long as possible because (1) the older the child the larger the anastomosed vessels with less chance for reobstruction, and (2) splenectomy, if part of the surgical procedure, is tolerated better in the older child. A single gastrointestinal hemorrhage, even if massive, is not sufficient indication for a shunt procedure; children can go for long periods of time between bleeding episodes and lead perfectly normal lives. The shunt procedures which are available include splenorenal shunts (including, by necessity, a splenectomy) and various types of anastomosis between the portal system and inferior vena cava. Portacaval shunts can be car-

* Manufacturer's precaution: Pitressin is not approved for intravenous use.

ried out in very young children; splenorenal shunts are limited, because of the size of the vessels, to children 10 years or older. Even if the initial operation is unsatisfactory because of obstruction of the anastomosis, a second or even third procedure is still possible and may be successful.

Portal hypertension and congestive splenomegaly secondary to intrahepatic disease presents a much more complicated problem. In addition to bleeding due to esophageal varices, the compromised liver function may also lead to a reduction in plasma clotting factor levels, which may contribute to the bleeding diathesis. Thrombocytopenia is also occasionally a problem. Shunt operations in these patients are often poorly tolerated because a further reduction in hepatic blood flow can (1) be associated with increasing signs of toxic encephalopathy, and (2) lead to increased hepatic ischemic necrosis with a further decline in liver function. If the progression of the underlying liver disease can be halted, as is often the case (for example, in Wilson's disease), and the patient has massive ascites or recurring hemorrhages, a shunt procedure should be seriously considered, especially if the child is old enough for a splenorenal procedure. If, on the other hand, the patient has progressive liver disease, little is to be gained from subjecting him to as serious a procedure as a shunt operation.

SPLENIC CYTOPENIA

Splenic cytopenia occurs when the rate of splenic sequestration of one or more formed elements of the blood exceeds the capacity of the bone marrow to replace them. It is dangerous to make the diagnosis of hypersplenism in the absence of both a palpably enlarged spleen and a hyperactive bone marrow. Signs of hypersplenism can evolve in any chronically enlarged spleen. Many patients have a moderate degree of hypersplenism which can remain stable for many years; it is only in the face of progressive decrease in blood counts (white cell count of 4000 per cubic mm. or less, a platelet count of less than 75,000 per cubic mm. or a hematocrit below 30 ml. per 100 ml.) that one becomes concerned. These patients must, however, be followed carefully, since any decrease in bone marrow function (for example, that associated with a viral infection) may be followed by a sudden marked drop in the peripheral blood counts with potentially disastrous sequelae. A relative folate deficiency, where the folate requirements of a hyperactive bone marrow outstrip the normally adequate dietary intake, is another cause for the development of rapidly progressive anemia. Folic acid supplementation (5 mg. per day by mouth) is therefore routinely prescribed for such patients.

Splenectomy becomes necessary when the marrow is no longer capable of keeping up with the rate of splenic sequestration and, in the case of children with a hemolytic process, the need for transfusions progressively increases. Surgery is delayed, if possible, until the child is at least four or five years old. Little or no special preparation is required prior to surgery. Transfusions are indicated only if the patient is markedly anemic; and platelet infusions are rarely needed, even in the face of marked thrombocytopenia. The hematologic response to surgery is usually prompt, in part because of autotransfusion of sequestered cells and in part because of decreased cell destruction. Splenectomy is routinely followed by a thrombocytosis, with platelet counts of 500,000 per cubic mm. not unusual. Thrombotic phenomena in children are, however, rare and the platelet count usually returns to normal within four to six weeks. Because of the hazards of serious postsplenectomy infection (see below), the patients are usually treated with prophylactic penicillin (200,000 units two times a day) for at least two years following surgery.

SPLENIC TRAUMA

Splenic trauma is usually considered a surgical emergency. It is not an uncommon injury in the four- to eight-year-old age group and is frequently the result of automobile accidents involving blunt trauma to the abdomen. In one series, almost 50 per cent of children with blunt injury to the abdomen had associated rupture of the spleen. Fifty per cent of those with splenic rupture had also sustained additional injuries. Patients with enlarged spleens are particularly susceptible to splenic rupture. This may be seen with even seemingly minor trauma and has been known to occur during palpation of the enlarged spleen in infectious mononucleosis.

COMPLICATIONS OF SPLENECTOMY

Complications of splenectomy can be divided into immediate and remote. The most obvious immediate complication is operative morbidity and mortality. Operative morbidity is difficult to evaluate and varies considerably with the underlying disease. The most frequent postoperative complications are pulmonary atelectasis and pneumonia, usually of the left lower lobe. Thrombophlebitis and thromboembolic phenomena are frequently seen in adults but are rare in children. Wound infections are also an occasional problem. The overall morbidity in children is probably no greater than 10 per cent. Operative mortality is considerably lower; in experienced hands it is probably less than 1 per cent. This, too, varies considerably with the selection of patients undergoing splenectomy, but at our institution we have had no deaths in the immediate postoperative period in the last 100 patients, many of whom were quite sick at the time of surgery.

The most important long-term complication of splenectomy is the risk of overwhelming sepsis. Such episodes are characterized by an extremely rapid clinical course and a high mortality; 50 per cent of affected patients are dead within 12 hours after the onset of symptoms. Sepsis in these patients is frequently complicated by disseminated intravascular coagulation contributing to the rapid, often irreversible, downhill course. Most of the infections are due to common pathogens; fully 50 per cent are pneumococcal. They are particularly frequent in patients with underlying hematologic disorders not "cured" by splenectomy (thalassemia, for example), and in patients less than four or five years of age. Most occur within two years of surgery. It has therefore been the policy in many institutions to treat children who have undergone splenectomy with prophylactic penicillin (200,000 units two times a day) for two years following surgery. Prophylactic therapy, in general, has been limited to patients less than five years of age who have underlying hematologic disease. However, we have seen a number of patients who have undergone splenectomy for splenic trauma or for hereditary spherocytosis and who developed the typical picture of overwhelming sepsis up to 12 years following surgery. All of these patients have had pneumococcal septicemia complicated by disseminated intravascular coagulation. We therefore feel that penicillin prophylaxis should be instituted in all patients (who are not allergic to the antibiotic) undergoing this operation and should be continued indefinitely. It is important to remember that splenectomy is not without risks and should be undertaken only for definite indications.

Lymphangitis

RICHARD H. MEADE, III, M.D.

The systemic infection erysipelas is the most obvious form of lymphangitis and is discussed under Streptococcal Infections. It is also caused by other bacteria, though uncommonly. Failure of response to penicillin should alert the physician to the possibility of other penicillin-resistant causes, specifically *Staphylococcus aureus.* Streptococci are recovered from the skin lesions only rarely; however, aspiration of the advancing border, using a tuberculin syringe with a 25 gauge needle, will usually disclose *S. aureus* on smear and on culture. This form of erysipelas is treated with parenteral antibiotics if there is fever and evidence of rapid advance. Cephalothin (100 mg. per kilogram per day in divided doses, dissolved in 50 ml. of normal saline, given intravenously every 3 hours until the temperature is normal), oxacillin (100 mg. per kilogram per day in divided doses at 4-hour intervals) or lincomycin* (25 to 50 mg. per kilogram per day in intramuscular or intravenous doses given at 6-hour intervals) is effective Lincomycin and oxacillin can be given by mouth to the afebrile patient in doses of 25 mg. and 50 mg. per kilogram daily, respectively, at intervals of 6 hours.

Lymphangitis in the form of red streaks on the skin arising from a focus of suppuration is visible evidence of the extension of a previously confined infection that previously may not have warranted antibiotic therapy. *Streptococcus pyogenes* is the most common cause, but *S. aureus* is also capable of producing this lesion. If the infection is streptococcal, penicillin is the most effective antibiotic. It is given orally. Penicillin V (phenoxymethyl penicillin) can be used in doses of 250 mg. every 6 hours for children under the age of 10 years. Older children can tolerate larger doses without developing diarrhea and should receive up to 500 mg. per dose. If there is a large area of skin involved and if there is also regional lymphadenitis and fever, parenteral penicillin should be used.

The total daily dose of aqueous benzyl penicillin G (not procaine penicillin) given intramuscularly or intravenously is one million to five million units; it should be given in saline solution. If intramuscular injections are used, the solution should be 250,000 units per ml. to avoid unnecessary muscle irritation. If the intravenous route is preferred, it should be given by rapid drip of saline solution (100,000 units per ml.) in doses no further apart than 3 hours.

Staphylococcal infections of the skin or of subcutaneous tissues can also produce lymphangitis and can be treated with penicillin if the

* Manufacturer's precaution: Lincomycin is not indicated in the newborn up to one month of age.

organism is known to be susceptible, or with the agents listed above if the organism is not susceptible to penicillin. If staphylococcal infection is presumed, it should be treated as if it were resistant to penicillin. The alternative antibiotics are equally effective in the treatment of streptococcal disease, so that both possible etiologic agents can be dealt with simultaneously.

Lymphangitic streaks from suppurative skin lesions are not always the result of infection with these two gram-positive bacteria. In cases where there is doubt, as in infections acquired as a complication of surgery or of trauma with a contaminated object, the physician must use a Gram-stained smear of available exudate to inform him of the shape and tinctorial characteristics of the causative organism. This will guide him to the selection of antibiotics effective against mouth organisms if there was a bite, or against bowel bacteria if there was surgery. Lymphangitis of this sort is uncommon and, unless due to mouth bacteria, is insensitive to penicillin. Ampicillin, 50 mg. per kilogram daily in four divided doses, can be used orally; or 100 to 200 mg. per kilogram daily intravenously at intervals of 3 hours is likely to be effective against *E. Coli* and Proteus strains.

Ulceroglandular tularemia is another cause of lymphangitis for which streptomycin, 20 mg. per kilogram per day by intramuscular injection every 12 hours, or chloramphenicol, 50 mg. per kilogram per day orally in divided doses every 6 hours, is effective.

Lymphedema

H. HARLAN STONE, M.D.

Lymphedema (or regional edema secondary to inadequacy of lymphatics) occurs as the result of several different conditions. More commonly it is a sequel to the destruction of lymphatic valves and channels by a bacterial lymphangitis. This may follow an extensive thermal burn or an unremitting episode of thrombophlebitis. Acquired lymphedema can also be caused by the removal of interposed lymph nodes, as with axillary or groin dissection, especially when complicated by local infection. The congenital variety appears shortly after birth or develops at some time during puberty (*lymphedema praecox*).

No form of therapy is uniformly successful. If infection plays a role, as is obvious during any acute recurrence of lymphangitis, a systemic antibiotic (penicillin) should be administered and continued for several weeks. Cultures of the portal for bacterial entry or, in the absence of such, of the lymphedema fluid itself should be used for antibiotic sensitivity testing and thus as an indication of which antimicrobial agents will be most effective. Likewise, any responsible wound in the periphery must be drained and/or cleansed and treated with a topical antibiotic (Neosporin or gentamicin cream).

Other measures are primarily directed at improving lymphatic drainage. The part (usually an extremity) is elevated during as much of the day as possible and continually throughout the night. Support hose or elastic stockings (or sleeves) may be worn during daylight hours; however, these appliances for external tissue support may lead to local ulceration through pressure necrosis or shearing of skin. Often the patient is forced to change his way of life because of an unwieldy or unsightly extremity.

Surgery may be indicated, particularly when the process is confined to the skin and subcutaneous tissues. Some modification of the Kondoleon operation is frequently beneficial. This entails (1) taking split thickness grafts from the skin of the involved extremity, (2) excision of all residual skin, subcutaneous tissue and deep enveloping fascia and (3) final wound closure by application of the previously harvested skin grafts. Recurrences are common but usually can be controlled by use of proper support stockings.

For deeper and more extensive lymphedema, a pedicled flap of veins and lymphatics can be constructed from the greater omentum. This structure is then tunneled into the deeper planes of the extremity to establish venous and lymphatic anastomoses with unobstructed proximal channels. The results of this operation are inconsistent but have occasionally produced dramatic improvement.

As a last resort to rid the patient of an ulcerated monstrosity, particularly if a foot alone or possibly a foot and lower leg are involved, amputation followed by expert fitting with a well-mounted prosthesis may be preferable to continuation of unsuccessful efforts at preservation of an unwanted extremity.

Lymph Node Infections

RICHARD H. MEADE, III, M.D.

Bacterial lymphadenitis can usually be treated with antibiotics alone. If suppuration is already present, surgical drainage is essential;

antimicrobial drugs are needed for control of the surrounding inflammation and to reduce to the minimum the time needed for healing. Palpation of superficially located lymph nodes is sufficient to determine whether surgical drainage is needed; for more deeply situated nodes, especially if they are under fascial layers such as in the neck, it is often necessary to aspirate to determine if there is central liquefaction. Infection of the lymph nodes overlying the psoas muscle, within the peritoneal cavity or within the mediastinum, constitutes a more complex therapeutic problem. For such infection, antibiotic treatment has to be given parenterally and the course of the disease followed closely to determine whether surgical drainage will also be needed.

Superficial lymph gland infection (that is, within the subcutaneous space) if due to bacteria is associated with inflammation of the overlying skin and usually with a visible primary focus. The primary lesion should be cleaned and dressed and systemic treatment initiated. Penicillin G, 200,000 to 400,000 units no less than 30 minutes before each meal and at bedtime for a period of 10 days, is sufficient therapy for infections due to streptococci. *Staphylococcus aureus* is less commonly a pathogen for such infection and is often insensitive to penicillin. Oxacillin (50 mg. per kilogram per day in four doses), erythromycin (50 mg. per kilogram per day in four doses) or lincomycin* (25 mg. per kilogram per day in four doses) should be used for this.

Infection of lymph nodes in the cervical chains often reaches substantial size before recognition and usually produces fever. Aspiration of the contents of the infected gland will help determine the cause as well as the presence or absence of suppuration. In children under the age of two years, *S. aureus* is the most common pathogen; for those old enough to have fully developed teeth, *Streptococcus pyogenes* is more common. Parenteral antibiotic treatment is required for children with high fever and associated cellulitis. Its use even when surgical drainage is necessary will return the temperature to normal and confine the overlying cellulitis usually within 24 hours. The antibiotics required for staphylococcal adenitis of this type have to be effective against penicillin-resistant strains (unless the drug sensitivity pattern has already been determined). They are as follows: Oxacillin, 50 to 100 mg. per kilogram per day can be given in divided doses every 4 to 6 hours intravenously or intramuscularly. Intravenous doses should be diluted in 50 ml. of normal saline and allowed to drip in rapidly over the space of 20 to 30 minutes. Cephalothin can also be used in doses that have to be administered every 3 hours intravenously using 100 mg. per kilogram per day. Lincomycin, 50 mg. per kilogram per day, can be given by intramuscular injection every 6 hours, or intravenously diluted in 5 per cent dextrose solution or in normal saline, 50 ml. per dose. Each of these drugs is useful in the treatment of streptococcal infection as well. For older children, or for any child with streptococcal adenitis, aqueous benzyl penicillin G (not procaine penicillin) is used in the dose of one million to two million units per day. Intravenous doses should be spaced at intervals of no more than 3 hours, and should be dissolved in normal saline in a concentration of 100,000 units per ml. Intramuscular injections must be spaced at 4 to 6 hours and injected in saline solution, using no more than 250,000 units per ml. to avoid undue local pain. The duration of treatment is determined by the speed of response. If surgical drainage can be carried out promptly and if there is quick resolution of the surrounding cellulitis, a week of treatment is sufficient. It is necessary to treat for periods of up to a month in cases with widespread cellulitis, induration and deep suppuration. Dental consultation is important if periodontal or periapical infection is present and believed responsible for the lymphadenitis.

The same principles of treatment are used in the management of axillary and inguinal adenitis. Postauricular adenitis is usually associated with middle ear infection and responds to therapy directed at the otitis (penicillin G or ampicillin), whereas parotid lymph node infection is due to streptoccocci.

Iliac lymphadenitis is uncommon. It produces lower quadrant abdominal pain, psoas irritation so that the thigh is flexed on the involved side, and often high fever. It is ordinarily caused by group A streptococci and is treated with penicillin G parenterally. Failure of response to medical therapy is an indication for surgical drainage.

Lymph node inflammation occurs as a response to a number of processes that are not treatable with antibiotics, as in the axillary adenitis resulting from smallpox vaccination, the inguinal adenitis resulting from epidermophytosis or the lymph node swelling that is associated with eczema. Inguinal adenitis in the older boy requires consideration of the possibility of primary syphilis or of gonorrheal urethritis. Primary syphilis is treated with 600,000 units of procaine penicillin a day for a

* Manufacturer's precaution: Lincomycin is not indicated in the newborn up to one month of age.

period of nine days (tetracycline in the dose of 1 Gr. a day for nine days for those allergic to penicillin),† and gonorrheal urethritis is treated with 2,400,000 units of procaine penicillin intramuscularly daily for two days.

Indolent and relatively painless swelling of lymph nodes in the neck or the groin may be due to tuberculosis, the treatment for which is outlined in another part of this volume. Cat scratch disease produces similar lymphadenitis in inguinal, axillary, cervical, preauricular, parotid and subpectoral glands. No specific therapy is available or usually required. Prolonged and uncomfortable swelling can be dealt with by surgical removal of the involved nodes, a procedure of both diagnostic and therapeutic value.

Children in the western and southwestern portions of the United States with high fever and enlargement particularly of inguinal nodes, and of axillary and cervical glands as well, require consideration of plague.

Yersinia pestis infection can be treated with streptomycin (20 mg. per kilogram per day in two doses intramuscularly) or chloramphenicol‡ (50 mg. per kilogram per day intravenously in doses 6 hours apart). Chloramphenicol should be the drug of first choice for anyone with severe systemic signs, since this infection may be complicated by the blood stream invasion of other bacteria as well, particularly group A hemolytic streptococci.

Tularemia is also the cause of local lymph node involvement usually in association with a cutaneous ulcer or with ocular infection. Treatment for this infection has been discussed under Lymphangitis. Tularemia is ordinarily seen in rural areas of the country but is confined to no geographical section.

Lymphangioma

H. HARLAN STONE, M.D.

The lymphangioma is a multilocular, cystic mass of non-neoplastic origin. It is composed of blind and dilated lymph channels that have been congenitally sequestered from their otherwise normal endothelial connections for lymph outflow.

Lymphangiomas vary in number and massiveness of the cystic locules. When the cysts are huge, the lesion is generally referred to as a *hygroma.* The fluid contained within is clear lymph, unless clouded by blood extruded because of local trauma or by purulent exudate from an adjacent infection. On occasion there is a hemangiomatous component. True malignant degeneration into lymphangiosarcoma has never been documented prior to the age of puberty.

Lymphangiomas usually appear at the time of birth or shortly thereafter. The majority develop in the vicinity of the head and neck, with prevalent sites being the posterior cervical triangle, the parotid region, the tongue, the floor of the mouth and the pterygoid fossa. Involvement of the axilla may be either a separate process or merely an extension down the brachial plexus from a similar lesion in the neck above. Other common sites of occurrence include the mediastinum, the retroperitoneal space, the bowel mesentery, pelvis and groin.

Physical findings are quite characteristic. A soft, multilocular cyst discovered in those areas of predilection is almost certainly a lymphangioma. The mass is usually attached to the deep fascia, is nontender, readily transilluminates light and is seldom associated with any other anomaly. Extension into the mediastinum should be looked for on the routine chest x-ray.

Complications of the lymphangioma are (1) infection, (2) airway obstruction and (3) physical disfigurement. *Streptococcal* lymphangitis may lead to infection of a neighboring lymphangioma and should be treated promptly with penicillin. Other types of infection generally follow needle aspiration or unwitting incision and must be managed by antibiotics specific for the bacterium thus inoculated. Airway obstruction is a more serious complication. It occurs primarily when there is involvement by lymphangioma of the base of the tongue, pharynx or larynx. Occasionally external compression of the larynx or trachea from a deeply seated hygroma can cause respiratory distress.

The only successful form of *therapy* is total or near-total surgical excision. Injection of a caustic agent merely leads to tissue necrosis, infection, and external fistulization; such procedures are strongly condemned. Drainage is indicated only as a means to unroof pharyngeal or laryngeal cysts that create a significant obstruction to the upper airway. Tracheostomy has been required at times to prevent actual strangulation by the occluding mass.

Lymphangiomas in the parotid gland or body of the tongue are managed by excision of

† Manufacturer's note: The use of tetracyclines during tooth development (last half of pregnancy, infancy and childhood to age eight years) may cause discoloration of teeth. This adverse reaction is more common during long-term use of the drug but has been observed following repeated short-term courses.

‡ Manufacturer's precaution: Chloramphenicol is not recommended for intramuscular or intravenous pediatric use. Chloramphenicol sodium succinate has been approved for intravenous pediatric use.

the lesion in continuity with the attached organ (parotidectomy or partial glossectomy, respectively). Elsewhere, the mass is resected as completely as possible. During operation, great care should be taken to preserve the cyst intact, for once ruptured there is loss of a definite plane for dissection and thus lymphangiomatous remnants are left behind. Special efforts are also taken to preserve all nerves and arteries that pass through or near the lesion, although adjacent venous channels and fascial sheaths can be sacrificed without regard to local attachments. If complete removal is impossible, all remaining cysts that have been exposed should be at least partially excised to ensure their direct drainage into adjacent tissues and thereby allow the possibility for establishment of an anastomosis to new lymphatic channels.

The incidence of lymphangioma recurrence is relatively low (less than 10 per cent) and is directly related to the thoroughness of the initial excision.

Lymphoma

AUDREY E. EVANS, M.D., *and*
GIULIO J. D'ANGIO, M.D.

In this category of diseases are included Hodgkin's disease, lymphosarcoma and reticulum cell sarcoma. The term "malignant lymphoma" is sometimes used for lesions which cannot be classified into any of these categories. Rappaport has suggested an encompassing classification and the interested reader is referred to his publication (see References).

The treatment of the lymphomatous diseases is unsettled, and there is continuous debate as to the relative value of surgery, radiation therapy and chemotherapy. Individual patients and the course of the disease vary greatly, making it difficult to find comparable groups to evaluate the results of therapy. Most authorities, however, agree that the bulwark of treatment in most cases of localized disease lies in radiation therapy given in adequate dosage. Chemotherapy has proved effective in many instances of generalized diseases. The value of combination radiation therapy and chemotherapy in cases of intermediate disease is not yet known, and opinions differ regarding their relative merits. Since the stage of the disease at diagnosis influences the selection of treatment, the most recent staging of Hodgkin's disease—the so-called Ann Arbor classification—is given below. This form of disease staging can also be used for other lymphomas but is less reliable since the progression of disease is more variable, including the pronounced tendency of localized lymphosarcoma in childhood to transform to lymphocytic leukemia.

Staging of Hodgkin's Disease—Ann Arbor Classification.* The earlier (Rye) staging system has been modified. Staging now includes designations for the presence of extralymphatic disease localized and related to adjacent involved lymph nodes. It also includes the additional information obtained from patients who undergo a staging laparotomy and splenectomy. Two methods of staging are used, Clinical Staging (CS) and Pathological Staging (PS), retaining the designations of A and B, depending on the absence or presence of systemic symptoms. Subscripts indicate the presence or absence of disease in specific sites; e.g., an asymptomatic patient with a single cluster of positive lymph nodes in the neck and nonpalpable spleen is designated stage CS IA, but PS III_{S+} if the spleen is found to be positive for Hodgkin's disease at laparotomy.

Stage I—Involvement of a single lymph node region (I) or a single extralymphatic organ or site (I_E).

Stage II—Involvement of two or more lymph node regions on the same side of the diaphragm (II) or localized involvement of extralymphatic organ or site and one or more lymph node regions on the same side of the diaphragm (II_E).

Stage III—Involvement of lymph node regions on both sides of the diaphragm (III), which may also be accompanied by localized involvement of extralymphatic organ or site (III_E), or by the spleen (III_S), or by both (III_{SE}).

Stage IV—Diffuse or disseminated involvement of one or more extralymphatic organs or tissues with or without associated lymph node involvement.

The pathologic staging follows the same classification and denotes which areas other than the primary disease were subjected to biopsy and are positive or negative for Hodgkin's disease. The abbreviations used are as follows: N+ or N− for lymph nodes other than the primary site, positive or negative for disease on biopsy. In similar fashion, H, S, L, M, P, O and D are used for liver, spleen, lung, bone marrow, pleura, bone and skin, respectively.

Staging of Non-Hodgkin's Lymphoma. The four stages used for Hodgkin's disease can be used to classify other lymphomas but do not have the same prognostic accuracy. For exam-

* Carbone et al.

ple, a patient with a stage II_E lymphosarcoma with a mediastinal mass and a pleural effusion has a very poor prognosis and can be expected to develop generalized disease early.

INVESTIGATIONS NECESSARY TO DIAGNOSE AND STAGE PATIENTS WITH LYMPHOMA. Biopsy of the primary lesion should be followed by a complete blood count, bone marrow aspiration (and biopsy for patients with Hodgkin's disease), liver function tests, chest and abdominal x-ray films, inferior vena cavagram and excretory urogram. For patients with localized Hodgkin's disease in whom treatment will be directed toward cure, a bilateral lymphangiogram to outline the pelvic and retroperitoneal lymph nodes should be followed by a laparotomy with liver and lymph node biopsies. Splenectomy is recommended for children six years of age or older with Hodgkin's disease. Girls should have the ovaries repositioned outside the radiation therapy field if treatment of the pelvis is likely.

Treatment of Hodgkin's Disease. RADIATION THERAPY. *Stages I and II, A and B.* The longest disease-free intervals in adults have been obtained by use of large field radiation therapy. An example of such a field is one designated to include all lymph node drainage areas from the tips of the mastoid processes down to the level of L4-L5. The fields are shaped to include the entire neck, trunk and shoulder girdle, excluding only the lungs. Megavoltage apparatus is used, and doses of 3500 to 4000 rads are given in 3½ to 4 weeks.

A controlled clinical trial that includes older children and adults has been under way for some time to evaluate the relative efficiency of local field irradiation versus the larger or extended field (EF) in patients with early Hodgkin's disease. In this investigation, the involved field (IF) is defined as that portal which will include all the diseased lymph nodes plus a margin of 7 cm. in any direction. Only preliminary data are available from this trial. Recurrence rates are higher in the IF group requiring re-treatment, but no clear-cut difference insofar as survival is concerned has been detected between the two groups. Thus, it would seem that patients with early disease and relapse can be salvaged by re-treatment. Very preliminary information from Memorial Hospital in a small group of children tends to confirm this observation. Bearing in mind the disadvantages of large field radiation therapy in childhood, the results of the national study are awaited with great interest. Meanwhile, it would seem reasonable to treat the EF in older children and the IF in younger patients who have considerable growth and development potential remaining.

Stage III, Types A and B. Data are being accumulated regarding the difference in prognostic significance, if any, between types A and B. Oncologists of considerable experience differ in their opinion on this point. We believe that patients with pronounced systemic signs have a poorer prognosis than those who have marginal signs and symptoms or none at all.

Radiation therapy is the mainstay of treatment. Large fields are employed. The pelvic, inguinal and femoral lymph nodes are included in appropriately shaped fields, and these zones are added to the EF described above. The dose is 3500 to 4000 rads given to all regions in 3½ to 4 weeks. Techniques to achieve these goals vary. One method that has been found useful at Memorial Hospital is the "3 and 2" technique, wherein multiple-shaped fields are used with suitable rest periods interposed (Nisce and D'Angio). All radiation therapy techniques involved in the treatment of patients with Hodgkin's disease are demanding and intricate, and should be employed only by experienced radiation therapists in centers which are equipped to perform the necessary dosimetry and in which modern treatment apparatus is available.

Stage IV. The Ann Arbor modification has helped to clarify some of the ambiguities of the Rye staging system. It has long been known that involvement of some extranodal sites is of less grave import than involvement of others. Disease in the liver is generally conceded to be a poor prognostic sign, whereas lung, bone and gastrointestinal tract disease is not as ominous. For this reason, the Ann Arbor classification makes provision for contiguous involvement of some of these structures, in which case the patients are no longer considered stage IV. For example, if a vertebral body adjacent to a diseased lymph node shows roentgenographic evidence of involvement, the prognosis is more nearly that of a patient with stage I disease than with stage IV.

Gastrointestinal tract involvement poses a more severe problem. Surgical removal of the affected part should be followed by irradiation of at least the lymph node drainage areas if not the total abdomen. Treatment under the latter circumstances is similar to that employed for those patients with liver involvement. The portal extends from the dome of the diaphragm to the femoral triangles. Two thousand rads are given to this entire volume. Kidney blocks are inserted from the beginning so that no more than 1500 rads are received by these structures.

The fields are then narrowed to include the para-aortic and pelvic lymph node chains, which receive an additional 1500 to 2000 rads. All of the above treatments are given in daily fractions of 150 to 200 rads.

CHEMOTHERAPY. The treatment of patients with Hodgkin's disease stages I and II does not at present include the use of drugs. Their place in stage III has yet to be determined. It is our practice to prescribe chemotherapy for six months in patients with stage IV disease. The regimen used (COPP) is as follows: Cyclophosphamide (*C*ytoxan), 10 mg. per kilogram intravenously, days one and eight; vincristine (VCR) (*O*ncovin)† 1.5 mg. per square meter intravenously, days one and eight; methylhydrazine (*P*rocarbazine), 50 mg. per square meter daily orally, for 15 days; *p*rednisone, 2 mg. per kilogram per day orally for 15 days and "tapered" over seven days. The course can be repeated at intervals of six weeks. A similar program can be used for patients with stage III disease who have pronounced systemic signs and symptoms. Treatment regimens employing both large field radiation therapy and multiple agent chemotherapy are vigorous and demanding. Toxicity and late deleterious consequences are such that management should be undertaken only by teams thoroughly familiar with the disease and with the exigencies of the radical therapy entailed.

Other agents can be tried if there is no response to COPP or if there is relapse after its use. Velban (0.1 to 0.2 mg. per kilogram intravenously) is a useful agent and can be continued as long as marrow tolerance allows. Nitrogen mustard (0.2 mg. per kilogram for two daily injections) is sometimes effective even in patients resistant to cyclophosphamide, and can be repeated in six weeks if marrow tolerance permits (e.g., peripheral blood neutrophil count). The two related antibiotics, daunorubicin (previously called daunomycin) and adriamycin, have shown some effect in the treatment of Hodgkin's disease, as has bleomycin, but all are still available only for therapeutic trials.

Non-Hodgkin's Lymphoma. The largest group of non-Hodgkin's lymphomas are lymphosarcomas, with reticulum cell sarcoma less often seen.

RADIATION THERAPY. Lymphosarcoma is very responsive to radiation therapy. High dose irradiation to the child with a large mediastinal mass (thymic involvement) is of doubtful value since such patients almost always have, or soon develop, bone marrow evidence of lymphosarcoma. Disease progression is not altered by intensive irradiation. Localized lymphosarcoma arising in the gut can be treated surgically. Even if the resection of the disease area appears complete, total abdominal radiation therapy is given to a dose of 3000 rads in three weeks, shielding the kidneys and liver, as described above for Hodgkin's disease.

Patients with localized reticulum cell sarcoma require more intensive radiation therapy. Doses of 4500 rads delivered at the rate of 1000 rads per week are given; even then, the local disease can recur.

Radiation for stage III or IV lymphosarcoma is usually given only for palliative purposes, though Jenkin recommends its use in the postoperative period for those patients with resected lesions of the gastrointestinal tract. Investigations are under way to determine whether better survival can be obtained by combining irradiation with chemotherapy; for instance, large fields, similar to those used for Hodgkin's disease and designed to include certain areas prone to relapse (such as the central nervous system), are being treated in these endeavors.

CHEMOTHERAPY. Lymphosarcoma is sensitive to alkylating agents, antimetabolites and corticosteroids, though frequently the response is short. The place of chemotherapy in the treatment of localized reticulum cell sarcoma and lymphosarcoma has yet to be determined. In view of the tendency of these forms of lymphoma to become generalized, vigorous treatment is probably indicated.

A multiple drug regimen has been shown to be more effective than single agents in the treatment of lymphosarcoma. Initial treatment should be with prednisone, 2 mg. per kilogram orally daily for 28 days; vincristine,† 2 mg. per square meter intravenously weekly for four weeks; and cyclophosphamide, 10 mg. per kilogram intravenously weekly, for four weeks. In the presence of massive disease or an elevated blood uric acid level, allopurinol, 150 to 400 mg. per day, should be commenced the day prior to the antilymphoma treatment, and attention should be directed toward maintenance of an adequate urinary output. The allopurinol can be discontinued at the end of one week if the renal function is normal. During or at the end of the initial one-month induction regimen, consideration should be given to the addition of radiation therapy. If large fields

† Manufacturer's precaution: Vincristine sulfate (Oncovin) is recommended only for treatment of acute leukemia in childhood.

are planned, treatment can be started on the completion of the first month course of chemotherapy. So-called prophylactic radiation therapy to the skull to control meningeal implants can be done at this time. Radiation therapy can be delivered to more localized areas, such as lesions causing tracheal or spinal cord compression, concomitant with the initial chemotherapy. The maintenance regimen should be with multiple drug cyclic therapy similar to the following program: 6-mercaptopurine (6-MP), 75 mg. per square meter orally daily; methotrexate, 30 mg. per square meter orally weekly; cyclophosphamide, 300 mg. per square meter orally weekly; vincristine,‡ 2 mg. per square meter intravenously monthly; and prednisone, 60 mg. per square meter daily for seven days each month for two years. Some patients will not respond to the above regimen, or the disease will recur in a short period. Other agents which have caused responses in lymphosarcoma and reticulum cell sarcoma are nitrogen mustard, 0.2 mg. per kilogram intravenously for two days every four to six weeks; Velban, 0.1 to 0.25 mg. per kilogram intravenously weekly; L-asparaginase, 6000 units per square meter intramuscularly three times a week for 12 weeks; and daunorubicin, 15 mg. per square meter intravenously daily for three to five days every four weeks. L-Asparaginase§ should be accompanied by prednisone or 6-MP to reduce the anaphylactic reactions, and if response is obtained, remission maintenance should be with agents such as methotrexate, 6-MP or cyclophosphamide, since continued treatment with L-asparaginase does not prolong the disease-free interval. Responses have also been seen following adriamycin and bleomycin (investigational).

The vigorous use of chemotherapy and radiation therapy in a curative attempt carries with it the same hazards that exist in the treatment of leukemia. Such programs will lead to bone marrow suppression and altered immunity in some patients with the attendant risks of infection. Adequate facilities and personnel should be available to support patients through such episodes.

‡ Manufacturer's precaution: Vincristine is recommended only for treatment of acute leukemia in childhood.

§ L-Asparaginase is an investigational drug.

References

Carbone, P. P., et al.: Report of the Committee on Hodgkin's Disease Staging Classification. *Cancer Res.*, 31:1860, 1971.

Jenkin, D.: Management of Malignant Lymphoma in Childhood; in T. J. Deeley (ed.): *Modern Radio-Therapy—Malignant Diseases in Children.* London, Butterworth & Co., Ltd. In Press.

Nisce, L. Z., and D'Angio, G. J.: A New Technique for the Irradiation of Large Fields in Patients with Lymphoma. *Radiology,* 106:641–644, 1973.

Rappaport, H.: In *Atlas of Tumor Pathology III, Tumors of the Hematopoietic System.* Washington, D. C., Armed Forces Institute of Pathology, 1966, pp. 91–206.

9

Endocrine System

Hypopituitarism

SOLOMON A. KAPLAN, M.D.

The method of treatment depends upon the nature of the disease and which pituitary hormones are affected. Successful therapy can only be achieved if the nature of the defect is properly ascertained. Adequate and careful testing must first be performed to determine which hormonal functions are disturbed and which require replacement therapy. It is beyond the scope of this chapter to deal with the signs, symptoms and methods for testing for hormonal deficiencies which are covered elsewhere (Lippe et al.). The testing must yield precise information on the capacity of the pituitary gland to secrete growth hormone (GH), adrenocorticotropic hormone (ACTH), thyroid-stimulating hormone (TSH), follicle-stimulating hormone (FSH), luteinizing hormone (LH) and vasopressin. Testing for other hormones, such as prolactin, melanocyte-stimulating hormone and vasotocin, is rarely required in pediatric practice and these will not be dealt with here. In addition, if hormonal abnormalities are suspected or proved, the nature of the underlying cause must be ascertained, such as tumor (e.g., craniopharyngioma), histiocytosis, granuloma, trauma, anorexia nervosa, vascular insufficiency and so forth. Methods for diagnosis of these *organic disorders* are also beyond the scope of this section and the reader is referred elsewhere for their discussion (Kaplan). In the absence of a clearly defined organic lesion which itself needs therapy, hormonal therapy may be the only form of treatment necessary. Idiopathic processes, insofar as they affect the anterior pituitary, are now considered as usually being hypothalamic in origin. They may comprise isolated or multiple hormonal deficiencies. For example, a patient may suffer from isolated GH deficiency or from combined deficiency of GH, TSH, ACTH, LH and FSH. Any combination of deficiencies may occur, as may isolated deficiency of any hormone. Vasopressin deficiency itself may also occur as an isolated finding or in combination with anterior pituitary insufficiency.

Therapy for GH Deficiency. Two factors are of paramount importance in determining the effectiveness of GH therapy. The first is species specificity, which requires that humans receive GH from human or anthropoid sources. The only practical source for GH is pituitary material obtained at autopsy. Although the complex human GH molecule has been synthesized in the laboratory, it is not yet available from this source for therapeutic purposes. The amount of GH available for treatment thus remains seriously limited. The second factor of great importance in GH therapy is that, with few exceptions, GH administration effectively increases growth for sustained periods of time only in those few children whose growth retardation is caused by GH deficiency. With occasional exceptions, only children with GH deficiency should undergo therapy with GH.

Human GH is administered by intramuscular injection usually in a dosage of 2 to 3 International Units (I.U.) three times weekly.* (Generally, 1 mg. is approximately 1 I.U.) Optimal dosages have not been determined because limited supplies of growth hormone prohibit extensive, well-controlled, therapeutic studies. The response may be better if higher

* Note: This therapy is still considered experimental and can only be carried out under a specific, approved research protocol.

doses than 2 to 3 I.U. are used. Generally, the response is better in the earlier months of treatment. The response is also generally better when treatment is given to younger children in whom growth increments in excess of 10 cm. per year are often seen. Although treatment may be beneficial at any time prior to epiphyseal fusion, it tends to be less effective in older children.

Administration of growth hormone results in some increase in skeletal maturation but, generally, advance in height age is equal to or greater than acceleration of skeletal age. The ultimate height achieved is therefore at least as great as that to be anticipated from the growth potential estimated from the delay in skeletal age. Failure of anticipated enhancement of growth rate with therapy may be ascribed to one of several causes: (1) If the diagnosis of GH deficiency is incorrect and shortness of stature is the result of other factors, GH administration will generally be ineffective. (2) As mentioned above, with passage of time, therapy tends to become less effective. Sometimes this deteriorating response is the result of development of antibodies to growth hormone. However, such antibodies are rarely neutralizing, and little correlation exists between development of these antibodies and diminution of growth response. (3) Generally, the growth response tends to be less marked in subjects with pituitary tumors than in those whose hormonal deficiency is of the idiopathic type. (4) If TSH deficiency coexists with GH deficiency, adequate growth will not occur unless thyroid hormone is administered in addition to GH. At the time of this writing, however, the role of thyroid hormone in the therapy of hypopituitarism is not completely understood. It has been suggested that if thyroid hormone and cortisone are administered concomitantly with GH, epiphyseal maturation may be accelerated excessively. Thus, it appears that thyroid hormone should not be part of the regimen unless the existence of hypothyroidism is established. Even if hypothyroidism is not present prior to therapy with GH, diminution in thyroid function may occur after GH therapy is initiated. For this reason it is important to monitor thyroid hormone levels in the blood at regular intervals after beginning GH therapy. If the level of thyroxine in the blood falls, and particularly if the growth rate also decelerates sharply, thyroid hormone should be administered in addition to GH. (5) Administration of ACTH or glucocorticoids tends to diminish responsiveness to GH even if the subject suffers from deficiency of ACTH. There is little evidence of adrenal deficiency in subjects with hypopituitarism, even if ACTH deficiency is demonstrable by laboratory testing. It is recommended that the patient with ACTH and GH deficiency receive only GH therapy but that he be observed carefully to determine if adrenal insufficiency develops. ACTH or glucocorticoids should be administered only if signs or symptoms of adrenal insufficiency develop.

Therapy for TSH Deficiency. In cases of deficiency of thyroid function due either to hypothalamic dysfunction [thyrotropin-releasing hormone (TRH) deficiency] or pituitary dysfunction (TSH deficiency), the therapy of choice is thyroid hormone. Desiccated thyroid, L-thyroxine or tri-iodothyronine is used in doses appropriate for treatment of hypothyroidism. The dose of thyroid hormone used for the treatment of secondary hypothyroidism is similar to that used for treatment of primary hypothyroidism and the reader is referred to the section on Thyroid Disease for details.

Therapy for ACTH Deficiency. In cases of ACTH deficiency, therapy with glucocorticoids is generally the simplest and most effective form of therapy. ACTH and its derivatives are generally less desirable because they have to be administered by injection. The dosage of glucocorticoids used in subjects with secondary hypoadrenocorticism is generally equivalent to that used in subjects with primary adrenal insufficiency; for details the reader is referred to the section on Adrenal Disorders. Generally, glucocorticoids are administered orally two or three times daily in dosage of 5 to 15 mg. per square meter per day of cortisone equivalent. To obviate growth impairment, the smallest dose of glucocorticoid which counteracts symptoms of hypoadrenocorticism is used. Therapy with mineralocorticoids is usually unnecessary, but should the need arise Florinef may be used in a dosage of 0.05 to 0.1 mg. daily by mouth.

Therapy for Gonadotropin Deficiency. With isolated GH deficiency, puberty is usually delayed and therapy for gonadotropin deficiency need not be undertaken until it is clear that neither time nor GH administration will produce gonadotropin secretion. When it is clear that permanent gonadotropin deficiency exists, a choice must be made between therapy with gonadotropins, androgens or estrogens.

GONADOTROPIN THERAPY. Gonadotropin therapy is potentially more effective than therapy with androgenic steroids because it may result in stimulation of spermatogenesis or oogenesis. Androgenic steroid therapy can produce only those effects which normally result from elaboration of testosterone, and this does not include spermatogenesis or oogenesis. Gonadotropin therapy, however, has important disadvantages. Aside from the inconvenience of intramuscular injections, long-term human chorionic gonadotropin (HCG) therapy is considerably less effective than androgenic hormones in stimulating development of secondary sexual characteristics (Hochman et al.).

Two kinds of preparations are available: (1) HCG produces effects largely by virtue of its luteinizing hormone (LH) type of action. It is administered by intramuscular injection two or three times weekly in a dosage of 500 to 2000 I.U. per injection. Dosage and frequency of injection are determined by the response of the patient. (2) Treatment with HCG by itself will not produce spermatogenesis, however. When promotion of fertility is considered desirable, injections of human menopausal gonadotropin (HMG), marketed as Pergonal,* will be necessary. This material, prepared from the urine of postmenopausal women, has an action comparable to FSH.

Androgenic (Anabolic) Steroid Therapy. Patients with hypothalamic (or pituitary) hypogonadism who also have GH deficiency should undergo therapy with GH initially. If GH is not available, androgenic steroids may be used to promote growth. It is not clear if long-term therapy with testosterone will ultimately impair capacity for spermatogenesis, and this consideration must be borne in mind if long-term androgenic steroid therapy is contemplated. In the prepubertal child with GH deficiency, gonadotropin deficiency is a normal physiologic state and no means are yet at hand for predicting if gonadotropin or releasing-factor deficiency will ultimately develop.

The prepubertal child with GH deficiency, for whom GH is not available, may be a suitable candidate for therapy with androgenic (anabolic) steroids. The dose used must be very carefully chosen, however, to obviate acceleration of skeletal age in excess of height age. Frequent checks of the skeletal age must be made (three to four times yearly) to determine if adverse effects have been produced. In addition, a search must be made for other undesirable effects, such as pubic hair growth, penile or clitoral enlargement, facial hair growth and so forth. In my opinion, anabolic steroids are all more or less equally androgenic when therapeutic dosages are used. Claims that a particular anabolic steroid is less likely to advance skeletal age have generally not been substantiated.

In the prepubertal child with GH deficiency, methyltestosterone, 2.5 to 5 mg. daily, may be administered sublingually or by mouth. Absorption is about twice as complete via the sublingual route. If untoward signs or symptoms do not develop, the dose may be increased gradually, but the prepubertal child should rarely receive more than 5 mg. sublingually or 10 mg. by mouth. Other anabolic steroids may be used in equivalent dosage.

When the normal age of puberty is reached, puberty may be delayed in the child with GH deficiency. When it is determined that permanent gonadotropin deficiency exists and (for reasons given above) it is elected to use long-term therapy with androgenic steroids rather than with gonadotropins, full replacement doses may be used (25 to 50 mg. daily of an oral preparation such as Oreton). More convenient may be the administration of 200 mg. of testosterone enanthate or cyclopentylpropionate by intramuscular injection once every two, three or four weeks, depending on the patient's response.

Estrogen and Progestin Therapy. Because estrogens tend to accelerate epiphyseal fusion when given in doses necessary to promote sexual development in patients with hypogonadotropic hypogonadism, treatment with estrogens should be deferred until growth retardation is no longer a serious problem. If estrogens are administered before adequate growth has occurred, careful attention must be paid to epiphyseal development and to the minimum dosage used which is compatible with maximum growth potential.

Numerous estrogen preparations are available. Premarin tablets, 0.325 to 1.25 mg., may be given daily for three to six months, and then cyclical therapy may be instituted to induce regular menses. The above dose of Premarin is given from day 1 to day 23 of each calendar month. From day 16 to day 23, a progestational agent (e.g., Provera, 2.5 to 10 mg. daily) is taken also. It is advantageous to have the patient follow such a regimen and to have regular menses. In this way, irregular or intermenstrual bleeding may have the same significance as the harbinger of genital tract malignancy for the gonadotropin-deficient woman as it has for the woman with normal hypothalamic pituitary function. Eventually, attempts at induction of fertility may be made with administration of combinations or preparations of FSH and LH as outlined above.

* Manufacturer's precaution: Pergonal is investigational for pituitary disorders.

Therapy for Vasopressin Deficiency. Vasopressin deficiency may be transitory (e.g., following removal of a pituitary tumor) or partial. Generally, however, once established it is permanent. After the diagnosis is established, treatment may consist of administration either of vasopressin or of other agents which are unrelated structurally to vasopressin.

VASOPRESSIN THERAPY. Vasopressin is generally administered by intramuscular injection or by nasal insufflation. The preparation used for intramuscular injection is Pitressin tannate suspended in oil (5 units per ml.). This material produces antidiuretic activity for 36 to 72 hours. The usual dosage regimen for children and adolescents is 2.5 to 5 units administered every other day. Infants often require smaller doses. The dosage varies with the individual subject and must be adjusted to his needs. The suspension must always be warmed and shaken vigorously before use to ensure that the small volume of the active principle is well mixed with the vehicle.

In recent years, a stable aqueous preparation of lysine vasopressin (Diapid) has become available. This material, dispensed in plastic compressible containers, is insufflated into either one or both nostrils three to six times daily. Frequency of administration and number of insufflations per administration must be determined for each individual. Provided that careful attention is paid to the method of insufflation, use of this preparation can often replace the need for intramuscular injection of Pitressin. One insufflation may produce antidiuretic activity for 3 to 6 hours. In our experience it has been particularly useful in children who are old enough to administer the preparation to themselves. The material is dispensed in 5 ml. vials which contain enough material for about 50 insufflations. One vial will last for five to seven days, especially if the patient is able to administer the preparation, or have it administered, properly.

Lysine vasopressin spray may be less effective during times when the nasal mucosa is inflamed. At this time it may be necessary to fall back on the use of Pitressin Tannate in Oil. The lysine vasopressin spray is not to be confused with Pituitrin Powder, also administered by nasal insufflation. This material is more irritating to the nasal mucosa than is the aqueous spray and, in our experience, is much less effective.

CHLORPROPAMIDE THERAPY. Chlorpropamide, administered orally, may be useful in some children with diabetes insipidus. Used widely as an oral hypoglycemic agent, it also appears to sensitize the renal tubules to the action of circulating vasopressin. It may be effective, then, in those subjects in whom small quantities of vasopressin can still be secreted by the neurohypophysis. The major advantage of chlorpropamide therapy is the ease of administration, but occurrence of hypoglycemia may seriously limit its usefulness. It has been suggested that the initial dose should be 250 mg. per square meter a day, in three divided doses (Vallet et al.). The dosage may then be increased or decreased, depending on the occurrence of untoward symptoms. Initial adjustment of dosage should probably be carried out under carefully controlled conditions, such as in a hospital.

References

Hochman, I. H., Laron, Z., Karp, M., Pertzelan, A., and Dolberg, L.: Effect of Gonadotropin Therapy on Testicular Volume and Sexual Development in Adolescent Boys with Hypogonadotropic Hypogonadism. *Arch. Dis. Child.*, 46:378, 1971.

Kaplan, S. A.: Hypopituitarism; in L. I. Gardner (ed.): *Endocrine and Genetic Diseases of Childhood.* Philadelphia, W. B. Saunders Company, 1969, p. 98.

Lippe, B. M., Wong, S.-L., R., and Kaplan, S. A.: Simultaneous Assessment of Growth Hormone and ACTH Reserve in Children Pretreated with Diethylstilbestrol. *J. Clin. Endocr.*, 33: 949, 1971.

Vallet, H. L., Prasad, M., and Goldbloom, R. B.: Chlorpropamide Treatment of Diabetes Insipidus in Children. *Pediatrics*, 45:246, 1970.

Disorders of the Ovaries

See page 424: Disorders of the Uterus, Uterine Tubes and Ovaries; and Tumors of the Uterus, Tubes and Ovaries.

Excessively Tall Stature in Adolescent Girls

JOHN D. CRAWFORD, M.D.

In our society the tall girl is admired. Her stature is an asset for a number of prestigious careers. Nonetheless, excessive tallness can be a handicap. It makes for difficulty in purchase of smart clothes; the victim is ineligible for certain professional positions, such as airline hostess; it poses problems in selection of a suitable dancing partner. But foremost is the injury of self-consciousness in the early teenage years when girls are so exquisitely sensitive.

Unusually tall stature is most often the result of abundant good health, a high plane of nutrition and certain normal predisposing genetic factors. Although tallness in close relatives, particularly parents, favors excess statural growth, tallness in the mother is of greater consequence than that occurring in the father. The frequency with which one finds that both parents are the tallest members of their sibships (heights being expressed as centiles to eliminate sex differences) suggests that what would be termed, in agriculture, "selective breeding," plays an important role. Unduly tall stature is also associated with a number of pathologic conditions, all rare, but of importance to consider when confronted by a young lady concerned about her height. These include the Marfan syndrome, homocystinuria, acromegaly, latent diabetes mellitus, thyrotoxicosis, neurofibromatosis, cerebral gigantism, anovarism (not gonadal dysgenesis) and the feminizing testis syndrome. The list does not include precocious puberty, for the excessive growth in this disorder is seen in the midportion of the first decade; at maturity, short stature is the rule. Nonetheless, it was this "experiment of nature" which gave the clue to appropriate therapy of girls who early in the second decade face the prospect of ultimately achieving a degree of lineal growth which will pose a handicap in adulthood.

It is well to consider therapy before growth has already progressed to an ultimately undesirable extent, for stature can be reduced only through drastic surgical measures. Prediction tables based on height, age and bone maturation provide a reliable means of assessing ultimate statural achievement (Bayley and Pinneau, Greulich and Pyle). Accordingly, such an estimate of adult stature should always be made in a girl presenting herself for treatment, and this should be coupled with careful serial measurements to determine the current growth rate and how closely the estimate is being realized. Height measurements must be carefully taken without footwear and under standardized conditions if they are to prove useful in estimating growth velocity over short intervals. At any one time, three measurements are desirable, and height is taken as the mean of these if the spread is not greater than ½ inch. One's height on arising in the morning is as much as an inch greater than at the end of the day because of the gradual compression of the intervertebral discs. Accordingly, an estimate of growth velocity over a month's interval could be erroneously low if the initial measurements are obtained in the morning, the latter in the afternoon.

Because there is no definition of what constitutes too tall stature, this must be discussed between patients, parents and physician, and a "ceiling" set. Choice of a figure less than 68 inches would seem inappropriate in most of our societies. Experience suggests, however, that the majority of women whose height has exceeded 70 inches consider themselves at a disadvantage. Conversations prior to instituting therapy should stress that treatment is demanding. To be effective it must be continued over many months and administered in accord with an exacting schedule. Certain undesirable side effects, especially morning sickness at the start and, later, undue weight gain, may be encountered. Safety can be assured both from the health and fertility records of women with idiopathic sexual precocity (Novak) and from observations during and following treatment of patients of the type presently being considered. This is not to deny that there are risks. The newspapers carry so many stories about the hazards of estrogen-containing contraceptive medications and stilbestrol that to avoid, at the least, mental anguish, the physician must discuss openly what is known and not known about the relationship between the drugs employed and unpleasant possible sequelae, such as tumors and vascular catastrophe. Doubts over whether it is right to "interfere with nature" must be resolved. Unwise is the physician who presses treatment on the unprepared family or less than a highly motivated patient.

Treatment. The treatment recommended in our clinic is sustained high dosage estrogen. Although it was the drug of choice for many years, the unfavorable notoriety given stilbestrol following its association with vaginal adenocarcinoma (Herbst et al.) has led us to substitute other drugs since 1971. The primary mode of estrogen action is inhibition of hepatic elaboration of sulfation factor (somatomedin) under the influence of pituitary growth hormone (Wiedemann and Schwartz). Growth hormone itself has no direct influence on the skeleton but exerts its stimulation through this "second messenger." Because growth during treatment slows or ceases long before epiphyses close, the hastening of epiphyseal fusion is a secondary manifestation of therapy. Table 1 gives the estrogenic preparations with which there has been substantial experience, and our recommended dosages. Also shown are the progestational agents which have been principally employed, their purpose being to promote regular menses. Experience suggests that it is easier for the teenage girl to remember to take her progesterone pills on the first five calendar days of each month than to attempt a lunar cycle. It would appear unwise to recommend that estrogen be omitted at the end of the progesterone course and for the duration of

TABLE 1. Preparations Employed in the Treatment of Excessively Tall Stature in Adolescent Girls

Estrogen (daily, every day)*	
Ethinyl estradiol	0.30 mg.
Diethylstilbestrol	5.00 mg.
Conjugated estrogens (Premarin)	10.00 mg.
Progesterone (taken with estrogen on first five calendar days each month)	
Norethindrone (Norlutin)	5.00 mg.
Medroxyprogesterone acetate (Provera)	5.00 mg.
Ethisterone (Pranone)	25.00 mg.

REGIMEN

1. Start with approximately one-quarter the ultimate recommended estrogen dose and increase to one-half at the end of the first week, three-quarters at the end of the second week and to the full treatment dose at the end of the third week. (In the post-menarchial girl begin four days after the start of menses.)
2. Progesterone in full dosage is given along with estrogen on the first five days of every month.
3. Continue with the above until skeletal maturation is equal to that of a 16-year-old girl (hand and wrist films) and bony union of the epiphyses at the distal femora and proximal tibiae is well underway. Terminate medication after combined course of estrogen and progesterone.

* These doses are approximately 10-fold larger than those necessary for replacement therapy in ovarian deficiency states or those used in contraceptive medications. Nevertheless, they are the lowest doses that will achieve the desired results in this particular application.

menses, because there is indication that rapid "escape growth" is thereby favored (Wettenhall and Roche).

Desirable and untoward effects of treatment are shown in Table 2. Acceleration of secondary sexual development in the relatively immature patient is listed as a desirable influence of medication, because treatment should be held in abeyance until this inevitable consequence is viewed with favor. Virtual freedom from adolescent acne is shown as a dividend of treatment. It should not be construed, however, that the hormonal therapy, at least the use of estrogen at such high levels, is recommended for treatment of acne. The pigmentation of the nipples, areolae, labia minora, linea alba and café-au-lait nevi is less marked with ethinyl estradiol and conjugated estrogens than with diethylstilbestrol. Occasionally, pigmentation will involve the creases of the neck giving rise to what we have termed "the dirty neck syndrome." Morning nausea is transient, seldom lasting in excess of one week. It has been experienced by 17 per cent of girls in our series, but in only 4 per cent has the symptom been severe enough to warrant loss of a day from school. A slow build-up of medication, ingestion of crackers and orange juice before arising and Dramamine (dimenhydrinate), 50 mg. as necessary, will avert distressing symptoms. Night cramps are increased in frequency during treatment. Once brought to our attention, 18 per cent of girls responded affirmatively to questioning about this symptom. Urticaria due to norethisterone has been seen twice; in both instances the problem was solved by changing to another progesterone preparation.

TABLE 2. Effects of Treatment

DESIRABLE

- Rapid slowing and cessation of lineal growth
- Accelerated epiphyseal closure: two years' maturation per calendar year
- Accelerated development of secondary sexual characteristics
- Amelioration of adolescent acne

UNDESIRABLE

- "Morning sickness":
  - Start estrogen slowly
  - Dramamine, 50 mg. p.r.n.
- Pigmentation (less with ethinyl estradiol than with diethylstilbestrol)
- Night cramps
- Urticaria due to progesterone
- Menometrorrhagia
- Obesity
- Hypertension

POTENTIAL HAZARDS

- Thromboembolism; vascular catastrophe
- Precipitation of diabetes mellitus and hyperlipemia
- Neoplasms of the genital tract
- Breast cancer

Intermenstrual bleeding has been encountered in 9 per cent of girls during treatment. In each instance it has responded promptly to temporary doubling of the estrogen dosage. The usual treatment level can be reinstituted immediately following the next course of progesterone, which is properly postponed one month if bleeding has been prolonged and profuse. Because mild menometrorrhagic episodes are not unusual in untreated adolescent girls, it is difficult to assess the importance of this complication. A tendency to excessive weight gain during treatment has been noted both in this clinic and by Wettenhall and Roche. Weight control during treatment is more troublesome for girls already plump at the start. In our series the mean weight gain rose from 2.75 kg. for the last six months before therapy to 4.31 kg. during the first six months of treatment. Fluid retention has not been clinically evident. A slight elevation of blood pressure has been evident in 37 per cent of girls during treatment. Thromboembolic phenomena have not been seen, although experience with the contraceptive medications indicates that these must be considered a potential hazard. Because of the inherent structural abnormalities of the aorta and other large vessels in the Marfan syndrome and the increased susceptibility, especially during pregnancy, to dissecting aneurysms and thromboembolic disease, estrogen therapy for control of the tendency to excessive statural growth must be undertaken with great caution (Manalo-Estrella and Barker). In any patient the possibility of increasing the risk of stroke by estrogen therapy must be considered (Collaborative Group for the Study of Stroke in Young Women).

The two potential hazards most worrisome for parents are the induction of tumors of the breast and genital tract. The report by Herbst et al. of clear cell vaginal adenocarcinoma in young women of mothers who received large doses of stilbestrol or one of its congeners during pregnancy has received widespread publicity. If, as seems to be the case, this is the result of a drug-induced developmental anomaly, the entrapment of mullerian tissue in a "hostile" environment beneath the vaginal epithelium, the hazard is not germane to the treatment under discussion. Possibly of much more importance is the risk of late development of adenosquamous carcinoma of the endometrium. Five instances of this unusual disorder, also possibly a phenomenon of entrapment of tissue in an ectopic location, were reported by Cutler et al. in relatively young women on long-term estrogen therapy for gonadal dysgenesis. Although aneuploidy may have been more important than the drugs employed (stilbestrol), the authors stress the possibility that "prolonged unopposed action of estrogen may have a role in endometrial carcinogenesis." This possibility, as well as the more effective control of growth and lesser incidence of menstrual irregularities, has led us to advocate the use of cyclic progesterone to ensure a more complete monthly shedding of the decidua than may be the case in schedules such as that of Schoen et al., where estrogen alone is employed and menses are the product of intermittent withdrawal.

Two cases of ovarian cyst were detected by Wettenhall, one during treatment and one at post-treatment follow-up (personal communication) in his series of over 100 Australian girls; one has been encountered in the Boston experience. A fibroadenoma of the breast was detected in a patient after four months of treatment, but the tumor was probably unrelated to medication inasmuch as breast asymmetry had been noted prior to commencing therapy. There is as yet no unanimity of medical opinion in regard to the potential of estrogen as used in this application or as employed by the vastly larger group of young women for contraception to augment the risk of late development of breast carcinoma (Vessey et al.).

When growth in the individual patient has progressed to within 2 inches or less of the "ceiling" set in preliminary discussions, its velocity is high, the prediction tables suggest a greater than desired ultimate stature and both patient and parents are enthusiastic to proceed, therapy should be initiated irrespective of the stage of adolescent development. It is best, if the child is premenarchial, if she is growing rapidly and if the estimate of ultimate achievement is much in excess of desired height, to commence treatment while there is yet more than an inch of leeway. Whitelaw et al. have suggested that in such instances estrogen acts initially to stimulate growth. We have not seen this in the present context, in all probability because we reserve treatment for an older age group. Estrogen in the prepubertal girl or the child with gonadal dysgenesis appears to stimulate the adrenal activity responsible for the so-called adolescent growth spurt. The mechanism, a relative blockade in the adrenal 3 β-hydroxysteroid dehydrogenase activity, has recently been elucidated by Sobrinho et al. In postmenarchial girls whose growth is already slowing, treatment can be withheld until they reach ½ inch or less of the desired limit, particularly when their predicted mature height is not far above this. In many of these girls, growth will cease short of the "ceiling," making intervention unnecessary.

Treatment is initiated with approximately one-quarter the ultimate recommended daily estrogen dose and moved up by equal increments at weekly intervals until the final, steady level is reached. In the postmenarchial girl it is well to commence treatment within four to six days after the beginning of menses.

Once undertaken, treatment should be continued until skeletal maturation has advanced to equal that of the average 16-year-old girl. Films are generally obtained at six-month intervals. A single view of the hand suffices if it includes all structures from the distal ends of the radius and ulna to the tips of the terminal phalanges and is taken with the palm flat on the cassette and the fingers slightly spread. Maturation ordinarily proceeds during therapy at a rate of two years' advance for each chronologic year. Even at the point when maturation has progressed to the 16-year level as judged by films of the hand, medication should not be discontinued until an anterior radiographic view of the knees shows bony union

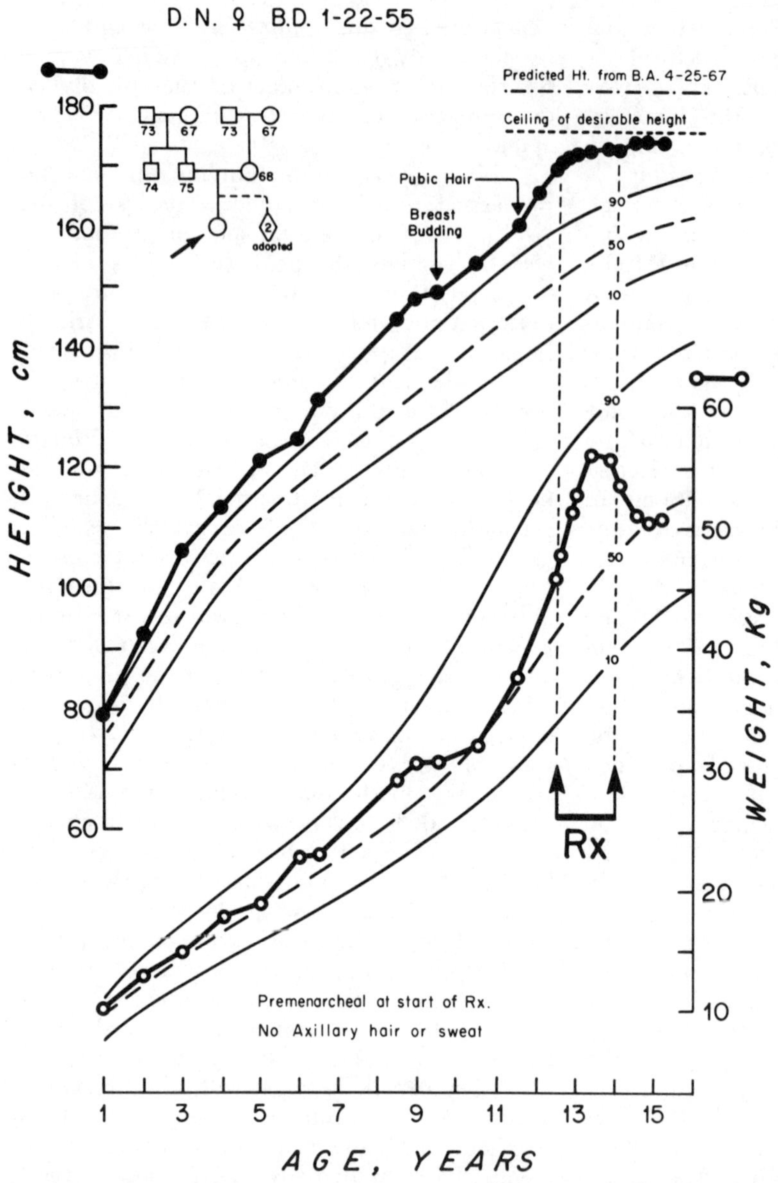

FIGURE 1. Effect of stilbestrol and cyclic norethindrone treatment in a 12-year, seven-month-old girl with unusually tall stature. Pubertal changes with acceleration of lineal growth and weight gain began at 10 years, 8 months. The bone age at onset of treatment was 12 years and predicted adult height was 72.0 inches (183 cm.). The first menstrual period occurred following the initial course of progesterone. Lineal growth began to slow promptly after beginning treatment. The 20-month course was terminated when bone age reached 16 years and closure of the epiphyses at the knees was well advanced. Spontaneous menses and a midcycle elevation of basal body temperature indicating ovulation were resumed when treatment was discontinued. Note the accelerated weight gain during therapy and weight loss on its completion, as well as the brief period during which statural growth was resumed at the end of treatment.

of the epiphyses at the distal femora and proximal tibiae, because these are the last areas which contribute substantially to statural growth. Medication should be terminated following a final regular course of progesterone. The first spontaneous period ordinarily is seen within six weeks of that which immediately follows withdrawal of medication. We have not encountered significant post-treatment menstrual irregularities, and basal body temperature records indicate prompt appearance of normal ovulatory cycles. Eleven girls have married and have in aggregate 16 children, suggesting no impairment of fertility.

An example of response to treatment is shown in Figure 1. Although such an abrupt slowing of growth while epiphyses remain open may rarely take place spontaneously, its general occurrence with the type of therapy recommended here attests to the efficacy of the treatment. This is further indicated by the fact that in three patients therapy has been prematurely interrupted with prompt resumption of growth at the pretreatment velocity.

In view of the undesirable side effects and potential hazards, girls should be closely followed during treatment and kept track of for a prolonged period thereafter. We schedule a return for examination at six weeks after initiation of treatment and at three-month intervals thereafter, through a visit three months following termination of therapy. A final return is scheduled one year later and reports sought by letter or telephone subsequently at five-year intervals. In addition to inquiries about menstruation, each visit should include measurements of height, weight and blood pressure and palpation of the breasts. Rectal examinations are done on all girls prior to treatment and repeated annually; there should be no hesitation to undertake a pelvic examination if circumstances warrant.

It remains to be considered whether there are other modes of treatment to weigh against that outlined here. Epiphyseal stapling or other direct orthopedic measures would appear less desirable because of the surgical scars and the hazards of asymmetric responses. The danger of late neoplasia interdicts use of selective epiphyseal radiation. Although the effectiveness of cortisone in slowing statural growth is all too well documented, other undesirable side effects disqualify its use. Pituitary irradiation, although useful in acromegaly, merits no consideration in the present context (Saxena and Crawford, Beck et al., Linfoot and Greenwood).

Finally, the method recommended is safe and has given satisfactory and virtually identical results in this clinic and in that of Wettenhall. In both, well over 100 girls have been treated (Table 3). Another experience has also been similar: far more girls have presented for treatment than it has been necessary or desirable to subject to this program.

TABLE 3. Results of Treatment*

Age at beginning of treatment	12.9 yr.†
Skeletal age	13.2 yr.
Pre- vs. postmenarchial patients	58:42
Height at start of treatment	68.5 in.
Predicted mature height	71.9 in.
Actual mature height	69.5 in.‡
Duration of treatment	17.2 mo.
Total cases	100.0

* Uniform regimen: Diethylstilbestrol, 5 mg. daily without interruption; norethindrone, 5 mg. daily on first five calendar days of month.

† Figures indicate averages.

‡ Based on measurements one year after termination of treatment.

References

Bayley, N., and Pinneau, S. R.: Tables for Predicting Adult Height from Skeletal Age: Revised for Use with the Greulich-Pyle Hand Standards. *J. Pediat.*, 40:423, 1952. (Reprinted in Greulich and Pyle, pp. 231–251; see below.)

Beck, P., Schalch, D. S., Parker, M. L., Kipnis, D. L., and Daughaday, W. A.: Correlative Studies of Growth Hormone and Insulin Plasma Concentrations with Metabolic Abnormalities in Acromegaly. *J. Lab. & Clin. Med.*, 66:366, 1965.

Collaborative Group for the Study of Stroke in Young Women: Oral Contraception and Increased Risk of Cerebral Ischemia or Thrombosis. *New England J. Med.*, 288:871, 1973.

Cutler, B. S., Forbes, A. P., Ingersoll, F. M., and Scully, R. E.: Endometrial Carcinoma after Stilbestrol Therapy in Gonadal Dysgenesis. *New England J. Med.*, 287:628, 1972.

Greulich, W. W., and Pyle, S. I.: *Radiographic Atlas of Skeletal Development of the Hand and Wrist.* 2nd ed. Stanford, California, Stanford University Press, 1959.

Herbst, A. L., Ulfelder, H., and Poskanzer, D. C.: Adenocarcinoma of the Vagina: Association of Maternal Stilbestrol Therapy with Tumor Appearance in Young Women. *New England J. Med.*, 284: 878, 1971.

Linfoot, J. A., and Greenwood, F. C.: Growth Hormone in Acromegaly; Effect of Heavy Particle Pituitary Irradiation. *J. Clin. Endocrin.*, 25:1515, 1965.

Manalo-Estrella, P., and Barker, A. E.: Histopathologic Findings in Human Aortic Media Associated with Pregnancy: A Study of 16 Cases. *Arch. Path.*, 83: 336, 1967.

Novak, E.: The Constitutional Type of Female Precocious Puberty with a Report of 9 cases. *Am. J. Obstet. & Gynec.*, 47:20, 1944.

Saxena, K. M., and Crawford, J. D.: Acromegalic Gigantism in an Adolescent Girl. *J. Pediat.*, 62:660, 1963.

Schoen, E. J., Solomon, I. L., Warner, O., and Wingerd, J.: Estrogen Treatment of Tall Girls. *Am. J. Dis. Child.*, 125:71, 1973.

Sobrinho, L. G., Kase, N., and Grunt, J. A.: Changes in Adrenocortical Function of Patients with Gonadal Dysgenesis after Treatment with Estrogen. *J. Clin. Endocrin.*, 33:110, 1971.

Vessey, M. P., Doll, R., and Sutton, P. M.: Oral Contraceptives and Breast Neoplasia: A Retrospective Study. *Brit. J. Med.*, 3:719, 1972.

Wettenhall, H. N. B., and Roche, A. F.: Tall Girls: Assessment and Management. *Aust. Paediat. J.*, 1:210, 1965.

Whitelaw, M. J., Foster, T. N., and Graham, W. H.: Estradiol Valerate: Its Effects on Anabolism and Skeletal Age in the Prepubertal Girl. *J. Clin. Endocrin.*, 23:1125, 1963.

Wiedemann, E., and Schwartz, E.: Suppression of Growth Hormone-Dependent Human Serum Sulfation Factor by Estrogen. *J. Clin. Endocrin.*, 34:51, 1972.

Thyroid Disease

BORIS SENIOR, M.D.

The management of thyroid disorders in children requires as much diagnostic precision as in adults as well as an appreciation of the vagaries imposed by the pediatric setting. In the adult, lack of thyroid hormone produces a distressing yet reversible disease, but in infancy the same lack may result in permanent curtailment of intellect. Hyperthyroidism in the newborn is of limited and relatively brief duration but may pose a threat to life, whereas in the older child it runs an inordinately tenacious and prolonged course. Treatment based solely on the nature of the drug to be employed and its dose does not suffice.

THYROID DISEASE IN THE NEWBORN

Except in areas of severe iodine deficiency, thyroid disease in the newborn is in most instances consequent upon maternal drug ingestion, maternal thyroid disease or a combination of both. Iodides readily cross the placenta and, if taken by the mother usually for the treatment of asthma, may produce a goiter in the newborn. Such a goiter may be exceedingly large and occasionally may produce respiratory embarrassment. In addition, iodide-induced hypothyroidism may be present. If the airway is compromised, surgical intervention may be necessary. Either partial thyroidectomy or tracheostomy has been performed in such patients. In most cases, however, simple extension of the neck over a sandbag relieves the respiratory difficulty. Tracheal intubation has also proved successful. Close observation is essential for the initial few days.

Both the enlargement of the thyroid and the hypothyroidism, if present, spontaneously remit over a period of weeks. Recovery is hastened by the administration of U.S.P. thyroid extract in a dose of 30 mg. once daily for two or three weeks.

Hyperthyroidism in the newborn rarely arises de novo, maternal hyperthyroidism being present during pregnancy or preceding it. It is thought that a humoral agent, which may be long-acting thyroid stimulator, crosses the placenta and produces hyperthyroidism in the newborn. If an antithyroid drug, such as propylthiouracil, has been used for treatment of the mother during pregnancy, it, too, will pass across the placenta and affect the fetal thyroid. Depending upon the transplacental passage of long-acting thyroid stimulator and the treatment of the mother, the infant may have hyperthyroidism or be euthyroid or even hypothyroid.

Hyperthyroidism may range in severity from a mild illness almost escaping recognition to a state resembling thyroid storm. Congestive heart failure may occur and fatalities have been reported. In mild cases treatment may consist of iodides alone, such as a saturated solution of potassium iodide, 0.05 ml. (1 drop) three times daily. Improvement should be seen within 48 hours and treatment should be continued for a week or two. Propylthiouracil in a dose of 10 mg. every 8 hours should be administered to infants with more severe hyperthyroidism. Treatment with propylthiouracil may be needed for several weeks, by which time permanent remission occurs. Digitalis, oxygen and parenteral fluids may also be required. In the extremely ill infant there are theoretical grounds for the use of adrenergic blocking agents, such as guanethidine.

HYPOTHYROIDISM IN INFANCY

The major factor influencing the success of therapy of hypothyroidism in infancy is the promptness with which the diagnosis is made and adequate treatment begun rather than the use of one form of hormonal therapy as opposed to another. Commonly the diagnosis in such children is first made at three to four months of age, by which time the physical signs resulting from thyroid deficiency are gross. Regardless of whether the hormonal deficiency results from absence of the thyroid, functional inadequacy of a displaced thyroid or a metabolic disorder involving the synthesis of hormone, the treatment is the same, i.e., U.S.P. thyroid extract, 15 mg., is given once daily by mouth with incremental increases of 15 mg. every fourth day to 45 mg. The dose by six months is usually 60 mg. daily; 90 mg., once daily, may be given between nine months and a year. The eventual maintenance dose of thyroid extract is 120 to 180 mg. per day. Following initiation of treatment the dosage level is adjusted on the bases of the clinical state of the child and the results of measurement of the protein-bound iodine, which should be in the range of 6 to 8 micrograms per 100 ml. The use of triiodothyronine or of levothyroxine offers little therapeutic advantage over U.S.P. thyroid extract and complicates management by changing the protein-bound iodine values from the accustomed range.

A large goiter may be present in infants who have metabolic defects which cause impairment of synthesis of thyroid hormone. With the replacement therapy as outlined, the goiter usually regresses and hypothyroidism, if present, is corrected. However, if treatment is unduly delayed, a disfiguring mass may remain and surgical excision may be needed.

It is essential that the mother know that therapy must be lifelong. Patients should be seen at regular intervals and the level of protein-bound iodine measured at least once annually. Despite excellent results in terms of physical development, the majority of these patients have already suffered irreparable intellectual damage. Psychometric examinations are desirable so that appropriate schooling may be planned from the beginning.

JUVENILE HYPOTHYROIDISM

Rarely hypothyroidism may occur spontaneously in children. More often it appears to follow the inability of a misplaced and maldeveloped thyroid to produce enough hormone for the needs of the growing child. This problem may be rendered more acute by ill-advised surgical excision. Later onset of hypothyroidism renders damage to the central nervous system less likely, but impairment of growth may be marked. The dose of thyroid extract for the older child is approximately 120 to 180 mg.

daily. Regular visits with estimations of the protein-bound iodine are needed to ensure adherence to the dosage schedule.

HYPERTHYROIDISM

There are three forms of therapy that may be employed for hyperthyroidism in childhood. No single form of treatment has universal support, which indicates that none is without disadvantage.

In adults the efficacy of radioiodine in the treatment of hyperthyroidism has been repeatedly demonstrated. An increased incidence of malignancy attributable to the treatment has not been found. Many hold, however, that sufficient time has not elapsed since its introduction to absolve it as a potential carcinogen. With 60 years or more as the expected life of the child after treatment, it seems that concern about the long-range effects of ^{131}iodine will take many years to abate. Of more practical note is the observation that hypothyroidism, long known to occur in 10 per cent of treated patients in the first two years, continued to appear in about 3 per cent of patients each succeeding year. Projection of this figure suggests that hypothyroidism would be almost inevitable in the child so treated.

Together, these two factors make one reluctant to use radioiodine as the first choice of treatment for childhood hyperthyroidism.

Surgery produces permanent remission in the majority of cases of hyperthyroidism of childhood. Unfortunately, a substantial minority fare less well. Figures vary with the type of operation performed, but about 20 per cent have a recurrence or develop hypothyroidism. A very much smaller but not negligible number may develop hypoparathyroidism or suffer section of the recurrent laryngeal nerve. With adequate preoperative medical preparation, fatalities are extremely rare.

Because reports tend to emanate from the larger centers, published figures may in fact be the best and the hazard may be greater in centers where such patients are less frequently treated. The inclination, therefore, is to reserve surgery or radioiodine for patients who are unwilling or unable to adhere to the rigorous schedule and prolonged course imposed by medical management, or for whom such medical treatment has manifestly failed. However, if surgery is decided upon, medical management in preparation for the operation should include treatment with an antithyroid drug, such as propylthiouracil, approximately 5 mg. per kilogram per day in three equally spaced doses for two weeks, at which time 0.1 ml. of saturated solution of potassium iodide three times daily is added for the 10 days immediately preceding the operation.

Antithyroid drugs remain the first choice for treatment of hyperthyroidism in childhood, the two most widely used being propylthiouracil and methimazole (Tapazole). Disadvantages include the necessity for extending the treatment over two years or more and the need for administering the drug at spaced intervals. When close supervision is not possible and the family is unwilling or unable to assume the burden of such responsibility, treatment with antithyroid drugs should not be undertaken. Untoward reactions, such as rashes and joint pains, may occur in approximately 5 per cent of patients treated with either propylthiouracil or methimazole, and necessitate changing from the one drug to the other. Agranulocytosis occurs in a much smaller percentage.

The initial dose of propylthiouracil is 5 mg. per kilogram per day divided into three equally spaced doses; the initial dose of methimazole is 0.3 to 0.4 mg. per kilogram per day, also in three spaced doses. Once control is achieved, the dose should be reduced but still given in divided portions. If very small amounts suffice, administration twice or even once daily may be satisfactory. Initially visits should be made at monthly intervals and later bimonthly. Clinical assessment and measurement of the protein-bound iodine enable appropriate adjustment of the drug dose. Allowance must be made for the emotional lability which is so often present in hyperthyroidism and the stresses it imposes on the family.

If hypothyroidism is induced by the treatment, the gland will enlarge under the influence of secreted thyroid-stimulating hormone (TSH). This normally necessitates a prompt reduction of dosage. A reduction in gland size during treatment augurs well for a lasting remission, as does suppression of ^{131}iodine uptake after three weeks of therapy with thyroid extract.

When treatment is stopped, the induced remission may be indefinitely sustained. Unfortunately approximately 50 per cent of patients have a relapse and of that group a majority will have a relapse again following re-treatment. It is apparent that the medical management of childhood hyperthyroidism is not simple, swift or necessarily successful, and it is essential that this be fully understood by the family.

SUBACUTE THYROIDITIS

The patient with subacute thyroiditis presents with tenderness and often enlargement of the thyroid. A history of recent streptococcal infection, of mumps or of a nonspecific febrile illness may be obtained. The sedimentation rate is often elevated and the ^{131}iodine uptake low. Thyroglobulin antibodies may be present. In some the illness is mild and subsides without the need for special measures. In others the administration of thyroid extract, 4 mg. per kilogram, will cause marked improvement. Treatment may be continued for three to six months. If symptoms recur when treatment is discontinued, thyroid extract may again be given. Patients who are refractory to thyroid extract or who experience marked pain and tenderness may be helped by the addition of prednisone, 3 mg. per kilogram, administered as a single dose on alternate days. Occasionally hypothyroidism ensues and maintenance therapy with thyroid extract is required.

CHRONIC LYMPHOCYTIC THYROIDITIS (HASHIMOTO'S DISEASE)

Chronic lymphocytic thyroiditis is probably the most common cause of thyroid enlargement in the adolescent girl. The diagnosis is supported by finding thyroglobulin antibodies and a BEI (butanol-extractable iodine) that is disproportionately low in relation to the level of protein-bound iodine. Most patients are euthyroid when first observed. Treatment with thyroid extract, 120 to 180 mg. administered for months, will in most patients effect regression of the goiter. Hypothyroidism is a not uncommon sequela of this disorder and requires continued therapy with thyroid extract.

SIMPLE GOITER

The term simple goiter is often used to refer to the thyroid enlargement observed in girls during early adolescence. Because chronic lymphocytic thyroiditis is the most common cause of such enlargement, it appears that the diagnosis is often erroneous. In many the enlargement is slight, and one suspects that a physiologic variation rather than a pathologic process is the cause. If the enlargement is slight and the patient euthyroid, a conservative approach is warranted because spontaneous regression may occur. Cosmetic considerations apply when the goiter is larger, and thyroid extract, 120 to 180 mg., may then be used. Occasionally the goiter is a later manifestation of a congenital impairment of synthesis of hormone and the patient is hypothyroid. Thyroid extract is indicated and should be continued.

CARCINOMA

The controversy surrounding the treatment of hyperthyroidism pales before the conflict attendant on the management of thyroid carcinoma.

By far the greatest number of cases of this rare childhood disease are of the papillary variety, with follicular carcinoma making up most of the remainder. The natural progression of the malignancies is extremely slow, and survival for scores of years is documented. It appears that both these tumors are exquisitely thyrotropin-dependent, and regression of tumor mass and of metastases has been repeatedly observed to follow suppression of thyrotropin secretion by the administration of thyroid extract. Furthermore, simple excision of the tumor, which is rarely complete because of its multifocal origin within the thyroid, may stimulate secretion of thyroid-stimulating hormone (TSH) and more rapid tumor growth.

It is believed by some that the beneficial effects claimed for excision of the thyroid may actually result from the concomitant substitution therapy with thyroid extract. Few now favor the extensive and mutilating excisions performed in the past. The present disagreement then is whether thyroid therapy alone is best or whether a limited excision should also be done. Regardless of the decision made, thyroid therapy should be continued, and the dose administered should be sufficient to reduce the uptake of a tracer dose of radioiodine to 10 per cent or less, ensuring suppression of secretion of TSH.

The extremely rare undifferentiated carcinomas do not respond to thyroid therapy, and the prognosis is poor regardless of the treatment.

References

Astwood, E. B.: Problem of Nodules in Thyroid Gland. *Pediatrics,* 18:501, 1956.

Astwood, E. B., and Cassidy, C. E.: Treatment of Goiter and Thyroid Nodules with Thyroid. *J.A.M.A.,* 174: 459, 1960.

Hayek, A., Chapman, E. M., and Crawford, J. D.: Long-term Results of Treatment of Thyrotoxicosis in Children and Adolescents with Radioactive Iodine. *New England J. Med.,* 283:949, 1970.

Man, E. B., Mermann, A. C., and Cooke, R. E.: The Development of Children with Congenital Hypothyroidism. *J. Pediat.,* 63:926, 1963.

Root, A. W.: Cancer of the Thyroid in Childhood and Adolescence. *Am. J. Med. Sci.,* 246:734, 1963.

Rosenberg, D., Grand, M. J. H., and Silbert, D.: Neonatal Hyperthyroidism. *New England J. Med.,* 268: 292, 1963.

Saxena, K. M., Crawford, J. D., and Talbot, N. B.: Childhood Thyrotoxicosis: A Long-Term Perspective. *Brit. Med. J.,* 2:1153, 1964.

Parathyroid Disease

SHUN M. LING, M.D.

HYPOPARATHYROIDISM

Successful long-term management of hypoparathyroidism and associated disorders depends on early diagnosis and therapy.

I have found the following treatment regimen for acute symptomatic hypocalcemia to be safe and adequate, regardless of etiology, if renal function is normal, and if hypokalemia, hypomagnesemia, hypoglycemia or hypoalbuminemia is not coexisting. Acute tetany or seizures should be treated with intravenous administration of 10 per cent calcium gluconate given slowly over 20 minutes by syringe while monitoring apical pulse for bradycardia or cardiac arrhythmia. The following doses are recommended: for premature and newborn infants of less than 3000 Gm. body weight, give 5 ml.; for newborn infants of more than 3000 Gm. body weight, give 5 to 10 ml.; for infants more than one month of age and older children give 10 ml. Serum for calcium, potassium and glucose determinations should have been drawn just before therapy and therapy begun before results return if seizures are occurring. Intravenous administration of 50 per cent dextrose in water at 1 ml. per kilogram of body weight by syringe may need to be given if hypoglycemia is suspected in the neonate or infant, because coexisting hypoglycemia and hypocalcemia is not uncommon. The initial dose of intravenous calcium may be given again in 30 minutes if tetany or seizures continue.

Intramuscular injection of calcium salts should never be given. Infiltration of any calcium salts into the soft tissues should be strictly avoided, because the salts are irritating, sclerosing and poorly absorbed, and can cause tissue slough.

Coexisting hypokalemia and hypomagnesemia can produce paresthesias, muscle cramps, tetany and even seizures, and complicate the treatment of hypocalcemia. Hypokalemia tends to protect hypocalcemic and hypomagnesemic persons from overt tetany. If one elevates the serum potassium level in these patients by administration of intravenous potassium salts alone, this may precipitate overt tetany and seizures. Correction of hypocalcemia should precede correction of hypokalemia. Simultaneous intravenous calcium gluconate can be given with slower gradual correction of hypokalemia with low amounts of potassium chloride intravenously at 1 mEq. of potassium per kilogram of body weight or 20 to 30 mEq. of potassium per square meter of body surface area.

Attempts to correct hypokalemia or hypocalcemia only may aggravate symptomatic hypomagnesemia. Therefore, if serum levels of all three cations are low, one should first correct hypomagnesemia, then hypocalcemia and, last, hypokalemia. Intramuscular administration of 50 per cent magnesium sulfate (50 per cent $MgSO_4 \cdot 7H_2O$ contains 4 mEq. of magnesium per ml.) is preferred at 0.2 ml. per kilogram of body weight or 5 ml. per square meter every 12 hours initially, then once daily for seven to 10 days for older children. Serum magnesium should be monitored daily initially, then every few days to avoid hypermagnesemia. In infants, the initial dose should be 0.5 ml. of 50 per cent magnesium sulfate daily to a 4- to 7-kilogram infant and 1 ml. daily to a larger infant followed by 0.5 to 1.0 ml. daily for seven to 10 days.

Continuous intravenous calcium or multiple intermittent injections of 10 per cent calcium gluconate may be avoided by early administration of oral calcium chloride in concentrations less than 2 per cent to avoid gastric irritation at doses varying from 1 to 3 Gm. in divided dosage daily. In neonates, a dose of 1.5 Gm. of calcium chloride or 15 ml. of 10 per cent calcium chloride has usually been adequate and well tolerated if given for two days only by adding and mixing 2.5 ml. of the 10 per cent salt solution in each 4-hour bottle of formula. Oral calcium chloride is an acidifying agent and can be administered usually for only two days before causing hyperchloremic acidosis.

Hydrous calcium chloride contains 27.26 per cent calcium and is more readily absorbed by the intestinal tract probably because of its acidifying effect. Further oral maintenance therapy can be provided by administering calcium gluconate or calcium lactate daily in four to five divided doses for more efficient absorption. Hydrous calcium gluconate contains 9.31 per cent calcium and hydrous calcium lactate contains 18.37 per cent calcium.

Dietary calcium usually has to be doubled or tripled over the normal requirements for the patient's age before intestinal absorption of calcium is increased sufficiently to elevate the level of serum calcium. Therefore, in neonates, 400 to 600 mg. of supplementary calcium as 4 to 6 Gm. of calcium gluconate or lactate is necessary. In older children and adults, as much as 2 Gm. of supplementary calcium may be necessary as 20 tablets of calcium gluconate or lactate. Serum calcium should be monitored daily early, then every week thereafter. The duration of this therapy depends upon the etiology of hypocalcemia. Vitamin D therapy should not be administered for acute symptomatic hypocalcemia until the cause is known and indications for its use are established.

Neonatal tetany is a self-limiting condition that occurs usually at one to two days of age or after five to 10 days of age when formula feeding has begun. Prematurity, placental dysfunction, low birth weight, maternal diabetes and toxemia and abnormal labor are predisposing factors in patients in whom it has an early onset. Both groups can be differentiated from permanent congenital hypoparathyroidism or pseudohypoparathyroidism by maintenance of normal serum calcium levels after oral calcium therapy had been stopped. A gradual decrease in oral calcium over two to three weeks is advised to avoid tetany resulting from abrupt or rapid withdrawal of oral calcium.

Transient congenital hypoparathyroidism may be found in as many as 50 per cent of infants of mothers with hyperparathyroidism. This condition is self-limiting with return of parathyroid function usually to normal after three to four weeks of oral calcium supplement. Permanent hypoparathyroidism at the age of one year has occurred in one such infant. Spontaneous abortions and stillbirths may occur in 25 per cent of women with hyperparathyroidism. Some women may be asymptomatic, and the diagnosis of hyperparathyroidism may be missed. Therefore, serum calcium and phosphorus determinations should be made on all mothers of infants with neonatal tetany. Proper treatment of these mothers may prevent fetal mortality and neonatal tetany in future offspring.

Transient congenital idiopathic hypoparathyroidism has also been described by several groups in infants with persistent hypocalcemia until three to 12 months of age. These infants may present with tetany at any time during the first two months of age. Their response to the usual intravenous and oral calcium therapy is poor. Vitamin D in small doses of 1000 units daily or dihydrotachysterol, 0.5 mg. daily, has been given for several months and then discontinued. Some infants have responded to intramuscular injection of parathyroid extract with an increase in serum calcium and a decrease in serum phosphorus. Transient hypoparathyroidism is nonfamilial and reversible after six to 12 months of age without any further therapy.

Infants with congenital absence of the parathyroids and thymus (diGeorge's syndrome) present with neonatal tetany, hypocalcemia and even hypomagnesemia. The condition is also called pharyngeal III and IV pouch syndrome. Death has almost uniformly occurred within the first two years of life from overwhelming infection or cardiac arrest. Congenital malformations of the great vessels and facial features and nephrocalcinosis are common. Thymus-dependent cellular immunity, such as delayed hypersensitivity, is impaired. Management is difficult. Those patients respond to parathyroid extract. Their response to the usual intravenous and oral calcium therapy is poor. Magnesium therapy may help if hypomagnesemia is present. Vitamin D therapy should be given. Thymus and parathyroid transplants would be ideal therapy in these infants. Thymus transplant has been reported to restore immunologic function to normal in one infant.

Diagnosis of either idiopathic hypoparathyroidism or pseudohypoparathyroidism should be made before undertaking long-term management of either condition. Pseudohypoparathyroid patients differ from idiopathic hypoparathyroid patients by being refractory to the administration of exogenous parathyroid extract intramuscularly over five days and to the infusion of intravenous calcium. Parathyroid extract will cause an increase in serum calcium and a decrease in serum phosphorus and at least a fivefold increase in urinary phosphorus excretion in hypoparathyroid patients. Intravenous calcium given at 15 mg. per kilogram over 4 hours in 0.45 per cent normal saline (as 150 mg. of calcium gluconate per kilogram over 4 hours) usually produces an increase in serum calcium and phosphorus and a profound increase in urinary calcium and phosphorus excretion in hypoparathyroid subjects.

I have used the following doses of parathyroid extract safely. As soon as the serum calcium reaches 10 mg. per 100 ml., the extract is stopped. Parathyroid extract will wear off within 24 hours. The total daily dose is given in divided doses every 8 hours intramuscularly for as long as five days, if necessary. Newborn babies and infants less than six months of age are given 60 to 100 units daily, and older children and adolescents are given 600 units per square meter of body surface area up to a maximum of 600 units daily. Long-term therapy with crude parathyroid extract is not feasible because of the expense, need for daily injections and variable potency of various lots. Antibodies to the extract or hormone have not been a major problem with intramuscular usage.

The results, recently, of parathyroid hormone assays indicate increased parathyroid hormone secretion in peripheral blood, parathyroid glands and urine from patients with pseudohypoparathyroidism. Recently, thyrocalcitonin, a hypocalcemic polypeptide secreted by the thyroid gland in mammals, was found in high concentrations in thyroid glands of untreated pseudohypoparathyroid patients. Excessive thyrocalcitonin in the thyroid gland may not be the cause of hypocalcemia but the result of interference with hormone release as an adaptation to chronic hypocalcemia. Subtotal and total thyroidectomies have been reported in at least two children and two adults in an attempt to test whether thyrocalcitonin excess causes chronic tetany and secondary hyperparathyroidism. The results were poor in one group and encouraging in another. Therefore, I would strongly recommend withholding thyroidectomies as treatment of pseudohypoparathyroid patients and await further studies of its value by centers that can assay both parathyroid hormone and thyrocalcitonin.

Current therapy for pseudohypoparathyroidism is still similar to that for hypoparathyroidism, with large doses of vitamin D and oral calcium supplement. Clinically, it would appear that progression of enamel hypoplasia, subcutaneous and basal ganglia calcifications and mental retardation may be slowed or prevented. Early dietary counseling can prevent progression of exogenous obesity if started as early as possible in these children. Hypothyroidism may develop in these patients with or without overt myxedema and may or may not be associated with selective deficiency of thyrotropin secretion. Long-term therapy with desiccated thyroid is indicated in this group. However, one should be aware that protein-bound iodine and thyroxine iodine levels will usually remain low in spite of adequate therapy with exogenous thyroid in these patients.

Enamel hypoplasia and shallow, underdeveloped roots are causes of poor dentition in both hypoparathyroid and pseudohypoparathyroid patients. Proper dental hygiene and care should be continually stressed.

Patients with pseudopseudohypoparathyroidism present with the clinical and physical findings of pseudohypoparathyroid patients, but they do not have tetany, hypocalcemia or hyperphosphatemia. Subjects with both syndromes may occur in the same family, and adequate studies are necessary to separate them. Treatment with vitamin D and oral calcium is not necessary in pseudopseudohypoparathyroidism. Hypothyroidism may also be present and needs therapy with desiccated thyroid. Long-term follow-up and continued assessment of serum calcium and phosphorus is necessary in treating pseudohypoparathyroidism with vitamin D not only to avoid hypercalcemia but also because patients have spontaneously developed normocalcemia and normophosphatemia and evolved into pseudopseudohypoparathyroidism.

If hypoparathyroidism is the only problem, long-term management of hypocalcemia is with vitamin D and oral calcium supplement. I find that elevation of the serum calcium level to normal by vitamin D provides an excellent diagnostic-therapeutic differentiation of idiopathic hypoparathyroid from pseudohypoparathyroid patients. Since parathyroid hormone causes an increase in renal tubular reabsorption of calcium, the former group tends to have mild to marked hypercalciuria above normal levels of 2.4 mg. per kilogram per day when the serum calcium level rises above 9 to 10 mg. per 100 ml., whereas the latter group continues to have low to low-normal urinary calcium excretion. Therefore, periodic follow-up of serum calcium and 24-hour urinary calcium at least every two to three months is necessary while on maintenance vitamin D therapy to avoid hypercalciuria, renal stones, nephrocalcinosis and hypercalcemia. High fluid intake should be emphasized.

The usual vitamin D preparation prescribed is calciferol or ergocalciferol (vitamin D_2), which is available in 50,000-unit capsules or can be made up in vegetable oil in any concentration. One milligram of vitamin D contains 40,000 units. It is also available dissolved in propylene glycol (Drisdol suspension), which is water-soluble and recommended for patients with coexisting malabsorption syndrome with steatorrhea. Vitamin D is a fat-soluble vitamin, and its absorption is impaired when steatorrhea is present, as are vitamins K, A and E. The dose of vitamin D_2 varies in patients. The dose for an infant varies from 10,000 to 50,000 units and for an older child between 50,000 and 200,000 units daily. Increments of 10,000 to 50,000 units should be made no sooner than at two-week intervals until serum calcium and phosphorus levels reach normal. Pure crystalline dihydrotachysterol* has three times the potency of calciferol. Dihydrotachysterol has been effective in patients resistant to conventional vitamin D_2 therapy. Vitamin D_2 is stored in the liver and may take as long as a year to be metabolized in patients who have received

* Pure crystalline dihydrotachysterol can be obtained from Philips Roxane Company, New York, New York; it is now available as 0.2-mg. tablets.

an excess of it. Dihydrotachysterol is metabolized within a few weeks.

Oral calcium supplements are usually necessary during rapid growth but may be tapered off in some patients with normal milk intake. Phosphorus restriction and the use of aluminum hydroxide gel to bind dietary phosphorus is unnecessary in maintenance therapy. Normal calcium and phosphorus intake is necessary for normal growth while on vitamin D.

If malabsorption syndrome with steatorrhea occurs with hypoparathyroidism, avid retention of intravenous calcium and lack of response may occur temporarily with exogenous parathyroid hormone administration. Relative or absolute vitamin D deficiency due to the steatorrhea impairs the action of endogenous or exogenous parathyroid hormone. This lack of response reverses with administration of sufficient vitamin D. Chronic hypocalcemia may be a factor in development of steatorrhea, because correction of serum calcium has caused reversal of the steatorrhea in some patients. Similarly, chronic hypocalcemia is thought to be partly responsible for development of chronic atrophic gastritis, hypochlorhydria or achlorhydria. Malabsorption of vitamin B_{12} and folate, and pernicious anemia have developed in hypoparathyroid patients and may be familial. Therapeutic doses of oral vitamin B_{12} and folate or intramuscular vitamin B_{12} may be necessary after adequate diagnosis. Because of impairment in absorption of fat-soluble vitamins with steatorrhea, water-soluble multivitamins should be given at three times the minimal recommended daily requirements.

Hypoparathyroidism may occur with varying combinations of associated endocrinopathy, including adrenal insufficiency, thyroid disease, diabetes mellitus, pernicious anemia and candidiasis. There may or may not be a familial pattern. Therapy becomes more complex. Sudden hypercalcemia developing in a stable hypoparathyroid on previously satisfactory maintenance doses of vitamin D should lead one to suspect adrenal insufficiency. The need for vitamin D is usually increased considerably after adrenal insufficiency has been compensated by physiologic replacement doses of hydrocortisone (between 20 and 30 mg. per square meter daily). Although it may be necessary to treat candidiasis, the organisms have not been found in the glands. The current view is that candidiasis is not causally related to the syndrome but that these patients are susceptible to developing atrophic autoimmune diseases and candidiasis.

Long-term overall management of a patient with hypoparathyroidism or any of the associated disorders should, therefore, include continual surveillance for occult development of any of the other potential coexisting disorders. Circulating autoantibodies against a specific tissue are presumed to reflect subclinical disease of that tissue. Presence of specific circulating autoantibodies to thyroid epithelial cell cytoplasm or thyroglobulin may be followed by clinical manifestations of chronic lymphocytic thyroiditis with formation of a nontoxic goiter or hypothyroidism. Hypothyroidism causes decreased bone turnover of calcium and impaired mobilization of calcium from bone similar to that in hypoparathyroidism. Therefore, exceptionally large doses of vitamin D may be required to correct hypocalcemia in a patient with coexisting hypoparathyroidism and untreated hypothyroidism. A similar situation occurs in coexisting pseudohypoparathyroidism and hypothyroidism. Correction of hypothyroidism lowers the vitamin D requirements to more reasonable and safer doses.

The use of adrenal glucocorticosteroids and immunosuppressive drugs has been disappointing in the few available reports and is not recommended. Replacement therapy of specific deficiencies should be provided after appropriate tests of organ function. Complete family assessment and care of any affected siblings and other family members should be a necessary and important part of the overall long-term management of any patient with hypoparathyroidism or other endocrinopathy. An adequate well-balanced diet for age, normal calcium and phosphorus intake and appropriate multivitamin therapy are important for optimal growth and development of these children and adolescents. Psychologic or emotional support should be part of the chronic therapy plan for such patients and their family.

Permanent hypoparathyroidism may occur at any time after neck surgery, such as thyroidectomy or parathyroidectomy. If severe bone disease, such as osteoporosis or osteitis fibrosa, occurred preoperatively, temporary hypocalcemia may occur postoperatively. When the avidity of bone uptake of calcium and phosphate has diminished and healing of bone has presumably occurred, the temporary need for oral calcium supplement and large doses of vitamin D_2 may diminish or become unnecessary. Transient postoperative hypocalcemia and hypoparathyroidism is more common than the permanent form. Continued long-term follow-up and periodic measurement of serum calcium and phosphorus are therefore necessary in order to avoid not only hypercalcemia or unnecessary vitamin D therapy but also the delayed diagnosis of permanent hypoparathyroidism.

Treated or well-controlled maternal hypoparathyroidism had no deleterious effects on pregnancies or newborn infants in the few reported cases in the literature. Inadequately treated or untreated maternal hypoparathyroidism has been associated with intrauterine hyperparathyroidism in infants.

HYPERPARATHYROIDISM

Primary Hyperparathyroidism

Successful and ideal management of primary hyperparathyroidism depends on a high index of suspicion that will lead to its early diagnosis during the stage of uncomplicated hypercalcemia. In children and adolescents, the reported cases have been predominantly parathyroid adenomas manifesting with bone disease in about 74 per cent of cases and nephrolithiasis in about 9 per cent of cases. Primary chief-cell hyperplasia has been reported less commonly in children; its presence is often familial and associated with multiple endocrine adenomatosis, including pancreatic islet, parathyroid and adrenal cortex. Definitive treatment of primary hyperparathyroidism involves careful exploration of the neck and at times the substernal area by an experienced surgeon until all four parathyroid glands are found. Removal of an adenoma is sufficient. If diffuse primary hyperplasia is present, three of the glands and part of the fourth should be resected.

The following causes of hypercalcemia in children and adolescents should be ruled out before concluding that primary hyperparathyroidism exists, because treatment would not be parathyroidectomy. These causes include spurious laboratory errors, hypervitaminosis D, sarcoidosis, adrenal insufficiency (primary idiopathic and congenital adrenal hyperplasia with salt-losing syndrome), disuse osteoporosis with immobilization and bed rest, hyperthyroidism, milk-alkali syndrome, malignancies and idiopathic hypercalcemia. In most of these conditions, hypercalciuria is uniformly present and may be greater than with primary hyperparathyroidism. Other signs and symptoms and diagnostic tests should help provide the accurate diagnosis and treatment of the underlying disease. A therapeutic-diagnostic trial with hydrocortisone (100 to 200 mg. per square meter) for five days almost never lowers the serum calcium level in primary hyperparathyroidism, but it does lower the serum calcium level in the other conditions.

Acute hypercalcemic crises may necessitate attempts to lower the serum calcium level by other means if steroids do not work and exploration of the neck is questionable or undesirable. High intravenous fluid infusion with normal saline as tolerated should be attempted first to increase calcium excretion. Intravenous and oral buffered phosphate and intravenous sodium sulfate solution have had variable success and would be preferable to the use of disodium EDTA (disodium salt of ethylenediamine tetraacetic acid). Peritoneal dialysis with calcium-free dialysate has had variable success.

SECONDARY HYPERPARATHYROIDISM

Malabsorption of calcium or vitamin D by the intestine in patients with steatorrhea or celiac syndrome, chronic renal disease, vitamin D deficiency, vitamin D refractory states with rickets or osteomalacia and renal tubular disease are all associated with secondary hyperparathyroidism. Therapy consists of the water-soluble form of vitamin D, preferably, at 2000 to 5000 units for vitamin D deficiency and malabsorption syndrome, 10,000 to 50,000 units for chronic renal disease and larger amounts for vitamin D refractory states.

TERTIARY HYPERPARATHYROIDISM

During the past decade, a severe, debilitating form of renal osteodystrophy and derangement of calcium and phosphorus metabolism has appeared in various renal hemodialysis and transplantation centers. This form of secondary hyperparathyroidism manifests in a more virulent form after improvement of renal function by chronic hemodialysis or peritoneal dialysis and following renal hemotransplantation. This condition has been called tertiary hyperparathyroidism and is thought to be due to an autonomous state of parathyroid hyperfunction and the formation of chief cell adenomatous hyperplasia. High vitamin D therapy and dietary adjustment of calcium-phosphorus intake may help if begun early during the course of chronic renal failure. Subtotal parathyroidectomy has been performed at various centers before transplantation to prevent nephrocalcinosis, nephrolithiasis and other aspects of the syndrome from appearing.

Adrenal Disorders

BORIS SENIOR, M.D.

A number of disorders due to impairment of enzyme systems involved in the production of cortisol and aldosterone from cholesterol have been described. As a result of a decrease in the formation of cortisol, secretion of adrenocorticotropic hormone (ACTH) is stimulated and hyperplasia of the adrenal gland occurs. Depending on the site of the enzymatic block, the hyperplastic adrenal gland may succeed in secreting more cortisol but, in most cases, only at the expense of forming excessive quantities of other corticoids which produce virilization and which may impair the conservation of sodium.

In essence, the management of these disorders, which vary in severity from mild virilization to a state in which life is in jeopardy, is the provision of corticoids which are deficient. Not only are the effects of hormone deficiency corrected, but also the excessive secretion of ACTH is halted and the production of undesirable adrenal compounds abates.

The therapeutic outline which follows should be modified according to the needs of the individual patient.

SALT-LOSING CONGENITAL VIRILIZING ADRENAL HYPERPLASIA (SEVERE 21-HYDROXYLASE DEFICIENCY)

The infant is usually between one and three weeks of age with a history of vomiting and weight loss. Commonly, dehydration, hyponatremia and hyperkalemia are present. Restitution of sodium and of water by the administration of desoxycorticosterone acetate in oil, 1 to 4 mg. intramuscularly per day, and isotonic saline in 5 per cent dextrose solution should allow sufficient time for the collection of urine for confirmation of the diagnosis by measurement of the steroid excretory products. If such collection is delayed until therapy with glucocorticoids is begun, the diagnosis may be obscured.

Initial Therapy. A solution of 0.9 per cent sodium chloride in 5 per cent dextrose in water, 150 ml. per kilogram per day, is administered intravenously. Desoxycorticosterone acetate in oil is administered intramuscularly once daily in a dose of 1 to 4 mg. If the need for glucocorticoids is urgent, hydrocortisone hemisuccinate (Solu-Cortef) may be added to the intravenous solution in a dose of 50 mg. per kilogram per 24 hours. Hydrocortisone hemisuccinate is also rapidly effective when administered intramuscularly, for which purpose the 24-hour dose, 50 mg. per kilogram, is given in four divided doses.

Depending on the condition of the patient, one may begin glucocorticoid therapy with the long-acting cortisone acetate or change to it from hydrocortisone hemisuccinate. Cortisone acetate is administered initially in a dose of 5 to 10 mg. per kilogram intramuscularly once daily. When administered intramuscularly, cortisone acetate has a much longer duration of action than when taken by mouth—as much as 72 hours versus approximately 8 hours.

In addition to this treatment, once feedings are taken, the patient may require 2 Gm. or more of sodium chloride per day as supplements in the formula.

Despite extremely high concentrations of potassium in the blood, which if present in other disorders would be an urgent indication for therapy, ill effects are extremely rare. If treatment of the hyperkalemia is needed, one may administer intravenously a solution containing 50 mEq. of sodium bicarbonate per liter of 10 per cent dextrose in water. In addition, a cation exchange resin, such as Kayexalate, may be given as a retention enema—1 Gm. of resin per kilogram of body weight in a mixture of 50 ml. of 70 per cent Sorbitol and 100 ml. of tap water.

Maintenance Therapy. GLUCOCORTICOIDS. After one to two weeks of daily injections of cortisone acetate intramuscularly, maintenance therapy may be continued by administering the cortisone acetate in a dose of 3 to 5 mg. per kilogram intramuscularly every second or third day. The precise dose and the frequency of injection depend on the patient's progress as assessed by linear growth and the excretion of 17-ketosteroids or pregnanetriol in the urine.

Several considerations affect the age, six months to two years, at which the administration of cortisone acetate is changed from the intramuscular to the oral route. If the mother is intelligent and responsible and has access to the pediatrician, oral medication may be introduced earlier. When the patient is on oral replacement medication only, a relatively minor illness accompanied by vomiting may be catastrophic. Because of this danger the parents are instructed to have hydrocortisone hemisuccinate available and in case of emergency, if there is a delay in obtaining medical assistance, to administer it intramuscularly in a dose of 100 mg.

When the decision has been made to administer the glucocorticoids by mouth, cortisone acetate may be prescribed in a dose of 1 to 2 mg. per kilogram per day. To imitate the normal circadian cycle of adrenal secretion, half the amount is given in the morning and the remainder is divided into equal portions and given in the middle of the day and on going to bed. When the patient is of school age, the inconvenience of taking medication in the middle of the day may require omission of that dose. Accordingly one may prescribe a longer-acting glucocorticoid. Prednisone may then be given in a dosage of 0.2 to 0.3 mg. per kilogram per day divided into two equal doses.

The parents and patient must clearly understand that the treatment is lifelong.

Mineralocorticoids. After treatment of the initial phase of the illness, the relatively short-acting desoxycorticosterone acetate in oil should be replaced by a longer-acting agent. For this purpose one may prescribe desoxycorticosterone pivalate, which is administered in a dose of 25 mg. monthly by intramuscular injection. This, too, can be replaced by oral medication as the child grows older. An effective oral agent for this purpose is fludrocortisone acetate (Florinef), which is taken once daily in a dose of 0.1 to 0.3 mg. The less severely affected patients may eventually dispense with mineralocorticoid therapy, but in other patients administration must be continued.

These patients will salt their food heavily and it should be freely available at meal times. In addition, particularly during infancy, it may be desirable to prescribe extra salt to be added to the formula in a dose of 2 to 4 Gm. daily.

Intercurrent Illnesses. Since maintenance therapy with glucocorticoids is at a physiologic level, provision must be made for the need for additional glucocorticoids during stress. The daily dose may be doubled or tripled during an illness and, if indicated, hydrocortisone hemisuccinate intramuscularly in a dose of 100 mg. may also be used.

The parents must understand that any concern about the patient's well-being should be immediately communicated to the physician.

Surgery. The ambiguous genitalia of the female should be corrected before the psychologic consequences become imprinted. Corrective surgery is performed before the age of two years. Recession of the clitoris may be preferable to amputation, since therapy and the growth of the patient renders it less conspicuous.

The patient is prepared for the stress of surgery by administering cortisone acetate intramuscularly in a dose of 5 to 10 mg. per kilogram daily, beginning two days prior to operation and including the day after surgery, following which the dose is halved for two days and then discontinued when the patient is able to retain maintenance medication by mouth. Hydrocortisone hemisuccinate should be available in the operating room and, if needed, may be given intravenously in a dose of 100 mg.

If surgery is required for any other reason, the same principles of management apply.

Counseling. It is extremely stressful for parents to cope with the problem of a child with ambiguous genitalia. An informed discussion with the pediatrician can do much to lessen their anxiety.

The genetic basis of the disorder must be explained, since future offspring may be affected. The possibility must be considered, particularly in simple virilizing hyperplasia, that the same disorder may be present but unrecognized in siblings.

SIMPLE VIRILIZING ADRENAL HYPERPLASIA (PARTIAL 21-HYDROXYLASE DEFICIENCY)

The management of this disorder is directed at suppression of adrenal hyperactivity by the administration of glucocorticoids. Depending on the age at which the diagnosis is made, adrenal suppression is achieved by administering cortisone acetate, 3 to 5 mg. per kilogram per day either orally in divided doses or intramuscularly in one dose and then continuing with glucocorticoid maintenance therapy as outlined for salt-losing virilizing adrenal hyperplasia.

Adequacy of dosage is judged by linear growth and urinary 17-ketosteroids or pregnanetriol. Growth is impaired if the dose of glucocorticoids is too high, whereas an inadequate dose results in excessive growth, increased concentrations of 17-ketosteroids in the urine and abnormally rapid maturation of the skeleton as judged by roentgenograms of the hand.

HYPERTENSIVE ADRENAL HYPERPLASIA (11-HYDROXYLASE DEFICIENCY)

This disorder is treated with physiologic doses of glucocorticoids as outlined previously. With adequate therapy the blood pressure should be restored to normal levels.

RARE BIOCHEMICAL VARIANTS OF ADRENAL HYPERPLASIA

The exceedingly rare congenital disorders of the adrenal glands which result from enzymatic defects of 20,22-desmolase, 3-beta-hydroxydehydrogenase and 17-hydroxylase pose difficult problems in diagnosis; their management follows the same principles of replacement therapy.

ADRENAL INSUFFICIENCY AND ADDISON'S DISEASE

The most common cause of adrenal insufficiency is the abrupt cessation of long-term therapy with glucocorticoids administered in daily divided pharmacologic doses. If glucocorticoids are administered as a single dose at longer intervals, once in 48 hours, the adrenal gland retains the ability to function adequately when treatment is halted. If glucocorticoids have been administered in daily divided doses, changing the treatment to a single dose at intervals of 48 hours before discontinuation may enable adrenal function to return.

The management of acute adrenal insufficiency is the same as for severe, salt-losing adrenal hyperplasia: an intravenous solution of 0.9 per cent sodium chloride in 5 per cent dextrose in water, 50 to 100 ml. per kilogram per 24 hours; hydrocortisone hemisuccinate, 100 mg. intravenously as needed; and desoxycorticosterone acetate in oil, 1 to 5 mg. daily.

Once the acute phase is controlled, maintenance therapy for Addison's disease consists of the provision of replacement doses of glucocorticoids and mineralocorticoids plus supplements of salt. The need for increased doses of glucocorticoids during periods of stress must be emphasized.

CUSHING'S SYNDROME

This disorder is most often brought about by the administration of pharmacologic doses of glucocorticoids. If the underlying illness for which the treatment is given can be controlled only by large daily divided doses of glucocorticoids, Cushing's syndrome will be inevitable and unavoidable. On the other hand, if satisfactory control of the illness can be achieved by single doses of glucocorticoids administered at longer intervals, once in 48 hours, Cushing's syndrome may be avoided.

If glucocorticoid treatment is to be discontinued after divided daily doses have been administered for a prolonged period, one may test the functional ability of the adrenal glands by measuring the increase in the concentrations of cortisol in the blood in response to the induction of hypoglycemia with insulin. Regular insulin, 0.1 unit per kilogram, is administered intravenously and blood samples are drawn just before and 30 and 60 minutes after the injection. Care must be exercised since severe hypoglycemia may result if adrenal insufficiency is present. An increase of the concentration of cortisol to 20 micrograms or more per 100 ml. indicates that the adrenal gland has retained a reasonable degree of function.

Cushing's syndrome due to bilateral hyperplasia of the adrenal glands is an indication for bilateral adrenalectomy.

Cushing's syndrome may also result from a unilateral adenoma or carcinoma. The treatment for either condition would be unilateral adrenalectomy. In the cases of carcinoma, the contralateral gland will be functionally depressed and atrophied. Thus, even if only one adrenal gland is excised, acute adrenal insufficiency will ensue.

In all cases, prior to surgery cortisone acetate is administered intramuscularly once daily in a dose of 5 to 10 mg. per kilogram per day, beginning 48 hours before operation. On the day of surgery hydrocortisone hemisuccinate is administered intramuscularly, 10 mg. per kilogram in four divided doses. Hydrocortisone hemisuccinate should also be available in the operating room and may be given intravenously in a dose of 100 mg. as required.

If a bilateral adrenalectomy is to be performed, in addition to the glucocorticoid therapy already outlined, 2 mg. of desoxycorticosterone acetate in oil is given intramuscularly on the morning of the operation. The subsequent management of the patient who has had a bilateral adrenalectomy involves a gradual reduction in the dose of intramuscular cortisone acetate over a period of days and then maintenance therapy with cortisone acetate by mouth, 1 to 2 mg. per kilogram per day in three divided doses. After several days, the long-acting desoxycorticosterone pivalate, 25 mg. monthly by intramuscular injection, may be substituted for the daily injections of desoxycorticosterone acetate in oil, and finally maintenance may be continued with fludrocortisone acetate, 0.1 to 0.3 mg. once daily by mouth.

Replacement therapy is, of course, lifelong and increased amounts of administered glucocorticoids are needed during periods of stress. The possibility of the appearance of a pituitary tumor in later years must be borne in mind.

After removal of a single adrenal gland for tumor, the administration of glucocorticoids is gradually reduced in amount and spaced at longer intervals so that the remaining adrenal gland will resume functioning. If one is uncertain whether the adrenal gland is able to secrete sufficient cortisol, one may cautiously administer insulin and measure the increase in cortisol in the serum, as for patients who have been maintained on long-term glucocorticoid therapy.

If an adrenal carcinoma has spread and is no longer curable by surgery, the metastases may be treated by administration of the investigational adrenocorticolytic agent *o, p'*-DDD [2,2-bis (2-chlorophenyl-4-chlorophenyl)-1,1-dichloroethane].

PHEOCHROMOCYTOMA

The treatment of a pheochromocytoma is surgical excision. However, the hypertension may be so severe that measures must be taken to control it before surgery can be undertaken. Phenoxybenzamine, an alpha-adrenergic blocking agent, may be administered for this purpose in a dose of 1 to 2 mg. per kilogram by mouth every 12 hours.

During surgery, manipulation of the tumor

may produce a sudden rise in the blood pressure, which can be controlled by the administration of a short-acting alpha-adrenergic blocker, phentolamine, in a dose of 1 to 2 mg. intravenously as required.

If precipitous hypotension ensues after removal of the tumor, the blood pressure may be restored by the administration of levarterenol (Levophed) in amounts of 1 mg. A slow infusion of 5 per cent dextrose in water throughout the surgical procedure facilitates the intravenous administration of either phentolamine or levarterenol.

It should be remembered, particularly in children, that more than one tumor may be present.

Endocrine Disorders of the Testes

ZVI LARON, M.D.

CONTRALATERAL (COMPENSATORY) HYPERTROPHY

A unilateral tumor should be differentiated from compensatory hypertrophy of the testis, which develops in unilateral testicular maldevelopment or hypofunction. Longitudinal measurements of both testes make this diagnosis unmistakable.

BILATERAL TESTICULAR HYPERTROPHY

This occurs in true precocious puberty and longstanding primary hypothyroidism. Measurement of the testes will help diagnose this disorder even at at prepubertal age. Institution of therapy in hypothyroidism leads to a decrease in the testicular size. In rare cases there may be testicular enlargement in congenital adrenocortical virilism, which is caused by hyperplasia of ectopic adrenal cells in the testes. The diagnosis is easily established and the institution of cortisol therapy results in a decrease in testicular size.

HYPOGONADISM

Hypogonadism, i.e., small testes for age, can be diagnosed even prepubertally when testicular measurements are recorded regularly. At puberty, blood and urinary gonadotropins rise to higher than normal concentrations. Primary hypogonadism may be due to testicular maldevelopment of known or unknown cause. Hypogonadism in true chromatin-negative males with a normal male karyotype should be distinguished from hypogonadal patients with Klinefelter's syndrome who have a positive chromatin pattern and a karyotype with one or more extra X chromosomes. The Del Castillo syndrome is characterized by germinal cell aplasia (Sertoli-cell syndrome). Reifenstein's syndrome may also present with smaller than normal testes, with biopsy showing minimal spermatogenic activity and normal Leydig cells, in addition to hypospadias and gynecomastia. In both Klinefelter's syndrome and Reifenstein's syndrome there may be a postpuberal testicular atrophy.

The leading signs may be retarded sexual development, depending on the degree of Leydig cell activity, and/or infertility. Treatment is based on replacing the endogenous androgens. Long-acting testosterone preparations, such as cyclopentyl propionate or enanthate testosterone, or others, 200 to 250 mg. once a month intramuscularly started at around age 14, produce normal male virilization and erection and make possible a normal sex life. The use of oral methyl testosterone is not advised because it causes gynecomastia, may lead to cholestasis and reduces prothrombin synthesis.

Secondary hypogonadism is caused by pituitary failure to synthesize or secrete follicle-stimulating hormone (FSH) or luteinizing hormone (LH = interstitial cell-stimulating hormone [ICSH]), whereas tertiary hypogonadism is the result of lack of hypothalamic gonadotropin-releasing hormones (Gn-RH). Clinically, both these conditions present as a lack of normal puberty. Growth may be either normal or retarded, depending on whether only the gonadotropins or other pituitary hormones are involved. Tertiary hypogonadism can be differentiated from secondary hypogonadism by the normal rise in plasma LH and FSH which takes place during intravenous administration of LH-RH (50 milliunits per square meter). In pituitary failure there is no rise. The most frequent syndromes are isolated gonadotropin deficiency (RH lack), which may be hereditary; Kallmann's syndrome (hypogonadotropic hypogonadism associated with anosmia); Rosewater's syndrome associated with gynecomastia; and Laurence-Moon-Biedl syndrome with mental retardation, retinitis pigmentosa, obesity and polydactyly.

The ideal treatment in hypothalmic (tertiary) hypogonadism would be Depo-LH-FSH-RH, a preparation which it is hoped will soon be available. Until then, Depo-testosterone, 200 to 250 mg. once a month intramuscularly, is indicated to induce or complete sexual maturation. Attempts to induce fertility can be made when adulthood is reached by using a scheme of human chorionic gonadotropin (ICSH-like) and human menopausal gonadotropin (FSH) combined therapy.

In panhypopituitarism, induction of sexual signs is usually postponed until an adequate height has been attained. In order to postpone epiphyseal closure in long bones, it is recommended that anabolic steroids such as methandrostenolone (0.04 to 0.05 mg. per kilogram per day) be administered initially.* These are slightly virilizing and have a growth-promoting effect. Later, Depo-testosterone should be used to complete the virilization.

ASSOCIATION BETWEEN TESTICULAR CHANGES AND OTHER DISEASES

Hypogonadism occurs with congenital and longstanding growth-hormone deficiency. Primary unilateral or bilateral hypogonadism or undescended testes have been described in association with various congenital anomalies of the urinary tract, the Prader-Labhart-Willi-Fanconi syndrome, Klinefelter's syndrome, a syndrome characterized by testicular tubular insufficiency, normal virilization (i.e., normal Leydig's cell function), blindness, deafness and metabolic abnormalities, and in children with undefined but congenital mental retardation.

PSYCHOLOGIC ASPECTS

The various disturbances associated with the male gonads—e.g., malformed scrotum, abnormal size of the testes for the corresponding age, delayed or retarded puberty caused by Leydig cell insufficiency, sterility due to tubular dysfunction—may give rise to psychologic reactions, in both the patient and his parents. Early and correct counseling of the parents and later of the patient is of the utmost importance.

Gynecomastia

H. D. MOSIER, M.D.

Gynecomastia or enlargement of the male breast may occur at any age. A variety of clinical types exist: neonatal breast enlargement secondary to maternal hormones; ingestion or percutaneous absorption of estrogens; feminizing adrenal tumor; adolescent gynecomastia; poly X chromosomal syndromes, e.g., Klinefelter's syndrome; Reifenstein's syndrome; familial gynecomastia with or without hypogonadism; unilateral or asymmetric adolescent gynecomastia; and gynecomastia secondary to treatment with androgens or chorionic gonadotropins.

Certain other forms of gynecomastia which have been observed in the adult, such as those associated with recovery from undernutrition, diffuse liver disease, hyperthyroidism, bronchogenic carcinoma and Leydig cell tumors, are seldom, if ever, observed in children or adolescents.

Adolescent gynecomastia is by far the most common form, occurring in over 50 per cent of normal males. It may begin in the prepubertal period prior to the development of coarse pubic hair. Management should consist of assurance and temporization, since in two or three years most cases of adolescent gynecomastia regress to cosmetically acceptable breast enlargement. In any instance in which there is severe psychologic disturbance or inadequate regression, surgical removal of the breast glandular tissue is recommended. The surgeon should be one skilled in cosmetic surgery of the breasts. Under no circumstances should androgens or gonadotropins be administered as treatment for gynecomastia.

Hermaphroditism and Intersex

BARBARA M. LIPPE, M.D.

The management of the infant or child with intersex involves the following principles: (1) prompt diagnosis, including establishment of the nature of the abnormality, (2) early assignment of sex of rearing, (3) early medical and/or surgical care, (4) appropriate hormonal therapy at the time of puberty, if indicated, and (5) completion of reconstruction of the internal and external genitalia at the time of full sexual maturation.

Diagnosis. If there is any ambiguity in the external genitalia of a neonate or any other evidence (such as family history) that the infant may have an intersex problem, initiation of the diagnostic work up should be started in the neonatal period. Twenty-four-hour urine collection for 17-ketosteroids and pregnanetriol should be obtained and chromosomal karyotyping should be done on lymphocytes. In selected cases, contrast urography may be helpful. Early exploration of the internal organs, with gonadal biopsies, should be carried out if the diagnosis is still unclear and sex assignment uncertain. Definitive removal of any structures can be undertaken somewhat later. Finally, no infant who may have congenital adrenal hyperplasia should be discharged from close follow-up before the question of the development of a salt-losing state has been resolved.

Sex of Rearing. The assignment of the appropriate sex of rearing should be made as early as possible. This should be based on the assessment of the best possible cosmetic and sex-

* Manufacturer's precaution: Methandrostenolone is not recommended in prepubertal children, although it may be used in selected cases in older children and adults with pituitary dwarfism in which there is evidence of marked maturational delay and growth hormone is not available.

ually functional result that can be obtained from repair of the external genitalia. Where possible, this should concur with the gonadal and chromosomal genotype. However, neither factor, nor the possibility of retaining fertility, should be given overriding consideration if it means raising the child with grossly ambiguous genitalia or subjecting it to many surgical procedures with crippling psychologic consequences. In many cases of virilized genotypic females, assignment of the female gender can be made promptly since surgical repair will often restore the individual to virtually normal status. Inadequately virilized males, males with agenesis of the phallus or infants with a streak ovary and hemiuterus but an apparently normal testis (mixed gonadal dysgenesis) present a more difficult problem because they may be considered potentially fertile. However, it is our experience that multiple and extensive surgical repairs for the creation of a less-than-adequate phallus sometimes make gonadectomy and assignment of the female sex a preferable choice.

At the time of sex assignment, psychologic support for the family should be initiated. It is important to emphasize that appropriate phenotypic psychosocial attitudes will develop. Often the fear of future development of homosexual attitudes or behavior will exist in the parents' minds but will not be verbalized. Continuous reassurance is often necessary regarding this fear. It has been our policy to offer a full explanation to the parents regarding the disorder and the nature of the chromosomes and gonads. Our explanations to the patients, however, never include revelation of the presence of chromosomes or gonads of the opposite sex.

Initial Medical and Surgical Care. In cases of congenital adrenal hyperplasia, continuous corticosteroid therapy under close supervision is required. The dosage of cortisone or hydrocortisone should be individualized according to variation in growth, urinary steroid excretion and bone age. Using these criteria, we find adequate control in most patients with the use of 25 mg. of cortisone per square meter, or two times the cortisol production rate (12 mg. per square meter), when given orally in divided doses. If salt loss is present, Florinef, 0.05 to 0.1 mg. orally, is added. We have not found it necessary or advantageous to use intramuscular or Depo preparations.

In patients where the disorder is not progressive, hormonal therapy is usually not indicated until the expected time of puberty. However, surgical management of all patients needing surgical correction should be initiated early. There is good evidence to suggest that gender identity is established by the end of the second year and some repair of the externalia should be undertaken by 18 to 24 months of age so that phenotypic identity is preserved. In the progressive virilizing syndromes, clitorectomy may have to be considered because the stimulus for excessive growth of the clitoris may recur if the patient is not adequately controlled at all times. Recession and relocation of the clitoris as an alternative have been used, but these procedures may result in significant pain when the organ becomes engorged and erectile. We also feel that if the internal structures (such as a gonad or müllerian remnant) need removal, it can be done at this time. There is no good evidence to support the concept that the gonads are necessary for normal prepubertal growth or psychosocial development. On the contrary, it has been our experience that parental anxiety about the possible effects of a heterosexual gonadal structure and the traumatic experience of laparotomy in a teenager makes early removal preferable.

Hormonal Therapy. At the expected time of puberty, institution of hormonal replacement will be necessary in the gonadectomized child. If one gonad is intact, physical examination and measurement of plasma gonadotropins (follicle-stimulating hormone and luteinizing hormone) and plasma sex steroids may be used to assess its potential function and obviate the necessity to institute replacement therapy. If replacement is indicated in the female, we use small doses of Premarin (0.625 to 1.25 mg. daily). Initially, even lower doses may be used to prevent too rapid epiphyseal fusion. The estrogen is given in a cyclic fashion (three weeks per month). If a uterine structure is present, a progestational agent is added during the last six days. We have found that 2.5 to 10 mg. of Provera per day is necessary for adequate withdrawal bleeding. At present there is some question that the continuous long-term administration of artificial estrogen preparations may have a carcinogenic potential, but neither compound in the doses listed has been so implicated to date. Continuous unopposed estrogen in itself, however, may not be innocuous, and for this reason we recommend its cyclic administration even in children who will not have withdrawal bleeding. Whether a progestational agent should be given to these children as well has not been established.

In the case of the male, androgen therapy may be administered as methyl testosterone tablets or linguets, or as a Depo preparation, testosterone cyclopentyl propionate or enanthate. The dose is increased from 10 to 50 mg. orally in an effort to produce normal pubertal staging and to yield a pubertal growth spurt without rapid epiphyseal fusion. Final maintenance is usually 25 to 50 mg. daily of oral testosterone, or 200 mg. every two to four weeks of an intramuscular preparation.

In rare cases a hypothalamic or pituitary lesion may have been responsible for failure of adequate virilization in the male. If this is the case and the gonads are intact, intramuscular administration of gonadotropins may result in both sexual development and fertility. The use of these preparations has been described elsewhere in this text (see Hypopituitarism).

Reconstructive Surgery. As much of the surgery as possible should be done at an early age. However, complete vaginal reconstruction is usually not practical until hormonal therapy has been instituted and sexual intercourse is anticipated. Testicular prostheses are not inserted until puberty has been initiated in the male. This allows not only for some growth of the scrotum but also for the placement of an appropriately sized adult prosthesis.

References

Gardner, L. I.: *Adrenal Function in Infants and Children—A Symposium.* New York, Grune & Stratton, Inc., 1956.

Walkins, L., Blizzard, R. M., and Migeon, C. J.: *The Diagnosis and Treatment of Endocrine Disorders in Childhood and Adolescence.* 3rd ed. Springfield, Illinois, Charles C Thomas, Publisher, 1965.

10

Metabolic Disorders

Infants Born to Diabetic Women

RONALD L. GUTBERLET, M.D., *and*
MARVIN CORNBLATH, M.D.

Therapy of infants born to diabetic women begins with conception. Meticulous metabolic control of the diabetes is important in all insulin-dependent pregnant women. This necessitates careful and frequent medical supervision and full cooperation of the pregnant woman. Ketosis, acidosis, excessive and fluctuating hyperglycemia and coma must be avoided or treated promptly. Prompt recognition and treatment of the complications of pregnancy, such as pyuria, pyelonephritis, excessive weight gain and toxemia, are important to the health of the infant. The effect of maternal hypoglycemia or polyhydramnios on the infant's outcome is less certain.

At our hospital, these babies have been delivered about three weeks prior to term if the woman has insulin-dependent diabetes mellitus, and at term if she has gestational diabetes mellitus. Indications for immediate delivery include a sudden change in insulin requirement, a change in the infant's activity in utero, failure to grow or a decrease in maternal urinary estriol excretion. Vaginal delivery is induced if conditions are proper; otherwise a cesarean section is done. When preterm delivery becomes necessary and the fetus will tolerate a 24- to 48-hour delay, and if examination of amniotic fluid for surfactant components or activity reveals fetal lung immaturity, administration of glucocorticoid to the mother for 24 to 48 hours prior to delivery may in certain circumstances prevent hyaline membrane disease (Liggins and Howie). Further experience is required with this form of therapy before recommending its use other than in controlled trials. Careful control of the blood sugar with avoidance of ketosis or acidosis is important prior to and during induction of labor and delivery.

A physician who is expert in the resuscitation of the newborn should be present during the birth. Although 40 to 60 per cent of these babies have an uneventful course, the infant who is sick demands prompt, expert attention.

Initially, respirations must be established utilizing immediate and active resuscitation as necessary. An Apgar score at 1 and 5 minutes aids in predicting infants at high risk. However, all are given 1 mg. of vitamin K_1 oxide intramuscularly and are then transferred to the intensive care nursery. All infants are placed unclothed in an incubator or radiant heated crib under servo-temperature control to create a neutral thermal environment (90 to 95° F., depending on weight of the infant). Oxygen is administered only as required for visible cyanosis or hypoxemia. A careful and complete examination for abnormalities should be done at this time, with particular attention to palpation of both flanks for kidney size. A search for congenital anomalies that may require immediate surgical correction is important.

Blood obtained from the placenta is used for baseline chemical determinations, including glucose, blood urea nitrogen, sodium, bilirubin, calcium and phosphorus. An initial roentgenogram of the chest and an electrocardiogram are obtained in any infant who is not entirely well. A complete blood count and hematocrit as well as a urinalysis are obtained shortly after birth. Screening for hypoglycemia is done at 1, 4, 6, 12, 24, 36 and 48 hours. Dextrostix are used (Swiatek et al.), and low values confirmed with laboratory determination of whole blood or serum glucose. A urinalysis is repeated prior to discharge. All these determinations are to assist in detecting the multiple problems these babies may have.

Careful clinical observations are critical in the first hours to first day of life to detect early signs or manifestations of distress. Respiratory difficulties (e.g., tachypnea, apneic spells or retractions), cyanotic spells or periods of tremulousness or lethargy may suggest impending trouble.

If well, the infant is allowed to recover from birth (4 to 8 hours) and then breast fed or given one to two feedings of sterile water followed by formula. The uneventful course of the infant born to a diabetic mother may be characterized by periods of poor feeding, mild jaundice and overactivity or underactivity. However, all of these clinical manifestations are of brief duration, and the infant is ready to go home with his mother.

On the other hand, about 50 per cent of these infants may have complications in the neonatal period. Their approximate incidence in infants of gestational diabetic mothers and of insulin-dependent mothers and our specific therapy for each are as follows:

1. Respiratory distress syndrome or hyaline membrane disease: (Infants of insulin-dependent mothers = 30 per cent; infants of gestational diabetic mothers = 10 per cent.)

Arterial oxygen and acid-base status are monitored via an umbilical artery catheter. The management of metabolic and respiratory acidosis, hypoxemia, body temperature, hydration and salt balance is detailed elsewhere (see Respiratory Distress Syndrome).

2. Hypoglycemia: <30 mg. per 100 ml. (Infants of insulin-dependent mothers = 50 per cent; infants of gestational diabetic mothers = 20 per cent.) Symptomatic, e.g., apnea, listlessness, tachypnea, bounding precordium or convulsions (infants of insulin-dependent mothers = 20 per cent, infants of gestational diabetic mothers = 10 per cent).

When a blood glucose <30 mg. per 100 ml. is obtained, draw a second sample for confirmation. If the patient is asymptomatic, glucagon, 0.3 mg. per kilogram, is given intravenously or subcutaneously. If symptomatic, do not wait for result but immediately give 2 to 4 ml. per kilogram of 25 per cent glucose in water at a rate of 1 to 2 ml. per minute by intravenous injection. The initial treatment is followed by 80 to 100 ml. per kilogram of 15 per cent glucose in water per kilogram per 24 hours (8 to 10 mg. per kilogram per minute). Glucose intake is adjusted to maintain values over 30 mg. per 100 ml. (monitored every 3 to 6 hours).

If the blood glucose remains over 40 mg. per 100 ml., the concentration of the infusion is decreased by 5 per cent every 24 hours.

If the blood glucose falls below 30 mg. per 100 ml., repeat the bolus infusion and start hydrocortisone, 5 mg. per kilogram per 24 hours in two or more divided doses. This dose is tapered as glucose requirements are decreased.

ALWAYS DISCONTINUE HYPERTONIC GLUCOSE BY REDUCING THE CONCENTRATION OF GLUCOSE TO 5 PER CENT AND DECREASING THE RATE OF ADMINISTRATION TO AVOID REACTIVE HYPOGLYCEMIA.

3. **Hypocalcemia:** <7.0 mg. per 100 ml. or <3.5 mEq. per liter. (Infants of insulin-dependent mothers = 25 per cent; infants of gestational diabetic mother = 15 per cent.) This has been attributed to relative maternal hyperparathyroidism leading to fetal hypoparathyroidism (Tsang et al.). If symptomatic:

(a) 5 to 10 ml. of 10 per cent calcium gluconate administered by slow intravenous injection, with constant monitoring of the heart rate.

(b) 4:1 calcium:phosphorus ratio formula for the first week and then gradually revert to standard formula. Calcium lactate (13 per cent calcium ion) can be added to make this ratio.

4. **Hyperbilirubinemia:** >12 mg. per 100 ml. (Infants of insulin-dependent mothers = 50 per cent; infants of gestational diabetic mothers = 23 per cent.)

Levels of bilirubin at which phototherapy (5 to 15 mg. per 100 ml.) or exchange transfusion (12 to 20 mg. per 100 ml.) should be done have not been established in the infant of a diabetic mother or in the infant of a gestational diabetic mother. Therefore, the decision will depend on the maturity and clinical status of the infant (increased risk of kernicterus with pre-maturity, asphyxia, hypoalbuminemia, acidosis, respiratory distress syndrome), and changing neurologic signs, e.g., loss of the Moro reflex and failure to suck.

5. **Polycythemia:** Hematocrit >70 per cent, or hemoglobin >20 Gm. per 100 ml. (Infants of insulin-dependent mothers = 40 per cent; infants of gestational diabetic mothers = 30 per cent.)

(a) If the patient is asymptomatic, just observe.

(b) If the disease is associated with otherwise unexplained periods of tachypnea, cyanosis, restlessness or irritability, remove 10 ml. of whole blood per kilogram and replace it with 10 ml. of plasma per kilogram to reduce hematocrit to 60 ml. per 100 mg.

6. **Heart Failure:** (Infants of insulin-dependent mothers = 10 per cent; infants of gestational diabetic mothers = ?)

Digoxin (.04 to .05 mg. per kilogram digitalizing dose) and diuretics (furosemide* 0.5 to 1 mg. per kilogram) by the route and frequency indicated. (See Congestive Heart Failure.)

7. **Renal Vein Thrombosis:** Frequency is unknown. Diagnosed by flank mass, hematuria, intra-

---

*** Manufacturer's precaution: Furosemide should not be given to children until further experience is accumulated.**

venous pyelogram and thrombocytopenia. Although prompt surgical intervention has been advocated in the past, supportive treatment alone may be indicated in some instances (Belman et al.).

It should be noted that two infants of gestational diabetic mothers (8 per cent) and one infant of an insulin-dependent mother (8 per cent) in a recent series had transient hematuria with no sequelae (Warrner and Cornblath).

In conclusion, careful metabolic control during pregnancy, labor and delivery and prevention and prompt treatment of any complications of pregnancy permit the best possible environment for the fetus of a diabetic person. After birth, careful observations, both clinical and laboratory, and appropriate therapy for the multiple problems these infants may encounter are critical for intact survival.

References

Belman, A. B., Susmano, D. F., Burden, J. J., Kaplan, G. W.: Nonoperative Treatment of Unilateral Renal Vein Thrombosis in the Newborn. *J.A.M.A.*, 211: 1165, 1970.

Cornblath, M., and Schwartz, R.: *Disorders of Carbohydrate Metabolism in Infancy. Major Problems in Clinical Pediatrics Series.* Vol. 3, Chap. 4. Philadelphia, W. B. Saunders Company, 1966.

Liggins, G. C., and Howie, R. N.: A Controlled Trial of Antepartum Glucocorticoid Treatment for Prevention of the Respiratory Distress Syndrome in Premature Infants. *Pediatrics,* 50:515, 1972.

Swiatek, K. R., Leubben, G., and Cornblath, M.: Screening Method for Determining Glucose in Blood and Cerebrospinal Fluid, *Am. J. Dis. Child.,* 117:672, 1969.

Tsang, R. C., Kleinman, L. I., Sutherland, J. M., and Light, I. J.: Hypocalcemia in Infants of Diabetic Mothers. *Pediatrics,* 80:384–395, 1972.

Warrner, R. A., and Cornblath, M.: Infants of Gestational Diabetic Mothers. *Am. J. Dis. Child.,* 117:678, 1969.

Diabetes Mellitus

LUTHER B. TRAVIS, M.D.,
WILLIAM B. LORENTZ, M.D., *and*
HUGO F. CARVAJAL, M.D.

All chronic illnesses present difficult therapeutic problems when they become manifest in the growing and ever-changing child. Diabetes mellitus is no exception and, in fact, the perplexity of this condition may exceed that of all others. In part, this is due to the fact that although the usual diabetic child does not appear ill, his daily routine (insulin shots, dietary attention, urine tests and so forth) is a constant reminder of his state of subnormal health. In planning optimum therapy, adequate attention must be given to the metabolic abnormality, while commensurate consideration is accorded his physical growth and emotional development.

Diabetes mellitus is a metabolic disorder which is thought to be inherited as an autosomal recessive trait. The childhood form of the disease may make its clinical appearance at any age but most commonly is precipitated by periods of rapid growth or by environmental situations such as infections or emotional stress. The degree of carbohydrate intolerance (i.e., insulin deficiency) determines the immediate severity of the clinical disease and thus will partially dictate the type of therapeutic program. Although patients presenting with ketoacidosis are becoming more uncommon, the following discussion will start with this consideration and then proceed to the more important, although less dramatic, long-term aspects of diabetic care.

KETOACIDOSIS

When acute insulin deficiency occurs, profound metabolic abnormalities result. Since insufficient insulin is available to transport glucose into the cell, the level of this sugar increases in the extracellular fluid (ECF). High concentrations of glucose in the ECF contribute to an elevated osmolality and water moves out of the cell to equalize this osmolality. The volume of the intracellular fluid (ICF) is thus reduced. The transiently expanded ECF with its high glucose level presents a larger "filtered load" to the kidney and an osmotic diuresis occurs (polyuria). The exaggerated loss of urinary water and electrolyte (particularly sodium and potassium) produces dehydration and evokes the stimulus of thirst (polydipsia). The cell, deprived of its prime metabolic fuel (glucose), is subjected to starvation and must begin to rely on substitutes for its energy demands. Breakdown of fats and fatty acids (lipolysis) occurs to meet these demands. However, there is incomplete utilization of these fatty acids, and ketone bodies (or ketoacids) accumulate in the ECF and are partially excreted in the urine. The increase in ketoacids causes an increase in free hydrogen ions and a reduction in bicarbonate concentration, both depressing blood pH. There is stimulation of the respiratory center and deep, pauseless respirations (Kussmaul) occur, increasing insensible water loss and furthering dehydration. In response to this acute situation, the elaboration of "stress hormones" (cortisol, epinephrine) is increased, furthering the rise in blood glucose by gluconeogenesis and glycogenolysis and increasing the rate of fat catabolism.

Ketoacidosis may occur at the onset of diabetes and thus be the presenting picture; or it may develop during the course of the disease. In the latter situation, the ketoacidosis is usually either preceded by a period of poor carbohydrate control or is precipitated by an acute period of stress such as an infection. Whatever the circumstance, the principles of therapy are the same: (1) aggressive treatment with insulin in amounts sufficient to promote glucose transport, (2) administration of sufficient fluids to correct the dehydration and (3) treatment of any associated conditions which may have precipitated the problem.

Insulin. Insulin is the cornerstone of treatment for ketoacidosis. No matter how skillfully intravenous fluids are selected, they will be of little value in the absence of insulin.

The type of insulin used should be plain or crystalline–usually referred to as regular insulin. The onset of action of this insulin after intramuscular injection is about ½ hour with a peak action being achieved in about 1½ to 2 hours. If administered by the intravenous route, the peak action is within the first hour but a considerable portion is excreted in the urine without exerting any biologic effect.

The amount of insulin given will depend on the severity of the clinical state; thus, the more severe the ketoacidosis and dehydration, the greater the initial dose of insulin. The height of the blood sugar *cannot* be used in determining this initial dose but may be useful in determining subsequent doses. Since the degree of central nervous system depression closely parallels the severity of the dehydration and acidosis, it is our practice to use this symptom to guide the selection of initial insulin dose as follows:

1. Diabetic ketoacidosis with mild CNS depression (lethargy or somnolence)–1 to 2 units per kilogram body weight.
2. Diabetic ketoacidosis with moderate CNS depression (semicoma)–2 to 3 units per kilogram body weight.
3. Diabetic ketoacidosis with severe CNS depression (coma, with or without shock)–3 to 5 units per kilogram body weight.

Many factors (presence of "stress" hormones, degree of acidosis, presence of ketoacids and so forth) contribute to a relative insulin resistance at this stage and large doses of insulin must be administered. The amount of insulin "recommended" by this plan compares closely to other methods (such as serum acetone) in selection of initial dosage.

The *route of administration* of the initial insulin will depend on the state of circulation. If the patient is in shock, it should be given intravenously. If the patient is not in shock, it is preferable to give the full dose intramuscularly. This route is chosen because the rate of absorption is rapid and relatively constant and, most importantly, because we use the change in blood glucose following this initial injection to determine the second dose of insulin.

Subsequent doses of insulin: virtually all the change in blood glucose will have been achieved in 3 to 4 hours after the insulin dose is administered. If the second blood glucose level is unchanged or increased, the initial dose is repeated. If the blood glucose level has decreased, a proportionate decrease is made in the insulin dosage. The third and subsequent doses of insulin are similarly based on the response to the previous insulin dose.

EXAMPLE. A 30 kilogram child presents with severe ketoacidosis and coma. Blood is obtained and 120 units (4 units per kilogram) of regular insulin is given intramuscularly. The initial blood glucose level is subsequently reported as 800 mg. per 100 ml.

Three hours later a second blood glucose is 600 mg. per 100 ml. and the child is given 90 units of insulin intramuscularly. (Blood glucose decreased by 25 per cent; thus, insulin dose was reduced by 25 per cent.) Three hours later, the blood glucose level is 300 mg. per 100 ml. and 45 units of regular insulin are administered (50 per cent reduction in both).

Intravenous Fluids. Virtually all patients with ketoacidosis will require intravenous fluids. The depressed sensorium and the frequency with which vomiting is present usually precludes the oral route. Since the presenting acute dehydration is mainly intracellular (due to the fact that the nontransportable glucose maintains an osmotic gradient toward the extracellular fluid), many of the usual signs of dehydration may be missing. Hypovolemic shock is being averted due to the relative maintenance of the ECF volume. The child may have severe depression of his sensorium–secondary both to the dehydration and to the effect of the acidosis and ketosis on brain function. Rehydrating fluids must be selected with concern for volume, type of fluid and rate of administration.

The volume of fluid to be administered in the first 24 hours will depend on the *antecedent loss* (degree of dehydration) and will usually exceed 10 per cent of the total body weight. We have used the status of the sensorium to roughly assess (estimate) the degree of dehydration and as an aid in estimating the initial volume of fluid to be administered:

1. Mild to moderate depression of the sensorium–10 to 12 per cent dehydration.

2. Moderate to severe depression of the sensorium—13 to 15 per cent dehydration.

3. Extreme depression of sensorium; signs of shock—> 15 per cent dehydration.

In determining the volume of fluid replacement for antecedent losses, a good "rule of thumb" is as follows:

100 ml./body surface area (M^2)/degree dehydration (%)/24 hours
or
3 to 4 ml./body weight (kg.)/degree dehydration (%)/24 hours

To this volume must be added the *maintenance fluid* for each 24-hour period of treatment. Because insensible and renal water losses are likely to be high, it is desirable to "aim" high. Suggested amounts are:

2500 to 3000 ml./M^2 of body surface area/24 hours
or
85 to 100 ml./kg. of body weight/24 hours

Consequently, the total fluid replacement for the first 24 hours in a 30-kilogram (1 square meter) child who has moderate to severe depression of the sensorium (13 to 15 per cent dehydration) might be:

4500 ml. (1500 ml. for antecedent loss plus 3000 ml. for projected maintenance)

It should be kept in mind that these volumes are estimates and that actual volumes must be appropriately altered to the patient's clinical condition.

The *rate of fluid administration* has to be most rapid in the early stages when the need is greatest. It has been our practice to give approximately one-half of the total volume in the first 8 hours and to administer the remaining one-half in the last 16 hours. It is well to remember that a larger proportion of the replacement for antecedent deficit will be needed in the first 1 to 2 hours. After the first 8 hours, the fluids can generally be given at a constant hourly rate. Essentially this means replacement of the acute volume deficit in the first 8 hours and administration of maintenance fluids over the last 16 hours.

The *type of fluids* to be administered usually produces the greatest controversy and the following remarks are simply guidelines that may be followed:

1. *Initial fluids* (first 2 to 4 hours) should approximate isotonicity with respect to salts (sodium and its anions). This is absolutely essential if one is to "protect" the ECF from contraction when glucose begins its move into the cell. It is our practice to use either isotonic sodium chloride (0.9 per cent NaCl) or a solution containing about three-quarters normal saline (116 mEq. Na and Cl per liter), to which is added 30 mEq. per liter of sodium bicarbonate.

2. *Maintenance fluid* administration begins when antecedent deficits are largely replaced and, as noted earlier, should be reached in about 8 hours. For the majority of children recovering from an episode of diabetic ketoacidosis, maintenance requirements are most closely approximated with a sodium concentration of approximately 50 mEq. per liter. This can be given as a ⅓ normal sodium chloride (0.3 per cent NaCl) solution or a prepared formula in which the concentration is altered by the addition of sodium bicarbonate.

3. *Intermediate fluid* administration refers to that period occurring between the two former solutions—usually commencing at 2 to 4 hours after institution of fluid replacement and continuing through the eighth hour. These fluids should continue to replace the antecedent deficits of water and electrolytes, but since electrolyte deficit is not generally as great as water deficit (and is thus replaced earlier), the intermediate fluids should become progressively more dilute with the passage of time.

4. Additional factors to be considered in fluid replacement in the diabetic patient are carbohydrate administration, potassium administration and bicarbonate administration.

(a) *Carbohydrate administration* as a 5 per cent glucose solution should be started as soon as a significant drop has occurred in the initial blood glucose. Glucose-containing solutions should always be started by the time the blood glucose reaches 200 mg. per 100 ml. or the urine glucose drops below a 5 per cent reaction by the 2-drop Clinitest method.

(b) *Potassium administration* should be initiated as soon as continuing urine output is assured. Total body potassium depletion is usually marked, despite the fact that initial plasma potassium may be normal. As glucose and insulin are given and acidosis is corrected, potassium moves back into the cell and profound hypokalemia may occur. Generally, the concentration of potassium should approximate 40 mEq. per liter of the infused fluids, but in cases of severe hypokalemia, concentrations in excess of this may be necessary.

(c) *Bicarbonate administration* must be approached with some caution and attempts at rapid correction of the acidosis should not be undertaken. Studies have shown that following the rapid administration of sodium bicarbonate, there is a depression in the respiratory rate with a rise in pCO_2. Carbon dioxide diffuses into the CNS much more rapidly than does the bicarbonate ion, thus further reducing the pH and potentially worsening the condition. On the other hand, the buffer capacity of the ECF is diminished and the administration of bicarbonate in concentrations of 20 to 30 mEq. per liter of infused fluids may be used with profit.

5. Oral fluid administration should be initiated as soon as the patient is alert and capable of taking and retaining these fluids. This is generally within 12 to 18 hours in patients with severe ketoacidosis and considerably sooner in the mild to moderate cases.

CHRONIC OR LONG-RANGE THERAPY

General Philosophy of Care. Treatment programs for diabetic ketoacidosis are relatively standard, and differences between any two regimens are often minor. In sharp contrast, there are often significant differences between the various approaches to the long-term care of the diabetic child. These differences have led to controversy and confusion among both physicians and their patients. Part of the reason for this conflict lies in the failure of some physicians to distinguish clearly between growth-onset and maturity-onset diabetes mellitus. Failure to appreciate this difference leads the physician to approach the management of the "total" diabetic (juvenile or growth onset) just as he would the "partial" diabetic (adult or maturity-onset). The basic long-term care needs of the two conditions are so distinctly dissimilar that they defy therapeutic comparison.

Treatment of the whole child is of paramount importance in this disease, as it is with any chronic condition. The physician must resist the temptation to emphasize treatment of the blood and urine glucose to the exclusion of proper emphasis on physical growth and emotional development. Diabetes mellitus forces the child to be different from those in his peer group. It should, consequently, be expected that the child will resist acceptance of his disease and may openly defy certain therapeutic programs which magnify these differences. The physician must be aware that the child is immature and must appreciate the child's desire to be similar to his peers.

Reasonable and realistic goals are essential and it should be recognized that what constitutes realistic goals at one age will not necessarily be realistic at another. A 17-year-old diabetic should be expected to exercise greater control over his diabetes than should a 7-year-old. The goals are different because the problems are different. The diabetic child and his family must understand that goals and treatment programs will change as the child changes, never losing sight of the fact that the "optimum" program is one which parallels the non-diabetic child of comparable age as closely as possible.

Education of the diabetic child and his family is, perhaps, the single most important therapeutic aspect of long-term care. The child with diabetes is constantly changing and is continually being subjected to environmental factors which influence his disease. It is virtually impossible for the physician to cope effectively with all of these factors—partially due to his lack of immediate availability. It is our practice to utilize the initial hospitalization for extensive education. The "depth" of these instructional sessions will depend on the educational background of the family, but we have found that *all* families can be helped by providing them with reasons and explanations for proposed therapy. We use the booklet *An Instructional Aid on Juvenile Diabetes Mellitus** as our basic educational aid for all families. The material in this booklet is augmented by other prepared material (texts, questionnaires and so forth) and by a scheduled dialogue with the members of the diabetic health team (physician, dietitian, nurse).

Education of the diabetic should never be a "one-shot" affair but should be a continuing process throughout life. As the diabetic matures and accepts more responsibility for his disease, he should receive "new" tools which will allow future growth. Periodic refresher courses are mandatory if the diabetic youngster is to remain aware of his goals in management. Some families will never be able to comprehend fully the needs of day-to-day care, but most will be able to assume responsibility for care with the aid of a periodic review of their understanding and therapeutic goals.

General Goals of Therapy. It is important that the physician clearly establish the

* Obtained from the South Texas Diabetes Association, P. O. Box 1638, Pasadena, Texas 77501.

overall goals for his diabetic patient. The specific goals (and methods of achieving them) may vary somewhat from patient to patient, but these broader objectives should not waver.

1. *Freedom from the majority of the symptoms and signs referable to diabetes* is the first of our objectives. This statement does not merely mean that the child should elude ketoacidosis and/or hypoglycemia. It also implies that he should escape the more subtle symptomatology, such as polyuria, enuresis, transient visual disturbances, school absenteeism, vaginitis and skin infections. It should also include "freedom" from undue concern that each period of stress will evoke ketosis or that even minor activity will precipitate hypoglycemia.

2. *Normal physical growth and development* is also important, and instances can be cited where poor diabetic care has led to delayed statural growth and sexual maturation. On the other hand, the mere presence of normal statural growth and development does not indicate that the degree of diabetic control is optimum, for examples can be cited where statural growth and sexual development have progressed normally despite multiple episodes of ketoacidosis and hypoglycemia.

3. *Normal emotional development* may be most difficult to achieve in the diabetic child. The diabetic is often overprotected and has been shown to have a lower self-esteem and a higher anxiety level than his nondiabetic peer. Unnecessary restraints and curbs must be actively avoided and his diabetes should never be used as a threat to gain compliance. Attention must always be directed to the patient as a child with diabetes, rather than to the diabetic child.

4. *Delay or prevention of the consequences of diabetes* would be the major consideration *if* there were clear evidence that control of the carbohydrate metabolism (i.e., blood and urine glucose) affects these degenerative changes. While it may be true that poor carbohydrate control hastens the progression of these changes, there is no evidence that excellent control delays or prevents them. However, because the possibility of a cause-effect relationship continues to exist and because of the other problems inherent with poor control, reasonable efforts at good control should be of paramount concern to the physician and the diabetic.

Specific Items of Care. *Urine testing for carbohydrate* is an essential element of diabetic care, and the more often the diabetic checks his urine, the more will be known about the level of carbohydrate control. It is our policy to regulate the insulin dosage by the degree of glycosuria, raising the dosage when glycosuria is excessive and lowering the dosage when there is consistently no glycosuria. In the very young child (less than 4 years), we strive to have minimal glycosuria in all urine samples. In the mature adolescent diabetic, we may strive for aglycosuria much of the time if this can be attained without hypoglycemia. In the ages between these extremes, we generally attempt to have approximately half of the urine samples free of sugar, while the other half can contain small amounts. For routine use, we prefer the Clinitest tablets, and in the younger child we have found the "2-drop method" preferable to the standard 5-drop technique (a scale for the 2-drop technique may be obtained from the Ames Company). This method allows one to separate clearly 2 per cent glycosuria from 3 per cent and 5 per cent glycosuria. The recent introduction of Diastix to the market has given the diabetic greater flexibility, in that it is more convenient and has a scale which is similar to that of the Clinitest. We do not recommend the other paper-strip tests for glucose (Tes-Tape and Clinistix), since they have little visual gradation between small and large amounts of glucose.

Initially, we start all children on four urine sugar checks daily (before meals and at bedtime) and urge that each test be performed on a revoided or fresh urine. When the child enters school, we delete the before-lunch check and, gradually, will alter the program so that only the before-breakfast urine is a revoided sample. With increasing resistance to urine testing during adolescence, we may compromise on some of the afternoon and evening urines. It is our practice however to resist strongly any alteration in the revoided, before-breakfast sample, for we believe it to be the single most important test for the child receiving one daily injection of insulin.

During periods of stress, such as infections, we ask the children to check their urine more frequently. Likewise, at times when there are problems with diabetic control, we may ask them to check fresh, before-and-after meal samples; or to collect one or more timed samples for quantitation. The diabetic should be made aware of the fact that certain drugs will produce a positive test for sugar and invalidate the urine tests. Among these are NegGram and Keflex.

Urine testing for acetone or ketones may be performed with either the Acetest tablets or with Ketostix. A positive test (purple color) in the presence of excessive glycosuria indicates insulin deficiency of considerable magnitude and usually dictates the need for supplemental insulin. The diabetic must be aware that starvation and certain drugs (e.g., salicylates) may give positive reactions for ketone bodies. We generally ask our diabetic children to check urine ketones only when the urine sugar is 2 per cent (4+) or above.

Blood sugar or glucose determinations are not a matter of routine with us in the management of diabetic children and we generally use them only as an aid in delineating certain problems. At these times, we may perform several blood sugar determinations per day, with each sample being carefully planned to give maximum information (i.e., to measure peak of insulin action, or duration of action).

Insulin is the cornerstone of therapy and, following the initial period of stabilization, it is our aim to manage the majority of children with a single daily injection. In our experience, this is possible in approximately seventy-five per cent of the children. Either of the two intermediate-acting insulins, Lente or NPH (isophane), may be the principal insulin used and may be employed alone or in combination with regular (crystalline) insulin. When regular insulin is added to either Lente or NPH, it should constitute no more than 20 per cent of the total dose and may be given in the same syringe. Semilente insulin is occasionally given in combination with Lente. In the management of some of our very young children (less than 2 years), it has been our practice to use two daily injections of Semilente alone. We feel that there is little, if any, cause to utilize either PZI or Ultralente insulin in the management of children, since the use of these compounds is often accompanied by episodes of nocturnal hypoglycemia.

The amount of insulin to be given is the amount necessary to accomplish optimum glucose utilization without leading to either frequent hypoglycemia or obesity. The insulin requirement varies at different stages of diabetes and one must alter the dose depending on the results obtained from urine glucose analysis. In the early stages (particularly with ketosis), the demand for insulin is high; subsequently, the requirement drops markedly and generally reaches its lowest level about four to six weeks after onset, only to return gradually to a higher level which eventually averages about 1 unit per kilogram of body weight per day.

If the diabetic has initially been ketotic and has required regular insulin, the initial dose of Lente (or NPH) might be approximated by giving 3/4 to 4/5 of the amount of regular insulin given to achieve control during the previous 24 hours. If, on the other hand, the diabetes was preketotic (with no signs of CNS depression), the initial dose of NPH (or Lente) might range between 1/3 and 1 unit per kilogram of body weight.

Our diabetic children (or their families) are taught how to alter their daily insulin depending on the results of their urine tests. In general, changes in dose should not be made more often than every three to four days. When changes are made, it is generally recommended that the magnitude of change (either up or down) be about 10 per cent. This is a safe and usually effective change.

Dietary therapy is an integral part of any diabetic program. Unless some attention is paid to constancy of the diet, the blood and urine sugars will fluctuate widely and it will be difficult to predict an appropriate insulin dose. We attempt to arrive at two "constants" in our approach to diet: constancy in time of eating and constancy in amount of carbohydrate consumed at each meal or snack. In approaching the latter, we utilize the concept of the exchange diet system but apply this concept more broadly. Any food can be integrated into our diet plan as soon as its carbohydrate content is known or can be closely estimated. For our purposes, we divide sugar-containing foods into those that are (1) simple (pure sugars or fruit exchanges), (2) those that are complex (starches or bread exchanges) and (3) milk. A single fruit exchange contains 10 Gm. of carbohydrate, and equivalent servings of similar types of food are equivalent; e.g., a small apple equals 4 ounces of orange juice, 3 ounces of coke, 2 teaspoons of table sugar or 2 tablespoons of syrup. Similarly, bread exchanges can be expanded from the more traditional foods to include items such as cakes and candies merely by knowing their approximate carbohydrate content. Our patients are taught that simple sugars are rapidly absorbed from the intestinal tract and thus can produce rapid fluctuations in blood and urine sugars. Complex sugars (bread and milk exchanges) are absorbed more slowly, thus producing slower but more lasting changes in blood sugar. Since meat and fat exchanges have little, if any, immediate effect on blood glucose, we allow considerable latitude in their use. Thus, if a diet specified one hamburger at lunch (usually consisting of 2 bread exchanges, 2 fat exchanges and 3 meat exchanges), the bread exchanges would make the only significant contribution to a rise in blood sugar. If, after eating, this child were still hungry, he might have a second hamburger pattie (another 3 meat exchanges) without significantly influencing his diabetic control.

In the initial planning of the diet, we rely heavily on the dietetic history of the particular family to ensure that the food selected for the diet is similar to that usually consumed by his family. The diabetic should eat neither better nor worse than the other family members. We discourage the use of "dietetic" foods for this reason, as well as because of their expense. Low calorie (low carbohydrate) items such as soft drinks, candies and gums may be used as "extras" for times when the child wishes to participate and yet does not need additional calories.

Problems – Prevention and Treatment. *Hypoglycemia* of some degree is common in the diabetic youngster. It occurs in two recognizable forms: the first and most common is related to a rapid fall in blood glucose and associated with the warning signs and symptoms of counterregulatory hormones (shakiness, pallor, sweating, rapid pulse). The second variety of hypoglycemia follows a slower fall in blood glucose, and these warning symptoms are more subtle. With both, mental confusion and personality change may be prominent features. The diabetic should try to prevent hypoglycemia by (1) regulation of insulin dosage so that there is some protective range of safety and (2) knowledge of the environmental factors that can produce hypoglycemia (peak in insulin action, exercise, missed meals and so forth) in order to prevent their simultaneous occurrence. For example if planned physical activity occurs at the peak of insulin action, the dose of insulin might be reduced in an anticipatory manner. By contrast, if unpredicted and increased physical activity occurs, the diabetic should eat additional carbohydrate-containing foods before or during the activity.

If preventive measures are not successful, it is important that hypoglycemia be recognized early and aborted. The exercising child should stop and consume a rapid acting carbohydrate (fruit exchange items). Sugar cubes (wrapped in foil) should be carried at all times by the diabetic for these emergencies. Sugar cubes appear to be better than candy, for there is not as great a temptation to eat the sugar cubes for a social snack.

Profound hypoglycemia will occur occasionally and should be terminated as quickly as possible. If the child is conscious enough to swallow, sugar cubes should be administered. If the child cannot swallow or is convulsing, other therapy may be necessary. Instant Glucose† (containing 25 Gm. of glucose in a squeezable tube) can be absorbed directly through the buccal mucosa and is quite useful. Glucagon, in doses of 1 mg. intramuscularly, is generally quite effective in releasing hepatic glycogen and raising blood glucose. It is our practice to equip the homes of our diabetic children with both these agents and to recommend that the school nurse also have both available.

Ketoacidosis can generally be prevented by appropriate treatment of ketosis. Ketosis may occur during infection or other stress and should be treated promptly to prevent more serious illness, perhaps culminating in hospitalization. Ketone (or acetone) excretion in the presence of heavy glycosuria demands the prompt administration of regular insulin. It is our practice to have patients give themselves supplemental regular insulin injections as soon as this condition is recognized (using an individual dose equal to 1/5 of the usual daily dose of insulin). On most occasions, two or three supplemental doses (given at 2- to 3-hour intervals) will be sufficient to "break" the ketosis and prevent further worsening of the condition. This dose of insulin is chosen because it is usually effective but, more importantly, it is also safe.

Perhaps the most troublesome acute illness complicating diabetes is the one accompanied by *nausea and vomiting.* The risk of serious disturbance is magnified as early dehydration (secondary to diminished intake and vomiting) compromises the body's usual defenses against acidosis. In addition, with protracted anorexia and vomiting, there is the possibility of starvation ketosis making its appearance at a time when insulin activity is still present. Our diabetic patients are instructed to manage the diabetic state in the usual fashion—administration of their ordinary insulin dosage and supplementation of this with additional regular insulin whenever the urine dictates a need (heavy glycosuria with ketonuria). Antiemetic drugs (suppositories) are utilized and the children are instructed to take small (and gradually increasing) amounts of carbonated beverages, coke syrup or Emetrol (15 to 30 ml. every 15 to 30 minutes) until the vomiting ceases.

Adolescent adjustment reactions appear to be somewhat more common in the diabetic child than in the nondiabetic. This is partially because the diabetic is subjected to a greater

---

† Obtained from the Cleveland Diabetes Association, 10205 Carnegie Avenue, Cleveland, Ohio 44106.

number of emotional stresses on a continuing basis. He is often overprotected and dependent. Increased anxiety and decreased self-esteem commonly follow. If diabetes has been the dominant feature in his life, the child may actually rebel against this "figure" of authority. The physician has an obligation to place all diabetic therapy in its proper perspective and thus to aid in circumventing some of these problems. Summer camps for diabetics are frequently helpful in this respect.

Hypoglycemia

MARVIN CORNBLATH, M.D., *and*
NOEL KEITH MACLAREN, M.D.

Clinical hypoglycemia is the association of an abnormally low blood sugar with a variety of signs and symptoms which are improved with glucose administration or food. The clinical state results from decreased glucose availability to the central nervous system and the induced catecholamine response, and includes weakness, apathy, irritability, hunger, bizarre behavior, mental confusion, apnea, cyanosis, hypothermia, convulsions and coma, together with pallor, sweating, tremulousness, tachycardia and shock.

The use of Dextrostix is a useful bedside diagnostic aid, but in every patient a reliable laboratory sugar determination of blood and/or cerebrospinal fluid must be done before initiating therapy. Serum or plasma should be frozen and saved for insulin measurement.

NEONATAL HYPOGLYCEMIA

Hypoglycemia in the neonate has been defined statistically on the basis of extensive clinical studies, such as replicate blood sugar values of less than 20 mg. per 100 ml. in the infant of low birth weight (less than 2500 Gm.), and of less than 30 mg. per 100 ml. in full-sized infants during the first 72 hours of life and less than 40 mg. per 100 ml. thereafter. Most infants with hypoglycemia have clinical manifestations, such as twitching, jitteriness, apathy, cyanotic spells, hypothermia, pallor, sweating or convulsions (Cornblath et al.). Symptomatic infants should be treated if the Dextrostix reads under 30 mg. per 100 ml. (Swiatek et al.), while waiting for laboratory blood glucose results.

Give 2 to 4 ml. per kilogram (0.5 to 1 Gm. per kilogram) of 25 per cent glucose intravenously as a slow push, and continue the infusion as 15 per cent glucose in water to provide 10 mg. per kilogram per minute for at least 24 hours or until 48 hours of age. Then, continue the infusion with 10 per cent glucose in 0.22 per cent saline at a rate to maintain a normal glucose level (4 to 6 mg. per kilogram per minute). Oral feedings should be introduced as soon as clinical manifestations subside. Therapy can be tapered off after blood sugar levels have remained over 30 to 40 mg. per 100 ml. for 24 to 48 hours by changing to 5 per cent glucose and then stopping.

Never discontinue hypertonic glucose abruptly, or a reactive hypoglycemia may ensue. If symptoms persist beyond 2 to 4 hours despite a sustained elevation in blood sugar, blood calcium and magnesium determinations are indicated.

If blood sugar levels remain under 30 mg. per 100 ml. with adequate glucose therapy, start hydrocortisone (Solu-Cortef), 5 mg. per kilogram per day every 8 hours by the oral, intramuscular or intravenous route. Hydrocortisone can be tapered when the blood sugar has remained over 30 mg. per 100 ml. for 48 hours, and stopped after three days. During treatment, blood sugars should be monitored at 2- to 6-hour intervals.

Glucagon (0.3 mg. per kilogram intramuscularly or intravenously) can be used with effect in asymptomatic infants of diabetic mothers. However, glucagon and epinephrine are not recommended for treating any other neonate with hypoglycemia.

HYPOGLYCEMIA OF INFANCY

Inborn Errors of Carbohydrate Metabolism

Hypoglycemia may present in the neonatal period or in early infancy.

GLYCOGEN STORAGE DISEASE. *Cori Type I (Glucose-6-Phosphatase Deficiency).* Since the production of glucose from the liver is severely restricted, frequent glucose-containing feeds should be given from early infancy. Diets limited in lactose are usually recommended to minimize glycogen storage from galactose. Glucose should replace sucrose as a dietary sugar. Oral bicarbonate therapy is often required for the associated lactic acidosis. A diet containing medium-chain triglycerides may be used to reduce hyperlipemia.

Cori Type III (Amylo-1, 6-Glycosidase or Debrancher Deficiency).

Cori Type VI (Deficiency of the Phosphorylase System).

Synthetase Deficiency. Hypoglycemia may be less severe and tends to ameliorate with increasing age. Dietary management as outlined for type I generally applies. Hormone therapies are probably ineffectual. (See Disorders of Carbohydrate Metabolism.)

Galactose Intolerance (Galactose–1–Phosphate Uridyl Transferase of Galactokinase Deficiency). Strict avoidance of lactose-containing milk, foods and sweets is essential. (See Disorders of Carbohydrate Metabolism.)

Fructose Intolerance (Fructose–1–Phosphate Aldolase Deficiency). Hypoglycemic attacks date from the introduction of fructose (often as sucrose) into the diet. Give a fructose-free diet, avoiding sucrose (table sugar) and fruits. Substitute glucose as a dietary sugar. (See Disorders of Carbohydrate Metabolism.)

Fructose-1, 6-Diphosphatase Deficiency. Glycerol and sucrose precipitate hypoglycemia and must be minimized in the diet. A special diet consisting of 65 per cent carbohydrate (excluding sucrose and fructose), 15 per cent protein and 20 per cent fat has been reported to be effective (Pagliara et al.). Lactic acidosis associated with the hypoglycemia may require alkali therapy.

Endocrine Deficiencies

Hypoglycemia rarely complicates congenital virilizing adrenal hyperplasia. Replacement doses of cortisone acetate (usually near 25 mg. per square meter per day) are usually effective in controlling such episodes.

Creatinism may be associated with hypoglycemia, and replacement therapy with desiccated thyroid usually controls symptoms.

Growth hormone deficiency may manifest as early hypoglycemia, and may occur in a syndrome with underdeveloped genitalia in infant boys. Intermittent replacement therapy with growth hormone is indicated (1 to 2 units three times a week).

Hyperinsulinism may occur in infancy, associated with "infant giant" syndrome, beta-cell hyperplasia, nesidioblastosis and beta-cell tumors of the pancreas. Surgery is indicated in such cases and should not be delayed in infants with recurrent or persistent hypoglycemia. If a discrete tumor is not palpated at laparotomy, a subtotal pancreatectomy should be carried out, removing 80 per cent or more of the pancreas (Baker et al.). Diazoxide and streptozotocin are supportive drugs useful in some cases (see below).

Idiopathic

Frequently, no specific cause for the hypoglycemia is found. Emergency treatment with intravenous glucose is given as outlined under Neonatal Hypoglycemia. Dietary management with frequent carbohydrate-containing feedings, avoiding prolonged fasts, is basic.

Leucine Sensitivity. Infants exhibiting hypoglycemia after oral leucine should be managed with low leucine diets. The diet must be adequate in leucine for growth, but divided into three or more meals to provide small amounts of leucine (Roth and Segal). Offer carbohydrate feeding 30 minutes after meals, on arising and before sleep. For infants, S-14 (Wyeth) is recommended, but SMA-26, Enfamil, Bremil or Similac can be used (see Marbry et al. for details).

Drug Therapy. For many infants, regular feeding schedules and avoidance of whole-night fasting are adequate. For others, attacks become recurrent and further measures are necessary.

Steroids. Oral cortisone acetate (5 mg. per kilogram per day) or prednisone (1 to 2 mg. per kilogram per day) in two to three divided doses is often effective. The steroid dosage should be reduced by approximately 20 per cent weekly until the lowest dose level compatible with freedom from hypoglycemia is reached. Steroids will retard growth, as well as cause other problems, and should be slowly withdrawn after prolonged use.

Adrenergic Drugs. These compounds offer the theoretical advantages of inhibiting insulin release, mobilizing fat stores and promoting hyperglycemia. Sus-phrine or epinephrine, 0.3 mg. subcutaneously, may be useful in treating an acute episode and can be given by parents in an emergency. Ephedrine may be used in long-term management, particularly in patients who fail to respond to hypoglycemia with increased catecholamine output (Zetterstrom).

Diazoxide. This drug is a thiazide derivative. It has a major action in inhibiting insulin secretion. Its side effects include hypotension, salt retention, hyperuricemia and low IgG levels. In practice, hirsutism (hypertrichiasis lanuginosa) is frequently encountered, and parents should be warned about this.

Start with 4 mg. per kilogram per day in 8- to 12-hour doses, and increase as necessary to 20 to 25 mg. per day.* Doses under 10 mg. per kilogram per day are usually effective. Diazoxide should *not* be discontinued *suddenly* after prolonged use.

Glucagon. In infants with hyperinsulinism, glucagon may produce a dramatic response. Give 0.03 to 0.10 mg. per kilogram intravenously or intramuscularly. If the infant responds to glucagon, parents should be shown how to administer it at home in an emergency.

---

* Manufacturer's precaution: The safety of the intravenous use of diazoxide in children has not yet been established.

HYPOGLYCEMIA IN LATE INFANCY AND CHILDHOOD

The frequency of *islet cell tumor* increases with age, but it remains a rare cause of hypoglycemia at any age. Treatment is surgical. In patients who have persistent hypoglycemia after partial pancreatectomy, *streptozotocin* may be considered. Streptozotocin selectivity destroys the pancreatic beta-cell in animals. Experience in humans is limited but it has been effective in some cases of beta-cell carcinoma and *intractable hyperinsulinism*. For adults, 2 to 5 Gm. have been given at one- to four-week intervals for two to three doses given as an intravenous infusion. Nausea and vomiting are usual. This drug is experimental.

Overdoses of insulin or hypoglycemic drugs may respond to glucagon (0.5 to 1 mg. by injection). Alcohol taken during fasting can cause serious hypoglycemia by inhibiting hepatic gluconeogenesis. In all cases of *alcohol ingestion* the child should have his stomach washed out and be admitted to the hospital for monitoring blood sugar levels. If the child is drowsy, intravenous glucose is given at a rate of 0.5 Gm. per kilogram per hour. Hypoglycemia may complicate severe aspirin overdose. Glucose therapy as outlined previously is given for hypoglycemia occurring in Reye's syndrome, hypothermia, malnutrition states and diarrheal disorders.

Idiopathic Hypoglycemia of Childhood

Ketotic hypoglycemia (Colle and Ulstrom) is the most common syndrome of hypoglycemia in childhood. It rarely occurs before one year of age and attacks seldom persist into puberty. Hypoglycemic episodes are widely spaced and can be largely prevented with frequent low fat, high protein, high carbohydrate meals coupled with the routine testing for ketonuria on rising or at times of illness. If ketonuria is found, attacks may be prevented with sugar in the form of candy, carbonated drinks or sweetened juices. This must be continued until the ketonuria clears. If vomiting, coma or convulsions occur, give 0.5 to 1 Gm. of intravenous glucose per kilogram by push, followed by 0.5 Gm. per kilogram per hour until food can be taken. Glucagon is characteristically ineffective and the poor response is often diagnostic. Treatment with glucose is essential. Steroids have been shown to prevent attacks but are seldom required since most children respond to dietary measures.

Hypoglycemia often constitutes a medical emergency and glucose administration is required, although some patients will respond to glucagon or epinephrine. Rational therapy subsequently depends on identification of the cause.

References

Baker, L., and Winegrad, A. I.: Fasting Hypoglycemia and Metabolic Acidosis Associated with Deficiency of Hepatic Fructose-1,6-Diphosphatase Activity. *Lancet,* 2:13, 1970.

Colle, E., and Ulstrom, R. A.: Ketotic Hypoglycemia. *J. Pediat.,* 64:632, 1964.

Cornblath, M., and Schwartz, R.: *Disorders of Carbohydrate Metabolism in Infancy*. Philadelphia, W. B. Saunders Company, 1966.

Cornblath, M., et al.: Symptomatic neonatal hypoglycemia. Studies of carbohydrate metabolism in the newborn infant. *Pediatrics,* 33:338, 1964.

Cunningham, G., Quickel, K., and Lebowitz, H.: The Use of Insulin Dynamics in the Evaluation of Streptozotocin Therapy in Malignant Insulinomas. *J. Clin. Endocr.,* 33:530, 1971.

Mabry, C. C., DiGeorge, A. M., and Auerback, V. H.: Leucine-Induced Hypoglycemia. Clinical Observations and Diagnostic Considerations. *J. Pediat.,* 57: 526, 1960.

Maclaren, N., Valman, B., Levin, B.: Alcohol Induced Hypoglycemia in Childhood. *Brit. Med. J.,* 1:278, 1970.

Pagliara, A. S., Karl, I. E., Keating, J. P., Brown, B. I., and Kipnis, D. M.: Hepatic Fructose-1, 6-diphosphatase Deficiency. *J. Clin. Invest.,* 51:2115, 1972.

Roth, H., and Segal, S.: The Dietary Management of Leucine-Sensitive Hypoglycemia, with Report of a Case. *Pediatrics,* 34:831, 1964.

Swiatek, K., Luebben, G., and Cornblath, M.: Screening Method for Determining Glucose in Blood and Cerebrospinal Fluid. *Am. J. Dis. Child.* 117:672, 1969.

Underwood, L. E., Van der Brande, J. L., Antony, G. J., Voina, S. J., and Van Wy, K. J.: Islet Cell Function and Glucose Homeostasis in Hypopituitary Dwarfism. Synergism Between Growth and Cortisone. *J. Pediat.,* 82:128, 1973.

Weyer, E. M. (ed.): Diazoxide and the Treatment of Hypoglycemia. *Ann. N.Y. Acad. Sci.,* 150:191, 1968.

Rickets

HAROLD E. HARRISON, M.D.

PREVENTION

Vitamin D–Deficiency Rickets. This can be prevented by the recommended intake of 400 I.U. of vitamin D daily, which is provided by one quart of fortified homogenized cow's milk or the equivalent amount of evaporated milk or prepared infant feeding preparations. Small, prematurely born or immature infants who for one or two months will not be taking an amount of milk sufficient to provide the necessary vitamin D requirement should receive a vitamin D–containing concentrate to increase their vitamin D intake to 400 I.U. daily. They do not need greater amounts of vitamin D than this. Breast fed infants also should be given a vitamin D preparation providing 400 I.U. of vitamin D daily, since human milk does not contain sufficient vitamin D for the infant's needs.

The vitamin D requirement of children beyond infancy is also assumed to be 400 I.U. per day. In this age group, exposure to sunshine and the vitamin D intake in foods, such as tuna fish, salmon, sardines and eggs, may provide most of the vitamin D needs. However, vitamin D fortified milk should still be recommended. There is no need for other vitamin D preparations unless there is a known defect of absorption or metabolism of vitamin D.

Infants and children with fat malabsorption, whether due to biliary atresia or other causes, require an increased intake of vitamin D because of the excessive losses in feces. Patients with hepatocellular injury (neonatal hepatitis, cytomegalic inclusion body hepatitis and so forth) also require increased amounts of vitamin D, presumably because of impaired liver metabolism of vitamin D to 25-hydroxy vitamin D. These patients should be given 2000 to 5000 I.U. of vitamin D daily in the form of a propylene glycol solution of ergocalciferol (Drisdol, 10,000 I.U. vitamin D per Gm., 250 I.U. per drop). Patients on large doses of anticonvulsant drugs may also need increased amounts of vitamin D and should also be given 2000 to 5000 I.U. per day.

TREATMENT

Vitamin D–Deficiency Rickets. Simple deficiency rickets can be rapidly healed by oral, massive dose treatment, i.e., 600,000 I.U. of vitamin D in a single dose or in several divided doses over a 24-hour period. A concentrated calciferol in oil preparation is necessary if this treatment is to be used, since this amount of vitamin D in the propylene glycol solution (Drisdol, 10,000 I.U. per Gm.) would produce propylene glycol intoxication with prolonged stupor. Alternatively, 5000 to 10,000 I.U. of vitamin D daily for six to eight weeks will suffice to heal the rickets. Following this, the child should be maintained on preventive amounts of vitamin D, 400 I.U. per day.

Rickets Due to Malabsorption of Vitamin D or Hepatic Disease. This can be treated with oral vitamin D if given in increased amounts, 10,000 to 25,000 I.U. daily, the dose being controlled by serial determinations of serum calcium, phosphorus and alkaline phosphatase concentrations as well as by roentgenographic examinations of wrists and knees for healing. Parenteral administration of vitamin D is not necessary even in the face of fat malabsorption if vitamin D in propylene glycol is given in sufficient amount. With marked malabsorption the vitamin D can be given with a medium-chain triglyceride preparation. When healing is evident, the dose of vitamin D can be reduced to the necessary maintenance dose.

Primary Hypophosphatemic Vitamin D–Resistant Rickets. The fundamental abnormality in this disorder is in the transport of phosphate, leading to impaired intestinal absorption of phosphate and wastage of phosphate in the urine. The basis for treatment in this disease is oral phosphate. Sufficient phosphate must be given to raise the serum phosphate at least transiently to levels at which mineralization of bone can occur (serum P greater than 4 mg. per 100 ml.). Very large amounts of phosphate salts, equivalent to at least 1.5 to 2 Gm. of phosphorus per day in divided doses, are required. The pharmaceutical preparation Neutra-Phos is a buffered mixture of phosphate salts. When the salts are dissolved as directed, 300 ml. provides 1 Gm. of phosphorus. A total of 450 to 600 ml. of solution per day divided into four or five portions spread out through the day is necessary for adequate therapy. A high phosphate intake interferes with calcium absorption and lowers serum calcium ion concentration, leading to secondary hyperparathyroidism. It is necessary, therefore, to increase calcium absorption by high doses of vitamin D, 25,000 to 100,000 I.U. per day, or dihydrotachysterol, 0.2 to 1 mg. per day. The proper dose is the amount of activated sterol which will maintain normal serum calcium concentrations and normal urine calcium excretion, 50 to 150 mg. per 24 hours. In our clinic, dihydrotachysterol is preferred because it is more rapidly excreted or inactivated in the body than is vitamin D, and therefore is less cumulative in its action. If hypercalcemia or hypercalciuria supervenes during treatment, the activated sterol should be discontinued until the urine excretion of calcium returns to normal values; administration of sterol is then resumed at a lower dose.

Vitamin D–Dependent Rickets. This is an abnormality of vitamin D requirement in which unusually large amounts of vitamin D are needed, but when suitable doses are given a complete physiologic response is obtained with return of serum calcium and phosphate concentrations to normal. The large doses of vitamin D must be continued or rickets will return. The necessary dose must be determined in the individual patient by monitoring serum calcium, phosphate and alkaline phosphatase concentrations. Doses as high as 25,000 to 50,000 I.U. have been required in some patients.

Rickets Associated with Renal Tubular Acidosis. In this disorder, correction of the acidosis leads to return to normal of the serum phosphate concentrations and healing of the rickets. Excessive amounts of vitamin D are not required. Correction of the acidosis can usually be achieved by administration of excess cation. A convenient preparation is a solution of sodium and potassium citrates (Polycitra). The dosage must be determined by monitoring serum bicarbonate concentrations. In most patients, 20 to 60 ml. per day in divided doses have been sufficient.

Rickets Associated with Fanconi Syndrome. In this disorder, whether due to cystinosis or other metabolic disorders, there are multiple renal tubular dysfunctions, including impaired renal tubular reabsorption of phosphate. Treatment must include correction of acidosis, potassium supplementation and phosphate administration. In some patients, renal tubular reabsorption of phosphate is improved by increased amounts of vitamin D, up to 25,000 to 50,000 I.U. as in patients with vitamin D–dependent rickets.

References

Harrison, H. E., and Harrison, H. C.: Hereditary Metabolic Bone Diseases. *Clin. Orthop.*, 33:147, 1964.

Harrison, H. E., Lifshitz, F., and Blizzard, R. M.: Comparison Between Crystalline Dihydrotachysterol and Calciferol in Patients Requiring Pharmacologic Vitamin D Therapy. *New England J. Med.* 276:894, 1967.

Tetany

HAROLD E. HARRISON, M.D.

Tetany is a state of heightened excitability of the peripheral and central nervous system due to altered concentrations of certain ions in extracellular fluid. Treatment is based on the three major categories of ionic deficiency; hypocalcemia, hypomagnesemia and hydrogen ion deficiency (alkalosis).

HYPOCALCEMIC TETANY

Vitamin D Deficiency. Treatment of hypocalcemia due to vitamin D deficiency consists in the administration of vitamin D. We prefer a large oral dose of vitamin D, 600,000 I.U. total, given in divided doses within a 24-hour period. This must be in the form of a highly concentrated vitamin D preparation and not the dilute vitamin D in propylene glycol (Drisdol, 10,000 I.U. per Gm.), since the required volume of propylene glycol would produce central nervous system depression similar to that produced by alcohol. If the infant is actively convulsing or having laryngeal spasm, immediate elevation of serum calcium ion concentration is mandatory and is obtained by intravenous injection of 10 per cent calcium gluconate, approximately 2 ml. per kg., up to a total of 10 ml. This is given at a rate which does not depress the sinus node and is controlled by monitoring the heart rate during the injection. If bradycardia occurs, the injection is stopped and then resumed as soon as circulatory mixing occurs and the heart rate returns to normal. This intravenous dose can be repeated at 6- to 8-hour intervals if necessary until the effect of vitamin D begins. Calcium solutions must never be given intramuscularly and care must be taken to avoid extravascular infiltration, since severe necrosis and calcification can occur at the site of infiltration.

HYPOPARATHYROID HYPOCALCEMIA

Early Hypocalcemia of Stressed Newborn, Such as Infants of Diabetic Mothers. This is usually a self-limited hypocalcemia which is treated with intravenous injection of 10 per cent calcium gluconate as described above. (See also p. 237.)

Transient Physiologic Hypoparathyroidism of the Neonatal Period. This hypocalcemia is the result of relative deficiency of parathyroid hormone in the face of the hyperphosphatemia of high phosphate feedings based on cow's milk. This can be corrected by reduction of the serum phosphorus through sequestration of phosphate in the intestine as calcium phosphate, which prevents phosphate absorption. A large excess of a calcium salt must be dissolved in the infant feeding so that the calcium-to-phosphorus ratio in the feed is raised to 4:1 by weight. The calcium can be added as calcium lactate powder, calcium gluconate powder or calcium gluconate solution (Neo-Calglucon Syrup). Calcium chloride should not be used because it is irritating to the gastric mucosa and will produce hyperchloremic acidosis if continued for several days. Calcium lactate powder is 13 per cent calcium, calcium gluconate powder is 9 per cent calcium, and Neo-Calglucon Syrup contains 92 mg. of calcium per 4-ml. teaspoon. A sample calculation is as follows:

The food intake of calcium and phosphorus is estimated to be 500 and 300 mg. per day, respectively. To achieve a Ca:P ratio of 4:1, 700 mg. of calcium must be added per 24-hour feed. This is provided by 5.4 Gm. of calcium lactate, 7.8 Gm. of calcium gluconate, or 8 teaspoons of Neo-Calglucon Syrup.

After the serum phosphorus concentration

is reduced and the serum calcium concentration restored to normal, the calcium supplement is reduced in stages until the infant can take an unsupplemented feeding without hypocalcemia. This may take from one week to several weeks and must be individualized.

Congenital and Idiopathic Hypoparathyroidism. This is a more complete deficiency of parathyroid hormone and cannot be treated simply by calcium supplementation. Large amounts either of vitamin D or of vitamin D–like steroids must be used to replace the lacking parathyroid hormone. We believe the most suitable steroid to be dihydrotachysterol, which is available as a pure steroid isolated from irradiated ergosterol. It is more potent than vitamin D as a pharmacologic substitute for parathyroid hormone, and it has a shorter biologic half-life than vitamin D, so that there is less danger of cumulative effects. A daily dose of 0.25 to 1 mg. is effective in most patients with hypoparathyroidism, but the dosage must be determined for each patient by serum calcium determinations. If vitamin D is used, doses of 50,000 to 200,000 I.U. may be required. In the growing child, serum calcium concentrations should be maintained close to the normal range to prevent the ectodermal defects of hypocalcemia, particularly lenticular opacities. Supplemental calcium salts are not needed if adequate amounts of dihydrotachysterol or vitamin D are given. In postthyroidectomy hypoparathyroidism, there may be sufficient residual parathyroid function; consequently, treatment with oral calcium salts may be sufficient, as in the patient with transient hypoparathyroidism of the neonatal period. In older children, calcium carbonate in suspension or tablet form can be given for this purpose. Calcium carbonate is 40 per cent calcium, and 10 Gm. of calcium carbonate (4 Gm. calcium) in divided doses can be tried before treatment with dihydrotachysterol or vitamin D is begun.

HYPOMAGNESEMIC TETANY

Hypomagnesemia can be associated with hypocalcemia in infants with transient hypoparathyroidism and does not require specific treatment, since it responds as does the serum calcium to reduction of serum phosphorus concentrations.

Primary hypomagnesemia of infancy can result from impaired intestinal absorption of magnesium due either to a congenital deficiency of a magnesium transport system or to a complication of chronic diarrhea and intestinal malabsorption. Acute hypomagnesemic tetany can be treated by intramuscular injection of a 50 per cent solution of $MgSO_4 \cdot 12H_2O$ in a dosage of 0.2 ml. per kilogram. This will elevate the serum magnesium for several hours. Supplementation of the diet with magnesium lactate or a magnesium chloride–magnesium citrate mixture is required in patients with chronic magnesium malabsorption (500 to 2000 mg. magnesium per day in divided doses).

TETANY OF ALKALOSIS

If alkalosis is the result of hyperventilation, the tetany can be controlled by rebreathing into a paper bag or anesthesia mask and balloon. The alkalosis of hydrochloric acid loss in patients with pyloric obstruction is rarely associated with tetany. The treatment is replacement of the chloride deficit by sodium chloride solution with potassium chloride added.

References

Harrison, H. E.; in R. E. Cooke (ed.): *The Biologic Basis of Pediatric Practice.* New York, McGraw-Hill Book Company, 1968, pp. 134 and 1137.

Paunier, L., Radde, I. C., Kooh, S. W., Cohen, P. E., and Fraser, D.: Primary Hypomagnesemia with Secondary Hypocalcemia in an Infant. *Pediatrics,* 41:385, 1968.

The Idiopathic Hypercalcemic Syndrome: Infantile Hypercalcemia

REGINALD LIGHTWOOD, M.D., F.R.C.P.

VARIETIES

1. Idiopathic hypercalcemia with failure to thrive is a syndrome manifesting anorexia, vomiting, constipation, polyuria, thirst, recurring dehydration and muscular hypotonia. It is usually transient and relatively benign; with good nursing care and increased fluid intake, most affected infants recover gradually. Recovery can be hastened by appropriate treatment.

2. Patients with the syndrome described as the *severe* type of hypercalcemia usually present with the same initial symptoms as the milder cases, but the characteristic facies of hypercalcemia is present and there may be osteosclerosis, renal and cardiovascular damage and mental impairment. As for the prognosis, some of these cases are fatal, often between one and three years of age.

3. The third syndrome has been called the triad of Williams. It comprises cases usually passing unrecognized until the late normocalcemic stage is reached. Williams' triad consists of

dwarfing and mental retardation, the peculiar facies of hypercalcemia and supravalvular aortic stenosis.

TO WHAT EXTENT CAN THESE SYNDROMES BE INFLUENCED BY TREATMENT?

In the active phase of infantile hypercalcemia, laboratory data indicate that, relative to skeletal growth, there is an excessive intestinal absorption of calcium with a strongly positive calcium balance. Therefore, treatment consists of stopping any supplementation with vitamin D and giving a diet sufficient for growth but low in calcium, or adding substances that inhibit calcium absorption. In the mild uncomplicated cases, calcium balance then becomes negative (Stapleton et al., 1956), symptoms disappear rather promptly and hypercalcemia gradually subsides, but azotemia usually persists somewhat longer. The evidence in these cases is that the pathologic changes are wholly reversible, and there are no sequelae.

In severe cases, however, not all the pathologic changes are reversible and the prognosis for complete recovery is poor; consequently, treatment may be of limited value.

There are, however, cases which are intermediate, between the mild or pathologically reversible cases and the severe or irreversible ones. Do the mild and the severe syndromes in fact represent the opposite ends of a clinical spectrum of the same pathologic process? Or are they separate entities? In this context, an observation first made by Butler is significant. He found that in most of the severe cases personally studied, the birth weight was below the average, whereas in the mild cases it was within the normal range. This was later confirmed by Fraser et al., who reported that the mean birth weight of a group of 25 patients (mild form) was not below that of a normal population, but the mean birth weight of a group of 36 "severe" cases was below the mean. In their report, data concerning the maternal intake of vitamin D during pregnancy were not available. Nevertheless, there are clear grounds for suspecting that in some cases, at least in the severe ones, the metabolic insult of hypercalcemia may begin to affect the fetus before birth. Thus, if we are to prevent all the severe cases, specific investigations of nutrition and vitamin supplementation in pregnancy are needed.

ETIOLOGY

Curative and preventive treatment should take account of the causal factors. Apart from obvious cases of vitamin D poisoning, there are a number of summating factors to consider: actual intake of vitamin D (from all sources), individual reactivity to vitamin D (including racial differences), vehicle of administration, type of feeding and rate of growth.

Intake of Vitamin D. Because of the influence of the other four factors, it is not possible to determine any fixed prophylactic dose capable of protecting all infants from rickets and harming none. Repeated administration of sufficiently large doses of vitamin D will result in symptoms of poisoning, and these symptoms are in general similar to those of the mild type of idiopathic hypercalcemia, sometimes including concurrent renal tubular acidosis and metastatic calcification. However, long-continued exposure may lead to the severe type of hypercalcemia.

Individual Reactivity. In cases of idiopathic hypercalcemia, is there a specific abnormality in the metabolism of vitamin D? Most healthy infants can tolerate intakes of vitamin D far in excess of so-called normal requirements, whereas, in contrast, a small minority exhibit intolerance to ordinary prophylactic doses. Not enough is known about the physiologic mechanisms by which the body protects itself against unwanted vitamin D, except that, as also in experimental animals, bile is a major route of excretion for vitamin D and its metabolites and these are found in the feces; however, the chemical structure of these fecal vitamin D sterols has not been defined; nor has there been a study of possible differences in this excretion in vitamin D intolerance. Furthermore, the phenomenon of vitamin intolerance has not been elucidated by the many recent research findings, which have now gone a long way in defining metabolic changes in vitamin D_3 after absorption, and mechanisms of action at the molecular level (DeLuca and Suttie).

RACIAL DIFFERENCES IN REACTION TO VITAMIN D. Geographic differences in the distribution of rickets are mainly due to environmental and dietary factors, but perhaps there are racial differences as well. Some North American Negro infants are more liable to rickets (and require larger therapeutic doses) than children of Northern European stock. A comparison of the vitamin D activity in the blood in white and Negro children demonstrated that some of the former had significantly higher serum levels (Warkany and Mabon). From reports in the literature it seems that the hypercalcemic syndromes occur predominantly and with very few exceptions in white children.

Vehicle of Administration. The antirachitic activity of vitamin D in infants is reportedly increased three or more times when milk, as compared with oil, is the vehicle. If these findings are correct, then the administration of, say, 400 I.U. in milk could be equivalent in vitamin D activity to several times that amount of vitamin when dissolved in oil (Seelig).

Type of Feeding–Human or Cow's Milk. Infantile hypercalcemia is very rare in breast fed infants, and this difference has been ascribed to the higher concentration of calcium in cow's milk, but a more likely explanation is the fact that vitamin D is usually incorporated in dried and evaporated milks but cannot be artificially added to breast milk.

Rate of Growth. Cessation or slowing of growth implies a reduced rate of calcium accretion in bone, and a vicious circle could develop of hypercalcemia leading to growth arrest leading to increased hypercalcemia. It may also be significant that hypercalcemia has been reported in a few cretins.

One of our aims in the treatment of hypercalcemia is to feed a sufficient amount of calories so that normal growth can be resumed.

TREATMENT

Preventive

In view of the individual variations in response to vitamin D, which depend on the several factors that have been described previously, it is obvious that the eradication of rickets is not simply a matter of administering a uniform prophylactic dose. Ideally the prophylactic dose should be not more than is safe for infants who are hyperreactive to the vitamin. Until this problem has been reinvestigated, it is advised that a daily intake of 400 I.U. (from all sources) should not be exceeded, except in the case of infants who show increased susceptibility to rickets. The enhancement of the potency of vitamin D in milk, in comparison to oil as the vehicle, should not be forgotten. During periods of arrested growth (e.g., acute infections) it is wise to stop vitamin D for the time being.

A mother's dietary intake of vitamin D during pregnancy should usually not exceed 400 I.U. per day (all sources).

Curative

During the active phase (hypercalcemia) management should provide for (1) a reduction of intestinal absorption of calcium, attained by eliminating vitamin D from the diet and giving a low intake of calcium, and (2) efforts to increase utilization and excretion of calcium, i.e., sufficient calories for resumption of growth, increased intake of fluid and increased physical activity.

Low Calcium Diet. Breast milk, if available, with its lesser calcium content and no added vitamin D, can be valuable. In formula fed infants with hypercalcemia, ordinary cow's milk and its products must be excluded and a special diet containing less than 100 mg. of calcium per day should be provided: Locasol (Trufood Ltd., London, England), a low calcium milk substitute in powder form containing not more than 0.05 per cent of calcium; Low Calcium Milk Food (Cow & Gate Ltd., London), containing not more than 0.1 per cent calcium; a soya bean formula without supplemental calcium to replace milk; or a meat formula to replace milk. Distilled water can be used for the formula in areas where the tap water is hard.

Calcium-Binding. With the object of reducing the amount of absorbable calcium, sodium sulfate can be added in molar quantities roughly equivalent to the calcium in cow's milk (approximately 1 Gm. per liter); in practice, 20 millimols of sodium sulfate per liter of milk is enough. Another method (in the case of babies of 7 to 10 kilograms) is to add 0.2 to 0.3 Gm. of sodium phytate to each milk feeding. These devices are not as effective as the low calcium diet.

Cortisone. When given as an adjuvant to the vitamin D–reduced low calcium regimen, prednisone, 2 to 6 mg. daily by mouth, speedily reduces the level of calcium in the serum. This is a measure especially indicated in patients with serum calcium levels of 14 mg. or above (potentially dangerous). When prednisone is used by itself, the serum calcium is apt to rise again on withdrawal; this is less likely to occur once the low calcium dietary regimen has been established. Prolonged treatment with corticosteroid is not advised.

Calcitonin.* Milhaud and Job were the first to report on treatment of infantile hypercalcemia with the hormone calcitonin. They administered 100 units daily by intramuscular injection and reported an immediate decrease in the plasma calcium level in both of three-month-old twins with the mild type of infantile hypercalcemia. This observation was substantiated in London by West and his colleagues, who presented a well-documented account of an infant with hypercalcemia due to vitamin

* Treatment with calcitonin is investigational in the United States.

D given in excessive doses at the age of seven months. In their report, it seemed that calcitonin was superior to a low calcium diet with cortisone acetate. After an initial intravenous test dose of porcine calcitonin, 50 units in 5 per cent dextrose, had reduced the serum calcium within 4 hours, daily intramuscular injections of the same dose in 16 per cent gelatin were given for seven days and normocalcemia was thus established.

A disadvantage of treatment with calcitonin is the necessity of giving it by injection. Vitamin D has a long biologic half-life. Porcine calcitonin acts rapidly and its half-life in the circulation of man is a matter of minutes (Buckle et al., 1972). Its value lies in the initiation of treatment when the level of calcium is high, e.g., 15 mg. per 100 ml. or more. Short-term treatment with porcine calcitonin does not have the disadvantage of the problem of antibody formation. Human calcitonin is available if long-term treatment is required, which is very unlikely.

Duration of Regimen

The natural duration of hypercalcemia in untreated patients varies from two weeks to four years, persisting longest in severe cases. The length of time that a strict dietary regimen needs to be continued depends on the case. Fraser et al. have suggested that a low calcium diet should be followed and exposure to direct sunshine avoided for at least nine months after normalization of the serum calcium. However, in many cases there is no necessity for such a prolonged regimen, especially in mild ones. I think that the oral calcium-loading test (Barr and Forfar) provides a convenient method for determining the point at which a low calcium diet can safely be discontinued, because the result of this test seems able to detect latent activity of the disease process.

Oral Calcium-Loading Test

This test is carried out after a short period of fasting. Then a blood specimen is taken for determination of total serum calcium (fasting level). Next, the loading dose of calcium lactate is given over a period of 10 to 15 minutes. The amount used is 385 mg. per kilogram of body weight, and it is dissolved by warming in 5 per cent dextrose solution (30 ml. per Gm. of calcium lactate). After the test feed, four or five blood specimens are taken at hourly intervals. The total serum calcium is conveniently measured by the microtechnique described by Wilkinson, which is performed on capillary blood samples taken by heel stab. The program for the test is as follows:

Fasting specimen (1) is taken at 0 time.
Test feeding started at 0 + 15 minutes and continued until completed—usually 10 to 15 minutes.
Specimen 2 is taken at 0 + 60 minutes—that is, 45 minutes after start of feeding.
Specimen 3 is taken at 0 + 120 minutes.
Specimen 4 is taken at 0 + 180 minutes.
Specimen 5 is taken at 0 + 240 minutes.

In Barr and Forfar's control group, the mean increase in total serum calcium, from the mean fasting level of 9.7 mg. per 100 ml., was approximately 1 mg. at 2 hours, with a subsequent decrease to 10.0 mg. per 100 ml. at 4 hours. But in patients with minimal hypercalcemia, the peak levels at 2 hours were considerably higher than in the control group, and the decline following the peak was slower. Typical curves for the test are included in the paper by Barr and Forfar.

If the fasting level of serum calcium is 12 mg. per 100 ml. or greater, the calcium-loading test gives little practical information and may increase the serum calcium to a dangerously high level.

References

Barr, D. G. D., and Forfar, J. O.: Oral Calcium-Loading Test in Infancy, with Particular Reference to Idiopathic Hypercalcaemia. *Brit. Med. J.*, 1:477, 1969.
Buckle, R. M., Gamlen, T. R., and Pullen, I. M.: Vitamin D Intoxication Treated with Porcine Calcitonin. *Brit. Med. J.*, 3:205, 1972.
Butler, N. R.: Personal communication, 1956.
DeLuca, H. F., and Suttie, J. W. (eds.): *The Fat-Soluble Vitamins.* Madison, University of Wisconsin Press, 1970.
Fraser, D., Kidd, B. S. L., Kooh, S. W., and Paunier, L.: A New Look at Infantile Hypercalcemia. *Pediat. Clin. N. Amer.*, 13:503, 1966.
Kenny, E. M., Aceto, J. R., Purisch, M., Harrison, H. E., Harrison, H. C., and Blizzard, R. M.: Metabolic Studies in a Patient with Idiopathic Hypercalcemia of Infancy. *J. Pediat.*, 62:531, 1963.
Lightwood, R.: Idiopathic Hypercalcemia with Failure to Thrive. *Proc. Roy. Soc. Med.*, 45:401, 1952.
Milhaud, G., and Job, J. C.: Thyrocalcitonin: Effect on Idiopathic Hypercalcemia. *Science*, 154:794, 1966.
Seelig, M.: Vitamin D and Cardiovascular, Renal, and Brain Damage in Infancy and Childhood. *Ann. New York Acad. Sci.*, 147:537-582, 1969.
Stapleton, T., MacDonald, W. B., and Lightwood, R.: Management of Idiopathic Hypercalcemia in Infancy. *Lancet*, 1:932, 1956.
Stapleton, T., MacDonald, W. B., and Lightwood, R.: The Pathogenesis of Idiopathic Hypercalcemia in Infancy. *Am. J. Clin. Nutr.*, 5:533, 1957.
Warkany, J., and Mabon, H. E.: Estimation of Vitamin D in Blood Serum: II. Level of Vitamin D in Human Blood Serums. *Am. J. Dis. Child.*, 60:606, 1940.
West, T. E. T., et al.: Treatment of hypercalcaemia with calcitonin. *Lancet*, 1:675, 1971.
Wilkinson, R. H.: A Micro-method for Serum Calcium and Serum Magnesium. *J. Clin. Path.*, 10:126, 1957.

Magnesium Deficiency

DONOUGH O'BRIEN, M.D., F.R.C.P.

Primary magnesium deficiency occurs most frequently as a complication of malabsorption syndromes, malnutrition, prolonged vomiting or gastric aspiration, and in situations involving extended parenteral therapy where replacement may be inadequate. In addition, deficiency may result from enteric losses in acute and chronic diarrheas, and from the kidney in chronic renal disease, hyperaldosteronism, vitamin D intoxication, excessive use of diuretics and diabetic acidosis. Much more rarely, body magnesium stores may be depleted because of inherited transport defects across either the bowel wall or the renal tubular epithelium or after removal of a parathyroid tumor when increased bone utilization of magnesium may lead to extracellular water depletion. Neonatal hypomagnesemia is also recognized in association with intrauterine undernutrition and difficult deliveries.

The condition is generally diagnosed clinically on the basis of tetany and convulsions, and in the laboratory by finding serum magnesium levels of less than 1.0 mEq. per liter, depending somewhat on the method. Confirmatory tests include a striated muscle biopsy magnesium of less than 1.2 mEq. per 100 Gm. wet fat-free tissue (normal 1.6 to 2.3 mg.) and a positive Thoren test (Harris and Wilkinson)—failure to excrete within 24 hours in the urine more than 40 per cent of an 0.5 mEq. per kilogram dose of magnesium chloride given intravenously over 1 to 1 ½ hours. Magnesium deficiency has in common with potassium deficiency the problem that serum (extracellular water) levels may be low in the presence of normal muscle levels and vice versa. A red cell magnesium of less than 3.0 mEq. per liter (normal 3.7 to 5.7) is sometimes a better indication of deficiency than is the serum level. Consequently, treatment is in some measure empirical in that the rate of intracellular migration cannot be accurately predicted and has to be monitored by repeating the serum level measurement.

The treatment of magnesium depletion is by supplementation, and by resolution of the primary condition (e.g., malnutrition, chronic renal disease) where that is possible.

Acute episodes of hypomagnesemic tetany and convulsions can be controlled by administering approximately 2 mEq. per kilogram body weight (0.5 ml. $MgSO_4$, 50 per cent weight per volume aqueous solution, U.S.P.) of magnesium intramuscularly twice daily. In neonatal hypomagnesia, oral treatment can be started 48 hours after intramuscular or intravenous therapy or as soon as the convulsions have stopped and the baby's intake can include an oral supplement. In familial hypomagnesemia, intramuscular treatment for five to seven days is usually wise prior to starting oral therapy.

The need for and duration of continuing oral therapy depend on the underlying problem and rate at which normal magnesium levels in the serum can be restored. Progress can be checked by repeated serum magnesium ion levels, and the probability and consequences of overdosage are negligible. A suitable initial objective is 3 mEq. per kilogram per 24 hours, but unpalatability can limit intake. Magnesium gluconate is the most suitable salt to use: 42 Gm. made up to 1000 ml. with ion-free water will give 1 mEq. per 5 ml.

The questions as to whether subclinical magnesium deficiency is undesirable and whether it should therefore be looked for in the absence of clinical signs are unanswered. Nonetheless, it seems reasonable to suggest that serum levels be occasionally checked in chronic diarrheas, in diabetic acidosis and during prolonged intravenous therapy, and that in the latter two situations the parenteral solutions contain approximately 2 mEq. per liter of magnesium.

Reference

Harris, I., and Wilkinson, A. W.: Magnesium Depletion in Children. *Lancet,* 2:735, 1971.

Hepatolenticular Degeneration
(Wilson's Disease)

HUGO R. TAPIA, M.D.,
DAVID M. WILSON, M.D., *and*
NORMAN P. GOLDSTEIN, M.D.

Available therapy for the amelioration of manifestations of hepatolenticular degeneration (HLD) makes an early diagnosis important; irreversible damage to the liver or brain lessens the success of therapy. Treatment for HLD can be divided into two types: specific and symptomatic.

Specific Therapy. To reduce the concentration of copper in critical organs, therapy consists of the use of chelating agents to increase the excretion of copper and measures to decrease the absorption of copper.

CHELATING AGENTS. These agents probably

act by preventing or reversing the binding of copper to enzymatic systems in body tissue, and by increasing the urinary excretion of copper. D–Penicillamine (Cuprimine) is the most effective chelating agent for copper at present.

Penicillamine (*β, β*–dimethylcysteine), introduced by Walshe in 1956, represented a great advance in the treatment of HLD. Several reports have confirmed the oral effectiveness of this drug (Boudin et al., Goldstein et al., Katsuki and Okumura, and Walshe). In vitro studies have indicated that two molecules of penicillamine combine with one atom of copper in its cupric state (Cu^{++}) to produce the cupriuretic effect. However, McCall et al., using chemical techniques, found that urinary copper is excreted as a copper-protein complex, suggesting that the influence of penicillamine in cupriuresis is not simple chelation; the mechanism of action requires further investigation.

In order to judge the efficacy of treatment with D–penicillamine, clinical observation, liver function tests, periodic liver biopsies to measure hepatic copper concentration when feasible, and copper balance studies are used. With long-term treatment, a slow but significant increase in the uptake of radiocopper by the liver has developed in symptomatic HLD patients (Goldstein et al.). Administration of D–penicillamine to asymptomatic patients with the biochemical abnormalities of HLD modifies the natural course of the disease by preventing the development of serious hepatic or neurologic manifestations (Sternlieb and Scheinberg). Tubular and glomerular defects also have been reversed by penicillamine (Leu et al.).

During treatment with D–penicillamine, the patient should undergo periodic urinalyses, complete blood counts including platelet count, and liver and renal function tests. Every three months is the preferred interval during the first year of treatment; annual measurements thereafter are sufficient. If toxicity appears, D–penicillamine should be discontinued until the reaction subsides. Subsequently, its use should be reinstituted in a small dose (250 mg. per day) and gradually increased until full dosage is attained. If repeated use of D–penicillamine always results in some toxic reaction, administration of corticosteroid medication for short periods (one or two months) may be necessary and is usually helpful. The eyes should be examined for cataracts and optic neuritis at least twice a year during the first year of treatment and yearly thereafter. Because of its affinity for metals and cystine and the possible effect on collagen, D–penicillamine should not be used during pregnancy.

D–Penicillamine can cause some adverse reactions of which physicians should be aware. The most common reaction is a maculopapular or erythematous rash with or without fever, arthralgia or lymphadenopathy. Patients allergic to penicillin may react to D–penicillamine, since there is cross-sensitivity between these two drugs, and may require desensitization. Other less common adverse reactions include the nephrotic syndrome (Adams et al.), hepatic dysfunction, tinnitus, loss of hair, eosinophilia, monocytosis, leukocytosis, thrombocytopenia and leukopenia. Rarely, thrombophlebitis, pancreatitis, cheilosis and gingivostomatitis can complicate its use. A lupus erythematosus-like syndrome (Harpey et al.) and polymyositis (Schroeder et al.) occasionally may develop. Focal glomerulonephritis is said to occur in HLD patients who are receiving D–penicillamine (Hayslett et al.). Because of its effect in increasing the amount of soluble collagen, this medication can cause increased skin friability at sites subject to pressure or trauma, such as the shoulders, elbows, knees, toes and buttocks. Purpuric lesions may appear, but they usually regress after the dosage of D–penicillamine is reduced.

D–Penicillamine is supplied in 250-mg. capsules. The dosage should be approximately 0.02 Gm. per kilogram of body weight, divided into four doses and given approximately 30 minutes before each meal and at bedtime. Most of our HLD patients require 750 to 1500 mg. of D–penicillamine daily, and it is rarely necessary to exceed 2000 mg. Determinations of copper in a 24-hour collection of urine and its concentration in the liver, with or without copper balance studies, help in evaluating the need for modification of the long-term program of treatment by increasing the dosage of penicillamine or by reducing the copper in the diet to maintain the patient in negative copper balance. Frequent reasons for failure in the treatment of HLD with D–penicillamine have included too low a dosage, too short periods of therapy and too much copper in the diet.

If the use of D–penicillamine is contraindicated, dimercaprol (BAL; British anti-lewisite) can be given intramuscularly in daily doses of 50 to 100 mg. The inconveniences of this drug are its parenteral administration and the frequent secondary effects of severe pain and abscess in the area of injection, nausea, vomiting, headaches, dizziness, leukopenia and thrombocytopenia. With less success, ethylenediaminetetraacetic acid salt (Versene) has been given intravenously in doses of 1 Gm. per day. More recently, Dixon et al. suggested that triethylenetetramine dihydrochloride (400-mg. capsules) in doses of 1.2 to 1.6 Gm. daily is a valuable alternative treatment for HLD patients who are intolerant to penicillamine.

MEASURES TO MINIMIZE COPPER ABSORPTION. In order to complement any attempt to reduce the copper stored in the tissues, a diet low in copper (1 to 2 mg. per day) is recommended. Foods high in copper, such as shellfish, liver, nuts, cocoa, chocolate, mushrooms, dried fruit and whiskey, are excluded. Drinking water should not contain more than 0.1 mg. of copper per liter and, if necessary, deionized water should be used for drinking and cooking. Sulfurated potash (potassium sulfide) is no longer used routinely because of its ineffectiveness in binding copper in the diet and its corrosive ability.

A diet low in copper and the oral administration of D-penicillamine have been successful in keeping our HLD patients in negative copper balance. In addition, cation exchange resins, such as carbacrylamine (Carbo-Resin), in doses of 1 to 2 tablespoons in water with each meal, have been used with success in reducing the amount of absorbable copper in the diet. Many patients, however, preferred to stop taking this medication because of its taste and consistency or because of constipation or diarrhea associated with its use. Therefore, we no longer routinely use carbacrylamine.

INCREASING LEVELS OF CERULOPLASMIN OR PROTEIN OR BOTH. Both the administration of estrogens to increase endogenous synthesis of ceruloplasmin (German and Bearn) and the infusion of purified ceruloplasmin (Bickel) have been unsuccessful in the treatment of HLD. The effect of growth hormone on protein synthesis needs further investigation.

Symptomatic Therapy. NEUROLOGIC MANIFESTATIONS. For the different forms of movement disorder, agitation and irritability, 2 or 5 mg. diazepam (Valium) * orally three times a day, with or without 1 to 2 mg. of trihexyphenidyl (Artane) orally three times daily, is helpful. Caution must be observed during the use of these drugs since excessive sedation may occur. Other drugs, such as thioridazine hydrochloride (Mellaril) † and chlorpromazine (Thorazine),‡ can be used for treatment of anxiety and agitation, but they can also cause an exacerbation of the dystonic movements (Tapia and Cavazos). Although poor results from surgical treatment of the central nervous system for neurologic manifestations of HLD have been reported (Boudin et al.), chemopallidectomy satisfactorily controlled involuntary movements in one patient (Tapia and Cavazos), and ventrolateral thalamic coagulation abolished flapping intention tremor in another (Denny-Brown). These operations, however, should be performed only on adults in whom treatment with chelating agents has been ineffective and in whom the movement disorder is disabling.

HEPATIC MANIFESTATIONS. Hepatic insufficiency is treated according to the complications that are present. For edema and ascites, a diet that contains 45 to 90 mEq. of sodium a day and is high in carbohydrate and moderately low in protein (0.6 Gm. per kilogram of body weight) should be prescribed. If the prothrombin time is prolonged, 4 mg. per day of synthetic vitamin K (Synkamin) given orally or intramuscularly can be helpful. All patients are given oral doses of multivitamins, such as hexavitamin (N.F.), 1 tablet daily. For life-threatening hemorrhage from esophageal varices, splenectomy and splenorenal or portal-systemic shunting could be carried out, with careful observation for possible exacerbation or appearance of neurologic abnormalities (Hallenbeck et al.). Orthotopic liver transplantation has been reported in a patient prior to hepatic coma (Starzl et al.).

The most fruitful result of therapy undoubtedly lies in the arrest and reversibility of the disease in its earliest stage, before irreparable damage is done, as well as in the prevention of symptoms in the preclinical (asymptomatic) patient.

* Manufacturer's precaution: Oral diazepam (Valium) is not for use in children under six months of age.

† Manufacturer's precaution: Thioridazine hydrochloride (Mellaril) is not recommended for children under two years of age.

‡ Manufacturer's precaution: Chlorpromazine (Thorazine) is not recommended for children under six months of age except when lifesaving.

References

Adams, D. A., et al.: Nephrotic Syndrome Associated with Penicillamine Therapy of Wilson's Disease. *Am. J. Med.,* 36:330–336, 1964.

Bickel, H.: Attempts at Ceruloplasmin Substitution in Wilson's Disease; in J. M. Walshe and J. M. Cumings (eds.): *Wilson's Disease: Some Current Concepts.* Oxford, Blackwell Scientific Publications, 1961, p. 273.

Boudin, G., Pépin, B., and Barraine, R.: Nôtre Expérience du Traitement de la Maladie de Wilson par la Pénicillamine. *Bull. Soc. Med. Hosp. Paris,* 1:631–641, 1963.

Denny-Brown, D.: Hepatolenticular Degeneration (Wilson's Disease): Two Different Components. *New England J. Med.,* 270:1149–1156, 1964.

Dixon, H. B. F., Gibbs, K., and Walshe, J. M.: Preparation of Triethylenetetramine Dihydrochloride for the Treatment of Wilson's Disease. *Lancet,* 1:853, 1972.

German, J. L., III, and Bearn, A. G.: Effect of Estrogens on Copper Metabolism in Wilson's Disease. *J. Clin. Invest.*, 40:445–453, 1961.

Goldstein, N. P., et al.: Wilson's Disease (Hepatolenticular Degeneration): Treatment with Penicillamine and Changes in Hepatic Trapping of Radioactive Copper. *Arch. Neurol.*, 24:391–400, 1971.

Hallenbeck, G. A., et al.: Results after Portal-Systemic Shunts in 120 Patients with Cirrhosis of the Liver. *Surg. Gynec. Obstet.*, 116:435–442, 1963.

Harpey, J. P., et al.: Lupus-like Syndrome Induced by D-Penicillamine in Wilson's Disease (letter to the editor). *Lancet*, 1:292, 1971.

Hayslett, J. P., et al.: Focal Glomerulitis due to Penicillamine. *Lab. Invest.*, 19:376–381, 1968.

Katsuki, S., and Okumura, M.: Treatment of Wilson's Disease. *Birth Defects*, *4*:136–138, 1968.

Leu, M. L., Strickland, G. T., and Gutman, R. A.: Renal Function in Wilson's Disease: Response to Penicillamine Therapy. *Am. J. Med. Sci.*, 260:381–398, 1970.

McCall, J. T., et al.: Comparative Metabolism of Copper and Zinc in Patients with Wilson's Disease (Hepatolenticular Degeneration). *Am. J. Med. Sci.*, 254:13–23, 1967.

Schroeder, P. L., Peters, H. A., and Dahl, D. S.: Polymyositis and Penicillamine. *Arch. Neurol.*, 27:456–457, 1972.

Starzl, T. E., et al.: Indications for Orthotopic Liver Transplantation: With Particular Reference to Hepatomas, Biliary Atresia, Cirrhosis, Wilson's Disease and Serum Hepatitis. *Transplant Proc.*, 3:308–312, 1971.

Sternlieb, I., and Scheinberg, I. H.: Prevention of Wilson's Disease in Asymptomatic Patients. *New England J. Med.*, 278:352–359, 1968.

Tapia, H. R., Cavazos, N.: Hepatolenticular Degeneration (Wilson's Disease): Observations in 7 Cases and Review of the Literature. *South. Med. J.*, 63:82–89, 1970.

Walshe, J. M.: Penicillamine, a New Oral Therapy for Wilson's Disease. *Am. J. Med.*, 21:487–495, 1956.

Phenylketonuria

MARY G. AMPOLA, M.D.

With the advent of statewide screening programs to detect metabolic diseases shortly after birth, it is now possible to begin treatment in the symptom-free period before irreversible damage has been done. As these programs, originally set up to detect only phenylketonuria, are expanded to include other testing of both blood and urine, we may expect an increase in the number of patients presenting for treatment with a wide variety of inborn errors.

In practice, a number of specialists are necessary to provide optimal care for these children. These include nutritionists to plan fully nourishing, although specialized, diets, and laboratories capable of performing the assays necessary for management. In addition, social workers and nurses are helpful in supporting and instructing the parents, as are psychologists to evaluate the child's mental status periodically. For these reasons, an experienced medical center team is strongly recommended for the overall disease management whenever possible.

Since phenylketonuria (PKU) is the most common disease being successfully treated at present, it is important that pediatricians involved in the care of such patients understand the goals and principles of therapy being used. In this way, they can work closely with the specialists primarily responsible for the child's treatment.

GOALS OF DIETARY TREATMENT

It is now generally accepted that dietary control is markedly beneficial in treating phenylketonuria, and that this is one of the few situations in which prevention of mental retardation is possible. Untreated institutionalized patients with this disorder have an IQ with a mean of 25 and a standard deviation of 15, although there have certainly been a number of documented reports of normal or near-normal intelligence. In "atypical PKU," where the phenylalanine blood level tends to be lower than in the classic form, a significant negative correlation exists between phenylalanine blood level and the eventual IQ. Indeed, many of the patients reported in the literature to have relatively normal intelligence may represent this milder variant.

The point to be kept in mind is that although there are rare patients with high blood phenylalanine levels who will develop normally without the special diet, these patients cannot be identified in early infancy, when the dietary treatment must be begun if any degree of success is to be expected.

The basic goal of treatment is to limit the phenylalanine intake to avoid the grossly elevated phenylalanine levels which lead to mental retardation. On the other hand, it is unwise to limit the phenylalanine intake so severely as to maintain the blood levels in the so-called physiologic range (1 to 2 mg. per 100 ml.), in part because of the lack of any reserves with which to deal with stress situations. Overtreatment, with resulting phenylalanine deficiency, is now one of the well-recognized hazards of the diet. If any one of the essential amino acids is deficient, protein synthesis cannot occur. Initially, a growth lag and dermatitis appear. If the deprivation continues, hypoproteinemia, refractory megaloblastic anemia, dystrophic bony changes, hypoglycemia and even death can occur.

A more subtle degree of phenylalanine deficiency, especially early in life, may explain why some "adequately" treated PKU's failed to achieve an IQ comparable to that of their unaffected siblings in the early days of the treatment program, when "physiologic levels" were routinely maintained. The latest evidence indicates that the final IQ is significantly higher on the average if phenylalanine blood levels are kept in a higher range, i.e., 5 to 10 mg. per 100 ml. Indeed, there is some indirect evidence that it may be safe to allow the level to go into the 10 to 15 mg. per 100 ml. range without adverse effects. The overall aim, therefore, is not to achieve "normal" levels, but instead to ensure that growth is not limited by overtreatment while at the same time avoiding the marked elevations seen in untreated phenylketonuria.

MANAGING THE DIET

Once the diagnosis has been established with certainty, most investigators suggest hospitalization for one to two weeks for dietary regulation. It is occasionally possible, however, to avoid this additional emotional and financial trauma to the family. The baby is seen on an outpatient basis every day or two during this period to check the blood phenylalanine level and to examine and weigh him.

In infancy, the treatment of phenylketonuria consists primarily of a casein hydrolysate which has had most of the phenylalanine removed and which is purchased in the dry state. In the United States, this preparation is Lofenalac, available from Mead-Johnson; in England, Albumaid is used. When one cup of Lofenalac powder is added to one quart of water, the formula contains the standard 20 calories per ounce, but only about 4 mg. of phenylalanine per ounce compared to 50 mg. from most common milk preparations. All other nutrients are present in comparable amounts.

The formula is given alone initially to lower the phenylalanine blood level to about 5 mg. per 100 ml. Once this has been achieved, another phenylalanine source must be provided, since there is too little in the Lofenalac formula to fulfill growth requirements; the amount is geared to achieve the desired blood level of 5 to 10 mg. per 100 ml. At first, the supplement is whole cow's milk in small amounts, the daily supply being divided in order to distribute the phenylalanine intake throughout the day.

After the newborn period, cereals, fruits and vegetables, sugars and fats become major supplements to the Lofenalac formula, replacing the whole milk by about four months of age. Breads, macaroni, cookies, cakes and puddings are made from special low-protein flour and are added later. High protein foods, such as meat, cheese, fish, and eggs are included in very small amounts, allowing the child to become accustomed to their taste and thus avoiding later problems of acceptance. In general, the various foods are introduced in the same sequence and at the same age for PKU babies as for normal children; amounts of some items are simply more limited for these children.

Before adding any new food, its phenylalanine content must be checked, and a number of references are available for this purpose. Particular caution is urged with canned or bottled products, including puréed infant foods; many have added protein not obvious from examination of the label. For some products, the phenylalanine content is not available, but this can be estimated by calculating 5 per cent of the total protein content. The older child is provided chewing food, for good dentition, in the form of raw vegetables and low protein cookies. Imaginative recipes have been devised using allowable foods.

Recent careful studies (Berry et al.) have been made of periods of "inconstant growth" (defined as a pattern of growth varying in a range greater than 1 standard deviation during the period considered). These periods correlate with clinical symptoms of irritability, fatigue, behavior changes, anorexia and a sallow appearance of the skin; frank anemia and hypoproteinemia appear if the causes are not recognized and corrected. Linear growth is more severely affected than the rate of weight gain. Detailed analysis of these data leads to the conclusion that these growth problems and clinical symptoms are caused by a poor balance between the amount of phenylalanine being given (primarily from natural food sources) and that of other essential amino acids (primarily from Lofenalac). Phenylalanine is utilizable to build protein only if sufficient amounts of other essential amino acids are provided. Conversely, if not enough phenylalanine is being given, the other amino acids are "wasted" in terms of their ability to be used to build tissue. Growth is optimal if the Lofenalac is given in amounts geared to, but no greater than, the child's protein requirement at that age and weight. Total phenylalanine is then given in an amount to balance the essential amino acids being given in the Lofenalac.

In practice, this goal is achieved as follows: The major source of essential amino acids other than phenylalanine is Lofenalac. The child's protein requirement is 2.5 Gm. per kilogram per day until age three years, 2.4 Gm. until age four and 2.2 Gm. up to eight years of age. This amount is calculated to be met *entirely* from Lofenalac; a small additional amount is of course provided by natural food supplements, but this is not considered in the calculations; rather, it is desirable to have this as a small excess.

On the other hand, the phenylalanine provided must be totaled from all sources; i.e., that amount being given in Lofenalac is subtracted from the total desired (Table 1), and enough natural foods are given to provide the difference. The figures quoted are of course meant to be guidelines; considerable individual variation is encountered and diet adjustments are made as indicated by the blood phenylalanine level.

The Lofenalac is prescribed in tablespoons per day rather than in fluid ounces; this allows flexibility in the amount of water in which the Lofenalac is dissolved, so that intake does not drop with the child's diminishing desire for fluids, particularly at the time of transition from bottle to cup. Indeed, some of the powder can be mixed into the child's food or incorporated into gelatin.

In writing the prescription, a *range* of phenylalanine intake is indicated, allowing for day-to-day fluctuations in appetite and promoting a somewhat less rigid attitude on the part of the mother. The daily prescription reads *X* tablespoons of Lofenalac powder and *Y* mg. of phenylalanine (± 25 mg.) from natural foods. The mother is given a list of foods with their phenylalanine content from which to select. One need not be overly concerned about caloric intake; if the diet is calculated as indicated, no growth lags occur because caloric needs are not being met.

Elevated blood phenylalanine levels are

TABLE 1. Protein and Phenylalanine Requirements (and Amount of Phenylalanine to Be Provided by Lofenalac* and by Natural Foods) at Various Ages

AGE	LOFENALAC TO PROVIDE DESIRED PHENYLALANINE INTAKE (*Tbsp./day*)	TOTAL PHENYLALANINE REQUIREMENT (*mg./day*)	PHENYLALANINE INTAKE	
			From Lofenalac (mg./day)	*From Natural Foods (mg./day)*
2 weeks	7.0	290	50	240
1 month	7.5	315	55	265
2 months	9.0	350	65	285
3 months	10.5	385	80	305
4 months	11.5	390	90	300
5 months	13.0	390	95	295
6 months	14.0	390	105	285
7 months	15.0	385	110	275
8 months	15.0	390	115	275
9 months	16.0	365	120	245
10 months	17.0	360	125	235
11 months	17.0	360	130	230
12 months	18.0	350	135	215
15 months	19.0	375	140	235
18 months	20.0	400	150	250
21 months	21.0	420	155	265
24 months	22.0	440	165	275
30 months	23.0	475	170	305
36 months	24.0	475	180	295
42 months	25.0	510	185	325
48 months	26.0	540	195	345
54 months	27.5	570	205	365
5 years	29.0	580	215	365
6 years	33.0	640	250	390
7 years	37.0	650	275	375
8 years	41.0	680	310	370
9 years	42.0	755	315	440
10 years	43.0	825	325	500

* Composition of Lofenalac: 1 tablespoon (1 scoop) contains 1.4 Gm. protein, 7.5 mg. phenylalanine and 43 calories. (After the work reported in Berry, H. K., et al.: Amino Acid Balance in the Treatment of Phenylketonuria. *J. Am. Diet. Assoc.*, 58:210, 1971. Reproduced by permission of the copyright owner and the authors.)

usually due to excessive intake of phenylalanine over the child's growth requirements at that time, provided enough of the other essential amino acids are being given to allow full utilization of the phenylalanine for building tissue. The other major cause of elevation is illness (infection or trauma). Catabolism of tissues releases phenylalanine rapidly; even minor respiratory infections may double or triple the previously stable blood level. Whenever a significant elevation occurs because of infection, the approach is to lower the phenylalanine intake temporarily. Lofenalac is continued and supplemented with low phenylalanine fluids and other sources of calories. Appropriate antibiotic and other therapy is vigorously pursued to keep the severity and duration of illness to a minimum. This regimen is continued until the serum phenylalanine has returned to the desired level, and the previous diet is then gradually resumed.

Iron supplements are necessary until about nine months of age, when the child generally begins taking enough Lofenalac to provide for his iron needs. Vitamin supplements are given as usual, as are routine immunizations.

In summary, there are several key points to be kept in mind concerning treatment. First, PKU children do not all have the same phenylalanine tolerance at the same age. Second, frequent monitoring of blood levels is essential, since the requirements change frequently. In fact, as the child becomes older he will be able to tolerate less phenylalanine per kilogram of body weight, since he is incorporating less into tissue protein as the growth rate slows. Finally, early and vigorous attention to infections is essential to avoid prolonged and dangerous rises in blood phenylalanine levels.

In the treatment of "atypical phenylketonuria" a similar regimen is followed, but with some modifications. Patients with this variant have phenylalanine levels in a borderline range (15 to 25 mg. per 100 ml.), and generally tolerate more dietary phenylalanine than do classic phenylketonurics of the same age. Indeed, later in childhood many can tolerate a diet containing normal amounts of protein with little or no increase in serum phenylalanine levels. Although the degree of mental retardation without treatment is usually less than in classic PKU, this is not always the case; dangerously high phenylalanine levels can be present in the critical periods of infancy and early childhood. Thus, in terms of treatment, it is generally agreed that all patients with levels of 20 mg. per 100 ml. or more, regardless of the type of PKU, should be given dietary treatment as long as necessary to maintain "safe" blood levels. Less agreement is to be found in the literature concerning the necessity of treating patients with blood levels in the 10 to 20 mg. per 100 ml. range. Most investigators appear to favor a modified low protein diet for atypical phenylketonurics. They are given as much phenylalanine as can be tolerated at all times, thus assuring that if the patient no longer needs restriction it will become obvious.

In addition to the classic and atypical forms of phenylketonuria, a third variant has been discovered. This has been called "persistent mild hyperphenylalaninemia," and patients' blood levels remain in the range of 6 to 8 mg. per 100 ml. Follow-up of these untreated patients (Levy, et al.) revealed their IQ's to be comparable to those of unaffected siblings, with adequate school performance. No dietary treatment is necessary for this group of children.

FAMILY GUIDANCE IN PHENYLKETONURIA

After the diagnosis of PKU has been made, the parents will require support as feelings of guilt and hostility become manifest. With time, most parents are grateful for the screening program which in most cases detected the problem, and for the quality of care the child is receiving in the attempt to prevent mental retardation. Genetic counseling with careful explanation of the autosomal recessive nature of the disorder and thus of the one-in-four risk of recurrence in future pregnancies is essential, as is screening of all siblings for the disease. The parents must understand that the basic problem is the accumulation of phenylalanine and of its metabolites, and that treatment is directed toward lowering the intake of this amino acid. Lofenalac is simply one of the means to this end.

To the mother of the phenylketonuric child falls the day-to-day problem of managing the low phenylalanine diet. Good initial counseling and constant support are essential if the long-term treatment is to be successful. The mother is asked to keep daily records of the child's intake, and these are reviewed by the physician and the dietitian at each appointment. Parents should also make note of any illnesses, immunizations or other unusual situations which may affect the phenylalanine level. An occasional visit to the home by the dietitian, as well as ready availability by phone as questions arise, is also helpful.

Problems commonly reported by mothers include the lack of variety in the menus, the apparently small size of the servings and the frequent need for preparing a separate meal for these children. The parents are reassured that the kinds and amounts of food, although limited, are adequate for proper nutrition and therefore for growth. The child is taught that his food is "special" and that he must eat only what is given to him by the parents. Siblings, relatives, neighbors and teachers must be instructed not to offer food without checking with the parents. It is not recommended that the child be told that forbidden foods will make him sick; if he tries them secretly, he will discover they do not, and problems of dietary control will worsen. Hunger between meals is a common complaint; items such as cookies made with a low protein flour, such as Paygel P (General Mills), can be given. After infancy, some of the Lofenalac powder can be prepared as thick mush with water (as intake decreases with age) and mixed with strained fruits or served with honey, sugar or fruit juice. Alternatively, the liquid preparation itself can be flavored with banana, pineapple, chocolate or vanilla extracts or with various flavors of Kool-Aid.

Conflicts concerning the diet may well occur. The older child may use the diet as a device against his parents, once he has sensed their anxieties about his intake. In counseling parents, a balance must be struck between an overly cautious, chronically anxious approach to the diet and a laxity which endangers the child. It is helpful to point out the contrast between the low phenylalanine diet, to which the parents are expected to adhere carefully and which allows no "cheating," and the reducing diet, which is often safely broken. The child is fully expected to remain in good general health and should not be overprotected.

There is accumulating evidence that the eventual IQ achieved even in normal children is enhanced by maximal mental stimulation in the preschool years, indeed from earliest infancy. It is helpful to acquaint the parents of phenylketonuric children under treatment with this concept and to suggest reading material on the subject. While carefully avoiding situations where undue pressure is exerted on the child, it is possible to encourage a highly stimulating milieu in the home, so that every possible opportunity is provided for maximal mental development.

RESULTS OF TREATMENT

Parental IQ, degree of environmental stimulation and the presence of other congenital abnormalities or of emotional problems also affect the eventual intelligence of the phenylketonuric. Even when all these unrelated factors are considered, the IQ's achieved and reported vary considerably. Three major points emerge from the literature. First, the earlier the treatment is begun, preferably before one month of age, the higher the average expected IQ. Second, the more comprehensive the overall management during early childhood (i.e., the more frequently the blood levels are checked and the diet adjusted, and the more ancillary services provided), the better the eventual results. Finally, overtreatment must be avoided. Subtle malnutrition, especially in the first year of life, may contribute to developmental as well as growth retardation. Again, this may explain the disappointing results with earlier groups of children, who were considered to be under "excellent" control (blood phenylalanine levels consistently 1 to 2 mg. per 100 ml.), yet who achieved lower than expected IQ's and often manifested cognitive, behavioral and learning problems of various kinds.

Results in more recent series, where overtreatment has been scrupulously avoided and blood levels maintained in the range of 5 to 10 mg. per 100 ml., have been more satisfactory. When this is done, the results are gratifying. For example, in a series of 27 patients (Kang) in whom treatment was begun before three weeks of age and who were reported at 1 3/12 to 7 2/12 years of age, the IQ results were as follows:

Average of 27 patients: Mean IQ = 99.4
(range 62 to 124)

Average of 16 unaffected siblings: Mean IQ = 102.8
(range 72 to 138)

In the same series, less satisfactory results were obtained when treatment was begun between three and six weeks of age:

Average of 12 patients: Mean IQ = 89.2
(range 71 to 109)

Average of 16 unaffected siblings: Mean IQ = 102.8
(range 72 to 138)

In 17 patients who were treated after eight months of age, the mean IQ did not differ from the mean of 11 untreated patients, even though a number of them made significant gains during therapy. As had been reported in previous series, there is a negative correlation between age of onset of treatment and eventual IQ.

Although very little gain in IQ can be achieved if treatment is begun after infancy, some children may benefit in other ways. Seizures may abate if they have not responded to the usual measures. Hyperactivity, autistic behavior and poor attention span may all improve somewhat. Abnormally blond hair may darken. When instituting the diet after infancy, a longer period (up to several weeks) is required to achieve desired blood levels, presumably because of large tissue stores of phenylalanine.

STOPPING THE DIET

In recent years, many workers have discontinued the diet when the patient has reached the age of four to six years. There is good evidence that after this age, the intellectual level which has already been achieved is maintained. Presumably this is because the brain has completed a critical growth phase during which it is sensitive to damage by elevated levels of phenylalanine and its metabolites. In the series described above, for example, the 11 children whose treatment was begun at less than six weeks of age were weaned from the diet at an average age of four years and three months. They showed no IQ deterioration 2½ to 3½ years after the diet was stopped. In the near future, the accumulation of similar follow-up data may provide further reassurance that some gradual minor loss in IQ does not continue to occur.

When patients are placed on a normal protein diet, behavior often improves because of removal of the rigid dietary restrictions and consequent easing of family tensions. However, adverse changes have also been noted, particularly when a high protein diet is suddenly offered without gradual introduction. These include increased irritability, shortened attention span, inability to concentrate, seizures, mental disorganization or (rarely) autistic behavior. Many of the changes are subtle. In most cases, these symptoms are transient and gradually disappear despite continuation of the normal diet.

At present, the best evidence indicates that intellectual potential, as measured by the IQ, does not deteriorate significantly if the diet is stopped after the age of four to six years, though behavior may do so transiently.

References

Berry, H. K., Hunt, M. M., and Sutherland, B. K.: Amino Acid Balance in the Treatment of Phenylketonuria. *J. Am. Diet. Ass.*, 58:210, 1971.

Church, C. F., and Church, H. N.: *Bowes and Church's Food Values of Portions Commonly Used.* 11th ed. Philadelphia, J. B. Lippincott Co., 1970.

Dobson, J., Koch, R., Williamson, M., Spector, R., Frankenburg, W., O'Flynn, M., Warner, R., and Hudson, F.: Cognitive Development and Dietary Therapy in Phenylketonuric Children. *New England S. Med.*, 278:1142, 1968.

Hudson, F. P., Mordaunt, V. L.. and Leahy, I.: Evaluation of Treatment Begun in First Three Months of Life in 184 Cases of Phenylketonuria. *Arch. Dis. Child.*, 45:5, 1970.

Kang, E. S., Sollee, N. D., and Gerald, P. S.: Results of Treatment and Termination of the Diet in Phenylketonuria (PKU). *Pediatrics,* 46:881, 1970.

Levy, H. L., Shih, V. E., Karolkewicz, V., French, W. A., Carr, J. R., Cass, V., Kennedy, J. L., Jr., and MacCready, R. A.: Persistent Mild Hyperphenylalaninemia in the Untreated State. *New England J. Med.*, 285:424, 1971.

Lonsdale, D., and Forest, M.: Normal Mental Development in Treated Phenylketonuria. *Am. J. Dis. Child.*, 119:440, 1970.

McCarthy, M. A., Orr, M. L., and Watt, B. K.: Phenylalanine and Tyrosine in Vegetables and Fruits. *J. Am. Diet. Ass.*, 52:130, 1968.

Nutritional Data. 6th ed. Pittsburgh, H. J. Heinz Co., 1972.

Recent Advances in Therapeutic Diets. Edited by the Nutrition Department of the University of Iowa. Iowa State University Press, 1970, p. 140.

Sutherland, B. S., Berry, H. K., and Umbarger, B.: Growth and Nutrition in Treated Phenylketonuric Patients. *J.A.M.A.*, 211:270, 1970.

Watt, B. K., and Merrill, A.: *Composition of Foods.* Agricultural Handbook #8. U.S. Government Printing Office, 1963.

Amino Acid Disorders

MARY G. AMPOLA, M.D.

See tables on following pages.

TABLE 1. Amino Acid Disorders

DISEASE (AND APPROXIMATE INCIDENCE)*	CLINICAL FEATURES	ABNORMAL ENZYME	AMINO ACIDS INCREASED IN BLOOD	AMINO ACIDS INCREASED IN URINE	COMMENTS	TREATMENT
PHENYLKETONURIA						
Phenylketonuria, classic. (1:15,000)	Mental retardation; also seizures, eczema and fair skin, eyes, and hair in some patients.	Phenylalanine hydroxylase (virtually total absence).	Phenylalanine—levels usually over 30 mg./100 ml.	Phenylalanine; phenylpyruvic, -lactic and -acetic acids, orthohydroxyphenylacetic acid also increased.	Treatment can probably be stopped at about age 4–6 without intellectual deterioration.	Low phenylalanine diet.
Phenylketonuria, atypical. (1:90,000)	Mental retardation; often less severe than in classic form.	Phenylalanine hydroxylase (partial defect).	Phenylalanine—levels not as high as in classic form, about 20 mg./100 ml.	Same as in the classic form but often in smaller amounts.	May not need treatment to maintain normal blood phenylalanine after early childhood.	Low phenylalanine diet to tolerance.
Hyperphenylalaninemia, persistent mild. (1:20,000)	Normal in all respects.	(Probable) Phenylalanine hydroxylase (partial defect—more enzyme remains).	Phenylalanine—levels in range of 6–8 mg./100 ml.	None.	Mental and physical development normal.	None necessary.
DISORDERS OF AMMONIA METABOLISM			**NOTE:** Glutamine elevated in blood and urine in all hyperammonemia situations, but often difficult to detect on screening.			
A. Urea Cycle Diseases						
Carbamyl phosphate synthetase deficiency. (Rare)	Episodic vomiting, acidosis, cyclic neutropenia.	Carbamyl phosphate synthetase.	Glycine.	Glycine.	Postprandial hyperammonemia.	Low protein diet (1 Gm./kg./day).
Ornithine transcarbamylase deficiency. (Rare)	Episodic vomiting and stupor, failure to thrive, hepatomegaly, seizures; mental retardation usually.	Ornithine transcarbamylase (also some decrease in carbamylphosphate synthetase).	—	—	Postprandial hyperammonemia.	Low protein diet (1 Gm./kg./day).
Citrullinemia. (Rare)	Vomiting, seizures, failure to thrive, mental retardation; may die in neonatal period.	Argininosuccinic acid synthetase.	Citrulline.	Citrulline.	Postprandial hyperammonemia.	Low protein diet (1 – 1.5 Gm./kg./day).

TABLE 1. Continued

DISEASE (AND APPROXIMATE INCIDENCE)*	CLINICAL FEATURES	ABNORMAL ENZYME	AMINO ACIDS INCREASED IN BLOOD	AMINO ACIDS INCREASED IN URINE	COMMENTS	TREATMENT
Argininosuccinic aciduria. (1:150,000)	Ataxia, seizures, mental retardation, friable hair, hepatomegaly; may die in neonatal period.	Argininosuccinase.	Argininosuccinic acid.	Argininosuccinic acid.	Postprandial hyperammonemia.	Low protein diet (1 – 1.5 Gm./kg./day).
Hyperargininemia. (Rare)	Seizures, spasticity, mental retardation.	Arginase.	Arginine.	Arginine; lysine ornithine and cystine also present.	Postprandial hyperammonemia.	Low protein diet (1.5 Gm./kg./day).
B. Other Hyperammonemias						
"Hyperglycinemia, ketotic form." (1:300,000)	Periodic vomiting, lethargy, ketosis, myoclonic jerks, osteoporosis, neutropenia and thrombocytopenia.	Not specific; deficiencies of the following are known: (1) carbamyl PO_4 synthetase, (2) methylmalonyl-CoA carbonylmutase and (3) propionyl-CoA carboxylase.	Glycine.	Glycine.	Hyperammonemia in (1) and (2); propionic acidemia in (3).	Low protein diet (1 – 1.5 Gm./kg./day).
Congenital lysine intolerance. (Rare)	Episodic vomiting, seizures and coma.	? Lysine NAD oxidoreductase.	Lysine, arginine.	Lysine.	Hyperammonemia.	Low protein diet (1.5 Gm./kg./day).
Ornithinemia (Type I) (with homocitrullinuria). (Rare)	Irritability, ataxia, myoclonic seizures, aversion to protein, mental retardation.	Unknown.	Ornithine.	Homocitrulline; ornithine may be normal.	Hyperammonemia.	Low protein diet (1.5 Gm./kg./day).
Familial protein intolerance with hyperdibasic aminoaciduria. (Rare)	Vomiting and diarrhea, failure to thrive, neutropenia, aversion to protein, progressive cirrhosis.	Defective transport of dibasic amino acids in kidney and intestine.	–	Arginine, lysine.	Usually normal intelligence. Ammonia intoxication after high protein intake.	Low protein diet (1 Gm./kg./day); arginine supplement (2 Gm./day) to improve urea formation from ammonia.

TABLE 1. Amino Acid Disorders (continued)

DISEASE (AND APPROXIMATE INCIDENCE)*	CLINICAL FEATURES	ABNORMAL ENZYME	AMINO ACIDS INCREASED IN BLOOD	AMINO ACIDS INCREASED IN URINE	COMMENTS	TREATMENT
OTHER AMINO ACID DISORDERS						
Cystathioninurea (1:150,000)	Probably benign.	Cystathionase.	Trace of cystathionine.	Cystathionine.	—	None necessary (although pyridoxine, 25–100 mg. daily, will clear cystathionine).
Cystinosis, nephropathic. (Rare)	Fanconi syndrome in urine, failure to thrive, vitamin D – resistant rickets.	Unknown.	Essentially normal, including cystine and cysteine.	Generalized aminoaciduria.	Phosphaturia, glycosuria; cystine deposits in many tissues.	Symptomatic; vitamin D (10,000–15,000 U./day); ? dithiothreitol. Low cystine diets and D-penicillamine tried with limited success.
Cystinuria. (1:16,000)	Renal calculi; ? mental retardation in some.	Defective transport of cystine and the dibasic amino acids in kidney and intestine.	—	Cystine and dibasic amino acids.	—	High fluid intake, D-penicillamine. Alkalization of urine and low methionine diet also effective but difficult to maintain.
Hyperglycinemia, nonketotic form. (1:150,000)	Lethargy, seizures, spasticity, mental retardation, failure to thrive.	Defect in an enzyme catalyzing conversion of glycine to CO_2, NH_3 and a one-carbon tetrahydrofolate derivative.	Glycine.	Glycine; occasionally not elevated.	—	Low glycine, low serine diet; supplemental methionine (? effectiveness).
Hartnup disease. (1:17,000)	May be benign; light-sensitive rash, ataxia, psychosis, mental retardation in some.	Defective transport of neutral amino acids in kidney and intestine.	None; indeed, neutral amino acids about 30 per cent less than normal.	Neutral amino acids.	Indoles produced by intestinal bacteria from tryptophan are absorbed and excreted into the urine.	None necessary in some; nicotinamide for rash (up to 400 mg./day); high protein diet for general nutrition.

TABLE 1. Continued

DISEASE (AND APPROXIMATE INCIDENCE)*	CLINICAL FEATURES	ABNORMAL ENZYME	AMINO ACIDS INCREASED IN BLOOD	AMINO ACIDS INCREASED IN URINE	COMMENTS	TREATMENT
Histidinemia. (1:20,000)	May be benign; speech defects and mental retardation in some.	Histidase.	Histidine.	Histidine.	Urocanic acid absent in skin homogenates and sweat; low serotonin in serum.	Low histidine diets tried without clinical improvement, even though so limited that growth lagged.
Homocystinuria. (1:200,000)	Dislocated lenses (downward), malar flush, intravascular thromboses, long, thin extremities, osteoporosis; mental retardation in some.	Cystathionine synthetase.	Methionine; small amount of homocysteine.	Homocystine.	Two variants: pyridoxine-responsive and nonresponsive.	Up to 500 mg. daily of pyridoxine for responders; otherwise, low methionine diet with cystine, homoserine, and choline supplements.
Hyperlysinemia. (1:300,000)	May be benign in some; mental retardation and other minor features in others.	Lysine - ketoglutarate reductase in some patients; ? saccharopine dehydrogenase in others.	Lysine.	Lysine; some also have increased saccharopine.	—	Therapy may not be necessary; low protein diet (1–1.5 Gm./kg./day).
Maple syrup urine disease (severe infantile form). (1:270,000)	Vomiting, progressive hypertonicity, acidosis, coma, early death.	Branched-chain keto acid decarboxylase (absence virtually complete).	Leucine, isoleucine, valine.	Leucine, isoleucine, valine (with their three corresponding keto acids.	Urine has odor of maple syrup.	Partially synthetic diet low in leucine, isoleucine and valine; exchange transfusions or peritoneal dialysis during crises.
Maple syrup urine disease (intermittent form). (Rare)	Episodic vomiting, lethargy, and coma, often with infections; normal between episodes, including IQ.	Branched-chain keto acid decarboxylase (activity 12–18% of normal).	Leucine, isoleucine, valine only during acute attacks.	Leucine, isoleucine, valine (with their three corresponding keto acids) only during acute attacks.	Odor of maple syrup when ill; disease may be fatal during crises.	Low protein diet during exacerbations (1–1.5 Gm./kg./day).
Ornithinemia (Type II). (Rare)	Prolonged neonatal jaundice, failure to thrive, liver cirrhosis, mental retardation.	Ornithine ketoacid transaminase.	Ornithine.	Ornithine may be normal; generalized aminoaciduria, glycosuria.	Normal serum ammonia even after protein loading.	Low protein diet (1 Gm./kg./day).

TABLE 1. Continued

DISEASE (AND APPROXIMATE INCIDENCE)*	CLINICAL FEATURES	ABNORMAL ENZYME	AMINO ACIDS INCREASED IN BLOOD	AMINO ACIDS INCREASED IN URINE	COMMENTS	TREATMENT
Hyperprolinemia (Type I). (Rare)	May have seizures, mental retardation, hereditary nephritis and deafness; others completely normal.	Proline oxidase.	Proline.	Proline; hydroxyproline and glycine may also be elevated.	–	? necessary; low proline, low protein diet tried with some success.
Hyperprolinemia (Type II). (Rare)	Seizures, mental retardation in some; others completely normal.	Δ^1-pyrroline-5-carboxylate dehydrogenase.	Proline.	Proline, Δ^1-pyrroline-5-carboxylate, hydroxyproline and glycine.	–	? necessary; low protein, low proline diet tried with some success.
Sarcosinemia. (Rare)	? Mild mental retardation; variable clinical picture in patients reported.	? Sarcosine dehydrogenase.	Sarcosine.	Sarcosine.	–	? necessary; no special diet tried.
Tyrosinemia. (Rare)	Failure to thrive, vomiting, diarrhea, liver cirrhosis, renal tubular defects, vitamin D-resistant rickets.	Unknown; ? parahydroxyphenylpyruvic acid oxidase.	Tyrosine, methionine.	Generalized aminoaciduria with especially large amounts of tyrosine.	Glucosuria, phosphaturia, hypophosphatemia.	Low phenylalanine, low tyrosine diet.

* Incidence figures are from the State of Massachusetts Metabolic Screening Program as of October, 1972 (courtesy of Dr. Harvey Levy) and from review of the literature. The figures presented are approximations; in many cases the disease is not detectable on routine screening and true incidence is unknown.

Disorders of Carbohydrate Metabolism

GEORGE N. DONNELL, M.D., *and*
MAURICE D. KOGUT, M.D.

GALACTOSEMIA

Galactosemia most often results in severe and life-threatening signs and symptoms early in infancy. Jaundice, hepatomegaly, edema and ascites, bleeding tendency, susceptibility to infection and failure to thrive are the most common manifestations. If galactosemia is suspected, it is preferable to institute treatment rather than risk irreversible damage or death while awaiting confirmation of the diagnosis. In the small number of galactosemic patients who survive the early severe manifestations, cataracts and retarded physical and mental development are usually seen.

Immediate attention must be given to the frequently fulminant secondary manifestations, but specific treatment of infections, bleeding tendency and other problems in these patients is rarely successful unless the primary disease is being cared for concurrently. The basic problem presented by these infants is the control of tissue accumulation of galactose metabolites which results from the absence of activity of galactose-l-phosphate uridyl transferase, an enzyme essential in galactose metabolism. At present, no way is known to provide a functional enzyme system, and the alternative must be exclusion of galactose from the diet. Dietary control of galactose intake is crucial in the management of galactosemia, but *dietary restriction alone is insufficient therapy of the fulminant secondary manifestations.*

Diet Therapy. Exclusion of galactose from the diet prevents or reverses many manifestations. The most important step is elimination of milk and milk products from the diet. In our clinic the substitution of a commercially prepared casein hydrolysate (Nutramigen), soya or meat base formulas has been successful. Nutramigen, used in powder form, contains a balanced mixture of amino acids, fats and carbohydrates. During the years that this preparation has been used in our clinic, progress of patients has been satisfactory, although the formula does contain a very small amount of free galactose (less than 70 mg. per 8-ounce feeding). In standard dilution (1 measure to 2 ounces of water) it provides 20 calories per ounce of formula.

In the rare infant who does not accept Nutramigen, or who has loose stools, a soy milk or meat base formula can be used. The formula may be the sole source of calories until the usual baby foods are added. Many "baby dinners," soups and puddings contain some form of milk and should not be offered. Manufacturers should be consulted if there is any doubt about the composition of their products.

Cereals, vegetables, fruits and meat are safe to administer. There previously was some question about the advisability of feeding legumes. Peas and beans contain oligosaccharides, of which galactose is a constituent. Presumably these more complex sugars cannot be digested to free galactose and their intake in limited quantities is permissible.

In the past there was concern about the oligosaccharide content of soya formulas. Recently, soy formulas have been prepared from soy protein isolate rather than from whole soy flour. The isolate reduces the oligosaccharide content and the potential source of galactose. Experience during the last years with these formulas has not resulted in increased erythrocyte galactose-l-phosphate levels and we regard these products as safe for galactosemic children.

As the child grows older and the diet becomes more varied, caution should be used in the selection of new foods. Milk is commonly found in bread, cake, some canned puddings and various chocolate candies. Accordingly, the labels of all food packages must be carefully examined. Another potential problem is the use of lactose as a sweetening agent in canned syrups or as a compounding agent in medications. Another common use of lactose is as a coating in frozen ready-to-eat foods. Nonfat milk solids are often added to prepared cereals to fortify the protein content of grains.

The parents will need periodic advice to ensure that the diet is well balanced and contains the nutrients needed for growth and development. Parents tend to be overcautious, and meal patterns often become monotonous and distasteful. Table 1 shows that food restrictions actually are minimal, and, for the most part, the galactosemic child can participate in family meals. This facilitates menu planning and avoids exclusion of the child from the family circle.

As these children reach school age, they will tend to reduce disproportionately their intake of Nutramigen. Water or fruit and vegetable juices may be substituted. If the Nutramigen intake decreases, it may become necessary to give a calcium supplement. (The same caution should be observed with infants whose

TABLE 1. Foods Which May Be Included in and Excluded from the Galactose-Restricted Diet

TYPE OF FOOD	FOODS INCLUDED	FOODS EXCLUDED
Milk and milk products	Isomil Nutramigen ProSobee Meat base formula Cream substitutes free of milk or milk derivatives	Breast milk Cow's milk or goat's milk or any other milk from an animal source in any form: whole, nonfat, evaporated, condensed; whey, casein, dry milk solids, curds, lactose Cream, butter, all cheeses, yogurt, ice cream, ice milk, sherbet, chocolate milk
Legumes	All may be included if laboratory facilities are available for periodic testing of blood (erythrocyte galactose-1-phosphate)	
Meat	Plain meats, fish, poultry Eggs	Liver, pancreas, brain or any organ meats Creamed, breaded, processed meats, fish, poultry which may contain lactose
Bread and cereal foods	Cooked and dry cereals without milk or lactose added *Bread or crackers without milk or lactose added; saltines, graham crackers Macaroni, spaghetti, noodles, rice	Cereals, breads, crackers which have milk, milk products or lactose added
Fats	Vegetable oils, such as soybean, corn, cottonseed, safflower, olive, peanut oils Shortening, lard, margarines which do not contain milk or milk products Olives, nuts, bacon	Butter, cream Margarine unless listed
Fruits and vegetables	Any fresh, frozen, canned or dried fruits, unless processed with lactose Any vegetable unless excluded, or if processed with lactose White potatoes, sweet potatoes, yams	Fruits processed with lactose Peas; vegetables processed with lactose Most brands of instant mashed potatoes
Soups	Clear soups; vegetable soups which do not contain peas; cream soups made with milk substitutes listed	Cream soups, chowders, commercially prepared soups containing lactose
Desserts	Water and fruit ices; gelatin, angel food cake, homemade cakes, pies and cookies made from acceptable ingredients; fruit-flavored cornstarch pudding made with water	Ice cream, ice milk, sherbet, custard Most commercial mixes for cakes and cookies
Miscellaneous	Unbuttered popcorn, marshmallows, sugar, corn syrup, molasses, honey, carbonated beverages, colas, root beer, instant coffee, unsweetened cocoa, unsweetened cooking chocolate, semi-sweet chocolate Pure spices, punch base without lactose	Caramels, toffee Milk chocolate Presweetened punch base with lactose

* Bread companies and markets should be contacted in each geographic area.

intake is low.) Meat, poultry, fish and eggs are excellent protein sources, but certain galactose-storing organs, such as liver, pancreas and brain, must be avoided. Labels on cold cuts and other meats commonly containing fillers should be carefully scrutinized to make sure that no milk or milk products are included. Creamed and breaded meats, poultry and fish should also be excluded from the diet.

Mothers must exercise care in keeping milk, bread, cake and other galactose-containing foods out of reach of the child. Parents must interpret the nature of the disease to neighbors, relatives, school personnel and others who associate with the child so that they may understand and cooperate. As the child grows older, he must be taught his diet and encouraged to take the responsibility for observing the restrictions. Generally, if school-age children avoid dairy products, they may eat the same foods as their schoolmates without fear of increased blood levels of galactose.

The question arises as to how long the diet should be continued. It is essential to exclude lactose during the years of rapid growth and development. Whether or not tolerance to galactose occurs with increasing age is still unclear. Unless an objective means, such as periodic monitoring with erythrocyte galactose-1-phosphate levels, is available, one should err on the conservative side and continue to control the diet.

Treatment of Complications. FLUID AND ELECTROLYTE DISTURBANCES. Vomiting, diarrhea, dehydration and acidosis are not unusual in the untreated patient, especially the infant. The indications for fluid therapy are the same as those in other disorders in which similar symptoms are present. The intravenous route is always preferred. Regardless of the details of procedure, it is essential to consider normal maintenance requirements, replacement of previously incurred deficits and meeting abnormal continuing losses. In the galactosemic patient with acidosis there is no contraindication to the usual administration of alkali.

INFECTION. Untreated galactosemic infants are extremely susceptible to infection. Septicemia, pyelonephritis and bronchopneumonia are the most common. Since gram-negative organisms predominate, it has been our practice to use broad-spectrum treatment until culture reports are available. Kanamycin has now become the drug of choice for initial therapy until reports of culture and sensitivity testing are known. Choice of drugs will then depend on these results.

JAUNDICE. Hepatomegaly is an invariable finding in infants with untreated galactosemia, although icterus develops in only two-thirds. Onset of icterus is generally during the first week of life, but it appears later than the hyperbilirubinemia associated with blood group incompatibilities. Only in rare instances has a sufficiently high level of indirect bilirubin warranted consideration for exchange transfusion. Removal of galactose from the diet and supportive treatment of infection are followed by rapid clearing of the jaundice. Liver size is reduced at a slower rate, but the liver usually returns to normal size by three to four months.

EDEMA. Liver damage may also be reflected in hypoalbuminemia, which in turn may result in generalized edema and ascites. Whole blood, plasma or human albumin may be administered intravenously to correct the hypoproteinemia.

BLEEDING TENDENCY. Bleeding manifestations in the untreated infant are due to prothrombin deficiency secondary to liver damage. Usually there is a rapid response to the exclusion of lactose from the diet and to the parenteral administration of phytonadione (vitamin K_1, Mephyton). When a diagnosis of galactosemia is suspected, even minor surgical procedures (such as percutaneous liver biopsy) should be avoided until the coagulation defect has been corrected.

CATARACTS. Cataracts of varying degrees of severity occur in the majority of untreated patients. Although cataracts usually become apparent during the first year of life, their detection in the early stages may be difficult. In the untreated patient progression to mature cataracts is variable. Patients with a late diagnosis or those improperly treated may require corrective surgery. When the diagnosis is made early, lesions become arrested or may even improve.

MENTAL RETARDATION. Retardation occurs in untreated patients. It would appear that the development of irreversible brain damage depends on the time interval before therapy and the *degree* of adherence to the diet. Although further mental impairment is arrested by treatment, the possibility of improvement with therapy depends on the age of the child. The need for early diagnosis and careful management is evident.

Assessment of Progress. If treatment is carried out properly, satisfactory progress can be expected. The principal problem is the ingestion of unsuspected sources of galactose, either in dietary materials or in foods consumed by the child under circumstances unknown to the parent. Objective assessment of improvement should include the pattern of growth and development and the child's intellectual progress. Reliance on clinical observation alone may not be adequate, since changes leading to irreversible damage are subtle and may be overlooked. Laboratory evaluation can be helpful. Only ingestion of relatively large quantities of galactose are reflected in galactosuria. At present, in our opinion, periodic measurement of erythrocyte galactose-1-phosphate levels is a useful procedure.

Genetic Counseling. With increasing frequency the physician is called upon to advise parents of an affected child on the problem of continued childbearing. To be effective, the physician should have at hand a well-confirmed diagnosis and a detailed family history. It is essential, furthermore, that he be familiar with the genetic transmission of the particular disease.

In galactosemia, the defect is transmitted as a simple mendelian autosomal recessive character. In view of the polymorphism described for a number of enzymes, it might have been anticipated that variant forms of transferase would be discovered.

Beutler has reported a transferase variant (Duarte variant) for which homozygotes are entirely asymptomatic. Homozygotes for the Duarte variant have about half of the normal erythrocyte transferase activity. Because galactosemic heterozygotes also have approximately half the normal transferase activity it is not possible to distinguish between galactosemia carriers and the Duarte variant homozygotes solely by means of measuring enzyme activity. Fortunately, it is now possible to distinguish the Duarte variant from the galactose heterozygote by their differences in migration on starch gel. Counseling of suspected carriers of the galactosemic gene must take this into account.

The problem of presenting to parents the known factors and risks is relatively simple. On statistical grounds, if one considers a large population of affected families, one-quarter of the children born will be affected homozygotes, one-quarter will be normal and one-half will be carriers of the trait. In any individual family, however, in each pregnancy the probability of an affected child being born remains one in four, regardless of the previous birth history. It has been our practice to avoid giving direct advice, but rather to present the known risks and to stimulate the parents to make their own decision. The need for prompt examination of any future newborn in galactosemic families should be emphasized as part of genetic counseling.

GALACTOKINASE DEFICIENCY

A second rare genetic disorder of galactose metabolism has been reported in which a deficiency of galactokinase is responsible for the clinical and laboratory findings. The inability to phosphorylate galactose results in the accumulation of galactose in blood and the appearance of galactose in urine. In contrast to the well-known transferase defect type of galactosemia, the only important clinical manifestation of galactokinase deficiency recognized to date is cataract formation. Diet therapy is identical to that described for galactosemia. Although experience is still limited, it appears that treatment instituted early not only limits progression of cataracts but also may result in their improvement.

GLYCOGEN STORAGE DISEASE

The term glycogen storage disease has been applied to a number of disorders in which excessive amounts of glycogen are found in various tissues. In most cases these are associated with specific enzyme defects. In our experience, as well as that throughout the United States, the most common type is *von Gierke's* disease or the hepatorenal form. It is associated with a deficiency in glucose-6-phosphatase activity; glycogen can be broken down, but conversion of glucose-6-phosphate to free glucose is impaired. Less common types include absence of phosphorylase activity, with the result that breakdown of glycogen cannot be initiated, and absence of debrancher enzyme (amylo-1,6-glucosidase), which prevents completion of glycogenolysis. In a limited number of cases the problem is in the synthesis of glycogen (brancher enzyme defect). In the cardiac form of generalized glycogenosis (*Pompe's disease*) a deficiency in alpha-glucosidase has been identified.

Glycogen storage diseases result from intracellular enzyme defects; consequently, at least for the present, therapy must be restricted to supportive measures. In some forms of glycogenosis it has been possible to prevent early death by appropriate therapeutic programs.

This group of diseases is rare, and no extensive experience with therapy has been accumulated in any particular institution. Principles of diet therapy are generally accepted, but the value of supportive medications (glucagon, thyroxin, androgens, human growth hormone and others) remains in doubt.

Glucose-6-Phosphatase Deficiency (von Gierke's Disease)

It has been our experience, and that of others, that some children with von Gierke's disease improve as they grow older, and scrupulous attention to management can be rewarding. Understanding of the metabolic mechanisms involved makes it possible to outline a rational therapeutic program.

Hypoglycemia. DIET. The critical management problem presented by the infant or young child with von Gierke's disease is hypoglycemia. In this age group, in addition to the risk of death, there is a possibility of brain damage. The metabolic error results in a tendency to low blood sugar levels. Acute episodes must be controlled as described in the following paragraphs, but can be minimized by a continuing therapeutic program directed at supporting blood sugar levels.

A liberal carbohydrate intake, divided into portions fed at frequent intervals, is prescribed. The young infant may require 3-hour feedings both day and night. It is our practice to recommend lactose-free milk substitutes (Nutramigen, soya bean milk) to which additional glucose is added to a final concentration of 5 to 10 per cent. Milk substitutes are used, since galactose theoretically would tend to increase liver glycogen, but not circulating glucose. Glucose water may be offered between feedings as needed.

As the child grows older, the interval between feedings may usually be lengthened and the night feedings may be omitted. As a general principle, however, a bedtime snack is always recommended. Since hyperlipemia is a feature of the von Gierke type of glycogenosis, low fat diets have been advocated. In our experience the course of the disease has not been appreciably influenced by restricted fat intake. In practice, when the diet is adjusted for a high carbohydrate intake, there is a reciprocal decrease in the amounts of fat and protein prescribed.

In the *phosphorylase deficiency* and *debrancher deficiency* types, as opposed to von Gierke's disease, a high protein diet offers theoretical advantages. Through gluconeogenesis, amino acids can provide phosphorylated sugars, physiologically useful in the presence of glucose-6-phosphatase. Since this is not the situation in von Gierke's disease, emphasis is placed on frequent carbohydrate feedings.

Severe hypoglycemic episodes are often precipitated by reduced food intake or by infection. It is important that each family be instructed as to the natural course of the disease and be prepared to initiate emergency care. Increased irritability, fretfulness and twitching are indications for administration of glucose by mouth or by proctoclysis if the oral route is not feasible. Parents should be instructed to contact their physician at once, regardless of the outcome of home emergency treatment. When convulsions occur, intravenous administration of glucose may be necessary.

INFECTIONS AND ACIDOSIS. These children are highly susceptible to infection, which may precipitate and aggravate episodes of hypoglycemia. The selection of antibiotics is without reference to the underlying disease, but depends on the nature of the infection. Early correction of dehydration, acidosis and hypoglycemia is mandatory. Fluids are calculated in the usual manner to meet maintenance and replacement requirements. Sufficient glucose must be provided in the fluids (10 to 15 per cent solutions) to prevent recurrence of hypoglycemia until oral intake can be resumed. Furthermore, glucose administration helps to prevent further lactic acid accumulation and is a major step in correction of the acidosis.

If the acidosis is moderate or severe, correction is accelerated by administration of sodium bicarbonate, 0.25 Gm. per kilogram, over a 12-hour period (3.3 ml. of 7.5 per cent sodium bicarbonate per kilogram will raise the carbon dioxide level approximately 5 mEq. per liter). Sodium lactate is inadvisable because of the hyperlactacidemia.

Bleeding Tendency. Patients with von Gierke's disease are known to have a bleeding diathesis, which is usually manifested by recurrent epistaxis. Studies in our hospital have demonstrated a decrease in platelet adhesiveness in patients with types I and IV glycogen storage disease. The cause of the change in platelet adhesiveness is not known. The common therapeutic approaches are usually successful in controlling the epistaxis, and only rarely are posterior nasal packs and blood transfusions necessary. Caution must be exercised when major surgical procedures, particularly tonsillectomy and adenoidectomy, are contemplated; if hemorrhage occurs, platelet transfusions may be considered.

Hyperuricemia. Increase in the serum uric acid levels occurs early in patients with glycogen storage disease type I, whereas the clinical manifestations of gouty arthritis and nephropathy do not appear until late adolescence. Hyperuricemia in glycogen storage disease type I results from both increased production and decreased excretion.

Acute uric acid nephropathy is treated with intravenous fluids to produce a diuresis and with intravenous sodium bicarbonate for alkalinization of the urine to reduce uric acid crystallization. Intravenous fluids should consist of at least 10 per cent dextrose to reduce hyperlactacidemia.

Gouty arthritis has been treated with probenecid† and colchicine with beneficial results. We have had no experience with these drugs in this disease. Since excess uric acid is present, investigational treatment with allopurinol,‡ a xanthine oxidase inhibitor, has been of value. Patients with hyperuricemia and uric acid calculi have benefited from allopurinol in a dose of 5 to 10 mg. per kilogram, with a maximum of 300 mg. per day.

† Manufacturer's precaution: Probenecid is not recommended for children under two years of age.

‡ Manufacturer's precaution: Allopurinol is contraindicated for use in children except for hyperuricemia secondary to malignancy.

Other Types of Glycogenosis

In the less common types of glycogen storage disease the same principles of supportive therapy apply as have been already outlined. In the hepatic phosphorylase or debrancher types, a high protein diet is used. Care is taken to ensure adequate carbohydrate intake. In all the conditions in which muscle is involved, exercise is restricted, especially when cardiac muscle involvement is suspected.

Genetic Counseling

The genetic transmission of the glycogen storage diseases is not well understood. Present information would suggest that they are transmitted as simple mendelian recessive characters. The general principles of genetic counseling have been outlined in the discussion of galactosemia.

INBORN ERRORS OF FRUCTOSE METABOLISM

Normal persons may have small amounts of fructose in the urine after ingestion of large amounts of food containing fructose. Small amounts of fructose also may be found in association with disease states. In contrast, there appear to be two clinically distinguishable forms of inborn errors of fructose metabolism in which the amounts of fructose in urine are relatively large. *Essential fructosuria* is a benign condition inherited as an autosomal recessive trait causing no symptoms, and its importance is in distinguishing it from diabetes mellitus and from hereditary fructose intolerance. The defect is due to a lack of hepatic fructokinase. These patients should not receive insulin, and there is no need for dietary management.

On the other hand, *hereditary fructose intolerance* is associated with a severe symptom complex and cannot be treated unless dietary fructose is removed. The defect is due to gross diminution or absence of activity of the hepatic enzyme fructose-1-phosphate aldolase. The onset of symptoms is determined by the age at which fructose-containing substances, e.g., cane sugar, are first included in the diet. Sucrose splits into fructose and glucose following ingestion and, consequently, cane sugar is the most common source of fructose in formula-fed infants.

In early infancy the symptoms are vomiting, anorexia, failure to thrive, retardation of growth, hepatomegaly, a Fanconi type of syndrome, fructosuria and, occasionally, hypoglycemic convulsions following the ingestion of fructose-containing foods. Splenomegaly, ascites, varying degrees of jaundice and a bleeding tendency may occur. If fructose ingestion persists, death may occur. Other metabolic abnormalities include hypophosphatemia and hypomagnesemia. Since blood fructose levels are elevated, a low blood glucose level will be masked unless a specific glucose oxidase method is used.

Patients who manifest the disease at an older age are more mildly affected and their only symptom may be mild hypoglycemia with seizures. Almost all affected persons develop an aversion to sweet food.

The immediate treatment is to correct hypoglycemia and other metabolic manifestations with the prompt intravenous administration of glucose and appropriate electrolytes. The long-term therapy of this condition is strict avoidance of fructose and sucrose-containing foods (Table 2). Care must be taken to ensure that vitamin supplements and medications are free of sucrose.

Treatment of complications, such as jaundice, edema and bleeding tendency, is the same as that discussed for galactosemia. Mental retardation appears to be uncommon.

The mode of inheritance in hereditary fructose intolerance is believed to be an autosomal recessive trait. No satisfactory test has been devised to detect the heterozygote. Liver fructose-1-phosphate activities are normal even in parents of affected children. In general, the counseling would be similar to that discussed for galactosemia.

TABLE 2. Common Foods Containing Fructose and Sucrose in Amounts Exceeding 1 Per Cent of the Edible Portion*

FRUITS	VEGETABLES	LEGUMES
Apples	Asparagus	Beans
Apricots	Beets	Peas
Bananas	Sweet potatoes	Lentils
Blackberries		Soya beans
Cherries		
Dates		
Figs		
Grapes		
Citrus fruits		
Melons		
Pineapples		SYRUPS
Plums		Sweet chocolate
MILK PRODUCTS	CEREALS	Honey
Ice cream	Corn	Maple syrup
Condensed milk	Rice bran	Molasses

* The polysaccharides and disaccharides which do not contain fructose and which, therefore, can safely be ingested include starch, glycogen, maltose, isomaltose and lactose.

PENTOSURIA

The pentoses, arabinose and xylose, are sometimes found in urine after ingestion of large amounts of fruit juices and fruits such as cherries, plums and grapes. With the exception of a minimal ribosuria as a secondary manifestation of muscular wasting diseases such as muscular dystrophy, no disease entity so far has been associated with pentose excretion.

There is, however, an inherited metabolic error characterized by a constant excretion of 1 to 4 Gm. per day of L-xylose. This disorder is found primarily in Jewish people of Central European origin and is inherited as a recessive character. The biochemical defect appears to be related to a defect in the glucuronic acid oxidation pathway. The primary problem is to differentiate this condition from the glucosuria of diabetes, since affected persons are most often asymptomatic and the condition is recognized during the course of a routine physical examination. No treatment is needed.

SUCROSURIA

Sucrose may be absorbed whole if it is not first split by intestinal enzymatic action. Its presence, however, will not be detected on routine urine testing, since it is not a reducing sugar. Sucrosuria has been described in association with a variety of gastrointestinal lesions, including gastroenteritis. Sucrosuria in itself is an asymptomatic condition and requires no therapy, but it may point to an intrinsic gastrointestinal lesion which requires attention.

CARBOHYDRATE MALABSORPTION

Intestinal malabsorption of carbohydrates results from decreased activity of one or more enzymes concerned with the hydrolysis or transport of various dietary sugars. Such conditions can occur either as a genetic defect or in association with other conditions affecting the intestinal tract. The inherited problems are rare, whereas deficiencies associated with celiac disease, severe gastroenteritis, surgery of the intestinal tract and similar disorders are more common.

The diagnosis of carbohydrate malabsorption may be suspected from a careful dietary history, and the characteristics of the stools, which are frothy, are acid in pH and contain the offending sugar.

Regardless of whether the specific condition is due to a genetic defect or is associated with another intestinal condition, treatment is the same except for the duration. Although the diagnosis may be suspected, confirmation must await stabilization of the patient after empirical treatment. The results of loading tests with various carbohydrates cannot be interpreted in the presence of continued diarrhea. Intestinal biopsies are not readily available for the determination of specific enzyme defects.

The treatment of the malabsorption is the removal of the offending carbohydrates from the diet if identification is possible. In the absence of a definitive diagnosis, treatment remains empirical and a dextrose based formula is substituted. Ordinarily, diarrhea diminishes within one week. In rare instances with glucose and galactose malabsorption, fructose must be used as the sole source of carbohydrate. As in any diet with limitation of components, sufficient daily intake of vitamins, minerals and trace elements must be provided.

It must be emphasized that when carbohydrate malabsorption is secondary to another intestinal problem, removal of the offending carbohydrate alone is insufficient to alleviate the diarrhea without treatment of the primary problem.

Lactose Malabsorption

Congenital lactose intolerance is a rare and isolated defect which becomes manifest soon after milk feedings are begun. A lactose-free milk substitute is used in treatment. Suitable preparations include a protein hydrolysate fortified with sucrose as a source of carbohydrate (Nutramigen), various soya bean products and a meat based formula containing sucrose. As solid foods are introduced, it is important to avoid major sources of lactose. As the child grows older, a small intake of lactose, such as that in cheeses or butter, is acceptable, but milk cannot be tolerated.

Lactose intolerance more commonly results from another intestinal problem. For example, lactose intolerance is often present in celiac disease, and its treatment should include dietary lactose restriction. Intolerance to sucrose may also be present. If, on the lactose-free diet, the child continues to have diarrhea and acid stools, a formula based on dextrose should be used (such as Borden's carbohydrate-free formula with dextrose added). Alternatively, addition of dextrose to a meat base is suitable, such as a modification of that originally described by McQuarrie and Ziegler. Cautious attempts to introduce the offending sugar can be made after a few months.

Sucrose and Isomaltose Malabsorption

In this condition, there is malabsorption of both sucrose and isomaltose. Isomaltose, plus maltose, results from the digestion of starch in the gastrointestinal tract. Dietary treatment involves avoidance of sucrose, as already described, and limitation of starch intake on a trial and error basis. In this particular disorder, lactose can be tolerated as a source of carbohydrate with, if necessary, additional carbohydrate calories provided as dextrose.

Glucose and Galactose Malabsorption

In rare instances the patient cannot tolerate either glucose or galactose. Carbohydrate must then be supplied entirely as fructose. Lactose, maltose and sucrose are to be avoided, since glucose results from the hydrolysis of each of these sugars and, in addition, galactose is produced from lactose. The diet used is a sugar-free soya bean or meat base preparation to which fructose is added to a maximum of 10 per cent.

Complete Carbohydrate Intolerance

A few infants may demonstrate a temporary intolerance to all carbohydrates, which may result from severe gastroenteritis. Initially these patients require fluid and caloric support parenterally. When foods are again used, a carbohydrate-free protein formula may be offered, but a carbohydrate-free diet is not acceptable for more than a short period of time. Fructose or glucose should be added cautiously after the child appears to have been stabilized. If there are no ill effects, the amount of carbohydrate can be increased gradually.

References

Beutler, E., et al.: A New Genetic Abnormality Resulting in Glucose-1-Phosphate Uridyltransferase Deficiency. *Lancet,* 1:353, 1965.

Fine, R. N., Frasier, S. D., and Donnell, G. N.: Growth in Glycogen-Storage Disease Type I. *Am. J. Dis. Child.,* 117:169-177, 1969.

Froesch, E. R., et al.: Hereditary Fructose Intolerance. An Inborn Defect of Hepatic Fructose-1-Phosphate Splitting Aldolase. *Am. J. Med.,* 34:151, 1963.

Gitzelmann, R.: Hereditary Galactokinase Deficiency, a Newly Recognized Cause of Juvenile Cataracts. *Pediat. Res.,* 1:14, 1967.

Laron, Z.: Essential Benign Fructosuria. *Arch. Dis. Child.,* 36:273, 1961.

McQuarrie, I., and Ziegler, M. R.: Comparison of Nutritive Value of Mineral-Enriched Meat and Milk. *Pediatrics,* 5:210, 1950.

Stanbury, J. B., Wyngaarten, J. B., and Frederickson, D. S.: *The Metabolic Basis of Inherited Disease.* 2nd ed. New York, McGraw-Hill Book Company, 1966.

Inborn Errors of Lipid Metabolism

ALLEN C. CROCKER, M.D.

THE HYPERLIPIDEMIAS (HYPERLIPOPROTEINEMIAS); FAMILIAL SYNDROMES WITH AN INCREASE IN BLOOD LIPIDS

Considered in this section are those children with a significant hyperlipidemia, in which the blood abnormality is not secondary to diabetes mellitus, von Gierke's disease, the nephrotic syndrome or obstructive liver disease.

Familial Hypercholesteremia

The most common of the genetically transmitted hyperlipidemias is the syndrome of "familial hypercholesteremia" (type II in the Fredrickson schema), in which there is a clear serum (normal triglycerides) but a moderate increase in cholesterol level (and beta-lipoprotein). Childhood cholesterol levels here range from 270 to 400 mg. per 100 ml. It is believed by some workers that the abnormality can be detected by analysis of cord blood specimens obtained at birth (cholesterol then over 100 mg. per 100 ml.), but it appears that the only reliable technique is demonstration of elevation of low-density lipoprotein. The trait is dominantly transmitted (usually from one parent only), with biochemical expression in the heterozygously involved individual. Such children, however, are asymptomatic, showing tendon and eyelid xanthomas, corneal arcus and early coronary disease only in young adult life. For the more infrequent homozygously involved child (both parents being hypercholesteremic), serum cholesterol levels are higher (600 to 1000 mg. per 100 ml.) and death usually occurs in adolescence, with coronary and valvular atheromas (of a soft, nonsclerotic type).

If children of either of these types are identified—by newborn screening, random sampling or search in a known pedigree—it is generally agreed that an obligation exists to attempt modification of the hyperlipidemia. There is no proof that this will circumvent the eventual cardiac complications, but such is the hope. It is certainly true that efforts to lower the serum cholesterol level are much more successful in children than in their similarly involved adult relatives. Hence, the pediatrician has the opportunity to intervene in the sequence of early onset and long duration of the biochemical abnormality, at least as this is reflected in the serum lipid levels.

For children with this syndrome, *dietary modifications* represent the first approach, with the promise of significant effects even if complete rectification is not achieved. It is advisable to reduce the intake of dairy fats (no cream, substitution of vegetable margarine for butter and of skimmed for whole milk, use of substitute ice creams and use of cottage cheese) and fatty meats (pork products especially). Corn oil and other unsaturated vegetable oils should be used for frying, salads and other food preparations. Fish and poultry should have priority over other meats. Extreme dietary manipulations, on the other hand, such as complete vegetarianism, do not provide sufficient further value to justify their disturbing psychologic effect. The child should develop customs which he can live with for decades, with moderation in the intake of fatty foods as the keynote; he should not be so constrained that serious adjustment problems result. Involved families of this sort are usually sufficiently motivated to modify the kitchen practices for all members, including those not definitely involved.

Chemotherapy. Chemotherapeutic agents which may affect the serum cholesterol level can be added, after the results from dietary change alone have been established. In certain instances the use of drug treatment can be postponed for some years if modification of diet has given a major corrective effect. Six medications are currently available, each of which will, in some individuals, induce important lowering of the serum cholesterol level (usually in the order of a 20 to 30 per cent change). These can be tried for six-month intervals, to assay their usefulness for members of the pedigree under discussion. They are as follows:

D-Thyroxine (Choloxin), 1 to 4 mg. once a day by mouth, the dosage increased step-wise, with avoidance of hypermetabolic side effects.

Clofibrate (Atromid-S),* ½ to 1 Gm. twice a day by mouth.

Cholestyramine (Questran),† a sterol-binding resin, in fractions of the adult dose of 20 Gm. per day, taken in divided doses with meals.

Beta-sitosterol (Cytellin), an emulsion of soy sterols which inhibit cholesterol absorption, up to 1 ounce before meals and at bedtime.

Nicotinic acid, 3 Gm. per day in divided doses by mouth, or increasing from this if the side effects (facial flushing, rashes) can be tolerated.

Neomycin, based on the adult dose of 0.5 to 2 Gm. per day in divided doses orally.

Using one or another of these drugs, the heterozygously involved child is likely to achieve normal serum lipid levels. For the homozygously affected child the final effects will still be disappointing. In these instances, specially controlled combinations should be considered, as well as the experimental surgical approaches (such as the ileal by-pass operation).

Idiopathic Familial Hyperlipemia

Occasionally one encounters children with heavily lipemic (lactescent) serum, where the neutral fat is massively increased (2000 to 6000 mg. per 100 ml.), with only mild elevations of serum cholesterol and phospholipid (Fredrickson type I).

These patients show lipemia retinalis, often have some enlargement of the liver or spleen and may have eruptive skin xanthomas and recurrent, self-limited "abdominal crises" of vomiting, fever, abdominal pain and prostration. A few instances of multiple involvement in siblings have been reported, but the family history is otherwise normal. This abnormality is sensitive to the level of dietary fat intake. The prognosis for cardiovascular disease is not serious.

Treatment of the hyperlipemia is motivated by a desire to limit the abdominal pain episodes or the eruptive xanthomas. No drugs are available which will modify the abnormal metabolism of this syndrome. *Dietary restriction* is theoretically adequate to produce lowering of the lipemia to near-normal levels, but it is difficult to achieve the continuing cooperation of the pediatric patient to a degree which will be effective. Reduction of the daily intake of fatty foods of all types to a point at which fat represents less than 20 per cent of the total calories is reasonable, and further restriction can be useful in special instances.

Other Hyperlipemic Syndromes

Additional patients are found with hyperlipemic serum, not conforming to the two classic patterns previously mentioned. Features which suggest this other type of involvement are a tendency for a less consistent degree of the lipemia, absence of a definite correlation of the lipemia to the level of dietary fat, a family history of diabetes mellitus without involvement of the child under consideration and relatives showing early cardiovascular disease. By the Fredrickson classification (based on lipoprotein electrophoretic patterns), three other phenotypes have been identified in adults (III,

---

* Manufacturer's precaution: Atromid-S is not recommended for use in children, since studies in this age group have been insufficient.

† Manufacturer's precaution: Dosage of cholestyramine resin (Questran) for children under six years of age has not been established.

IV and V), with important amounts of "pre-beta"-lipoprotein present, apparent sensitivity of the blood fat level to carbohydrate intake and poor cardiovascular prognosis. The situation for children in these pedigrees remains unclear, and careful individual studies are required before treatment is begun. Some of the medications listed previously may be of use, especially clofibrate. Restriction of carbohydrate intake is difficult to implement for a pediatric patient.

THE LIPIDOSES; SYNDROMES WITH SPECIAL TISSUE LIPID ACCUMULATION

The past decade has seen identification of deficiencies in the activity of specific lysosomal enzymes for virtually all of the lipidoses. From these studies one could conclude that the ideal treatment plan would be an enzyme replacement program, but this basically reasonable contention has to date proved unattainable in practice. Provision of active enzyme in high concentration, sufficiently early in the course of the disease, and at the critical tissue site, has been technically impossible. Infusion of fresh plasma, transfusions of living white blood cells, organ transplant and administration of tissue concentrates have not as yet been successful in children with these inborn errors. Use of the enzyme assay is pertinent, however, in prenatal diagnosis (on cultures of amniotic fluid cells) for the prevention of the birth of such children in families who are known to be involved. Population screening for the identification of parents at risk has become feasible at least in the instance of Tay-Sachs disease, by assay of serum hexosaminidase-A levels in young adults of Ashkenazi Jewish ancestry. For all of these syndromes, autosomal recessive inheritance patterns are seen.

Tay-Sachs Disease

The major responsibility for the pediatrician in the family with a Tay-Sachs child is provision of continuing support for the parents. This includes informed counseling about the genetic issues, assistance in the formation of long-term care plans (now usually at home, with professional back-up) and contact with appropriate parents' groups. During the second year of life the Tay-Sachs child begins to present important care problems. Seizures and irritability are usually modified by treatment with Dilantin, phenobarbital and/or chloral hydrate. Poorer feeding becomes a challenge and often must be ultimately solved by teaching parents gavage techniques. Constipation is relieved by a mineral oil–magnesia mixture, or enemas. Difficulty in the handling of respiratory mucus, complicated by infections of the respiratory tract, can be assisted by postural drainage after the use of expectorants. Portable suction machines can be rented by the family. Antibiotic use should be restricted to discrete episodes of acute infection. During the late phases of the disease the skin requires special attention to prevent the formation of decubitus ulcers. After the second birthday, the child characteristically is almost totally out of contact, with blindness, stiffness, inactivity and chronic pulmonary difficulties. Death usually occurs when the patient is between three and four years of age.

Niemann-Pick Disease

There are several, genetically unrelated types of Niemann-Pick disease with varying degrees of personal handicap. Most common are the children with signs of cerebral pathology in infancy and early childhood. Again, the management is largely supportive, with many of the same issues present as discussed under Tay-Sachs disease. In some pedigrees the children show neurologic abnormality only in middle or late childhood (emotional instability, intellectual plateauing, cerebellar signs); they require special education programs and personal support. Some children have normal central nervous system function but important visceral signs of disease (hepatosplenomegaly, pulmonary infiltration and so forth). In any of these phenotypes, splenectomy may be advisable because of blood cell suppression.

Gaucher's Disease

The majority of Gaucher's disease patients have the so-called "chronic" syndrome, which usually includes enlargement of the abdominal organs in the early years and bone pain as well. The ultimate length of life of these patients is normal, but clinical difficulties occur in two principal areas:

1. Enlargement of the spleen may effect a reduction in the levels of platelets, white blood cells and hemoglobin. Particularly for the control of thrombocytopenic bleeding, splenectomy may be required; this treatment will result in permanent cure of these problems. Postsplenectomy infections have not been more notable than in other hematologic syndromes.

2. Gaucher's disease patients often have bizarre spontaneous episodes of pain in the bones and, especially, the joints. These may be rheumatic-like in appearance, but frequently seem to represent cortical microfractures (in areas where there is already altered bone texture visible by x-ray). Current films should be

reviewed, and when no new or special lesion is found the management should be conservative, with avoidance of weight-bearing until the pain has ceased. There may also be more critical osseous complications, particularly pathologic fracture of the femoral neck. This commonly results in progressive deterioration of the condition of the femoral head. Compression may also occur in one or more lumbar or dorsal vertebral bodies. Special orthopedic assistance is necessary for the management of these difficulties. Chronic arthropathy of the hip may eventually require major operative intervention.

The much more infrequently found, genetically unrelated "infantile Gaucher's disease" patient has early serious central nervous system handicaps (especially those pertaining to cranial nerve function), and supportive care for him is similar to that listed for the Tay-Sachs infant.

Other Syndromes

The rarer lipidoses present specialized difficulties which are appropriately handled in particular clinics where there has been experience in these areas. This includes Wolman's disease, Farber's disease (lipogranulomatosis), generalized gangliosidosis, metachromatic leukodystrophy, I-cell disease, fucosidosis and so forth.

References

Crocker, A. C., and Farber, S.: Therapeutic Approaches to the Lipidoses; in S. M. Aronson and B. W. Volk (eds.): *Cerebral Sphingolipidoses.* New York, Academic Press, Inc., 1962, p. 421.

Fredrickson, D. S.: Diseases Characterized by Evidence of Abnormal Lipid Metabolism; in J. B. Stanbury, J. B. Wyngaarden and D. S. Fredrickson (eds.): *The Metabolic Basis of Inherited Disease.* 3rd ed. New York, McGraw-Hill Book Company, 1972, p. 493.

Congenital Unconjugated Hyperbilirubinemia and Benign Recurrent Cholestasis

M. JEFFREY MAISELS, M.B., B.CH.

CONGENITAL UNCONJUGATED HYPERBILIRUBINEMIA

Gilbert's Disease. The serum bilirubin levels in this condition (up to 6 mg. per 100 ml.) are not dangerous, but some patients experience intermittent malaise and abdominal discomfort. It may be desirable, for cosmetic reasons to reduce scleral icterus, and this can be achieved with phenobarbital (3 to 5 mg. per kilogram per day). In a minority of patients the gastrointestinal symptoms will also respond to this regimen. The clinical response is variable, and since the disease is benign, continuous therapy is not usually indicated.

Crigler-Najjar Syndrome. The marked elevation of serum unconjugated bilirubin will nearly always necessitate exchange transfusion in the first two weeks of life. Together with this, phenobarbital or phototherapy may be used and continued as long-term therapy to keep serum bilirubin at safe levels. In type I syndrome (complete absence of the glucuronyl transferase enzyme) the serum bilirubin level will be unaffected by phenobarbital, but phototherapy has been effective in maintaining acceptable serum bilirubin levels in two patients. In one child, who continues to develop normally both mentally and physically, it has been used for over four years. Twelve hours of daily phototherapy using daylight fluorescent lamps were effective in maintaining acceptable serum bilirubin levels for three years. Subsequently, the use of special blue (F20T12/BB, Westinghouse) narrow-spectrum lamps has been necessary to keep serum bilirubin levels at 12 to 13 mg. per 100 ml. Whether this will continue to be effective in later childhood and adolescence is unknown.

The type II syndrome (incomplete enzymatic defect) will respond well to the continuous administration of phenobarbital (3 to 5 mg. per kilogram per day). A fall in serum bilirubin will be seen after a week to 10 days of therapy and will reach the minimum level attainable within about a month. Continuous therapy is then necessary to maintain these bilirubin levels.

BENIGN, RECURRENT CHOLESTASIS

Therapy is directed against the recurrent episodes of obstructive jaundice with pruritus, anorexia and steatorrhea. Cholestyramine,* which binds bile acids, is effective in relieving symptoms. The drug is best administered in powder form mixed with puréed fruit in a dose of 8 to 16 Gm. per day. Higher doses may be necessary and as much as 24 Gm. per day has been given without adverse gastrointestinal effects.

Recently, phenobarbital (3 to 10 mg. per kilogram per day) has been used with considerable success to reduce serum bilirubin and bile acid concentrations and thus relieve pruritus. Since the disease is episodic, treatment can usu-

* Manufacturer's precaution: Dosage of cholestyramine resin for children under six years of age has not been established.

ally be instituted as soon as an exacerbation occurs, although in some cases continuous therapy may be necessary.

References

Black, M., and Sherlock, S.: Treatment of Gilbert's Syndrome with Phenobarbitone. *Lancet,* 1:1359, 1970.

Ertel, I. J., and Newton, W. A.: Therapy in Congenital Hyperbilirubinemia: Phenobarbital and Diethylnicotinamide. *Pediatrics,* 44:43, 1969.

Karon, M., Imach, D., and Schwartz, A.: Effective Phototherapy in Congenital Nonobstructive, Nonhemolytic Jaundice. *New England J. Med.,* 282:377, 1970.

Powell, L. W., Hemingway, E., Billing, B. H., and Sherlock, S.: Idiopathic Unconjugated hyperbilirubinemia (Gilbert's Syndrome). *New England J. Med.,* 277:1108, 1967.

Sharp, H. S., Carey, J. B., White, J. G., and Krivit, W.: Cholestyramine Therapy in Patients with a Paucity of Intrahepatic Bile Ducts. *J. Pediat.,* 71:723, 1967.

Stiehl, A., Thaler, M. M., and Admirand, W. H.: The Effects of Phenobarbital on Bile Salts and Bilirubin in Patients with Intrahepatic and Extrahepatic Cholestasis. *New England J. Med.,* 286:858, 1972.

Disorders of Porphyrin, Hemoglobin and Purine Metabolism

RICHARD D. LEVERE, M.D., *and*
STANLEY L. WALLACE, M.D.

THE PORPHYRIAS

Congenital Erythropoietic Porphyria. This rare type of porphyria usually first makes its clinical appearance shortly after birth. Severe photosensitivity is the most disabling manifestation of this disorder of erythrocyte porphyrin metabolism, and avoidance of direct sunlight is mandatory. Also helpful is the use of protective clothing and barrier creams to shield out incident ultraviolet light. When cutaneous bullae and vesicles occur they frequently become infected and should be treated with local and systemic antibiotics as indicated by the appropriate cultures.

Congenital erythropoietic porphyria is frequently complicated by hemolytic anemia, and the resulting anemia often requires blood transfusion. The transfusion requirement may be alleviated by splenectomy, but this procedure should be postponed until as late in childhood as is possible because of the repeated exposure to skin infections and the possibility of resultant sepsis.

Erythrodontia (pinkish-brown discoloration of the teeth due to porphyrin deposition) is another cardinal manifestation of this disease. If cosmetically disturbing it may be treated with jacket crowns, but this treatment may prove difficult because of the frequently associated gingivitis which may lead to loss of the crowns.

Congenital Erythropoietic Protoporphyria. This disorder of erythroid porphyrin metabolism is less rare than erythropoietic porphyria, but the symptomatology is much milder. Photosensitivity is the most disturbing manifestation, and protection from sunlight, coupled with protective clothing and barrier creams, is essential. The production of carotenemia with the daily oral administration of 30 mg. of beta-carotene as beadlets has been reported as being useful in the management of the photosensitivity. Hemolytic anemia is a rare complication of this disease, but when it does occur it may be ameliorated by splenectomy.

Acute Intermittent Porphyria. Development of clinical symptomatology in this form of hepatic porphyria is frequently precipitated by exposure to various exogenous agents. Specifically, barbiturates, sulfonamides, ethyl sulfones, griseofulvin and sulfonylureas have been known to produce acute exacerbations of acute porphyria and are, therefore, contraindicated in anyone with a personal or family history of the disease. During periods of remission, strict attention should be directed toward the maintenance of good nutrition, since a diet deficient in carbohydrate can predispose the patient to an acute attack.

Large quantities of carbohydrate, in the form of glucose in water, should be used to treat the acute attack. This requires the placement of a catheter into one of the great veins to permit infusion of 10 to 15 per cent glucose solutions in order to reach a goal of 450 to 600 Gm. of glucose administered in each 24-hour period. Pain and distress are best treated with chlorpromazine,* opiates should be discouraged because of the possibility of addiction. Inappropriate secretion of antidiuretic hormone is a not infrequently associated feature of the acute attack. The resultant hyponatremia should be managed with fluid restriction and, if refractory, by the cautious intravenous administration of hypertonic sodium chloride solution. Severe hypertension may occasionally accompany the acute attack and this should be managed in the same manner as primary malignant hypertension.

Paralysis of the muscles of respiration with resultant respiratory insufficiency is a common

* Manufacturer's precaution: Chlorpromazine is not recommended for children under six months of age except when lifesaving.

mode of death in this disorder. Since paresis is often reversible in acute porphyria, this manifestation should be treated vigorously with the hope of maintaining life until remission occurs. The patient is best treated in a respiratory care unit, with a tracheostomy, a mechanical respirator and constant blood gases monitoring.

Congenital Cutaneous Hepatic Porphyria (Porphyria Variegata). This disorder of porphyrin metabolism is often exacerbated by the same drugs which adversely affect acute intermittent porphyria; they are therefore contraindicated in these patients as well. Photosensitivity is a cardinal manifestation of congenital cutaneous hepatic porphyria and, as in the erythropoietic porphyrias, should be managed by barrier creams and by protection from exposure to sunlight. Oral administration of the resin cholestyramine† in a dose of 12 Gm. per day may prove helpful in the management of the cutaneous lesions because of its ability to bind porphyrins in the intestinal tract and prevent their reabsorption. Caution must be exercised when using cholestyramine to make sure that the patient does not become depleted of fat-soluble vitamins. When acute neurologic symptoms develop in this form of porphyria, they are managed as described under acute intermittent porphyria.

Acquired Hepatic Porphyria (Porphyria Cutanea Tarda Symptomatica.) This type of porphyria may be seen in patients with alcoholic cirrhosis or in individuals with chronic exposure to certain chemicals, such as hexachlorobenzene, ethyl sulfone, stilbestrol, griseofulvin and sulfonylureas. The majority of these patients have associated chronic liver disease which requires dietary management. The photosensitivity should be managed as outlined for the congenital porphyrias. In addition, iron-unloading, by repeated phlebotomies, has proven helpful in those patients who have demonstrated evidence of hepatic hemosiderosis. The goal of this venisection therapy is to remove a total of from 3 to 3.5 Gm. of iron.

METHEMOGLOBINEMIA AND SULFHEMOGLOBINEMIA

Hereditary Methemoglobinemia with Normal Hemoglobin Structure

Congenital Methemoglobin Reductase (Diaphorase) Deficiency. Methemoglobinemia of this type is usually due to a deficiency of NADH-methemoglobin reductase (diaphorase I). Hereditary deficiency of NADPH-methemoglobin reductase (diaphorase II) is not associated with methemoglobinemia unless the patient is exposed to oxidant drugs. A transient deficiency of NADH-methemoglobin reductase may occasionally be seen in newborn infants of mothers who had received prilocaine during caudal anesthesia.

Patients with methemoglobin reductase deficiency usually do not require treatment except for cosmetic reasons to decrease the associated cyanosis. Chronic oral administration of either ascorbic acid or methylene blue will decrease the cyanosis and can be useful in alleviating any associated symptoms such as headache. Ascorbic acid is given in a dose of 300 to 600 mg. per day and methylene blue at a dose of 60 mg. four times a day. Care should be taken when administering methylene blue, since excessive doses may be toxic and cause an increase in methemoglobinemia.

Towne's Variant of Hereditary Methemoglobinemia. This rare disorder is associated with normal levels of methemoglobin reductase but manifests a decrease in total erythrocyte glutathione content. These patients also respond to orally administered ascorbic acid.

Hereditary Methemoglobinemia with Abnormal Hemoglobin Structure. Methemoglobinemia is also seen in association with hemoglobin M and the unstable hemoglobins (Zürich, Köln and so forth). Patients with unstable hemoglobins are particularly sensitive to oxidant drugs and these should be avoided. Ascorbic acid and methylene blue are of no value in treating these defects in globin structure. Transfusion may be necessary if hemolysis and the associated anemia are severe.

Congenital Sulfhemoglobinemia. This extremely rare disorder is relatively benign and requires no therapy.

Acquired Methemoglobinemia

A number of drugs are capable of activating the oxidation of ferrous hemoglobin to ferric hemoglobin, leading to methemoglobinemia. Nitrites, sulfonamides and aniline derivatives have been the most frequently incriminated drugs. Other compounds include acetanilide, phenacetin, chlorates, quinones, sulfones and nitrobenzene. Infants and children may acquire methemoglobinemia from aniline dyes used in marking inks on diapers or other clothing. Aniline dyes may also be absorbed from recently dyed blankets or shoes. Benzocaine ointments have also been implicated in the production of methemoglobinemia

† Manufacturer's precaution: Dosage of cholestyramine resin for children under six years of age has not been established.

in children. Children may also be affected by drinking well-water with a high nitrite content.

Acute and severe drug-induced methemoglobinemia requires treatment with intravenous methylene blue. The recommended dosage for infants is 2 mg. per kilogram of body weight, 1.5 mg. per kilogram for older children and 1.0 mg. per kilogram for adults. The methylene blue is given as a 1 per cent aqueous solution and is readily available in ampules. If cyanosis persists the dose may be repeated in 1 to 2 hours. In extremely severe cases transfusion may be indicated. Milder cases may require only discontinuance of exposure to the offending agent. If mild symptoms are present, oral ascorbic acid or methylene blue should be administered as described in the section dealing with hereditary methemoglobinemia.

Acquired Sulfhemoglobinemia. The same drugs which cause methemoglobinemia may also lead to sulfhemoglobinemia. However, sulfhemoglobin cannot be reduced and treatment with ascorbic acid or methylene blue is of no value. Treatment consists of removal of any causative agent and correction of constipation when present. If anoxia occurs, transfusion is indicated.

MYOGLOBINURIA

Familial Myoglobinuria (Meyer-Betz Disease). Infection or severe exertion may precipitate acute episodes of this disease and strenuous activity is therefore contraindicated in susceptible individuals. Acute attacks may be associated with severe muscle weakness and respiratory paralysis which should be treated with a mechanical respirator. The degree of associated renal insufficiency usually determines the ultimate prognosis in this disorder and this complication should be treated in the usual manner.

Secondary Myoglobinuria. Myoglobinuria may be seen in association with crush injuries, high voltage electric shock, extensive infarction as in the main artery of a limb, alcoholic polymyopathy and polymyositis. If respiratory failure occurs, this requires supported respiration. Among the above predisposing factors, crush injury is the most common cause of associated renal failure, which snould be treated in the usual manner.

Myoglobinuria in McArdle's Syndrome. Severe exertion may cause myoglobinuria in McArdle's syndrome (myophosphorylase deficiency glycogenosis). Patients should be instructed to limit activities, avoid tight garments and increase carbohydrate intake before attempting increased physical exertion.

GOUT

Traditionally, the treatment of gout is divided into three parts: (1) control of the acute episode, (2) prevention of subsequent attacks and (3) dissolution of tophaceous deposits or stones by reducing the serum urate level to normal. Juvenile and adolescent gout is almost always associated with significant urate overproduction. For this reason, the prevention of recurrences and the treatment of deposited urate can be considered together.

The four most effective agents in the treatment of acute attacks of gout are colchicine, phenylbutazone, indomethacin and adrenocorticotropic hormone. The earlier in the course of the acute attack any of these drugs is used, the more effective it is in eradicating the episode.

Colchicine has both diagnostic and therapeutic value in acute gout. A dramatic, objective response in an inflamed joint strongly suggests that the patient has had acute gout. The drug is given by mouth as a single 0.5-mg. or 0.6-mg. tablet once hourly, until one of three eventualities occurs: objective improvement, gastrointestinal side effects or, if neither of the preceding occurs first, an arbitrary maximum dose. For the adolescent, oral colchicine doses should not exceed 6 mg. as total therapy for an attack. However, about 80 per cent of patients given oral colchicine develop major gastrointestinal side effects, including abdominal cramping, diarrhea, nausea and vomiting. For this reason, colchicine should be given intravenously, if possible, rather than by mouth. The effective dose is 1 to 3 mg. as a single total dose. Gastrointestinal side effects occur very rarely after intravenous colchicine. Colchicine solutions are strong chemical irritants, so that it is vital to be certain that the material is being given well into the vein, and slowly.

Phenylbutazone is effective in 90 per cent of patients with acute gout. Once the diagnosis of gout is made, phenylbutazone is the orally administered drug of choice. Doses vary with body size, ranging from 200 to 500 mg. per day for three days, in divided doses. Indomethacin‡ is about as effective as phenylbutazone, in divided doses of 75 mg. to 200 mg. per day for five days. However, with these doses, frequent gastrointestinal and central nervous system side effects occur. Adrenocorticotropic hormone, in doses of 100 mg. of the gel intramuscularly daily for five days, is effective in the treatment of acute gout. However, as many as one-third

‡ Manufacturer's precaution: Indomethacin is contraindicated in children 14 years of age and under.

of the patients so treated rebound with an acute gouty recurrence after therapy. Adrenocorticotropic hormone therefore must be given with, and must be followed by, colchicine therapy, 0.6 mg. per day for 14 days, to prevent the flare-up.

Treatment to prevent recurrences and to dissolve tophi and stones involves the return of the miscible pool of urate to normal. The miscible pool can be considered normal several months after the last recognized tophus has disappeared, or in the patient without visible tophi, after about one year of normal serum urate level.

Drugs capable of lowering serum urate levels include a xanthine oxidase inhibitor and several uricosuric drugs. Allopurinol,§ the xanthine oxidase inhibitor, lowers both serum and urinary urate levels. Doses must be titrated to accomplish the urate level reduction needed. Such doses range from 100 mg. to 500 mg. per day. Toxic effects are infrequent. Severe disseminated vasculitis has been reported. Mild cutaneous vasculitides, hepatocellular chemical changes, and nausea and diarrhea may occur. Allopurinol has also been shown to alter enzyme function in liver microsomes, prolonging the half-life of bishydroxycoumarin and antipyrine by inhibiting their biotransformation.

When allopurinol has reduced the serum level to normal, but deposited urate still persists, there is an increased potential for new attacks of acute gout. Colchicine is necessary, in doses of 0.6 mg. once daily, to prevent these, and must be given with allopurinol until the urate miscible pool is normal (see above).

For those rare patients with juvenile or adolescent gout unable to tolerate allopurinol, the uricosuric drugs, probenecid|| and sulfinpyrazone, are available. These reduce serum levels but increase urinary urate content. Probenecid doses range from 0.5 Gm. to 2 Gm. per day, while sulfinpyrazone doses range from 100 mg. to 400 mg. per day. The major risk in the use of either of these agents is the precipitation of renal calculi. A large fluid intake and urinary output are imperative in conjunction with their use. Triggering of fresh attacks of gout is also possible with these agents; colchicine, 0.6 mg. per day, should be given along with them.

Dietary restrictions can be mild, with the elimination only of foods high in purine content, such as organ meats (kidneys, sweetbreads, brain and liver), anchovies, sardines, meat extracts and gravies and wild game.

HYPERURICEMIA DUE TO HEMATOLOGIC NEOPLASMS

Hyperuricemia occurs frequently in association with leukemia and lymphoma; the treatment of these disorders with cytolytic agents leads to major overproduction of uric acid due to the rapid breakdown of cellular nucleic acids. This in turn may result in the precipitation of uric acid in the upper and lower urinary tract, and sometimes in total urinary obstruction.

The treatment of choice in the prevention of such precipitation is the use of allopurinol. Since it takes about 72 hours for allopurinol to reach its maximal inhibition of xanthine oxidase, with the consequent maximal lowering of serum and urinary urate concentrations, allopurinol therapy in these disorders should precede cytotoxic therapy by at least three days or, preferably, by five to seven days if possible. In situations where pretreatment is not feasible, allopurinol should be used concurrently with cytotoxic agents. Optimal doses range from 100 mg. to 500 mg. per day, roughly according to body weight. However, individual measurement of serum urate is necessary to accomplish the appropriate reduction.

Mercaptopurine is also degraded by xanthine oxidase. For this reason, when the cytotoxic agents mercaptopurine and azathioprine are used in conjunction with allopurinol, doses of the former agents must be reduced sharply. Potential toxic manifestations of allopurinol are described above.

Other therapeutic approaches to minimizing uric acid lithiasis during treatment of hematologic neoplasms include the following:

1. Cautious initiation of cytolytic therapy.
2. Vigorous administration of fluids.
3. Administration of alkali or acetazolamide in an attempt to alkalinize the urine, thus increasing solubility of uric acid.

If uric acid is already precipitated, allopurinol, fluid and alkali therapy may not be adequate, and peritoneal or hemodialysis may be required.

HYPERURICEMIA ASSOCIATED WITH CHOREOATHETOSIS, MENTAL RETARDATION AND SELF-MUTILATION (LESCH-NYHAN SYNDROME)

The profound uric acid overproduction in the Lesch-Nyhan syndrome, caused by severe deficiency of the enzyme hypoxanthine-guanine phosphoribosyltransferase, is characteristically

---

§ Manufacturer's precaution: Allopurinol is contraindicated for use in children except for hyperuricemia secondary to malignancy.

|| Manufacturer's precaution: Probenecid is not recommended for children under two years of age.

associated with hyperuricosuria and urate gravel or stone. Optimal therapy must include allopurinol, in doses sufficient to return the serum urate level and urinary excretion of urate to normal. Customary doses range from 100 mg. to 300 mg. of allopurinol** per day in divided amounts, but must be individually titrated to accomplish the desired reduction in serum and urinary urate levels. Increasing the fluid intake and urinary output (diluting the excreted uric acid) also is of value.

There is no evidence that allopurinol can prevent the neurologic manifestations of the syndrome, even if therapy is initiated at birth.

OROTIC ACIDURIA

Uridine, in divided doses totaling 150 mg. per kilogram per day, has resulted in hematologic remission in orotic aciduria, with decreased urinary excretion of orotic acid. Glucocorticoid therapy can produce a partial hematologic remission without reversal of the megaloblastic marrow. Prednisone, in doses of 10 to 20 mg. per day by mouth, will accomplish this result. A large fluid intake will dilute urinary orotic acid and minimize the likelihood of precipitation. Uracil has been shown to be therapeutically ineffective.

XANTHINURIA

The purpose of treatment in xanthinuria is to inhibit the formation of xanthine stones. Reducing the concentration of xanthine in the urine in patients with xanthinuria can be accomplished by restricting the content of purine in the diet or by increasing the fluid intake, or preferably both. Foods high in purine content include the organ meats, meat extracts and concentrates (gravies and so forth), anchovies, sardines and wild game.

Xanthine has limited solubility in acid urine, so that alkalinization of the urine may be necessary in selected cases. However, the hazards of continuous alkalinization of the urine (calcium stones, infection with certain alkaline-preferring organisms) must be considered.

Allopurinol does not seem to influence the urinary excretion of xanthine or of hypoxanthine in xanthinuric individuals.

** Manufacturer's precaution: Allopurinol is contraindicated for use in children except for hyperuricemia secondary to malignancy.

11

The Histiocytosis Syndromes

The Histiocytosis Syndromes

ALLEN C. CROCKER

Twenty-five years of continued effort in the chemotherapy of children with the histiocytosis syndromes has allowed the formulation of some useful treatment recommendations but has failed to produce a single management routine which is uniformly successful for all patients. This correlates, one can assume, with the fact that now more than 40 years of scientific study of these bewildering clinical disease pictures have not yet provided a cohesive hypothesis about the basic pathogenetic mechanism (or mechanisms). At the present time it is possible to say only that the natural history and histopathology of the lesions in these syndromes suggest that a reactive phenomenon is demonstrated, of a nature which is presumably specialized to the host under discussion, and which must be qualified by unknown environmental and personal factors.

There is a continuum of degrees of expressed involvement in children with this acquired granuloma formation, referred to as a histiocytosis (or reticuloendotheliosis). The term *eosinophilic granuloma* is commonly used for localized lesions in the medullary cavity of bone; *Schüller-Christian syndrome* for a more protracted, multiple-site involvement; and *Letterer-Siwe syndrome* when deeper visceral lesions are found (skin, liver, lung, lymph nodes, spleen and so forth). Microorganisms have not been isolated from these granulomas, and antibiotics do not give any basic control. In many regards the lesions are fundamentally reversible; in younger patients, however, there is a tendency for the disease process to become widespread and develop complications. The ultimate prognosis is generally evident from the nature of the progress during the first year of involvement. Recently, a number of disease pictures bearing partial resemblance to Letterer–Siwe syndrome have been described which have familial involvement and often generalized nervous system lesions; these are of separate origin and should be viewed individually.

For patients with *localized lesions in bone* only, the management is not difficult. *Surgical curettage* of a lesion (e.g., during the original procurement of a biopsy specimen) usually results in the induction of healing; vigorous surgical attack is not required. *Radiotherapy,* in relatively low dosage (400 to 600 R at depth) will also produce control of local lesions. This is advised for inducing rapid suppression of granulomas in particular circumstances: (1) for lesions in weight-bearing bones where pathologic fracture is feared, (2) for unusually large, painful or cosmetically threatening bone lesions, (3) for the pituitary-hypothalamic lesions which cause diabetes insipidus and (4) to gain temporary improvement in troublesome cutaneous lesions or symptomatic adenopathy.

For the child with *multiple lesions, and especially with generalized visceral involvement, chemotherapy* holds the best promise of control of disease. As mentioned above, a number of agents, either antitumor or anti-inflammatory in nature, are available, each of which can be expected to produce favorable responses in a portion of the treated children. The vigor of their use depends on the urgency suggested by the clinical course of the patient. Trial with one agent is appropriately continued for three or four months; failure by that time to achieve objective evidence of favorable effect justifies discontinuance and proceeding to a medication from another class of agents. Combination therapy, as often practiced in the management of the leukemias and lymphomas, should be pursued cautiously; the resultant marrow depletion and predisposition for unusual infections can prove more threatening than the original disease. According to present experience, children with moderately extensive involvement will often receive critical assistance from chemotherapy, while the infant with a brisk petechial eruption, splenomegaly, sustained fever and other signs of advanced disease will not be saved. The current recommendations are as follows:

Alkylating Agents. These medications have achieved a notable record of usefulness in the management of the histiocytoses. Nitrogen mustard may be given for rapid effect (a course of one or two intravenous injections, totaling 0.5 to 0.6 mg. per kilogram for the course). For continuing use, chlorambucil (Leukeran) is advised (0.1 to 0.2 mg. per kilogram per day orally), given for many months, with dosage regulation based on weekly white blood cell counts. A common practice is to discontinue chlorambucil therapy only after several months have passed beyond the last signs of new disease activity. Cyclophosphamide (Cytoxan) appears to offer comparable granuloma-suppressive action (1 to 3 mg. per kilogram per day orally), but the experience with it is less extensive.

The only distinct side effect of the alkylating agents in children is that of temporary depression of hematopoeisis in bone marrow. There is little specific information available regarding long-term effects on gonads and endocrine organs, and these theoretical risks must be weighed against the clinical urgency for chemotherapy.

* Manufacturer's precaution: Vincristine sulfate (Oncovin) is recommended only for the treatment of acute leukemia in childhood.

Periwinkle Alkaloids. Vinblastine (Velban) and vincristine (Oncovin)* have now also been shown to have a distinctly useful effect against the histiocytosis process in patients, including some children in whom alkylating agents have given limited response. The usual method of administration is as a weekly (or at first semiweekly) intravenous injection, 0.1 to 0.3 mg. per kilogram for vinblastine and 0.025 to 0.1 mg. per kilogram for vincristine, monitored for safety by the white cell level and other side effects (neuropathy and loss of hair). This is usually continued for an 8- to 10-week course, if possible.

Prednisone and Other Corticosteroids. There is disagreement about the role of the corticosteroids in the chemotherapy of the histocytosis syndromes. It does appear that prednisone (1 to 2 mg. per kilogram per day orally) does give symptomatic assistance to the patient with disseminated disease, especially regarding irritability, fever, cutaneous eruptions and so forth). It is probable that double dosage on an every-other-day basis is equally effective. Present recommendations are for the use of these drugs as adjuvants to the more basic antitumor agent program.

Other chemotherapeutic agents should be cautiously explored in poorly responsive patients. The antimetabolites (folic acid antagonists and 6-mercaptopurine) have not proved effective.

References

Crocker, A. C.: The Histiocytosis Syndromes; in W. E. Nelson, V. C. Vaughan, III, and R. J. McKay (eds.): *Textbook of Pediatrics*. 9th ed. Philadelphia, W. B. Saunders Company, 1969, p. 1479.

Lucaya, J.: Histiocytosis X. *Amer. J. Dis. Child.*, 121: 289, 1971.

Starling, K. A.: Therapy of Histiocytosis X with Vincristine, Vinblastine, and Cyclophosphamide. *Amer. J. Dis. Child.*, 123:105, 1972.

12

Diseases of Connective Tissue

Diseases of Connective Tissue
(The So-Called Collagen Diseases)

JOHN J. CALABRO, M.D., F.A.C.P.

These systemic rheumatic disorders are grouped together because they are characterized by inflammatory changes of connective tissue in various parts of the body and have many similarities in their initial signs and symptoms. Nevertheless, each disease will pose different problems in management, and failure to perceive the exact diagnosis can delay specific, often lifesaving, treatment. A further challenge, even after institution of appropriate therapy, is the need to enlist full parental cooperation in home care, for without this vital collaboration, complete and sustained treatment is impossible.

JUVENILE RHEUMATOID ARTHRITIS

Any chronic disease of children that might kill, cripple or blind must be recognized promptly and treated comprehensively. Early diagnosis is facilitated by considering juvenile rheumatoid arthritis as having three distinct modes of onset. These are *acute febrile,* with prominence of high fever and other systemic features but with variable articular manifestations, often only arthralgia, *polyarticular,* and *monarticular.* Details of management will depend to a large extent on the type of onset. For example, death from myocardial failure is a constant threat in acute febrile onset, while blindness from asymptomatic iridocyclitis is a major hazard in the child with involvement of a single joint. Quite soon, therefore, one sees the urgent necessity for a spectrum of care involving the primary physician, various specialists, school and social services, and parents in a collaborative effort that may last a score of years.

Treatment for the individual child may be difficult because the long course of disease is so unpredictable and may change at any time. Consequently, management must include an active treatment program and regular follow-up care which are often best obtained from an arthritis clinic. From the outset, the physician must recognize that he can only initiate and supervise therapy. The actual treatment will be done at home by the parents, and results will depend on establishing a working collaboration with them. Therefore, the physician must educate and motivate the parents; they must know all about their child's disease, what they must do and what they may expect.* This is perhaps the best way to reassure parents and to overcome unreasonable expectations of an immediate or decisive "cure." This approach can be reinforced by the knowledge that in a setting of comprehensive care, at least 85 per cent of children achieve normal growth and development. Cooperation usually follows when parents realize that their child's well-being depends primarily on a family approach to home care. The most important part of home care is physical therapy, which can be made possible only by the use of antirheumatic drugs that suppress both joint inflammation and systemic manifestations.

Drug Therapy. Aspirin (acetylsalicylic

* A helpful pamphlet entitled *What Parents Need To Know About Juvenile Arthritis* can be obtained from the Arthritis Foundation, 1212 Avenue of the Americas, New York, New York 10036.

acid) is the drug of choice for treating all modes of onset. Strict analgesics (acetaminophen, codeine, propoxyphene and so forth) are unsatisfactory alternates because they lack the necessary antirheumatic effect. The amount of aspirin required by individual patients may be difficult to determine from serum salicylate levels, which should ideally be maintained between 25 and 30 mg. per 100 ml. Nevertheless, active disease can be suppressed in the majority of children by four to six daily doses that total 90 to 130 mg. per kilogram (⅔ to 1 grain per pound).† Patients with acute febrile disease require the more frequent and higher doses. Once active disease is suppressed, 90 to 100 mg. per kilogram of aspirin daily must be continued for months before it is gradually withdrawn. Acute aspirin toxicity may cause intense ketosis, acidosis and hyperpyrexia in infants and younger children. Older children (like adults) usually develop respiratory alkalosis. Since early signs of chronic salicylate intoxication are easily overlooked, parents should be taught to watch for the occurrence of lethargy and episodic hyperpnea, changes that are especially important in the child too young to complain of tinnitus. When they occur, aspirin should be stopped for 24 hours, then reinstituted at a slightly lower dosage.

Corticosteroids are indicated only for the seriously ill child or when disease threatens life or sight. These drugs are used in heart failure due to myocarditis, and in pericarditis, since undetectable myocarditis may coexist. They are vital for protracted iridocyclitis and vasculitis. For these conditions, 0.5 to 1.0 mg. per kilogram of prednisone (or its equivalent) daily should provide adequate therapy.‡ For short periods, moderate doses of prednisone, 0.2 to 0.4 mg. per kilogram daily, may also be given to patients with acute febrile disease or to those who do not tolerate or who fail to respond to aspirin. Generally, alternate-day steroid therapy is not as effective as three or four divided doses daily. If prolonged steroid therapy is unavoidable, every effort must be made to reduce the dosage to the lowest one possible. Steroids should never be stopped abruptly but withdrawn only gradually and always in conjunction with adequate salicylate therapy. A rare adverse reaction to steroids is pseudotumor cerebri, a form of intracranial hypertension causing headache, nausea, vomiting and papilledema. It occurs primarily in children on long-term steroid therapy and is due either to an abrupt decrease in maintenance dosage or to a change from one steroid compound to another. Should it occur, one must return to the previous maintenance dosage or resume treatment with the original drug.

While steroids can provide symptomatic relief for children with continuous polyarthritis, they do not alter the underlying disease. In fact, the long-term use of steroids in progressive hip involvement may be risky, since these drugs can produce avascular necrosis of the femoral head. Clearly, the major drawback of prolonged steroid therapy is the appreciable increase in the mortality rate in children so treated. Other risks include retardation of statural growth and skeletal maturation, vertebral collapse, glaucoma, cataract, myopathy, psychosis and hypertension.

Intrasynovial steroid injections may be helpful when one or two joints are so seriously affected that exercise and rehabilitation are compromised. One may use 5 to 20 mg. of long-acting preparations of prednisolone or triamcinolone, the amount depending on the size of the joint. I prefer not to inject the same joint more often than every three or four months, because more frequent injections encourage abuse of joints that are still actively diseased.

Gold therapy may be useful in patients with polyarthritis who fail to respond to aspirin. Gold requires at least three months to exert any beneficial effects, and one cannot predict which patients will respond. Gold salts are injected intramuscularly at weekly intervals in a dosage of less than 1 mg. per kilogram, or closer to 0.5 mg. per kilogram in children under six years. Weekly therapy is continued for six months and stopped at this point if there has been no response. With a favorable effect, the intervals are gradually reduced until injections are given monthly. *Only the physician experienced with gold administration and the potentially serious adverse reactions should undertake this form of treatment.* Major complications, more frequent in children under six, include nephrotoxicity and various blood dyscrasias. It is therefore vital to monitor a patient's progress with blood and urine tests, which must be evaluated before each injection.

There are several other drugs, the therapeutic value of which has not yet been determined. These include the immunosuppressive or cytotoxic agents. The antimalarial drugs

---

† This dose exceeds that generally recommended for acetylsalicylic acid, but we believe it is warranted in this situation.

‡ This dose exceeds that generally recommended for corticosteroids, but we believe it is warranted in this situation.

and phenylbutazone are rarely used because serious toxic effects are observed more often in children than in adults. Indomethacin, too, is currently contraindicated in children 14 years of age and under.

Supportive Measures. Appropriate rest, splinting and exercise are fundamental to the prevention and correction of deformity. Moderate use of rest (8 to 10 hours of sleep at night and a nap during the day) facilitate resolution of synovial inflammation. Complete bed rest must be avoided, since this may cause flexion contractures because children will automatically flex inflamed joints to ease pain and spasm. Lightweight bivalved splints, usually made of plaster of paris but preferably made of plastic, are used not only to rest inflamed joints but also to correct deformities. Resting splints for the hand, wrist or knee are generally used for no more than one to three weeks. Traction, sandbags or other methods of keeping joints in proper alignment are alternatives to resting splints. However, for immobilization of a hip, traction is preferred to splinting. If a joint deformity has been sustained (a flexion contracture of a knee, for example), serial splinting may be useful. A new bivalved splint is applied every 10 to 14 days as the range of motion improves. It may be removed to permit daily exercise and then replaced.

A physiatrist or physical therapist must teach the patient or parents a program of regular daily exercises that can be performed in the home. Daily activities, in addition to formal exercise, should be those that maintain strength and move joints primarily through motions of extension. Recreation and sports can help to achieve these goals, but those which involve sharp impact to the joints (basketball, football) must be avoided. Swimming is an excellent sport, since it requires mainly extension-type movement with the added advantage of the positive buoyancy of water. Keeping the child in school also assures that mental activities are maintained. However, provisions must be made to allow the patient more freedom than other students.

Eye Care. The recognition and therapy of iridocyclitis should be entrusted to an ophthalmologist. Iridocyclitis often smolders quietly, and it may not be detected with an ophthalmoscope. Periodic slit-lamp examinations are thereby the only means of early iridocyclitis detection. These should be carried out at six-month intervals in all patients. Children with involvement of only one to three joints (the most susceptible group) and those with previous iridocyclitis require examination every three months, even if the arthritis is in remission.

Surgery. Established deformities can be successfully corrected by a variety of procedures, even in the presence of active disease. However, early synovectomy, or the removal of granulation tissue early enough to prevent erosion of cartilage and bone, is an area of current controversy. The correct timing of the procedure and the proper selection of patients are the issues at the moment. Generally, children six years or younger are poor surgical risks because of their inability to cooperate fully with important postoperative measures.

SYSTEMIC LUPUS ERYTHEMATOSUS

About 15 per cent of cases begin in childhood, but the disease is rare under the age of five years. Disease in children differs somewhat from that observed in adults, in that children more frequently have hemolytic anemia, splenomegaly, generalized lymphadenopathy, high fever and leukocytosis. Patients should be carefully studied for major organ involvement, particularly for the presence of nephritis, which is the major cause of death.

Corticosteroids may be lifesaving, especially in severely ill children with nephritis, vasculitis, psychosis, hemolytic anemia or pericarditis. As much as 1 to 2 mg. per kilogram daily of prednisone may be needed.§ Steroids are more effective when the daily requirement is given three or four times and not in a single dose or on alternate days. Mental changes may occur secondary to steroids or from the disease itself. Should this occur in a patient already on steroids one may increase the dose of steroids greatly; failure to help the patient will implicate the steroids. Patients with severe nephritis who fail to respond to adequate steroids after several months may benefit from the addition of immunosuppressive drugs. However, these agents are extremely toxic and should be administered only by a specialist.

Children with mild disease, such as those with predominantly arthritis, may require only aspirin or minimal doses of steroids. Topical steroid ointments help in treatment of the rash, as do the antimalarial drugs. Sunlight may exacerbate the rash or systemic manifestations; these patients should avoid the sun and apply a sun-screen preparation to protect the face and other exposed areas of the body. Children should avoid fatigue but should be encouraged

§ This dose exceeds that generally recommended for prednisone, but we believe it is warranted in this situation.

to lead reasonably active lives. All require careful follow-up, usually with the help of a specialist. Serial measurements of serum complement levels may provide a useful measure of disease control.

POLYARTERITIS AND HYPERSENSITIVITY ANGIITIS

It is difficult to distinguish true polyarteritis from hypersensitivity angiitis, both of which are rare in children. Marked cutaneous involvement suggests hypersensitivity angiitis, which is often caused by drugs, notably sulfonamides and penicillin. The toxic appearance of patients with either disorder reflects the variable and widespread organ involvement that results from diffuse vascular occlusion. Prompt treatment is vital and is best provided by a specialist who can render critical supportive care. High doses of steroids (prednisone, 1.0 to 2.0 mg. per kilogram daily§) may benefit some patients. Immunosuppressive drugs may be added, but this approach is still investigational. The prognosis is poor; surviving patients should avoid any implicating drugs.

HENOCH-SCHONLEIN (ANAPHYLACTOID) PURPURA

Unlike polyarteritis, this disease is usually benign and occurs primarily in children, chiefly boys. It is characterized by a distinctive rash (erythematous papules followed by purpura), abdominal pain and joint symptoms. Renal disease occurs frequently, but other organ involvement is unusual. Generally, the disease subsides within a few weeks, but occasionally serious sequelae may emerge.

Most patients need only supportive care, such as aspirin for arthritis. If the illness seems related to a particular food, drug or allergen, these should be avoided. All children should be carefully monitored for serious complications. Rare gastrointestinal complications include hemorrhage, intussusception and perforation. These may require surgical intervention, but bleeding usually subsides promptly in response to a brief course of steroids (prednisone, 0.5 to 1 mg. per kilogram daily§). Steroids are also indicated for central nervous system manifestations and for acute renal failure. If chronic renal disease develops, steroids and even the experimental immunosuppressive drugs may be tried, but their efficacy in this situation is uncertain.

§ This dose exceeds that generally recommended for prednisone, but we believe it is warranted in this situation.

DERMATOMYOSITIS (POLYMYOSITIS)

The insidious onset of progressive muscle weakness in a child may go unnoticed until fever, rash or muscle pain prompts medical attention. The single most useful diagnostic aid is assessment of the serum muscle enzymes. Prompt treatment with corticosteroids has undoubtedly contributed to the currently improved prognosis.

Management consists of the use of systemic corticosteroids, general supportive care and individualized physical therapy. The initial dose of prednisone is 1 to 2 mg. per kilogram per day administered in four divided doses.|| After four weeks this amount can usually be reduced by one-half, depending on clinical improvement and reversal of serum enzyme abnormalities. At eight weeks the steroid dosage may be reduced further at a rate averaging 1 mg. every one to two weeks until a maintenance level is achieved that permits both clinical and serum enzyme control. If palatorespiratory muscles are affected, great care is needed to prevent aspiration and to ensure adequate respiration. A program aimed at preventing deformity and increasing muscle strength should be initiated early.

PROGRESSIVE SYSTEMIC SCLEROSIS (SCLERODERMA)

Progressive systemic sclerosis is rare in children. Localized scleroderma (morphea) occurs more frequently but can occasionally progress to the systemic form.

Therapy is primarily supportive. One may use corticosteroid ointments or injections for patches of morphea, vasoactive drugs and protection from the cold for Raynaud's phenomenon, and physical therapy for the prevention and correction of contractures. Arthritis responds to aspirin in amounts similar to those used in rheumatoid arthritis. Esophagitis secondary to gastric reflux may be managed by elevating the head of the bed and by the use of antacids. Malabsorption syndrome secondary to decreased gastrointestinal motility may improve with tetracycline,** 125 mg. three times daily, given for one month. Corticosteroids may be used for serious extracutaneous manifesta-

|| This dose exceeds that generally recommended for prednisone, but we believe it is warranted in this situation.

** Manufacturer's note: The use of tetracyclines during tooth development (last half of pregnancy, infancy and childhood to age eight years) may cause permanent discoloration of teeth. This adverse reaction is more common during long-term use of the drugs but has been observed following repeated short-term courses.

tions, but only under the close supervision of a specialist.

References

Calabro, J. J., and Marchesano, J. M.: Fever Associated with Juvenile Rheumatoid Arthritis. *New England J. Med.*, 276:11, 1967.

Calabro, J. J.: Management of Juvenile Rheumatoid Arthritis. *J. Pediat.*, 77:355, 1970.

Calabro, J. J., Parrino, G. R., Atchoo, P. D., Marchesano, J. M., and Goldberg, L. S.: Chronic Iridocyclitis in Juvenile Rheumatoid Arthritis. *Arthritis Rheum.*, 13:406, 1970.

Hanson, V., and Kornrich, H.: Systemic Rheumatic Disorders ("Collagen Disease") in Childhood: Lupus Erythematosus, Anaphylactoid Purpura, Dermatomyositis, and Scleroderma. *Bull. Rheum. Dis.*, 17: 435, 441 (Parts I and II), 1967.

Sullivan, D. B., Cassidy, J. T., Petty, R. E., and Burt, A.: Prognosis in Childhood Dermatomyositis. *J. Pediat.*, 80:555, 1972.

13

Genitourinary Tract

Cystic Disease of the Kidney

GUNNAR B. STICKLER, M.D., *and*
PANAYOTIS P. KELALIS, M.D.

Because morphologic classifications of cystic disease of the kidney lack uniformity, it seems appropriate here to consider cystic disease of the kidney in terms of clinical and genetic entities. Cystic renal disease may be a part of several syndromes, such as Zellweger's syndrome (cerebrohepatorenal syndrome), Meckel's syndrome (dysencephalia splanchocystica), Ivemark's familial dysplasia, tuberous sclerosis, von Hippel–Lindau's disease and the trisomy syndromes D (13, 14 and 15), E (16, 17 and 18) and G (21). With the trisomy syndromes, often gross structural defects, such as horseshoe kidneys and larger renal cysts or cystic dysplasias, are found.

Simple cysts of the kidney are uncommon in children. Specific symptoms are unusual, though occasionally there may be gastrointestinal complaints. Diagnosis of the cyst may be made by the discovery of a renal mass during routine physical examination or by roentgenographic studies made for another purpose. Intravenous nephrotomography has led to a more accurate diagnosis. Simple cysts should be excised because they tend to enlarge as the child grows older.

Multilocular cysts of the kidney, though usually large and loculated, are difficult to distinguish from simple cysts urographically; they do not require any different therapy.

Pyelogenic cysts generally form from a small cystic enlargement communicating with the calyceal system. Lack of free communication between the cyst and the calyx may result in infection and stone formation. Excision of the cyst, usually by partial nephrectomy, is indicated only if the cyst is responsible for recurrent pain, stone formation or infection.

Multicystic dysplasia of the kidney is a congenital cystic degeneration with persistence of primitive renal elements. The lesion is almost always unilateral. The kidney may be small or be so enlarged as to fill the whole flank. An important sign is the inability to obtain a retrograde pyelogram; the ureter or the pelvis, or both, are atretic or obliterated. Since this type of cyst tends to enlarge early, nephrectomy is necessary. It is essential that bilateral disease be excluded.

Polycystic disease occurs in an infantile and an adult form. In infants it usually is inherited as an autosomal recessive disorder. It was once reported to be fatal in the neonatal period, but such reports were based on autopsy series. Many patients have been known to survive beyond infancy. Usually both kidneys are massively enlarged. This form of polycystic disease is associated also with enlargement of the liver lesions, such as cystic proliferation or dilation of the bile ducts and marked portal fibrosis. Most of the patients are admitted in infancy, the precipitating factor being respiratory distress due to compression of thoracic viscera by the enlargement of liver and kidney, atelectasis, congestive heart failure or pneumonia. An excretory urogram and renal biopsy (open rather than percutaneous) confirm the diagnosis.

Treatment consists first in correction of respiratory distress with oxygen and, if necessary, other respiratory aids, such as intubation and continuous positive airway pressure (CPAP) breathing. Congestive failure is treated promptly with digitalis and diuretics (see p. 136), and pneumonia should be treated with appropriate antibiotics. After the age of one month, hypertension may be the major complication of this disease and this will require specific treatment (see pp. 151 and 387).

If renal insufficiency progresses, renal transplantation may be considered. The liver involvement may cause portal hypertension, with esophageal varices and splenomegaly; portacaval shunt then is indicated.

Lieberman and associates (1971) have suggested that patients with *congenital fibrosis of the liver* differ from those with the infantile form of polycystic disease. It is true that most of these patients with congenital fibrosis of the liver have cystic or polycystic renal changes. These children, however, usually have no renal functional impairment and only occasionally do they require treatment for hypertension or renal failure.

More important in these cases of congenital fibrosis of the liver is the need to treat portal hypertension, which may cause bleeding from esophageal varices or symptoms of hypersplenism, such as leukopenia and thrombocytopenia. Portacaval shunt is the preferred management.

Children with the so-called adult form of polycystic disease most often come to the pediatrician's attention during a pedigree study of a parent in whom this disease has been identified. The disease is transmitted as an autosomal dominant trait and the children are asymptomatic. The diagnosis is made by excretory urography. No treatment is necessary during childhood and early adult life, but transplantation may later be required in cases of renal failure. The pediatrician must give appropriate genetic counseling, because 50 per cent of the offspring of an affected person also become affected.

Medullary cystic disease or *juvenile nephronophthisis,* in its azotemic form, is rare. It is transmitted as an autosomal recessive. It is manifested by early onset of polydipsia and polyuria, anemia, impaired renal function and renal osteodystrophy with growth failure. The clinical diagnosis is confirmed by renal biopsy. It is usually fatal in the early teens. Renal osteodystrophy requires early treatment with the appropriate doses of vitamin D (see p. 7), and if renal failure progresses, renal transplantation becomes necessary.

Reference

Lieberman, E., et al.: Infantile Polycystic Disease of the Kidneys and Liver: Clinical, Pathological and Radiological Correlations and Comparison With Congenital Hepatic Fibrosis. *Medicine,* 50:277, 1971.

Hydronephrosis and Disorders of the Ureter

PANAYOTIS P. KELALIS, M.D., *and*
GUNNAR B. STICKLER, M.D.

Aberrations in the development of the kidney and ureter and obstruction to the flow of urine constitute the vast majority of disorders of the kidney and ureter in children. Often, many different parts of the urinary tract may be affected.

The ureteropelvic junction is the most common site of primary ureteral obstruction. Obstruction usually is the result of intrinsic stenosis in an aperistaltic segment of ureter, but other causes of obstruction include high insertion of the ureter into the pelvis, formation of periureteric adhesions with kinking and aberrant position of renal vessels. Vesicoureteral reflux often may simulate apparent ureteropelvic obstruction, and this should be excluded from the differential diagnosis. Unless the entire ureter is satisfactorily visualized in an excretory urogram, a retrograde ureterogram is necessary; it can be done as a preliminary to surgical exploration after induction of anesthesia for the scheduled operation, in order to minimize the calculated risk of iatrogenic infection.

The aim of surgery is to achieve a dependent, funnel-shaped ureteropelvic junction of good caliber. The surgical approach is extraperitoneal, through a flank incision. If renal function virtually has been destroyed, and if the thin parenchyma collapses upon release of the obstruction, nephrectomy is necessary. If, in cases of ureteropelvic obstruction, urography has shown that the kidneys are functionless and the cortex is relatively normal, a reparative procedure is indicated because function is likely to return. Before the correction of the obstruction, the renal pelvis is distended by injecting saline. This stimulates peristalsis and helps the surgeon to define the stenotic segment of ureter in which peristalsis is either erratic or absent.

Ureteropyelostomy is the most versatile operation, but Foley Y-V-plasty and spiral flap operations sometimes are performed. In ureteropyelostomy the narrowed segment of ureter is excised. Obstruction in other parts of the ureter or at the ureterovesical angle is excluded by calibration of the ureter with Braasch bulbs. Next, the ureter is spatulated for 0.5 to 1 cm. and anastomosed to the obliquely cut pelvis with 5–0 interrupted chromic catgut. For the primary repair, no vents, stents or nephrostomy tubes are used; the anastomotic site is merely drained. In some cases the narrow segment of ureter is too long to allow its excision and subsequent ureteropyelostomy without tension; pyeloplasty (using the Y-V Foley principle or a spiral flap) then is indicated. The pelvic flap of tissue is rotated downward and anastomosed to the edges of the incised narrow ureteral segment, thus increasing its caliber. When the stenosed segments of ureter are longer, pyeloplasty combined with a Davis intubated ureterotomy is indicated. A ureteral stent (size 10 French or larger) is brought through the lower pole of the kidney, together with a nephrostomy tube, to the outside. The stent and the nephrostomy tube usually are left indwelling for three weeks.

Frequently an aberrant vessel is intimately related to the ureteropelvic junction. This, however, rarely is the sole cause of obstruction, and it almost always is associated with intrinsic stenosis of the ureter. In these cases, the pathologic segment of the ureter is excised, the ureter is transposed anteriorly to the vessel and a ureteropyelostomy is performed. The vessel is left undisturbed.

A localized stricture of the ureter at any other level is excised, and ureteroureterostomy is performed by spatulating the cut ends of the ureter in opposite directions; stents are not used. If the disparity in caliber between the proximal dilated segment and the normal distal segment of ureter is great, a Z-plasty type of anastomosis is necessary. Multiple strictures of the ureter are incised and an intubated ureterotomy is performed.

Patients who have functional or anatomic strictures of the intramural ureter without reflux—unless associated with progressive hydroureteronephrosis, deteriorating renal function or infection—are followed closely. Both the dilatation and tortuosity of the ureter may lessen with growth and the hydronephrosis may regress. Surgical correction necessitates excision of the narrowed segment of ureter, ureteroneocystostomy and, when the diameter of the ureter is greater than 1 cm., simultaneous reduction of its caliber. For massively dilated and tortuous ureters, with or without reflux, dissection of the ureter all the way to the renal pelvis is necessary, with careful preservation of the blood supply. Once the ureter is straightened, the redundant portion is resected and the caliber of the distal ureter is reduced, commensurate with the age of the patient. Such reduction will then permit satisfactory antireflux surgery. When the renal function is decreased or when there is unrelenting infection, preliminary diversion of urine via cutaneous pyelostomy or loop ureterostomy is required.

A ureter which opens outside the posterolateral extremity of the trigone is ectopic. It is frequently associated with ureteral duplication. The ureter associated with the lower segment is likely to reflux, whereas the one leading to the upper segment may become ectopic or develop a ureterocele. In girls, when the ectopic ureter opens at the vesical neck or proximal urethra, continence will be preserved but there may be reflux on voiding. The associated kidney segment almost always is affected by pyelonephritic atrophy or even dysplastic changes, and therefore heminephrectomy and subtotal ureterectomy is the operation of choice. The ureter is not removed in its entirety because of the likelihood of compromising the blood supply of the ipsilateral ureter to the lower segment. If reflux is associated with the ectopic ureteral stump, this then acts as a urethral diverticulum, perpetuating urinary infection; in such instances excision of the stump is undertaken four to six months later. In boys, the ectopic ureter always drains proximal to the external sphincter in the prostatic urethra or seminal vesicle. Nephrectomy (or heminephrectomy if complete ureteral duplication is present) with total ureterectomy is essential. Urinary incontinence in such patients is caused by associated sphincteric deficiency and should diminish with age. When the ectopic ureter drains outside the sphincteric mechanism in the vestibule or distal urethra in girls, voiding is normal but urinary incontinence is also taking place.

The ectopic ureteral orifice in the periurethral area may be identified with the aid of an intravenous injection of indigo carmine. The associated renal segment may be normal, and therefore reimplantation of the ectopic ureter into the bladder is justifiable. Often, however, the segment may show dysplastic changes; heminephrectomy or nephrectomy then is the best treatment.

Ureterocele in most cases also is associated with complete ureteral duplication. This may be intravesical or ectopic. The former, if small, may be left undisturbed; otherwise, the ureterocele is excised, followed by meatoplasty and ureteral reimplantation of the associated ureter. Ectopic ureteroceles are treated according to the same surgical principles as the ectopic ureter without ureterocele.

Paraureteral diverticula often distort the

ureterovesical angle during filling of the bladder, thereby producing incompetence leading to vesicoureteral reflux. Occasionally they may cause obstruction to the ureter. Their size varies. If small, they are left undisturbed since they usually diminish with age. Otherwise, excision through a transvesical approach and concomitant ureteroneocystostomy are done.

A multicystic kidney is seldom drained by an intact ureter; and since the kidney is functionless and tends to enlarge, best treatment is early nephrectomy. Appropriate studies are necessary to exclude disease in the opposite kidney, the incidence of which is quite high.

Anomalies of shape (horseshoe kidney) or position (pelvic kidney, or crossed renal ectopia with or without fusion) themselves need no treatment. Treatment, however, is necessary if there are associated disorders such as hydronephrosis. In horseshoe kidneys, hydronephrosis may be the result of obstruction or dysfunction at the ureteropelvic junction, and its surgical revision combined with symphysiotomy may be indicated. Frequently such changes are more apparent than real and may be the result of vesicoureteral reflux whose incidence in horseshoe kidney is high. In such instances, primary surgical treatment must be directed to the ureterovesical junction, even though both conditions may coexist.

The pelvic kidney frequently is pathologic or, despite its normal appearance, responsible for pain; nephrectomy then may be justified. In more than 50 per cent of such cases the normally placed kidney also is abnormal or it may even be absent; thorough preoperative investigation therefore is mandatory.

Malignant Tumors of the Kidney

PANAYOTIS P. KELALIS, M.D., *and*
GUNNAR B. STICKLER, M.D.

Primary malignant tumors of the kidney in children are nearly always Wilms' tumors; adenocarcinoma (hypernephroma) and malignancies of the renal capsule are exceedingly rare. Malignant tumors of the retroperitoneum arising from the adrenal or sympathetic chain (perirenal neuroblastoma) also may involve the kidney intimately. In such instances, nephrectomy may be necessary to achieve removal of the intact tumor.

For adenocarcinoma of the kidney (hypernephroma), radical nephrectomy suffices. For Wilms' tumors, radical surgical removal is but one facet of the treatment, and irradiation and oncolytic agents, in various combinations, are necessary.

The discovery of Wilms' tumor is not considered a surgical emergency, but all diagnostic studies are performed promptly. In addition to the routine hematologic studies–which include white cell and platelet counts—serum glutamic oxaloacetic transaminase (SGOT) and alkaline phosphatase are measured to serve as a base line for future comparison of liver function. Roentgenograms of the chest and the complete skeletal survey are done; if metastases to the bone are found, marrow aspiration is necessary to assess tumor infiltration. Urinary excretion of the catecholamines (vanillylmandelic acid and homovanillic acid) is measured in every patient having an abdominal tumor; increased excretion suggests that the tumor is a neuroblastoma. Liver scanning also is advisable, but this is not absolutely necessary prior to primary surgical treatment.

Urograms are indicated in all cases. For small tumors no further radiologic studies are necessary. Larger functionless renal masses are the result of obstruction and rarely tumor; a retrograde pyelogram will settle the issue. For larger tumors, which may involve many contiguous structures, retrograde aortography and selective renal arteriography are indicated, and an inferior venacavogram is also desirable. The last can be done as a preliminary to the excretory urogram.

If these preoperative studies reveal involvement of the great vessels, complete surgical removal is unlikely. Therefore, irradiation (dose, 800 to 1250 r) over a period of six to nine days is preferred before surgical excision. Expected tumor shrinkage after two to three weeks should make subsequent surgical exploration easier.

Removal of Wilms' tumor presents special considerations in anesthetic management in relation to blood loss, occlusion of the inferior vena cava during the operation, opening of the pleural cavity and maintenance of normal body temperature. For blood replacement, one needle is placed in an arm vein so that transfusion is not impeded by a partially or completely occluded inferior vena cava, and a second is placed in the external jugular vein as a supplemental route for blood replacement and for monitoring central venous pressure. If the pleural cavity needs to be opened during the operation, use of controlled ventilation will prevent any problems associated with open pneumothorax. To prevent hypothermia, use of a warming mattress, transfusion of warm blood and temperature monitoring are essential.

A transabdominal transperitoneal incision, with a thoracic extension if necessary, is used. The abdominal contents are examined carefully. A biopsy is made of any suspicious lesions, and if tumor is diagnosed the areas are marked with metallic vascular clips. The opposite kidney is examined adequately to rule out bilateral involvement. Palpation usually suffices, but if there is any doubt about involvement of the other kidney, visual inspection is necessary. The lateral peritoneal reflection is opened and the colon reflected medially. Before the tumor is mobilized, the renal vessels are exposed and ligated; this, however, may not be possible or even safely undertaken. The renal vein is palpated to exclude extension of the tumor to the vein; should extension be evident, the vein is opened and the tumor removed, preferably prior to ligation. Rupture of the tumor is avoided by establishing a plane of cleavage outside Gerota's fascia, thus allowing removal of the kidney and tumor with all its investing tissues. All perforating vessels are ligated individually, and a biopsy of their distal ends is made for evidence of tumor spread. A radical periaortic node dissection is included. When the tumor arises in the upper pole, the adrenal gland should be removed with the neoplasm. Any surrounding structures, such as the spleen, colon, tail of the pancreas, diaphragm or psoas muscle, which are involved are resected in continuity. Such radical dissection is indicated only if in this way all tumor tissue can be completely removed. If residual tumor tissue must be left behind, it is subjected to biopsy and marked with silver clips.

In infants, nephrectomy and careful follow-up usually suffice. Tumors in infants are probably variants of Wilms' tumor containing fibromatous elements with little malignant potential. Beyond this age, radiotherapy and chemotherapy with dactinomycin and vincristine* are used as adjuvants to the surgical extirpation of the tumor.

In cases of tumors that have not penetrated the renal capsule and do not involve the renal vein—and therefore are completely resectable—the treatment is dactinomycin and irradiation to the renal bed. If the tumor has penetrated the capsule or has involved the renal vessels or para-aortic nodes, irradiation treatment and both oncolytic agents are preferred, irrespective of the completeness of the surgical treatment. If distant metastases are present initially, oncolytic drugs (vincristine* or dactinomycin) in combination with radiotherapy are given to assess the response of the tumor to therapy. If the metastases regress, the primary tumor is removed and all modalities of treatment are continued. For bilateral tumors, a combination of nephrectomy on one side with partial nephrectomy on the other may be possible. Even renal transplantation in such a situation has been reported.

Irradiation, using a high-energy source, is started within 48 hours of surgical exploration. The frequency of treatment is five to six days a week, the weekly dose is 1000 to 1200 r and the route is through opposing anteroposterior portals. As to the total dose, for infants and children up to 18 months of age it is 1800 to 2400 r; for children between 1½ and 2½ years of age it is 2400 to 3000 r, and for older children it is 3000 to 4000 r. The field includes the entire area of kidney and tumor and it extends across the midline to include all the vertebral bodies in such a way that scoliosis may be prevented but the opposite kidney remains unaffected.

Dactinomycin is given first in the operating room once the diagnosis has been visually confirmed (biopsy is contraindicated) and prior to any manipulation of the tumor mass. It is injected intravenously, the dosage being 15 micrograms per kilogram to a maximum of 500 micrograms. After operation, dactinomycin is given daily in the same manner for a total of five days; and the treatment is repeated at six weeks, and at 3, 6, 9, 12 and 15 months thereafter. Vincristine also is injected intravenously; the dosage is 1.5 mg. per square meter, but a single dose must not exceed 2 mg. Vincristine is given weekly for six doses after operation, then in single doses at three-month intervals up to and including 15 months. Because of possible drug toxicity, careful supervision is necessary, and it may be necessary to discontinue the treatment program or decrease the dose if toxic reactions occur.†

The combination of dactinomycin and vincristine increases the hazards of toxicity. Dactinomycin may cause reactions of the alimentary tract, including stomatitis, ulceration of the mouth and vomiting; hematopoietic depression evidenced as thrombocytopenia or leukopenia; and accelerated cutaneous radiation reaction or alopecia. Frequent leukocyte and

* Manufacturer's precaution: Vincristine sulfate is recommended only for treatment of acute leukemia in childhood.

† Manufacturer's precaution: Vincristine is recommended only for treatment of acute leukemia in childhood.

platelet counts are necessary before each administration of the drug. Granulocyte counts of less than 1500 per cubic mm. or platelet counts of less than 100,000 per cubic mm. are indications for cessation of treatment with dactinomycin.

Vincristine toxicity includes muscular weakness, hyporeflexia and neuropathy (recovery from which may be slow); constipation, which may be severe, suggesting intestinal obstruction or paralytic ileus; depression of all hematopoietic elements; and, commonly, alopecia.

All children are seen frequently for periodic evaluation, since oncolytic agents may at times delay the appearance of metastases. For the first two years, a physical examination is done every three months; and thereafter, for the next three years, physical examination is given every six months. A chest roentgenogram is taken at three-month intervals for the first two years, and then repeated yearly for three more years. Skeletal roentgenograms of irradiated parts every two to three years indefinitely are necessary. Urographic examination of the kidney on a yearly basis for five years and a liver scan at six-month intervals also are recommended.

If pulmonary metastases develop, both lungs are treated by irradiation (1400 r) and by oncolytic agents irrespective of the number and location of metastases. Solitary persisting metastases are excised. Only those liver metastases that are not surgically removable should be irradiated; the dose of radiation ranges, according to volume, from 500 to 3000 r. Metastases of the brain, bone, lymph nodes and other parts are irradiated using doses comparable to those delivered to the liver.

Glomerulonephritis

WALLACE W. McCRORY, M.D., *and*
MADOKA SHIBUYA, M.D.

The clinical manifestations of glomerulonephritis are as varied as the diverse group of conditions that can be associated with glomerular disease. Acute glomerulonephritis is most commonly poststreptococcal but can be associated with anaphylactoid purpura, viral infections (ECHO, mumps), hemolytic-uremic syndrome, lupus erythematosus, polyarteritis, drug reactions and so forth. Until we have a complete understanding of the pathogenetic mechanisms causing this disease, no specific therapy can be developed. Therapy is directed at management of those pathophysiologic problems that arise as consequences of disturbances in renal function caused by the primary disease process. The aim of treatment is to carry the patient through the acute episode into the period of convalescence. With the availability of techniques for peritoneal dialysis and hemodialysis, death in the acute stage should now be avoidable in most instances even in the presence of rapidly progressive nephritis with massive irreversible glomerular damage. This section is concerned only with problems encountered in patients presenting with signs of sudden onset of glomerulonephritis.

EDEMA

When edema of mild to moderate degree is present, salt intake should be limited to 1 Gm. per square meter of surface area per day. If edema is severe or is progressive in spite of restriction of salt intake, diuretic therapy should be initiated. In the absence of acute renal failure (oliguria or anuria), fluid intake (nonsodium-containing) is generally not restricted, especially when a diuretic is used. Although the manufacturer does not recommend its use in children because of current limited experience, furosemide (Lasix), 1 to 2 mg. per kilogram intravenously or 2 to 4 mg. per kilogram orally per day, can be effective (Repetto et al.). Other diuretics (thiazides and so forth) are usually ineffective. Since profound sodium and potassium diuresis may result, careful monitoring of fluid and electrolyte intake and blood and urine chemistry values are needed to guide therapy. Edema is usually a manifestation of other problems, especially hypoproteinemia, azotemia, acute renal failure and/or cardiac failure, and its relief may require correction of the underlying primary problem. A trial of diuretics can be employed in the presence of oliguria but not when there is anuria.

HYPERTENSION

In patients seven years of age or less, hypertension is present when several consecutive diastolic pressure readings of 90 mm. Hg or above are obtained. In patients over seven years of age, the critical value is 100 mm. Hg. In cases in which this is the only abnormal finding, bed rest, salt restriction and sedation with phenobarbital in a single oral dose of 1 to 5 mg. per kilogram will usually suffice. More vigorous antihypertensive therapy is indicated in the presence of rising blood pressure or when hypertension is associated with signs of encephalopathy or cardiac failure.

Antihypertensive therapy in acute nephritis involves three components: control of sodium balance. avoidance of or reduction of hypervolemia, and use of specific antihypertensive drugs. Sodium intake should be limited to 1 Gm. of salt per square meter of surface area per day as long as hypertension is present.

Hypervolemia may be associated with hypertension in acute nephritis. Its presence contributes to the development of cardiac failure. Treatment with a natriuretic (furosemide) is helpful if adequate renal function is present (as described under the section on edema). If anuria (acute renal failure) is present with cardiac failure, hypervolemia and hypertension, removal of extracellular fluid by peritoneal dialysis or hemodialysis should be employed. Rarely, phlebotomy has been used with benefit.

The choice of antihypertensive drugs is still largely a matter of individual experience. The combination of hydralazine (Apresoline), 0.1 to 0.15 mg. per kilogram, and reserpine (Serpasil), at an initial dose of 0.07 mg. per kilogram, administered intramuscularly is usually effective. Hydralazine can be repeated in 6 to 8 hours as needed. Reserpinization is usually accomplished by the initial dose. Reserpine in large dosage causes marked somnolence. When its use is without effect in 6 to 8 hours, repeated administration is unlikely to improve the situation. Its hypotensive effects can be maintained for as long as desired when administered at 12- to 24-hour intervals at one-third to one-half the initial dose.

For hypertensive crisis unresponsive to combined hydralazine and reserpine therapy, alpha-methyldopa (Aldomet), administered intravenously in a dose of 4 to 15 mg. per kilogram during a 5- to 10-minute period, may be effective. This dose may be repeated at 6-hour intervals when the desired effect is obtained; conversion to oral therapy at a dose of 6 to 25 mg. per kilogram every 6 to 8 hours may be desirable to maintain long-term effects. Aldomet is largely excreted by the kidney. Untoward effects may include mild sedation during the first 48 hours of therapy, dry mouth, edema, weight gain, drug fever, abnormal liver function tests, dizziness, arthralgia, psychic depression, toxic encephalopathy, parkinsonism and reversible reduction of the white blood cell count.

Guanethidine (Ismelin) may be helpful in patients with severe hypertension unresponsive to the above therapy. The usual starting oral dose is 10 mg. daily. Guanethidine is administered once a day. If necessary, the dose may be increased every four to five days. The effective daily dosage varies from 10 to 100 mg. Side effects include dizziness, weakness and syncope resulting from postural or exertional hypotension, bradycardia, diarrhea, rise in blood urea nitrogen and fluid retention and edema.

We have occasionally employed diazoxide (Hyperstat). This drug has been approved by the Food and Drug Administration, but its safety in children has not been established. Intravenous diazoxide results in rapid, effective lowering of both systolic and diastolic blood pressure. It is to be used only when satisfactory control has not been obtained by the measures mentioned previously. It should be considered only when the patient's condition at the time justifies a rapid lowering of the blood pressure to more normal levels. Diazoxide works by a relaxing effect on peripheral arteriolar smooth muscle with consequent decrease in peripheral resistance, and is excreted in the urine. The dose varies between 2 to 10 mg. per kilogram, usually 5 mg. per kilogram, and is given as a single intravenous bolus as rapidly as possible (10 seconds) (McLaine and Drummond). If no effect is observed, either the dose was inadequate or the rate of intravenous administration was too slow. The maximum response is seen 10 minutes after administration. During administration, vital signs must be carefully monitored. Side effects include lowering of the diastolic blood pressure to zero without signs of reduced cerebral blood flow, transient hyperglycemia, hypertrichosis, burning sensation at the site of injection, vague gastrointestinal upsets, edema and hyponatremia, transient hyperuricemia, cardiac arrhythmia and orthostatic hypotension. No refractoriness has been noted on repeated use. In most cases, after one or two doses of diazoxide, the usual antihypertensive drugs can then be used effectively.

RENAL FAILURE

Various derangements of fluid and electrolyte balance may arise secondary to impairment of renal function. The severity of each problem (azotemia, oliguria, anuria with uremia, hyperkalemia, hyperphosphatemia, hypocalcemia, cardiac failure and/or hypertensive or metabolic encephalopathy) may vary from mild, requiring only careful observation with dietary restrictions, to severe, necessitating specific intervention (Dobrin et al.). Oral intake, urine output, weight and blood pressure should be recorded daily in all cases to stay abreast of the clinical course of the patient's disease in the acute stage.

The most serious complications associated with acute renal failure include anuria, cardiac failure, edema, hyperkalemia and hypertensive or metabolic encephalopathy. Anuria is always preceded by some period of oliguria (urine volume less than 350 ml. per square meter per day when fluid intake has been normal). Recognition of its occurrence can alert the physician to the likelihood of impending complete renal failure and allow appropriate prophylactic measures (e.g., diet restriction) to be instituted before anuria develops. Infusion of hypertonic mannitol at the onset of oliguria may be considered if the possibility of reversible functional renal failure secondary to fluid and electrolyte depletion (prerenal azotemia) cannot be excluded. Mannitol, once filtered, cannot be reabsorbed by the renal tubular epithelium, and it increases urine flow in proportion to its concentration in the glomerular filtrate. If filtration is adequate, an osmotic diuresis can thus be produced. The recommended test dose of mannitol is 0.5 Gm. per kilogram of a 20 per cent aqueous solution infused intravenously during a 3- to 5-minute interval. The patient must be adequately hydrated before injection of mannitol. One repeat dose may be indicated if it is observed that for each 0.5 Gm. of mannitol administered there is an increase in urine flow of 6 to 10 ml. in the ensuing 1 to 4 hours. (Note: The use of mannitol in pediatric patients has not yet been studied comprehensively, but this schedule has been effective in our experience.)

Once renal failure is present, overhydration with resultant hypervolemia must be avoided. However, if the history of decreased urinary output is not associated with physical signs of overhydration, and if there is a history of vomiting or an unknown fluid intake, a normal fluid intake should be provided for the initial 12 to 24 hours with observation of its effect on weight, output and electrolytes in order to ensure that dehydration (prerenal azotemia) is not a factor contributing to oliguria. Thereafter, with evidence of oliguria, total fluid intake should be restricted to an amount sufficient to prevent weight gain and to cover existing nonrenal losses of water (about 350 ml. per square meter per day) plus measured urine output in the preceding 24 hours. Water resulting from oxidation of ingested food or from body fat, carbohydrate and protein can be estimated to be 100 ml. per square meter per day in the average patient. The aim of treatment is to stabilize the patient's condition, avoid weight gain and anticipate return of improved renal function.

Daily determination of the patient's weight, recording intake and output and serial measurements of serum and urine electrolyte concentrations are necessary for proper management. Serious degrees of acidosis should be partially corrected with lactate or bicarbonate solutions. The minimal basal caloric need for the patient's age should be estimated and an attempt made to provide it daily in the form of carbohydrate and fat to limit endogenous catabolism which contributes to azotemia and hyperkalemia.

When hyperkalemia (serum potassium of 6.5 mEq. or more per liter) exists, further potassium administration by any route must be avoided. An effective measure for reducing serum potassium levels is the administration of cation-exchange resin, sodium polystyrene sulfonate (Kayexalate). A dose of 1 Gm. per kilogram lowers serum potassium concentration approximately 1 mEq. per liter. The desired amount of resin can be administered rectally or orally as a 20 to 30 per cent suspension. The desired therapeutic effect when the rectal route is used is usually evident in 1 to 3 hours. If needed, a repeat dose of resin may be administered 6 to 12 hours later, after redetermination of the serum potassium concentration. When the serum potassium level falls below 4 mEq. per liter, resin should no longer be administered. Serum calcium concentration must be checked for hypocalcemia if cation exchange resin is used for more than three days.

If this is ineffective and serum potassium continues to rise, other forms of treatment of hyperkalemia include infusion of calcium gluconate (100 to 200 mg. per kilogram), insulin and glucose (1 unit of insulin to 3 Gm. of glucose) or hypertonic sodium lactate or bicarbonate solutions (3 mEq. per kilogram). These procedures result in only transitory relief. Persistent hyperkalemia refractory to treatment outlined above is a clear indication for hemodialysis or peritoneal dialysis.

Patients with hypocalcemia should receive calcium gluconate at a dose of 4 to 8 Gm. per day by mouth or smaller amounts intravenously. Efforts to raise the serum calcium level in the presence of hyperphosphatemia will be ineffective unless the hyperphosphatemia can also be corrected. Aluminum hydroxide gel in a dose of 1 to 2 tablespoons orally three to four times a day is effective in reducing phosphate absorption from the intestinal tract, and this will facilitate lowering of the serum phosphorus concentration. Temporary restriction or elimination of milk and other phosphate-rich foods from the diet is also indicated.

The onset of diuresis following a period of prolonged oliguria or anuria may be accompanied by transitory excessive renal loss of water and/or electrolytes. Careful monitoring of fluid and electrolyte balance is essential during this recovery period.

ANEMIA

A mild normochromic normocytic anemia (hemoglobin 8 to 10 Gm. per 100 ml.) may be found in some cases. If anemia is more marked (hemoglobin less than 8 Gm. per 100 ml.), studies should be done to identify the cause. The presence of the hemolytic-uremic syndrome is suggested when there is a hemolytic anemia with red cell fragmentation, thrombocytopenia (100,000 platelets per cubic mm.) and uremia. When further diagnostic studies are indicated, they should be done prior to blood replacement therapy. Transfusions with buffy coat poor red blood cells or thawed frozen red blood cells are safest if the patient is a possible candidate for renal transplantation and the anemia requires correction. Although anemia does occur in association with uremia, it requires two to four weeks to develop after the onset of azotemia.

CARDIAC FAILURE

In glomerulonephritis, cardiac failure with pulmonary edema is usually associated with hypervolemia and hypertension. Therapy for these has been mentioned. The treatment of cardiac failure requires oxygen, sedation with opiates and digitalis. Digitalis may be a difficult drug to use in patients with acute nephritis and renal failure, since changing serum potassium levels may modify considerably the response to digitalis. The maintenance doses must also be reduced below those employed in patients without the complication of renal failure.

LETHARGY AND CONVULSIONS

Lethargy may be secondary to azotemia and an early sign of encephalopathy. Convulsions may occur in association with hypocalcemia and hyperphosphatemia, hypertension and/or uremia. Immediate therapy for convulsions always requires provision of an adequate airway and adequate oxygenation. We have found three anticonvulsant drugs to be of value in achieving immediate control of seizures: Phenobarbital administered intramuscularly at dose of 3 to 5 mg. per kilogram per dose as needed; diazepam (Valium)* given intravenously at a very slow rate in a dose of 0.05 to 0.1 mg. per kilogram per minute (6 to 10 mg. per square meter per minute; and diphenylhydantoin sodium (Dilantin) given intravenously in a dose of 10 to 20 mg. per kilogram. The normal daily maintenance dose of Dilantin is 3 to 8 mg. per kilogram per day. It must be remembered that all anticonvulsant drugs when given intravenously at too rapid a rate may result in respiratory arrest. When renal failure is present, repeated administration of drugs removed by renal excretion should be avoided. Maintenance anticonvulsant therapy is usually essential. In patients with convulsions and severe uremia (BUN greater than 100 mg. per 100 ml.) with renal failure, dialysis may result in an improved sensorium and relief of seizures.

* Manufacturer's precaution: Safety and efficacy of injectable diazepam (Valium) in children under 12 years of age have not been established.

NAUSEA AND VOMITING

Nausea and vomiting are uncommon in glomerulonephritis, but may contribute to oliguria and become sufficiently severe to require intravenous replacement fluid therapy. Careful daily monitoring of body weight and serum electrolyte values (Na^+, K^+, CO_2, Cl^-) and BUN or creatinine is essential during intravenous therapy in patients with vomiting and renal failure. Gastrointestinal disorders are likely to be present when nephritis is associated with the hemolytic-uremic syndrome or anaphylactoid purpura or complicated by cardiac failure and hypertensive or metabolic encephalopathy.

PROTEIN INTAKE

No dietary restriction need be imposed on patients with acute glomerulonephritis who show no or only mild evidence of impaired renal function. The amount of protein in the diet should be restricted to (0.5 to 1.0 Gm. protein per kilogram per day or less) only in patients with persistent azotemia (BUN greater than 60 mg. per 100 ml. or creatinine greater than 2.5 per 100 ml.).

RASH

Rashes seen in association with acute nephritis do not pose a therapeutic problem except for impetigo (pyoderma), which requires specific antibiotic therapy. Their presence may be helpful in reaching an etiologic diagnosis. History of generalized erythematous rash followed by peeling, especially of the hands and fingers, is suggestive of a preceding beta-hemolytic streptococcal infection. A facial butterfly rash is diagnostic of systemic lupus erythematosus. A purpuric rash is seen in patients with anaphylactoid purpura or periarteritis nodosa; however, among patients with the latter diagnosis, subcutaneous pea-sized nodules are often palpable, which may be superficial and painless or red and tender. A fine, sometimes purpuric, morbilliform maculopapular erythematous exanthem of the face and upper trunk and especially the lower extremities is often seen with ECHO virus infections.

RESTRICTION OF PHYSICAL ACTIVITY

While bed rest is desirable in the early stage of acute nephritis, it is not indicated after gross hematuria, hypertension and edema are no longer evident. The convalescent patient can be reambulated slowly, provided the above signs do not recur. Return to normal physical activity is usually feasible within two months after the acute onset of nephritis.

IMMUNOSUPPRESSIVE THERAPY

The majority of cases of acute nephritis (over 90 per cent) recover from the acute stage without benefit of adrenocortical steroid therapy or use of cytotoxic agents, such as cyclophosphamide and azathioprine, or heparin therapy. Accordingly, the need for or value, if any, of the use of these agents in acute nephritis is yet to be demonstrated. In those instances when edema due to the nephrotic syndrome (hypoalbuminemia and significant proteinuria 1 Gm. per square meter per day) persists beyond the first two to three weeks of the disease, a trial of adrenocortical steroid therapy may be warranted. There is no clear-cut evidence that steroid therapy is of long-term value, and its use may be harmful. The experience of some nephrologists suggests that in rapidly progressive forms of acute glomerulonephritis associated with evidence of progressively decreasing renal function, combined treatment with adrenocortical steroids and azathioprine or cyclophosphamide may be of some value in arresting the progression of the disease. The opinion of a nephrologist should be sought before initiating such therapy. The use of heparin or other anticoagulant therapy has no demonstrated value in the treatment of children at this time, and its use can be harmful.

RENAL BIOPSY

A specific morphologic diagnosis is possible only by histopathologic examination of a renal biopsy. This is not essential for treatment when the diagnosis is evident by the typical clinical and laboratory findings. If the presentation is equivocal or glomerulonephritis could represent a manifestation of a systemic disease such as lupus erythematosus, polyarteritis, toxic nephropathy and so forth, renal biopsy is indicated. A renal biopsy should certainly be done before immunosuppressive therapy or chronic renal dialysis is instituted, in order to establish whether there is a possibility of therapeutic benefit from such therapy. The persistence of abnormal urinary findings for two years or longer after a well-documented initial attack of presumably typical acute glomerulonephritis (failure to heal) is another indication for renal biopsy. Percutaneous renal biopsy is now a safe procedure when done by an experienced pediatric nephrologist, and the services of such an expert should be sought when needed.

References

Dobrin, R. S., Larsen, C. D., and Holliday, M. A.: Diagnosis and Treatment. The Critically Ill Child: Acute Renal Failure. *Pediatrics,* 48:286–293, 1971.

McLaine, P. N., and Drummond, K. N.: Intravenous Diazoxide for Severe Hypertension in Childhood. *J. Pediat.,* 79:829–832, 1972.

Repetto, H. A., Lewy, J. E., Brando, J. L., et al.: The Renal Functional Response to Furosemide in Children with Acute Glomerulonephritis. *J. Pediat.,* 80:660–666, 1972.

The Nephrotic Syndrome

CHESTER M. EDELMANN, Jr., M.D.; *and* IRA GREIFER, M.D.

The nephrotic syndrome in childhood may occur as a manifestation of a systemic or generalized disease (such as lupus erythematosus or Henoch-Schönlein purpura), or during the course of virtually any form of glomerulonephritis. In the absence of identifiable systemic or renal disease, it is referred to as the *idiopathic nephrotic syndrome of childhood* or pure lipoid nephrosis. The discussion presented here will deal mainly with the latter two groups of children, in 80 per cent of whom the disease is idiopathic.

Treatment of children with the nephrotic syndrome must include measures directed toward control of the outstanding clinical feature, edema and, more importantly, toward attempts to modify favorably the course of the disease and its ultimate prognosis. In addition, because of the chronicity of the disease and the uncertainty of the outcome, the parents of a child with nephrosis need more than the usual amount of psychologic support from the physician.

General Measures. The *diet* of the nephrotic child is that suitable for the normal child. Salt needs to be restricted only during periods of edema, at which time foods are not salted during cooking, a shaker is not provided and excessively salty foods are avoided. The protein content of the diet is not altered. No restrictions are placed on the activity of the child beyond those which he may impose during periods of edema.

It is important to maintain associations with other children, but because exacerbations of proteinuria and edema may follow common upper respiratory tract infections, some limitations are advisable. For example, when contacts with other children during visits or playtimes are planned, more than the usual amount of attention is paid to the possibility of infection in the other children. Although exposure to large groups is best avoided, patients are allowed to attend kindergarten and regular school classes.

Serious intercurrent infections are a real hazard for the nephrotic child. Although continuous prophylaxis with antibiotics is not recommended, it is advisable to administer antibiotics after definite exposure to bacterial infection and to use these agents promptly and more liberally for possible bacterial infection, particularly during periods of edema. In the past, most serious infections were due to pneumococcus, but at present they are caused more frequently by other organisms, particularly gram-negative bacilli and staphylococci. Until the infecting organism can be identified, a broad-spectrum antibiotic is indicated.

Infection of the urinary tract is encountered not infrequently. The first indication of such infection may be failure of a child to respond to adrenocortical steroid therapy. Therefore, the urine should be repeatedly examined in nephrotic children, particularly in the previously responsive child who fails to show his usual prompt response to treatment.

Adrenocortical Steroids. In approximately 95 per cent of children with the idiopathic nephrotic syndrome, adrenocortical steroid therapy induces a complete clinical and biochemical remission within six to eight weeks. In this group of patients, therefore, the adrenocortical steroids remain the drugs of choice for initial therapy. In contrast, it is uncertain whether patients with progressive glomerulonephritis respond to such treatment. Moreover, children with some types of disease, such as membranoproliferative or mesangiocapillary glomerulonephritis, are extremely sensitive to steroid therapy and are unusually susceptible to development of severe toxicity.

It is recommended by many nephrologists, therefore, that nephrotic children with other than "minimal change" disease not be given adrenocortical steroid therapy, but rather be treated with one of the immunosuppressant cytotoxic drugs. However, we are uncertain enough about the efficacy of these drugs in children with membranous and proliferative glomerulonephritis, and at the same time concerned enough about their potential toxicity, that we recommend that all nephrotic children be given an initial trial of steroids. In patients with glomerulonephritis, this is done with extreme caution, and often with lower dosages than those described in this discussion for patients with the idiopathic nephrotic syndrome and minimal change disease.

Although recommendations for specific adrenocortical steroids and dosage schedules vary considerably, the basic aim of all regimens is to maintain the patient free from proteinuria* with the minimal dosage of adrenocortical steroids. We are not convinced that any one of the suggested therapeutic regimens for adrenocortical steroids has any clear advantage over the others, including the following plan, which has been used for the past several years by the International Study of Kidney Disease in Children. This plan is relatively easy to follow, it utilizes one of the less expensive drugs and it involves oral medication exclusively.

Initial Treatment. Adrenocortical steroid therapy is started as soon as the diagnosis is established, prednisone being given orally in a daily dosage of 60 mg. per square meter of body surface area (approximately 2 mg. per kilogram, based on "dry" weight). The drug is given in divided doses; a maximal daily dose of 80 mg. is not exceeded. Treatment is continued for 28 days regardless of response.

Following the initial four weeks of treatment, the daily dosage of prednisone is reduced by one-third, and the drug is given intermittently, three consecutive days of each week. Intermittent therapy is given for a total of four weeks to the patient whose urine became free of protein during the initial 28 days of treatment. In the patient whose urine becomes

* Patients are followed up in our clinic with periodic (1) Addis counts (2) measurements of urea and creatinine clearances, (3) determinations of serum concentrations of urea, creatinine, cholesterol and total protein, (4) analysis of electrophoretic distribution of the various serum protein components and (5) bacterial colony counts of clean-voided urine specimens. More important than these, however, in regulating therapy with adrenocortical hormones is the daily determination of urinary protein concentration performed at home by the parents on the first urine specimen in the morning, using 10 per cent sulfosalicylic acid or Albustix. This test is the simplest and yet indicates the most important manifestation of disease activity. It has been extremely valuable in judging adequacy of treatment.

protein-free while receiving intermittent therapy, four more weeks of intermittent therapy are given from the time of response. Patients who continue to have proteinuria after four weeks of daily and four weeks of intermittent therapy are defined as steroid-nonresponsive and are considered candidates for other drugs.

Treatment of Relapse. The treatment of a relapse (recurrence of proteinuria) is similar to the initial treatment, except that the daily administration of prednisone in a dosage of 60 mg. per square meter is continued only until the urine has been free from protein for three days. At this point prednisone is given intermittently for four weeks, as already described. Patients having frequent relapses are treated in a similar fashion, unless the quantity of steroid required becomes excessive and steroid toxicity develops. In such instances, patients are considered candidates for treatment with other drugs (see below).

Alternate-day steroid therapy, in which a single dose, equivalent to twice the usual daily dose, is given once every 48 hours, has not in our experience been successful in inducing or sustaining remissions, although good results have been reported by others. In a few patients in whom it was not possible to taper the daily dosage of adrenocortical steroid below a particular level without recurrence of proteinuria, gradual elimination of treatment was successfully accomplished by omitting the dosage first one day and then an additional day each week. Although these methods have been used in only a few children and therefore cannot be adequately evaluated, they are mentioned to indicate that any regimen, such as the one we have recommended, is arbitrary and may have to be varied.

In addition to hypothalamic-pituitary-adrenocortical suppression, the many and varied side effects of adrenocortical steroid therapy are frequently seen in children with the nephrotic syndrome who are treated with relatively large dosages over prolonged periods. Extensive experience indicates, however, that serious side effects are uncommon and are not seen more frequently in children with the nephrotic syndrome than in children receiving steroids for other reasons.

An occasional child is encountered in whom tapering of steroids after many months of therapy at large dosage is associated with headache, lethargy, weakness, anorexia and vomiting. Treatment is accomplished by providing the minimal dosage of steroid which is adequate to alleviate the symptoms. After two to three months, therapy is stopped. If symptoms reappear, treatment is given for another two to three months. In rare instances, supportive therapy may be required for as long as one year before treatment can be discontinued completely.

Immunosuppressant Drugs. A variety of drugs has been used for the treatment of patients with the nephrotic syndrome who are steroid-nonresponsive or who do respond but relapse frequently. The value of these agents in such patients has not been established, and recommendations for their use are under constant revision. Our recent experience suggests that the two most widely used of these drugs, azathioprine and cyclophosphamide, are of no value in patients with any form of chronic glomerulonephritis. The unusual patient with minimal-change disease who fails to respond to initial steroid therapy seems to attain remission more rapidly when treated with cyclophosphamide than with continued steroid. This drug has also been shown to be very effective in delaying and decreasing the frequency of relapses in steroid-dependent, frequently relapsing patients. However, serious potential side effects, such as aspermia, limit the use of cyclophosphamide to patients with severe steroid toxicity or life-threatening disease.

Since the use of the newer immunosuppressant drugs must still be considered experimental, it is suggested that patients considered candidates for such treatment be managed by or in consultation with investigators actively engaged in studying the effect of these drugs in patients with the nephrotic syndrome.

Diuretics. Sodium restriction, though capable of slowing accumulation of edema during an exacerbation of the nephrotic syndrome, is usually not successful in eliminating edema. In recent years numerous diuretic agents have become available which, combined with moderate sodium restriction, contribute significantly to control of edema.

Since the majority of patients diurese satisfactorily one to four weeks after beginning adrenocortical steroid therapy, diuretic agents are not given initially. Diuretics may provide important symptomatic relief in refractory patients, or before diuresis has occurred in very edematous patients who become more edematous during treatment.

Hydrochlorothiazide in a dosage of 2 to 4 mg. per kilogram per day may be used initially. The thiazide drugs are relatively nontoxic. Hypokalemia is usually not seen if a child is eating a normal diet, but it may be avoided by giving potassium supplements. Elevated serum concentration of uric acid is frequent. The other side effects, including thrombocytopenia, skin rashes, jaundice, pancreatitis and hyperglycemia, either are extremely rare or have not been reported in children.

In the patient who does not respond to hydrochlorothiazide—a common experience in the severely edematous child—a more potent diluretic is indicated. In this situation we have had excellent results with furosemide.* Patients are pretreated with salt-poor albumin, in a dosage of 0.5 or 1.0 Gm. per kilogram of body weight, depending on whether the serum albumin is above or below 1.5 Gm. per 100 ml. The albumin is infused over 30 minutes. After a further 30 minutes to permit equilibration, furosemide is given intravenously in a dosage of 1 mg. per kilogram. This therapeutic schedule may be repeated every 4 to 6 hours as necessary. Attempts are *not* made to increase the concentration of albumin in plasma to the normal range. However, administration of albumin in the dosage mentioned maintains the integrity of the circulation and avoids the circulatory insufficiency that may result when a vigorous diuresis is produced in a severely hypoalbuminemic subject with a contracted vascular volume.

THE NEPHROTIC SYNDROME AS PART OF OTHER RECOGNIZABLE DISEASES

The rare instance of the nephrotic syndrome associated with *renal vein thrombosis* or *constrictive pericarditis* can be treated only by alleviation of the underlying condition.

Adrenocortical steroid therapy of congenital or infantile nephrosis thus far not only has been ineffective, but also may have caused a more rapid progression of the disease. Since this form of nephrosis has been invariably fatal, one is strongly tempted to try to influence its relentless course. Nevertheless, present knowledge contraindicates the use of adrenocortical steroids in infants with this form of the disease.

The renal disease associated with *disseminated lupus erythematosus,* which may present as the nephrotic syndrome, formerly was considered to be uninfluenced by therapy. Recent experience with intensive therapy, however, indicates that steroids alone or in combination with an immunosuppressant drug have a decidedly beneficial effect.

The nephrotic syndrome related etiologically to certain drugs, such as trimethadione, usually resolves after discontinuation of the offending agent. If not, it is questionable whether adrenocortical steroids should be used. At present we would tend not to give them until several weeks or even months after the drug has been stopped. Drugs implicated in producing the nephrotic syndrome should be withheld permanently, since their repeated administration may subsequently result in irreversible disease.

* Although there has been extensive experience with this drug in children, both in Europe and in the United States, to date such use has not been approved by the Food and Drug Administration.

References

Abramowicz, M., Arneil, G. C., Barnett, H. L., et al.: Controlled Clinical Trial of Azathioprine in Children with Nephrotic Syndrome. *Lancet,* 1:959, 1970.

Spitzer, A.: Cyclophosphamide in the Treatment of the Nephrotic Syndrome in Childhood. *Pediatrics,* 50: 358, 1972.

Chronic Renal Insufficiency
Chronic Uremia

CHESTER M. EDELMANN, Jr., M.D., *and* ADRIAN SPITZER, M.D.

Treatment of patients with chronic renal insufficiency is nonspecific unless there is a recognizable and treatable underlying condition. It is extremely important, therefore, whenever possible, to make a precise diagnosis of the cause of this condition. Successful treatment of infants and children with impairment of renal function due to pyelonephritis, particularly when associated with correctable forms of obstructive uropathy, is a striking example of the importance of this principle. In this article, however, aspects of treatment which apply to patients with chronic uremia and its complications will be considered irrespective of the cause. Although in most instances such treatment does not influence the underlying kidney disease favorably, it is often effective symptomatically and should be applied diligently.

With appropriate dietary and pharmacologic management, patients with renal disease can be maintained surprisingly well despite advanced degrees of renal insufficiency. It must be appreciated, however, that therapy becomes more and more complicated for both patient and physician as renal insufficiency progresses. At the same time, it becomes easier and easier to do harm. Therapeutic decisons must be carefully planned, physiologically based and individualized to the needs of each patient.

Diet. Regulation of the diet is a primary means of treating disturbances, such as chronic uremia, in which there is a decreased ability to handle some of the end-products of the metabolism of foods. Arbitrary, unnecessary restrictions should be avoided. Although these patients frequently grow slowly, a palatable, well-balanced diet, adequate to meet caloric and other nutritional needs, should be provided.

In the asymptomatic infant or child with chronic renal disease who, except for some elevation in the concentrations of urea and creatinine, has sufficient renal function to maintain other blood chemical values within the range of normal, no change should be made in the usual well-balanced diet. Patients with more severe degrees of renal insufficiency require dietary regulation, involving particularly their intake of protein, osmotically active solutes and certain electrolytes and minerals, such as sodium, calcium and phosphate.

Each 100 Gm. of dietary protein, essential in the maintenance of a positive nitrogen balance, requires renal excretion of approximately 70 mEq. of hydrogen ion. In order to provide essential protein and yet not induce metabolic acidosis in patients with severe renal insufficiency, dietary protein should be limited initially to 0.3 to 0.5 Gm. per kilogram of body weight per day. This amount can be increased empirically as tolerated. Protein-containing foods should be restricted mainly to those of high biologic value—meat, fish, eggs, cheese and milk. The intake of high protein vegetables, particularly those of the bean family, should be markedly curtailed.

Owing to its high solute content, milk is a poor source of protein in advanced renal insufficiency; however, infants with renal insufficiency often do very well on "humanized milk" formulas with low concentrations of both electrolyte and protein (PM 60/40 and SMA S-26).

Experience is beginning to accumulate in the treatment of patients with advanced renal insufficiency (rates of glomerular filtration as low as 5 ml. per minute) by means of synthetic diets designed to maintain adequate nutritional intake, with proteins of high biologic value and virtually no electrolytes. The application of these extreme measures to children is limited because such diets are unpalatable. Nevertheless the principles underlying this type of therapy have been applied with success to infants and small children with lesser degrees of renal failure, using naturally available foods and less vigorous attempts at dietary control.

One of the major limitations in imposing severe dietary restrictions is the difficulty in maintaining adequate caloric intake. Low protein, low electrolyte products, such as Controlyte and Resource Baking Mix, may be of considerable value in this regard by providing calories in the form of bread, cookies, milk shakes and other foods.

Arbitrary restriction of dietary sodium is one of the most common errors in treatment of patients with renal disease. The child with hypertension, edema or salt intolerance may need restriction of dietary sodium to as little as 0.2 mEq. per kilogram per day. In many patients with renal insufficiency, a low sodium intake results in a negative sodium balance, depletion of extracellular volume and further deterioration of renal function. Unless there are clear indications for either sodium restriction or supplementation, a normal sodium intake should be allowed. Certain milks with low sodium content, e.g., Lonalac, which are excellent for infants and children with cardiac impairment, may be dangerous to children with renal disease, owing to their high potassium content.

Most patients with renal insufficiency can be allowed to ingest water ad libitum, their water intake being regulated by their own thirst mechanisms. There may be a decrease, however, in the renal ability to conserve water, requiring the provision of adequate water to prevent dehydration and hemoconcentration, particularly in hot weather and during febrile illnesses. Children allowed free access to water usually present no problem, but disturbances in water balance may occur in the infant and the sick child whose water intake is regulated by the physician.

Anorexia, nausea and vomiting are frequent disturbances in chronic uremia. Early in the course of renal insufficiency, gastrointestinal symptoms usually respond well to simple restriction of dietary protein; in the more advanced stages they may be exceedingly resistant to treatment. Phenothiazines, such as prochlorperazine* (0.4 mg. per kilogram per 24 hours) or chlorpromazine† (2 mg. per kilogram per 24 hours), given in three or four oral doses, may be very effective.

Acidosis. Patients with mild acidosis are usually asymptomatic; nevertheless they should be treated. Mild degrees of acidosis usually respond to restriction of dietary protein. The child who remains acidotic despite this may require more specific therapy.

Correction of acidosis requires administration of alkali, given usually in the form of

---

* Manufacturer's precaution: Prochlorperazine is not recommended for children under 20 pounds or under two years of age.

† Manufacturer's precaution: Chlorpromazine is not recommended for children under six months of age except when lifesaving.

sodium bicarbonate or sodium citrate in a dosage of 1 to 3 mEq. per kilogram per day. After prolonged ingestion of diets low in protein and high in carbohydrate, patients with chronic acidosis may have potassium depletion (despite normal blood levels) and therefore may require a mixture of sodium and potassium salts, as in the following formula, which provides 25 mEq. of each cation per 15 ml.:

Sodium citrate ($Na_3C_6H_5O_7 \cdot 5H_2O$)	97 Gm.
Potassium citrate ($K_3C_6H_5O_7 \cdot H_2O$)	90 Gm.
Water q.s.	500 ml.

If there is severe reduction in glomerular filtration rate, potassium depletion is less likely and the potassium load of this solution may be excessive. In these instances a solution of sodium citrate alone can be given.† Some acidotic patients may be unable to excrete the amount of sodium in this mixture and may not tolerate it. Aluminum and magnesium hydroxide, used primarily to correct hyperphosphatemia, may also serve to correct acidosis. A dosage of 50 to 150 mg. per kilogram per day can be given.

Respiratory compensation of metabolic acidosis, resulting in low pCO_2 in blood, may be of extreme importance in preventing severe acidosis in the patient with impaired renal mechanisms for hydrogen ion excretion. Interference with alveolar ventilation secondary to pneumonia, sedatives or thoracic surgery may result in profound acidosis and sudden death.

Disturbances in Handling of Water and Solutes. The unusual patient requiring sodium supplementation to combat excessive salt losses has been mentioned. More common, however, is the child whose ability to excrete sodium is reduced to the level that ingestion of normal amounts of dietary sodium is excessive and results in edema. Frequently, it is corrected by restriction of sodium intake to 0.2 to 1 mEq. per kilogram per day. When this measure is not successful, diuretic therapy may be given. Hydrochlorothiazide is a useful drug and is given orally in a dosage of 2 to 4 mg. per kilogram per day. If this is not successful, more potent diuretics are used. We have had good results with furosemide, which is given orally in a dosage of 1 to 2 mg. per kilogram, once or twice per day. It should be noted that although there has been extensive experience with this drug in patients of all ages, it has not been approved by the Food and Drug Administration for use in children.

Hyperkalemia and Hypokalemia. Significant elevation of extracellular potassium concentration is not common in patients with chronic renal sufficiency unless there is a severe reduction in glomerular filtration rate, oliguria or acidosis. In these instances, exogenous sources of potassium, such as drugs and antibiotics, candy and fruits, must be carefully controlled. Hydrochlorothiazide (see previously) may be useful in promoting urinary losses of potassium. Kayexalate, a sodium-potassium exchange resin, is especially effective. It can be given orally or rectally in starting dosage of 0.5 to 1.5 Gm. per kilogram per day with subsequent adjustment of the dosage according to need. It should be appreciated that with this form of therapy the patient receives an amount of sodium equal to that of the potassium removed. Prolonged treatment with Kayexalate, therefore, may result in administration of excessive sodium.

Hypokalemia, due to anorexia, diarrhea, vomiting or the use of diuretic drugs, also occurs in patients with chronic uremia. Increase in potassium intake is a simple corrective measure and may be given in a dosage calculated to provide a daily supplement of 3 to 5 mEq. per kilogram.‡

Hypocalcemia and Bone Disease. Hypocalcemia is common in patients with chronic renal disease. Although it usually causes no symptoms, muscle cramps, weakness, tetany and convulsions may be seen occasionally. Therapy is aimed at symptomatic control and consists of a diet low in phosphate and of oral administration of aluminum hydroxide and calcium. The calcium is usually given in the form of calcium lactate,§ calculated to provide 10 to 20 mg. of calcium per kilogram per day. Without supplemental vitamin D, patients with chronic renal insufficiency usually remain in negative calcium balance despite oral calcium supplementation. Therefore, the use of vitamin D to promote calcium absorption from the gut has been advocated. Vitamin D may induce hypercalcemia and metastatic calcification, however, and therefore should be used with caution. We recommend its use in patients in whom other measures have not been successful, and then only with careful monitoring of concentrations

† Although not tolerated by all patients, some find sodium bicarbonate (baking soda) to be a convenient form of therapy: 1 Gm. contains 11.9 mEq. of sodium. One measuring teaspoon is approximately 3.7 Gm., and thus provides about 44 mEq.

‡ One gram of potassium chloride contains 13.4 mEq. of potassium; Potassium Triplex is a palatable liquid preparation which contains 15 mEq. per 5 ml.

§ One gram of calcium lactate, $Ca(C_3H_5O_3)_2 \cdot 5H_2O$, contains 130 mg. of calcium. A variety of proprietary preparations is available.

of calcium and phosphate in serum. Attempts to restore calcium values to normal are hazardous, in that hypercalcemia is easily produced. A dosage of 10,000 to 20,000 units of vitamin D daily may be given initially, but higher dosage levels may be necessary.

The bone disease of chronic renal insufficiency generally falls into one of two categories: rickets (or osteomalacia) or osteitis fibrosa. Vitamin D is the treatment of choice for the former. In osteitis fibrosa, serum calcium levels may be normal or slightly reduced, suggesting that an unusually severe degree of secondary hyperparathyroidism may play a main role. Doses of vitamin D adequate to cause healing may result in dangerous degrees of hypercalcemia. Partial parathyroidectomy has been carried out on a limited number of patients, including children and adults, with apparently beneficial results.

Hypertension. Control of hypertension can be an important factor in prolonging survival in patients with chronic renal disease. Therapy is empirical, the particular drug and effective dose being determined by trial in each patient.

Hydrochlorothiazide, discussed previously, may be successful in controlling mild elevations in blood pressure, especially in patients with a tendency toward sodium retention.

Reserpine is perhaps the safest and simplest antihypertensive agent available. A dosage of 0.01 to 0.02 mg. per kilogram per day orally in one or two divided doses is often effective and usually completely without side effects, although somnolence, headaches, nasal stuffiness and diarrhea may be seen at higher dosage levels. When hypertension is not controlled satisfactorily by reserpine alone, hydralazine is given in addition. The effective dosage of this drug varies enormously. Therapy should be initiated at low dosage levels and adjusted over a period of days to weeks until the desired response or side effects are noted. An initial dosage of 1 to 2 mg. per kilogram per day orally in four divided doses can be tried with careful monitoring of the blood pressure. Doses as high as 20 mg. per kilogram may be required. Side effects include nausea, hypotension, headaches and tachycardia.

Often it is not possible to return the blood pressure to normal with either or both of these agents. In such cases, guanethidine or alpha-methyldopa can be employed orally, in starting dosages of 0.2 mg. per kilogram per day and 10 mg. per kilogram per day, respectively. Guanethidine is given as a single daily dose; alpha-methyldopa is divided into two or three doses daily. The major side effect of guanethidine is postural hypotension. Other side effects include bradycardia and diarrhea. Methyldopa should not be given in the presence of liver disease. Side effects include hemolytic anemia, leukopenia and fever.

Anemia. The anemia of chronic renal disease is rarely symptomatic, although it may be persistent and severe. In advanced uremia the hematocrit usually stabilizes between 15 and 20 ml. per 100 ml.; such low levels are well tolerated in most instances. There is no specific therapy, assuming that iron deficiency and other nutritional insufficiencies, such as vitamin D, folic acid and vitamin B_{12}, have been ruled out. Blood transfusions are of only temporary value, depress the bone marrow and are not without hazards. Severe hypertension is often observed. Sudden, unexpected and unexplained deaths have followed transfusions of whole blood in patients with chronic renal insufficiency. If anemia is severe and symptomatic, we recommend the slow, cautious infusion of previously frozen washed red blood cells, which appear to cause fewer reactions than whole blood. Transfusion of blood containing leukocytes may cause sensitization, which may be of considerable importance with regard to subsequent renal transplantation.

Growth Failure. The cause of growth failure in chronic renal disease is uncertain, although poor nutrition, chronic acidosis, negative calcium balance, anemia and chronic infection may play important roles. Therapy is directed toward each separate problem or complication in an attempt to provide as healthy a milieu as possible for growth. The possible beneficial effect of growth hormone or of anabolic steroids has not been established.

Neuromuscular and Psychologic Disturbances. It is important to realize that the irritative neuromuscular phenomena commonly seen in patients with chronic uremia, including muscle twitching and convulsions, are rarely due to hypocalcemia and thus respond poorly to calcium therapy. This is probably because of the protective effect of the associated acidosis and elevated level of serum magnesium. Other than the rare instance in which hypocalcemia can be implicated, therapy is nonspecific and unsatisfactory, consisting merely of sedation.

Other types of neurologic disturbances include a variety of mental symptoms, ranging from depression to psychosis, and peripheral neuropathy. Treatment other than dialysis is not available.

Management of a child with chronic renal insufficiency must include psychologic support not only of the child but also of his family. Considerable understanding of child development and of the defenses used by children of different ages is required for this aspect of treatment. As in other serious diseases in which the cause is not known, the parents and older patients need to be reassured repeatedly that they are not responsible for the disease. In an illness such as chronic uremia, in which medical treatment is usually inadequate, it is important also for the physician to examine repeatedly how his own feelings may be affecting his relations with the patient and family.

The Effect of Chronic Uremia on Unrelated Intercurrent Disturbances. The presence of chronic renal insufficiency in an infant or child must be taken into account in the treatment of unrelated intercurrent disturbances. For example, toxic amounts of potassium may inadvertently be given in the form of potassium penicillin, and the concentration of other drugs excreted by the kidneys may reach abnormally high levels if they are given in the usual dosage. Also, there is the recurrent and difficult problem of trying to assess how much chronic renal insufficiency may be contributing to common events such as recurrent respiratory infections and particularly psychologic disturbances.

Immunosuppressant Drugs. At present there are only limited data on the value of these drugs in the treatment of patients with chronic renal insufficiency. Earlier experience indicated that adrenocortical steroids were of little, if any, value, and there was even some suspicion that in addition to their known undesirable side effects they accelerated loss of kidney function in some patients. Other reports have indicated that unexpected improvement has occurred in some patients given adrenocortical steroids.

At present, with the possible exception of patients with lupus nephritis, we do not recommend adrenocortical steroids in the treatment of infants and children with chronic renal insufficiency. Moreover, there is very little evidence that treatment with other immunosuppressant drugs, such as 6-thioguanine, azathioprine and cyclophosphamide, arrests or retards progression of any of the various types of chronic glomerulonephritis. Similarly, firm evidence is lacking for any beneficial effect of chronic therapy with heparin. Nevertheless, the patient who is progressing toward chronic renal insufficiency often is treated empirically with one of these drugs in the continued hope that some benefit may ensue. Since their use remains experimental, children considered candidates for such therapy should be evaluated by investigators actively engaged in studying the effects of these drugs in patients with chronic renal disease.

Dialysis. Peritoneal dialysis has been used frequently in the treatment of infants and children with acute renal failure, but to a lesser degree in patients with chronic renal failure. The procedure, which is technically simpler than hemodialysis, is tolerated even by small infants. Commercially available catheters (such as the Baxter Trocath) are suitable for use in children, and are inserted after distending the abdomen by instilling, through a number 18 needle, a volume of fluid equal to that of one exchange. The site of insertion is in the midline, halfway between the symphysis pubis and the umbilicus.

Commercially prepared dialysis fluid (e.g., Dianeal and Inpersol) is used, with 1.5 per cent dextrose and appropriate amounts of potassium, plus 5 mg. of heparin per liter. We do not recommend the addition of antibiotics. The volume of exchange is 1 liter in older children, and 50 to 100 ml. per kilogram in younger children. We have used a 30- to 60-minute cycle of exchange, although recommendations regarding optimal dwell time vary considerably.

Dialysis can be continued for 48, 72 or more hours, although the risk of peritonitis increases as the duration of dialysis is prolonged.

Adults with terminal renal failure have been maintained with chronic hemodialysis for many years. Attempts at such therapy in children, although initially discouraging, more recently have met with considerable success. The technical problems are greater than in adults, particularly with regard to maintenance of cannulas. Recent experience with surgically created internal arteriovenous fistulas, which obviate the need for cannulization, is encouraging. In children, special attention must be paid to nutritional requirements, and in many instances nutritional supplements may be necessary. Despite the improved success with chronic hemodialysis in children, its major role, apart from the treatment of acute renal failure, remains the maintenance and preparation of children for renal allotransplantation.

Renal Allotransplantation. As survival figures following renal homotransplantation steadily improve, this procedure becomes increasingly the one of choice in the management of terminal renal failure. This is particularly true for children in whom chronic dialysis as definitive therapy has generally been unsuccessful. Recent experience indicates that remarkably good results can be anticipated when the donor is a living relative with good histocompatibility. Since children are likely to have healthy, young parents or siblings who are ideal donors, transplantation may have its greatest success in the pediatric age group. In addition, children appear to develop less toxicity during immunosuppressive therapy, and they are more likely to be free from diseases of other body systems.

Any discussion of the treatment of chronic renal insufficiency in infants and children forces the physician to recognize its inadequacy. The final solution to the problems presented by these patients will come not from the brilliant advances either in dialysis or even in kidney homografts, but rather from more complete knowledge of etiology and from prevention of the diseases and conditions which lead to chronic uremia.

References

Fine, R. N., et al.: Hemodialysis in Children. *Am. J. Dis. Child.*, 119:498, 1970.

Fine, R. N., et al.: Renal Homotransplantation in Children. *J. Pediat.*, 76:347, 1970.

Korsch, B. M., et al.: Experiences with Children and Their Families during Extended Hemodialysis and Kidney Transplantation. *Pediat. Clin. N. Am.*, 18: May, 1971.

Lilly, J. R., et al.: Renal Homotransplantation in Pediatric Patients. *Pediatrics*, 47:548, 1971.

Merrill, J. P.: *The Treatment of Renal Failure.* 2nd ed. New York, Grune & Stratton, Inc., 1965.

Merrill, J. P.: Uremia. *New England J. Med.*, 282:953, 1970.

Potter, D., et al.: The Treatment of Chronic Uremia in Childhood. I. Transplantation. *Pediatrics*, 45: 432, 1970.

Potter, D., et al.: Treatment of Chronic Uremia in Childhood. II. Hemodialysis. *Pediatrics*, 46:678, 1970.

Simmons, J. M., Wilson, C. J., Potter, D. E., and Holliday, M. A.: Relation of Calorie Deficiency to Growth Failure in Children on Hemodialysis and the Growth Response to Calorie Supplementation. *New England J. Med.*, 285:653, 1971.

Welt, L. G.: Symposium on Uremia. *Am. J. Med.*, 44: 653, 1968.

The Hemolytic-Uremic Syndrome

GERALD S. GILCHRIST, M.B., B.CH., *and* ELLIN LIEBERMAN, M.D.

The hemolytic-uremic syndrome is characterized by acute renal failure, microangiopathic hemolytic anemia and thrombocytopenia. The vast majority of affected children are less than two years old, with the peak incidence in those less than one year old. The search for an etiologic agent has been unsuccessful although a viral cause has been suggested. No single virus or group of viruses has been implicated, and the disorder may be a nonspecific response to various viral, bacterial or rickettsia-like pathogens. Most affected children have been in apparent good health and well nourished. A history of a preceding gastroenteritis-like illness is commonly elicited, and the stools are occasionally bloody. Neurologic abnormalities, particularly seizures, have been a prominent prodromal feature.

The clinical and laboratory features of the syndrome vary considerably from patient to patient, and the severity may vary in different geographic areas. At one extreme are the patients with profound anemia, life-threatening thrombocytopenia and complete anuria, whereas at the other are patients that may manifest only a slight decrease in hemoglobin level and platelet count, with little reduction in urine output. At diagnosis, the phase of the illness that the patient is presenting is difficult to ascertain, because the mildly affected patient can be in either the early or the recovery phase of his illness at presentation. Currently, no laboratory tests can answer this question. This variability in clinical severity is compounded by a poor understanding of the pathogenesis of the disease. Intravascular coagulation with deposition of fibrin and platelets in the renal microvasculature occurs at some time during the course of the disease, but some patients fail to show laboratory evidence of accelerated intravascular clotting at the time of diagnosis, suggesting that the process is no longer active.

Inasmuch as no etiologic agent has been found, therapy is essentially supportive and is mainly directed at the management of the renal failure, correction of anemia, control of hypertension and treatment of cardiac failure, if present. The use of anticoagulants or fibrinolytic agents is based on an analysis of clinical and pathologic studies, suggesting that intrarenal vascular thrombosis is a major contribution in the pathogenesis of the disease. However, not all patients require this type of therapy, and a well-designed controlled study should be carried out to evaluate the role of anticoagulant and fibrinolytic agents in the treatment of this condition. Until this is done, we consider the use of anticoagulants in all patients, particularly those with severe oliguria or anuria, in the hope of preventing further fibrin deposition in the kidney and retarding the development or extension of renal cortical necrosis. There is no evidence to suggest that corticosteroids are of use in this disorder, and they may, in fact, be contraindicated because of their ability to enhance the generalized Shwartzman reaction.

Management of Renal Failure. FLUID AND ELECTROLYTE THERAPY. Fluid balance must be carefully monitored. Many patients are overloaded at the time of diagnosis because of prior therapy and failure to recognize the renal shutdown. In the mildly affected patient, fluid balance and adequate caloric intake may be maintained through routine peripheral vein infusions, but the severely oliguric or anuric patient should have a venous catheter inserted into either the superior vena cava or the saphenous vein. The catheter allows for infusion of solutions high in glucose content and provides a means for monitoring central venous pressure, for administering transfusions and for securing blood samples. Insensible water loss is calculated on the basis of 300 ml. per square meter per day, but this value should be increased to 500 or 600 ml. if the patient is febrile. Caloric intake should be adjusted to 100 Gm. of carbohydrate per square meter per day to reduce protein breakdown to a minimum. This may involve using intravenous glucose concentrations as high as 30 per cent. Serum sodium and potassium levels should be monitored frequently because hyponatremia is common, particularly in the anuric patient. Correction of hyponatremia, using hypertonic solutions, carries the risk of producing congestive heart failure, particularly in hypertensive patients, and in these situations dialysis may be indicated. Similarly, in the severely acidotic patient, the administration of sodium bicarbonate may produce tetany and cardiorespiratory arrest. Dialysis may be indicated to avoid the risk associated with infusion of concentrated sodium bicarbonate. During diuresis, an increase in fluid requirements should be anticipated, and supplemental potassium should be administered in anticipation of hypokalemia. The fluid and electrolyte requirements vary considerably, depending on the degree of renal failure and the type of therapy previously given. Body weight should be monitored because, under optimal conditions, loss of 1 to 2 per cent in body weight per day can be anticipated. Changes outside these limits suggest that the patient is not in acceptable fluid balance.

HYPERKALEMIA. Prompt treatment is indicated when serum potassium levels exceed 7 mEq. per liter or when there is electrocardiographic evidence of hyperkalemia. A 10 per cent solution of calcium gluconate in a dose of 20 ml. per square meter is administered by slow intravenous push, with stethoscopic monitoring of the heart. If there is no response, a 7½ per cent solution of sodium bicarbonate is injected intravenously in a dose of 100 ml. per square meter, but if there is no response, this dose should not be repeated. The next approach is to infuse a solution of 50 per cent glucose (3 ml. per kilogram body weight) and administer a single dose of insulin intravenously (½ unit per kilogram). Blood glucose levels should be monitored for evidence of hypoglycemia. In less urgent situations in which hyperkalemia is anticipated and the electrocardiogram is normal, a sodium-potassium exchange resin (Kayexalate) can be given orally or by enema. One gram of Kayexalate is diluted in 4 ml. of 10 per cent dextrose, and a dose of 1 Gm. per kilogram body weight should lower the serum potassium level by 1 mEq. per liter. If there has been no response to these measures in 2 to 3 hours, dialysis should be undertaken.

PERITONEAL DIALYSIS. Peritoneal dialysis is indicated in the following situations: (1) anuria for 24 hours or more; (2) pulmonary edema or other evidence of circulatory overload; (3) blood urea nitrogen level higher than 150 mg. per 100 ml. or serum creatinine above 10 mg. per 100 ml. and increasing; (4) hyperkalemia that has not responded to other measures; (5) hypocalcemia; (6) hypernatremia; and (7) increasing neurologic problems as manifested by irritability, stupor, opisthotonus, and convulsions.

Wherever possible, dialysis is begun before anticoagulant therapy is instituted, but in most patients who are already receiving heparin, the use of the drug is temporarily discontinued and the coagulation status is allowed to return to normal over 4 or 5 hours so that the peritoneal catheter can be inserted without the risk of hemorrhage. As soon as the dialysis is in progress, heparin can be restarted. We have observed peritoneal hemorrhage in only one patient, but have cross-matched blood available in case this type of emergency should arise.

Correction of Anemia. Because hemolysis is a prominent feature of this disorder, the hemoglobin level must be carefully monitored, and corrected if the level falls below 7 Gm. per 100 ml. In order to minimize the circulatory overload, sedimented or packed red cells are used for transfusion, and these should be the freshest possible in order to reduce the potassium load in the infusion. The blood should be administered slowly over 2 to 3 hours, and a single transfusion should not exceed 10 ml. per kilogram body weight. The patient should be carefully observed for evidence of secondary encephalopathy, congestive heart failure or a precipitous increase in blood pressure. If the serum potassium level is higher than 6 mEq. per liter, Kayexalate should be given prior to the transfusion.

Correction of Thrombocytopenia. We have not found it necessary to transfuse platelets in patients with the hemolytic-uremic syndrome, particularly because the platelet count is rarely less than 20,000 per cubic mm., and in situations in which active intravascular coagulation is taking place, platelet transfusions could aggravate this process.

Control of Hypertension. Severe cardiac and neurologic complications can occur in the acute phase if hypertension is not controlled. We administer hydralazine (Apresoline) intravenously in a dose of 0.4 to 0.85 mg. per kilogram. Intramuscular injections should be avoided in the heparinized patient, and hydralazine should be administered by a physician, with careful monitoring of the blood pressure so that the diastolic pressure is less than 100 mm. Hg. This dose may be repeated every 4 to 6 hours.

Anticoagulation. Heparin is the anticoagulant of choice, and one aims at prolonging the clotting time to 2 to 2½ times the control value. These figures hold true whether one uses the Lee-White whole blood clotting time or the activated partial thromboplastin time. An initial loading dose of 100 units per kilogram body weight is administered by rapid intravenous push. For the first 4 hours thereafter, heparin (100 units per kilogram) is added to the intravenous fluids, and thereafter the dosage is regulated according to the clotting time. During the early phase of treatment, we have observed that a high dose of heparin (usually up to 200 units per kilogram) every 4 hours is necessary, but the heparin requirements may decrease dramatically during diuresis. We have found that this method of administration is easier to control than intermittent intravenous administration because continuous infusion provides a more uniform blood level of heparin; then one is not faced with the problem of profound hypocoagulability immediately after administration, with relatively little heparin effect at the end of the 4-hour period.

Heparin therapy is continued until diuresis is firmly established and the blood urea nitrogen or serum creatinine level has begun to decrease. We discontinue the use of the drug irrespective of the platelet count, and only 5 or 6 days of heparin therapy are usually necessary. This approach is based on the concept that the major effect of fibrin deposition is within the kidneys, and once this has been overcome, there is is no particular need to maintain anticoagulation, particularly because complications secondary to thrombocytopenia beyond the acute phase of the disease are rare.

Other Forms of Therapy. Antifibrinolytic therapy with or without heparin has been reported to be successful on some occasions and may be a logical way to treat this disease. At the present time, streptokinase and urokinase, two agents capable of promoting the activation of plasminogen, are still investigational in the United States and should not be utilized until further information on their safety and efficacy is available.

Similarly, exchange transfusion has been successful, but prompt peritoneal dialysis probably is a much more efficient means for reducing the blood levels of toxic metabolites, and heparin is a more logical treatment for control of intravascular coagulation.

Peritoneal Dialysis

RICHARD N. FINE, M.D.

Peritoneal dialysis is based on the principle that the peritoneum acts as a semipermeable membrane facilitating the movement of water and solutes of small molecular size across the membrane according to the concentration on either side of the membrane. Although peritoneal dialysis was utilized to treat the uremic state in man in 1903, its widespread use was prevented by technical difficulties until the publication of Maxwell et al., in 1959, initiated the presently accepted technique. Simultaneously, the availability of commercial dialysis solutions and the development of disposable plastic catheters popularized this therapeutic modality.

Indications. Peritoneal dialysis has been employed with success in pediatric patients to treat renal failure—both acute and chronic—accidental poisonings, intractable congestive heart failure, hypernatremia, severe acidosis in children with disorders of amino acid metabolism (maple sugar urine disease, hyperglycinemia) and severe hyperkalemia associated with congenital adrenal hyperplasia. It has been utilized in children with hepatic coma, respiratory distress syndrome and Reye's syndrome without uniform beneficial results.

The indications for the institution of peritoneal dialysis in children with acute renal failure are variable and dependent on the clinical status of the patient. Absolute indications are evidence of deteriorating central nervous system function (coma) and congestive heart failure unresponsive to diuretics and control of hypertension. Various biochemical parameters are useful in indicating the propitious time to commence dialysis: blood urea nitrogen value greater than 150 mg. per 100 ml.; carbon dioxide content less than 12 mEq. per liter; potassium greater than 6.0 mEq. per liter; and a falling hematocrit (less than 20 ml. per 100 ml.) necessitating transfusion in the face of hyperkalemia and hypertension. However, it must be stressed that each of the above abnormalities can be managed without dialysis. The decision to institute dialysis should be based on the clinical status of the child.

Although intermittent peritoneal dialysis has been used to prolong life in children with chronic renal failure, this method is far less acceptable to the children than is intermittent hemodialysis, and the clinical results are inferior. Presently, peritoneal dialysis is employed at our institution in patients with chronic renal failure in preparation for cannula insertion or fistula creation prior to the institution of intermittent hemodialysis, or for acute symptoms of uremia superimposed on chronic renal failure.

Peritoneal dialysis has proven beneficial in the treatment of accidental poisoning in children. In general, any substance which is water-soluble is potentially dialyzable. The efficacy of dialysis generally depends on the degree of protein-binding. Fat-soluble substances do not lend themselves to peritoneal dialysis. The indications for dialysis are dependent on the poison ingested, the blood level of the poison and the clinical status of the patient.* The routine use of peritoneal dialysis in the management of children with salicylate intoxication is probably superfluous if an adequate diuresis and alkalinization of the urine can be obtained. However, with severe intoxication, dialysis using a 5 per cent Albumisol solution is beneficial.

Congestive heart failure in a child with normal renal function which is unresponsive to digitalis and diuretics may be improved by fluid removal during peritoneal dialysis. Such circumstances are rare, but temporary improvement has been reported.

Severe hypernatremia can lead to irreversible central nervous system damage and is a pediatric emergency. When the serum sodium level approaches 200 mEq. per liter, dialysis is indicated. More efficient correction of hypernatremia can result from peritoneal dialysis than with intravenous fluid administration when severe hypernatremia is present. The beneficial effects of peritoneal dialysis in children with respiratory distress syndrome, hepatic coma and Reye's syndrome have not been consistent, and the use of alternative modes of therapy in the latter two entities, such as exchange transfusion, are probably more efficacious.

Contraindications. The only contraindication to the use of peritoneal dialysis is intra-abdominal bleeding consequent to a coagulopathy. Patients with peritonitis and pancreatitis have undergone successful peritoneal dialysis. Recent abdominal surgery, even in the presence of drains, is not a contraindication to commencing peritoneal dialysis, although the efficiency of the procedure may be decreased in this circumstance.

Technique. Prior to starting dialysis, a well-functioning site for delivery of intravenous solutions should be present, and one to two units of whole blood should be available in case of trochar-induced hemorrhage.

If the patient is not comatose, intramuscular or intravenous analgesic is administered approximately ½ hour prior to dialysis. Analgesic drugs which are respiratory depressants should be administered with caution, since the general status of the patient may affect respiratory depression, and the elevation of the diaphragms with the institution of dialysis may further compromise the respiration efforts. The bladder is then catheterized if the patient has not voided within the hour or cannot void voluntarily. This is to avoid the inadvertent puncturing of a distended bladder with the trochar. A surgical preparation of the abdomen from the xiphoid to the pubis is then performed.

Commercially prepared dialysis solutions are available with glucose concentrations of 1.5 per cent and 4.25 per cent and contain no potassium. Both the 1.5 per cent and 4.25 per cent solutions are hypertonic with respect to plasma osmolarity to effect fluid removal during dialysis. Depending on the patient's serum potassium level, 3 to 4 mEq. per liter of potassium are added to the dialysis solution. It is dangerous to dialyze with a potassium free solution because of the potential of precipitating hypokalemia. Heparin (1 ml. of 1000-U.S.P.-units-per-ml. of aqueous heparin) is added to each liter of dialysis fluid used for the initial two passes to prevent clotting in the catheter. If the dialysate fluid is persistently blood-tinged, producing clot formation in the catheter, heparin can be continued in subsequent passes. Each bottle of dialysate solution is warmed to

---

* For a detailed analysis of this subject, one should consult Dialysis of Poisons and Drugs—Annual Review. *Trans. Am. Soc. Artif. Int. Organs*, vol. 17, 1971.

37° C. prior to instillation in the peritoneal cavity to prevent hypothermia. The amount of dialysate solution instilled into the peritoneal cavity is generally 1200 ml. per square meter; however, if the 4.25 per cent solution is used, only one-half to three-fourths of this amount should be instilled, since the hypertonicity of the solution will produce an egress of fluid into the peritoneal cavity producing uncomfortable abdominal distention and elevation of the diaphragms, precipitating respiratory difficulty.

After the abdomen is prepared, a puncture site 1½ to 3 cm. below the umbilicus is selected and is anesthetized with a local anesthetic (Xylocaine 1 per cent). A 14-gauge long needle is then inserted into the peritoneal cavity at the previously anesthetized site. Previously warmed dialysis solution containing 1.5 per cent glucose, 4 mEq. per liter potassium and 1 ml. of 1000-U.S.P.-units-per-ml. of aqueous heparin is instilled into the peritoneal cavity until the abdomen is tense; the tense abdomen facilitates insertion of the trochar. The needle is then removed and a 0.5 cm. stab wound through the skin is made at the puncture site to permit insertion of trochar and catheter. Cautiously, the trochar and catheter are inserted into the peritoneal cavity with a steady circular motion. Once the trochar and catheter are in the peritoneal cavity, the trochar is removed and the catheter is maneuvered into either lower quadrant. The fluid in the peritoneal cavity is removed and the dialysis commences. Generally, each pass takes 1 hour: 15 minutes for the fluid to flow into the peritoneal cavity, 30 minutes for dialysis and 15 minutes for removal. Equilibration between the plasma and dialysis fluid usually is maximum at 30 minutes, and longer periods of instillation are inefficient. If excessive fluid removal is desirable, the 1.5 per cent and 4.25 per cent solutions can be utilized alternately. Generally, 48 hours is sufficient for dialysis; however, if dialysis is being performed for hyperkalemia only, such as in the child with congenital adrenal hyperplasia, shorter periods of dialysis will suffice, and if dialysis is being performed to remove a toxic substance, longer periods may be desirable. The risk of infection increases considerably after 48 to 72 hours.

Prophylactic antibiotics are not used either locally or systemically. If fever or clinical evidence of septicemia or peritonitis develops, blood and peritoneal fluid cultures are obtained and, depending on the clinical status of the patient, systemic ampicillin therapy is started.

Complications. TROCHAR INSERTION. Bladder perforation will be evident if the returning dialysate solution has a urine odor. If the catheter is placed in the bladder via the trochar perforation, the patient will void large amounts shortly after each pass. Insertion of a Foley catheter for 7 to 10 days is generally curative. Dialysis can continue after insertion of the Foley catheter.

Bowel perforation is usually evident by the appearance of fecal material in the returning dialysis solution. If possible, dialysis should be discontinued and the perforation repaired surgically.

Vessel perforation can lead to catastrophic consequences. If an artery is punctured, shock is the initial finding. Shock should be treated with blood replacement and the perforation repaired immediately. With venous perforation the dialysis fluid is darker and shock may not occur.

In patients with a coagulopathy, such as the hemolytic-uremic syndrome, generalized peritoneal bleeding may mimic venous perforation. Since it is difficult at times to discern the degree of intraperitoneal bleeding by visual inspection, the performance of a hematocrit on the dialysis fluid may be helpful. If the hematocrit is greater than 5 ml. per 100 ml., significant bleeding is present and dialysis should be discontinued. Subsequent therapy will depend on serial blood hematocrit determinations.

TROCHAR REMOVAL. Fat and/or omental herniation occasionally occurs when the attendant trochar is removed. Since it is difficult to discern whether subcutaneous fat or omentum is present, surgical replacement of the herniated tissue is advisable.

SHOCK (HYPOTENSION). Excess fluid removal can precipitate hypotension. This is usually easily reversed with saline administration. In the child with edema and severe hypoalbuminemia, fluid removal from the interstitium may not occur until the serum albumin level is raised above 3.0 Gm. per 100 ml. with the use of intravenous Albumisol.

DISEQUILIBRIUM SYNDROME. Seizures occur with some frequency during the course of peritoneal dialysis. Persistent hypocalcemia after correction of acidosis is occasionally responsible; however, the disequilibrium syndrome is more frequently implicated. A more rapid decrease in the extracellular (as opposed to the intracellular) urea level leading to an osmotic gradient, which necessitates water imbibition by the cells and eventual water intoxication, has been implicated in the causation of this syndrome. Treatment with intravenous Valium,† 2 to 5 mg., usually terminates the seizure, and maintenance phenobarbital, 3 to 5 mg. per kilogram per 24 hours, is advisable for at least 24 to 48 hours after discontinuation of dialysis to prevent recurrence.

HYPERGLYCEMIA. Because the dialysis solutions contain higher glucose concentrations than does plasma, hyperglycemia occasionally results. Hyperosmolar coma can develop. Treatment with insulin may be necessary, and if dialysis must be continued, substitution of sorbitol for glucose is advisable.

Renal Vein Thrombosis

S. MICHAEL MAUER, M.D.

IN INFANCY

Management of babies with renal vein thrombosis (RVT) requires attention to etiologic factors, reversal of metabolic disturbances, precise delineation of the extent of involvement and control of the thrombotic process.

In infants with RVT associated with evidence of sepsis, it should be remembered that fulminant renal parenchymal infection may have initiated the thrombotic process. Cultures of the urine, blood and cerebrospinal fluid should be obtained and the infant begun on appropriate antimicrobial therapy. RVT in the infant of a diabetic mother requires management of the metabolic and respiratory complications of the underlying condition. Babies with severe dehydration should have rapid correction of their fluid and electrolyte imbalances. It is important to withhold potassium administration in these infants until the adequacy of renal function has been established. Fluid overload in the uremic infant with RVT is usually iatrogenic. With little or no renal function, diuretics are generally ineffective. Extreme pulmonary edema may require positive pressure ventilation and immediate phlebotomy (removing 10 to 15 ml. of blood per kilogram). Sorbitol administered repeatedly at 2- to 4-hour intervals is effective in producing osmotic diarrhea. It is used in a dose of 2 ml. per kilogram of the 70 per cent solution by mouth, or 10 ml. per kilogram of the 20 per cent solution by enema retained for 45 minutes. Peritoneal dialysis with a hypertonic solution such as Peridial or Dianeal, containing 7 Gm. per 100 ml. dextrose, or hemodialysis with aggressive ultrafiltration are also extremely effective methods of fluid removal. Severe uremia associated with RVT usually signifies bilateral acute renal venous obstruction. With uremia, particularly if associated with hyperelectrolytemia, an extreme hyperosmolar state may develop. This state is most efficiently managed by peritoneal dialysis or hemodialysis. In the hypernatremic uremic infant, dialysis should be carried out prior to obtaining contrast radiograms (intravenous pyelography or angiography), since the extreme hypertonicity of the contrast agents may precipitate intracranial bleeding, convulsions and coma, and may produce renal papillary necrosis. The kidney with acute venous obstruction is prone to spontaneous rupture, and massive subcapsular or retroperitoneal hemorrhage may develop, requiring whole blood administration for the control of shock and immediate surgical intervention to stem the bleeding. Bleeding associated with severe thrombocytopenia may be helped by a 10 ml. per kilogram infusion of platelet-rich plasma.

Precise definition of the extent of the thrombotic process is best achieved by angiography. The choice between arteriography and venography will depend on the experience and preference of the radiologist. In the newborn infant, renal arteriography via an umbilical artery is relatively easy to accomplish. If the process is unilateral and is unassociated with infection or uremia, a trial of medical management of the RVT is indicated and is usually successful, since extension of the process to involve the other kidney does not tend to occur.

Although its efficacy is unproved, anticoagulation therapy is the mainstay of the primary medical management of RVT. This therapy demands meticulous attention to details. Heparin is given as an initial intravenous injection of 20 units per kilogram followed immediately by a constant intravenous infusion at 20 units per kilogram per hour. The effect of heparin is noted by both the thrombin time (TT), which is very sensitive to low heparin concentrations, and by the activated partial thromboplastin time (APTT), which has a linear relationship to heparin levels.* The aim is to modulate the heparin infusion rate so as to maintain the TT at greater than 2 minutes *and* the APTT at approximately 10 seconds

† Manufacturer's precaution: The safety and efficacy of injectable Valium in children under 12 years of age have not been established.

* Use reagents of Hyland Laboratories (Costa Mesa, California) for APTT, and use great care in the blood sampling technique to avoid contamination with tissue fluid (use double syringe technique) or with heparin infusate (avoid heparin line).

above the base line value. This provides small but definite heparin effect without, particularly postoperatively, the major risk of bleeding which even moderate heparin concentrations may cause. After one or two days of therapy, as control of the process of intravascular coagulation is achieved with the heparin, the APTT may have to be maintained at 20 to 30 seconds above base line in order to maintain the TT at greater than 2 minutes. This is because the intravascular clotting process may be associated with a hypercoagulable state and thus a short APTT. Heparin therapy is continued for 10 to 14 days.

Fibrinolytic therapy (streptokinase) followed by heparinization has been used, reportedly with success, in RVT. This is a complex and risky form of treatment with which experience is limited; thus, it cannot be recommended for general use at this time.

Surgery is the treatment of choice for acute bilateral RVT, since survival by means of medical management is unusual. Bilateral RVT in infancy is almost always associated with inferior vena caval thrombosis; with this sudden loss of most avenues for collateral renal venous drainage, it becomes a race to remove the obstruction before bilateral renal infarction occurs. The infant with bilateral RVT should be prepared for surgery by the rapid correction of fluid, electrolyte and uremic abnormalities as outlined above. With incision of the inferior vena cava, the thrombus can be removed from this vessel and from the renal veins. Following removal of the renal vein clots, particularly if brisk bleeding from the renal vein does not occur, the kidney should be flushed via its artery with 25 to 50 ml. of 0.9 M saline containing 2 units heparin per ml.; this will dislodge many tiny thrombi from the intrarenal venous radicles. If oliguria is present, the infant should receive furosemide (Lasix),† 1 mg. per kilogram, and mannitol,‡ 1 Gm. per kilogram intravenously immediately after thrombectomy to increase renal perfusion and to establish good urinary flow. Anticoagulation with heparin should be started at surgery to prevent recurrence of thrombosis. The anticoagulation should then be maintained for 10 to 14 days as described above.

Surgery is mandatory if sepsis is present, since the infected thrombosed kidney must be removed.

† Manufacturer's precaution: Furosemide (Lasix) should not be given to children until further experience is accumulated.

‡ Manufacturer's precaution: Use of mannitol in pediatric patients has not been studied comprehensively.

Complete or segmental renal infarction following unilateral RVT may result in hypertension, requiring nephrectomy months to years after the acute thrombotic event. If bilateral renal cortical scarring results, medical therapy of the hypertension is the only course available.

IN OLDER CHILDREN

In older children, RVT has been associated with the nephrotic syndrome of any cause including congenital and nil lesion nephrosis, membranous nephropathy and systemic lupus erythematosus. Other causes include invasive renal tumors, trauma and local surgical intervention including renal transplantation. Thus, therapy must include the underlying disease as well as the thrombus per se. Further, in the older child, RVT often develops gradually, providing time for a marked increase in collateral renal venous drainage. Infarction is thus less common and uremia may be absent even with bilateral involvement. However, thromboembolism is more common. The basic principles of management outlined for infants apply to these children except that one may elect to manage bilateral RVT medically as long as renal function remains intact. If the underlying cause of the RVT cannot be eliminated (e.g., nephrotic syndrome which is resistant to therapy) long-term treatment with Coumadin is indicated.

Perinephritis and Perirenal Abscess

C. W. DAESCHNER, M.D.

Bacterial infection of the perirenal tissue is characterized by the acute onset of high septic fever, chills, malaise and *intense* local pain. The pain is unilateral, but localization to the flank, hip, psoas or abdominal area depends upon the site and distribution of the primary process. The infection may originate from rupture of a septic renal cortical abscess, primary cellulitis of the perirenal tissue or penetrating trauma. Although etiologic bacteria may vary widely, the Staphylococcus is the most common offender. Broad antibiotic coverage is indicated unless the specific etiologic agent is known. Frequently surgical drainage will be necessary to release loculated pus before signs and symptoms are relieved. In recent years perinephritic infections have been uncommon.

Urinary Tract Infections

HUGO F. CARVAJAL, M.D., *and*
C. W. DAESCHNER, M.D.

For the purpose of this discussion, it is assumed that infection of the urinary tract represents widespread bacterial contamination of the kidney and urinary collecting system. Present methodology does not readily permit exact definition, and signs and symptoms are unreliable guides to localization. It is desirable then to use generic terms such as "urinary tract infection" and reserve the specific diagnosis of "pyelonephritis," "cystitis" or "pyelitis" until the histologic specimen can be examined or until other similarly valid confirmatory evidence is found.

The successful management of patients with urinary tract infections evolves from fulfillment of four major therapeutic principles:

1. Correct establishment of diagnosis.
2. Selection of proper antimicrobial agents and therapeutic regimens.
3. Early correction of predisposing anatomic defects.
4. Adequate follow-up.

Establishment of Diagnosis. One of the most common therapeutic errors is the initiation of antibiotic therapy without documentation of infection. This does not imply that antibiotics need to be withheld until the responsible organism has been identified; it means that the institution of specific therapy should be preceded by careful examination of the urinary sediment for bacteria and that a "properly collected" urine specimen is obtained for culture and antibiotic sensitivity testing before treatment is started. Whenever possible, one should await the bacteriologic report and obtain additional cultures for confirmation.

Bacteria are not filtered by the glomerulus; hence the urine formed by the kidneys under normal circumstances is sterile. If the normal architecture of the urinary tract is maintained, bladder urine should likewise be sterile. During the act of voiding, however, the urine is frequently contaminated with bacteria from the urethra, glans, labia, vagina, skin and so forth. Careful washing of the external genitalia and surrounding structures minimizes the likelihood of contamination but does not ensure sterility.

To establish the diagnosis, one must demonstrate that the pathogenic organism is present in quantities not likely to be the result of contamination. Colony counts of 100,000 per ml. of urine or greater are generally accepted as evidence of infection. Colony counts below this level, however, need to be interpreted according to the method and technique used for urine collection. If the sample was obtained by spontaneous voiding, a colony count less than 10,000 can be regarded as being the result of contamination. Colony counts in the 10,000 to 100,000 range, however, should be viewed with concern as they may represent either infection or contamination (faulty technique).

When the urine is obtained by catheterization or suprapubic aspiration of the bladder, the possibility of contamination at the time of collection is practically eliminated and counts below 10,000 can be indicative of significant infection.

Regardless of the methodology, falsely low counts may be the result of prior antimicrobial therapy, polyuria or an obstructed ureter. The examination of at least two urine samples is therefore needed before a high level of reliability is assumed.

When facilities for quantitative cultures are not convenient, a relatively reliable evaluation can be accompanied by microscopic examination of the urinary sediment after Gram or methylene blue staining. The latter is perhaps better for defining morphology. The presence of clearly defined bacteria in each field is highly suggestive of a significant colony count, but failure to identify bacteria by this means does not exclude infection. Semiquantitative culture methods for office use are now available as inexpensive and relatively reliable disposable units (Testuria or slide culture methods).

Selection of Antimicrobial Agent. General measures include a generous fluid intake, both to replace enteric and febrile losses and to ensure a large urine volume. The latter may reduce stasis in the urinary tract and relieve signs and symptoms, but it is unwise to assume that such patients are cured. It seems reasonable to recommend bed rest during febrile and other acute phases of the illness, but prolonged bed rest is not indicated. The role of good perineal hygiene in the female is unknown, but again it seems reasonable to encourage this. Some advocate the substitution of shower for tub bathing in females who show recurrent urinary tract infection.

Antibiotic treatment is indicated in all patients and must be initiated as soon as the diagnosis is well established. In some cases it may be necessary to begin therapy before confirmatory evidence of infection is available or the antibiotic sensitivity spectrum of the infecting organism is known. Under these circumstances, the selection of the antibiotic to be used must be based on recent and reliable epidemiologic data.

Since *Escherichia coli* continues to be responsible for most initial urinary tract infections, the antibiotic of choice should be one that will eradicate this organism.

Nitrofurantoin* is particularly useful in *E. coli* urinary tract infections and is effective against most other urinary pathogens. At the usual recommended dose of 5 to 7 mg. per kilogram per day, disproportionately high concentrations of the drug develop in the kidney. This is apparently related to the recycling of the drug by the renal tubule and perhaps explains the greater effectiveness of this drug in urinary as contrasted to systemic bacterial infections. It is our habit to begin treatment with this drug in patients with symptomatic but not systemic evidence of urinary tract infection. It is well tolerated orally except for mild gastrointestinal irritation and the latter usually disappears when the dose is reduced. The fact that it does not modify stool flora makes it suitable for prolonged suppressive therapy as well.

Judging from recent reports, *E. coli* sensitivity to the sulfonamides is changing, and today a significant percentage of common urinary pathogens may be resistant to this agent. Treatment of urinary tract infections with sulfonamides, best represented by sufisoxazole (Gantrisin), however, continues to offer certain advantages. These include the good tissue and urine levels of drug, the relative freedom from toxic side effects and the low cost to the patient. In the case of sulfisoxazole,† an initial loading dose of 0.1 Gm. per kilogram followed by .05 Gm. per kilogram every 8 hours for a total of two to three weeks, is usually sufficient to eradicate most sensitive urinary pathogens.

For several years, ampicillin enjoyed an excellent reputation in urinary tract infections and was considered by many to be the antibiotic of choice. However, in recent years, the report of *E. coli* strains resistant to this agent have increased to the point that it is estimated that 20 to 30 per cent of urinary *E. coli* strains are now highly resistant. Although no longer considered a drug of primary choice, ampicillin is a well-tolerated antibiotic, gives excellent blood and tissue levels, and is still a very useful drug in the management of selected patients with urinary tract infections. The drug is bactericidal and, when given orally in doses of 100 mg. per kilogram of body weight per day (four divided doses), adequate urinary levels are attained.

In patients requiring parenteral antibiotics, gentamicin and kanamycin are certainly the leaders. The former, having replaced polymyxin B, currently enjoys the greater popularity.

Although considerable controversy remains and proponents of different therapeutic programs argue as to what should be "adequate length of therapy," the truth of the matter is that the recurrence rate, particularly in females, continues to be high, regardless of the therapeutic program used.

Although we currently favor the two-week course, and in most cases adhere to it, we are the first to recognize the need for well-designed double blind prospective studies to answer this particular question.

Correction of Predisposing Anatomic Defects. Although considerable controversy surrounds the indication for complete urologic studies, most physicians and surgeons agree that the initial evaluation should be radiologic. An intravenous pyelogram and a voiding cystogram are definitely indicated, if not in all children with urinary tract infections, certainly in all males after the first infection and in all females after the second infection. It is well accepted that this initial evaluation should be performed after the patient has been adequately treated (four to six weeks after diagnosis) and has recovered from the effects of the inflammatory process which may otherwise be difficult to differentiate from true anatomic defects.

Additional urologic investigations are indicated if the radiologic studies disclose significant abnormalities or if the patient continues to have recurrent infections despite what on x-ray appears to be an intact genitourinary system.

The purpose of this investigation is early detection of surgically correctable anatomic defects; institution of appropriate therapy should follow the diagnosis.

Obstruction, whether functional or anatomic, must be promptly corrected if recurrent infection and progressive deterioration of kidney function are to be prevented.

Follow-up. More important than length of initial therapy is adequate follow-up. Judging from various prospective studies, 25 to 75 per cent of female patients with initial urinary tract infections will have a recurrence within two to three years from onset. The physician's responsibility is to promptly detect and eradicate these infections. This can best be accomplished through well-organized follow-up programs in

---

* Manufacturer's precaution: Nitrofurantoin should not be administered to infants under one month of age.

† Manufacturer's precaution: Sulfisoxazole (Gantrisin) is contraindicated in infants under two months of age except in the treatment of congenital toxoplasmosis as adjunctive therapy with pyrimethamine.

which cultures are obtained routinely at fixed intervals.

It is appropriate to begin therapy with an antibiotic likely to be effective, but soon thereafter one must demonstrate its efficacy or recognize its failure. If the antimicrobial agent selected is an effective one, the patient's urine should be sterile in 48 to 72 hours. It is therefore good practice to obtain a culture two or three days after the initiation of treatment either to confirm the suitability of the therapeutic choice or to provide a basis for making a new selection. The patient should not be dismissed until post-treatment cultures or the stained urine sediment at approximately four weeks after treatment is negative. Subsequent cultures at 3, 6, 9, 15, 24 and 36 months after the last infection are in order if the at-risk patient is to be identified early and the number of chronic infections reduced.

Recurrent Infections. These patients present quite a different problem. Not infrequently they have multiple acute episodes, and some require years of intermittent or continuous therapy. It is essential that the etiologic bacteria be identified and tested for antibiotic sensitivity. Use of the specific antibiotic in full therapeutic dose for two to three weeks should be followed by sulfonamide‡ (or nitrofurantoin)§ for four to six additional weeks. If recurrences become numerous, the physician may reasonably elect to continue antimicrobial treatment for months or even years.

A detailed discussion of all the antibiotics is unnecessary here; however, some characteristics of certain less commonly required agents should be mentioned. The tetracyclines have a broad antibacterial spectrum, which includes most of the common urinary pathogens with the exception of Proteus and Pseudomonas. The latter are common in uncomplicated urinary tract infections. Since the tetracyclines are well absorbed following oral administration and produce good tissue and urine concentrations of active drug, they might be expected to be highly desirable agents for the management of urinary tract infections. However, experience indicates that during therapy, resistant strains emerge rapidly and that when prolonged or repeated administration is necessary there is a tendency for the original sensitive organisms to be replaced by more resistant strains or species (e.g., Proteus or Pseudomonas). Their marked tendency, when given to small children, to cause permanent dental staining further detracts from their usefulness in pediatrics.

The cephalosporins now available (cephaloridine‖ and cephalothin) are quite effective against all coliform bacteria except Aerobacter and Pseudomonas. They are excreted in the urine in an unmodified, active form. Their renal toxicity limits their use to patients with good renal function and good hydration. Oral forms, particularly cephalexin, now undergoing clinical trial, show promise in long-term management of urinary tract infection.

Carbenicillin is a broad-spectrum penicillin which has been shown to be effective in Pseudomonas and Proteus infections of the urinary tract. At present, the drug is only available for parenteral use, but oral forms are being investigated. Carbenicillin offers the advantage of producing excellent urinary levels and low toxicity and should form a part of the physician's armamentarium for the treatment of acute or chronic infections.

Gentamicin is a relatively new parenteral antibiotic which appears to have a significant role in the management of Pseudomonas urinary tract infections. The propensity of this agent to both ototoxicity and nephrotoxicity (particularly in the presence of impaired renal function) requires that it be reserved for serious infections and for resistant infections not amenable to other antimicrobial agents. The patient must be observed carefully to ensure that good hydration is maintained and to detect early signs of drug toxicity.

Finally, it should be remembered that in vitro sensitivity testing generally may be misleading, and an in vivo trial of an agent is often indicated when its therapeutic spectrum includes the etiologic organism.

Chronic Infection. Chronic infection of the urinary tract is frequently silent and is most often associated with significant anatomic or functional abnormalities. When the functional abnormalities can be eradicated, the hope for cure is reasonable; when they cannot, cure is infrequent. Culture and sensitivity testing are particularly important, because the etiologic organism is less predictable, and not infrequently mixed infection exists. Initial treatment in these patients should be similar to that for acute recurrent infections, and good symptomatic relief can be expected; however, the frequent recurrence of symptoms or persisting silent bacteriuria

‡ Manufacturer's precaution: Sulfonamide is contraindicated in infants under two months of age.

§ Manufacturer's precaution: Nitrofurantoin should not be administered to infants under one month of age.

‖ Manufacturer's precaution: The safety of cephaloridine in premature infants and infants under one month of age has not been established.

following cessation of therapy may encourage the physician to give prolonged periods of antimicrobial therapy.

As renal insufficiency develops, supportive therapy to combat hypertension and hypoplastic anemia should be added as appropriate clinical indications appear. Unilateral pyelonephritis with renal atrophy and hypertension may indicate nephrectomy, but only when the other kidney is uninvolved and function in the infected kidney is negligible.

Renal Tuberculosis. This is an infrequent but serious form of urinary tract infection both because it usually implies significant involvement of the kidney, and because if untreated it is quite contagious. The diagnosis is usually suspected by the presence of a positive tuberculin test or chest radiogram in a patient with painless gross hematuria or "sterile" pyuria. It can be confirmed by urine culture and requires prolonged therapy (p. 621).

Hemorrhagic Cystitis. This occurs infrequently in children and may represent chemical, mechanical or infectious inflammation of the urinary bladder. There is usually fever, acute suprapubic pain, dysuria, urgency and frequency, together with grossly hematuric urine—sometimes containing clots, but never erythrocyte or hemoglobin casts.

The causative bacterium is frequently *E. coli*, and treatment with a sulfonamide, nitrofurantoin or ampicillin, as for acute urinary tract infection, is effective. In many of these patients the illness is self-limited and no bacterial agent is found; therefore a viral etiology is assumed.

Foreign bodies, calculi and tumors may also present the clinical syndrome of hemorrhagic cystitis. Cyclophosphamide therapy may produce an acute hemorrhagic cystitis and in some cases lead to permanent vascular changes (telangiectasia) in the bladder mucosa. When possible, removal of the offending agent is the obvious treatment for these patients.

Urolithiasis

A. BARRY BELMAN, M.D., M.S.

Recent reports from the United States and Britain note that urinary tract stones are responsible for only one in 6000 hospital admissions (Bass and Emanuel, Myers, and Wenzl et al.). Of particular note is the complete absence of uric acid calculi in patients recently reviewed, and the low incidence in the Negro population.

Patients with urinary calculi present most frequently with hematuria or symptoms of urinary tract infection. Abdominal pain may also be the primary complaint, particularly in the presence of obstruction. The diagnosis of urinary tract calculi is made secondarily, i.e., when patients with hematuria, urinary tract infections or abdominal discomfort undergo urography in an effort to ascertain the cause of their presenting complaints. The necessity for complete evaluation of patients with hematuria or urinary tract infection is underscored by the high incidence of anatomic abnormalities noted when such screening is carried out.

Approximately half the patients with stones who are seen by the physician will have an anatomic abnormality, usually of an obstructive type, as the underlying cause. Most of these present with infection, and the stones are generally calcium ammonium phosphate. Obstruction resulting in renal calculi may occur at the ureteropelvic junction, along the course of the ureter (most often at the ureterovesical junction), at the bladder outlet or intraurethrally. Stones may be lodged at any point proximal to the obstruction. Patients with stone disease in association with obstruction frequently have severe damage to the involved renal unit, particularly if the obstruction has been present for a long time.

Identifiable metabolic disorders are the underlying cause of stones in 10 to 20 per cent of children. Idiopathic hypercalciuria or hypercalciuria secondary to hyperparathyroidism or hypercortisonism produce radiopaque calcium stones. Familial forms of oxaluria, cystinuria or other forms of aminoaciduria may result in calculi, the composition of which is related to the metabolic disorder. We recently removed a xanthine calculus from the renal pelvis of a girl whose serum uric acid was zero. A younger sister was evaluated and was also noted to have a serum uric acid of zero; however, she had not developed stones. Neither child was taking medication prior to diagnosis.

Iatrogenic calculi may result from the milk alkali syndrome or excessive vitamin D ingestion. Foreign bodies in the urinary tract produce stones and are usually seen in the bladders of little girls, though boys are not immune. Immobilization occurring with prolonged orthopedic manipulations also may be associated with stone disease in children, but is nowhere nearly as frequent as in immobilized adults. Urinary calculi have not been associated with metabolic bone disease in children in any of the recent reviews. Nephrocalcinosis has been noted with renal tubular acidosis, oxalosis and patients on long-term exogenous steroids.

Stones associated with infection and obstruction are best treated by finding the underlying cause of the obstruction and correcting it. Calculi are removed simultaneously, such as removal of a renal pelvic stone in conjunction with repair of a ureteropelvic junction obstruction. It is imperative that all of the calculus be removed at the time of operation, since any residual fragments serve as a nidus for recurrence. In the absence of a known underlying cause which can be treated, maintenance of a dilute urine may be the only therapeutic device possible. This usually requires that the patient awaken during the night to drink additional water in an effort to avoid nocturnal urinary concentration. Additionally, aluminum gels have been used in the treatment of phosphatic calculi (Shorr and Carter).

Patients with cystine stones are treated with alkalinization of the urine or with penicillamine under careful supervision, since the side effects are multiple. Alkalinization is attained with an oral citrate mixture (Polycitra) and is verified by frequent monitoring of the urinary pH. It has recently been suggested that the urine need not be continuously alkaline in these patients. Since cystine is highly soluble, intermittent alkalinity during each 24-hour period prevents stone formation. Stone formation secondary to hyperoxaluria has been successfully controlled with oral magnesium oxide (Silver and Brendler), and our two sisters who are unable to convert xanthine to uric acid are on a regimen of urinary alkalinization. No further stones have formed. Though uric acid calculi have not been noted in children recently, allopurinol* should be considered in the therapeutic regimen in such a patient.

References

Bass, H. N., and Emanuel, B.: Nephrolithiasis in Children. *J. Urol.*, 95:749, 1966.

Myers, N. A. A.: Urolithiasis in Childhood. *Arch. Dis. Child.*, 32:48, 1957.

Shorr, E., and Carter, A. C.: Aluminum Gels in the Management of Renal Phosphatic Calculi. *J.A.M.A.*, 144:1549, 1950.

Silver, L., and Brendler, H.: Use of Magnesium Oxide in the Management of Familial Oxaluria. *J. Urol.*, 106:274, 1971.

Wenzl, J. E., Burke, E. C., Stickler, G. B., and Utz, D. C.: Nephrolithiasis and Nephrocalcinosis in Children. *Pediatrics,* 41:57, 1968.

* Manufacturer's precaution: Allopurinol is contraindicated for use in children except for hyperuricemia secondary to malignancy.

Exstrophy of the Urinary Bladder

JOHN K. LATTIMER, M.D.

The best therapy for exstrophy varies with the patient. For example, some patients are born with large elastic bladders which evert and stretch with crying, and which can be completely inverted into the abdomen with the pressure of a finger. Such bladders could obviously be formed into an elastic sac with a possibility for detrusor action, and anatomic closure should certainly be attempted, assuming that the ureters and kidneys are intact and functioning well. At the other extreme are children born with a tiny fibrotic disk of bladder remnant, no larger than 2 cm. in diameter, which has absolutely no elasticity and cannot be inverted into the abdomen at all by pressure of the probing finger. Such cases should be diverted with an ileal conduit or ureterostomy, and the anatomic reconstruction confined to the prostatic urethra and penis, or the vulva and clitoris.

Between these two extremes is a group of patients with bladders of intermediate size, some of which may grow to adequate size if they are reinserted into the abdomen. This has been the experience of both Dr. Williams of England and ourselves. If there is some indication of elasticity in the bladder remnant, we are inclined to give it a chance by reinserting it into the abdomen to see whether it will then grow and become elastic.

Other associated features may detract from the suitability of some patients for simple anatomic closure, and must be taken into account. For example, severe dilation of the lower ureteral segment on either side, or of the entire ureter and kidney, seen on intravenous urograms, would certainly argue against immediate anatomic reimplantation. If these conditions could be remedied first, then closure might be considered. The presence of a large omphalocele, or deformities of the rectum or other organs such as the heart, might argue against extensive multiple reconstructive procedures. Simple rectal prolapse, common in children with exstrophy, can be remedied easily and is not a contraindication.

Practically all exstrophic bladders that have been put back into the abdomen lack a valve mechanism to prevent the reflux of the urine up to the kidneys. Thus, antireflux operations must be anticipated to cope with the reflux problem as well as to repair the epispadias.

No attempt to make these children truly continent can be permitted until after the reflux has been corrected. This will mean a delay of some years in all probability, during which time the patient will remain wet because of constant urinary leakage through the urethra.

The accumulated experience of several clinics seems to indicate that the optimum course with these children is to place the bladders back in the abdomen in those cases which have some elasticity, leaving the patient totally incontinent for a period of years, until the bladder has a chance to grow sufficiently to accommodate antireflux operations. If these are successful, then an effort can be made to make the patient completely continent. If the patient is rendered continent at too early an age, dilation of the ureters and kidneys occurs and chronic infection compels conversion of the case to an ileal conduit type of diversion. The possibility that investigative workers can devise a practical bladder substitute, either from bowel or using a prosthesis, is not too promising at this moment, but could evolve rapidly and should be kept in mind.

After experience with approximately 170 cases of exstrophy, treated by various methods, it is my opinion that the majority should have the benefit of at least one attempt at anatomic closure, according to the foregoing precepts. If complications arise, or if it does not work out satisfactorily, the case can always be converted to ileal conduit or other diversion, before too much harm can be done.

Vesicoureteral Reflux

ALAN B. RETIK, M.D.

Vesicoureteral reflux is an abnormal condition which has been detected in from 30 to 70 per cent of children undergoing urologic investigation for recurrent urinary tract infections. The treatment of reflux depends to a large extent upon the etiologic factors involved. A systematic evaluation of the child with urinary tract infection is essential for accurate diagnosis, prognosis and therapy. The diagnostic tools employed are the excretory urogram, voiding cystourethrogram and cystoscopy.

It is well documented that urinary infection may be a cause as well as a result of reflux. Radiologic evaluation of a child with a urinary tract infection should be delayed until the urine has been sterile for three to four weeks. This will usually eliminate the group of children with reflux secondary to inflammatory changes. However, if there is difficulty sterilizing the urine or if the child remains symptomatic, these investigations should be performed sooner because a serious disorder may be present.

Anatomic lesions of the ureterovesical junction associated with reflux include absence or partial absence of the intravesical ureter, a paraureteral diverticulum in which the intravesical ureter lacks muscular support, and a markedly underdeveloped trigone with laterally placed patulous ureteral orifices. Reflux is often seen in children with autonomous neurogenic bladders and is associated with loss of tone in the bladder detrusor. A small percentage of children may have reflux secondary to obstruction at or distal to the bladder neck. Children with bladder exstrophy and those born with the syndrome of absence of abdominal musculature, cryptorchidism and urinary tract abnormalities often exhibit reflux associated with one of the previously mentioned primary abnormalities at the ureterovesical junction.

Treatment. Treatment must be individualized; such factors as length of history, age at onset, number of infections and the ease with which they are controlled should be considered in deciding whether surgery should be performed.

Operative. The indications for antireflux surgery are recurrent urinary infection despite continuous chemotherapy, radiologic evidence of chronic pyelonephritis, or persistent reflux associated with a basic anatomic abnormality at the ureterovesical junction. Obstructions at or distal to the bladder neck associated with reflux should be corrected. Surgical correction of the reflux should be performed as well if the ureterovesical junction is anatomically abnormal. Antireflux surgery in children with neurogenic bladder dysfunction is not recommended because results have been disappointing. This problem is best handled by a nonoperative program or, more likely, by ileal diversion.

The type of antireflux procedure most often employed is the Politano–Leadbetter operation with the creation of an adequate submucosal tunnel.

Nonoperative. It is generally agreed that reflux in the absence of infection does not cause renal damage. Therefore, if it is decided to pursue a nonoperative program, it is imperative that continuous chemotherapy be employed as long as reflux persists. The drugs most often used for this purpose are sulfisoxazole,* nitro-

* Manufacturer's precaution: Sulfisoxazole is contraindicated in infants less than two months of age except in the treatment of congenital toxoplasmosis as adjunctive therapy with pyrimethamine.

furantoin† and methenamine mandelate. Urinalysis and culture with colony count should be obtained at four- to eight-week intervals. Excretory urograms and voiding cystourethrograms are repeated at 6- to 12-month intervals. In the infant and young child with severe vesicoureteral reflux, pyelonephritis may progress rapidly and x-ray studies should be performed at more frequent intervals. Other measures designed to reduce the incidence of urinary stasis and infection should be encouraged. These include adequate hydration, attention to proper perineal hygiene, a frequent voiding schedule and double voiding in the older cooperative child. Measures designed to reduce outlet resistance, such as urethral dilatation, meatotomy or internal urethrotomy, may be helpful in eliminating minor degrees of reflux or in reducing the severity of reflux.

The ultimate goal of nonoperative management is the cessation of reflux. This has been reported to occur by maturation of the trigone or by healing of a chronically inflamed ureterovesical junction. When reflux is still present at puberty, it is likely to persist and surgical intervention should be recommended.

Neurogenic Vesical Dysfunction

ALAN B. RETIK, M.D.

Neurogenic vesical dysfunction in childhood is most often due to spina bifida with myelomeningocele or sacral deformities. It is but one aspect of the difficult problem confronting the pediatrician, neurosurgeon, orthopedic surgeon, urologist and psychiatrist. However, the ultimate prognosis in those children who have survived the early hazards of meningitis and hydrocephalus depends upon the severity of their renal disease. Progressive renal dilatation and deterioration may occur over a period of years in urinary tracts which initially appear to be anatomically and functionally normal. Not only does renal failure cause serious morbidity, but urinary incontinence plays an important role in the social acceptability of the child. In general, the bladder disturbance is of the lower motor neuron type, although it is difficult to correlate bladder behavior with the level of the spinal lesion and the degree of paralysis of other functions.

The goals of therapy in the neurogenic bladder are preservation of renal function and urinary continence. Infants and children are managed by conservative means—providing that chemical and radiologic evidence of renal deterioration is not present, urinary infection is controlled, and Credé and other maneuvers produce reasonably dry intervals. The bladder must be evacuated by manual expression at regular intervals to ensure a low residual urine and reduce dribbling incontinence. Older children readily learn to perform the Credé maneuver on themselves. Fecal impaction must be avoided to aid bladder expression. This is most readily achieved by the use of bowel softeners, but often enemas two or three times a week or even digital assistance may be necessary.

An excretory urogram should be performed during the first month of life and repeated at regular intervals. Urinalysis and urine culture with colony counts must be obtained every two to four months. Severe vesicoureteral reflux, demonstrated by voiding cystourethrography, occurs frequently and may lead to chronic urinary infection and severe pyelonephritis. Continuous chemotherapy is often necessary in these children.

When the bladder fails to empty properly following conservative measures, operations designed to lower urethral resistance may be undertaken. Anterior vesicourethroplasty, transurethral resection of the bladder neck or pudendal neurectomy may be of occasional benefit in the boy. These procedures are usually doomed to failure in girls. Anticholinergic drugs such as Pro-Banthine (7.5 to 15 mg. three times a day) may be of some help in the spastic bladder. Similarly, Urecholine (0.6 mg. per kilogram per day) may help evacuate a large atonic bladder.

Many children have some degree of incontinence, requiring an external collecting apparatus or urinary diversion. In the boy, incontinence can often be managed with a penile urinal, providing that the phallus is large enough. In the girl, unfortunately, an external collecting device is not feasible.

Indications for urinary diversion are hydronephrosis, progressively decreasing renal function, repeated attacks of pyelonephritis or urinary incontinence. The most satisfactory form of diversion is the ileal conduit, which has as the advantage over other methods of drainage, a lower incidence of urinary tract infection. In the severely uremic child with dilated, tortuous ureters, ureterostomy should be strongly considered as an alternative and simpler procedure. Stomal problems are not uncommon with all methods of tubeless urinary diversion, and stomal revisions may be necessary.

† Manufacturer's precaution: Nitrofurantoin should not be administered to children under one month of age.

Patent Urachus and Urachal Cyst

JOHN K. LATTIMER, M.D.

The treatment for these two conditions is surgical. The principal questions are, "Why is the urachus patent?" and "When is the patient in optimal condition for the operation?" Simple excision of the patent urachus or urachal cyst with exploration of the dome of the bladder is easily done, and the opening should be closed by inverting sutures. Before any such operation is undertaken, the reason for the patent urachus must be determined and eliminated.

One of the most common causes is obstruction of the prostatic urethra by so-called urethral valves. These valves are, in truth, a membrane which starts at the verumontanum on the floor of the prostatic urethra and extends from the floor to the roof of the urethra, with the attachment at the roof slightly farther out in the urethra, distal to the verumontanum, in the direction of the external sphincter. This membrane commonly splits in the midline or is broken by the passage of a catheter or instrument, but the partially obstructing remnants remain and can be seen through the cystoscope as two cusplike sacs, which bulge toward the tip of the penis, owing to the pressure of the urine flowing out from the bladder. As a result of this obstruction, the prostatic urethra is greatly lengthened and expanded, causing a spool-shaped dilation of the prostatic urethra which is readily seen on a voiding urethrogram. It also displaces the verumontanum from its normal infantile position at the lip of the bladder, outward for a distance of an inch or more. The rim of the detrusor can be seen through the urethroscope as a prominent ring, which has the appearance of an obstruction, but is usually not truly obstructive. The bladder wall is usually greatly thickened and heavily trabeculated as a result of the back pressure, and the ureters may be dilated, with severe damage to the kidneys due to such back pressure.

The back pressure in utero may also keep the urachus patent, and whenever a patent urachus is found, a search for urethral valves should be made both with the cystourethroscope and by voiding cystourethrograms. If a catheter cannot be inserted through the urethra, then a suprapubic puncture may be attempted, with filling of the bladder through a tiny polyethylene tube, threaded over a stylet which has been inserted suprapubically, through a fine needle. A solution of 50 ml. of Hypaque (diatrizoate sodium) in 250 ml. of normal saline solution (sterile) containing 100 mg. of fresh Achromycin is injected, and pictures are taken at intervals until there is good visualization or until a pressure of 24 inches of water is achieved. As a child voids, a urethrogram can be taken. It should be remembered that any instrumentation may introduce infection which could prove fatal within a few hours in a debilitated child who has been obstructed. Thus the means for open drainage should be instantly available. Urethral valves can usually be resected with a resectoscope or cut away retropubically (if absolutely necessary). Drainage of secondary points of obstruction which may have resulted from the kinking of dilated ureters or hypertrophy of the muscle at the bladder outlet--must be dealt with when they are encountered.

Other causes for urethral obstruction which might bring about patent urachus are severe meatal stricture or severe atresia of the urethra. Congenital deficiencies of the abdominal musculature with associated genitourinary anomalies frequently have urethral valves of a severe degree, with patent urachus in approximately half of the reported cases. The absence of abdominal musculature in the region of the urachus in these patients is something of a hazard to a strong closure of the abdominal wound after operation, and extra precautions such as stay sutures and support with binders must be utilized in the postoperative care of this condition.

For intravenous pyelography, we use Renografin (methylglucamine diatrizoate), 2 ml. per kilogram of body weight with *no* dehydration.

Tumors of the Bladder and Prostate

JOHN K. LATTIMER, M.D.

TUMORS OF THE BLADDER

There have been occasional rare reports of papillary tumors of low grades of malignancy in the urinary bladders of children. These are usually heralded by gross hematuria. If the child's urethra is large enough to accommodate a number 16 or 21 French cystoscope, which is almost always true of even infant females, then the tumor can be fulgurated cystoscopically with anticipation of cure. Conscientious follow-up cystoscopic examinations, always done under anesthesia, at intervals of three months at first, and at increasing intervals of four, six, nine and 12 months thereafter, are essential to detect recurrences, or multifocal tumors too small to see on the first examination.

Recurrences have not been reported on any great scale in the few children known to have had such bladder tumors. In males, if the urethra is too small to accommodate a number 16 cystoscope, a suprapubic approach with fulguration of the bladder tumor should be done. Fill the bladder, by way of an inlying catheter, with an effective topical anticancer agent such as Thio-TEPA (60 mg. in 60 ml. of sterile water) immediately before opening the bladder, and empty it within five minutes so that there will be no overflow and spillage of contaminated urine. The catheter can be drained just before the bladder is opened suprapubically.

A search should be made for carcinogenic factors in the diet and environment of the child. Recurrences should be treated locally with topical Thio-TEPA and fulguration if minor, or by open surgery if major.

Ascorbic acid, 500 mg. three times a day orally, has been suggested as a possible means of reducing potential carcinogens in the urine.

SARCOMA BOTRYOIDES (RHABDOMYOSARCOMA) OF THE BLADDER OR PROSTATE

This is occasionally seen in children, especially females, appearing like a large bunch of grapes projecting up into the bladder; it sometimes originates from the urethra or vagina. This condition is best treated by immediate radical excision of the tumor and node-bearing areas, up to the bifurcation of the iliac vessels. Pelvic exenteration may be indicated if the rectal or uterine area is invaded.

Diversion of the urine by ileal conduit may permit radiotherapy of the tumor-bearing area without excessive irradiation of the ileal conduit itself. The prognosis is poor, radical surgery offering the only hope. Palliation may be obtained in some inoperable cases by the use of moderate exposures to radiation.

The role of chemotherapy, as in other forms of rhabdomyosarcoma, requires further evaluation in view of the generally poor outlook.

TUMORS OF THE PROSTATE

Sarcomas of the prostate have been reported in young boys, which are usually detected as a large mass growing with startling rapidity. These can be treated only by an attempt at excision in the widest possible manner, taking all of the genitals, with high ileal conduit diversion, and excision of possible node-bearing areas up to the bifurcation of the iliac vessels. Excision of a thick layer of the undersurface of the pubic and iliac bones, contiguous with the tumor, is necessary in an effort to prevent local recurrences.

If the tumor tissue indicated radiosensitivity by autoradiographic studies, radiotherapy might be attempted, although the likelihood of radiosensitivity is small.

If the child is approaching puberty, certainly bilateral orchidectomy and androgen assays of the urine should be done, seeking any possible excessive secretion of these hormones. If so, estrogens such as stilbestrol, 2 mg. daily, could be given orally, even though it has not been clearly shown that antiandrogenic therapy helps sarcomas of the prostate. If the tumor proves to be an *adenocarcinoma* of the prostate, excision plus castration should be performed, and estrogen (2 mg. of stilbestrol daily by mouth) should be given.

Disorders of the Bladder, Prostate and Urethra

LOWELL R. KING, M.D.

Children often require urologic evaluation because of urinary tract infection, abdominal mass, hematuria, poor urinary stream, voiding at inappropriate times during the day and other, less frequent and sometimes less compelling reasons. In general, diagnostic studies should be systematically performed so that no significant abnormality is overlooked. A micturition cystourethrogram, which may be followed by intravenous pyelography, is usually the first special study done, and it is the single test most likely to establish the presence of a significant anatomic abnormality, allowing one to make the diagnosis of vesicoureteral reflux and some types of bladder outlet obstruction. Cystoscopy and urethral calibration are useful when the radiographic studies do not reveal a cause for the presenting symptomatology, and may also, of course, be necessary as a therapeutic measure.

Bladder outlet obstruction initiates compensatory hypertrophy of the detrusor, manifest as bladder trabeculation – in many instances, the earliest objective sign of outlet obstruction. If obstruction persists, hydroureteronephrosis begins, and bladder decompensation occurs, resulting in the presence of residual urine in the bladder after voiding. These diagnostic criteria must be kept in mind, because the reliable diagnosis of obstruction early in the course of the disease is often difficult.

Meatal stenosis, in boys, is treated by meatotomy. Except in the case of infants, a general anesthesia is required. In girls, the distal urethral ring is more commonly the narrowest point in the urethra than is the meatus. This is detected under anesthesia by urethral calibration with bulbous bougies of increasing size. The caliber of the meatus and distal urethral ring may be enlarged by dilatation of the urethra to 26 French or greater, or by internal urethrotomy.

A congenital obstructing circumferential fold in the mucous membrane of the male urethra may be ruptured by urethral dilatation. Leaflet or cusp-shaped valves of the posterior urethra are engaged in the working element of the miniature resectoscope and are excised or fulgurated endoscopically. Leaflet valves in the anterior urethra may be treated in like manner but more often require precise open excision. Obstructing polyps of the verumontanum are excised endoscopically, with care to excise the tissue at the base of the stalk so that the polyp will not regrow.

Primary bladder neck obstruction is relatively rare, and it is most often seen in infant males with severe secondary hydronephrosis. Prompt cystostomy or cutaneous ureterostomy may be necessary to protect residual renal function. Open *anterior* Y-V-plasty of the bladder neck is the treatment of choice to enlarge the bladder outlet. The obstructing tissue in the posterior aspect of the bladder neck is usually not excised, because retrograde ejaculation is likely to occur after this maneuver.

The treatment of hypospadias varies, depending on the location of the meatus and the degree of chordee present. When the chordee is severe, a buccal smear should be performed to ascertain that the patient is a genetic male. Correction is performed, or staged repairs begun, at about two years of age. When the meatus is at the coronal sulcus, and chordee is absent or involves only the glans, no treatment is required. Dorsal meatotomy and circumcision to remove the dorsal hood improve the appearance of the penis, however.

When the hypospadiac urethral orifice is more proximal than the midpenile shaft level, staged urethroplasty or, alternatively, utilization of a full-thickness free skin graft is necessary. The graft should be from a nonhair-bearing area, such as the prepuce or the inside of the arm.

Chordee is first released, and the hypospadiac meatus is detached. The graft is rolled into a tube over a piece of rubber catheter or other suitable stent. The graft is sewn to the meatus and to the ventral aspect of the glans. This newly formed urethra is then covered by the skin of the lateral aspect of the penis and the remainder of the dorsal hood, which is transposed to the ventral surface of the penis. Urinary diversion is required for seven to 14 days.

Chordee without hypospadias is treated by Z-plasty of the skin of the ventral penile shaft to allow the penis to straighten.

Duplications of the urethra are treated by urethrourethrostomy, complete excision of the more hypoplastic member or, in instances in which one hypospadiac orifice is present, anastomosis of the short urethra to the urethra ending in a glandular orifice.

Epispadias with incontinence in girls is treated by transvaginal plication of the bladder neck and urethra using urethroscopic control. Layers of plicating sutures are placed until the internal vesical sphincter becomes competent and can be seen to close as the urethroscope is withdrawn.

Epispadias with incontinence in boys is treated by formation of additional urethral length from muscle of the posterior aspect of the bladder base. To make this feasible, the ureters must usually be reimplanted into the bladder well above the trigone. A midline strip of trigone, 3 to 5 cm. in length, is then rolled into a tube 16 to 20 French in caliber. This healthy bladder muscle now serves as a urethral sphincter. The distal urethra is buried, and a more cylindrical appearance is given to the penis by approximating the corpora cavernosa anteriorly.

Diverticula of the bladder are excised, if sizable. Because about half are due to bladder outlet obstruction, the child should be carefully studied to ascertain if obstruction is present. Diverticula are most common in close association with the ureteral orifices, and in these instances, concomitant ureteral reimplantation, by an antireflux technique, should be carried out.

Neurogenic bladder is always present in children with myelomeningocele and sacral agenesis and occurs after cord transection and in certain paralytic states. When it is the result of congenital lesions, hydronephrosis may be present at birth. An intravenous pyelogram is obtained as soon as possible. In instances in which severe hydronephrosis is present, prompt high urinary diversion by cutaneous pyelostomy or cutaneous ureterostomy may be necessary to protect kidney function. In most cases, the upper urinary tract is normal. These children are followed by frequent urinalysis to detect infection promptly when it occurs, with pyelography at yearly intervals. Residual urine determinations and cystourethrography are done if infection occurs or if hydronephrosis develops, or, in stable children, at age four to five years to evaluate the possibility of toilet training.

Children with total incontinence, dribbling constantly from an empty bladder, tend to have normal upper urinary tracts and stable kidney function with little or no tendency toward infection. However, urinary diversion, usually by ileal conduit, is required to permit urine collection. In boys, an external urine collecting device, such as a condom catheter, sometimes suffices.

Children in whom the bladder retains urine can sometimes be taught to empty it, often with the help of the Credé maneuver. These patients may eventually stay dry by "voiding by the clock" once the interval between emptying and the onset of overflow incontinence has been established. Most such patients do not empty completely, and hence remain susceptible to urinary infection. Many also develop vesicoureteral reflux. The overriding consideration in treatment must always be preservation of kidney function; hence, some children who achieve some urinary control must still undergo supravesical urinary diversion. Patients who do achieve useful bladder function must always be kept under urologic surveillance, because infection may occur or hydronephrosis worsen after a seemingly stable balance has been achieved.

Sarcoma of the prostate is highly malignant in boys, and radical surgical extirpation is necessary. The bladder, prostate, urethral bulb and periprostate musculature of the perineum should be removed en bloc. Actinomycin-D and high voltage x-ray therapy together should be employed postoperatively; radiotherapy alone has proved ineffectual in the past.

Sarcoma of the bladder is treated by radical cystectomy, and in boys the prostate must also be removed in continuity or an adequate margin around the tumor cannot be obtained. Actinomycin-D, alone or in combination with radiation, should be given in the postoperative period.

The treatment of exstrophy depends, in part, upon the size of the exstrophic bladder. When relatively small – less than 1½ inches in diameter at birth – the bladder when closed will not hold enough urine to function as a reservoir. Such patients are best treated by excision of the exstrophic bladder and ureterosigmoidostomy. This is usually deferred until 18 to 24 months of age in order to facilitate accurate ureterocolic anastomosis, which must be done by an antireflux technique to prevent reflux of fecal material, and pyelonephritis. Should these complications occur, an ileal conduit is necessary to forestall severe renal damage.

Larger exstrophic bladders are closed when the child is about six months of age. Bilateral iliac osteotomies are first performed so that the bony pelvis will be more stable and so that the defect in the abdominal wall can be closed. A few days later, the exstrophic bladder is freed from circumferential attachments to the skin and abdominal wall and is turned in. Care is taken that the bladder neck and the urethra are 14 to 16 French in caliber, so that bladder outlet obstruction is not produced. The epispadiac penis is repaired at the same time.

Most patients with exstrophy initially closed in this manner remain incontinent, although 10 to 20 per cent develop adequate urinary control. After an attempt at toilet training at age four to five, those in whom incontinence persists are reevaluated. If renal function remains normal, a second operative procedure is tried, at which time a urethral sphincter is formed from a strip of trigonal muscle 3 to 5 cm. in length. This strip is rolled into a tube 16 to 20 French in caliber. The bladder muscle, thus employed, then serves as a urethral sphincter. Ordinarily, some degree of voluntary control of urination is possible after this maneuver; indeed, perfect continence may be achieved. When incontinence or near incontinence persists, urinary diversion, by ureterosigmoidostomy if the upper tracts are normal, or by ileal conduit, is elected to permit urine collection and to prevent upper urinary tract dilatation.

Disorders of the Penis and Testes

ALAN B. RETIK, M.D.

PENIS

Balanitis. Balanitis is an inflammation of the glans penis which is almost invariably associated with infection in the coronal sulcus in uncircumcised males. The acute infection is best treated by adequate hygienic measures and the application of topical antibiotic ointments such as bacitracin. However, balanitis tends to recur if phimosis is present, and circumcision should be performed. Occasionally, balanitis may lead to severe cellulitis and septicemia. This should be treated with a broad-spectrum antibiotic.

Phimosis. Phimosis, or an abnormal narrowing of the preputial outlet, may prevent the glans penis from being adequately cleansed and therefore may be responsible for balanitis. Severe phimosis may cause difficulty in voiding and, in rare instances, secondary obstruction. If the prepuce cannot be retracted to permit adequate cleansing of the glans or if balanitis is a problem, circumcision should be performed.

Paraphimosis. Paraphimosis results when the retracted foreskin cannot be brought back over the glans and becomes fixed in the coronal sulcus. This may result in marked edema, pain and ischemia to the glans penis. The foreskin can usually be reduced manually. If reduction cannot be accomplished, immediate circumcision should be performed. This can usually be accomplished even in the face of marked edema and is preferable to doing just a dorsal slit with a circumcision at a later date.

Preputial Adhesions. Preputial adhesions are adhesions between the foreskin and glans which prevent complete retraction of the foreskin. This condition may lead to a collection of smegma beneath the adhesions with resultant infection. Treatment consists of forceable retraction of the foreskin, thus lysing the adhesions manually. The area should be cleansed with aqueous benzalkonium (Zephiran). In this situation the prepuce should be retracted daily and the area lubricated with petrolatum jelly. In severe cases the adhesions may have to be lysed under anesthesia.

Meatal Ulcer and Stenosis. Meatal ulcer usually results from inflammation of the urethral meatus from urinary irritation in the diaper age group. Repeated inflammation and ulceration may lead to fibrosis and a narrowed meatus. Meatal ulcer and stenosis are almost exclusively seen in circumcised males. Meatal stenosis may cause symptoms of decreased urinary stream, frequency and straining to void. Severe meatal stenosis may cause urinary retention. Treatment of meatal ulcer consists of exposure, avoidance of rubber pants and the application of an antibiotic ointment such as bacitracin. Meatal stenosis is treated by urethral meatotomy, which I prefer to do with the patient anesthetized. Dilatation of the meatus by the parents or child for 10 days postoperatively should prevent recurrence.

Hypospadias. In children with hypospadias, the urethral meatus may be located on the ventral surface of the penis anywhere from the corona to the perineum. Deficient foreskin on the ventral surface gives the penis a characteristic hooded appearance. There is usually an associated chordee which results in a ventral angulation of the penile shaft. Coronal hypospadias does not usually require surgical correction, although there is a significant incidence of meatal stenosis with this condition. I prefer to advance the meatus toward the tip of the glans at the same time the meatotomy is performed.

Hypospadias repair should be complete by the time the child goes to school. In the more severe degrees of hypospadias, staged repair is done first by excising the chordee and straightening the penis and then by constructing the new urethra. Staged repairs are usually started when the child is between 18 and 24 months old. I prefer one-stage repairs (correction of chordee and construction of a new urethra) in the less severe degrees of hypospadias.

Infants with severe hypospadias should have an excretory urogram because of an increased incidence of urinary tract anomalies.

Epispadias and Exstrophy. Epispadias is a rare anomaly resulting from failure of fusion of the dorsum of the urethra and penis. The milder degrees of the anomaly are confined to the shaft of the penis and urinary incontinence is not a problem. Surgical repair is readily accomplished. Urinary incontinence accompanies the more severe degrees of epispadias. In addition to surgical correction of the penile defect, a procedure at the bladder neck is also performed to increase urethral resistance at this level. I use a modification of the Young-Dees procedure. If the penis is extremely short, a penile lengthening procedure is done as a preliminary measure. Surgery should be performed when the child is between the ages of three and four.

In affected children, the degree of exstrophy of the bladder may vary. In general, we attempt to close the bladder, especially if there is a reasonable bladder capacity. Closure is usually performed between 6 and 18 months of age following bilateral iliac osteotomies. In some children, penile lengthening procedures are done according to need. If it is decided that closure is not feasible and anal sphincter tone is normal, ureterosigmoidostomy may be the procedure of choice. Ilial conduit diversion is usually reserved for the child in whom reconstructive surgery is not successful. Even following successful closure, some degree of urinary incontinence may be a problem.

SPERMATIC CORD AND TESTES

Torsion of the Testis. Torsion of the spermatic cord must be differentiated from other causes of acute scrotal swelling, such as torsion of the appendix testis, acute epididymitis, orchitis and trauma. Treatment is immediate exploration and detorsion of the testis. The testis should always be left in place even if gangrenous, because it may contribute to hormonal production and also have some cosmetic value. At the time of surgery, the contralateral testis should also be pexed.

Torsion of the Appendix Testis. The swelling and discomfort of torsion of the testicular appendages are not usually as extreme as seen with torsion of the testis. When seen early, the twisted organ is usually palpated and may be seen through the skin as a bluish discoloration. When seen late, however, it may be difficult to differentiate from torsion of the testis. I prefer exploration of the scrotum if there is the slightest doubt as to the diagnosis. The twisted appendix is removed. If the diagnosis is certain, one may elect a nonoperative approach. Symptoms will usually subside in 5 to 10 days. Even in this situation, pain may be severe enough to necessitate surgery.

Epididymitis. Epididymitis is very unusual in the prepubertal boy. It must be differentiated from other causes of acute scrotal swelling. Treatment consists of bed rest, elevation and the application of ice packs. I also employ a broad-spectrum antibiotic, such as tetracycline* or ampicillin, administered in therapeutic doses by weight, for 10 days. An excretory urogram should be obtained to determine whether there is some preexisting urinary pathology.

Orchitis. Orchitis in children is rare. Mumps orchitis may occasionally be seen and is sometimes difficult to differentiate from torsion of the testis. Mumps orchitis is best treated by bed rest and elevation of the scrotum. On several occasions with very severe swelling, I have operated upon children with mumps orchitis and performed cruciate incisions in the tunica albuginea to lessen compression of the organ.

Trauma. Trauma to the testis may cause varying degrees of swelling, ecchymosis and discomfort. In general these symptoms are treated by rest and elevation. If the trauma is severe and swelling increases, exploration of the scrotum is advisable to decompress the hematoma, secure any bleeding points and repair any possible testicular injury.

Cryptorchidism. (See page 419.)

Tumors. Tumors of the testes in infants and children present as firm scrotal masses which do not transilluminate. Preoperative studies employed include excretory urography, chest x-ray and metastatic series. Through a generous inguinal incision, a rubber-shod clamp is placed across the spermatic cord at the region of the internal inguinal ring. The testis is then retracted into the incision and examined. If the mass is obviously a tumor, a radical orchiectomy is performed, ligating the spermatic cord above the internal inguinal ring. If there is some question as to the diagnosis, a frozen section is performed.

Malignant tumors in the pediatric age group are usually embryonal cell carcinoma, endodermal sinus tumor or teratoma. Seminoma and adenocarcinoma are rare. Following radical orchiectomy, further therapy depends on histologic diagnosis. If the tumor is a seminoma, radiation therapy of the retroperineal lymph nodes is performed. Retroperitoneal lymph node dissection is performed for the other malignant tumors. If retroperitoneal nodes show no evidence of metastatic disease, further therapy is not necessary although careful follow-up is indicated. If the nodes are positive, chemotherapy is indicated. We have used a variety of chemotherapeutic agents. The most common agents are actinomycin D or Cytoxan used in therapeutic doses by weight. Recurrent courses of therapy at three- to six-month intervals for several years have been employed.

Benign tumors of the testicle are uncommon and may be either a benign teratoma or an interstitial tumor. Treatment consists of simple excision.

Hernia and Hydrocele

ALAN B. RETIK, M.D.

INGUINAL HERNIA

The main indication for correction of inguinal hernia is prevention of incarceration. Hernias should be corrected surgically shortly after the diagnosis is made. The operative procedure consists of high ligation of the hernia sac at the internal inguinal ring. Bilateral inguinal hernias are both repaired during the same operation. The infant or child is usually discharged from the hospital the following day.

---

* Manufacturer's note: The use of tetracyclines during tooth development (last half of pregnancy, infancy and childhood to age eight years) may cause permanent discoloration of teeth. This adverse reaction is more common during long-term use of the drugs but has been observed following repeated short-term courses.

Correction is occasionally done as an outpatient procedure.

INCARCERATED INGUINAL HERNIA

Reduction of an incarcerated hernia should be attempted, rather than emergency surgery, which carries an increased morbidity and complication rate. Most incarcerated hernias can be reduced by gentle manual pressure following sedation. If reduction is unsuccessful, immediate surgery is indicated. Following successful reduction of an incarcerated inguinal hernia, elective surgery should be delayed for 48 to 72 hours to allow edema and inflammation to subside.

HYDROCELE

Hydroceles of the tunica vaginalis, canal of Nuck or the spermatic cord seldom require operation within the first year of life. Small accumulations of fluid will often disappear without treatment. However, hydroceles which persist or develop after the first year of life will not usually regress spontaneously and therefore will require surgical correction.

Hydroceles are invariably associated with a hernia and approached surgically through the inguinal region. High ligation of the hernia sac is performed and only a small rim of the hydrocele sac need be excised. Hydrocele of the spermatic cord is completely removed along with the hernia sac.

Undescended Testis

ALFRED M. BONGIOVANNI, M.D.

Cryptorchidism may be unilateral or bilateral. There is less reason for concern in the unilateral failure of descent because one normal testis should be adequate to assure fertility. It is important to distinguish true cryptorchidism from the retractable testis.

The treatment of cryptorchidism remains controversial, and there is no solid proof that any special form of therapy is always successful. In some cases there is primary gonadal dysgenesis, under which circumstances an inherent defect is present which probably cannot be corrected.

Since spontaneous descent occurs in the first year of life, treatment always should be deferred until after this time. Skilled surgical correction is the treatment of choice, and it is usually wise to perform this after the fifth year but well before puberty. I do not favor hormonal therapy. However, if the practitioner feels compelled to employ this type of therapy, it is recommended that he administer one intramuscular dose of human chorionic gonadotropin, 1000 I.U. three times weekly for three weeks in a total dosage not exceeding 10,000 I.U. If descent does not occur within a few weeks of completing treatment, no further hormonal therapy should be employed.

When surgical exploration reveals the absence of gonads, prostheses should be placed in the scrotum. In most cases, although the germinal elements of the testis may be compromised, the Leydig cells are preserved and the secretion of sex hormone is adequate at puberty. However, if there is a failure of development of secondary sexual characteristics at the time of puberty, methyl testosterone, 10 to 20 mg. orally daily, may be prescribed.

Disorders of the Vulva and Vagina

RAYMOND H. KAUFMAN, M.D., *and*
PETER K. THOMPSON, M.D.

TRAUMATIC LESIONS

Lacerations. Treatment should be directed toward the restoration of normal anatomic relationships. Lacerations should always be repaired under general anesthesia. After the wounds are clean and foreign bodies looked for and removed, bleeding vessels should be ligated and the tissue edges carefully approximated. Large traumatic areas should be thoroughly irrigated with sterile saline, and necrotic tissue debrided. Adjacent organs, such as the bladder and rectum, should be examined for evidence of damage, and if any is found it should be repaired. If the peritoneal cavity has been penetrated, it should be explored for evidence of visceral laceration and intra-abdominal bleeding. If loss of blood is significant, it should be replaced. Reassurance should be given to the parents that the injury will not impair their child's ability to have children normally, if this is true.

Hematomas. Small hematomas require merely the use of analgesics, careful observation for evidence of continued enlargement and, if possible, local application of ice shortly after their occurrence. A large fluctuant collection of blood should be incised and evacuated. In the latter circumstances, bleeding points should be located and ligated, if possible. Extensive exploration for obscure bleeding vessels, however, is inadvisable. In the presence of considerable generalized oozing, the cavity of the hematoma should be carefully packed.

Rape. Injuries usually associated with rape include laceration or hematomas, and their treatment is outlined above. When bleeding is extensive in a young child or the extent of the injury is difficult to determine, the patient should be given an anesthetic before hemostasis and repair of the lacerated tissues are undertaken. Since the examining physician is frequently called upon to give testimony in a court of law, it is essential that an accurate history and careful documentation of his findings be obtained. The following procedures are suggested:

1. Consent of the parents or guardian for the examination should be obtained before the child is looked at.
2. The time and place of the examination should be recorded and, also, the length of time since the assault took place.
3. Physical examination of the child should include a detailed notation of where the lacerations and hematomas were found. Bruises and scratches on the face, extremities and trunk should be recorded. Foreign hairs that may be found on the patient should be saved and labeled.
4. Laboratory studies should be made. It is preferable that all material obtained for laboratory examination be given directly to the clinical pathologist who will examine the specimens. If this is not feasible, a signed receipt should be given for each specimen delivered to the laboratory by the technician who will make the test.

   (a) When the child is examined under anesthesia, a wet mount of secretions should be obtained from the vagina to determine the presence of sperm. If the vagina is dry, it may be irrigated with saline and the preparation made from the solution. Motile sperm should be looked for. A dry smear stained with methylene blue or Wright's, or Gram's stain, should also be studied for spermatozoa.

   (b) The absence of sperm does not preclude intercourse, since the assailant may have been azoospermic or may have withdrawn. Dried stains on the clothing or the pubic hair may be examined for the presence of seminal fluid. Ultraviolet light produces a bluish fluorescence on seminal fluid stains quite unlike that observed on material from the bladder or rectum. A vaginal aspirate and dried stains may be studied for acid phosphatase, which presumes the presence of seminal fluid. The finding of a positive fluorescence, together with a high acid phosphatase (Phosphatabs-acid, Warner–Chilcott Laboratories, may be used), provides good presumptive evidence of seminal fluid.

   (c) Secretors of A and B substances will have these in their seminal fluid. If they are present, A or B blood group can be determined and compared with the blood group of the alleged assailant.

   (d) Dried stains of blood on the victim should be typed and compared with the blood of the suspected assailant as well as that of the victim.

   (e) Foreign hairs found on the clothing or body of the victim should be saved for comparison with the hair of the alleged assailant.

   (f) Smears, cultures and serology studies should be made as indicated.

5. If possible, photographs should be taken of any bruise marks on the body of the patient and lacerations and bruises of the genital areas.
6. If the child has already gone through the menarche and is menstruating regularly, the use of stilbestrol, 25 mg. daily for five days, will prevent a possible pregnancy.
7. The immediate physical and emotional needs of the child must be met as well as the emotional needs of the parents. The response of the parents to this tragic event may affect the psychosexual development of the child.

VAGINAL FOREIGN BODIES

Foreign bodies in the vagina must be removed. In the very young child who cannot be reasoned with, it is necessary to do this under a general anesthetic. Frequently, however, in older children this can be accomplished under local anesthesia. The topical use of such agents as Xylocaine Jelly (2 per cent lidocaine) is advisable under these circumstances. The method of removal of the foreign body depends on the shape, size and consistency of the object. Its manipulation toward the introitus with the finger in the rectum is often possible. A grasping instrument, such as those used by urologists, may be operated through a Kelly cystoscope or very small virginal speculum. Removal of such objects as safety pins or any hard substance that has become embedded in the vaginal wall will require general anesthesia and, under rare circumstances, a short, midline episiotomy.

PREMENARCHAL LEUKORRHEA

With the increased production of unopposed estrogen in the period of time immediately before the menarche, a physiologic type of leukorrhea may develop. Since its true nature is not understood by the child and mother, it may be interpreted as indicative of vaginal infection. The increased secretions result from proliferation and desquamation of vaginal epithelium and an increased production of mucus by the cervical glands. The only treatment usually required is reassurance of the patient and the parent and instructions regarding vulvar hygiene. On rare occasions when the patient has a profuse discharge, cryocautery of the cervix may be necessary. As a rule, this is best deferred until the child has reached full sexual and anatomic development.

INFECTIONS

Nonspecific Pediatric Vulvovaginitis. In view of the inability to assign definite causes to many cases of vulvovaginitis in children, this term is utilized. Any disease of unknown etiology can present therapeutic problems. Frequently, nonspecific pediatric vulvovaginitis will disappear following the institution of hygienic measures alone. Local cleansing with a mild soap and an abundance of water is helpful; medicated soaps may be helpful in some individuals but harmful in others. After a soapy water soaking and rinsing, the vulva should be gently dried, preferably by a blotting action instead of rubbing. The child should be taught to wipe from the front to the back after defecation to prevent fecal contamination of the vulva. The wearing of loose-fitting cotton panties instead of tight ones made of synthetic material will help to prevent the accumulation of moisture. Topical applications of anesthetics and germicides are essentially useless and might aggravate the disease. If the vulvovaginitis has not responded to hygienic measures, the use of topical estrogen is frequently of value. Premarin Vaginal Cream (0.625 mg. of equine-conjugated estrogens per Gm.) may be instilled into the vagina through a glass or rubber catheter. One gram of the cream may be instilled nightly for two weeks and thereafter every three to four nights for an additional six weeks. If the response to estrogen proves disappointing, the use of antibiotic or chemotherapeutic agents locally or systemically should be tried. One-half tablet of Sultrin may be gently inserted into the vagina nightly for two weeks. Furacin-E Urethral Inserts may also be used nightly for the same period of time.

Trichomoniasis, Candidiasis and *Hemophilus vaginalis* Vaginitis. These infections are unimportant in the overall problem of pediatric vulvovaginitis, especially in infants and young girls, since the immature vagina does not provide a suitable environment for growth of the causative organisms. In the rare case where they are found, treatment is as follows: For trichomoniasis, Flagyl, 250 mg., one tablet once or twice daily for five days, depending on the age of the child; for candidiasis, one-half of a nystatin vaginal suppository nightly for two weeks; and for *hemophilus vaginalis,* ampicillin in appropriate dosage depending on age and weight of the child, for five days.

Gonorrheal Vulvovaginitis. Although the dosage may be varied according to the age and weight of the patient, as a rule, 600,000 I.U. of procaine penicillin may be given intramuscularly daily for three days. If the child is allergic to penicillin, tetracycline may be utilized for a period of five days in a dose dependent on the age and size of the child. In addition, the usual hygienic measures previously outlined should be carried out.

Worm Infestation. For the treatment of *Oxyuris vermicularis* involving the vagina, some piperazine preparations, such as Antepar or Povan, may be used. Povan is given as a single oral dose, 5 mg. per kilogram of body weight.

Streptococcal Vulvovaginitis. The use of local antibiotics, such as tetracycline, penicillin or Mycitracin (polymyxin-neomycin-bacitracin mixture), may be used once nightly for two weeks. Furacin-E Urethral Inserts may also be used nightly for a two-week period of time. On occasion the systemic use of antibiotics, such as procaine penicillin, 600,000 units intramuscularly, or tetracycline, may be of value.

Herpes Genitalis. Infections due to type 2 herpes virus are rarely seen in the child, since this virus is usually transmitted by sexual contact. On rare occasions, when this infection does develop, treatment is primarily symptomatic. Hot sitz baths three to four times daily will speed healing and ease the discomfort. The local application of an antibiotic cream such as Neosporin-G. after the hot sitz baths will prevent secondary infection. Preliminary studies would suggest that photoinactivation of the virus using proflavine, 0.1 per cent, liberally applied to the ulcers, and exposing the ulcers to bright light for a period of 10 minutes, will speed up resolution of the infection. This should be done several times daily for two to three days and the medication can be applied by the child's mother. This treatment appears to be more effective in bringing about resolution of recurrent infections and also in preventing recurrences at the site of treatment.

CONGENITAL DISORDERS

Labial Adhesions. The application of a local estrogen cream such as Premarin Vaginal Cream or Dienestrol Cream (0.01 per cent) to the line of adhesions twice daily will usually result in separation of the labia within a period of two weeks.

Imperforate Hymen. This malformation is not likely to be suspected in young children unless their mucoid vaginal secretions distend the vagina and cause protrusion of the hymen. Under these circumstances, a wide cruciate incision should be made through the hymen, entering into the vagina, thereby allowing the mucoid secretions to escape. This naturally should be done under general anesthesia. If the imperforate hymen is found incidentally on general examination and there are no symptoms, nothing need be done until the child begins to approach the menarche. At this time, the hymen should be opened under general anesthesia. Naturally, this condition must be distinguished from congenital absence of the vagina.

Congenital Absence of the Vagina (Vaginal Agenesis). This congenital anomaly usually is not found until the child's mother becomes alarmed when her daughter does not begin to menstruate. Under these circumstances or if this congenital defect is found early in life, there is no urgency in its treatment—this is especially true if there is not a functioning uterus, which is the case in most instances. When there is a functioning uterus, definitive surgery consisting of construction of an artificial vagina should be carried out at the time of puberty or slightly thereafter. In the majority of cases, construction of an artificial vagina can be carried out immediately prior to anticipated marriage or other planned sexual activity. After the vagina is constructed, if the patient is not having frequent coitus, she must wear a vaginal obturator, and this inconvenience must be considered before repair is undertaken.

Female Pseudohermaphroditism with Ambiguous Genitalia. This usually is associated with clitoral hypertrophy and labial scrotal fusion accompanied by a scrotal appearance of the labia majora. In the majority of affected infants, this problem arises from congenital adrenal hyperplasia. The medical treatment for congenital adrenal hyperplasia consists of adequate substitution therapy with cortisone to suppress function of the adrenal gland and thus prevent further virilization. In severe forms of this disease process, particularly in the presence of the salt-losing syndrome, the treatment is considerably more complicated and is discussed elsewhere in this text. In rare cases, the external genitalia of the female fetus may be masculinized incidental to the presence of an androgen-secreting ovarian tumor or owing to the mother's ingestion of a virilizing hormone during pregnancy. The ambiguous external genitalia of the female pseudohermaphrodite should be treated surgically, in general, when abnormal genital development has been recognized in infancy. The precise diagnosis and cause must first be established. Surgical correction is not recommended until the child is 18 months to two years old. This is generally considered the age of memory; therefore, the child has no recollection of the genitalia prior to this time. Plastic repair can restore normal function and a reasonably normal appearance to the external genitalia. Growth and development, puberty, and sexual and reproductive capability should all be normal. The degree of the defect will determine the degree of success of the surgical procedure. Conservation of the clitoris is important; every attempt should be made to keep this organ as a functional unit of the external genitalia. Where the phallus is unusually large, only clitoridectomy is likely to afford a reasonable cosmetic result. When this is done, an anatomically shortened clitoris can be left. Exteriorization of the vagina with plastic repair of the labial scrotal folds to form an introitus can usually be performed when the child is 18 months to two years of age. The majority of patients with female pseudohermaphroditism, after treatment, should be able to participate in a satisfactory marriage, conceive and bear children.

Aside from those with female pseudohermaphroditism, most patients with ambiguous external genitalia are sterile. The choice of sex of rearing thus depends on the ease with which a functional sexual unit may be reconstructed from the anomalous organs. In general, it is easier to reconstruct the genitalia along female lines; fewer social problems arise and the long-term result is more acceptable if the patient is reared as a female. Ancillary procedures, such as construction of an artificial vagina and resection of the gonads because of harmful endocrine function or potentially malignant change, may be carried out before or at puberty.

PRECOCIOUS PUBERTY

The most common type of precocious puberty is idiopathic, and the most effective therapy is Depo–Provera in doses of 100 mg. to 200 mg. intramuscularly every two weeks (use of Depo-Provera for this disorder is investigational). This therapy should bring about cessation of breast development and menses but may not produce any decrease in the somatic or linear growth of the child. Precocious puberty due to an estrogen-secreting ovarian tumor should be suspected if a palpably enlarged ovary is present on physical examination. If such a tumor is found, laparotomy and resection of the tumor, along with bisection of the contralateral ovary, is the therapy of choice. If central nervous system lesions are suspected as the cause of the precociousness, neurologic or neurosurgic consultation is indicated. Other causes of precocious puberty could be exogenous estrogens or hypothyroidism. Elimination of the exogenous estrogen will cause disappearance of the signs of sexual precocity, though any epiphyseal changes induced by the estrogen will be permanent. Treatment of hypothyroidism is covered elsewhere.

LICHEN SCLEROSUS ET ATROPHICUS

The treatment of lichen sclerosus et atrophicus in children is directed primarily to the relief of pruritus. Usually this can be accomplished with topical corticosteroids, such as Synalar Cream, 0.01 per cent or 0.025 per cent, applied topically two to three times daily. Many of the lesions in children improve or disappear spontaneously during or after adolescence. Resolution usually leaves normal skin. The clearing of the lesions has no consistent relationship to the menarche, although there is a general correlation between improvement of the lesions and maturation of the child. In addition to the use of topical steroids for the relief of pruritus, the general hygienic measures already discussed should be followed.

BENIGN TUMORS OF THE VULVA AND VAGINA

Condylomata Acuminata. These wart-like growths are very rarely seen in children. Where present, they are usually isolated lesions and can easily be removed surgically under general anesthesia. Twenty per cent podophyllin in tincture of benzoin can be applied to the lesions and washed off in 3 to 4 hours; however, this preparation should be used in the child only with great caution.

Hemangiomas. The strawberry hemangioma is frequently observed shortly after birth. After an initial period of growth in early infancy, it frequently undergoes spontaneous involution over several years. In view of the possibility of their disappearance, treatment of these lesions may be unnecessary. Where, however, they persist beyond the age of five or six, or where they result in ulceration and bleeding, they should be treated. The simplest and most effective treatment is cryotherapy with the use of solid carbon dioxide or one of the currently available cryotherapy units which utilize carbon dioxide, Freon or liquid nitrogen. The lesion is frozen until it fully blanches down to the level of the skin. Treatment may be repeated after four to six weeks; on occasion, two to four treatments may be required.

Cavernous hemangiomas frequently appear during the first few months of life and increase in size until the child reaches the age of about 18 months; thereafter, they may remain static or they may begin to regress and eventually they almost disappear. Those lesions that rapidly enlarge during the first six to eight months of life are prone to spontaneous involution and thus should not be treated unless severely symptomatic. Hemangiomas present at birth that grow slowly seldom undergo spontaneous regression. Numerous factors influence the choice of treatment of these tumors in children. Treatment may be expectant and conservative unless ulceration and bleeding occur or unless the tumor grows rapidly and destroys the surrounding tissue. If treatment is deemed advisable, solid carbon dioxide or freezing, utilizing a cryosurgical unit, can be undertaken. The injection of sclerosing solutions into the tumor has also been suggested. Even though radium and x-ray have been recommended, it is preferable not to use this approach in the genital area. On rare occasions the hemangioma may require surgical extirpation by ligation of isolated vessels. Surgical removal of extensive, deep tumors is usually accompanied by severe blood loss and risk to the child.

Vulvar and Vaginal Cysts. The large majority of cysts found on the vulva and vagina of the child are congenital in nature and are of mesonephric or paramesonephric origin. Unless they produce symptoms, such as pressure and discomfort, they can be left alone.

MALIGNANT TUMORS OF THE VULVA AND VAGINA

Squamous cell carcinoma of the vulva and vagina, and adenocarcinoma of the Bartholin gland are literally unheard of in the child.

Clear Cell Adenocarcinoma of the Vagina. The pediatrician and gynecologist are becoming more aware of this lesion since information has become available relating its occurrence in areas of vaginal adenosis in children whose mothers received stilbestrol during their pregnancies. These tumors are malignant and locally invasive and should be treated aggressively with a surgical approach. In many instances, this will require radical hysterectomy or total pelvic exenteration, depending on the location of the lesion.

Sarcoma Botryoides. The only reported successful treatments of this lesion have entailed radical surgery, which in most instances involves total pelvic exenteration.

Disorders of the Uterus, Tubes and Ovaries

RAYMOND H. KAUFMAN, M.D., *and*
PETER K. THOMPSON, M.D.

CONGENITAL ANOMALIES

Only the very few anomalies affecting the premenarchal patient will be discussed.

Uterine Anomalies. Uterine anomalies, such as partial or complete duplication of the uterus, may be noticed incidentally at the time of abdominal surgery, but no therapy is indicated until such time in adult life when problems related to the abnormality arise.

Abnormal Ovarian Descent. This condition is frequently associated with inguinal hernia and the gonad must be returned to the peritoneal cavity. The patient should be evaluated for pseudohermaphroditism by preoperative buccal smear or by gonad biopsy at the time of surgery.

Accessory Ovaries. The small nodules of ovarian tissue lie along the path of ovarian descent and no therapy is necessary.

Ovarian Agenesis (Dysgenesis). This condition can be diagnosed before adolescence by the somatic characteristics and buccal smear revealing an absence of the Barr body and a typical XO chromosomal pattern, or the other mosaic patterns that have been described. By age 11 the patient should be started on low doses of estrogen in the form of conjugated estrogen, 0.625 mg., or ethinyl estradiol, 0.02 mg. This dose is small enough so that premature closure of the epiphyses does not occur. By age 12 or 13 the patient should be receiving conjugated estrogen, 2.5 mg., or ethinyl estradiol, 0.15 mg., daily for the first 25 days of each month. Withdrawal bleeding can be accomplished by using medroxyprogesterone acetate, 10 mg. daily from day 20 to day 25 of each month. A simplified regimen for withdrawal bleeding would be to use a sequential oral contraceptive, such as Oracon, Norquen or Ortho-Novum SQ. Roentgenologic evidence of unduly accelerated bone age is an indication to reduce the dosage of estrogen.

INFLAMMATION OF THE UTERUS, TUBES AND OVARIES

Cervicitis. Cervicitis is frequently seen in conjunction with vaginitis and will tend to heal spontaneously as the vaginitis is treated. No cauterization in the premenarchal child is indicated. A "congenital ectropion" need not be treated.

Salpingitis. Salpingitis is exceedingly rare in the premenarchal patient. Gonorrheal salpingitis in a child of this age is almost unheard of.

Mumps Oophoritis. The ovaries may swell to 6 to 8 cm. in diameter and treatment should consist of analgesics and supportive therapy.

TORSION OF THE ADNEXA

Torsion of the adnexa is confirmed at laparotomy. The strangulated tube and/or ovary may show gangrenous changes. Therapy should be removal of the involved organs without untwisting the pedicle.

Tumors of the Uterus, Tubes and Ovaries

RAYMOND H. KAUFMAN, M.D., *and*
PETER K. THOMPSON, M.D.

BENIGN UTERINE TUMORS

Cervical Papillomas. This rare condition is treated by local excision. The patient should be reexamined at frequent intervals for several years to make sure that the tumor has not recurred.

Myomas. Uterine myomas are very uncommon in the premenarchal patient. Surgical excision is not necessary unless a large pelvic tumor is found or unless the patient is symptomatic.

MALIGNANT UTERINE TUMORS

Carcinoma of the Cervix. In the premenarchal patient, adenocarcinoma is more frequent than is squamous cell carcinoma, although both conditions are quite uncommon. Radical surgery consisting of hysterectomy and partial vaginectomy, along with excision of the paracervical and paravaginal connective tissues and pelvic lymphadenectomy, offers the child the best chance of survival. In more advanced cervical carcinoma, wider excision including pelvic exenteration and total vaginectomy is necessary. Healthy ovaries should be preserved, unless this is impossible.

Mixed Mesodermal Sarcoma of the Cervix. Rarely, sarcoma botryoides will arise only from the cervix. Treatment of this condition should consist of at least hysterectomy and total vaginectomy with excision of the paravaginal connective tissue. Any evidence of extension beyond the cervix and paravaginal tissue demands also excision of the vulva, urethra, bladder, pelvic lymph nodes and occasionally excision of the rectum with urinary and fecal diversion. Most results show that radiation is of limited value as definitive treatment for this condition.

Carcinoma of the Uterine Corpus. These are usually adenocarcinomas probably of mesonephric origin. Complete hysterectomy is the preferred method of therapy.

TUMORS OF THE OVIDUCT

Tumors of the oviduct are exceedingly rare and salpingectomy is usually indicated unless malignant potential is seen. There have been no malignancies of the tube reported in the premenarchal girl.

TUMORS OF THE OVARY

Non-neoplastic Ovarian Tumors. Follicular cysts occasionally occur in the premenarchal patient and they should be removed if they exceed 5 to 6 cm. in size and persist for more than three to six months. The preferable means of excision is by shelling out the cyst, leaving the normal ovarian tissue behind.

Benign Neoplasms. The most common benign neoplasm is benign cystic teratoma. Other benign tumors in the premenarchal patient are cystadenomas, including the serous and mucinous type. Fibromas have also been discovered in children. Treatment of these tumors consists of exploratory laparotomy with adequate abdominal incision to remove the tumor without aspirating or rupturing it. If possible, the tumor should be separated from the normal ovary; this shelling-out process may allow for preservation of the ovary. The tumor should be submitted to the pathologist for preliminary report before closing the abdomen. The normal-appearing contralateral ovar
should always be bisected and inspected to r
out the presence of another tumor.

Malignant Ovarian Tumors. Dys
oma. If the tumor is well-circumscri
there is no gross evidence of extension
tasis, unilateral salpingo-oophorecto
be adequate therapy. After the
ovary is bivalved, the ovary should
out of the pelvis. Postoperative r
shielding of the remaining ovar

livered to the pelvic lymph nodes on the side from which the tumor was removed if there is evidence of nodal spread. If there is any evidence of extension or metastasis, total abdominal hysterectomy and bilateral salpingo-oophorectomy are necessary. Postoperative radiotherapy to the pelvis is indicated under these circumstances.

Carcinomas, Malignant Teratomas and Sarcomas. If the tumor is well-circumscribed without metastasis, a salpingo-oophorectomy on the involved side should be performed. The opposite ovary is bivalved, and if no tumor is present this therapy should be sufficient. Radiotherapy to the involved side after excision of the malignant tumor should be considered. In more advanced ovarian cancer in which other pelvic structures are involved, a complete hysterectomy and bilateral salpingo-oophorectomy are indicated. Chemotherapy is used in inoperable or widely metastatic cases but, unfortunately, improvement is only temporary.

Granulosa Cell Carcinoma. If this feminizing tumor is unilateral and well-encapsulated without evidence of extension, unilateral salpingo-oophorectomy is sufficient therapy. Again, the contralateral ovary should be bisected and inspected for small tumors. If there is evidence of spread of the tumor beyond the
ovary, complete hysterectomy with bilat
salpingo-oophorectomy is indicated. Sinc
losa cell carcinomas are sensitive t
postoperative radiotherapy to th
visable if residual tumor is
child should remain unde
rest of her life; vagi
used to show any
stimulation.

Embryona
malignant t
tube and
much
sh
t

ried out. If the tumor is well-encapsuled and there are no signs of extension to other organs, unilateral oophorectomy should be sufficient therapy. If metastasis or extension is present, hysterectomy and bilateral salpingo-oophorectomy should be performed. Also, the metastatic growth in the pelvic or abdominal cavity should be removed, since regression of distant metastases have been reported after excision of the primary tumor. In cases with metastatic disease, a trial of methotrexate is indicated although choriocarcinoma of the ovary is not very responsive to chemotherapeutic agents.

14

Bones and Joints

Craniostenosis, Crouzon's Disease and Apert's Syndrome

JACK H. RUBINSTEIN, M.D.

Craniostenosis or craniosynostosis refers to the premature closure of one or more of the sutures between the cranial bones. It may occur as an isolated primary cranial malformation, as a major component of certain syndromes (as in Crouzon's craniofacial dysostosis, Apert's syndrome and the other acrocephalosyndactyly and acrocephalopolysyndactyly syndromes) or in occasional association with or secondary to a number of other clinical conditions (as in idiopathic hypercalcemia and after ventriculovenous shunts).

The diagnosis of the various craniostenoses and associated syndromes is made on the basis of the type of cranial deformity, the presence or absence of facial abnormalities, and the presence or absence, degree and type of syndactyly, with or without polydactyly. The findings are confirmed with appropriate roentgenographic studies of the skull, hands and feet. Clinical and roentgenographic clues of intracranial hypertension are sought and evaluated (papilledema, bulging fontanelle if patent, separation of uninvolved sutures, cracked-pot percussion note and beaten-silver appearance). The possibility of associated hydrocephalus should be considered. The clinical and laboratory studies chosen are those that might pinpoint or exclude the various conditions that are occasionally associated with secondary craniostenosis, including primary microencephalic conditions. Consideration is given to the possibility of other hidden malformations, as well as to neurologic, intellectual, visual and auditory dysfunctions. Proper identification of the various syndrome complexes and a careful family history may facilitate genetic counseling.

There has been considerable unresolved debate during the past 10 years in the neurosurgical and pediatric literature over the indications, objectives and potential results of operative intervention on the closed sutures, especially where only a single suture is involved. Proponents argue that operation at four to six weeks of age, in the absence of any specific contraindication to surgery, such as a bleeding diathesis, offers the best chance for a good cosmetic result, and might possibly remove the risk of the synostosis causing brain damage by restricting normal brain growth. Opponents have argued that in the absence of increased intracranial pressure, there is no evidence that a single fused suture (especially the sagittal) carries any risk of impairing neurologic function, and that the risk of the procedure, albeit small (0.39 per cent mortality and 14 per cent morbidity in an excellent pediatric neurosurgical referral center), does not warrant the surgery being performed for only cosmetic reasons; some authors have even questioned the degree of cosmetic improvement that might be expected.

With multiple suture closure, if not secondary to microencephaly, the risk of increased intracranial pressure and the potential cosmetic gain may be greater. Intracranial hypertension, occasionally reported with single suture involvement, may be due to an undetected closure of a portion of another suture which functions as if the entire suture is closed. There appears to be no argument against surgery in the presence of intracranial hypertension and less debate over multiple synostoses even without signs of pressure. Other indications for operative intervention include progressive exophthalmos and possibly progressive visual, auditory or neurologic dysfunction.

The primary physician, responsible for assisting the family in decision making, must consider the availability or lack of a competent neurosurgeon thoroughly experienced with the techniques, pediatric anesthesiology and pediatric preoperative and postoperative care.

The surgical procedure for infants and toddlers is linear craniectomy, along or parallel to the absent suture, and covering the opposing bone edges with polyethylene film or Zenker's solution to prevent early refusion; bilateral parallel craniectomies are performed for sagittal suture involvement. There appears to be little evidence for surgical intervention in the older age group except for those patients with signs of increased intracranial pressure. Staged surgical procedures may be needed for multiple synostoses. Special attention must be paid to blood loss, compressing subgaleal hematoma and subgaleal infection from aspiration. A one-stage bilateral flap operation has been advocated for the child over three years of age with intracranial hypertension and craniostenosis.

Careful follow-up is indicated until the age of four years to determine if reoperation is required for relief of intracranial hypertension or for refused sutures. If the initial operation is performed for cosmetic reasons for single-suture synostosis, refusion at the craniectomy site probably would not produce a significant deformity and therefore would not warrant a second operation.

Early shunting procedures for alleviation of hydrocephalus may be indicated in the infant with the rare craniostenosis syndrome of cloverleaf skull (Kleeblattschädel syndrome), and occasionally with Apert's syndrome or the more common forms of craniostenosis.

It may be necessary in patients with coronal synostosis to repair a wide gap caused by an abnormal separation of the halves of the squamous portions of the frontal bone on each side of a wide metopic suture.

Various surgical procedures have been employed in attempts to improve the disfiguring facial deformities of Crouzon's and Apert's syndromes, and they have been aimed at the exophthalmos secondary to extremely shallow orbits, the maldevelopment of the middle third of the face and the relative prognathism. Orbital decompression may be indicated for severe exophthalmos associated with exposure keratitis or even luxation of the globes. Surgeons have attempted with split-rib grafts to build up the orbital floor, the supraorbital ridge and the maxillary and zygomatic regions. A rather radical system has been described for the "definitive correction" of the craniofacial deformities; it is carried out at 10 to 12 years of age and consists of total osteotomy together with postero-anterior movement of the middle third of the facial block. Appropriate dental, surgical and orthodontic management is needed for the oral and palatal anomalies that may be present. Awareness of the possibility of upper airway obstruction due to narrow nasopharyngeal and oropharyngeal passages, or even choanal atresia, with secondary pulmonary hypertension and cor pulmonale may necessitate remediation of the obstruction. Relief of this life-threatening complication by adenotonsillectomy has been reported.

In the acrocephalosyndactyly syndromes, appropriate and often multiple surgical procedures may be required to produce maximally functional hands and feet. Release of the thumb and little finger to permit a pincer grasp is indicated in the first year of life. Further procedures and goals must be determined by the nature and severity of the deformities and the skill and experience of the surgeon. Removal of one of the extra toes, usually one of the duplicated great toes, may be necessary in acrocephalopolysyndactyly to permit wearing normal shoes.

The complexities of the operative procedures; the lengthy, frequent and costly hospitalizations; the frequently associated problems of mental retardation, visual dysfunction, conductive or sensorineural hearing loss; the progressive synosteosis of affected bones of the feet and cervical spine; and the superimposed psychologic and emotional reactions to the deformities require for optimal habilitation a well-integrated team of medical, dental and health-related professionals who are capable of not only carrying out the technical aspects but also offering counseling and support to the family and later to the child. Early institutionalization of the child with Apert's or Crouzon's syndrome because of parental rejection precipitated by the severe disfigurement is certainly contrary to the best interests of the child.

References

Duggan, C. A., Keener, E. B., and Gay, B. B., Jr.: Secondary Craniosynostosis. *Am. J. Roentgen.* 109:277, 1970.

Fishman, M. A., Hogan, G. R., and Dodge, P. R.: The Concurrence of Hydrocephalus and Craniosynostosis. *J. Neurosurg.* 34:621, 1971.

Freeman, J. M., and Borkowf, S.: Craniostenosis: Review of the Literature and Report of Thirty-four Cases. *Pediatrics,* 30:57, 1962.

Hoover, G. H., Flatt, A. E., and Weiss, M. W.: The Hand and Apert's Syndrome. *J. Bone Joint Surg.,* 52-A: 878, 1970.

Shillito, J., Jr., and Matson, D. D.: Craniosynostosis: A Review of 519 Surgical Patients. *Pediatrics,* 41:829, 1968.
Tessier, P.: The Definitive Plastic Surgical Treatment of the Severe Facial Deformities of Craniofacial Dysostosis: Crouzon's and Apert's Disease. *Plast. Reconstr. Surg.* 48:419, 1971.

Hypertelorism and Hypotelorism

JACK H. RUBINSTEIN, M.D.

HYPERTELORISM

The term hypertelorism is often loosely employed in clinical situations in which the eyes appear further apart than normal. True hypertelorism, documented by appropriate measurements, such as interpupillary or interorbital distance, should be differentiated from apparent, illusory, false, suggested or pseudohypertelorism, in which the eyes appear to be far apart secondary to superficial anatomic features, such as epicanthi, lateral displacement of the medial canthi, flat nasal bridge, flat forehead, divergent strabismus, or blepharophimosis. The term telecanthus is used to describe any condition in which the distance between the medial canthi of the palpebral fissures is increased, with or without true hypertelorism.

Mild hypertelorism may occur alone as a variant of normal; in more marked degree it accompanies a wide variety of clinical syndromes and malformations (e.g., frontal encephalocele, certain craniotubular bone dysplasias and hyperostoses, and median cleft face syndrome or frontonasal dysplasia). It is also the hallmark of a relatively specific syndrome (Greig's syndrome). Rare occult malformations, such as transsphenoidal and transethmoidal basal encephaloceles, may manifest mild hypertelorism. Some of the conditions with hypertelorism appear to have a familial pattern, and some have associated mental retardation.

The management of hypertelorism requires a total evaluation of the child's physical, mental, psychologic and social assets and liabilities. Differentiation of true from apparent hypertelorism is important for the early identification of certain problems occurring in some of the syndromes associated with apparent hypertelorism and requiring early and appropriate management (e.g., deafness in the Waardenburg syndrome). In the same way, identification of a specific syndrome in which true hypertelorism is a feature may be useful in alerting the examiner to possible associated defects, as in the multiple lentigines syndrome, as well as in suggesting the degree of mental impairment and, possibly, facilitating genetic counseling. Unfortunately, a specific clinical syndrome usually is not identifiable; even when one may be identified, the evaluation and programming for each child must remain an individual matter.

Mild hypertelorism requires no specific treatment per se. Proper neurosurgical removal of frontal encephaloceles is usually indicated early in life for prevention of infection and for cosmetic reasons; however, inadequate preoperative diagnosis and attempts at local treatment can result in disaster in the management of what might have been a relatively benign lesion. If progressive hydrocephalus is present or develops, it must be controlled by adequate shunting procedures. Reconstructive correction of hypertelorism may involve several surgical approaches, including the correction of the true hypertelorism by reduction of the widened interocular distance by bone resections, as well as the reduction of the width (e.g., epicanthi) or building up of the component facial parts (e.g., flat nasal bridge) responsible for exaggeration of the appearance of far-apartness.

Some of the very severe disfiguring malformations, such as certain frontal meningoencephaloceles and some forms of the median cleft face syndrome, may be consistent with relatively intact intellectual development; therefore, the detection of these malformations in the newborn period does not necessarily warrant a pessimistic prognosis or recommendations for immediate placement of the patient outside the home. On the other hand, the extent of the neurosurgical and plastic surgical procedures, as well as the amount of hospitalization that may be required, may be tremendous. Frequently, a coordinated interdisciplinary team effort by a group of experienced medical, dental, surgical and health-related specialists is mandatory to achieve the necessary continuum of comprehensive care. This includes managing the complex decisions, techniques and complications. It also requires dealing with the associated psychologic, social and economic problems. The team must be able to offer emotional support for the family and later for the child. The cosmetic result must be matched by a reasonably well-adjusted patient and family.

HYPOTELORISM

As in hypertelorism, ocular hypotelorism may occur as a variant of normal. It may be found in syndromes, such as Down's syndrome, and with certain malformations, including the holoprosencephaly-arhinencephaly spectrum and trigonocephaly. There may be associated premature synostosis of the metopic suture, as in trigonocephaly. The more severe malformations are not compatible with life, e.g., cyclopia and ethmocephaly. Some cases in the holoprosencephaly-arhinencephaly spectrum are associated with trisomy 13–15 (D), others with deletion of the short arm of chromosome 18, and others with an apparently normal chromosome karyotype. Familial cases have been reported.

The management of children with ocular hypotelorism requires an evaluation of the more severe underlying brain pathology. Unlike hypertelorism, the more disfiguring syndromes with hypotelorism are usually accompanied by significant mental retardation; however, the severity of the facial anomalies usually, but not always, predicts the severity of the brain malformation. In addition to careful clinical evaluation of cranial and extracranial pathology, including clinical photography, cytogenetics, dermatoglyphics, transillumination of the skull and posteroanterior roentgenograms of the skull, other studies that may provide useful information include planigraphy, electroencephalography, echoencephalography and pneumoencephalography.

Initial efforts are directed toward maintenance of body temperature and nutrition. Seizures require adequate anticonvulsant control with phenobarbital, diphenylhydantoin (Dilantin) or other appropriate drugs. Occasionally there is accompanying hydrocephalus which requires shunting procedures. When the condition is compatible with life and the family understands the possible overall prognosis, consideration must be given to surgical repair of associated malformations, such as cleft lip and palate. In cases in which marked trigonocephaly appears to be the only obvious malformation, consideration may be given to neurosurgical repair of the prematurely fused metopic suture for cosmetic purposes (see the discussion under Craniostenosis). The comprehensive habilitation program should be conducted by an experienced and coordinated interdisciplinary team which can also render needed support and counseling for the family.

References

DeMyer, W.: The Median Cleft Face Syndrome: Differential Diagnosis of Cranium Bifidum Occultum, Hypertelorism, and Median Cleft Nose, Lip, and Palate. *Neurology,* 17:961, 1967.

DeMyer, W., Zeman, W., and Palmer, C. G.: The Face Predicts the Brain: Diagnostic Significance of Median Facial Anomalies for Holoprosencephaly (Arhinencephaly). *Pediatrics,* 34:256, 1964.

Gerald, B. E., and Silverman, F. N.: Normal and Abnormal Interorbital Distances, With Special Reference to Mongolism. *Am. J. Roentgen.,* 95:154, 1965.

Rogers, B. O.: Rare Craniofacial Deformities; in J. M. Converse (ed.): *Reconstructive Plastic Surgery: Principles and Procedures in Correction, Reconstruction and Transplantation.* Philadelphia, W. B. Saunders Company; 1964, vol. 3, p. 1213.

Schmid, E.: Surgical Management of Hypertelorism; in J. J. Longacre (ed.): *Craniofacial Anomalies: Pathogenesis and Repair.* Philadelphia, J. B. Lippincott Co., 1968, p. 155.

Sedano, H. O., Cohen, M. M., Jr., Jirasek, J., and Gorlin, R. J.: Frontonasal Dysplasia. *J. Pediat.,* 76:906, 1970.

Disorders of the Clavicle, Scapula and Spine

DAVID S. BRADFORD, M.D.

KLIPPEL-FEIL SYNDROME

Congenital synostosis of the cervical spine, better known as the Klippel-Feil syndrome, is a rare malformation characterized by failure of segmentation of the cervical vertebrae. Clinically, the neck is short and webbed, and motion is limited. No treatment will correct the deformity and surgery is rarely indicated. Plastic surgical procedures, such as Z-plasty of the skin with fascia and muscle releases, may in part overcome the webbing effect. Associated deformities, such as elevation of the scapula (Sprengel's deformity), cervical ribs and scoliosis may require surgical management (see below).

SPRENGEL'S DEFORMITY

Congenital high scapula, or Sprengel's deformity, is an anomaly secondary to failure of the scapula to descend from the neck to its normal location. The scapula rides very high and is distorted in shape. It may even be attached to the vertebral column by a fibrous, osseous or cartilaginous band extending from the superior angle of the scapula to the posterior elements of one of the cervical vertebrae. Associated abnormalities in the musculature of the shoulder girdle, as well as hemivertebrae, fused ribs and Klippel–Feil syndrome, are not uncommon. In fact, congenital scoliosis may be present in 50 per cent of patients with Sprengel deformity (see below).

Surgical intervention is determined by the severity of deformity or pain, or the limitation of shoulder motion. Surgery is best performed between the ages of four and seven. It consists of dividing soft tissue and bony attachments from the scapula to the trunk, transferring the scapula distally and maintaining the transfer with a traction wire and plaster cast until the soft tissue has healed.

SPONDYLOLISTHESIS AND LUMBAR INTERVERTEBRAL DISC HERNIATION

Spondylolisthesis is an acquired defect in the pars interarticularis, allowing slippage of the vertebral body anteriorly. Symptoms of back or radicular pain with hamstring tightness can often be managed conservatively by bed rest followed by a proper exercise program, as well as a brace or corset. Surgery is indicated for progressive slippage and symptoms unresponsive to conservative management. Radiographic evidence of spondylolisthesis may not in itself be an indication for an operation. The surgery consists of several approaches: (1) spinal fusion from the sacrum to the uninvolved vertebra above the spondylolisthesis; (2) a wide decompressive laminectomy, removing the fibrocartilaginous masses that impinge on the nerve roots; or (3) decompressive laminectomy combined with a spinal fusion.

Rupture of the intervertebral disc in children and adolescents presents a syndrome complex not markedly different from that in the adult. Frequently it may be missed because it is not suspected. Treatment for the most part is conservative and consists initially of strict bed rest and traction (which facilitates keeping the patient in bed if nothing else), analgesics and local heat to the back. This regimen is thought to decrease the inflammation around the nerve root and to allow regression of the disc protrusion. When the signs and symptoms have subsided, the patient is given an exercise program and a back brace if it is thought necessary. Surgery is occasionally indicated in patients who fail to respond to treatment, who have recurrent and intractable back pain and who develop persistent and progressive neurologic signs. Surgery consists of laminectomy with removal of the protruding disc. Spine fusion concomitant with the laminectomy is occasionally believed to be desirable.

KYPHOSIS AND SCOLIOSIS

The treatment of kyphosis and scoliosis in great part depends on the nature and severity of the curvature as well as the etiology of the deformity. For instance, kyphosis may be secondary to congenital deformity, tumor, trauma, infection, decompressive laminectomy, the chondrodystrophies, such as Morquio's syndrome and Hurler's disease, or cretinism and achondroplasia.

Kyphotic deformities that are minimal in severity and quite mobile can initially be managed successfully with Milwaukee braces. This is particularly applicable in cases secondary to juvenile kyphosis or Scheuermann's disease. This type of conservative treatment must be continued until maturity. Congenital kyphosis, on the other hand, is difficult to manage with a brace, and rapid progression is the rule. Early surgical intervention is recommended. This consists of a spine fusion over the involved area, sometimes anteriorly as well as posteriorly, followed by plaster immobilization until the fusion becomes solid. If neurologic compromise has developed secondary to the kyphosis, an anterior decompression may be necessary.

In the management of scoliosis, it is also important that every effort be made to determine the cause of the scoliosis, whether it be neuromuscular, paralytic, congenital, secondary to neurofibromatosis or idiopathic. For flexible curves of less than 45 degrees in growing children, the Milwaukee brace is the preferable method of treatment. The brace initially must be worn all the time and the treatment supervised closely with periodic x-rays during the growth period. A properly designed exercise program in the brace is desirable. As maturity approaches, the patient can be gradually weaned from the brace. It must be stressed that exercises alone without a brace have never been shown to be of any benefit in correcting a curvature. Curves greater than 20 degrees in the growing child must be properly treated to prevent their progression.

Operative treatment is indicated in patients with rapidly progressing curves not responding to brace treatment (patients with neurofibromatosis are poor candidates for brace treatment) and in patients with curves greater than 50 degrees who are far along in their development and present a deformity that is cosmetically unacceptable. Surgical treatment is often preceded by a period of distraction, followed by spine fusion and plaster immobilization for approximately nine months. The use of a Harrington distraction rod has facilitated correction of the curve and early ambulation following surgery, and has decreased the incidence of pseudarthrosis.

OSTEOMYELITIS OF THE SPINE

Before initiating treatment for osteomyelitis of the spine, every effort should be made to determine the type of organism, either by means of a needle biopsy or blood cultures. Treatment consists of appropriate antibiotics and bed rest with a brace or plaster cast immobilization. Treatment should continue until constitutional signs and symptoms of infection have subsided and there is radiographic evidence of healing.

Chest Wall Abnormalities

J. ALEX HALLER, JR., M.D.

The major chest wall abnormalities which are bothersome to both children and parents are funnel chest deformity (pectus excavatum), which is nearly always a central, bilaterally equal abnormality, and pigeon breast (pectus carinatum), which is frequently off the midline and may be unilateral.

Pectus excavatum is a disturbing chest deformity because of its cosmetic significance to parents and children. It also interferes with the functional pull of muscles of the shoulder and chest and may result in very striking postural abnormalities. There is little objective evidence that a child with pectus excavatum suffers any physiologic embarrassment to his heart and lungs, but there is growing suspicion that our tests are inadequate to detect some of these deficiencies. The cosmetic impact of this deformity on a child's developing personality may be of lasting importance; this, along with the problem of poor posture, characterized by slumping shoulders and protuberant abdomen, are the two major reasons for operative reconstruction of this abnormality.

The exact etiology of this condition remains unknown, although the abnormality is clearly related to the deformed anterior costal cartilages. Once these have been removed, the depressed sternum is usually easily elevated and may or may not be supported artificially in its new position.

Since pectus excavatum is usually asymptomatic in childhood, surgical correction is undertaken only because of a severe deformity. This attitude is justified if the surgeon is convinced that the child and his family are psychologically affected by the pectus deformity, and that the defect is significantly interfering with normal postural development. The decision to correct the deformity then must be based on thoughtful communication with the patient and his family. In our opinion, restoration of the anterior wall to its normal anatomy is reason enough to recommend surgical correction, if the operation is safely performed and the patient can be reasonably sure of a lasting satisfactory result. In our experience with more than 180 patients with pectus excavatum abnormalities undergoing operative repair, the absence of operative mortality and the very low morbidity with satisfactory late results offer strong recommendations for its continued use in selected patients. We prefer to operate on the child before he enters school and earlier if the pectus deformity is quite marked. The youngest child operated on in our experience was one year of age and he has gotten an excellent long-term result.

The operative procedure of choice in our experience has been a modification of the one developed by Dr. Mark Ravitch. This consists of a transverse skin incision, elevation of the pectoral muscles off the chest wall and resection of the abnormal costal cartilages, leaving the perichondrium behind for later regrowth. A transverse osteotomy of the sternum at the apex of the deformity is performed in conjunction with an oblique transsection of the highest normal costal cartilages, bringing the medial ends of these cartilages over their lateral extensions. Tripod-like internal fixation is achieved without the use of implanted foreign material. Approximately 90 per cent of patients undergoing this operative procedure have had excellent long-term results. The period of hospitalization is one week to 10 days, and the period of protection from strenuous exercise and contact sports is six weeks.

The operative procedure for *pectus carinatum* is similar in concept, in that the abnormal costal cartilages must be excised to allow the sternum to recede to a normal position. The indications for operation for pectus carinatum are not as clearly defined, because there is no postural abnormality associated with this condition. The indication is purely a cosmetic one. If the deformity is severe and the parents and child are anxious to have it corrected, we believe that this is a legitimate indication for such a procedure.

References

Adkins, P. C., Graff, D. B., and Blades, B.: Experiences with Metal Struts for Chest Wall Stabilization. *Ann. Thorac. Surg.*, 5:246, 1968.

Haller, J. A., Jr., Peters, G. N., and White, J. J.: Surgical Management of Funnel Chest (Pectus Excavatum). *Surg. Clin. N. Am.*, 50:929, 1970.

Ravitch, M. M.: Technical Problems in the Operative Correction of Pectus Excavatum. *Ann. Surg.*, 162:29, 1965.

Disorders of the Extremities

HENRY H. BANKS, M.D.

DEFORMITIES OF THE EXTREMITIES

Deformities of the extremities are either congenital or acquired during the growing period.

Congenital deformities may be due to failure of differentiation, defective segmentation, abnormal, or failure of, fusion of ossification centers, or incomplete migration. The principles of treatment involve early recognition and correction when feasible, beginning even in the nursery. Such correction must be maintained usually by exercises and night support during the growing period. The ultimate purpose of treatment is the achievement of a functional position of the involved upper or lower extremity, ambulation and self-sufficiency. Not only must the deformity be corrected, but also the psychologic needs of the child and parent must constantly be considered. All too frequently the education of the child may be grossly disturbed by multiple and prolonged hospitalizations.

Some congenital deformities, e.g., myelodysplasia, require the expertise of several disciplines, but unfortunately, some of these children are abandoned to the care of one. The pediatrician must assume a leadership role in such problems.

Acquired deformities of the extremities may develop at any time during the growing period, but they are less likely to be significant if the cause is amenable to surgery at the end of growth. In an actively growing musculoskeletal system, many factors may be responsible for deformity. Trauma, especially to an epiphyseal plate, may cause asymmetrical growth of an extremity. Muscle imbalance, regardless of whether due to myelodysplasia, cerebral palsy or other causes, with the added factors of active growth and gravity, may be responsible for significant deformity, as may metabolic defects affecting the conversion of cartilage to bone, e.g., resistant rickets. Infections of bone and joints as well as inflammatory joint disease may cause significant upper or lower extremity deformity. There are still other etiologic factors, such as posture and gait disturbance.

Treatment obviously involves early recognition of a potential etiologic factor and prevention of a deformity when possible. In muscle imbalance, for example, proper bracing, night support and exercises may be helpful in prevention. Muscle transplantation may be necessary to restore balance. This should be done only when the muscle to be transplanted is strong enough to function adequately and the deformity is corrected. Furthermore, a cooperative child and family, as well as a detailed postoperative regimen, are essential to obtain a satisfactory result.

In deformities due to metabolic bone disease, the metabolic defect requires adequate treatment if the deformity is to be prevented, minimized or corrected. The best example here is vitamin D–resistant rickets.

Leg length discrepancy need no longer be an accepted deformity and treated by an unsightly elevated shoe. Repeated special x-rays of the extremities during the growing period allow the surgeon to perform an epiphyseal arrest about the knee at the proper age, yielding equal or almost equal leg lengths in most patients. When the discrepancy is too great for correction by epiphyseal arrest alone, leg lengthening, especially of the tibia in paralytic disease, is a successful procedure in experienced hands.

Bowlegs. Bowlegs unrelated to classic or resistant rickets or epiphyseal injury are ordinarily congenital, familial or positional in origin. Asymmetrical epiphyseal growth may be a factor. Osteochondrosis of the medial aspect of the proximal tibial epiphysis (Blount's disease) may also be present. Bowing of the tibia, often with internal tibial torsion and normal genu valgum giving the impression of bowlegs, is more common than classic genu varum. There is usually associated foot pronation. Evaluation by roentgenograms is important to identify epiphyseal disturbances, i.e., classic, resistant or renal rickets. Successful treatment would then require proper management of the underlying condition.

Mild degrees of genu varum and tibia vara often resolve with growth. Arch support is important. An outer sole wedge of ⅛ inch is often used. Well-supervised daily manipulations may be helpful. The child should be encouraged to sleep on his back or side and not on his abdomen.

The correction of severe degrees of bowlegs (more than 6 inches between the femoral condyles with the medial malleoli touching) may be accelerated by a Denis Browne night shoe splint. It is important not to use a bar of more than 12 inches between the shoes to prevent the creation of valgus feet and undue genu valgum.

Operative correction – osteotomy – is reserved for severe degrees of deformity which do not respond significantly to conservative treatment. Ordinarily this approach is not considered before six or seven years of age.

Genu Valgum (Knock Knees). Genu valgum more than the usual physiologic 10 to 15 degrees and unrelated to rickets or epiphyseal injury may be familial and associated with pronated feet, ligamentous relaxation and overweight. Correcting the pronation with inner heel wedges and arch supports tends to correct knock knee as growth occurs. Weight reduction is important where this is a factor.

Severe degrees of genu valgum (12 inches or more between the medial malleoli with the femoral condyles touching) which do not respond to conservative measures may require osteotomy of the distal femur or proximal tibia, depending upon where the maximal deformity is. Ordinarily this approach is not considered before six or seven years of age.

Genu Recurvatum. This deformity, when present at birth, responds well to the early application of long leg casts changed weekly, and to gradually developing flexion. When range is developed, then maintenance of correction by night support and exercise is of value.

Genu recurvatum noted after infancy is related to ligamentous relaxation or quadriceps muscle weakness and a secondary growth disturbance at the knee. When due to ligamentous relaxation, the deformity is minimal, and no treatment is indicated other than would be done for the often-related foot pronation.

When recurvatum is related to muscle weakness and the deformity minimal, a long leg brace prevents progression of the deformity. Muscle transplants to strengthen the quadriceps function may be of value when feasible. When the deformity is severe (20 to 30 degrees or more), surgical osteotomy of the proximal tibia may be required. If there is muscle imbalance which cannot be corrected, then a long leg brace is needed after the osteotomy has healed, to prevent recurrence of the deformity during the growing period.

Recurrent Dislocation of the Patella. In childhood this condition, with or without precipitating trauma, may be associated with underdevelopment of the lateral condyle of the femur, genu valgum, external tibial torsion and ligamentous relaxation. Conservative treatment, including quadriceps strengthening, is usually ineffective. Surgical correction is important to prevent chondromalacia of the patella and lateral condyle of the femur as well as the formation of loose bodies in the knee joint. Prior to the completion of growth (even at four or five years of age), the patellaplasty of Green is effective in correcting recurrent dislocation of the patella. When growth has ceased, one may need to transplant the tibial tubercle medially and distally as well as to perform this patellaplasty.

Tibial Torsion. Most children with internal tibial torsion walk with a toe-in gait which disturbs parents, grandparents and neighbors. Most of these deformities resolve with growth. Arch support and outer sole wedges (1/8 inch or so) are helpful. When the child is old enough to cooperate, gait training daily by the mother is important. Often there is enough external rotation of the hips in extension to make it possible for the child to walk with a normal gait. The correction of severe degrees of internal tibial torsion often associated with tibia vara may be accelerated by wearing a Denis Browne night shoe splint. Here again, it is important not to use a wide bar between the shoes to prevent the development of undue genu valgum and flat feet. Surgical correction by osteotomy is rarely indicated.

Preventing the patient from sleeping on his abdomen or sitting with his hips in internal rotation is important.

External tibial torsion is usually less of a problem in management. Arch supports, inner heel wedges (1/8 inch) and gait training are ordinarily successful. Surgical correction by osteotomy is rarely indicated.

Toe-in Related to Deformity of the Hip. Some children have normally aligned lower extremities and toe-in because of rotational deformities of the hip. These children may have as much as 90 degrees of internal rotation of the hip in extension and sharply restricted external rotation. They often sit and sleep with their hips internally rotated. The deformity apparently is due to anteversion of the hip, although torsion of the femur may be present.

The problem in such children is usually resolved with growth. Attention to sitting and sleeping posture is important. Support of the feet for associated pronation is advisable. In some instances it is necessary to equip the child with external rotation twister braces because of the tendency to fall frequently. The few children who do not respond to the usual conservative measures by the age of 10 may require a subtrochanteric osteotomy to realign the femur.

AMPUTATIONS

Congenital and acquired amputations are best handled by a multidisciplinary team involved in the prescription, supervision and training in the use of prostheses. The type of prosthesis varies with the length of the stump and the extremity involved. A lower limb prosthesis is usually well accepted by the child and should be provided when attempts are being made to stand. Initially, a brace may be used because of the expense involved in repeated construction of prostheses during the growing period. The tendency now is to fit an upper limb prosthesis early (by six months) to encourage its use.

DEFORMITIES OF THE FEET

At birth, the most common foot deformities are *positional,* including talipes equinovarus, varus, valgus, calcaneus and calcaneovalgus. When there is passive flexibility, appropriate exercises beginning in the nursery correct these deformities. When there is no passive flexibility initially, a plaster of paris cast applied at least at weekly intervals corrects the deformity in four to six weeks. Night support in the form of removable bivalved casts and exercises may be necessary for several months to maintain the correction.

Adduction of the anterior part of the foot, when passively correctable, usually responds rapidly to stretching exercises performed at each diaper change. When it is not passively correctable, a plaster cast must be applied at frequent intervals. When treatment is delayed or fails, capsulotomy of the metatarsal-cuneiform joints or metatarsal osteotomy may be necessary. If surgical procedures are necessary (certainly not performed during the first few years of life), the correction must be maintained by straight last shoes, night support and exercises during most of the growing period.

Congenital Clubfoot. Although any deformity of the foot is classically called a clubfoot, the most common deformity given this name is talipes equinovarus. It is important to differentiate such a deformity from that due to muscle imbalance in myelodysplasia and arthrogryposis.

The treatment of the classic congenital clubfoot should begin as soon as possible, preferably in the nursery. One must be sure that there are no associated deformities, including torticollis, myelodysplasia, congenital dislocation of the hip and arthrogryposis. The treatment of choice is usually preceded by a short interval of manipulation into correction, followed by the application of a long leg cast in the most comfortable position of correction. Generally, the inversion and adduction of the anterior part of the foot responds more readily to the correction than does the talipes equinus. When the deformity of the foot responds to conservative measures, usually four to six months are required with repeated applications of casts at weekly intervals.

Once the deformity is corrected, it is important to maintain the correction throughout the growing period. This usually requires the use of a bivalved night cast, outflare shoes and exercises. There is a constant tendency for recurrence during the growing period, which may require repeated plaster cast correction. If the talipes equinus does not respond to conservative measures after a year or so of treatment, posterior capsulotomy of the ankle and subtalar joint, along with heel cord lengthening, is necessary. The correction must then be maintained throughout the growing period by the previously described measures. When there is muscle imbalance, tendon transplantation may be necessary to restore balance. However, such a procedure should not be done in the presence of deformity. At the end of the growing period when significant bony deformity is already present, a triple arthrodesis may be necessary to correct the deformed foot.

The Pronated Foot. The most common foot problem in childhood is pronation. Under the age of three, this is quite often seen in the normal child, particularly with his wide-based toe-out gait. During this interval, a child does well with a high shoe, including a hard sole and $\frac{1}{8}$-inch inner heel wedge. After this age, the child may also require a longitudinal arch support. Mild pronation does well with such treatment. Indeed, a normal arch may be apparent under such circumstances within a few years. In some children, particularly those who have relaxed ligaments, pronation may persist throughout the growing period. Such children are symptomatically better with longitudinal arch support and inner heel wedges. Even if they never develop an arch, at least the bones and joints of the feet will adapt to a normal position. Significant deformities may require lightweight Whitman support.

When the pronated foot is related to a contracted heel cord, exercises may be necessary for this structure as well. In the patient with spasticity, significant heel cord contracture may need surgery to correct significant talipes valgus of the foot. After the age of five, such patients may need a subtalar arthrodesis as well.

When muscle imbalance is a factor, attention must be directed to this problem as well as to proper support of the foot.

If peroneal spasm and a tarsal coalition are responsible for symptomatic flat feet, a triple arthrodesis may be required at the end of the growing period.

Cavus Feet. In a cavus foot, there is an abnormally high-arched contour. This may be familial or neurologic in origin. When the deformity is not progressive and not neurologic, the patient must wear shoes with metatarsal support and must do exercises to prevent contracture of the plantar fascia and to keep the toes in proper position. When the deformity is significant and does not respond to the usual conservative measures, plantar fasciotomy and transplant of the toe extensors to the neck of the metatarsal bones may be necessary. At the end of the growing period, the patient may also require a triple arthrodesis.

HEMIHYPERTROPHY

Hemihypertrophy may involve both upper and lower extremities on one side or just one lower extremity. Both upper and lower extremities on the one side are longer and larger in circumference than the ones on the other side. Although hemihypertrophy is more common than hemiatrophy, sometimes it is difficult to be sure which is the more prominent problem in any one patient. Usually the clinician bases his decision on which extremity seems to be more appropriate to the rest of the contour of the child. All structures in the involved extremity appear to be normal but larger.

When there is significant leg length discrepancy, the growth potential of the involved extremity must be recorded at regular intervals during the growing period, usually at the time of the child's birthday. If the discrepancy is minimal, a minor shoe elevation may be all that is required. When it is significant, an epiphyseal arrest may be performed about the knee at the appropriate time to equalize the leg lengths.

Whereas congenital hypertrophy is more common, one must be aware of the possible relationship of neurofibromatosis or vascular anomalies. The orthopedic treatment is essentially the same.

Diseases of the Hip

HENRY H. BANKS, M.D.

TOXIC OR NONSPECIFIC SYNOVITIS

This disease is a nonspecific inflammation of the synovium, which causes painful limited hip motion and limping. It is a diagnosis made by exclusion because the same complaints and physical signs may be present in other diseases, such as monarticular arthritis, tuberculosis and aseptic necrosis of the head of the femur. Other causes of synovitis of the hip must, therefore, be considered. The evaluation should include not only a careful history and physical examination but also adequate blood studies and x-rays. Aspiration and analysis of the hip joint fluid may be necessary.

The treatment consists of nonweightbearing. In mild cases, this may be with bed rest for a week or two. When the physical signs are more marked, traction, even in the hospital, may be required. In such circumstances, two to three weeks of treatment may be necessary for the physical signs to disappear. During this interval, the child must be repeatedly examined to be sure that other joints are not involved. Furthermore, the physician and family must be aware that radiologic changes of aseptic necrosis of the head of the femur (Legg-Calvé-Perthes disease) may appear within six months of onset of symptoms.

LEGG-CALVÉ-PERTHES DISEASE

Osteochondrosis of the hip (coxa plana or Legg-Calvé-Perthes disease) is an avascular necrosis of the proximal femoral capital epiphysis. It is a common cause of painful limited hip motion and limp between the ages of 4 and 10. This is a self-limited condition from which recovery is spontaneous. The problem is to maintain the normal contour of the femoral head during the course of the process. When there is painful limited hip motion because of an associated synovitis, nonweightbearing, usually with traction for one to three weeks, is necessary to develop a full range of motion. The standard treatment then consists of a nonweightbearing brace until the process is resolved within two to three years. Various braces designed to provide abduction and internal rotation are now available and appear to be helpful in this regard. It is important that the head of the femur remain covered by the acetabulum during the active phase of the condition. In some circumstances, an iliac osteotomy or subtrochanteric osteotomy may be necessary to better cover the femoral head by the acetabulum.

SLIPPED FEMORAL CAPITAL EPIPHYSIS

In slipped proximal femoral capital epiphysis, the femoral head is displaced from its normal relationship with the femoral neck. The physical findings may be classic with no internal rotation and limited abduction. In some patients, there may be hyperextension of the hip. Indeed, it is the only condition of the hip that may yield this physical finding and not a flexion deformity.

Surgical treatment is required to prevent further slipping of the femoral head off of the femoral neck. Bed rest with or without traction is insufficient because the femoral head may come off of the femoral neck even when the patient is in bed.

Once the diagnosis has been made, the

patient is hospitalized and placed in traction until the acute symptoms have subsided. If the displacement is a centimeter or less, in situ fixation with a vitallium wood screw or threaded pins will cause the epiphyseal plate to close within six months, preventing further slippage. When the slipping is more than a centimeter, anatomic restoration by intra-articular or extra-articular procedures is generally recommended. For the operator not thoroughly experienced in handling this disorder, particularly when dealing with a non-Caucasian patient, an extra-articular subtrochanteric osteotomy, plus measures to close the epiphyseal plate, is necessary. In more experienced hands, the deformity may be corrected in Caucasian patients by an intra-articular wedge osteotomy of the neck of the femur.

In all persons with a slipped femoral capital epiphysis, one must be aware of the possibility of this condition developing bilaterally. Furthermore, in renal rickets and abnormalities of the thyroid, a slipped epiphysis may be observed in the shoulders as well as in the hip joint.

In some patients with classic proximal slipped femoral capital epiphysis, acute chondrolysis of the acetabulum and the femoral head may occur. With prolonged heavy skeletal traction, physical therapy and nonweightbearing, the patient may effect his own arthroplasty. A joint space will be noted radiographically after a year of such treatment.

Disorders of Bone

HENRY H. BANKS, M.D.

FIBROUS DYSPLASIA OF BONE

Fibrous dysplasia is a disease characterized by cystlike areas in one or more bones, often combined with café au lait spots. Uncommonly it involves multiple bones and is associated with precocious sexual development and early skeletal maturation. It may be responsible for deformity because of weakened bone or a pathologic fracture, particularly in the vicinity of the hip.

Surgical curettage of the lesion and replacement by a bone graft is usually curative. When more than one lesion is present, surgery is reserved for those which are providing a clinical problem.

When there is extensive involvement of the proximal femur, attempts must be made to prevent coxa vara, often by nonweightbearing braces. Surgical correction as described is usually necessary.

When precocious puberty and premature skeletal maturation are present, the patient and family require a great deal of support from both surgeon and pediatrician.

PSEUDO-OSTEOCHONDROSES

Osteochondrosis of the vertebral body is also known as Scheuermann's disease. Treatment is required, not only because of pain and muscle spasm, but also because there may be progressive deformity of the vertebrae with wedging anteriorly.

When the process is mild, hyperextension exercises and a hyperextension brace are often sufficient. When symptoms are acute, plaster of paris immobilization and hyperextension may be necessary for a month or two prior to such treatment.

Osteochondrosis of the tibial tubercle, Osgood-Schlatter's disease, is usually noted in adolescence, affecting boys more often than girls. There is pain and swelling over the tibial tubercle.

In mild cases, the avoidance of kneeling, squatting and going up and down stairs may give relief during the course of this self-limited condition. When symptoms are significant and not responding to simple protection, plaster of paris immobilization for six to eight weeks is necessary. Surgical treatment is rarely indicated.

DISLOCATIONS

Cervical Subluxation. Rotatory subluxation of the first cervical vertebra on the second usually responds to a week or two of head traction in the hospital followed by a cervical collar. When the process is related to rheumatoid arthritis or tuberculosis, obviously measures must be directed toward these underlying conditions. When there is true dislocation due to rheumatoid arthritis, skull traction may be necessary to reduce the deformity.

Congenital Hip Dysplasia. Some children who have positional deformities of the lower extremities also have an underdeveloped acetabulum and a contracture of the adductor muscles on that side. Such children do very well with adductor stretching exercises and triple diapers. When the acetabular underdevelopment tends to persist, a Frejka pillow or abduction splint may be necessary.

Congenital Dislocation of the Hip. This disorder must be diagnosed early to obtain a good result from treatment. The principle of treatment involves placing the femoral head into the acetabulum and maintaining abduction until the point develops satisfactorily. Because the classic signs of dislocation are known to all pediatricians, the condition should be recognized in the nursery or at least in the first few months of life. Certainly, the diagnosis should be made prior to weightbearing.

In the newborn, maintaining the hip in abduction with a Frejka pillow or abduction splint is satisfactory. Within the first few months of life, closed reduction of the hip and maintenance of abduction with a plaster spica are necessary. In patients with significant adduction contracture, preliminary skin traction is often needed prior to closed reduction. When closed reduction is successful, plaster of paris immobilization for 6 to 12 months is necessary before the acetabulum is adequately developed. The cast must be changed every three months or so because of the growth of the child.

When closed reduction is not possible or is unstable, open reduction is necessary, again followed by plaster of paris immobilization until the acetabulum is well-developed. Early exercises, however, are required under these circumstances. When the acetabulum is slow in developing, an osteotomy of the ilium may be performed. Further surgery to correct anteversion may also be needed. Such children require careful follow-up throughout the growing period to ensure proper development of the hip joint. In some circumstances the proximal femoral capital epiphysis closes early and the greater trochanter continues to grow, limiting abduction. A significant incidence of aseptic necrosis appears to be inevitable in this condition, and requires the same treatment as aseptic necrosis in Legg-Calvé-Perthes disease.

Housemaid's Elbow. Housemaid's elbow or subluxation of the head of the radius may occur when someone lifts a young child or pulls his upper extremity. The child then cannot move his elbow and has pain in attempting motion. Treatment consists of gentle supination followed by flexion. There is usually immediate relief of symptoms. The child wears a sling for a few days and then resumes normal activities.

Infantile Cortical Hyperostosis

GERALD H. HOLMAN, M.D.

The child with this disorder presents with a classic triad of fever, irritability and local bone tenderness. (A good review outlines the clinical course and extent of usual involvement [Holman]).

Mild Involvement. Phenobarbital, 5 mg. per kilogram per day in three or four doses, is essential to allay anxiety. If significant fever is present, acetylsalicylic acid, 65 mg. per kilogram per 24 hours in four to six doses, is helpful. This should be avoided in the very young patient if possible. Careful handling of the affected part minimizes pain. The parents should feed the child gently because of frequent mandibular involvement.

Severe Involvement. Patients with severe hyperostosis require more vigorous therapy. Oral administration of glucocorticosteroids is the treatment of choice.

Hydrocortisone, 30 to 60 mg. per day in four divided doses orally, or prednisone, 10 to 15 mg. per day in three or four divided doses orally, is given. Usually there is a prompt response with normalization of the temperature within 72 hours. The corticoids should then be gradually reduced and may frequently be discontinued in 10 days. If symptoms recur, reinstitution of the foregoing is necessary, followed by reduction to the smallest dose which will maintain freedom from symptoms. This dose is continued until all clinical signs and laboratory evidence of disease have disappeared (including normalization of the sedimentation rate and radiologic evidence of no further disease progression). This may take several weeks to several months in some infants, but one must strive to discontinue steroid therapy as quickly as possible.

Long-term radiologic follow-up is advisable (up to 24 months after onset of the disease) for evaluation of possible permanent bone changes.

Complications. Some severely ill patients exhibit a rapid reduction in circulating hemoglobin. Even if response to glucorticoids is dramatic, restoration of normal red blood cell volume by blood transfusion may be necessary in rare instances.

Oral calcium gluconate, 500 mg. per kilogram per day in four doses, should be given for significant hypocalcemia.

Symptomatic thrombocythemia may require heparinization by continuous intravenous drip, 100 U.S.P. units per kilogram every 4 hours. Antimegakaryocyte therapy consisting of busulphan, 0.06 mg. per kilogram per day in two doses, maintains the platelet count at safe levels. Steroid therapy may be contraindicated in this situation.

Parental Counseling. Gerrard et al. have stressed the familial occurrence of this disease. Available data suggest that this disorder is transmitted as an autosomal dominant with variable penetrance. The possibility of another child having this disorder may be as high as 50 per cent. All subsequent children should be carefully followed during the first six months of life for evidence of disease, thus allowing for early management.

References:

Gerrard, J. W., et al.: Familial Infantile Cortical Hyperostosis. *J. Pediat.,* 49:543, 1961.
Holman, G. H.: Infantile Cortical Hyperostosis: A Review. *Quart. Rev. Pediat.,* 17:24, 1962.

Chondrodystrophia Calcificans Congenita

HENRY H. BANKS, M.D.

This is a rare but clinically recognizable generalized disorder of bone and other tissues. Constant signs include saddle nose, hypertelorism, frontal bossing, high arched palate, short neck and short stature. Variable signs include rhizomelia, flexion contractures of joints, congenital dislocation of the hip, cataracts, optic atrophy, mental retardation, skin rash, renal anomalies and congenital heart disease. Synonyms are stippled epiphyses and Conradi's disease.

The roentgenographic findings are classic and consist of discrete punctate calcific densities in the epiphyses (stippling) and in all bones preformed in hyaline cartilage. The larynx, trachea and hyoid may also be involved.

Half of the patients die within the first six months of life. The remainder tend to improve slowly. The roentgenographic appearance of the skeleton gradually approximates normal by three to four years of age.

Supportive therapy, including early diagnosis, is indicated. When mild flexion deformities of joints are present, gradual correction with exercises and splinting is effective. If the deformities are severe, repeated plaster casts may be necessary for correction.

The entity has an autosomal recessive mode of inheritance with a familial incidence of 10 per cent; if the parents are consanguineous the incidence is 12 to 30 per cent. Early diagnosis is essential to provide effective genetic counseling of the family.

Osteomyelitis and Suppurative Arthritis

RICHARD H. MEADE, III, M.D.

Osteomyelitis is often diagnosed by x-ray and can be treated after isolation of the causative bacteria. When it is accompanied by fever, inflammation of surrounding tissues and pain, treatment is usually given before the offending pathogen can be identified in order to halt the progress of a systemic infection as soon as possible. For this reason, it is occasionally necessary to change the antibiotic therapy if cultures show an unexpected etiology. As important as the initial drug choice, therefore, are the steps taken to identify the cause.

The following cultures and smears must be carried out as soon as the diagnosis of osteomyelitis is made, regardless of the severity of attendant systemic signs and symptoms: (1) At least three consecutive blood cultures should be obtained at intervals of not less than 20 minutes. This is necessary both as an adjunct to culture of the infected bone, since bacteremia is often present, and to distinguish between transient blood stream dissemination of bacteria from the osseous focus and endocarditis. The latter is identified by the presence of bacterial growth in all cultures. (2) Cultures and Gram-stained smears should be made from the exudate in adjacent muscle abscesses, if present. (3) Culture and Gram-stained smear examination should be made of material from the infected bone itself, whether obtained by percutaneous needle aspiration under fluoroscopic control, or by open biopsy. (4) The sensitivity of bacteria recovered from blood or from other cultures should be determined unless the organism is a group A streptococcus, pneumococcus or *Hemophilus influenza* bacillus whose antibiotic susceptibilities are known. It is of great importance for *Staphylococcus aureus,* for Salmonella, for enteric gram-negative bacilli and for Pseudomonas species. This test can be performed in vitro with antibiotic disks applied to plates of nutrient agar on which the pathogen has been inoculated.

Treatment is a combination of orthopedic and medical procedures:

1. Immobilization of the involved bone is necessary to ensure healing and to prevent injury to weakened bony plates. This can be provided by simple traction to an extremity if a long bone is involved or by the use of a cast to the extremity or to the trunk for vertebral osteomyelitis. Immobilization also ensures the great-

est possible comfort by preventing painful movement.

2. *Antibiotic selection before the cause is identified:* Osteomyelitis following injury, or blood stream dissemination from infection in the skin, or following no recognizable primary disease is commonly due to *Staphylococcus aureus* and less often to *Streptococcus pyogenes* group A. Treatment with any of the following antibiotics will be effective: Oxacillin (or other semisynthetic penicillinase-resistant penicillin) in a dose of 100 to 150 mg. per kilogram of body weight daily. This is divided into aliquots and given intravenously every 4 hours. The individual dose is diluted in 50 to 100 ml. of 0.9 per cent saline and allowed to flow in within 30 minutes. It can be mounted as a separate bottle beside another used for parenteral fluid administration, or given through a heparin lock device. Erythromycin in a dose of 100 mg. per kilogram per day can be used intravenously only, and at intervals of 6 hours. It is given in the same way as oxacillin. It produces severe phlebitis in some patients, and for this reason lincomycin* is often preferred. It is used in a dose of 50 mg. per kilogram daily. Cephalothin requires a larger dose than is used for more superficial infections. To ensure adequate bone concentration, 200 mg. per kilogram per day should be given if this antibiotic is chosen, and the interval between doses should be no longer than 3 hours.

Osteomyelitis developing in a patient with sickle cell anemia is due to Salmonella often enough (and to Shigella) to require empiric treatment directed against this organism even before it has been demonstrated in cultures. Because *Staphylococcus aureus* is also a potential pathogen, the drug used should be capable of inhibiting its growth as well. Chloramphenicol† would serve excellently until cultures were available to determine which pathogen was present, but its suppressive effect upon reticulocyte formation is such that it should not be given to the patient with hemoglobin S disease. Cephalothin in large doses, as listed above, will be sufficiently effective against Salmonella to permit its use here. Another drug, such as ampicillin (300 mg. per kilogram body weight daily, in doses divided to permit intravenous injection every 2 to 3 hours), can be substituted if Salmonellae are recovered on culture.

Osteomyelitis of the tarsal bones complicating infection following a perforating injury (as acquired by a child stepping on a nail) is commonly due to Pseudomonas. Unless exudate in the wound contains gram-positive cocci as seen on a Gram-stained smear, antibiotic therapy should be directed against this gram-negative bacillus. Until sensitivity tests show it to be susceptible to other drugs, polymyxin, colistimethate or gentamicin will have to be used parenterally (intramuscular and intravenous routes are equally useful). Polymyxin is used in the dose of 2.5 mg. per kilogram daily in three divided doses; colistimethate is used in the dose of 3 to 5 mg. per kilogram daily; and gentamicin in the dose of 3 to 5 mg. per kilogram of body weight daily. Each antibiotic can be given by either route. Since each can cause renal tubular damage, kidney function should be determined by obtaining a serum creatinine level before the drug is given, although this need not be known to give the first dose. If the value is elevated above normal, the next dose should be delayed and subsequent doses should be spaced to prevent further renal damage. Intervals of 12 to 18 or even 24 hours will have to be allowed, depending on the degree of functional impairment. Creatinine determination should be carried out daily in this situation, and twice a week if the value is normal. Gentamicin is ototoxic. If given intravenously, it should not be administered except by carefully regulated drip to ensure a 30-minute interval of injection. Hearing function should be monitored by testing before treatment has been under way for more than a day, and weekly thereafter. The danger to hearing is not as great in the child as it is in the adult and is not, therefore, a reason to prevent its use even in infants whose hearing cannot be determined accurately.

Certain additional clinical syndromes are of value in determining the pathogen before it is isolated. (1) Maxillary osteitis in infants in association with maxillary sinusitis is due to *S. aureus* and is treated with any of the four drugs listed above. (2) Hematogenous osteomyelitis in the newborn, or complicating bowel surgery in the older infant, is often due to enteric gram-negative bacilli. Unless antibiotic treatment has already been given because of sepsis before osteomyelitis is recognized, *E. coli* is the most common cause for this infection. In the absence of obvious abdominal or genitourinary infection, however, the neonate may be infected by either *S. aureus* or Pseudomonas. Cephalothin is the antibiotic of greatest general effectiveness for children in either category. Polymyxin or colis-

* Manufacturer's precaution: Lincomycin is not indicated in the newborn up to one month of age.

† Manufacturer's precaution: Chloramphenicol is not recommended for intravenous or intramuscular pediatric use. Chloramphenicol sodium succinate has been approved for intravenous pediatric use.

timethate should be added in treating the neonate, however, if for any reason it is considered that Pseudomonas infection is present, and should be continued until evidence as to the true cause is available.

Treatment for osteomyelitis in which the cause is known can be given according to the recommendations in Tables 1 and 2. In all cases, drug therapy must be sustained for a period of four weeks in full parenteral dose for the entire period. It has been recommended by some that the amount of antibiotic given can be safely reduced after fever has gone, and that oral preparations can be substituted for injected forms. I cannot agree with this as a recommendation because it is based on the observation that relapse and recrudescence do not occur very often. No one knows how well a patient will do until treatment has been completed and a follow-up period of at least 10 years has passed. Full treatment must be given to reduce the number in whom relapse will occur, and to give assurance that everything was done that was possible. Parenteral therapy may become impossible in some cases, and oral therapy will have to be substituted. This is necessary in some, but cannot be regarded as a safe recommendation for all. X-ray evidence of bone involvement will often continue to progress even while effective therapy is being administered. Longer treatment is necessary only in unusual cases in which there is persistent purulent drainage from bone or persistent muscle abscess. In this case the disease has become chronic and surgical excision of infected and necrotic bone must be carried out while antibiotic therapy is maintained.

The requirements for the treatment of suppurative arthritis unassociated with osteomyelitis are little different. Such additional pathogens as *Neisseria meningitidis, Neisseria gonorrhoeae* and *H. influenzae* are encountered and should therefore be considered before initiating drug therapy empirically. Diagnosis by aspiration of the joint is usually readily accomplished, thus making antibiotic choice easier at

TABLE 1. Antibiotic Choice for Specific Bacterial Pathogens in Osteomyelitis and Suppurative Arthritis

PATHOGEN	ANTIBIOTIC
S. aureus	Penicillin G*
S. pyogenes	Cephalothin
D. pneumoniae	Oxacillin
	Erythromycin
	Lincomycin
N. meningitidis	Penicillin G
	Ampicillin
	Chloramphenicol
H. influenza	Ampicillin
	Chloramphenicol
	Streptomycin with penicillin G
N. gonorrhoeae	Penicillin G
	Ampicillin
	Cephalothin
E. coli	Ampicillin
P. mirabilis	Chloramphenicol
	Kanamycin
	Gentamicin
Proteus species†	Kanamycin
Enterobacter	Gentamicin
	Chloramphenicol
Pseudomonas	Gentamicin
	Polymyxin, colistimethate

* For penicillin-sensitive *S. aureus.*

† This is not *Proteus mirabilis,* which is sensitive to penicillin, cephalothin, ampicillin and other antibiotics.

TABLE 2. Antibiotics and Dosages for Use in Treatment of Osteomyelitis and Suppurative Arthritis

DRUGS	DILUENT	DOSE	ROUTE	SCHEDULE
Penicillin G	Saline, 0.9% solution, 20,000 units/ml.	200,000 units/kg./day (infants) 10–20 million units/day (children)	I.M. or I.V.	8–12 doses/day except in neonates
Ampicillin	5% Dextrose, saline	200–400 mg./kg./day	I.V.	8–12 doses/day
Erythromycin	Dextrose solution, 10 mg./cm.	50–100 mg./kg./day	I.V.	4 doses/day
Lincomycin	Saline or dextrose	50–75 mg./kg./day	I.V. or I.M.	3 doses/day
Oxacillin	Saline	100–200 mg./kg./day	I.M. or I.V.	4–6 doses/day
Cephalothin	Saline or dextrose, 10 mg./ml.	100–200 mg./kg./day	I.V.	8–12 doses/day
Gentamicin	Saline for I.M., saline or dextrose for I.V.	3–5 mg./kg./day	I.M. or I.V.	3 doses/day
Polymyxin	Saline	2.5 mg./kg./day	I.M.* or I.V.	2–3 doses/day
Colistin	Saline	3–5 mg./kg./day	I.M.	3 doses/day
Chloramphenicol	Saline	50–100 mg./kg./day	I.V.	4 doses/day
Kanamycin	Saline	15 mg./kg./day	I.M. or I.V.	2–4 doses/day
Streptomycin	Saline	20–30 mg./kg./day	I.M. or I.V.	2–4 doses/day

* Manufacturer's note: Intramuscular administration is not routinely recommended because of severe pain at injection site, particularly in infants and children.

the beginning. Joint infection involving the ankles, wrists, knees or shoulders can usually be managed additionally with no more than the initial aspiration of the purulent fluid required both to relieve pressure upon articular cartilages and to discover the bacterial pathogen. Arthritis of the hip joint, however, requires open surgical drainage and the installation of a rubber drain. This should be kept in place for a week or longer if necessary for continued decompression.

Treatment for suppurative arthritis due to *S. aureus* should be continued for four weeks as in the therapy of osteomyelitis. Other bacterial species such as *S. pyogenes,* the Neisseria, *H. influenzae* and *Diplococcus pneumoniae* need be treated for only two weeks. It is not clear how long the less common examples of enteric bacillary infection need be treated. If response is rapid and healing is nearly complete at the end of two weeks, this is long enough. It should be continued longer if any doubt exists.

Bone Tumors

SEYMOUR ZIMBLER, M.D.

Bone tumors are divided into benign and malignant types. These are further separated into a number of categories, depending on their cells of origin.

The benign lesions cause symptoms and signs in a number of ways, including:

1. Local pain via cortical and periosteal expansion.
2. Irritation of contiguous structures including joints, tendons and neurovascular bundles.
3. Bony distortion of epiphyseal and apophyseal plates, with remodeling abnormalities and growth discrepancies.
4. Pathologic fractures through cystic lesions.
5. Malignant degeneration of basically benign lesions.

TUMORS OF CARTILAGE CELL ORIGIN

The *osteocartilaginous exostosis* (osteochondroma) is a cartilage-capped bony projection which arises from the cortex of bone, usually in the metaphyseal region. These are the most common benign neoplasms of bone and develop in any bone which forms by endochondral ossification. Most occur in the distal femur or proximal tibia; 80 per cent of the patients are under age 21. Most patients will present single lesions; 65 per cent of those with multiple osteocartilaginous exostoses are of the familial type.

All of these tumors are similar grossly. They are covered by periosteum and have a smooth cartilage cap; there is also a broad or pedunculated type of bony base. The cartilaginous cap can be relatively acellular, but the bone in the base of the lesion is normal microscopically.

The exostoses are not excised unless they are causing local pain or progressive bony deformity. Rapid increase in size, especially after puberty, is another firm indication for excision. Malignant degeneration is rare in patients with solitary exostoses; those with multiple lesions may have a 20 per cent incidence of malignant change.

An *enchondroma* is a benign cartilaginous neoplasm arising within the medullary cavity of a bone. Most patients are in the second decade of life. The commonly involved bones are the phalanges, metacarpals and metatarsals. These tumors are well localized and can thin the surrounding cortex. The lobules of cartilage show uniform cellular detail and lacunae by microscopic examination. Curettage with or without bone grafting is the accepted treatment.

The *chondroblastoma* is a benign tumor of cartilaginous origin. These lesions comprise less than 1 per cent of all bone tumors. Most patients are in the 20- and 30-year age group. The epiphyseal areas of the proximal femur and proximal humerus are the most commonly involved regions. Most lesions are 1.5 to 6 cm. in size, ovoid and lobulated with a surrounding sclerotic bony margin. The basic chondroblastic cell is polygonal with an oval nucleus. Spindle cells are also present with a chondroid substance as the stroma. Multinucleated giant cells and spotty calcification can be present.

The treatment for these lesions is curettage or local excision with or without bone grafting. The tumor must be clearly differentiated from the giant cell tumor.

The *chondromyxoid fibroma* is another benign, slowly growing tumor of bone. It occurs in young adults and in any long bone. It is usually in the metaphyseal region of long bones and eccentrically placed with a lobulated sclerotic margin and thinned overlying cortex.

Microscopically these tumors show a chondroid matrix with a lobular pattern. Myxomatous areas with multinucleated giant cells, mononuclear leukocytes, hemosiderin and focal calcification have been present in portions of all lesions.

Wide excision with bone grafting is required mechanically as the treatment of choice.

A *chondrosarcoma* is a malignant tumor of bone arising from the basic cartilage cell. These tumors can occur primarily or secondarily from a preexisting benign cartilage tumor. The primary lesions develop commonly in pelvic bones, ribs and the proximal femur. Chondrosarcomas arise centrally within the medullary canal or peripherally on a preexisting cartilaginous lesion. These tumors can grow to a large size, causing local destruction on this basis but eventually metastasizing via the venous route. Most patients are in the 30- to 50-year age group, but children can be affected.

The cartilage cells in these lesions show multiple atypical nuclei with mitotic figures and size variation.

Radical amputation is the treatment of choice once the diagnosis is made. The five-year survival in chondrosarcoma is approximately 20 to 30 per cent.

TUMORS OF OSTEOBLASTIC ORIGIN

The *osteoblastoma* is a relatively rare, benign osteoblastic lesion of bone which involves mainly the posterior elements of vertebrae and long bones. Local pain and tenderness of a chronic type are common in the presentation. The patients fall in the 10- to 35-year range. X-rays usually show a circumscribed lesion, 2 to 10 cm. in diameter with a surrounding sclerotic bony rim. The dense circumferential bone of the osteoid osteoma is usually not seen.

Microscopically these tumors show much cellularity with osteoid formation, osteoblasts, multinucleated giant cells and wide trabeculae.

Curettage and/or local excision is the treatment of choice.

The *osteoid osteoma* is a benign tumor consisting of a small core of osteoid and/or osseous tissue (so-called osteoid nidus) and a perinidal zone of bone sclerosis or thickening. The lesion can have been present for many years but the nidus will not exceed 1 cm. at its greatest diameter. Osteoid osteomas are found usually in older children and young adults. The most common site of the lesion is the femur, and in about 25 per cent of the cases it is also found in the tibia and less commonly in the fibula, humerus, vertebrae, talus and calcaneus. Involvement of the skull is rare. Clinical presentation of the osteoid osteoma consists of local or referred pain with many months of symptoms before X-ray evidence of the lesion is noted. The pain may be occasional, sometimes occurring only at night. Immobilization of the part may not relieve the symptoms, and activity does not necessarily increase the symptoms. The principle clinical finding is local tenderness if the lesion is in the area where palpation is possible. Local swelling and sometimes associated sympathetic synovitis can be noted. Neurologic complaints with atrophy and symptoms similar to nerve root compression in the lumbar region are associated with lesions in the upper end of the femur. The X-ray finding of osteoid osteoma is usually surrounding sclerosis with the nidus itself being mainly lucent. Microscopic examination of osteoid osteoma grossly reveals that the nidus is of granular, gritty consistency and red-brown in color. This consists microscopically of osteoid tissue with trabeculae of newly formed osseous tissue in a substratum of highly vascularized osteogenic tissue. The appropriate treatment for osteoid osteoma is block excision of the nidus and the surrounding sclerosis. Radiation therapy has been used in some lesions in inaccessible areas, but this is felt to be questionable treatment. There have been reports of cases of spontaneous resolution of symptoms, ranging from two to 24 years after onset with no treatment.

The *osteosarcoma* is the most common primary malignant tumor of bone. It is listed here with the tumors of osteoblastic derivation, but cells of origin may actually be primitive mesenchyme. The cellular elements of the tumor can be mainly osteogenic in type (54 per cent), but some variations of the basic tumor will present with either a fibroblastic (23 per cent) or chondroblastic (22 per cent) predominance. These neoplasms occur more commonly in the male (62 per cent), with those in the second decade being the most frequently involved group. Fifty-two per cent of the cases involve the distal femur or proximal tibia.

Grossly, these tumors cause bone destruction with periosteal new bone as well as tumor bone being formed. Intramedullary as well as soft tissue extension is common. Neoplastic osteoid with cell variation and atypism make the microscopic diagnoses in these patients.

Metastases are blood-borne and occur too rapidly in most cases: Four of five patients have occult metastases at the time of definitive treatment. The best results to date from large clinical series reveal only a 17.1 per cent five-year survival rate. This particular group of patients was treated by immediate amputation at the time of frozen-section diagnosis. A combination of supravoltage radiation, selective amputation surgery and high-dose combination chemotherapy is promising regarding increasing survival time. Possibly an immunologic approach may have more to offer in the future.

TUMORS OF FIBROUS CONNECTIVE TISSUE ORIGIN

The *fibrous cortical defect* is a localized benign lesion of bone consisting of a focus of fibrous connective tissue and giant cells. These lesions may develop as a "rest" from local periosteum, invading underlying bony cortex and creating a cystic, loculated eccentric, lytic lesion on X-ray. The distal femur and proximal tibia are the most commonly involved areas. Thirty per cent of children age four to eight present these lesions. The tumors may persist for only two years and then disappear.

In some instances the lesions enlarge and grow shaftward; in this situation they are called nonossifying fibromas. Local pain can be caused by cortical expansion or pathologic fracture. Curettage and bone grafting are indicated in these situations.

Giant cell tumors of bone appear to arise from the fibrous connective type stroma. These tumors can be locally aggressive or frankly malignant with peripheral metastases reported in several instances (questionably, 15 per cent). The lesions are found in the epiphyseal areas of long bones following skeletal maturity (age 10 to 30), particularly about the knee. The radiographic picture reveals a radiolucent, expansile lesion, eccentrically placed in the epiphyseal region of a long bone. Cortical infractions and periosteal reactions occur.

Microscopically, a vascular stroma with plump ovoid or spindle-shaped cells are found. Giant cells and foam cells are common. Atypism of the stromal cells should be graded as a progressively more malignant lesion histologically. Total excision is the treatment of choice where possible; amputation or joint replacement may be necessary in more aggressive lesions. Radiation has been questioned as a cause of malignant change in these tumors.

TUMORS OF MESENCHYMAL ORIGIN

Ewing's sarcoma is a rare primary malignant tumor of bone probably arising from the mesenchymal or endothelial cells within the medullary portion of bone. Lesions occur in all bones but 56 per cent have been found in the metaphysis or midshaft of long bones. Most patients are age 10 to 20; they present with local pain and swelling. Sometimes the lesions appear "inflammatory," with fever, anemia, increased sedimentation rate and rapid expansion in size. X-rays reveal a metaphyseal or diaphyseal lytic lesion with periosteal new bone formation about it ("onion skin" or spicules). Microscopically the lesions show sheets of round cells with a vascular stroma and some mitoses. Treatment of this tumor consists of a combination of supravoltage radiation with high-dose combination chemotherapy. The value of amputation, total body irradiation and pulmonary irradiation is being evaluated at this time. The five-year survival rate is no better than 12 per cent.

The *reticulum cell sarcoma* is a rare primary malignant tumor of bone, probably arising from reticulum cells within the medullary canal of bone. Local pain of a chronic nature is a common presenting symptom. Most patients are age 20 to 40, with some children definitely involved. Forty-five per cent of the lesions are in the femur or tibia. Multiple bones can be involved. Histologically these lesions show sheets of round cells with indistinct borders. Supravoltage x-ray plus combination chemotherapy probably offers the best chance for good results in treatment. A 32 per cent five-year survival rate has been quoted.

15

Muscles

Congenital Muscular Defects

PAUL W. HUGENBERGER, M.D.

The treatment of infants and children with congenital absence of muscles is largely dependent on the normal function of the particular muscle that is absent and whether its absence will result in some significant deformity, either as a result of muscle imbalance or of the combination of muscle imbalance and growth.

In the upper extremity, the *palmaris longus* is perhaps the most common muscle to be congenitally absent, and in this case no treatment is really indicated. It may be absent in one arm or both without any functional impairment.

The *pectoralis major* may be absent, creating some asymmetry of the two shoulders. This is of some significance cosmetically, especially in the case of a girl, with of course some weakness of the shoulder. However, through exercises and overdevelopment of the remaining shoulder girdle musculature the functional loss is not great. There is no operation or specific treatment for this condition of which I am aware, and the patient should receive reassurance.

A portion of the *sternocleidomastoid muscle* may be absent, which may result in a torticollis, or wryneck, deformity on the opposite side. This may require surgical treatment to make the two sides of the neck more symmetric. However, as a rule, with congenital absence of a muscle there seems to be spontaneous readjustment so that significant deformities do not occur. In these cases the treatment is occasional check-up with reassurance for the patient.

Congenital absence of *muscles about the eyes* may require surgical correction. Patients with this anomaly should be seen by an ophthalmologist.

Congenital absence of the *abdominal muscles* is apparently extremely rare, if it occurs at all. The abdominal muscles can be congenitally deficient and extremely weak, requiring a corset type of support with exercises and possibly surgery with reinforcement with fascia.

Congenital absence of the *thenar muscles* of the thumb can be treated by transplantation of the flexor digitorum sublimis from the fourth finger to the thumb to restore opposition, with fascial stabilization or fusion of appropriate joints.

In the lower extremity, congenital absence of the *peroneal muscles* associated with a paralytic type of clubfoot requires the usual treatment for the clubfoot deformity, namely, frequent daily gentle manipulations to correct the deformity, and maintenance of correction by the use of bivalved long-leg plaster casts, splints or braces. The tendon of the posterior tibial muscle can be transferred through the intermuscular septum into the dorsum of the foot, or the anterior tibial tendon can be transferred more laterally, or the tendon can be split and half inserted into the dorsolateral aspect of the foot to give better balance. In addition to possible tendon transplantation, the foot may require bony stabilization, possibly a triple arthrodesis plus the tendon transplantation when the child is older.

Congenital *arthrogryposis,* localized or diffuse, is often associated with congenital absence of muscles, in addition to stiff joints and other congenital deformities including clubfeet. A very early diagnosis is important in order to institute immediate, intensive but gentle physical therapy with emphasis on passive range of motion in all joints involved. Therapy should be started as soon as possible after the birth of the child; the gentle, manipulative types of exercises should be done many times a day and maintenance of correction should be accomplished by simple, light plaster splinting. Early active exercises should be encouraged, but since all muscles are poor and some are absent, muscle imbalance does exist; however, muscle transplantation is almost never indicated. Heel-cord lengthening and other soft tissue release operations might be indicated to improve a club-foot deformity. In severe cases astragalectomy may be the operation of choice. Corrective shoes, with or without lightweight bracing, with early physical therapy seems to give the best results.

Finally, the absence of individual muscles is relatively common, but if there is no interference with function, no treatment is indicated.

Torticollis

PAUL W. HUGENBERGER, M.D.

The ideal treatment for congenital muscular torticollis in infancy depends on early diagnosis and is nonoperative. A careful clinical examination will confirm the diagnosis by noting that the head is rotated to one side and tilted to the opposite side with slight extension. The sternocleidomastoid muscle on the side of the tilt and opposite the side of rotation either will be contracted and tight or will contain a nontender fusiform tumor mass in the lower half of the muscle. Passive and active range of motion will be limited, and the degree of limitation will depend on the severity of the involvement. Rotation of the head will be limited toward the involved side, and lateral flexion will be limited away from the involved side.

Gentle but frequent manipulations of the head to stretch out this tightness is essential. This is done by rotating the head toward the involved side so that the baby is looking over that shoulder, and then tilting the head, in neutral rotation, away from the involved side so that the ear approaches the opposite shoulder, at the same time the shoulder on the involved side is depressed by the mother's free hand. These manipulations should then be repeated slowly about five to ten times prior to each feeding, bathing and diaper change. It is absolutely necessary for the mother to be taught how to carry out the treatment, since only she or a full-time nurse is able to do the exercises as frequently as needed.

Proper positioning of the baby's head is likewise very important in aiding correction and in preventing flattening of the occiput and facial asymmetry. Whether the baby is prone or supine, the face should be rotated so as to be looking toward the side of the involved sternocleidomastoid muscle, and the head should be tilted away from that shoulder. These positions can be maintained by the use of sandbags or a little blanket roll. When the infant is placed in the crib on the side away from the involved muscle, a small pillow or a little blanket roll placed under the chest and shoulder will allow the head to fall away from the involved side, thus stretching the tight sternocleidomastoid muscle.

A special skullcap can be made with traction weights over either side of the crib to maintain the head in the corrected position. Since effective bracing of an infant's head in the corrected position is difficult and sometimes dangerous, passive stretching and early active corrective exercises with proper positioning of the head are essential in preventing cranial and facial deformities secondary to the torticollis. Within a few months the sternocleidomastoid "tumor" will disappear and the contractures will be corrected. Usually an excellent result will be obtained if treatment is started within a few days following birth.

If correction is not obtained or if treatment cannot be started in early infancy, active and passive stretching exercises plus the wearing of a well-fitted torticollis brace, which holds the head in the overcorrected position at all times except for bathing, exercises and meals, is recommended. If the torticollis is very severe or if the child is older, surgical correction may be necessary. Occasionally operation is indicated fairly early if the sternocleidomastoid muscle is very tight and fibrous, or if no progress is being made with stretching. However, it is preferable to delay operation until the infant is old enough for suitable bracing postoperatively, along with manipulations and active exercises, to ensure that the deformity will not recur.

If surgery is necessary, it is important to do the operation which will correct the specific deformity and at the same time maintain a good cosmetic appearance; this is particularly true for girls. If the sternocleidomastoid muscle is uniformly tight, it can be satisfactorily released by using a slightly curved incision in back of the ear which will not be visible from the front. The tight, fibrous mastoid portion of the muscle can be divided after delivering it into the wound with a blunt dissector or curved snap. Dividing the tendon should be done between snaps so that all bleeding can be controlled. The distal cut end will retract. The flattened occipital portion of the sternocleidomastoid muscle should then be identified and released. This portion of the muscle extends backward on the occiput for about an inch. Following the division of these two ends of the muscle, the head should be stretched gently to the opposite side to make sure that all tight structures in the area have been released and good correction has been obtained, with no tightness remaining at the sternal and clavicular ends. This small incision is closed with a single subcuticular suture tied over a sterile gauze dressing, with a collodion cocoon dressing over all. This will give a good cosmetic result, and it is easy to remove the single suture along with the dressing when the wound is healed, without disturbing the patient.

If the entire deformity is not satisfactorily corrected following division of both portions of the upper end of the muscle, I recommend making a small transverse incision in the skin crease just above the clavicle, over the clavicular portion of the sternocleidomastoid muscle, and dividing this portion and leaving the sternal end intact to preserve the normal neck contour. If the sternal portion is particularly tight, it can be divided in the case of a boy, or lengthened in the case of a girl, to maintain the normal sternal angle. The lower-end incision can also be closed with a subcuticular suture tied over a dressing; this keeps the dressing in place and leaves a minimal scar.

Immediately following operation the head should be tilted and rotated toward the normal side, and a long sandbag can be placed on the bed, with the end of the sandbag resting on the operative side of the neck to give pressure hemostasis and to keep the face turned to the opposite side while recovering from the anesthesia. Afterwards the head is placed in the overcorrected position, which is maintained by a brace made preoperatively or by some form of traction or splinting until the torticollis brace is available. The patient should be started on early gentle active exercises when the brace is removed three times a day for meals. Gentle passive stretching is started when the wounds are healed.

The brace should be worn during the day for at least three months, and during the night for six months, and even longer if asymmetry of the face and flattening of the occiput are marked. The brace is discontinued during the day when the patient has acquired the habit of maintaining slight overcorrection and is conscientious in doing the exercises, and when there is no residual tightness.

Occasionally, congenital muscular torticollis is bilateral, with the more severely affected muscle dominating the clinical picture. If this condition exists, the patient may develop a torticollis on the opposite side following surgery and this will require conservative treatment and possibly operation to obtain a satisfactory result.

If the torticollis in an infant or newborn is not associated with limitation of passive rotation or side bending, it most likely represents a postural type of torticollis, probably due to persistence of the position in utero. This should be treated by frequent changes of position so that flattening of the occiput with flattening of the face on the opposite side will not occur, thus making it difficult later to place the baby on the nonflat portion of the head. If the infant is permitted to roll back onto the flat side, secondary contractures of the neck may develop and require stretching exercises and maybe even a brace for a short period of time. Early recognition of this condition and early treatment provide an excellent prognosis.

Torticollis in infancy with limitation of passive motion but without tightness of the sternocleidomastoid muscle is probably due to hemivertebra or some abnormality of the cervical spine, either congenital or traumatic. The treatment largely depends on the x-ray findings and might include, in addition to some exercises and stretching, early support or cervical traction. A Milwaukee type of brace might be indicated in the older child, or even early operative fusion if there are hemivertebrae and congenital bars or fusion areas that would limit growth on the side to which the head is tilted.

If the torticollis is not congenital but acquired, the cause must be determined; specific treatment depends on the etiology. If there is a rotary subluxation of C1 on C2, cervical traction by means of a head halter or skeletal traction may be necessary to obtain reduction, after which immobilization in a cervical collar or a Minerva jacket may be necessary for several weeks or months. The patient is then started on active exercises until normal function of the cervical spine has been restored.

If the torticollis is due to an infection like lymphadenitis, treatment of the infection will suffice and spontaneous recovery of the torticollis will usually follow. Infections involving the cervical vertebrae, such as tuberculosis or arthritis, may require a fairly prolonged period of traction followed by immobilization and exercises, along with specific treatment for the specific condition.

Other neuromuscular conditions like cerebral palsy with unilateral hypertonia of the neck musculature can cause persistent rotational deformity of the head. The condition may be improved with muscle training, and I doubt if operation would be necessary.

Spasmodic torticollis is the most difficult of all these conditions to treat. It does not occur in infancy and only rarely in children. If the cause can be determined and corrected, cure may be expected. Otherwise, the treatment is questionable. Light mechanical support with active muscle exercises in the direction of correction, intermittent cervical traction plus corrective exercises for the neck, and psychotherapy might be tried. Neuropsychiatric and neurosurgical consultation should be obtained in persistent cases.

Congenital Hypotonia

EDWARD F. RABE, M.D.

Hypotonia in neonates and young infants is a symptom of many diseases. It implies decreased resistance to passive motion of limbs, trunk and neck, and this may be due to muscle weakness, abnormality in the reactivity of the gamma motor system of the spinal cord or abnormalities of viscoelastic properties of muscle, joint and tendon. Two large groups of diseases which are associated with hypotonia are neuromuscular disease and generalized medical disease affecting nutrition and the elasticity of collagen. Our discussion will be concerned with the neuromuscular diseases "causing" hypotonia in infants.

Because of the organization of the nervous system, disease at any level of the neuromuscular axis, brain, spinal cord, peripheral nerve or muscle system can cause hypotonia. Thus, the diagnostic approach to hypotonia should reveal whether hypotonia in the infant is due to disease of the brain, spinal cord, peripheral nerve, myoneural junction or muscle. Table 1 presents in outline the most commonly encountered diseases associated with neonatal and infantile hypotonia according to level of dysfunction. It also contains data concerning the inheritable diseases which occur at each anatomic level.

A systematic approach to the diagnostic examination is important, and it is mentioned only because it is so often neglected. Besides a thorough history and physical examination, a careful neurologic evaluation is a minimal requirement. Table 2 lists a number of tests which frequently are necessary to reach a diagnosis. Two comments are needed to enhance the usefulness of this table. First, the 24-hour urinary coefficients of creatine and creatinine are expressed in milligrams per kilogram per 24 hours. Whenever muscle is decreased in mass, as in neural atrophy, or function, as in dystrophy, there is an increase in the creatine coefficient and a decrease in the creatinine coefficient. The normal coefficients according to age are as shown at the bottom of this page.

Secondly, when myasthenia in the neonatal transient or congenital form is suspected, swallowing and breathing difficulty and decreased spontaneous movement can be improved with anticholinesterase. Thus, improvement should appear 15 to 30 minutes after intramuscular injection of neostigmine in a dose of 0.125 mg., or within a few minutes after intravenous injection of edrophonium hydrochloride (Tensilon). Intravenous edrophonium dosage is as follows: up to three months, 1.0 mg.; 3 to 12 months, 2.0 mg.; older infants and children, 0.15 mg. per kilogram of body weight to a maximal single dose of 10 mg. One-tenth of the total dose is given, and if no untoward effects (vomiting, diarrhea, bradycardia, shock or hypotension) are noted after a minute or two, the remainder is given by a slow syringe injection. Subcutaneous atropine is an antidote for the cholinergic overstimulation possible as the result of anticholinesterase medication. The dose for subcutaneous atropine is 0.01 mg. per kilogram of body weight, and may be repeated every 2 hours as needed.

Treatment of the infant with congenital hypotonia depends upon the associated or "causative" disease for which hypotonia is the presenting symptom. Since a number of diseases are inheritable, genetic counseling of the parents is an important part of management once the diagnosis is established. Reference to Table 1 will aid in this decision.

If myasthenia is diagnosed, it may be treated with intramuscular neostigmine, 0.125 mg. 10 to 15 minutes before every 4-hour feeding. Pyridostigmine (Mestinon), 15 mg. orally, may be used in the same interval in place of

	PREMATURE INFANT	FULL-TERM INFANT (BIRTH TO TWO YEARS)	CHILDREN 2 TO 18 YEARS
Creatine coefficient	0.08 to 1.0	0.12 to 5.15	0.7 to 9.2
Creatinine coefficient	9.9 to 14.0	14.2 to 32.0	16.3 to 36.2

TABLE 1. Etiology of Hypotonia in Neonates and Infants (Neuromuscular Disease)

DISEASE	GENETIC TRANSMISSION
Hypotonia due to diseases of the central nervous system	
Atonic diplegia	—
Congenital chorea and athetosis	—
Congenital cerebellar ataxia	—
Kernicterus	—
Ganglioside storage disease (Tay-Sachs)	Autosomal recessive
Down's syndrome	Depends on chromosomal pattern
Metachromatic leukodystrophy	Autosomal recessive
Hypotonia due to diseases of the spinal cord	
Werdnig-Hoffman disease	Autosomal recessive
Kugelberg-Welander disease	Autosomal recessive
Neonatal anterior poliomyelitis	—
Cervical spinal cord disease:	
Hematomyelia secondary to traumatic delivery	—
Metastatic neuroblastoma growing epidurally	Single family reports
Hypotonia due to disease of the peripheral nerves	
Acute infectious polyneuritis (Guillain-Barré disease)	—
Chronic idiopathic polyneuropathy	Single family reports
Metachromatic leukodystrophy	Autosomal recessive
Hypotonia due to disease of the myoneural junction	
Myasthenia gravis—transient	—
Myasthenia gravis—congenital	Single family reports
Hypotonia due to primary disease of muscle	
Benign congenital hypotonia	—
Universal muscular hypoplasia	Autosomal dominant
Congenital muscular dystrophy (primary infantile myopathy)	Autosomal recessive
Myotonic dystrophy	Autosomal dominant
Central core disease	Autosomal dominant
Nemaline (rod-body) myopathy	Autosomal dominant
Pleoconial myopathy	Single family reports
Megaconial myopathy	Autosomal recessive
Polymyositis	—
Glycogen storage disease	Autosomal recessive
Muscular dystrophy (Duchenne type)	Sex-linked recessive

TABLE 2. Tests Useful in Diagnosis of Possible Site of Pathology in Hypotonic Infants

TEST	SITE OF PATHOLOGY
Neurologic examination—focal or global deficit	Brain
24-hour urinary creatine and creatinine coefficients	Spinal cord, peripheral nerve, muscle
Neostigmine or edrophonium test	Neuromuscular junction
Serum enzyme—aldolase, creatine-phosphokinase	Muscle
Electromyography	Spinal cord, muscle
Nerve conduction time	Peripheral nerve
Lumbar puncture	Spinal cord, peripheral nerve
Radiography or vertebral column	Spinal cord

neostigmine. Continue anticholinesterase medication for seven days; then try omitting a dose since the symptoms may spontaneously subside within a period of a few days to as long as three months after onset in transient neonatal myasthenia. Symptoms, however, will continue in the congenital form, but their onset is later.

Infants with polymyositis or acute or chronic peripheral polyneuropathy should be given a trial of steroid therapy. Oral prednisone is given the first day in a dosage of 5 mg. per kilogram per 24 hours in divided doses. The dosage is then decreased daily by 1 mg. per kilogram until a maintenance dosage of 3 mg. per kilogram is reached. This is continued for seven days. If no benefit is apparent after 10 days of therapy, the dose is gradually tapered over five more days and prednisone is discontinued. If clinical benefit accrues, and the patient is not well, the daily dosage of 3 mg. per kilogram may be continued for another week. If further therapy is necessary, it is wise to give twice this dosage at two-day intervals. This decreases the likelihood of toxic side effects from the steroid.

Long-term management of certain diseases seen in infants with hypotonia is important, but too frequently neglected. Thirty per cent of infants with hypotonia and congenital encephalopathy with global retardation develop spasticity after 8 to 12 months of age. This symptom may be ameliorated by administering oral diazepam (Valium)* in a dose of 1 mg. per day for three days, followed by 1 mg. twice daily for three days, and then increasing the daily dose by 1 mg. per day every seven days until lethargy or mild sedation occurs. The dose is then decreased by 1 mg. per day, and this level is continued for as long as it is deemed necessary. Physiotherapy and, in some instances, orthopedic procedures, may be concomitantly beneficial.

Infants with hypotonia and arthrogryposis multiplex congenita, from intrauterine spinal cord disease or muscle disease, derive great benefit from an aggressive program of passive exercises under the care of a physiatrist. Joints with limited motion may be given full range, and, depending upon the degree of residual muscle strength, mobility may be almost completely provided.

Many infants with Werdnig-Hoffman disease whose symptoms begin after four months of age have moderately severe symptoms but a spontaneously arrested course. Such infants have normal intelligence, and although they are weak, they can be made quite mobile with devices such as electric wheelchairs. They may lead happy and satisfactory lives, but they are subject to severe contractures. Aggressive, persistent and well-planned physiotherapy should be given to these children to prevent the remarkable contracture deformities that some poorly cared for children with Werdnig-Hoffman disease do develop.

* Manufacturer's precaution: Oral diazepam is not for use in children under six months of age.

Infants with Kugelberg-Welander disease and the nonprogressive myopathies such as congenital myopathy and benign congenital hypotonia should be similarly supervised by physicians who are aware that in all these diseases contractural deformities can occur but that they do so very slowly. Repeated reevaluation, proper referrals for physiotherapy and assessment of the global function by a psychologist to assure parents and teachers that this crippled child with marked weakness and motor slowness is not also mentally retarded are all important facets in the long-term management of these patients.

Muscular Dystrophy and Related Myopathies

FREDERICK J. SAMAHA, M.D.

The primary inherited diseases of muscle in this group are presumably due to intrinsic metabolic abnormalities. However, the basic biochemical defect has not been elucidated for any of the several types of muscular dystrophy and related myopathies.

None of the specific medical therapies advocated over the past several years, including vitamin E, nonandrogenic anabolic steroids, cardiac glycosides, thyroid hormones, bamethan and various combinations of nucleotides, nucleosides and their precursors, has proved valuable. Their use in muscular dystrophy and related myopathies cannot be recommended.

Patients with myotonia congenita (Thomsen's disease) and occasionally those with myotonic dystrophy may be disabled. Partial relief of this symptom may be afforded by quinine (50 to 400 mg. per day) in divided doses orally. Quinine may damage the 8th nerve, producing tinnitus and deafness, and the drug should be discontinued if there is clinical or audiometric evidence of impaired hearing. If tinnitus is the only complaint, reduction in dosage may be all that is required. Rarely, quinine produces an optic neuropathy, another complication demanding cessation of treatment.

Procainamide hydrochloride, 250 to 2000 mg. a day in divided doses orally, also may prove beneficial in ameliorating the myotonia. Untoward side effects of this drug include anorexia, nausea, vomiting, pruritus, insomnia, mental depression and, rarely, agranulocytosis. This drug may also produce either a clinical picture resembling lupus erythematosus or a serologic picture seen in the lupus syndrome.

Corticosteroids and ion exchange resins have been used in myotonic dystrophy and myotonia congenita, but they are of questionable value.

Supportive Care. Despite the lack of curative medications, every effort should be made to establish a precise diagnosis, because the clinical course of the several types of muscular dystrophy varies considerably (Table 1).

If available data indicate that the patient has one of the relatively benign forms of dystrophy, this should be stressed in discussions with the parents. On the other hand, if the patient clearly has the Duchenne form of dystrophy, it is important that the family be apprised of the serious nature of the disease.

Genetic counseling is important. A realistic statement regarding the probability that other siblings or children of future generations may be affected should be made. Results of creatine phosphokinase levels may be helpful in counseling, because the level of this enzyme may be elevated in carrier, preclinical and clinical states.

Supportive management is essential. Affected children should be reexamined at regular intervals and the progress of the disease documented. Knowledge that a physician is interested affords immeasurable solace to the family. A reasonable amount of activity, including sports consistent with the child's limitations, should be encouraged. When weakness is severe, precluding a full range of voluntary movement about major joints, passive manipulation by the family or a professional physiotherapist may reduce the tendency to develop contractures and restricted joint motion; overzealous passive manipulation of muscles undergoing shortening and contracture may injure muscle fibers and hasten the very process one is attempting to avert.

Orthopedic procedures are of limited value in most cases of rapidly advancing muscular dystrophy, especially of the Duchenne variety. Lengthening of the Achilles tendon or the gastrocnemius recession procedure may permit the patient to walk less on the balls of his feet. This improvement is usually short-lived, however, and often disturbs an already tenuous balance

TABLE 1. Clinical Features of Muscular Dystrophy

TYPE OF DYSTROPHY	MODE OF INHERITANCE	USUAL AGE OF ONSET	MUSCLES INVOLVED	PROGNOSIS
Duchenne's	Sex-linked recessive	1 to 6 years	Pelvofemoral, gastrocnemius and shoulder girdle; pseudohypertrophy in 80% of cases; cardiac	Poor; severely handicapped or dead by third to fourth decade
Becker's	Sex-linked recessive	4 to 30 years	Pelvofemoral; pseudohypertrophy frequent	Relatively benign
Limb girdle	Autosomal recessive	10 to 30 years	Shoulder or pelvic girdle; occasional pseudohypertrophy	Slow progression; severe disability 20 years after onset
Facioscapulohumeral	Autosomal dominant	Childhood or early adult life	Face and shoulder girdle with spread to pelvic girdle	Most survive for full life
Myotonic	Autosomal dominant	Newborn period, childhood or early adult life	Distal arm and leg, temporalis, sternomastoid, eyelid, ocular and cardiac	Mildly to moderately disabled 15 to 20 years after onset
Ocular	Uncertain; familial incidence in 50% of cases	Adult life	Extraocular, lid, upper face and pharynx in 50% of cases; neck, trunk and limbs in 25% of cases	Restricted involvement and minimal disability

in walking. The same may be said for all orthopedic efforts to correct the patient's posture, including the use of crutches and braces. As the disease advances the patient falls when only slightly jostled. He is unable to negotiate anything but the smoothest terrain. Bed rest for more than a few days aggravates the patient's inability to walk and should be avoided if possible. Inevitably he eventually is unable to get about without falling repeatedly. At this point the advantages of a wheelchair should be discussed.

As the Duchenne dystrophy advances, the muscles of respiration become progressively involved. Particular attention must then be directed to the pulmonary toilet and avoidance or treatment of minor pulmonary infections. In the late stages, tracheostomy and assisted ventilation may be necessary. At times, with subsidence of pulmonary sepsis, the need for assisted respiration and tracheostomy disappears for a variable period of time. Cardiac failure, due to a myopathy of the heart muscle, is a late complication of the Duchenne and myotonic dystrophies. It is treated as are other forms of congestive failure (see Congestive Heart Failure).

References

Dodge, P. R., et al.: Myotonic Dystrophy in Infancy and Childhood. *Pediatrics,* 35:3, 1965.

Walton, J.: Progressive Muscular Dystrophy; in J. Walton (ed.): *Disorders of Voluntary Muscle.* Boston, Little, Brown and Company, 1969, pp. 455–459.

Zundel, W. S., and Tyler, F. H.: The Muscular Dystrophies. *New England J. Med.,* 273:537, 1965.

Myasthenia Gravis

DAVID GROB, M.D.

Myasthenia gravis is a chronic disease characterized by weakness and abnormal fatigability of skeletal muscle. The weakness is ameliorated, although to a variable degree, by anticholinesterase compounds, which increase the local concentration of acetylcholine by inhibiting muscle cholinesterase. This response to anticholinesterase compounds serves as the basis for diagnosis and management of the disease.

Anticholinesterase Compounds. The most useful medications are neostigmine (Prostigmin), pyridostigmine (Mestinon) and ambenonium (Mytelase).* Edrophonium (Tensilon) is useful in diagnosis and in evaluation of adequacy of dose of the longer acting compounds, but is too short acting for use in management. The maximum strength obtained after optimal doses of any of these compounds is approximately the same. The compounds differ mainly in their duration of action (ambenonium > pyridostigmine > neostigmine > edrophonium), and in the severity of their parasympathomimetic side effects (neostigmine > ambenonium > pyridostigmine > edrophonium). The administration of graded doses of any of these compounds results in an increase in strength in muscles affected by the disease, but the maximal strength attained is usually below normal, and may be far below normal.

Before regulation of a patient is attempted, the diagnosis should be established and the maximal strength determined by the response to the intravenous injection of edrophonium (0.2 mg. per kilogram) or the intramuscular injection of neostigmine (0.04 mg. per kilogram). The effect of intravenous edrophonium is manifest within 30 seconds, and of intramuscular neostigmine in 30 minutes. Atropine (0.01 mg. per kilogram) should be given with or prior to neostigmine to prevent parasympathomimetic side effects. The optimal oral dose of pyridostigmine, neostigmine or ambenonium may then be determined by gradually increasing the dose until the same degree of maximal improvement has occurred as after the test parenteral dose. Further increase in dose seldom results in further increase in strength, and excessive dosage, particularly of the longer acting compounds, is likely to produce generalized weakness—the so-called cholinergic crisis.

Regulation is initiated by the administration of a dose of anticholinesterase medication below that necessary to produce maximal strength. If the patient is able to swallow, pyridostigmine is the drug of choice, in an initial oral dose of 1 mg. per kilogram every 4 hours when awake. In patients with mild myasthenia, neostigmine bromide may be employed instead, in an initial dose of 0.3 mg. per kilogram every 3 hours when awake. In patients with predominantly peripheral weakness who have not been satisfactorily regulated on pyridostigmine, ambenonium may be tried in an initial oral dose of 0.1 mg. per kilogram. In patients who are unable to swallow, and in infants, the drug of choice is neostigmine methylsulfate administered intramuscularly in an initial dose of 0.025 mg. per kilogram every 2 to 3 hours. Measurements of strength are carried out, and the dose of anticholinesterase medication is then gradually increased by increments of one-fourth of the above amounts, until no further increase in strength occurs. The time between doses may be

* Manufacturer's precaution: Ambenonium (Mytelase) should never be used in infants because no blood-brain barrier exists for this drug, and even a slight overdose can cause convulsions.

decreased by ½ to 1 hour if this proves necessary to maintain strength. Since the duration of action of pyridostigmine and ambenonium is longer, adjustments in dose of these drugs should be made at intervals of one to two days, since increase in dose at shorter intervals may result in cumulation of drug and consequent overdose. The dose of neostigmine may be adjusted at shorter intervals, and when parenteral neostigmine is employed the dose may be adjusted several times a day if necessary. Whenever augmentation in dose of any anticholinesterase drug results in no further increase in strength, the dose should be reduced to the previous level in order to administer the least amount of drug necessary to produce a maximal level of strength.

Adjustment in the dose of any of the anticholinesterase compounds may be facilitated by the intravenous injection of 0.04 mg. per kilogram of edrophonium 1 hour after the last dose of anticholinesterase medication. If there are technical difficulties with intravenous administration, the intramuscular route may be used, in which case twice the intravenous dose is given. If the patient is in need of increased anticholinesterase medication, there will be transient increase in strength, beginning within ½ to 1 minute after intravenous injection or 2 to 5 minutes after intramuscular injection, and lasting a few minutes. If the patient is already overdosed, there will be a transient decrease in strength, sometimes accompanied by fasciculations, lacrimation, salivation, sweating, cramps or nausea. If none of these changes occurs, it can generally be assumed that the patient is at or near his optimal dosage level, although occasionally patients who are overdosed may exhibit no further change.

Atropine. Atropine sulfate (0.01 mg. per kilogram) may be administered orally or intramuscularly as needed to suppress or prevent the muscarine-like effects of anticholinesterase compounds, such as excessive salivation, bronchial secretion, sweating, nausea, vomiting, abdominal cramps, diarrhea, bradycardia and, rarely, hypotension. Myasthenic patients generally have a higher threshold for the development of these effects than do nonmyasthenic subjects. During the initial period of drug regulation, atropine is best administered only as needed to ameliorate these side effects, so that the occurrence of cumulation and overdose of anticholinesterase compound may be more easily detected. Atropine may be administered every 4 to 8 hours if necessary, but overatropinization should be avoided, since this may produce inspissation of bronchial secretions, atelectasis and increased risk of pulmonary infection, as well as tachycardia, flushing, urinary retention and disorientation.

Exacerbation of Myasthenia Gravis. This is characterized by increased weakness, often with dysphagia, weakness of cough, obstruction of the upper airway and respiratory weakness. Exacerbation may result from upper respiratory infection, other infectious illness, emotional tension or inadequate or excessive anticholinesterase medication. During severe exacerbation, the patient becomes less responsive to anticholinesterase medication, presumably because more muscle end-plates have become insensitive to acetylcholine. It is this insensitive state that constitutes the main problem in management of the disease, and often leads to the administration of large doses of anticholinesterase medication and confusion as to whether the patient is overdosed ("in cholinergic crisis") or underdosed ("in myasthenic crisis"). Many patients who are thought to be overdosed are in an insensitive state, and administration of large doses of anticholinesterase compound often renders the patient more insensitive. If respiration is being supported mechanically, the dose of anticholinesterase compound should be reduced to the smallest dose necessary to sustain respiration in case of failure of mechanical support. There may be some advantage to discontinuing all anticholinesterase medication for 48 to 72 hours, but this should be done only if there is constant observation of the patient.

Airway obstruction or impaired respiration is managed by inserting an endotracheal catheter and instituting mechanical respiration. The endotracheal tube should not be left in place more than 48 to 72 hours, since it produces edema of the larynx, which may result in airway obstruction when the tube is removed. Since most myasthenic patients continue to have severe dysphagia after withdrawal of the tube, it is usually best to perform a tracheostomy under local procaine anesthesia while the tube is still in place. The outer tracheostomy tube is not changed for the first four days to allow a tract to form, and then is changed every two to three days. The inner tube is changed at more frequent intervals. A short tube should be employed to prevent pressure on the tracheal wall. Suction should be carried out at frequent intervals, with 1 to 2 ml. of saline instilled every few hours. The inspired air should be humidified. The head should be turned from side to side to allow the catheter to be inserted into each bronchus. The cuff of the endotracheal tube or tracheostomy should be deflated for at least 5 minutes of every hour to prevent pressure necrosis of the trachea. Mechanical positive-pressure respiration can be maintained with humidified air unless the arterial pO_2 falls below 60 mm. Hg., in which case oxygen can be piggy-backed for short periods of time. Pure oxygen should be avoided, since it causes destruction of cilia, drying and atelectasis. Signs of anoxia may include elevation of pulse and blood pressure, sweating, confusion and arrhythmia. When these signs occur, intensive tracheal suctioning should be carried out. A pressure-cycled respirator usually suffices, since lung compliance is usually good. However, if inspissated secretions or chronic lung disease cause decreased compliance, a volume-cycled respirator is occasionally helpful. The lungs should be inflated periodically with an Ambu bag to prevent atelectasis, and back slapping and postural drainage employed.

Adequate fluid intake should be maintained to prevent dehydration and inspissation of mucus in the bronchioles. Atropine should be employed only if absolutely necessary to diminish excessive secretions, and then used in small doses to avoid overatropinization. Electrolyte balance should be maintained by intravenous administration of sodium chloride and potassium chloride. If the patient is unable to swallow by the third day, a nasogastric tube should be inserted and feeding begun to maintain an adequate nutritional state. Nasogastric feeding should be alternated with milk and antacid every hour to prevent peptic ulceration induced by anticholinesterase compounds, anoxia, stress or steroid administration. Although the value of prophylactic administration of antibiotics to patients on respirators has been questioned, it probably is helpful to administer penicillin or erythromycin parenterally, since the dysphagia and impairment of cough and respiration that precede institution of artificial respiration predispose to atelectasis and pneumonia. The tracheostomy can be utilized as long as dysphagia persists or recurs, for years if necessary. The overlying skin may be allowed to close whenever the patient's condition permits, but the sinus tract of the tracheostomy persists and can be utilized again if necessary.

Corticotropin and Corticosteroid. For patients with generalized, severe myasthenia gravis who are responding poorly to anticholinesterase medication, the next step in management is the administration of corticotropin (ACTH) or corticosteroid, or thymectomy. If the patient is severely weak, the risk of thymectomy can be reduced if the procedure is carried out after strength has been improved by the administration of corticotropin or corticosteroid.

Corticotropin is administered in short intensive courses of 2 units per kilogram of gel intramuscularly daily for 10 days. The hormone should be administered in an intensive care unit, since most patients become weaker during hormone administration and may require tracheostomy and assisted respiration. Most become stronger after the course, for an average of two months. Short intensive courses of methylprednisolone (1.5 mg. per kilogram intramuscularly daily for 10 days) have effects similar to those of corticotropin. During hormone administration, the dose of anticholinesterase medication should be reduced. Antacid medication should be administered through a nasogastric tube to prevent peptic ulceration.

Corticosteroid may also be administered orally for more prolonged periods of time in the form of prednisone, 1 to 2 mg. per kilogram daily or every other day. Some patients experience an exacerbation of weakness during the first week or two of hormone administration. Supplementary potassium chloride should be administered in a dose of 40 mg. per kilogram orally four times a day as a 10 per cent solution. Most patients improve over many months. Since prolonged use of corticosteroid may cause peptic ulcer, osteoporosis, aseptic necrosis of the femoral heads, cataracts and increased susceptibility to infection, this treatment should be limited to patients with disabling myasthenia, and the hormone should be reduced in dose and discontinued when possible.

Adjuvant Drugs. Approximately one-third of myasthenic patients experience a slight increase in strength following the oral administration of ephedrine sulfate (0.5 mg. per kilogram orally three times a day) as an adjuvant to anticholinesterase medication, and a smaller number have a similar response to potassium chloride (40 mg. per kilogram orally four times a day after meals, administered as a 10 per cent solution). Ephedrine should not be given after 4 P.M. since it may cause wakefulness. An occasional patient may improve when calcium gluconate (20 mg. per kilogram orally four times a day), theophylline, spironolactone, or triamterene is added to anticholinesterase medication. If there is no significant improvement after one to two weeks of trial with any of these drugs, they should be discontinued. Germine diacetate may enhance the action of anticholinesterase compounds and is under investigative study. Guanidine is seldom helpful. Certain drugs may increase neuromuscular block and should be avoided. These include streptomycin, colistimethate, colistin, neomycin, kanamycin, vancomycin, novobiocin, polymyxin-B, D-tubocurarine, succinylcholine, quinine, quinidine, procainamide and magnesium sulfate. Morphine should not be used. Sedatives are best avoided or prescribed in half the dose.

Thymectomy. This is performed through a transverse neck incision in patients with generalized myasthenia gravis who are not able to carry out normal activity on anticholinesterase medication. Tracheostomy should be performed over the endotracheal tube after removal of the thymus, and the patient should be cared for in an intensive care unit. Anticholinesterase medication produces more muscarine-like effects and fasciculations for several days after thymectomy, and should be reduced or discontinued during this time, with respiration supported mechanically if necessary. Most patients improve over a period of months or years after thymectomy. Patients with thymoma, which is rare in children, are less likely to improve, but the tumor should be removed. Radiation of the thymus is contraindicated in children, since thyroid carcinoma may develop later in life.

Immunosuppressive Drugs. In patients with disabling weakness who have failed to respond to thymectomy and to repeated courses of corticotropin and corticosteroid, immunosuppressive drugs, such as azathioprine, cyclophosphamide, methotrexate, and 6-mercaptopurine, may be administered on a trial basis. There have been some reports of improvement over a period of several months.

Ocular Myasthenia Gravis. In approximately 15 per cent of patients, myasthenia gravis is limited to the extraocular muscles. Ptosis is usually, though not always, relieved by anticholinesterase medication, while diplopia responds less satisfactorily. Lid crutches attached to the eye glasses may be more effective in relieving ptosis, and alternately patching one eye and then the other may be more helpful than anticholinesterase medication in relieving diplopia.

Myasthenia in the Infant. Approximately 10 per cent of children born to mothers with myasthenia gravis have neonatal myasthenia, which is manifested by weakness at birth, lasting one to six weeks and followed by complete recovery if the infant survives the transient weakness. If the infant has difficulty breathing, the bronchial tree must be aspirated thoroughly, and artificial respiration started, with endotracheal intubation if necessary. Neostigmine methylsulfate, 0.03 mg. per kilogram, is administered intramuscularly every 2 to 3 hours. If muscarine-like side effects develop, atropine sulfate, 0.01 mg. per kilogram, may be administered every 4 to 8 hours as needed, but overatropinization should be avoided. The dose of neostigmine may be adjusted after observing the response to edrophonium, 0.04 mg. per kilogram intravenously, or twice this amount intramuscularly, administered 1 hour after the last dose of neostigmine. Overtreatment with anticholinesterase medication may be heralded by the development of excessive salivation and bronchial secretion, diarrhea, vomiting, bradycardia, fasciculations and increased weakness, and requires reduction in dose. As the infant improves, parenteral anticholinesterase compound can be replaced by oral pyridostigmine bromide, 1 mg. per kilogram every 4 hours, or neostigmine bromide, 0.3 mg. per kilogram every 3 hours. Ambenonium is never used in infants, because even a slight overdose may cause convulsions. As the infant improves, the requirement for anticholinesterase medication will decrease, and the dose should be reduced and the drug discontinued when possible. If the mother is taking anticholinesterase medication, breast feeding is contraindicated, since the medication may be transferred through breast milk. Antibiotic administration may be needed to treat pneumonia.

Myasthenia gravis rarely develops in children of nonmyasthenic mothers at birth, and seldom before the age of one year. Infants born of nonmyasthenic mothers who have respiratory difficulty at birth are much more likely to be suffering from cerebral anoxia, brain damage, airway obstruction, pulmonary disease or the effect of sedative or hypnotic drugs administered to the mother, than from myasthenia gravis.

Periodic Paralysis

F. Q. VROOM, M.D.

A number of periodic paralysis syndromes have now been described. The most common forms are familial hypokalemic periodic paralysis (hypokalemic PP) and familial hyperkalemic periodic paralysis (hyperkalemic PP). The latter has a number of variants: adynamia episodica hereditaria, paramyotonia congenita, hyperkalemic periodic paralysis with hypocalcemic episode, hyperkalemic periodic paralysis and cardiac arrhythmia, and normokalemic periodic paralysis. All develop paralysis with potassium loading and therefore are likely to represent the same disorder. Rarely, other families have been reported (periodic muscle weakness, normokalemia, and tubular aggregates) that have no change in serum potassium or other electrolytes during attacks, are unaffected by induced hypo- or hyperkalemia and are refractory to therapy; they are of uncertain significance.

Attacks of weakness may be so mild that the casual observer is not aware of any disability, or so severe that the patient is quadriplegic and unable even to turn over in bed. Weakness usually begins in the proximal legs but may involve any limb especially if exercised; ocular motility, facial muscles, chewing, swallowing, respiration and cardiac muscle are usually spared; loss of consciousness and death are very rare. Tendon reflexes are reduced or absent during attacks. Severely affected individuals may have continuous weakness and may at middle-age have permanent proximal muscle weakness and wasting, but most are free from attacks at about the age of 40 years. Eyelid myotonia can occur in hypo- and hyperkalemic PP; however, localized myotonia of the face, tongue and distal arms probably occurs only in hyperkalemic PP. Myotonia is demonstrable both during and between attacks. Paresthesias may occur in some patients during attacks of hyperkalemic PP. Although these clinical features may suggest a specific type of periodic paralysis (Table 1), there is so much variation between families that precise diagnosis can be made only by determining serum potassium changes that occur with attacks. The changes in serum potassium in spontaneous attacks may be so slight that they can be discerned only by serial determinations during the attack, and even then some doubt as to the type of disease may remain. Unfortunately, electromyography and muscle biopsy will not distinguish between the types of periodic paralysis.

Sporadic cases are a relatively common occurrence in these rare diseases and either represent the first genetic mutation of the familial variety or are a manifestation of an associated disease. Few associated diseases will be overlooked if all the endocrine (thyrotoxicosis, Addison's disease, hyperaldosteronism, excessive licorice ingestion), renal (renal tubular acidosis, chlorothiazide diuretics) and gastrointestinal (diarrhea-producing hypokalemia, perhaps acute alcoholic myopathy) causes of hyper- and hypokalemia are considered. By the time serum electrolytes are sufficiently disturbed to cause an attack of paralysis in an otherwise normal individual, the underlying disorder is usually obvious. Most of these sporadic patients present with a single attack of severe acute weakness, and gradually recover over days to weeks as the underlying disorder is treated. One exception is thyrotoxic periodic paralysis. This is a form of hypokalemic periodic paralysis generally occurring in males, especially Japanese, and may result in repeated attacks identical to that produced by other forms of periodic paralysis. Treatment of thyrotoxicosis results in the disappearance of attacks of paralysis.

Induced paralysis is frequently necessary to determine the type of periodic paralysis once associated diseases have been excluded. Serum sodium, potassium, carbon dioxide, chloride and calcium should be determined initially and at the height of the attack. Serial serum potassium determinations should be made before, during and after paralysis. Induction of an attack has the obvious value of being scheduled at an opportune time as well as definitely determining the patient's response to a glucose or potassium load. This is of particular importance, since these medications could be given inadvertently in the emergency treatment of an accident victim with disastrous results. Once the response to these medications is determined, appropriate information should be carried by the patient, preferably by identification tags.

Induction of Attacks. Induced attacks of paralysis should be performed only in the hospital under constant medical supervision and with electrocardiographic (ECG) monitoring and provisions for respiratory assistance, such as having an anesthesiologist on call and appropriate respiratory assistance devices at the bedside. The risk under these circumstances is no greater than with spontaneous attacks; death during attacks is extremely rare and none has been reported during induced attacks.

Hypokalemia is generally produced with glucose and insulin. Generally, 1.75 Gm. per kilogram of oral glucose as Glucola and intramuscular regular insulin, 10 to 15 units in children, 20 to 30 units in adolescents, are used. If spontaneous attacks have been severe, then 1 Gm. per kilogram of oral glucose without insulin should be tried initially. Hyperglycemia produced by epinephrine or glucagon will cause hypokalemia and precipitate attacks. Attacks have also been produced by sodium chloride loading, a mineralocorticoid (fluorohydrocortisone) and adrenocorticotropic hormone (ACTH).

Hyperkalemic paralysis is usually produced by oral administration of potassium as potassium chloride, but is more palatable when flavored or as potassium citrate and/or potassium bicarbonate (e.g., K-Lyte). Although 4, 8 or even 12 Gm. of potassium have been given to adolescents, it is certainly preferable to start off with smaller doses, increasing them on separate days. Attacks are usually produced with 25 to 50 mg. of potassium per kilogram; only rarely is 75 to 100 mg. per kilogram required.

Induced attacks of paralysis usually begin in 1 to 2 hours and reach a maximum in 2 to 3 hours. Attacks can usually be terminated in 1 to 2 hours by activity but may take longer when severe. Both glucose and potassium loads are recommended, since the diagnosis could be confused by the occurrence of a spontaneous attack, and weakness induced by one preparation may be terminated by the other.

Repeated observations of strength and

TABLE 1. Characteristics and Management of Periodic Paralyses

DISEASE	HYPOKALEMIC PP	HYPERKALEMIC PP
AGE ONSET	Puberty	Infancy
INHERITANCE	Dominant	Dominant
FREQUENCY	*Weekly* to monthly	*Daily* (normokalemic—monthly)
DURATION	*Hours* to days	Hours (normokalemic—days to weeks)
SEVERITY	Intermediate	Mild (normokalemic—severe)
SERUM K AND DEGREE OF WEAKNESS	Weakness may occur with normal serum K in both disorders. 2.5 mEq./liter—moderate 2.0 mEq./liter—severe	5–6 mEq./liter—moderate 7 mEq./liter—severe
PRECIPITATING FACTORS	Prolonged inactivity (sleep, long distance driving, spectator sports), exercise followed by rest, anxiety, emotion, cold and alcohol are common to both disorders. Carbohydrates and NaCl precipitate only hypokalemic PP.	
INDUCED ATTACK	Glucose, 1.0–1.75 Gm./kg., with I.M. regular insulin, 10–15 units in children; 20–30 units in adolescents.	Potassium, 25, 50, 75 or 100 mg./kg. on separate days. 75 or 100 mg./kg. are rarely necessary.
PROPHYLAXIS EFFECTIVE IN:	*Hypokalemic and Hyperkalemic PP* Acetazolamide (Diamox), children: 125–1000 mg./day; adolescents: 250–1500 mg./day in single or divided doses.* or Chlorothiazide (Diuril), children: 125–500 mg./day; adolescents: 250–1000 mg./day in single or divided doses.	
EFFECTIVE IN:	*Hypokalemic PP* Spironolactone (Aldactone), 50–200 mg./day, or low salt diet (10 mEq./day), or low carbohydrate diet.	*Hyperkalemic PP* *Normokalemic PP:* High NaCl diet, or 0.1 mg. flurohydrocortisone daily.
TREATMENT OF ACUTE ATTACK	Usually unnecessary except for preparation to support respiration. Oral KCl or potassium bicarbonate (K-Lyte), adolescents: 5 Gm. every 1–2 hours (total = 10–15 Gm./day); children: 25 mg./kg. every 1–2 hours (total = 100 to 200 mg./kg./day).	Oral or I.V. glucose, 1.75 Gm./kg. with regular insulin, 10–15 units in children; 20–30 units in adolescents. Calcium gluconate, 1–2 Gm. slowly I.V. in adolescents; sometimes successful. *Normokalemic PP:* Oral NaCl, 5 Gm. every 1–2 hours (total = 15 Gm. in adolescents).
SERUM K AND DEGREE OF WEAKNESS	Weakness may occur with normal serum K in both disorders. 2.5 mEq./liter—moderate 2.0 mEq./liter—severe	5–6 mEq./liter—moderate 7 mEq./liter—severe
PRECIPITATING FACTORS		
INDUCED ATTACK	Glucose, 1.0–1.75 Gm./kg., with I.M. regular insulin, 10–15 units children; 20–30 units adolescents	Potassium 25, 50, 75 or 100 mg./kg. on separate days.

* Note: Some investigators believe that doses in excess of 1 Gm. do not produce any better results than doses of 1 Gm. Optimum dose is 375 to 1000 mg. per day.

tendon reflexes in proximal and distal limb muscles contralateral to the intravenous needle is sufficient. Vital capacity determinations are recommended and measurement of grip strength with a dynamometer is useful.

It is convenient to obtain blood samples at 30-minute intervals through a 17- to 19-gauge needle kept open by intermittent heparinized saline flushes given immediately after each blood sample. The initial few milliliters of each blood sample must be discarded to prevent contamination by saline or heparin, which could alter electrolyte determinations.

The electrocardiogram is a sensitive indicator of serum potassium concentrations and allows immediate estimation of the serum potassium. The ECG is normal with serum potassiums of 5 mEq. per liter. At 3.5 mEq. per liter, there is a prominent U-wave; at 3.0 mEq. per liter it is frequently higher than the T-wave. At 2.5 mEq. per liter there is a depressed ST segment along with a low T-wave and a high U-wave. At 7 mEq. per liter the T-wave is high and peaked. At 8 mEq. per liter there is a prolonged PR interval, high T-wave and depressed ST segment. At 9 mEq. per liter atrial standstill and interventricular block occur. At 10 mEq. per liter, ventricular fibrillation occurs.

Prophylactic Treatment. Since most patients have been having attacks daily to monthly for years, the greatest problem is prevention of further attacks. A number of therapeutic agents have been tried and have had variable success (Table 1). Potassium chloride, spironolactone, triamterene, low salt diet, avoidance of exercise and high carbohydrate loads have been variably successful in treating hypokalemic PP. In hyperkalemic PP, diuretics such as acetazolamide (Diamox) have been very successful in preventing attacks. Because of an error in diagnosis, acetazolamide was inadvertently given to patients with hypokalemic PP and surprisingly resulted in a striking reduction in attacks even in very refractory cases.

Acetazolamide, therefore, is the treatment of choice in both forms of the disease. It is a carbonic-anhydrase inhibitor which prevents the hydrolysis of carbon dioxide and hence prevents the production of carbonic acid. This, in turn, limits the number of hydrogen ions available for exchange in the distal convoluted tubule of the kidney. Since hydrogen ions cannot be exchanged for sodium ions, sodium output is increased. Similarly, hydrogen ions cannot be exchanged for potassium ions and urinary potassium output is transiently increased. As sodium and bicarbonate excretion increases, the urine becomes alkaline, which in turn lowers the ammonium excretion. Failure to excrete hydrogen ions results in a metabolic acidosis and a compensatory drop in plasma carbon dioxide. The means of prevention of attacks of paralysis remain uncertain; since carbonic anhydrase does not exist in muscle and acidosis is an unlikely mechanism. Acetazolamide is also an anticonvulsant, decreases intraocular pressure, produces paresthesias, gives carbonated beverages a metallic taste and rarely may cause fever, skin reactions and bone marrow depression; sulfonamide-like renal lesions have also been described. Calculus formation and ureteral colic have been attributed to reduced urinary citrate, but this is rare and may be fortuitous. Disorientation has been induced in patients with hepatic cirrhosis presumably because of decreased ammonia excretion. Acetazolamide is readily absorbed from the gastrointestinal tract, reaching a peak within 2 hours, and has a half-life in serum of approximately 8 hours. Attacks of paralysis are frequently controlled with 60 to 125 mg. one to three times a day in children, and with 250 mg. one to three times a day in adolescents. In refractory cases, 1 to 1.5 Gm. per day have been given in children and adolescents, respectively.* Some added benefit may be obtained by evenly divided doses or a single dose usually at bedtime. If attacks are still not controlled, the addition of previously tried therapies, such as potassium chloride, 1 to 10 Gm. per day in hypokalemic PP, or ad libitum salting of food in hyperkalemic PP, may add another measure of control. It is advisable to check for electrolyte disturbances at 1-, 3-, 6- and 12-month intervals initially. Many patients find they can skip treatment for one to two days without precipitating an attack. When an attack of weakness begins, the prompt reinstitution of oral therapy will abort or minimize an attack without inconvenience.

Dichlorphenamide (Daranide) is a newer carbonic-anhydrase inhibitor. It is one of the most potent carbonic-anhydrase inhibitors available and in dosages of 25 to 200 mg. per day has been effective in preventing attacks of hypokalemic PP; however, it has no clear advantage over acetazolamide.

Interestingly, chlorothiazide (Diuril), approximately 250 mg. daily, has been successful in treating both forms of periodic paralysis. Chlorothiazide inhibits carbonic anhydrase but also promotes excretion of sodium and chloride

* Note: Some investigators believe that doses in excess of 1 Gm. do not produce any better results than doses of 1 Gm. Optimum dose of acetazolamide is 375 to 1000 mg. per day.

and, to a lesser degree, of potassium and bicarbonate without affecting acid-base balance. Thiazide diuretics may produce hypokalemia through the renal loss of potassium; hyperuricemia also occurs, probably because thiazide diuretics and uric acid compete for the same tubular secretory mechanisms. Rarely, thiazide diuretics have caused acute pancreatitis, skin rash, thrombocytopenic purpura, agranulocytosis, photosensitive dermatitis, purpura and necrotizing vasculitis. Prolonged drug therapy may induce mild hyperglycemia, particularly in patients with latent diabetes mellitus. As with other carbonic-anhydrase inhibitors, hepatic coma may be precipitated with preexisting cirrhosis of the liver. Chlorothiazide is readily absorbed from the gastrointestinal tract; the diuretic effect begins within an hour and lasts 3 to 6 hours after a single oral dose.

Spironolactone (Aldactone) is a competitive inhibitor of aldosterone. It blocks the resorption of sodium, thus preventing the exchange for potassium and hydrogen ions. Presumably, the value of spironolactone in hypokalemic PP results from the promotion of sodium diuresis and potassium retention. In adolescents the usual daily dosage is 50 to 100 mg. orally in divided doses. Hyperkalemia is the only contraindication to the use of the drug, and serum potassiums should be monitored until the effects of the drug are determined.

Triamterene (Dyrenium) is a diuretic whose main site of action is the distal convoluted tubule; it promotes loss of sodium chloride and water with retention of potassium and slight alkalinization of the urine. Its exact mechanism of action is uncertain, but it does not appear to have any inhibition on carbonic anhydrase; its mechanism of action is also independent of aldosterone antagonism. The drug is readily absorbed from the gastrointestinal tract. Dosage in adolescents varies from 100 mg. every other day to 300 mg. a day in divided doses. The side effects are relatively few and consist mainly of nausea and vomiting, leg cramps and dizziness. Prerenal azotemia sometimes occurs and electrolytes should be checked to guard against severe hyperkalemia.

A low sodium chloride (10 mEq. per day) and/or a low carbohydrate diet has also been useful in hypokalemic PP, but is not as well tolerated as are other therapies.

Potassium chloride tablets are available in 300-mg. and 500-mg. sizes, but they cause considerable gastric irritation if they are not enteric-coated, and they may cause ulcerations of the gastrointestinal tract and gastrointestinal bleeding even when they are enteric-coated. Other potassium salts, such as potassium bicarbonate and citrate (K-Lyte), are more palatable, being available in flavored tablets containing 25 mEq. of potassium, and are readily dissolved in water. As with other potassium compounds, gastric irritation, nausea, vomiting, diarrhea and abdominal discomfort may occur; however, these effects are minimized when the tablets are taken slowly over 10 or more minutes with meals.

Some variants of hyperkalemic PP (normokalemic PP) have not responded to acetazolamide but have responded to a high salt diet and a fluorohydrocortisone (Florinef), which is the most potent synthetic mineralocorticoid. The usual adolescent daily dose is 0.1 mg. orally. Small doses produce marked sodium retention and increased urinary potassium excretion, as well as causing glucocorticoid effects. Because of side effects, glucocorticoids have not been given for more than a few months. If they must be given, it is probably best to try them on alternate days, in a single dose, watching for hypertension, aggravation of existing diabetes, activation of tuberculosis, iatrogenic adrenal insufficiency, suppression of growth in children and keratogenetic effects.

It appears likely that the chronic proximal muscle weakness which can occur in later years may be prevented or reduced by successful prophylactic therapy.

Treatment of the Acute Attack. This is rarely a problem, since respiratory muscles are generally spared and patients with severe attacks generally have had frequent attacks over a long period of time. If the type of periodic paralysis is known, the appropriate therapy is the opposite of that used to induce an attack. Potassium is indicated for hypokalemic PP (Table 1).

Calcium gluconate is effective in combating the effects of hyperkalemia on the myocardium as well as sometimes terminating an attack of hyperkalemic PP. Calcium gluconate may be administered intravenously in a 10 per cent solution with ECG monitoring. As much as 50 ml. can be administered safely in adolescents if given slowly, and another 50 ml. may be placed in a large volume of fluid, such as 5 per cent glucose and water, which will also help in lowering serum potassium by transiently promoting cellular uptake of potassium. Intramuscular administration of calcium gluconate should be avoided because of local abscess formation. Induced hyperglycemia is also useful in terminating an attack of hyperkalemic PP. Sodium chloride should be tried in refractory cases of hyperkalemic PP or the normokalemic variant.

If the type of periodic paralysis is not known, then ECG monitoring, serial electrolyte determinations and appropriate supportive measures are indicated until a definitive diagnosis is made. The administration of intravenous acetazolamide appears logical but has not yet been reported. In our only case so treated, an induced attack of hypokalemic PP was unaffected, but spontaneous attacks were abolished.

References

Burch, G. E., and Winsor, T.: *A Primer of Electrocardiography.* Philadelphia, Lea & Febiger, 1960.

Dyken, M. L., and Timmons, G. D.: Hyperkalemic Periodic Paralysis in Hypocalcemic Episode. *Arch. Neurol.,* 9:76, 1963.

Griggs, R. C., Engel, W. K., and Resnick, J. S.: Acetazolamide Treatment of Hypokalemic Periodic Paralysis. *Ann. Int. Med.,* 73:39–48, 1970.

Lisak, R. P., Lebeau, J. T. S. H., and Rowland, L. P.: Hyperkalemic Periodic Paralysis in Cardiac Arrhythmia. *Neurology,* 22:810–815, 1972.

McArdle, B.: Metabolic and Endocrine Myopathies; in John Walton (ed.): *Disorders of Voluntary Muscle.* London, J. & A. Churchill Ltd., 1969, pp. 607–616.

Meyers, A. R., Gilden, D. H., Rinaldi, C. F., and Hansen, J. L.: Periodic Muscle Weakness, Normokalemia and Tubular Aggregates. *Neurology,* 22:269–279, 1972.

Owen, E. E., and Verner, J. V.: Renal Tubular Disease with Muscle Paralysis and Hypokalemia. *Am. J. Med.,* 28:8–21, 1960.

Poskanzer, D. C., and Kerr, D.N.S.: A Third Type of Periodic Paralysis, with Normokalemia and Favourable Response to Sodium Chloride. *Am. J. Med.,* 31:328-342, 1961.

Resnick, J. S.: Episodic Muscle Weakness; in W. K. Engel (ed.): *Current Concepts of Myopathies.* 1965, pp. 63–68. Reprinted from Clinical Orthopedics and Related Research, No. 39.

Satoyoshi, E., Murakami, K., Kowa, H., Kinoshita, M., and Nishiyama Y.: Periodic Paralysis in Hyperthyroidism. *Neurology,* 13:746-752, 1963.

Myositis Ossificans

F. Q. VROOM, M.D.

Two types of myositis ossificans are recognized. One is localized and follows trauma; the other is widespread and progressive.

Traumatic myositis ossificans results from a single severe injury to skeletal muscle, such as being kicked by a horse; from repeated lesser injuries, such as to the brachialis and biceps brachii muscles in baseball pitchers from rapid stretching of these muscles; or from continuous minor trauma, such as to the thighs of horsemen. Following a single severe injury, there is tearing of tissue and hemorrhage which results in a firm, tender mass lasting several weeks. In repeated minor injuries there is often little or no discomfort. Both injuries may result in formation of bone and cartilage, presumably by osteoblasts which have been displaced by torn tendons; both produce progressive limitation of movement. Because of the nature of the injury, most occur in vigorous males and usually affect proximal limb muscles. No abnormalities of calcium, phosphorus, or phosphatase enzymes have been identified. Most patients improve spontaneously with avoidance of further trauma. In severe injuries, range of motion exercises to prevent complicating joint contractures should be initiated; care should be taken to avoid further trauma especially in the first few days. A few patients may require surgical removal of the mass if it remains painful. Diagnosis is by history of trauma and the presence of a firm mass with feathery calcifications on x-ray.

Progressive myositis ossificans is a rare disorder in which proliferation of connective tissue is followed by calcium deposition and bone formation. It has been described also in association with polyostotic fibrous dysplasia. The onset is usually between the first and tenth year of life but may be present at birth or occur as late as the twentieth year. There are usually other congenital anomalies, such as failure of development of the great toes, thumbs or other digits, leading to microdactyly. Other anomalies, such as exostoses or congenital hallux valgus, absence of ear lobes, absence of upper incisors and spina bifida may also occur. Progressive myositis ossificans and/or short thumbs in other family members suggest that genetic transmission probably occurs as an autosomal dominant and most cases represent a new mutation.

Spontaneously, or following minor trauma, soft fluctuant or firm masses may develop on any part of the body with or without associated redness and induration of the skin. The acute swelling and discomfort may subside over the next several weeks, leaving in their places a smaller, firm, often fixed, mass. Muscles of the neck, back and proximal limbs are most commonly affected; eventually the jaw, palmar, plantar and intercostal muscles may be affected, producing a "stone man" and death from restricted respiration. Cardiac, ocular, tongue, laryngeal, diaphragmatic and perineal muscles are usually spared. Ulcerations of the tense overlying skin may result in secondary infection. Pathologically there is little inflammatory response or hemorrhage; there is extensive proliferation of connective tissue and eventually new bone formation. New lesions tend to occur within 6 to 12 months and death generally occurs by the fourth to fifth decade.

The disorder should be distinguished from vitamin D calcinosis in which prolonged ingestion of large doses of vitamin D may also produce widespread calcium deposition in muscles, subcutaneous tissue and joints. The distinction between myositis ossificans and calcinosis universalis, which usually occurs with scleroderma or polymyositis, remains uncertain.

Because of the possible relationship of myositis ossificans to polymyositis and scleroderma, particularly in the more rapidly progressive cases, corticosteroid therapy may be worthwhile. If corticosteroids are given, high-dose, alternate-day, single-dose prednisone therapy (25 to 50 mg. in children and 100 mg. in adolescents) is recommended because the side effects are decreased. If a significant response is obtained, either acutely or with repeated trials, continued therapy of several months to years should be considered with gradual tapering. In this case, prophylactic antituberculin therapy is recommended if there is a positive PPD or evidence of tuberculosis on chest x-ray; sodium chloride and calories should be restricted to prevent hypertension, edema or obesity. Antacids should be given between meals and at bedtime to prevent gastrointestinal ulceration. Care should be taken to prevent aggravation of pre-existing diabetes or hypokalemia from urinary loss of potassium. Surgery is rarely indicated, since it usually provokes a larger mass. Similarly, diagnostic studies such as needle electromyography and muscle biopsy should be avoided, since they may trigger new lesions.

Disodium etidronate (EHDP),* 10 mg. per kilogram per day by mouth, has prevented further calcific deposits, caused regression of preexisting ossifications and produced improved joint mobility and resolution of painful skin lesions in both myositis ossificans progressiva and dermatomyositis over 12 to 18 months. EHDP decreases the rate of calcium deposition in the body, increases fecal calcium, has not caused known side effects, and has not prevented skeletal growth in the few cases so treated.

References

Bassett, C. A. L., Donath, A., Macagno, F., Preisig, R., Fleisch, H., and Francis, N. D.: Diphosphonates in the Treatment of Myositis Ossificans. *Lancet,* 2:845, 1969.

Cram, R. L., Barmada, R., Geho, W. D., and Ray, R. D.: Diphosphonate Treatment of Calcinosis Universalis. *New England J. Med.,* 285:1012–1013, 1971.

* EHDP is an experimental drug and is available only on this basis.

16

Skin

Alvin H. Jacobs, M.D., Editor

Topical Therapy: A Formulary for Pediatric Skin Disease

ROBERT M. ADAMS, M.D.

General Considerations

Choice of Active Ingredient. The fewer active ingredients the better; one usually is enough. Exceptions are mixtures containing steroids with tars, nystatin and, perhaps, neomycin, which may be useful in special situations. Avoid prescribing potent fluorinated steroids for use on the face over long periods of time, since atrophy and telangiectasia may result. Also avoid these agents for prolonged use in intertriginous areas because of the possible development of striae.

The concentration of the active ingredient is very important. Choose the smallest concentration which is effective. However, hydrocortisone in ¼ per cent concentration, for example, probably possesses little anti-inflammatory effect. A better choice is a ½ or 1 per cent concentration.

Choice of Vehicle. The vehicle is often as important as the active ingredient. Although pharmacologically inert, vehicles do possess therapeutic properties based on physical properties. Ointments, creams and pastes protect the skin and relieve dryness, while lotions and baths clean by removal of crusts, scales and exudate.

Greater penetration occurs with ointments than with creams, pastes and lotions, in decreasing order. Shake lotions, such as calamine, may "cake" on the skin, especially when used on acute, oozing dermatitides, and may thus lead to secondary bacterial or monilial infection.

Cosmetic Effect. The effect of treatment on the patient's appearance is always an important consideration. Iodochlorhydroxyquin may stain the skin yellow and must be used cautiously on the face and other visible areas. Other staining medications are potassium permanganate, gentian violet, silver nitrate, tars and anthralin.

Cost. Prescribe only the amount necessary to treat the disease. Written instructions as to proper application may help reduce the amount of medication wasted, since most patients apply far more topical medication than is necessary.

Basic Principles of Topical Therapy

Do Not Overtreat. Therapeutic aggressiveness should be inversely proportional to the acuteness of the disease. When treating acutely inflamed skin, use bland medications such as wet dressings and simple, almost inert lotions; creams should be used sparingly, and ointments must never be employed on acute oozing dermatitides. The irritant properties of the active ingredient(s) and the possibility of allergic sensitization must be considered. Overtreatment may induce a widespread or generalized dermatitis. Systemic absorption may occur from potent medications employed under plastic wrap occlusion, or when intertriginous areas such as the axilla and groin are treated.

Remove the Contributing Factors. Success or failure of topical therapy may hinge on the physician's recognition of the influence of environmental factors. In pediatric practice the most important of these are soaps, bubble baths and bath salts, rough or tight clothing, wool blankets, rugs, toys, dirt, sand, heat, cold, moisture and wind. Irritating or sensitizing home remedies used as self-medications are common causes of aggravation.

Decrease Itching. The most effective method of alleviating pruritus is by prompt and adequate treatment of the disease. Topical "caine" anesthetics may produce allergic sensitization. Systemic antihistamines and aspirin are the medications of choice. Menthol and phenol which are frequently found incorporated into topical medications as antipruritic agents may be systemically absorbed when applied to large areas of skin.

Recognize and Promptly Treat Secondary Infection. The appearance of secondary bacterial infection of dermatitic skin may be subtle and thus easily overlooked. Increased pruritus and pain, accompanied by yellow crusting, may signal its development. Children with atopic dermatitis are particularly likely to develop secondary pyogenic infection. Treatment of choice is the use of systemic antibiotics, such as erythromycin, often continued for two to three weeks. Topical antibiotics are less effective, and probably should not be employed without concomitant systemic antibiotics.

Individualize Treatment. In pediatrics, tailor the treatment carefully, not only to the patient and disease but also to the parents. Parental concerns which are most frequent are (1) contagiousness, (2) disfigurement, (3) malignancy and (4) inheritance. Reassurance in such matters may play an important role in the successful outcome of the therapeutic program.

FORMULARY

Open Wet Dressings

Open wet dressings, the mildest form of topical therapy, cool the skin by evaporation, relieve itching and clean the surface by loosening and removing crusts and debris. Used on acute blistered dermatitides, open wet dressings may often be the only treatment possible. The principle is based on cooling by evaporation.

Kerlix gauze, plain gauze without absorbent cotton, thin white handerchiefs or strips of bed linen are most commonly used. Moisten the dressings in the solution and apply them, wet but not runny, to the affected area. One layer is usually sufficient. Wrap fingers separately; wrap arms and legs so that the elbows and knees can bend. The patient must be comfortable during treatment and must be prepared so that he can still look at pictures, play with toys and so forth.

Apply the dressings flat and smooth against the skin and leave them uncovered. When evaporation begins to dry the cloth after 5 or 10 minutes, remove the entire dressing, resoak it in the solution and reapply it to the inflamed area. Never pour or syringe the solution directly over the dressings. The treatment ordinarily has a duration of 30 minutes to 1 hour, three to four times daily. Ordinary tap water is used and it is not necessary to sterilize the water or the dressings. Keep the solutions at room temperature and mix them immediately before each treatment. Do not keep the solutions overnight, since they may become unstable and more concentrated on standing.

Wet dressings are usually discontinued after 36 to 48 hours; if they are continued longer than this, drying of the skin can result. Do not cover more than one-third of the body at any one time, and avoid chilling the patient. After treatment, dry the skin by patting with a towel or washcloth. At this time a lotion or other medication may be applied.

Burow's Solution. (Domeboro powder, powder packets, tablets) (Dome Laboratories) Composition: aluminum sulfate and calcium acetate, which has an acid pH in solution. Prepare a 1:40 solution by mixing one packet of powder or one tablet in one quart of tap water. The more concentrated solutions indicated on the package directions may be irritating. Burow's solution is mildly astringent and antiseptic and leaves a fresh, dry feeling. It is supplied as tablets in boxes of 12 to 1000, and as powder in packets from 12 to 100. Bulk powder is also available in 4-ounce containers, in which ½ teaspoonful equals one Domeboro Powder Packet or Tablet.

Soyboro Powder Packets. (Dome Laboratories) One packet of powder in a quart of tap water provides a soothing and cleansing wet dressing combining Burow's solution with a soya protein complex. This preparation is highly acceptable to patients and should be used more frequently.

Potassium Permanganate. Potassium permanganate is available in 300-mg. tablets. A 1:15,000 solution may be prepared by pulverizing one 300-mg. tablet between spoons; add the powder to 4½ quarts of water. Be certain the entire tablet dissolves, since skin contact with particles of tablet may cause a chemical burn. Solutions of potassium permanganate are mildly antiseptic and drying, and are useful for vesicular, oozing dematitides. Potassium permanganate stains clothing and skin and should never be used on the face.

Dalibour Solution. (Dalidome powder packets) (Dome Laboratories) Composition: zinc sulfate, copper sulfate and camphor. Dalibour solution is an effective nonstaining wet dressing which can be used in place of potassium permanganate. Dissolve the contents of one powder packet in one quart of water, making a 1:16 solution. It is supplied in boxes of 12 and 100 packets.

Silver Nitrate. Silver nitrate is a very effective antiseptic, coagulant germicidal agent. Prepare a 0.5 per cent solution by adding two teaspoonfuls of a 50 per cent aqueous solution to one quart of cool tap water. The concentrated solution must be dispensed in a brown or other opaque bottle. Silver nitrate is expensive and stains the skin dark brown after exposure to light, and will also stain everything else with which it comes in contact, such as teaspoon, containers and floor. In 0.5 per cent concentration, silver nitrate does not irritate normal skin or inhibit epidermal proliferation; it is not antigenic. The chief disadvantages are its staining properties and its costliness.

Bluboro Powder. (Derm●Arts Laboratories) Composition: aluminum sulfate, calcium acetate, boric acid and FD&C blue dye number 1. The addition of boric acid contraindicates the use of this preparation in pediatric practice.

Boric Acid. Because of the possibility of systemic poisoning, boric acid should *never* be used.

Soaks and Paints

Formaldehyde Solution. For the treatment of hyperhidrosis of the feet and recurrent multiple plantar verrucae, 3 per cent aqueous formaldehyde solution has been advocated by some. The feet are soaked once or twice daily for 15 or 20 minutes. Formaldehyde solution must be freshly prepared prior to each use and may be sensitizing.

Glutaraldehyde. Glutaraldehyde in a 10 per cent solution may be painted on plantar skin with a cotton swab three times weekly for treatment of hyperhidrosis. Glutaraldehyde is an allergic sensitizer, and cross-reactions with formaldehyde may occur. Remember that the skin will stain yellow following its use. (Note: glutaraldehyde is investigational, not yet having been approved by the Food and Drug Administration. It is manufactured by Mathison, Coleman and Bell, Norwood, Ohio.)

Lotions and Solutions

Lotions are suspensions of a powder in liquid. As the liquid evaporates, a coating of powder remains on the skin surface. Evaporation cools the surface and the powder soothes, protects and dries the skin. Lotions are useful in the treatment of acute dermatitis but must be avoided on oozing surfaces and in hairy or intertriginous areas.

They are most often applied with the fingers or gauze, or with a small paint brush, in which case they should be dispensed in a wide-mouthed bottle. Apply evenly; remove by soaking in a portion of the compress solution, not by peeling the dried material from the skin. If used for more than three or four days, shake lotions may cause chapping. Addition of an oil and a dispersant forms an emulsion.

A BASIC SHAKE LOTION		TO WHICH ONE MAY ADD	
zinc oxide	15%	olive oil	10%
talc	15%	menthol	⅛–¼%
glycerin	10%	ichthammol	2–3%
sufficient water to make		liquor carbonis detergens	5–10%
		Vioform	1–3%
		hydrocortisone	½–1%

Do not add "caine-type" anesthetics or antihistamines.

Calamine Lotion U.S.P. Composition: zinc oxide, ferric oxide and yellow ferric oxide, with glycerine and bentonite magma and calcium hydroxide solution. Calamine solution is inexpensive and has a wide and well-deserved reputation. Its disadvantages are that it tends to dry and cake, especially in the presence of oozing.

Aveeno Lotion. (Cooper Laboratories) Composition: 10 per cent Aveeno colloidal oatmeal in an aqueous base consisting of propylene glycol, isopropyl myristate and liquid petrolatum. In acute and subacute dermatoses, Aveeno Lotion forms a flexible adherent coating which does not crack or flake off. It is supplied in 6-ounce plastic bottles.

Cetaphil Lotion. (Texas Pharmacal) Cetaphil Lotion is a lipid-free lotion and skin cleanser containing propylene glycol, cetyl alcohol, stearyl alcohol, sodium lauryl sulfate, butyl, methyl and propyl parabens and water. It may be used as a waterless cleaner, especially for atopic dermatitis, and also as a vehicle for various active ingredients, especially hydrocortisone, in the treatment of other forms of dermatitis. Apply by rubbing in two layers. It is dispensed in one-pint containers.

Steroid-Containing Lotions and Solutions.

SYNALAR SOLUTION, 0.01 PER CENT. (Fluocinolone acetonide) (Syntex Laboratories) The vehicle is propylene glycol with citric acid added as a preservative. It is especially useful in hairy and intertriginous areas, and can be used on the scalp overnight under a "Baggie" or a shower cap. It is available in 20- and 60-ml. plastic squeeze bottles.

CORDRAN LOTION. (Lilly) Composition: 0.05 per cent flurandrenolone in glycerine, stearic acid, cetyl alcohol, glycerile monostearate, mineral oil, polyoxyl 40 stearate, menthol, methyl and propyl parabens and water. Cordran Lotion is easy to apply and useful in acute and subacute dermatoses. Available in 15- and 60-ml. plastic squeeze bottles, but rather expensive.

KENALOG LOTION. (Squibb) Composition: 0.1 and 0.025 per cent triamcinolone acetonide. The base includes propylene glycol, cetyl and stearyl alcohols and methyl and propyl parabens. It is dispensed in 50- and 150-ml. plastic squeeze bottles. Kenalog Lotion is very effective for seborrheic dermatitis on the face and in intertriginous areas.

Special-Purpose Lotions. ANTIFUNGAL. *Dermatophytes. Tinactin Solution.* Composition: 1 per cent tolnaftate solution with butylated hydroxytoluene in a vehicle of polyethylene glycol. It is effective against Trichophyton, Microsporum and Epidermophyton species of fungi, as well as tinea versicolor. However, Tinactin Solution is impractical for the latter because of the large amount required. Remember that Tinactin is ineffective against Candida. It is dispensed as a 10-ml. plastic squeeze bottle and is also available as a cream or powder. Recently, Tinactin preparations have become available "over the counter."

Candida. Fungizone Lotion. (Amphotericin B) (Squibb) Composition: 3 per cent amphotericin B in a vehicle containing thimerosal, titanium dioxide, guar gum, propylene glycol, cetyl alcohol, stearyl alcohol and other ingredients, including methyl and propyl parabens. Apply two to four times daily. It is effective against *Candida albicans* infections. It is available in 30-ml. plastic squeeze bottles. Fungizone lotion discolors fabrics, but the stain may be removed by applying a standard cleaning fluid.

Gentian violet as a lotion must be freshly prepared in concentrations ranging from 1/4 to 2 per cent in water or 70 per cent alcohol. It is very messy and rarely used.

Tinea Versicolor. Tinver Solution. (Barnes-Hind) Composition: 25 per cent sodium thiosulfate, 1 per cent salicylic acid, 10 per cent isopropyl alcohol, propylene glycol, menthol, sodium edetate, colloidal albumina and water. Apply after showering, twice daily, for tinea versicolor only. However, it is less effective than Selsun in the treatment of tinea versicolor. It is dispensed in 5-ounce plastic squeeze bottles.

ANTIPARASITIC. *Kwell Lotion.* (Reed & Carnrick) Composition: 1 per cent gamma benzene hexachloride. Apply on four consecutive nights after showering for treatment of scabies and pediculosis pubis. It is supplied in 2- and 16-ounce bottles.

Eurax Lotion (Geigy) contains 10 per cent *N*-ethyl-o-crotonotoluide in a cream or emollient lotion base. It is used for treatment of scabies and is also an excellent antipruritic, but it should never be applied to acutely inflamed skin.

Thiabendazole (Merck, Sharp & Dohme) is a suspension containing 500 mg. of thiabendazole per 5 ml. Use for topical treatment of creeping eruption.

Baths

For treatment of a widespread dermatitis, baths are antipruritic and mildly anti-inflammatory. Fill the tub half full of lukewarm water and bathe the patient for 15 to 30 minutes. The bathroom must be well ventilated when volatile tars are used.

Aveeno Colloidal Oatmeal. (Cooper Laboratories) This preparation is a concentrated colloid fraction of oatmeal which is useful in the treatment of widespread poison ivy or oak dermatitis, diaper rash, atopic dermatitis and contact dermatitis. Add one cup to a tub of warm water once or twice daily. For infants, add one or two tablespoonfuls to the bathinette. It is available in 1-pound and 4-pound boxes, plain and "oilated." Do not use the oilated type for treatment of acute oozing dermatitis. Individual dose packets are also supplied.

Soyaloid Colloidal Bath. (Dome Laboratories) This is a colloidal soya protein complex with 2 per cent polyvinylpyrrolidone. It is very valuable for the treatment of diaper dermatitis, poison ivy or poison oak and sunburn. Dissolve one packet in a tub of warm water, or two to three tablespoonfuls to each gallon of warm water for an infant's bath.

Potassium Permanganate Baths. These are used for generalized weeping dermatoses; they have some deodorizing properties. Crush 12 300-mg. tablets between two spoons and dissolve the powder by shaking in one quart of lukewarm water. Pour the mixture into a tub of tepid water; this will produce a concentration of about 1:20,000. The particles of potassium permanganate must completely dissolve, since tiny crystals may burn the skin if sat upon; they will also stain any cracks in the porcelain.

Lubricating Baths. These include *Alpha-Keri* (Westwood), *Domol* (Dome Laboratories), *Aveenol* (Cooper Laboratories), *Lubath* (Texas Pharmacal) and *Nutraspa* (Owen Laboratories). Baths are very useful for treatment of dry and pruritic skin, such as from ichthyosis, psoriasis and atopic dermatitis. They can also be used after showering or sponge bathing, and also for general cleansing of dry skin.

Tars. Tar baths may be used for the treatment of widespread dermatoses such as psoriasis, atopic dermatitis, seborrheic dermatitis and other such diseases in older children and adolescents. The room must be kept well ventilated during treatment.

Liquor Carbonis Detergens (N. F.). This preparation contains crude coal tar with quillaja, a foaming agent also known as soap bark. Add ½ to 1 ounce to a tub full of water.

Zetar Emulsion. (Dermik Laboratories) Zetar emulsion contains 50 per cent colloidal crude coal tar. One or two tablespoonfuls placed directly under the open water tap usually suffice.

Polytar Bath. (Stiefel Laboratories) Polytar Bath is a combination of 25 per cent polytar, which is a blend of juniper tar, pine tar, coal tar solution, polyunsaturated vegetable oil and water-dispersible solubilized crude coal tar, with 25 per cent butyl stearate in a water-miscible emulsion base. It may be used for psoriasis and chronic atopic dermatitis, lichen planus and other dermatoses. It does not discolor the hair, skin or tub. Add two to three capfuls to an 8-inch tub of water.

Creams and Ointments

The most important characteristic of creams and ointments is their ability to be spread evenly over the skin. The fatty component may be composed of (1) animal fat, such as lard or wool fat; (2) mineral substances, such as petrolatum; or (3) vegetable oils. With the addition of emulsifiers, it is possible to incorporate large amounts of water. When rubbed onto the skin, the water evaporates slowly, producing a cooling effect. The cholesterolization of yellow petrolatum produces artificial lanolin-like materials. Aquaphor and Eucerin are the most frequently employed preparations of this type, and they have justifiably found wide acceptance as effective emollients.

Creams are cosmetically more attractive than ointments because they tend to "vanish" when rubbed into the skin. They are less occlusive than ointments, and also cannot be used in intertriginous or hairy areas or for treatment of acute weeping dermatitis.

The useful ointments and creams include the following: *Lubriderm Cream* (Texas Pharmacal), *Unibase* (Parke, Davis), *Aquaphor* (Duke Laboratories), *Nivea Cream* (Duke Laboratories), *Keri Cream* (Westwood Pharmaceuticals).

A useful tar-containing ointment is *Pragmatar* (Smith, Kline & French), which contains a coal tar distillate in a 4 per cent concentration, with near-colloidal sulfur and salicylic acid, in an oil-and-water emulsion base. Pragmatar is particularly useful in the treatment of dandruff and "cradle cap." For treatment of infants' scalps, it should be diluted by mixing in equal parts with either Aristocort Topical Cream 0.1 per cent, or a water-miscible vehicle.

Pastes

Pastes consist of semisolid mixtures of a powder and ointment base. In pediatrics the one most frequently prescribed is *Lassar's paste* U.S.P., also known as "zinc oxide ointment," which contains 25 Gm. each of zinc oxide and starch or talc, with 50 per cent white petrolatum.

Pastes absorb moisture and have a drying effect. They are best applied on gauze or to the skin with a spatula or tongue depressor.

Medications are released much more slowly from pastes than from creams and ointments. They are useful in the treatment of chronic dermatitis and have been extensively employed for diaper dermatitis.

Anthralin, 0.1 to 0.4 per cent, in plain zinc oxide paste "hardened" with the addition of 5 per cent hard paraffin and 0.2 to 0.4 per cent salicylic acid, has been found useful in treating individual lesions of psoriasis. Since anthralin stains the skin and can never be used around the eyes, it is impractical for infants and young children.

Powders

Powders are soothing, absorb moisture and protect the skin by reducing friction. They are chemically inert and are used chiefly for prophylaxis, as in intertriginous areas to prevent miliaria. Apply as a fine film which will not cake or form lumps when wet. Frequent application is advisable.

Kaolin and Talc. Kaolin and talc in equal parts, with the addition of 0.5 per cent spermaceti for added greasiness, is a valuable "general-use" powder.

ZeaSORB. (Stiefel Laboratories). This is a medicated powder containing 45 per cent microporous cellulose, 0.5 per cent hexacholorophene, 0.5 per cent parachlorometaxyenol, and 0.25 per cent aluminum dihydroxy allantoinate. ZeaSORB is useful for its water-absorbing capacity and also because it is mildly antibacterial and antifungal.

Neosporin Powder. (Burroughs Wellcome) This preparation contains polymixin B sulfate and zinc bacitracin in a powder base of lactose. It may be applied to raw surfaces after minor surgical procedures, such as following the electrodesiccation and curettage of warts and other lesions. It should not be used in intertriginous areas because of the likelihood of sensitization to neomycin. It is available in 10-Gm. shaker-top containers.

Mycostatin Topical Powder. (Squibb) Mycostatin Topical Powder contains nystatin, a specific antibiotic for moniliasis. Particularly useful in intertriginous areas for treatment of *Candida albicans,* it may also be used as a prophylactic measure. It is available in plastic squeeze bottles of 15 Gm.

Tinactin Powder. (Schering) Tinactin Powder contains 1 per cent tolnaftate in cornstarch and talc. It may be used for the daytime treatment of tinea pedis and also for prophylaxis. Apply two to three times daily. It is supplied in 45-Gm. plastic containers.

Corn Starch. Corn starch is useless as a therapeutic agent and tends to cake and irritate the skin, providing an excellent medium for growth of bacteria and fungi, especially *Candida albicans.* It should never be recommended and its use should be discouraged whenever possible.

Topical Steroids

These are probably the most overused class of medications today. They are, nevertheless, of undisputed value as anti-inflammatory and antipruritic agents.

The release of steroids by vehicles is extremely complex, and for this reason most "homemade" preparations made from compounding ground-up corticosteroid tablets and various vehicles are ineffective.

Triamcinolone Acetonide. (Aristocort, Lederle) (Kenalog, Squibb) This is available in 0.1 and 0.025 per cent cream, lotion or ointment. Aristocort is now available as a 0.5 per cent cream which is very useful for short-term treatment of small, stubborn lesions, especially lichen simplex chronicus and psoriasis. Kenalog Spray is also available.

Fluocinolone Acetonide. Synalar (Syntex) is available as cream (0.01 or 0.025 per cent, the latter also with neomycin), ointment (0.025 per cent) or solution (0.01 per cent). Synalar-HP cream contains 0.2 per cent fluocinolone acetonide.

Flurandrenolone Acetonide. Cordran (Lilly) is available as cream, ointment and lotion and also with neomycin. Cordran tape in two lengths is also available.

Betamethasone. Valisone (Schering), available as a cream, ointment or spray, is very effective.

Lidex. (Syntex) This is available as a cream or ointment.

Occlusive Dressings. Topical steroids are covered with a thin plastic film followed by a covering of stockinette, cotton glove, stocking, T-shirt, pair of shorts or Ace bandage. Occlusive dressings are very effective in the treatment of chronic dermatitis, such as psoriasis, lichen planus, lichen simplex chronicus (localized neurodermatitis), atopic dermatitis and other conditions. Treatment usually is overnight for a period of 8 to 12 hours. No more than 10 per cent of the body should be treated at any one time, since significant systemic absorption may occur, especially with the fluorinated corticosteroids. Complications include an objectionable odor, folliculitis, sweat retention, secondary irritation and infection. Late sequelae may include atrophy and striae.

For treatment of small and medium-sized lesions of psoriasis, lichen planus and other chronic dermatoses, Cordran Tape (Lilly) is useful. Before application the area must be cleansed gently to remove scales, crusts and dried exudate and any traces of medications. Dry the skin thoroughly and apply the tape smoothly against the skin, usually leaving it in place for about 12 hours. The adhesive consists of a synthetic copolymer of an acrylic ester.

Another very useful method of occlusive therapy is the use of a *plastic* suit, which retains body heat and causes slight maceration of the skin and thus greater penetration of medication. The suit material is a washable vinyl with elastic at the waist, ankles, neck and wrist. This form of treatment must be employed very cautiously in children, since significant systemic absorption of corticosteroid may occur. It is usually better to treat the upper half of the body one night and the lower half the next. A plastic suit is available from the Slim-Ez Company, Chattanooga, Tennessee, and sold in many sporting goods stores.

Topical Antibiotics

The most valuable topical antibiotics are those which are rarely used systemically; neomycin, bacitracin, polymyxin, and gramicidin are most commonly employed. Other therapeutic agents often classed with antibiotics are Vioform, Sterosan and Furacin.

Neosporin-G Cream. (Burroughs Wellcome) Neosporin-G Cream contains polymyxin B, neomycin sulfate and gramicidin in a water-miscible vanishing-cream base. Neosporin ointment contains polymyxin B, zinc bacitracin and neomycin sulfate in white petrolatum. Both the cream and ointment are useful for bacterial infections such as impetigo, ecthyma and secondarily infected dermatoses. The ointment is more effective in the treatment of impetigo than is the cream. Remember that neomycin is a fairly common skin sensitizer. It is available in tubes of 15 Gm.

Garamycin. (Schering) Garamycin contains 0.1 per cent gentamicin sulfate as cream or ointment. It is effective for topical treatment in primary and secondary bacterial infections of the skin. It is available in 15-gm. tubes.

Erythrocin Ointment. (Abbott) This contains 1 per cent erythromycin. Indicated against gram-positive cocci, this preparation is useful for superficial skin infections. Apply three or four times daily. It is available in 15- and 30-Gm. tubes.

Chloromycetin Cream. (Parke-Davis) Chloromycetin cream contains chloramphenicol in a water-miscible ointment base with 0.1 per cent propyl paraben. It is useful in superficial skin infections. It is supplied in 1-Gm. tubes.

Sterosan. (Geigy) This contains 3 per cent chlorquinaldol as cream or ointment. Chlorquinaldol is an iodine-free compound effective as a bacteriostatic and fungistatic agent. It may be used in the treatment of impetigo, ecthyma and other pyodermas. It is available with 1 per cent hydrocortisone.

Mycolog. (Squibb) Mycolog contains nystatin, neomycin sulfate, gramicidin and triamcinolone acetonide. It is one of the most overused preparations in dermatology today, and is often employed without clear-cut indications for its use. The cream contains several possible allergic sensitizers: neomycin and nystatin, ethylenediamine and parabens. Formerly it also contained thimerosal. Striae may result after prolonged use in intertriginous areas. Mycolog should be restricted to short-term use in treatment of conditions where it is clearly indicated, such as in *Candida albicans* infections (moniliasis).

Vioform. (Iodochlorhydroxyquin) (Ciba) Because of its iodine content (41 per cent) Vioform is fairly effective as a topical bactericidal and fungicidal agent. It has been greatly overused in the past, although this is less frequently the case today. It possesses three objectionable features: (1) it is a possible contact sensitizer; (2) it stains the skin and hair yellow; and (3) it is less effective as a germicidal agent than are many of the newer preparations available. Vioform is marketed as cream and ointment with or without hydrocortisone. Lotion, powder and vaginal inserts are also supplied.

Sunscreens

Sunscreens are topical preparations to protect the skin from the effects of ultraviolet light. They are either (1) "barriers," which generally impede the passage of ultraviolet light or (2) screens which absorb the light at a particular wavelength. They are extremely valuable for sun-sensitive persons and those with sunlight-aggravated diseases, such as porphyria, xeroderma pigmentosum, lupus erythematosus and polymorphous light eruptions.

A-Fil. (Texas Pharmacal) A-Fil contains 5 per cent titanium dioxide with 5 per cent menthyl anthranilate in a vanishing cream base tinted to blend with the skin color. The titanium dioxide physically screens out wavelengths of light up to 3900 Å, while menthyl anthranilate absorbs the sunburning wave lengths between 2950 and 3200 Å.

Pabafilm. (Owen Laboratories) This contains an amino benzoate in an ethyl alcohol base. It effectively blocks out ultraviolet radiation in the 2900 to 3250 Å range. The base is greaseless, dries quickly and will provide protection up to 2 to 3 hours after swimming and 8 to 12 hours in the absence of excessive moisture.

PreSun. (Westwood Pharmaceuticals) PreSun contains 5 per cent para-aminobenzoic acid in an alcohol base with moisturizers. As with Pabafilm, the patient will tan but not burn. PreSun may stain clothing.

RVP. (Paul B. Elder) RVP contains red petrolatum improved with 5 per cent surfactants for easy application. RVP absorbs the sunburn spectrum and additional ultraviolet to 3400 Å. It resists perspiration and water and can be used around the eyes and lips. It is, however, very greasy. RVPaque is skin tinted and contains zinc oxide, a physical barrier to sunlight. RVPlus contains titanium dioxide, also a physical barrier.

Solbar. (Person & Covey) This contains 3 per cent oxybenzone, a benzophenone. Solbar is a broad-spectrum ultraviolet sun protective lotion which, after application, dries to a transparent film which has high skin retention, but a "tight" feel which is objectionable to many patients.

Masking Preparations

Covermark. (Lydia O'Leary) Covermark is a neutral, opaque, greaseless cream which is a most effective agent for concealing birthmarks, many types of scars and skin discolorations. It is particularly useful for covering lesions of vitiligo, port wine stains and nevi. Ten shades are available and the company provides professional help in selecting the proper shade for the skin and instructing patients in its application. A Lydia O'Leary finishing powder is also available. When applied with skill, Covermark can be a very effective masking agent.

Soaps

Germicidal soaps provide adjunctive therapy for skin infections, especially in prophylaxis for recurrent furunculosis. They are also effective deodorants. Incorporated bactericidal agents include halogenated salicylanilides and carbanilides. The halogenated salicylanilides have occasionally been a cause of allergic contact photodermatitis. Soaps containing one or more of these substances include Dial (Armour), Lifebuoy (Lever Brothers), Safeguard (Procter & Gamble), Zest (Procter & Gamble) and Irish Spring (Colgate-Palmolive).

Betadine. (Purdue Frederick Company). Betadine is a topical microbiocide containing a detergent with iodine and polyvinyl pyrrolidine. It is also available as an aerosol spray, surgical scrub, douche, vaginal gel, mouthwash, gargle and skin cleanser. In pyodermas, Betadine Skin Cleanser is a useful topical adjunct to systemic antimicrobial therapy.

Super-Fatted Soaps. Addition of extra fat, such as lanolin, cold cream or mineral oil, to soap during manufacture makes a soap "super-fatted." The superfat is said to produce a soap somewhat less alkaline than ordinary soap, which hopefully will be less irritating to the skin.

In pediatric practice, super-fatted soaps are used most commonly in the treatment of children with atopic dermatitis and ichthyosis. The effectiveness of these soaps has been overemphasized, but when used in place of ordinary soap they may play a minor therapeutic role. Preparations include Basis (Texas Pharmacal), Oilatum (Stiefel), Emulave (Cooper Laboratories) and Lowila (Westwood).

Shampoos

Regular. Sebulex (Westwood), Ionil (Owen), Head & Shoulders (Procter & Gamble) and Fostex Cream (Westwood) are safe for the use in children. Selenium- and cadmium-containing shampoos are not indicated for use in pediatric patients.

Tar Shampoos. Tar shampoos are useful for treatment of scalp seborrhea and psoriasis. The most frequently used tar shampoos are Ionil T (Owen), Sebutone (Westwood), Polytar Shampoo (Stiefel) and Zetar Shampoo (Dermik). Remember that tar shampoos may stain the hair a yellowish color.

Antiparasitic Shampoos. Kwell Shampoo (Reed & Carnrick) is valuable for treatment of pediculosis capitis. Shampoo the hair for a full 4 minutes, rinse and then dry with a towel. Repeat after 24 hours and once or twice more if necessary.

Chemical Cautery

Cauterizing chemicals, such as salicylic acid, bichloroacetic acid, silver nitrate and cantharidin should be used with caution in children, but they are safe if the directions are carefully followed. Caustic agents such as phenol, fuming nitric acid and monochloroacetic acid should never be used in the treatment of children. Phenol especially is rapidly absorbed through intact skin and, following treatment of large areas, severe renal damage may result. Monochloroacetic acid is a highly reactive substance which is rapidly destructive to tissue.

Because chemical cautery may be relatively painless at the time of application, it can be preferable to other destructive methods of treatment, such as liquid nitrogen and electrodesiccation.

Salicylic Acid. Salicylic acid, 40 per cent, in an elastic adhesive plaster has been used in the treatment of plantar warts for a very long time. The plaster must be cut to the exact size of the wart, applied firmly and covered with a strip of adhesive tape. This should be allowed to remain against the skin for four days, after which the dressing is removed and the white keratotic tissue is pared using a number 15 blade. A new plaster may be applied at that time and the process repeated until the verruca disappears, usually after four to six treatments. Recurrences are common, however.

Silver Nitrate Sticks. Silver nitrate sticks (available from Arzol) are 75 per cent silver nitrate with 25 per cent potassium nitrate. Moisten the tip with tap water before use and apply to fissures and ulcers to remove excess granulation tissue.

Cantharone. (Cantharidin collodion) (Ingram) This preparation consists of 0.7 per cent cantharidin in an acetone and flexible collodion vehicle. Cantharidin is a colorless, crystalline scale obtained from cantharides or dried Spanish flies. It is used chiefly for removal of periungual and plantar warts and molluscum contagiosum. The method is relatively painless during application, but marked discomfort may be experienced after 24 hours. The method leaves no scar.

For periungual warts, apply the substance directly to the wart. After the film begins to dry and a white membrane appears, cover the wart with a nonporous adhesive. Keep this in place for 24 hours, after which the patient replaces the tape with a Band-Aid. In 10 to 12 days, pare off the dead tissue, first obtaining a cleavage line, which should be easily found at this time. Cantharone may be reapplied to any remaining wart tissue. Often one or two treatments suffice.

For plantar warts, pare away the keratotic dead tissue on the surface first, then apply Cantharone generously to the entire lesion. A cut-out cushion bandage made from moleskin is then applied and the whole dressing covered with nonporous tape. The patient should remove the dressing in two to three days, reapplying the cushion bandage for comfort. The patient returns to the physician in 10 to 14 days for paring of dead tissue and re-treatment if necessary. Two or three treatments often are sufficient.

For molluscum contagiosum, coat each lesion with Cantharone, using a small wooden stick, and cover with a small piece of tape. The patient should return in one week and any new lesions are treated in the same manner. The patient should remove the tape after about 6 hours, however.

Podophyllin. Although not a caustic, podophyllin is commonly used in the treatment of venereal warts or condylomata acuminata, which are increasingly seen among adolescents today. Podophyllum resin is derived from dried rhizomes and roots of *Podophyllum peltatum* or May apple. A specific treatment for condylomata, podophyllum is ineffective in the treatment of other types of warts.

Apply a 20 to 25 per cent solution in tincture of benzoin directly to the lesions with a wooden applicator stick. Take special care not to permit the liquid to extend to any extent over normal skin. Instruct the patient to wash the area thoroughly with soap and water using a washcloth in about 12 hours, and to return for re-treatment in four to five days. Usually three or four treatments suffice.

Podophyllin is an antimitotic agent, and, if transferred to eyes by the fingers, can cause severe keratitis. For this reason, perhaps one should use it only in adolescents and older children.

Cryosurgery

Liquid nitrogen is available from the suppliers of liquid gas and can be stored in loosely stoppered thermos bottles. One pint is sufficient to treat 30 to 40 patients and will last for two to three days. With long cotton applicator sticks the liquid is applied with *intermittent,* firm pressure for 10 to 30 seconds, until the lesion blanches and an areola of frozen tissue appears around the lesion. Within a few hours a blister will form which will carry the verrucous tissue into its roof. As sloughing occurs during the next two or three weeks the wart comes off, leaving no scar. Frequently a small "core" of verrucous tissue remains behind, which can be re-treated with liquid nitrogen in three or four weeks.

Skin Diseases in the Newborn

JOAN E. HODGMAN, M.D.,
ROBERT I. FREEDMAN, M.D., *and*
NORMAN E. LEVAN, M.D.

In this section we discuss the care of the normal newborn skin as well as a group of conditions in which specific therapy is unnecessary and often contraindicated.

CARE OF THE NEWBORN SKIN

The normal skin of the neonate needs no special care. It should be recalled that the significant protective barrier of the skin is limited almost entirely to its outermost layer, the dry stratum corneum. Creams or other emollients diminish this barrier capability by macerating or otherwise injuring the stratum corneum. In addition, emollients often encourage bacterial growth. Cleansing, chiefly for esthetic reasons, is acceptable if done gently with warm water. An initial cleansing should be postponed until the infant's temperature is stable. For routine subsequent cleansing, as of the diaper area or face, warm water is all that need be used. Until recently, daily bathing with detergents containing 3 per cent hexachlorophene has been recommended as a part of routine newborn skin care. The use of detergents containing hexachlorophene for routine bathing has been widely accepted as an effective method of reducing staphylococcal infections in the nursery. However, in December, 1971, both the Food and Drug Administration and the American Academy of Pediatrics warned against the routine use of 3 per cent hexachlorophene for this purpose because of the question of associated neurotoxicity. Shortly following this warning, many hospital nurseries, including our own, discontinued bathing newborn infants with 3 per cent hexachlorophene. Following withdrawal of this preparation, an increased incidence of staphylococcal outbreaks was reported throughout the country, and there has been an increase in staphylococcal colonization and infection in our own nurseries. When such outbreaks occur, daily bathing with 3 per cent hexachlorophene may be reinstituted as one of the measures for controlling the outbreak. Careful rinsing following the bath is recommended to limit the absorption of hexachlorophene from the skin. It is important to note that neither the question of neurotoxicity nor the appropriate minimum use of 3 per cent hexachlorophene to decrease staphylococcal colonization can be answered from data currently available. Consequently, the recommendation that 3 per cent hexachlorophene be restricted to use during outbreaks is tentative until more information becomes available. In the absence of routine use of hexachlorophene, strenuous measures must be directed toward reducing colonization. The primary source of colonization is by nursery personnel through personal contact. Meticulous handwashing by nursery personnel should be enforced, using soaps or detergents containing antibacterial preparations such as iodophors, or tricarbosalicylanilide analogs. The use of light cotton gloves, changed with each handling of an infant, will further decrease bacterial colonization.

CARE OF THE PREMATURE SKIN

The treatment of the skin of the premature infant does not differ essentially from that of the mature infant. However, it should be emphasized that the stratum corneum is particularly vulnerable and easily removed in the premature. As mentioned above, it is the stratum corneum which is the chief barrier to molecular diffusion and infection. Maceration is the most common factor which may cause disruption of this protective barrier. Many common practices in the nursery, such as the application of ointments or bandaging, produce maceration very rapidly. Even prolonged contact with a plastic mattress is an example of such occlusion which should be avoided. Other factors that may disrupt the epidermal barrier include failure to remove promptly antiseptic solutions used for preparation of the skin before diagnostic or therapeutic procedures, as well as the simple act of applying and removing adhesive tape.

MILIA

The term milia deserves definition, since it tends to be applied in a nondiscriminating fashion to at least three different lesions. As we use the term, milia are very superficial epidermal inclusion cysts. In the neonate they are spontaneously eliminated by normal desquamation. No intervention is required, and the family may be assured that no scarring ever results.

MILIARIA CRYSTALLINA

Miliaria crystallina is the most superficial form of sweat retention. The lesions are entirely intraepidermal and for the most part subcorneal. Miliaria crystallina is a result of two factors: increased sweat production and obstruction of the follicular ostia by hygroscopic swelling of the stratum corneum. Management includes attention to both the temperature and the humidity of the infant's immediate environment. Avoid occlusion due to clothing or emollients, allowing free evaporation from the surface of the skin. The lesions disappear spontaneously without sequelae and require no treatment.

TOXIC ERYTHEMA OF THE NEWBORN

Toxic erythema of the newborn (erythema toxicum neonatorum, fleabite dermatitis) is a benign self-limited dermatitis occurring in the first week of life. The lesions first appear as a blotchy macular erythema. Within the area of erythema, one or more small white papulovesicles or pustules may appear. Histologically, these pustules are perifollicular, subcorneal and filled almost exclusively with eosinophils. Eosinophils are also the predominant cell of the dermal infiltrate. This eosinophilia, demonstrable on smear, readily distinguishes the pustules of toxic erythema from infectious lesions in the neonate. The eruption may be limited to a few macules or may become widespread with confluent areas of involvement. The sites of most pronounced involvement are the buttocks, trunk, face and proximal extremities. In the rare case where lesions are present at birth, they appear less erythematous and more pustular and occur primarily on the extremities. The condition is self-limited and no therapy is indicated even for the pustular form.

BIRTH TRAUMA

Caput succedaneum implies swelling of the presenting part due to edema and occasionally hemorrhage into the subcutaneous tissues.

There is no necrosis of the overlying epidermis; in fact, if necrosis is observed the physician should be alert to a complicating infection such as herpes simplex. Except for such unusual instances, the edema subsides spontaneously within 48 hours. Treatment of the uncomplicated caput is unnecessary. Local measures, such as hot compresses or ointments, may aggravate the problem, since they promote maceration, infection and ulceration.

Cephalohematoma may occur independently or in conjunction with the preceding disorder. It is a subperiosteal hematoma limited by the sutures, and may overlie one or more of the skull bones. Its course differs from caput succedaneum in that there is an initial enlargement of the swelling during the first days of life followed by a slow resolution in the ensuing three to four weeks. Aspiration is contraindicated because it may introduce infection. Spontaneous infection occurs rarely but when present requires drainage and systemic antibiotics.

Birth trauma may produce a rare condition called *giant cephalohematoma,* actually a subgaleal hemorrhage. At times this hemorrhage may be severe enough to be exsanguinating. Treatment is supportive, including transfusion for symptoms of circulatory embarrassment or a hematocrit less than 40. Again, aspiration of this mass is contraindicated. Jaundice secondary to absorption of bilirubin may complicate the course.

Pressure necrosis is most common over the bony prominences of the head and face, particularly over the parietal bosses and less often over the zygomata. The latter is seen almost exclusively in large term infants of diabetic mothers. The involvement is primarily of the subcutaneous tissue but there may be necrosis of the overlying epidermis. The goals of treatment are prevention of infection and minimizing scar formation. It has been our practice to allow the lesion to reabsorb or drain spontaneously, and the resultant scars have been gratifyingly small. Smear and culture of the exudate from draining lesions will show polymorphonuclear leukocytes and normal scalp flora findings which are not per se indications for antibiotic treatment. In our experience, routine skin care suffices and antibiotics, either topical or systemic, have not been necessary. Isolation of these infants in the nursery is also unnecessary.

APLASIA CUTIS CONGENITA

This disorder represents congenital absence of the epidermis, dermis and sometimes subcutaneous tissue. It occurs most frequently on the scalp near the vertex, as either solitary or multiple lesions. In the scalp, the defect may involve underlying bone. Less frequently, the defect is present on the trunk or extremities, where it may be extensive and is bilateral and symmetrical. It appears as a sharply marginated area at birth which may be eroded or covered with a thin translucent membrane. With epithelialization, the raw area is replaced by an atrophic, smooth scar, devoid of adnexal structures. A number of familial cases have been reported; however, no final conclusions can be drawn as to the mode of inheritance. The presence of an apparent injury, especially on the scalp, at the time of birth may lead to false accusations of birth injury with medicolegal implications. The configuration and sharp outlines of the lesion should readily suggest the diagnosis of cutis aplasia. Healing produces an atrophic scar which may require later cosmetic surgery. No immediate therapy is indicated.

SCLEREMA NEONATORUM

Sclerema neonatorum is not a primary disease but rather a complication of a variety of life-threatening conditions, particularly in the premature. We feel that hypothermia may be significant in its pathogenesis, since, with prevention of hypothermia in the ill neonate, sclerema neonatorum has almost disappeared. Thus, management is primarily prevention. When this condition occurs, treatment is that of the underlying disorder. Measures aimed directly at the sclerema, including corticosteroids, are of no apparent value.

SUBCUTANEOUS FAT NECROSIS

Subcutaneous fat necrosis appears in apparently healthy term infants. It has been most commonly reported in the infants of diabetic mothers. The few cases we have seen have been marked by a febrile course of 10 to 14 days' duration, terminating without residual lipoatrophy. The absence of residual lipoatrophy suggests that the process may be panniculitis rather than a necrosis. Antibiotics are not indicated, but steroids may be useful. Our recommendation is oral prednisone in dosage of 2 mg. per kilogram per day in three divided doses every 8 hours for five to seven days.

Eruptions in the Diaper Area

ALVIN H. JACOBS, M.D.

Since many different skin disorders can cause eruptions in the diaper area, accurate diagnosis based upon history of onset, morphology and localization is essential.

Prophylactic Treatment. Much can be done to prevent diaper rashes in susceptible babies and to prevent recurrence in babies already treated. Most of these general measures should also be carried out in conjunction with specific therapy.

Prevention of excess heat and maceration is essential. This is accomplished by eliminating excess clothing and removal of impervious diaper covering. Frequent diaper changes are necessary. The use of additional diapers or of absorbent diaper covers with no waterproof material is permissible, since evaporation contributes to cooling.

Several steps can be taken to prevent ammonia production in the diapers. Most important is thorough laundering and sterilization of the diapers. Commercial diaper laundries accomplish this satisfactorily. Home-laundered diapers should be thoroughly rinsed to remove all possible irritants and allergens. They may be sterilized by boiling, drying in the sun, or prewash soaking in a quaternary ammonium compound, such as Diaparene.

Acidification of the diaper and the urine will also help to prevent ammonia production. Acidifying the diapers can be accomplished by using a vinegar rinse after washing. Acidifying the urine is easily done by giving the baby 1 or 2 ounces of cranberry juice once or twice daily.

Active Treatment. In addition to the above general measures, active treatment of specific disease processes must be carried out.

Seborrheic dermatitis and psoriasis are discussed in the article on papulosquamous disorders. It must be kept in mind that seborrheic dermatitis in the diaper area is nearly always complicated by infection with *Candida albicans.*

Atopic dermatitis is discussed in the Allergy section of this book.

Contact dermatitis is easily managed by removal of the primary irritants, or, in the case of allergic contactants, by patch testing to determine which allergens to remove.

Bacterial infections are covered in a separate article. A special caution in regard to infection in the diaper area is to avoid topical antibiotics in greasy ointment bases if the lesions are moist or macerated. Instead, use lotions or cream preparations. I feel that systemic antibiotics, such as penicillin or erythromycin, should also be used to assure thorough eradication of the bacteria, prevent complications and avoid frequent recurrence of the infection.

Contact Dermatitis

PETER J. KOBLENZER, M.D.

As the name implies, this is a skin eruption due to contact with an exogenous factor.

Two types are recognized: direct irritant contact dermatitis and allergic contact dermatitis. In the latter, prior exposure and ensuing sensitization are necessary to produce the rash. Most cases of diaper dermatitis are good examples of direct irritant contact dermatitis; poison ivy dermatitis is a classic example of allergic contact dermatitis.

In direct irritant contact dermatitis, the responsible agent is usually readily recognized, i.e., urine, feces, the rash of the chronic lip lickers or contact with a caustic or acid substance. In allergic contact dermatitis, by reason of delayed appearance, identification of the offending material is often difficult or impossible. In infancy or childhood, however, the spectrum of possible contact allergies is minimal compared to that for workers in certain industries. Poison ivy dermatitis and contact dermatitis from topical medications such as mercurochrome, surgical tape and Furacin, and from garments such as footwear, are probably the most frequently encountered.

Direct irritant contact dermatitis is treated by removal of the offending material. In mild cases a topical glucocorticoid cream followed by a lubricant is an entirely adequate approach. In more severe cases, application of the salve should be preceded by cool saline, Zephiran or aluminum acetate compresses.

In allergic contact dermatitis, again an attempt should be made by history and examination to identify the allergens. Thus, the telltale linear lesions in poison ivy dermatitis or the characteristic distribution of a shoe dermatitis will give valuable clues. However, attempts at patch testing should be deferred until the eruption is well under control.

Lesions are often weeping, crusted and extremely itchy. Cool compresses are the most valuable form of topical treatment which can be employed. Saline, Zephiran or aluminum acetate should be used in the most acute stage. Tar may be used in the more chronic and less exudative cases. Compresses are decidedly superior to baths or soaks because evaporation adds cooling—an important therapeutic modality in these cases. Crusts and dead skin should be gently removed, blisters unroofed and a glucocorticoid cream applied; this should be repeated three to four times daily in the acute stage. In more chronic stages, glucocorticoid cream under occlusion may hasten resolution of the problem. If infection is suspected, glucocorticoid/antibiotic cream should be used as well as an oral or parenteral antibiotic. Preferably, the infecting organism should be identified and its sensitivity determined. Oral antipruritics are often helpful. Especially severe or disseminated cases may require a short course of oral glucocorticoids.

POISON IVY DERMATITIS

Many practitioners do not seem to understand fully the sequence of events in poison ivy dermatitis. The allergen is an oleoresin present in the leaves, stems and roots of the vine. In susceptible persons, upon contact with the skin the oleoresin will produce an allergic contact dermatitis. Severity of the eruption will be determined by the dose of the antigen and the intensity of the contact, and by the thickness of the skin. For example, the rash may never occur on the palms and soles, and it may appear in the orbits or on the penis within only a few hours of exposure. Thus, in most cases there will be several contacts in different parts of the body—of varying intensity and on skin of differing thicknesses. Therefore, the eruption will not be simultaneous but sequential. This will give to the patient the appearance of a spreading eruption. This is not the case. Once the skin has been washed with soap, the oleoresin is removed and no further spread is possible. The fluid from bullae *does not* cause spread of the rash. Inadvertent repeated exposures may also cause "spread" of the eruption.

Topical treatment is of value in controlling the itch but does little to hasten involution. In many cases of Rhus dermatitis, only oral glucocorticoids will bring about speedy control and resolution. Prednisone or its equivalent should be used in a dosage of 2 mg. per kilogram per day and should be continued in full dosage for five to seven days. Decreasing the dosage will only deprive the patient of the benefit of adequate dosage and will not automatically diminish the risk of complications. There appears to be no contraindication to discontinuing the dosage abruptly, provided that the period of treatment has not exceeded the above-mentioned time limits. The usual precautions should be observed prior to use of this modality. A slight flare may follow discontinuance of the drug, but this usually settles rapidly.

Analgesics and antipruritics are occasionally needed. Desensitization procedures against poison ivy have been disappointing to date.

Nummular Eczema

PETER J. KOBLENZER, M.D.

This is probably a variant of atopic eczema. The name (*nummuss:* a coin) refers to the circular patches which characterize this condition. The treatment is that of atopic dermatitis.

DYSHIDROTIC ECZEMA

This term refers to an eczematous eruption of the palms and soles and areas immediately adjacent in subjects who also suffer from palmar and plantar hyperhidrosis. There is no evidence that there is abnormal function of the sweat glands. It is probably the most misunderstood and most misdiagnosed dermatologic condition. Although eventually, in most cases, both palms and soles become affected, initial involvement in childhood most frequently occurs on the feet.

The condition usually occurs in individuals who by birth or heredity are predisposed to atopy and palmar and plantar hyperhidrosis. When these patients are examined standing on their bare feet, they often show minor abnormalities of their feet, such as mild hallux valgus, pes planus or genu valgum, or they may have spina bifida or rheumatoid disease. The distribution of the eruption is characteristically at sites which have the most intimate contact with the shoes, such as the top and medial aspect of the big toes, or on any toes which project upward. It may be assumed that the combination of the predisposition to eczema, the constant sweating which moistens and softens the skin and the friction from footwear is chiefly responsible for the great chronicity and recalcitrance of this condition.

All of these factors must be taken into consideration when outlining curative and preventive therapy. The acute stage requires tepid soaks or compresses. Physiologic saline solution, Zephiran 1:10,000 or aluminum acetate solution are the most widely used preparations. This should be followed by gentle débridement. Large vesicles should be opened and unroofed. A glucocorticoid cream is then applied. Bed rest may initially be required in severe cases.

Subacute and chronic cases benefit by soaks in tar solutions or in a tar/oil mixture. This should be followed by an application of a glucocorticoid ointment, or a cream followed by a lubricant to deal with the painful fissures which occur so frequently about the fingers and heels. When soaking the feet, the toes should be kept apart with small corks, pledgets of cotton or styrofoam and the interdigital spaces carefully debrided.

Analgesics may be needed for pain and antihistamines for pruritus. Occasional severe cases, especially those which have begun to disseminate, may require a short course of oral glucocorticoids. Preventive treatment consists of the choice of proper footwear: cotton socks, two pairs in the winter if necessary, and all-leather shoes. These permit transmission and evaporation of the abundant perspiration. In the house, the patient should be bare-footed or wear socks or terrycloth scuffs. The latter should be worn at school in severe cases. Rubber and plastic shoes, including sneakers, are unsuitable.

Hyperhidrosis palmaris et plantaris is largely controlled by emotional factors, and this, together with the fact that patients who usually have worn sandals all summer begin wearing shoes in the fall, is probably responsible for the many instances of recurrence of this problem in the fall after school starts.

It should be borne in mind that tinea pedis (athlete's foot) almost never occurs in children and is responsible for only a small percentage of the vesicular eruption of feet even in adults.

Shoe contact dermatitis is rare, but may occur and this should be ruled out by patch tests in cases where this is suspected.

Interdigital infection with gram-negative bacteria may cause a secondary vesicular or bullous eruption of the feet. This infection is often readily recognized by its characteristic smell, and should be proved by culture and treated orally as well as with the usual topical creams.

Hand eruptions occur in children but are less frequent than in adults, where they are often precipitated by chronic exposure to soap and other detergents as well as to many other chemicals. In addition to appropriate topical treatment, which is similar to that for other eczematous eruptions, patients must be cautioned to protect their hands at all times. In cold weather, gloves should always be worn. When doing work of any kind, light cotton gloves or, where appropriate, leather or cotton work gloves should be worn. Wet work should be done only while wearing light cotton gloves with an additional pair of light unlined rubber or plastic gloves over them. The former absorbs the abundant moisture which is retained under the latter and prevents maceration. Emotional factors play a large part in precipitating and perpetuating hand and foot eruptions, and this aspect must be evaluated in recalcitrant and difficult cases. Psychologic counseling, sedatives or ataractics may prove to be valuable adjuvants here. "Id" eruption secondary to fungus infection is extremely rare in childhood.

Counseling in adolescents in regard to proper choice of jobs is important in these cases. It is obvious that in many jobs a tendency to recurrent hand eruptions would be a grave disadvantage.

Urticaria

WILLIAM A. AKERS, M.D.

ACUTE URTICARIA

Usually the cause of acute urticaria is inferred and not proved for obvious reasons. Consequently, symptomatic therapy against the hives is employed. Five drugs are commonly used:

1. Diphenhydramine hydrochloride (Benadryl) has a duration of 4 to 6 hours. The oral dosage is 5 mg. per kilogram of body weight divided into four doses during a 24-hour period (maximum dosage, 300 mg. per day). The popular elixir contains 2.5 mg. per ml., and capsules of 25 mg. and 50 mg. are available. The parenteral form for intramuscular or intravenous injection is available in sterile vials containing 10 mg. per ml. or 50 mg. per ml. Parenteral diphenhydramine hydrochloride is indicated as supplemental therapy to epinephrine in anaphylaxis and angioedema. Diphenhydramine hydrochloride should not be used in premature or newborn babies or during an asthmatic attack, since it has an atropine-like action. Over half of all children are sedated by the drug.

2. Tripelennamine U.S.P. (Pyribenzamine) exerts its effect for 4 to 6 hours. The oral dosage for infants is 10 to 20 mg. three to four times a day. Tripelennamine is available in

50-mg. tablets and in an elixir containing the equivalent of 5 mg. per ml. or 20 mg. per 4 ml.

3. Chlorpheniramine maleate (Chlor-Trimeton, Chlo-Amine, Chloramate, Drize) has a usual duration of 4 to 6 hours. Orally to children under one year, give 1 mg. twice a day; for children one to five years, give 1 or 2 mg. twice a day; for children over six years, give 2 mg. three to four times a day. Chlorpheniramine maleate is available in 4-mg. tablets and in a syrup containing 2 mg. per 5 ml.

4. Epinephrine offers the most rapid, although transient, relief for urticaria. Epinephrine injection U.S.P. (1:1000) contains 1 mg. per ml. and is available in 5-, 10-, and 30-ml. vials. The usual dosage for children is 0.1 to 0.3 ml. of the aqueous solution every 30 minutes for three to four doses until relief is obtained. Duration of action is 1 to 2 hours. Epinephrine in peanut oil (1:500) contains 2 mg. per ml. The dosage for children is 0.1 to 0.75 ml. intramuscularly. Relief may last from 4 to 24 hours; the usual duration is 8 to 16 hours.

5. Ephedrine sulfate is useful in treating urticaria; it is usually given with an antihistamine. Capsules containing 25 and 50 mg. of ephedrine sulfate are available, as well as syrup containing 4 mg. per ml. Usual dosage is 12.5 to 25 mg. every 3 to 4 hours. For severe symptoms, 3 mg. per kilogram daily, divided into 4 to 6 doses, may be given.

ANGIOEDEMA

Angioedema will occur at least once in most persons who have recurrent hives. Epinephrine usually affords faster relief than do antihistamines.

HEREDITARY ANGIOEDEMA

This disorder can be fatal when laryngeal edema occurs, and tracheostomy should be anticipated, rather than performed as an emergency procedure. Epinephrine solution (1:1000), 0.3 ml., is injected intramuscularly or subcutaneously and repeated every 15 minutes for three to five doses if necessary. Antihistamines are much too slow but are given for their longer-lasting action. Treatment with testosterone, 10 mg. sublingually per day, has prevented recurrent attacks. The use of testosterone for this condition is not included among the list of indications stated by the manufacturers, and endocrinologic consultation is advisable when embarking on a course of prophylaxis. The considerable side effects of testosterone on a growing child must be weighed against the lethality of the disease (approximately 20 per cent).

Applying a cold, wet washcloth or towel to an area of hives or angioedema offers a modicum of relief. For generalized hives, lying in a tub of comfortably warm water for 20 to 30 minutes helps relieve some of the pruritus. No beneficial topical therapy is available.

CHRONIC URTICARIA

Management of chronic urticaria requires patience and persistence, and depends upon finding the etiologic agents (usually several), eliminating the offending agents and avoiding future contact if possible.

Inhalant allergens are responsible for about 20 per cent of chronic urticaria; they require scratch and intradermal skin test for diagnosis; and they often require hyposensitization for control. Twelve common molds, animal danders, house dust, grass, tree and weed pollen mixes prepared for different geographic regions of the country generally suffice for diagnosis, while specific antigens are used for therapy. Infection—focal, systemic or topical—occurs in another 20 per cent of patients. Draining abscessed teeth and sinuses, treating urinary tract infections or culturing and treating fungal infections of the skin will usually afford prompt relief. Drugs, especially salicylates and penicillin, are responsible for approximately 15 per cent of urticaria and must be eliminated.

Two antihistamines are useful for treating chronic urticaria:

1. Cyproheptadine hydrochloride (Periactin), 4-mg. tablet, has a duration of action lasting for 4 to 6 hours. For children 2 to 6 years, give 2 mg. orally three times a day (do not exceed 12 mg. a day). For older children, usually 4 mg. three times daily suffice (do not exceed 16 mg. a day). Adjust the dosage according to the patient's response. If a fourth dose is needed, give it at bedtime.

2. Hydroxyzine hydrochloride (Atarax) or hydroxyzine pamoate (Vistaril) is a potent antihistamine; its action persists 4 to 6 hours. Hydroxyzine hydrochloride tablets are available in 10-, 25- and 50-mg. sizes, and in a syrup containing 2 mg. per ml. Hydroxyzine pamoate is available in 25- and 50-mg. capsules and in a suspension containing 5 mg. per ml. The usual children's oral dose is as follows: under 6 years of age, 50 mg. daily in four divided doses; over 6 years of age, 50 to 100 mg. in four divided doses (2 mg. per kilogram of body weight daily divided into four doses).

As with other antihistamines, one drug form or salt may be effective where others are not. With hydroxyzine, this occurs about 10 per cent of the time.

In my experience in treating chronic urticaria, giving cyproheptadine or hydroxyzine daily for 21 days usually clears the lesions for months if it is effective during the first few days of treatment; with shorter or interrupted therapy, the hives may persist.

Often, the lesions of patients with dry skin and persistent urticaria will not clear until the stratum corneum is made supple and soft. Stop using soap. Recommend a liquid petrolatum-based bath oil; or in atopic children, a cottonseed oil–based bath oil may be better tolerated. Follow the directions on the bottle as to the amount of oil to add to the bath. Choose a comfortably warm water temperature. Add the bath oil. Let the child play and soak in the bath for at least 20 minutes, preferably 25 to 30 minutes, which allows the stratum corneum to absorb water. Use a wash cloth to rub off any surface dirt. Remove and dry the child. Do not remove the bath oil with soap.

Avoiding rough textured clothing often helps eliminate chronic urticaria. Wool, Dacron, new denims and corduroys seem particularly abrasive to the hyperactive skin.

DERMOGRAPHIA

Test every patient with hives for dermographia. A small instrument can be made from a number 10 knitting needle inserted through a plastic pill vial containing 400 Gm. of lead shot. Pull the blunt tip over the patient's skin to test and retest his skin reactivity. Patients showing white dermographism with a white axon reflex (with or without the wheal) will have a markedly positive Mecholyl skin test. Cyproheptadine hydrochloride affords relief to the greatest number of patients. Adding ephedrine sulfate is beneficial in some cases.

CHOLINERGIC URTICARIA

Cholinergic urticaria accounts for 20 per cent of all patients with chronic urticaria. The typical pencil-eraser–sized lesion with the surrounding red axon flare suggests the diagnosis. An intradermal injection of methacholine (Mecholyl) confirms the diagnosis. The solution is prepared by adding 1 ampule (25 mg.) to 125 ml. of normal saline solution, making a 1:5000 dilution. Inject 0.1 ml. intradermally. A positive response is a halo of erythema, 20 mm. or greater in diameter. Pseudopods may or may not be present. The Mecholyl test may be negative for at least 4 hours after generalized urticarial eruptions because of a refractory state. Hydroxyzine drugs will relieve cholinergic urticaria in 95 per cent of the cases.

COLD URTICARIA

For primary acquired cold urticaria, cyproheptadine hydrochloride has afforded the best control in several recent reports. The patients and parents must be warned against swimming, since the danger of anaphylactic shock with fainting, urticaria and angioedema, occurs in about two-thirds of patients.

Familial cold urticaria is rare. To date, the only reported control of symptoms has been with pseudomonas polysaccharide complex (Piromen), given as weekly intravenous injections of 10 to 20 micrograms. Initially begin with 1 or 2 micrograms, with subsequent doses increased by 1 microgram every three days until the desired level is obtained; then give the injections weekly. The usual effective dose is about 0.5 microgram per kilogram body weight.

PAPULAR URTICARIA

Papular urticaria, or lichen urticatus, is urticarial only initially, and in childhood is generally caused by insect bites. Fleas, chiggers, mites, ticks, mosquitoes and bedbugs are common agents. Pruritus is intense. Topical crotamitom cream (Eurax) kills most chiggers and mites and relieves pruritus. Thoroughly massage the cream into the skin on the whole body from the chin down. A second application is advisable 24 hours later. Clothing and bed linen should be changed daily. A cleansing bath should be taken 48 hours after the last application. For pruritus, massage the cream gently into affected areas until the medication is completely absorbed. Repeat as needed. Diphemanil methyl sulfate cream (2 per cent Prantal Cream) seems particularly effective in relieving pruritus and shortening the course of papular urticaria resulting from mosquito, flea or tick bites. Massage the cream into the lesions until the medication is completely absorbed. Repeat as needed.

If secondary bacterial infection occurs, I use topical 1 per cent chloramphenicol cream (Chloromycetin Cream) containing 10 mg. per Gm. or 1 per cent erythromycin cream or ointment; this is rubbed into each infected lesion every 3 hours. If extensive impetiginous lesions occur, I use a systemic antibiotic for five days or give penicillin G, benzathine, injection, once at 300,000 units for children under 25 kilograms, and 600,000 units to children over 25 kilograms.

Certain individuals (about 20 per cent) with papular urticaria respond favorably to excess amounts of thiamine hydrochloride U.S.P.; usually 10 to 25 mg. is given orally three times a day. Presumably it acts as an insect repellent.

In some individuals, papular urticaria will last for months and will respond only to topical steroid preparations or will even require that steroids be injected into each lesion. Triamcinolone diacetate suspension for intralesional injections (Aristocort), 25 mg. per ml., is diluted one part to three parts (0.5 ml. to 1.5 ml.; total 2.0 ml.) with 1 per cent lidocaine N.D., U.S.P. (Xylocaine Hydrochloride) without epinephrine. This results in a working solution of 6 mg. per ml. Inject about 0.1 to 0.2 ml. directly into each lesion. Pruritus is usually relieved instantly, the lesion flattens in five to seven days and healing occurs by 14 days except for residual postinflammatory hyperpigmentation. Occasionally, local postinjection steroid atrophy occurs which may last four months. Attempting to find the offending insect is often frustrating. I emphasize to the parents that only some individuals react to bites with papular urticaria, while most members of the family will be unaffected. For dogs and cats, antiflea collars containing 2, 2-dichlorovinyl dimethyl phosphate are recommended. Spraying the house with an insecticide containing 5 per cent DDT or 1 per cent lindane, or hiring a professional exterminator, often becomes necessary, especially if rugs, furniture, books, automobiles or the yard becomes infested.

ERYTHEMA MULTIFORME

The mildest form of erythema multiforme is the most common. Treatment is symptomatic. Aspirin and diphenhydramine hydrochloride are given orally in the usual doses unless suspected as the etiologic agents for the attack. If painful oral lesions are present, diphenhydramine hydrochloride expectorant cough syrup stings less than the elixir and may be held in the mouth for 1 or 2 minutes to anesthetize any painful erosions. No topical medicament is helpful for the skin lesions, although steroid creams and ointments are sometimes prescribed.

The Stevens-Johnson syndrome is an emergency in severe cases. Systemic steroids are indicated, beginning with 40 to 50 mg. of prednisone daily in divided doses. For infants and small children, 30 mg. may suffice. After four days, if the response is satisfactory, the dose is gradually reduced. A systemic antibiotic is often combined to reduce secondary infection of denuded areas and to reduce pulmonary complications. Dyclonine hydrochloride (Dyclone Solution), 5 mg. per ml., or lidocaine hydrochloride viscous solution (Xylocaine Hydrochloride) swabbed, sprayed or gargled may relieve local oral discomfort to permit eating, drinking and cleansing the mouth. Skilled nursing care remains important.

ERYTHEMA NODOSUM

No adequate topical medication is available. Bed rest, aspirin and diphenhydramine hydrochloride* given orally in the usual doses provide symptomatic relief. A frame or box to keep the painful pressure of bedclothes off the skin lesions is helpful. Sometimes a heating pad or an ice bag applied locally offers comfort. The underlying cause is treated if identified: treat streptococcal infections with penicillin; treat coccidioidomycosis, histoplasmosis and tuberculosis appropriately, or avoid the responsible drug. Although systemic steroids offer prompt, temporary relief, they should not be used unless the etiology is proved and no contraindications to their use exist.

URTICARIA PIGMENTOSA

No satisfactory treatment for urticaria pigmentosa exists. Cryproheptadine or hydroxyzine given orally may decrease pruritus and the wheal and flare. Topical antibiotic ointment or cream may be necessary for secondarily infected bullae overlying solitary lesions. Some patients deliberately degranulate their mast cell tumors by taking a hot bath and toweling vigorously, thereby inducing a refractory period for 12 or more hours. Such a practice can cause severe hemorrhage in infants and small children owing to massive heparin release. Certain drugs, like codeine and polymyxin, may also cause mast cell degranulation, thereby producing flares.

Drug Eruptions
(Dermatitis Medicamentosa)

HERMAN BEERMAN, M.D.

A drug eruption is a cutaneous or mucocutaneous process incident to the administration of drugs or their split products which come in contact with the affected part by way of the

* Manufacturer's precaution: Diphenhydramine (Benadryl) should not be used in premature or newborn infants.

general circulation by whatever route of administration.

Treatment. Because of the variety of eruptions produced by numerous drugs, only general principles can be outlined for the management of the complex problem of drug eruptions.

The first and foremost principle is: *Withdraw the offending drug.* This usually effects cure of many drug eruptions in a reasonably short time. Notable exceptions are the bromide, iodide and arsenical eruptions, and the lupus erythematosus phenomenon, produced by drugs (hydralazine, and so forth). Also, the patient must avoid sunlight if drugs with high photosensitization potential are being taken [e.g., demethylchlortetracycline (Declomycin) and chlorothiazides (Diuril)].

SUPPORTIVE TREATMENT. In severe cases of quinacrine, sulfonamide and other eruptions, supportive treatment with liver extract, vitamin A, ascorbic acid and nicotinic acid may be of value.

BAL. As a by-product of the successful search for an antidote to the arsenical gases, it was found that 2,3-dimercaptopropanol (BAL, British antilewisite) is also effective in the therapy of certain metal intoxications.

ANTIHISTAMINICS. The antihistaminic drugs are of limited value against drug reactions of the skin, and dermatitis may occur as a result of their administration. Nevertheless they should be given a thorough trial in drug eruptions. Benadryl elixir, 1 to 2 teaspoons (14 to 30 ml.; 10 to 20 mg.) three or four times a day is the dosage for children up to 12 years of age.

SODIUM CHLORIDE. Sodium chloride is useful in the therapy of iodide and bromide eruptions.

EPINEPHRINE. Epinephrine, 1:1000 U.S.P. in small doses of 0.1 to 0.5 ml. subcutaneously and repeated in a few hours, is on occasion of use in anaphylaxis and certain urticarial eruptions (e.g., laryngeal edema).

EPHEDRINE. Ephedrine, 15 to 25 mg. orally every 4 to 6 hours according to age and weight of the child, has a limited usefulness in urticaria.

STEROIDS. These compounds are of considerable value in reducing the inflammatory element in dermatitis medicamentosa. They are especially useful in widespread eruptions. Cortisone and other steroid preparations are given with a high initial dose. Hydrocortisone, ACTH, prednisone or prednisolone may be used in proportionate dosage. As the process improves, the dosage may be reduced fairly rapidly. Corticotropin and prednisone may be responsible for eruptions (acneiform, dermatitis and others). These can be eliminated by stopping treatment. Except in certain patients with exfoliative dermatitis, treatment need not be prolonged.

Our preference, generally speaking, is for triamcinolone (Aristocort or Kenacort), in oral doses of 4 to 12 mg. a day for children under 60 pounds (28 kilograms). For children over 60 pounds, the adult dose of 8 to 32 mg. a day may be used. After a few days of therapy the dosage is reduced by 2 mg. every two to three days.

LOCAL TREATMENT. Local treatment for drug eruptions follows the principles and procedures of therapy for the type of eruption a particular drug produces. A simplified scheme of local management consists of the following: In acute cases relief is obtained by the use of simple local applications, such as a greaseless ointment base. Of value in the acute phase of dermatitis are Burow's solution, 10.0; lanolin, 20.0; Lassar's paste, to a sufficient quantity, 60.0; or 3 per cent ichthyol in zinc oxide ointment.

In patients sensitive to wool, one may use, cautiously, petrolatum or other nonlanolin-containing bases. Follow the constitutional treatment previously outlined. Do not vaccinate, inoculate or perform cutaneous tests during the acute phase.

Prevention. Prevention is not always easy, since drugs of a relatively high cutaneous sensitizing index are included in preparations in which their presence might not be suspected (e.g., phenolphthalein in cough syrup or effervescent salts; penicillin in milk, transplacental transmission or mother's milk), and such sensitizing medicaments are too often readily available on the open market. The best prophylactic for recurrent attacks is for the patient to avoid even minute quantities of the offending agent for either medicinal, testing or desensitizing purposes. Disregard of this caution may be fatal for the patient.

Important prophylactic procedures include a good history, especially of previous reactions, avoidance of sunlight if certain photosensitizing drugs are involved and, particularly, good clinical records.

Certain drugs have a high sensitizing index, which should be known to the physician. Such drugs include antibiotics, especially penicillin, tetracyclines, sulfonamides (including Diuril, Hydrodiuril, Esidrix, Diamox); antimalarials (Atabrine); ataractic drugs (all types); and antiepileptics (Dilantin).

Drug houses have been careful in the distribution of warnings and the recall of questionable drugs, but practitioners have often disregarded the facts, with serious medical and legal consequences.

Papulosquamous Disorders

ALVIN H. JACOBS, M.D.

PSORIASIS

Psoriasis is a chronic, constitutional disorder with a tendency to familial occurrence. No age is exempt; in fact, the onset is usually in childhood or adolescence, and it is even seen occasionally in infancy. Before embarking on treatment, it is of great importance that the patient and the parents understand that the child has a lifelong problem, although remissions are common; that general health is usually unaffected; and that with a persistent and concentrated treatment program much can be accomplished to minimize the problem.

General Therapeutic Measures. Assessment of the emotional status of the patient is important, since tensions and anxiety can exacerbate psoriasis. Attention to family difficulties and school problems may be important. The use of sedatives and tranquilizers should be considered. For daytime use, hydroxyzine hydrochloride (Atarax) is a satisfactory tranquilizer for children; it is given in doses of 5 to 20 mg. three times daily.

It is important that the parents of the patient completely understand the treatment and its rationale. It should also be brought to their attention that injury to the skin may result in more psoriasis (Koebner response). This means that bruises, abrasions, scratches, poorly fitting clothing or shoes may cause skin injury sufficient to generate a reaction.

Most psoriatics are benefited by exposure to sunlight and thus frequently are better in the summer. Advantage should be taken of this in planning the summer activities of the psoriatic child, although caution must be exercised, since sudden overexposure to sunlight can result in enough skin injury to cause an exacerbation.

Since acute guttate (drop-like) psoriasis frequently follows a streptococcal respiratory infection, it is especially important that psoriatic children receive adequate therapy for streptococcal disease. Children with guttate psoriasis should routinely have throat cultures taken, and if beta-hemolytic streptococci are found, a course of penicillin therapy should be instituted before more active therapy for the psoriasis is instituted. In many instances, the psoriasis will improve markedly with treatment only of the streptococcal disease.

Proper general hygiene should be emphasized, especially frequent removal of scales by means of warm tub baths with ordinary soaps or tar soap. A tar bath, made by the addition of 1 ounce of Zetar emulsion, Balnetar or liquor carbonis detergens to a tub of water, may be used.

Systemic Therapy. No systemic drugs currently available are safe for administration to children. Systemic corticosteroids clear psoriasis temporarily but should never be used for this purpose, since cessation of therapy is usually followed by a serious flare-up of the eruption.

Cytotoxic antimetabolite drugs, such as methotrexate, are used in the treatment of severe adult psoriasis. These are very toxic drugs, and although they suppress growth of hyperplastic epidermal cells, they are capable of producing the same effects on other rapidly growing cells. The use of such toxic agents for a nonmalignant disease in childhood is not indicated.

Topical Therapy. Since psoriasis is a chronic disorder with remissions and exacerbations, and since responsiveness to treatment may vary, it is necessary to have a variety of regimens available and to start with the simplest. The usual effective remedies include ammoniated mercury, salicylic acid, tars, anthralin compounds and topical corticosteroids. Many times in mild psoriasis it is sufficient to recommend frequent sunbaths (with proper caution) and the use of an emollient to supply adequate moisture to the skin. Eucerin cream is an excellent choice for this purpose, since it is composed of equal parts water and Aquaphor.

Localized Psoriasis

Two per cent ammoniated mercury in zinc oxide ointment massaged into involved areas three times daily may be all that is needed in mild cases and is not messy. If the scales are thick, 1 or 2 per cent salicylic acid may be added to the ammoniated mercury.

One to three per cent crude coal tar in zinc oxide ointment may be applied if the ammoniated mercury is ineffective. The addition of 0.5 per cent polysorbate 80 (Tween 80) permits the preparation to be washed off easily. If the use of crude coal tar proves too objectionable, 10 per cent liquor carbonis detergens (LCD) in hydrophilic ointment (U.S.P.) may be substituted.

Fluorinated steroids, such as 0.1 per cent

triamcinolone (Kenalog), 0.025 per cent fluocinolone (Synalar), 0.05 per cent flurandrenolid (Cordran), and 0.1 per cent betamethasone (Valisone) have proved to be the most effective of the topically applied corticosteroids. These preparations in a cream or ointment form should be rubbed into each lesion four or five times daily.

An effective method of treatment is the use of one of the fluorinated steroids in an ointment base with occlusive dressings. The fluorinated steroid is applied to the lesions, and the area is completely covered with an occlusive plastic, such as Saran Wrap, and then sealed with 3M Blenderm Tape. If necessary, an elastic bandage may be applied over the plastic to keep it in place. These occlusive dressings are applied at bedtime and left on throughout the night. In the morning when the dressings are removed, additional ointment should be rubbed in, since the formerly dry scaly lesions will be soft and somewhat macerated and will more easily absorb additional medication. It is best to treat only one upper or lower extremity or the trunk at any time in order to avoid systemic absorption. Those areas of the body not being actively treated by the occlusive method can be kept lubricated with an emollient, such as Eucerin cream or Lubriderm.

A very convenient method of occlusive therapy in localized areas is to apply Cordran Tape, which consists of flurandrenolid-impregnated plastic tape.

Generalized Psoriasis

Removal of scales by daily tar baths is often a necessary preliminary to adequate treatment.

Massage 1 per cent crude coal tar in zinc oxide ointment into all lesions at bedtime; according to the results, the concentration of tar may be increased to as much as 5 per cent. In intertriginous areas use 1 per cent liquor carbonis detergens in a base consisting of one part Unibase to nine parts water.

Remove the ointment in the morning with mineral oil followed by a cleansing bath or shower.

Ultraviolet light may be used in suberythema doses in the office once or twice weekly, or the patient may purchase a lamp for home use. Natural sunlight, when available, is superior to either. Great care must be exercised in any case, since exacerbation of the lesions can result if the skin is allowed to burn.

If prompt results are not evident, it is best to hospitalize the patient for two or three weeks during which the Goeckerman regimen can be carried out. This treatment consists of applying 5 per cent crude coal tar to the entire body every 2 or 3 hours. Each morning the ointment is removed with mineral oil and the patient is then given a tar bath. After the bath, ultraviolet light is used in suberythema doses and the crude coal tar is reapplied. A very satisfactory remission usually follows this type of therapy.

The length of hospital stay can be reduced by the use of anthralin paste in place of the crude coal tar. This treatment, however, is difficult to carry out and should be supervised by an experienced dermatologist.

Psoriasis of the Scalp

Removal of thick scales may be accomplished by daily warm oil applications. This is carried out by saturating the scalp with mineral oil and then applying hot towels in turban fashion every 10 minutes for half an hour before shampooing.

After several days, if the scales have been adequately removed, one can then use daily tar shampoos. Polytar shampoo is an effective and nonmessy preparation for this purpose.

Following the shampoo, Synalar Solution is rubbed into the scalp. It is best to avoid greasy preparations in hairy areas.

SEBORRHEIC DERMATITIS

Seborrheic dermatitis is an inflammatory, scaly, crusting eruption involving the body areas containing the greatest concentration of sebaceous glands, namely, the scalp, face, postauricular areas, presternal area and the intertriginous zones. It appears in infancy between 2 to 12 weeks of age and usually clears spontaneously by 8 to 12 months of age. It is not seen again until puberty, after which it remains as a chronic condition.

In infancy, seborrheic dermatitis involves primarily the scalp as well as flexural and intertriginous areas and is very frequently secondarily infected with *Candida albicans*.

Seborrheic Dermatitis of the Scalp

Treatment of cradle cap is best carried out by the use of one of the commercially available antiseborrheic shampoos, such as Sebulex or Ionil. The scalp should be washed thoroughly with the shampoo daily at first and later two or three times each week. If the scale has become too thick and adherent for easy removal by shampooing, it can be loosened first by massaging warm mineral oil into the scalp and allowing it to remain for 15 or 20 minutes followed by the therapeutic shampoo. Mother should be reassured that rubbing the infant's scalp vigorously will not injure the baby's fragile-feeling skull.

Adolescents with seborrheic dermatitis of the scalp may use the same type of shampoo and then rub a corticosteroid lotion, such as Synalar solution, into involved scalp areas after the shampoo.

Seborrheic Dermatitis of the Face

The use of corticosteroid creams will clear the facial and postauricular involvement in a very short time. For this, one of the fluorinated preparations is best (0.01 per cent Synalar cream, or 0.025 per cent Kenalog cream). Involvement of the eyelids with seborrheic blepharitis can be managed by first removing the marginal crusts with warm water twice daily followed by application of an ophthalmic corticosteroid ointment.

Seborrheic Dermatitis of the Diaper Area

In most instances, *Candida albicans* superinfection must be cleared first. This can be done by application of a nongreasy anticandidal agent, such as Mycostatin dusting powder or Fungizone Lotion. As the candidiasis subsides, one can change to one of the corticosteroid creams mentioned above. Combination treatment such as Nystaform-HC Lotion can also be used.

PARAPSORIASIS

The term parapsoriasis embraces a poorly defined group of rare maculopapular squamous eruptions of unknown origin. None of these disorders has any relationship to psoriasis. Three conditions which come under this heading can occur in childhood. Pityriasis lichenoides et varioliformis acuta occurs most commonly in childhood or early adult life. The course of the disease is usually a few weeks to several months and recovery is the rule.

Guttate parapsoriasis occurs mostly in young adults and has a longer course, usually from three months to seven years. The ultimate prognosis is good.

Treatment for the above two conditions is purely symptomatic. While awaiting recovery, antipruritic medication such as diphenhydramine (Benadryl),* 25 to 50 mg. three times a day orally, may be administered, and emollients, such as Lubriderm or Keri Lotion, applied.

Parapsoriasis en plaques, which may occur at any age, is regarded as an expression of a lymphoreticular disease. Approximately 25 per cent of these eventually progress to mycosis fungoides. Although treatment of parapsoriasis en plaque is symptomatic, careful long-term follow-up is essential.

PITYRIASIS ROSEA

Pityriasis rosea is a common, mild inflammatory skin disorder characterized by round or oval, discrete or confluent salmon-tinted, slightly scaly macules or rings. The disease is self-limited, lasting about four to six weeks. Treatment is directed toward allaying anxiety, speeding recovery and relieving pruritus.

Exposure to ultraviolet light to the point of producing erythema and exfoliation may hasten recovery.

Since soap is irritating in this condition, cleansing may be accomplished by colloidal starch baths (one cup of Linit starch to a tub of warm water) or by oatmeal baths, such as Aveeno.

Systemic antipruritic drugs are useful if itching is a problem. Temaril is given in divided doses three or four times daily, following the manufacturer's recommended schedule. If necessary, one to two teaspoonfuls of elixir of Benadryl* may be given at bedtime.

PITYRIASIS RUBRA PILARIS

Pityriasis rubra pilaris is a very rare disorder characterized by fine, acuminate, horny follicular papules. The hereditary form of the disorder may be present at birth or may develop during infancy. The acquired type may occur at any age. The disease tends to be lifelong.

Some patients have been reported to respond to large doses of vitamin A (150,000 to 200,000 units per day), but this is a toxic and dangerous therapy for use in childhood. More recently, it has been suggested that vitamin A acid (Retin-A) applied locally may be of help. Keratolytic ointments, such as 3 per cent salicylic acid, will result in some improvement.

LICHEN STRIATUS

Lichen striatus is a rare condition of unknown cause occurring in children as a linear band of scaling papules usually appearing suddenly on the extremities. Spontaneous resolution usually occurs in several months. Treatment is usually not necessary, but if desired, local application of topical corticosteroids will relieve pruritus and possibly hasten recovery.

LICHEN NITIDUS

This is an asymptomatic, rare, chronic eruption which consists of small, sharply de-

* Manufacturer's precaution: Diphenhydramine (Benadryl) should not be used for premature or newborn infants.

fined, flesh-colored papules localized on the penis, arms and abdomen. The disease is chronic, although spontaneous resolution after many years may occur. No method of treatment has been found to be effective.

Vesiculobullous Disorders

Dermatitis Herpetiformis, Drug-Induced Toxic Epidermal Necrolysis, Pemphigus Vulgaris and Bullous Pemphigoid

GUINTER KAHN, M.D.

Although the skin of children blisters more easily than that of adults, the chronic blistering diseases occur rarely in young people. Pemphigus vulgaris and bullous pemphigoid are almost unheard of before the teenage years. Drug-induced toxic epidermal necrolysis (TEN) is much less common than staphylococcal toxin–induced TEN in children, especially in infants. Dermatitis herpetiformis (DH) is very uncommon in children, but it does occur throughout the pediatric age group. It appears more often as a bullous eruption and more often in the groin among children than among adults. In the past DH has been called juvenile bullous pemphigoid, a misnomer rectified by the recent advent of diagnostic immunofluorescent tests for these diseases.

DERMATITIS HERPETIFORMIS

The sulfone, diaminodiphenyl sulfone (dapsone), and the sulfapyridines are the agents of choice for this affliction. Neither the cause of the disease nor the reason why these agents help is known. The dramatic relief of symptoms and signs by either of these drugs is almost therapeutically diagnostic of DH. The agent chosen as first therapy varies with the practitioner's experiences with each drug.

Sulfones

Dapsone (Avlosulfone) is available as 25- and 100-mg. tablets. It is better tolerated and more economical than sulfapyridine; however, its side effects can be serious.

Dose. Initially, 50 to 200 mg. per day should be given, increasing or decreasing about 50 mg. per day depending on response or side effects of therapy.

Cautions. (1) A glucose-6-phosphate dehydrogenase (G6PD) screening test should be done prior to giving this drug to Negroes or Caucasians of Mediterranean descent because of the increased incidence of severe hemolytic anemia in some of these people following the use of dapsone. (2) Order a urinalysis and complete blood count every month during the first year of therapy, then about every three months.

Side Effects. Methemoglobinemia is common and causes headaches and an ashy grey color. It is *not* an indication to stop medication if the G6PD test is normal. In weeks, these symptoms diminish while the drug's therapeutic activity continues.

Less frequent side effects include febrile reactions, hepatitis, peripheral neuropathy, psychoses, exfoliative erythroderma and agranulocytosis.

Pediatric Formulation. A liquid suspension can be tailored for children unable to swallow pills (25 to 100 mg. per teaspoon). Since its stability is unknown, it should be kept in a refrigerator and used within two weeks after formulation.

Maintenance. A dose which reduces signs and symptoms to a minimum is determined for each patient. About every three to six months, slow withdrawal should be attempted, since the disease may remit spontaneously after years.

Sulfapyridine

Sulfapyridine is available as 500-mg. enteric- or nonenteric-coated tablets. Some clinicians claim that it is more effective than dapsone. Proof is lacking.

Dose. Initially, 250 to 1000 mg. per day should be given, depending on the size of the patient. Increase the medication by doubling the dose about every other day until symptoms or signs abate or nausea occurs. Thereafter, tailor dosage weekly according to symptoms, signs and side effects.

Cautions. (1) The patient should be encouraged to consume large quantities of fluids to avoid renal crystalline aggregates. (2) The enteric-coated tablet causes much less nausea because often it is not absorbed. The patient should closely examine his stools for tablets. (3) When using nonenteric-coated tablets the dose must be kept extremely low initially and must be given with meals; otherwise, severe nausea often occurs. (4) Order a urinalysis and complete blood count monthly.

Side Effects. Nausea and vomiting are usually the first and most common side effects. Others include fever, headaches, leukopenia, agranulocytosis, hepatitis and renal damage (from sulfa crystal aggregates).

Maintenance and Pediatric Formulation. See dapsone.

Discussion

Some patients respond to one of these agents in preference to the other. Occasional patients need the combination of both medicines. Rarely, patients will be refractory to both drugs, and such patients are given large doses (4 to 6 mg. per kilogram per day) of prednisone to effect a remission.

DRUG-INDUCED TOXIC EPIDERMAL NECROLYSIS (TEN), THE SCALDED SKIN SYNDROME (LYELL'S DISEASE)

Staphylococcal-induced TEN is discussed elsewhere.

The extent of involvement varies from a few small, flaccid bullae to widespread denudation of skin and mucous membranes. Accordingly, therapy varies from cautious neglect and observation to that of a total body burn regimen. But basic to any therapy for this condition is to *avoid the provoking medication* and substances with which it may cross-react.

Caution. Children with recurrent TEN should make the physician suspicious of recurrent burns. The physician should look for any other signs or symptoms of neglect or cruelty (battered child syndrome).

Therapy. Death occurs in about 25 per cent of all patients, but much less often in children. Therapeutic measures will be described for the severest, generalized form, and the practitioner can scale down his therapy in proportion to the clinical presentation.

Death follows a pattern similar to that in burns, i.e., secondary infection, dehydration, decreased electrolytes and serum proteins. Therefore, when available, these patients should be transferred to a burn unit and be under the surveillance of a physician experienced with burn therapy and of a dermatologist.

TEN patients, however, differ from burn patients in that the remaining "normal" epidermis readily shears away from the underlying dermis (Nikolsky's sign) with the slightest trauma. Personnel must be warned to minimize trauma or handling of the patient's skin. A vibrating, flannel-covered mattress should be used to avoid creating local pressure zones. The patient's skin and mucosa must be observed daily, since the course of blistering can change suddenly and spread rampantly.

Blistered areas should be treated aseptically. Isolation techniques are advisable; blisters should be punctured with the covering left on. However, infected and necrotic tissue should be removed, the base cultured and systemic antibiotics chosen as needed on the basis of sensitivity studies. Silver nitrate wet dressing (0.5 per cent) should be applied to the involved skin daily or more often in the presence of purulence. Fluids and electrolytes must be monitored, especially since silver ion applications can rapidly deplete serum sodium.

An alternate, proved form of topical therapy is the application of warm, dry air, at 40° C. and 20 per cent humidity, through a gently vibrating, porous mattress. An air conditioner giving 2000 liters per minute of this air quickly dries the moist wound surfaces. The 40° C. ambient temperature relieves the body's metabolic need to produce heat as fluid is evaporated from the skin's surface.

The value of steroids here is not proved, but considering the severe possible prognosis, they commonly are used. Prednisone should be given in substantial doses (4 to 6 mg. per kilogram) and the dose doubled daily if the course of the disease is not abated. The author uses Solu-Medrol (sodium succinate methylprednisolone) intravenously for patients unable to swallow large doses of prednisone. He has successfully used doses as high as 8000 mg. a day in an adult. These dosages of prednisone are higher than those recommended by the manufacturers. However, they may be warranted in these cases, and they have worked well in our experience.

Mucosal Care. Topical steroid ointments should be applied about four times a day to involved mucosal surfaces. The involved eyes and vulvar surfaces should be separated widely after each application to avoid synechiae. Eye care should be controlled by an ophthalmologist. The patient with oral-pharyngeal pain should rinse his mouth with 4 per cent viscous lidocaine to encourage eating. Meals for such patients should be soft and not hot.

The family should be warned of possible sequelae even with successful treatment: pigmented scars, keloids, corneal scarring and, less often, ectropion and nail loss.

PEMPHIGUS

The vulgaris form is extremely rare in children, while the more superficial foliaceus form is more common and less severe. It is endemic to parts of Brazil. The youngest case reported was that of an 18-month-old girl who responded to 0.5 per cent triamcinolone cream applied four times a day. Nevertheless, we recommend systemic prednisone, 3 to 6 mg. per kilogram per day, depending on the severity of the process. These figures may have to be revised upward if the process is inadequately suppressed. When the progression of the disease has been checked and no new lesions have appeared for two weeks, the dosage may be reduced by about 20 per cent every two weeks. As one approaches maintenance dosage (2 to 5 months after onset of therapy for severe cases), alternate morning prednisone becomes the preferred therapy because steroid side effects are reduced. Alternate-morning prednisone is the initial therapy of choice for those mild to moderate forms of pemphigus that would require less than 100 mg. per day to control. The second choice would be to control the patient on a daily early morning (6 to 8 A.M.) prednisone regimen. Side effects are less than with the daily divided dose regimen, which is needed only in the acute stage of the severest form of the disease.*

Uncommonly, severe cases do not respond to large doses of steroids, so that the dose must be doubled about every week until the disorder is stabilized. For unknown reasons, in these rare instances, patients may respond to nominal ACTH dosage, about 80 units per day initially, while they appear refractory to systemically administered corticosteroids.

Once a maintenance dose is established for such difficult patients, immunosuppressives may be added to the regimen, since they allow for the further reduction of steroid dosage. Methotrexate, Imuran and Cytoxan have been used successfully in doses varying with the severity of the process. The physician should be cautious in the use of these drugs, which presently are experimental for the treatment of pemphigus and could be potential mutagens in a child. A basic dictum is the younger the patient, the shorter the course of drug, and contraceptive measures are used when indicated. Hepatic, renal and hematologic systems are monitored by the laboratory when antimetabolites become part of the regimen.

The local care of the skin and mucosa in severe cases is adequately described in the section Drug-Induced Toxic Epidermal Necrolysis.

PEMPHIGOID

Because the course is similar but less severe than that for pemphigus, treatment is similar and response is usually quicker than for pemphigus. Only one preteen patient with this disease is known to the author.

* A complete check list for physicians treating patients with systemic corticosteroids for prolonged periods of time is found in Lowney, E. D.: Anticipation of Problems of Systemic Corticosteroid Therapy. *Arch. Derm.*, 99:588, 1969.

Scleroderma

DENNY L. TUFFANELLI, M.D., *and*
ROBERT LaPERRIERE, M.D.

Scleroderma can be broadly classified into two categories, the localized cutaneous type, including morphea and linear scleroderma, and systemic scleroderma.

The onset of morphea is insidious and begins with a distinctly purplish area of skin. The lesions may be multiple and generally resolve in a three- to five-year period. In children morphea occurs in a 3:1 female-to-male ratio, the average age of onset being about five years. Systemic manifestations are rarely present.

Linear scleroderma usually involves the head or an extremity and is often associated with atrophy of underlying structures. "En coup de sabre" is linear scleroderma involving the scalp or face. Scleroderma patients with facial atrophy should have skull films and electroencephalographic and neurologic examinations as part of their work up. Other forms of linear scleroderma may be associated with bony defects of the spine.

Systemic scleroderma is quite rare in children. It can be seen in the edematous, sclerotic and atrophic phases. The earliest clinical sign usually is Raynaud's phenomenon. Other complaints may include arthralgias, thickening of the skin, ankylosis of the fingers and digital ulcerations. Gastrointestinal disturbances include dysphagia, constipation, regurgitation, weight loss and malabsorption. Calcinosis cutis is a late sequela.

Therapy. No specific treatment is available and therefore management is mainly supportive. In morphea and linear scleroderma, physiotherapy may be important, depending on the area of involvement. Whirlpool, deep heat, hot water baths, paraffin baths, casts, splints, massage and exercise have been utilized. Skin protection and lubrication are necessary.

In systemic scleroderma general measures are indicated, including avoidance of factors producing vasospasm (tension, fatigue, stress and cold weather) and minimizing trauma to the hands. Rest is also important. If mild polyarthritis is present, salicylates may be useful. Sympatholytics may be helpful early before damage to peripheral vessels occurs. Intra-arterial reserpine may be beneficial. Corticosteroids may be utilized, but only if absolutely necessary, such as in patients with debilitating arthritis, sclerodermatomyositis, cutaneous edema, severe recurrent digital ulcers and acute toxic phases of the disease. Many other pharmacologic treatments have been used without rewarding effect. Immunosuppressive drugs are still experimental. Treatment of gastrointestinal symptoms is aimed at controlling gastric acid content, using bland diet and antacids. Frequent small feedings and raising of the head of the bed are also helpful. The malabsorption syndrome should be treated with vitamins, antidiarrheal agents and broad-spectrum antibiotics. Sympathectomy is rarely, if ever, indicated.

Discoid Lupus Erythematosus

DENNY L. TUFFANELLI, M.D.

We consider "discoid" lupus to be the chronic cutaneous form of the disease lupus erythematosus. It is the same disease as systemic lupus erythematosus but represents the more benign ranges of the lupus erythematosus spectrum. The discoid form may transform into the systemic form. The recorded incidence varies from 2 to 20 per cent, and the incidence depends on the clinical group studied and the methods of analysis. Serologic and hematologic abnormalities are frequently noted in discoid lupus.

Cutaneous lesions are characterized by persistent erythema, adherent scales, follicular plugging, telangiectasia and, in the later stages, scarring and atrophy. Sun-exposed areas are most affected. Some lesions form permanent scars, while others resolve completely. Hyperpigmentation and hypopigmentation often occur, the latter being particularly distressing in Blacks.

Cutaneous lupus erythematosus may subside spontaneously, remain a minimal problem or progress with resultant scarring and disfigurement. Therapy should be as conservative as possible. A common error in management is to excessively frighten the patient who has minimal cutaneous lupus erythematosus. In only a small proportion of patients does chronic cutaneous lupus erythematosus progress to the life-threatening systemic form of the disease.

Patients in whom photosensitivity is a factor should avoid excessive sun exposure. Photosensitive patients should use sunscreens on exposed areas when excessive exposure is anticipated. Use of local corticosteroid creams and ointments is the simplest and most effective therapy, particularly for early erythematous plaques. Occlusion with a pliable plastic film increases absorption of the medication. Intralesional corticosteroids are occasionally useful in refractory lesions.

Antimalarial therapy is often useful in adults with cutaneous lupus erythematosus, but is hazardous in older children and should not be used in younger children.

Bacterial Infections of the Skin

ANDREW M. MARGILETH, M.D.

IMPETIGO

Impetigo is a superficial vesiculopurulent pyoderma involving the stratum corneum. Two common types are observed. *Bullous impetigo* occurs more often in the neonate and infant and is usually due to staphylococci. *Impetigo contagiosa,* characterized by thick yellowish crusts, is seen usually in the child and is caused by staphylococci and streptococci. Regional lymphadenopathy commonly occurs with secondary infection of insect bites, eczema, poison ivy, scabies, herpetic lesions and varicella.

Effective therapy is based on four factors: etiology and type of infection, local therapy, antibiotics and systemic disorders.

Etiology. The cause and type of the infection are determined by aspiration and culture of bullae, or by culture after removal of a crust. Knowledge of the bacteriologic characteristics of skin infections in the community will guide the physician in giving the appropriate antibiotic therapy. Sensitivity of the streptococcus to a Taxos A bacitracin disc applied directly on the blood agar plate is essential to determine whether the beta-hemolytic streptococci are group A. Coagulase determination of the staphylococci isolated and the antibiotic sensitivity tests are necessary only when the patient has had recurrent or severe skin infections. At the Children's Hospital of D.C. during 18 months (1971 to 1972) skin cultures were taken from 413 clinic children with impetigo. Group A beta-hemolytic streptococci were isolated in 57 per cent of cases, and beta-hemolytic *S. aureus* were isolated in 31 per cent of cases.

Local Therapy. Local therapy consists of cleansing the skin, with scrupulous removal of crusts by soaks and thorough scrubbing of lesions four or five times daily. A hexachlorophene solution or a Betadine surgical scrub is effective if used for five to seven days until no new lesions appear. Concomitantly, a bacitracin ointment, 500 units per Gm., should be applied locally.

Antibiotics. For severe, extensive or recurrent infections, especially in the newborn, parenteral antibiotics must be considered. The antibiotic of choice for the office patient is benzathine penicillin G, using one injection of Bicillin: 600,000 units for the child under 60 pounds and 1.2 million units for those over 60 pounds. Oral penicillin G therapy is effective provided that doses, 400,000 units three or four times daily, are not missed and that all medication is taken for 7 to 10 days. If group A beta-hemolytic streptococci are recovered, a full 10-day course is necessary. For severe infection in the newborn, hospitalization may be indicated.

In patients with penicillin sensitivity, oral erythromycin or cephalexin may be substituted. Dosage is the same for both drugs: 40 mg. per kilogram of body weight per day given every 6 hours for 7 to 10 days. Use of semisynthetic penicillinase-resistant penicillins should be reserved for seriously ill patients, when bacterial sensitivity studies indicate their need, and particularly if clinical response to Bicillin is not observed in two or three days. If group A beta-hemolytic streptococci are cultured, a urinalysis, performed two weeks after the infection, is indicated, since nephritis may occur in four per cent of patients.

Systemic Disorders. Any associated systemic disorders must be treated. Management of repeated skin cuts and breaks is best accomplished by reducing skin bacteria. A shower twice daily using a hexachlorophene solution or a Betadine surgical scrub will decrease the number of secondarily infected abrasions. Since impetigo is contagious, sibling contact must be avoided and separate washcloths and towels provided.

Ecthyma is a deeper form of impetigo in which the bacterial infection penetrates the epidermis. Since tissue is destroyed beyond the epithelium, ecthyma is usually followed by scars. Treatment is based on the principles outlined for impetigo. Systemic antibiotics necessarily are prescribed more frequently, especially if the lesions are extensive or if regional lymphadenitis is present. Insect bites with associated pruritus and secondary infection should not be overlooked as a basic underlying cause, particularly in recurrent or persistent cases.

Therapy for phagedenic ulcers due to Pseudomonas infection follows: For local lesions, polymyxin B, 0.1 per cent solution in 1 per cent acetic acid, may be useful. Soaks of 0.5 per cent silver nitrate are also effective. Soaks are applied locally two or three times daily for 7 to 10 days. For severe infections, carbenicillin and gentamicin are effective. The gentamicin dose is 4 to 5 mg. per kilogram per day intramuscularly in three doses; the carbenicillin dose is 500 to 600 mg. per kilogram per day intravenously in six divided doses for 10 to 14 days.

FURUNCLE

Furuncles, or boils, common in the summer, are infections of hair follicles or sweat glands usually due to staphylococci. One or two lesions are easily treated locally by using the principles outlined for impetigo and ecthyma. Essential therapy consists in soaking the lesions continuously or not less than four times daily for 1 hour with warm tap water or saline compresses. If spontaneous drainage, or resolution, does not occur, continuous compresses must be prescribed. Incision and drainage when the lesion becomes fluctuant should be followed by continuous moist compresses for several days. Dressings should be changed every 4 hours and should be cut small to avoid tissue maceration. Bacitracin ointment, 500 units per Gm., may be used locally.

Chronic recurring *furunculosis* is less common, but requires thorough investigation to reveal any underlying chronic disease. Often no disease is found; however, an epidemiologic survey must be made of the family. Cultures taken from the anterior nares (not nasopharynx) often show which family members in addition to the patient harbor beta-hemolytic staphylococci (rarely streptococci) in the nose. These organisms are usually coagulase-positive and penicillin-sensitive unless a member works in a hospital. Phage typing is not necessary.

All members found to be nasal carriers of the infecting strain should routinely use a hexachlorophene soap for bathing, and four times daily a bacitracin ointment (500 units per Gm.) should be applied to both anterior nares. This should be continued at least two weeks and followed by repeat cultures of both nares to be sure that treatment was effective. Fingernails must be trimmed short and nose-picking discontinued. Staphylococcal vaccines and toxoids are not recommended. Systemic administration of antibiotics is rarely necessary unless multiple furuncles are present or regional lymphadenitis occurs. For severe infections, especially if caused by penicillin-resistant *S. aureus,* cloxacillin* is preferred; the dose is 25 to 100 mg. per kilogram per day orally in divided doses every 6 hours given 1 to 2 hours before meals. In the penicillin-allergic patient,

* Manufacturer's note: Pediatric capsules have been removed from the market. Other forms of sodium cloxacillin monohydrate (Tegopen) are still available.

clindamycin, 8 to 20 mg. per kilogram per day orally in divided doses every 6 to 8 hours, is effective. Therapy is continued 10 to 14 days and occasionally in chronic cases may be continued for three to six weeks.

PARONYCHIA

Inflammation of the nail fold is usually due to a hemolytic staphylococcal or streptococcal infection secondary to local injury, e.g., nailbiting or thumbsucking. Occasionally Pseudomonas will be cultured in infants or children with a chronic systemic disease. Therapy consists of continuous tap water or saline compresses for one to three days to effect localization of infection and promote drainage. Incision and drainage may be necessary, however; with soaking and systemic antibiotic therapy (noted in the discussion of impetigo and furuncle), most lesions will heal completely over a 5- to 10-day period. If these measures are ineffective, repeat cultures should be performed, including fungal cultures for Candida.

CELLULITIS

Cellulitis, an acute inflammation of the skin and subcutaneous tissues, may be differentiated clinically from *erysipelas,* a superficial cellulitis of the skin with marked perilymphangitis. Group A (rarely G) beta-hemolytic streptococci and, very rarely, hemolytic *S. aureus* are the etiologic agents. The main difference between the two diseases is the margin of the lesion: in erysipelas, a raised, sharply demarcated advancing edge of inflammation is seen; in cellulitis, an indistinct, nonelevated area of acute inflammation blends with adjacent uninvolved skin. Erysipelas tends to occur most commonly in infants and very young children. Erysipelas tends to be self-limited with clearing over a 7- to 10-day period, whereas cellulitis spreads rapidly and sepsis may occur. Adequate and early administration of penicillin in the dosage noted for impetigo will be most effective. Bicillin Long-Acting Injection should suffice for the older child unless extensive lesions are present. Bicillin C-R Injection (600,000 units procaine penicillin, 600,000 units benzathine penicillin G) should be effective in young children or infants. If *S. aureus* resistant to penicillin is recovered, dicloxacillin, 12.5 to 50 mg. per kilogram per day orally in divided doses every 6 hours for 10 days, is effective. In serious infections, begin with 50 mg. per kilogram per day. Rarely, in a young child acute *Hemophilus influenzae* cellulitis (bluish-purple) will be seen involving the face or an extremity. After appropriate cultures, ampicillin, 150 mg. per kilogram per day in divided doses every 4 to 6 hours, should be given intravenously initially. Treatment should be given for 7 to 10 afebrile days.

TOXIC EPIDERMAL NECROLYSIS

Toxic epidermal necrolysis (Ritter-Lyell) is an acute painful generalized erythema with vesicobullae and intraepidermal peeling closely resembling scalded skin. This syndrome in children has been expanded by Melish and Glasgow to include Ritter's and Lyell's diseases, scarlatiniform eruption (staphylococcal scarlet fever) and bullous impetigo of infancy. Those authors consider all four diseases to be variants of the staphylococcal scalded skin syndrome. The first three disorders have generalized cutaneous involvement; bullous impetigo is usually localized. In all disorders, beta-hemolytic *S. aureus* can usually be isolated from the nose, throat, conjunctivae or skin. Bullae are usually sterile, since they result from an exfoliative exotoxin produced by *S. aureus.* We isolated *S. aureus* in 82 per cent of cases (37 of 45 children) observed at Children's Hospital of D.C. over a five-year period. The staphylococci are usually phage type, group II, and are reported as penicillin-resistant. In our series only 50 per cent of the *S. aureus* were resistant to penicillin.

Management of mild cases, especially the older infant or child, consists of thorough washing of lesions using pHisoHex, two or three times daily, with removal of excess hexachlorophene by rinsing; 0.1 per cent gentamicin cream, or bacitracin ointment, 500 units per Gm., especially for dry skin; and close observation by parents and physician. For moderate or severe cases, especially young infants, hospitalization is mandatory. Patients are placed in reverse isolation; penicillin or dicloxacillin or both are started (in doses noted in the discussion of cellulitis) after appropriate cultures are taken; fluids, electrolytes and temperature are monitored carefully; and lesions are washed thoroughly with a hexachlorophene soap three times daily. pHisoHex should not be used on extensively denuded areas, especially in neonates. Steroids are contraindicated. If lesions are extensive, compresses of sterile water or normal saline, to which 0.1 per cent silver nitrate has been added, will be effective. When antibiotic sensitivity results are known, the appropriate antibiotic should be continued for five to seven afebrile days. Recovery in most cases is complete in 9 or 10 days or less. Tepid baths twice daily followed by application of Cold Cream U.S.P. will be effective for dry skin in the healing phase. Sulfacetamide sodium solution, Bleph-10 or Bleph-30, 100 to 300 mg. per ml., or ointment, 100 mg. per Gm., applied four times a day is effective for conjunctivitis. Prognosis is excellent for patients under five years of age; death has been reported in 0 to 7 per cent of cases. We experienced one death in 39 patients; however, this patient had Pseudomonas cultured from the skin and blood both pre- and postmortem; steroid therapy was used.

HUMAN BITE

Management of a wound from a human bite depends on the nature of the wound, and the time elapsed between the bite and the physician's treatment. An accurate history of the circumstances and careful examination of the child and wound quickly determine the necessary therapy.

If the wound is minimal and is limited to a minor abrasion and contusion, thorough scrubbing with surgical soap (Betadine) or pHisoHex followed by a tetanus toxoid booster should suffice. Thereafter, parents should be instructed to watch closely for signs of inflammation or wound infection. If these occur, parenteral penicillin therapy should be started in addition to continuous moist compresses or soaks using tap water or saline solution.

In view of the contamination by bacterial flora of the mouth, scrupulous cleansing is essential for more extensive wounds. Wounds of the hand, especially those of the knuckles which were inflicted by teeth during a scuffle, must be carefully debrided. To facilitate debridement, a bloodless field may be effected by application of a tourniquet. If the child is uncooperative, sedation with chloral hydrate (50 mg. per kilogram per dose orally or rectally not to exceed 1 Gm. per dose) or a short-acting barbiturate (6 mg. per kilogram intramuscularly or rectally) may be necessary. Wet dressings of saline solution facilitate good drainage, and splinting of the involved part aids healing. Primary wound closure is not advised for human bites. If no evidence of infection has appeared after two or three days of careful observation, secondary closure may be performed.

If the wound is a penetrating or puncture type, or is deep and has devitalized tissue, particularly if soil or fragments of clothing are embedded, penicillin and a 0.5-ml. booster of fluid tetanus toxoid should be given. One injection of benzathine penicillin G (600,000 units for patients under 60 pounds; 1,200,000 units for those over 60 pounds) is sufficient. Erythromycin orally, 40 mg. per kilogram per day, given every 6 hours for one to three weeks, is equally effective for patients sensitive to penicillin. If this therapy is administered within 24 hours of injury, the use of antitoxin is unnecessary in most previously immunized persons.

In instances of extensive wounds in the presence of chronic debilitation or shock, antitoxin may be indicated. If the period is over 24 hours, especially if the patient has not had his basic series of tetanus toxoid, all three therapies (penicillin, fluid toxoid, human antitoxin) are necessary. Human tetanus antitoxin is given intramuscularly in a dose of 250 units regardless of weight. The toxoid and antitoxin should be injected at different sites using separate syringes. In highly contaminated wounds the dose of human antitoxin should be doubled. If a toxoid series had not previously been given, it is mandatory that two or more doses of toxoid (either fluid or alum) be given at four-week intervals and followed by a booster in 12 months.

One must never rely on the use of penicillin alone as a substitute for antitoxin, nor a toxoid booster, since tetanus has been known to occur in such cases apparently because of penicillin-resistant strains.

References

Fruste, W., Skudder, P. A., and Hampton, O. P., Jr.: Prophylaxis Against Tetanus in Wound Management. *J. Trauma,* 6:516, 1966.

Margileth, A. M., et al.: Streptococcal surveillance during April through October 1972. *Clin. Proc. Child. Hosp. Nat. Med. Ctr.,* 29:71, 1973.

Swartz, M. N., and Weinberg, A. N.: Infections Due to Gram-Positive Bacteria; in T. B. Fitzpatrick et al. (eds.): *Dermatology in General Medicine.* New York, McGraw-Hill Book Company, 1971, p. 1963.

Fungous Diseases

GAVIN HILDICK-SMITH, M.D.

CANDIDIASIS

Candidal infection in children can be associated with disease processes such as malnutrition, neoplastic diseases and diabetes mellitus, and every effort should be made to control these disorders. In addition, local factors, such as eczema, hyperhidrosis, maceration and damage to the skin, are commonly associated with candidal infection and should be corrected in the management of local candidal infection.

Intertriginous Candidal Infection

As pathogenic Candida species proliferate on the skin surface, they can be effectively treated by the topical application of preparations containing anticandidal agents, with lotions being used on exudative acute lesions, creams and ointments on drier lesions.

The topical application of nystatin (Mycostatin Cream or Ointment), amphotericin B (Fungizone Ointment or Cream), candicidin (Candeptin lotion, ointment or cream) or preparations containing glucocorticosteroids (Mycolog Cream or Ointment, Neo-Nysta-Cort Ointment) three or four times a day readily controls the infection. Other preparations containing anticandidal compounds can be used topically in the treatment of cutaneous candidiasis, but in general they are less effective than topically applied nystatin or amphotericin B. Such preparations are Vioform-Hydrocortisone and gentian violet.

In acute exudative lesions, amphotericin B or candicidin lotion is applied three or four times a day until the lesion is controlled, and products containing corticosteroids, such as Mycolog Lotion, readily control the inflammatory lesion.

Culture of the lesion under therapy for Candida species and examination of scrapings for mycelia indicate when the pathogen has been eradicated from the lesion and when medication can be withdrawn.

In some instances of cutaneous candidal infection, early withdrawal of therapy results in a relapse of infections; thus, medication should be administered initially for at least seven days, with a longer period of therapy indicated when relapse has occurred. In addition to the use of specific medication, consideration must be given to means of eradicating Candida species from other body sites, such as the vagina or intestinal tract. Oral administration of nystatin, one tablet three times a day, eliminates the organism from the bowel, with local daily or twice daily use of nystatin vaginal suppositories usually controlling the vaginitis. Correction of general and local factors predisposing to candidiasis or diseases associated with candidal infection must also be corrected when possible.

Nystatin is not absorbed from the intestinal tract and as such is ineffective when given orally for cutaneous infection. The topical application of nystatin or amphotericin B is singularly free of toxic manifestations, with local discomfort being occasionally reported and sensitization rarely encountered.

Candidal Diaper Dermatitis

Initially the diaper area must be kept dry, with moist diapers changed as soon as they are soiled. The topical application of nystatin, amphotericin B or candicidin (lotion or cream) two or three times a day for 7 to 10 days readily controls infection.

In acute lesions the concomitant local application of preparations containing nystatin or amphotericin B with glucocorticosteroids (Mycolog Cream or Lotion, Fungizone Lotion) rapidly controls the inflammatory lesion.

Candidal Paronychia

Paronychia in children is usually caused by a mixed infection of the area around the nail base, with Candida species frequently present. The lesion may be associated with excessive exposure of the hands to moisture. In association with specific therapy every effort must be made to keep the area as dry as possible.

In addition, chronic candidal paronychial infection is often associated with generalized superficial cutaneous infection or candidal infection of the bowel or mouth. In such cases every effort should be made to eliminate pathogenic Candida species from the intestine by oral administration of nystatin, one tablet three times a day, with the generalized form of candidal infection being treated with topical nystatin ointment or, if this fails, with intravenously administered amphotericin B.

Ointments, creams or lotions containing nystatin or amphotericin B should be applied topically three or four times a day until the lesion has resolved and the site is free of pathogenic Candida species. The concomitant local application of preparations containing neomycin helps control the local bacterial infection.

Generalized Cutaneous Candidiasis

The cutaneous candidal infection in generalized cutaneous Candida infection does not usually respond to topical therapy but will respond to the intravenous use of amphotericin B. The infection, however, tends to recur, and repeated courses of intravenous amphotericin B therapy may be required to control the infection. The use of transfer factor should be considered in persistent cases. In some cases alterations of the function of adrenal, thyroid or parathyroid glands may be present and call for appropriate therapy.

Vaginal Candidiasis

Vaginal candidiasis can be associated with diabetes mellitus or candidal infection in other body sites. Vaginal candidiasis is treated by the use of nystatin or candicidin vaginal tablet introduced into the vagina twice daily for two weeks. The infection may recur, calling for a further course of therapy. In addition, in instances of relapse the elimination of Candida species from the stools is indicated and may be achieved by orally utilizing nystatin oral tablets (500,000 units), one to two tablets three times a day for seven days or until the stools are free of Candida species.

Oral Candidiasis (Thrush), Candidal Glossitis

Oral candidiasis is treated readily by instillation of 1 to 2 ml. of nystatin for suspension in the mouth three or four times a day for 10 to 14 days, depending on the local response. The lesion usually responds to this form of therapy, but relapse is not uncommon and calls for a further course of medication. Other forms of therapy, such as the local application of gentian violet, are less effective than nystatin, and can discolor skin and clothing.

Gastrointestinal Candidiasis

The oral administration of 1 or 2 ml. of nystatin suspension three or four times a day for 10 to 14 days usually controls gastrointestinal candidiasis. In the older child, one or two nystatin tablets is administered three times a day for 10 days.

Repeated culture of the stools reveals the presence of Candida species, and medication may be withdrawn when the pathogen has been eradicated.

Systemic Candidiasis

In systemic candidiasis or candidal infection of the central nervous system, kidney, heart or other organs, intravenous amphotericin therapy is indicated. The instructions supplied by the manufacturer for administration should be closely followed.

Therapy is withdrawn when the pathogen is eradicated from the site of the infection or when the patient can no longer tolerate medication. The oral use of flucytosine (Ancobon) is advised if amphotericin B therapy is not successful.

DERMATOPHYTOSIS (RINGWORM INFECTIONS)

Tinea Capitis

Tinea capitis is caused by fungi, all of which are sensitive to griseofulvin. Orally administered griseofulvin is therefore the specific treatment for tinea capitis, with optimal therapeutic results obtained by daily oral administration. A daily oral dose of 250 mg. of microcrystalline griseofulvin (Grifulvin, Grisactin, Fulvicin) given to children up to 10 years, or 500 mg. a day in older children, should ensure a cure in most patients in four to eight weeks. In order to minimize the risk of cross infection by viable organisms present in the outgrowing hair, it is desirable to cut the hair short and apply topically each day antifungal preparations such as Whitfield's Ointment, tolnaftate (Tinactin Cream or Solution) or Desenex Ointment. For patients who fail to respond to an adequate therapeutic regimen, consideration must be given to points such as failure to take the medication, inadequate blood levels because of poor absorption and resistance of the infecting organism to the antibiotic.

Administration of the antibiotic two to three times a day in association with a high fat intake enhances absorption and therapeutic results. In cases of tinea capitis in which daily administration of griseofulvin is not practical, satisfactory therapeutic results have been obtained when the griseofulvin was administered either as one single large dose or in weekly doses.

One gram of regular griseofulvin given orally once a week, combined with topically applied keratinolytic medication (Whitfield's Ointment), cured 95 per cent of children infected with *T. violaceum* in six weeks. A single 3-Gm. dose of regular griseofulvin in conjunction with a daily application of Whitfield's Ointment cured 81 per cent of cases in four weeks, whereas this therapy cured only 50 per cent of children infected with *T. tonsurans* in a period of four weeks. Griseofulvin medication can be discontinued when clinical evidence of infection has disappeared, fluorescence is no longer present and repeated negative cultures are obtained.

Available data indicate that the microcrystalline form of griseofulvin is absorbed twice as readily from the bowel as the regular type of antibiotic, with concomitant oral administration of a high fat diet enhancing absorption of both forms. The administration of griseofulvin is singularly free of adverse reactions, which, when encountered, can present in the form of headache, nausea or vomiting. The use of the antibiotic is contraindicated in patients suffering from porphyria.

Tinea Corporis

Glabrous skin infection caused by dermatophytic fungi can be effectively treated by daily or twice daily topical application of antifungal preparations such as tolnaftate (Tinactin), cream or solution; haloprogin (Halotex), cream or solution; or miconazole cream (Daktarin).* Acute weeping lesions are treated with a lotion while creams are used on chronic lesions.

Tinea versicolor and candidal infection do not respond to oral griseofulvin therapy, and topical medicaments used in the treatment of dermatophyte infection are not effective in the treatment of candidal infection.

Tinea Cruris, Tinea Pedis and Tinea Manuum

The dermatophytes are causative organisms in most cases of tinea cruris and in some cases of tinea infection of the feet, with the latter lesion being most commonly caused by a mixed bacterial infection. The infection responds to local therapy with topically applied antifungal preparations such as haloprogin, miconazole or tolnaftate cream or solution, Desenex Ointment or Whitfield's Ointment.

In acute lesions, the topical application of tolnaftate or Desenex lotion two or three times a day, in combination with topical applications two to three times daily of glucocorticosteroids such as triamcinolone (Kenacort or Kenalog Lotion, Synalar or Decadron Ointments), rapidly controls the inflammatory process.

The topical application of tolnaftate, haloprogin, miconazole or Desenex Ointment two or three times a day usually controls infections in 2 to 10 weeks with clearing of the lesion, procurement of negative cultures from the lesion being indicative of the time for withdrawal of medication.

Tolnaftate, miconazole and haloprogin are efficacious against the dermatophytes when applied topically but have no value in the treatment of candidal infections. The topical application is singularly free of toxic manifestations, with local irritation occasionally encountered and sensitization rarely seen.

Because the fungal infection can recur, the daily prophylactic use of talc dusting powders alone or dusting powders containing antifungal agents, such as Desenex Powder, is indicated, with every effort being made to minimize local trauma and reduce hydration of the skin by wearing appropriately light, nonabrasive clothing and by maintaining good local hygiene.

Onychomycosis

Oral administration of griseofulvin cures most cases of nail infection due to dermatophytes, provided a satisfactory dose is given for a sufficient period. In small children a daily oral dose of 250 mg. of microcrystalline griseofulvin should be administered, with a dose of 500 mg. given daily in children over 10 years. The fingernails are usually cured in three to four months, with the toenails taking 6 to 12 months to cure. In patients failing to respond to therapy, evulsion of the nail with twice daily topical therapy with tolnaftate, administered in association with the oral administration of griseofulvin, is usually effective.

Tinea Versicolor

Tinea versicolor can be treated by the topical application of tolnaftate to the lesion two or three times each day until the lesion is cleared. However, the disease responds readily to application twice daily of 10 to 25 per cent aqueous solution of sodium thiosulfate, with cure obtained in two to four weeks.

FUNGAL INFECTION OF THE EYE

A wide variety of fungi can cause infection of the eye, and in all cases it is important to isolate and identify the pathogenic organism prior to treatment and to culture the lesion regularly during treatment, so that medication can be continued until the organism has been eradicated.

Keratomycosis

The local application of nystatin or amphotericin B is the treatment of choice in fungal infections of the cornea.

Amphotericin B has been introduced into the conjunctival sac initially at 1- to 2-hour intervals in a concentration of 1 to 4 mg. per 1 ml. of distilled water or 5 per cent dextrose in water.

Nystatin in a concentration of 10,000 to 20,000 units in 1 ml. of normal saline given at 1- to 2-hour intervals is also effective in controlling keratomycosis.

Therapy should be continued until the lesion is cleared and is free of the invading fungus.

Chorioretinitis

Fungal retinochoroiditis is occasionally seen in association with systemic fungal diseases such as histoplasmosis, and in such cases intravenous administration of amphotericin B is indicated.

FUNGAL INFECTION OF THE EAR

Mycotic Otitis

In the treatment of fungal external otitis it is important initially to clear the external canal of debris manually or by local instillation of 2 per cent thymol in 70 per cent alcohol. The local application of amphotericin B or

* Not available in the United States.

candicidin cream or lotion twice daily or nystatin ointment three or four times a day eradicates the fungi.

In cases caused by Aspergillus species, physical removal of fungal material, followed by insufflation of iodochlorhydroxyquin powder and application three times daily of iodochlorhydroxyquin lotion, is usually effective in one to two weeks of therapy.

Because most infections are mixed, the associated use of antibacterial antibiotics is indicated, and the local application of agents such as neomycin, polymyxin and bacitracin eradicates sensitive bacteria. In cases in which inflammation is significant, local use of glucocorticosteroids is indicated. In rare cases the lesion is caused by fungi sensitive to griseofulvin, in which case the oral administration of this antibiotic controls the infection.

Fungal Otitis Media

Fungal infection of the middle ear is treated by local application twice daily of amphotericin B or insufflation of iodochlorhydroxyquin powder twice daily. In cases that do not respond to this therapy, consideration should be given to the use of amphotericin B intravenously.

SYSTEMIC MYCOTIC DISEASES

The intravenous administration of amphotericin B is the first-order drug in treating systemic fungal disease. If amphotericin B therapy fails, oral flucytosine should be tried. The oral administration of amphotericin B or nystatin is ineffective owing to the failure of absorption of these antibiotics from the gastrointestinal tract.

Intravenous Administration of Amphotericin B. Because most systemic mycoses respond to the intravenous use of amphotericin B, a description of its method of use is indicated.

The antibiotic should be given only under close medical supervision and the manufacturer's instructions for use closely followed. Its success depends not only on the skill and tenacity of the physician but also on the fortitude and cooperation of the patient.

Intravenous amphotericin B is administered in a concentration of 1 mg. per 10 ml. of 5 per cent dextrose injection U.S.P. (pH above 5.0), utilizing an initial intravenous dose of 0.25 mg. per kilogram administered over a period of 6 hours. The dose is then gradually raised to the average optimal dose of 1 mg. per kilogram, with the maximal daily dose never exceeding 1.5 mg. per kilogram. The initial doses are given daily, with alternate-day administration instituted when the optimal dosage level is reached, and with all doses being given over a 6-hour period. Rapid administration of the antibiotic must be avoided, because the drug may produce convulsions, anaphylaxis, hypotension and cardiac fibrillation or arrest.

During intravenous therapy the amphotericin B solution should be gently agitated every 15 to 30 minutes to avoid precipitation of the drug, and the solution should be protected from light. Because the intravenous needle may become obstructed, a Y tube or three-way stopcock should be used so that the needle can be flushed or small amounts of medication administered. Heparin or the sodium succinate ester of hydrocortisone may be added to the infusion fluid to reduce the fever, chills and rigor that may occur.

Adverse reactions are encountered in most patients in association with medication, which usually consist of fever, chills, headache, nausea and vomiting, all of which can be treated symptomatically. In some cases premedication with analgesics, chlorpromazine† and antihistaminics may be of value. During courses of medication, liver, kidney and hematopoietic system function should be studied at regular intervals, with blood urea, sodium and potassium concentrations as well as creatinine clearance studies obtained at weekly intervals.

If the blood urea nitrogen level rises to over 40 mg. per 100 ml., the drug should be discontinued for two to seven days until the level falls to normal. A 50 per cent reduction in creatinine clearance indicates significant renal damage, and medication should be withheld with treatment reinstated if the test returns to normal in two to three weeks' time. Temporary withdrawal of medication may be indicated in association with intractable nausea, vomiting and anorexia. If medication has been withdrawn for seven days or more, the dose should be restarted at a level of 0.25 mg. per kilogram per day to avoid the severe reactions that can arise under such conditions.

Therapy should be continued for one to three months. Medication is withdrawn when the patient shows no signs of infection and is free of the invading organism, cannot tolerate the medication or shows signs of significant impairment of renal function. The information supplied by the manufacturer should be carefully studied by the physician before initiating a course of intravenous amphotericin B.

INTRATHECAL ADMINISTRATION OF AMPHO-

† Manufacturer's precaution: Chlorpromazine is not recommended for children under six months of age except when lifesaving.

TERICIN B. In seriously ill patients suffering from fungal meningitis or infection of the central nervous system, the intrathecal administration of amphotericin B is indicated, with a view to rapidly controlling the infection. The administration of amphotericin B by other than intravenous means is still investigational.

Adult intrathecal therapy is initiated with a dose of 0.1 mg. and is increased to a dose of 0.5 mg. given every 48 to 72 hours, depending on the state of the patient and acceptance of medication. Three to 5 ml. of cerebrospinal fluid is withdrawn, and the antibiotic is dissolved in it prior to slow introduction of this solution into the intrathecal space. Transient urinary retention, hyporeflexia, paresthesia, paralysis and relaxation of sphincters may occur, as may local arachnoiditis and transient myelitis. These conditions are usually reversed on withdrawal of medication. The administration of amphotericin B intravenously in meningitis may be needed for one to three months to provide a cure.

Flucytosine (Ancobon) inhibits the growth of *Cryptococcus neoformans* and Candida species and may be of value in cases systemically infected by these organisms. The drug is given orally in a dose of 150 mg. per kilogram per day in divided amounts at 6-hour intervals. Medication is maintained for six weeks or until the infection is eradicated.

Actinomycosis

Actinomyces israeli, the causative organism of the disease, is sensitive to antibiotics effective against gram-positive bacteria. Penicillin is the treatment of choice, and it should be given in daily intramuscular doses of 1 to 6 million units to ensure adequate concentration of the antibiotic within the actinomycotic lesions. Therapy is maintained for 6 to 12 weeks to avoid relapse. In severe cases the dose of penicillin should be increased and the antibiotic given intravenously.

In patients sensitive to penicillin, broad-spectrum antibiotics, such as tetracycline, erythromycin or chloramphenicol, should be given orally in adequate dosage. Appropriate surgical procedures, such as drainage of abscess, should be combined with chemotherapy.

Coccidioidomycosis

Primary Coccidioidomycosis. Intravenous amphotericin B should be given to patients who are severely ill, all infants under one year and those who have a racial predilection for systemic disease, such as Negroes, Filipinos, American Indians and Spanish Americans. All cases should be followed for daily body temperature and three-weekly sedimentation rate and complement fixation levels. If the complement fixation level reaches a titer of 1:32 or higher dilution, disseminated disease is liable to occur and amphotericin B should be given intravenously.

Disseminated Coccidioidomycoses. All patients should be given bed rest and supportive care, and the titer of the complement fixation test should be obtained weekly.

Intravenous amphotericin B should be given daily or on alternate days in a maximal tolerated dose not to exceed 1.5 mg. per kilogram per day. The course of the infection is closely observed, and medication is given for three or more months until the disease is controlled.

Decrease in the complement fixation titer and failure to isolate the pathogen from sites of infection are indications of control of the infection. Surgical removal of pulmonary cavitary lesions should be considered when the cavity is expanding, hemorrhage occurs in a cavity or an asymptomatic cavity fails to close. Intravenous amphotericin B should be given before and after surgery with a view to minimizing the risk of disseminating the infecting organism.

Cryptococcosis

The diagnosis of cryptococcal infection in any site calls for the administration of amphotericin B. For investigation in some cases of meningitis initial administration of amphotericin B has been intrathecal in association with intravenous therapy. Medication is given until the pathogen is eradicated from the central nervous system, usually occurring in two to four months of therapy.

Histoplasmosis

Primary Infection. Primary pulmonary histoplasmosis is usually a self-limiting disease in adults, but in children it is liable to progress to disseminated infection. Intravenous amphotericin B is accordingly recommended for use in children, with a short course of 7 to 21 days of therapy rapidly controlling the infection. Amphotericin B should be given to patients who are severely ill and those in whom the complement fixation titer reaches a dilution of 1:16, indicating the likelihood of disseminated infection.

Disseminated Disease. All patients with disseminated infection are treated with intravenous amphotericin B, given in the maximal tolerated dose for one to two months.

Mucormycosis

Because the disease is often rapidly progressive, intravenous amphotericin B therapy should be instituted without delay and maintained until the infection is controlled. Infection by Mucor species is often associated with poorly controlled diabetes mellitus, and every effort should be made to stabilize patients with this disease.

Nocardiosis

In cases of nocardiosis, the infecting organism should be isolated and its in vitro sensitivity to amphotericin B, penicillin, broad-spectrum antibiotics and sulfonamides determined. The appropriate antibiotics to which the organism is sensitive should be given in the maximal tolerated doses, with the clinical course of the patient closely followed. In addition, sulfonamide as sulfadiazine or sulfisoxazole (Gantrisin) should be given, 0.1 to 0.15 Gm. per kilogram, in daily divided doses for three to six months. Supportive measures should be provided for the patient and surgery utilized for removal or drainage of abscesses.

North American Blastomycosis

Blastomyces dermatitidis, the causative organism of North American blastomycosis, is sensitive to amphotericin B and hydroxystilbamidine. All patients with disseminated disease sould be initially treated with intravenous amphotericin B given for one to three months. In patients not able to tolerate or failing to respond to amphotericin B therapy, a course of hydroxystilbamidine is indicated. The total dose of 100 mg. per kilogram of hydroxystilbamidine should be given in divided daily doses over a 30-day period or in several shorter courses each of 10 to 14 days. Surgical procedures should be undertaken when indicated.

South American Blastomycosis (Paracoccidioidomycosis)

The oral administration of sulfonamides effectively suppresses infection by *Blastomyces brasiliensis.* If they are given for a sufficient period, cure of the infection may be obtained in half the patients treated. In disseminated cases, but not in premature or newborn infants, sulfadiazine or its analogues should be given every 6 hours in a total daily dose of 2 to 4 Gm. to ensure a blood level in excess of 5 mg. per 100 ml. The clinical course of the patient is closely followed; if improvement does not occur in one to two months of therapy, intravenous amphotericin B is given for one to three months, depending on the clinical response of the disease. Infection is liable to recur on withdrawal of medication, and a further course of amphotericin B is then indicated.

Sporotrichosis

Oral administration of potassium iodide is the treatment of choice in sporotrichosis. A saturated solution of potassium iodide is given orally in increasing doses, starting with 1 drop three times a day in a small child or 5 drops three times a day in a large child. The dose is increased by 1 to 3 drops per day until a final dose of 10 drops three times a day for a small child and 20 to 40 drops three times a day for a teenager is reached. A two- to three-week course controls the infection, but medication should be continued for one month more to avoid relapse.

A course of intravenous amphotericin B should be given initially in all cases of disseminated infection and in patients with primary lesions who cannot tolerate iodide therapy.

Surgical excision or incision of the lesion should be considered in appropriate cases.

References

Bindschadler, D. D., and Bennett, J. E.: A Pharmacologic Guide to the Clinical Use of Amphotericin. *Brit. J. Infect. Dis.,* 120:427, 1969.

Brugmans, J. P., van Cutsem, J. M., and Thienpont, D. C.: Treatment of Long-Term Tinea Pedis with Miconazole. *Arch. Derm.,* 102:428, 1970.

Carter, V. H.: A Controlled Study of Haloprogin and Tolnaftate in Tinea Pedis. *Curr. Ther. Res.,* 14: 307, 1972.

Epstein, W. L., et al.: Griseofulvin Levels in Stratum Corneum. Study After Oral Administration in Man. *Arch. Derm.,* 106:344, 1972.

Hildick-Smith, G., Blank, H., and Sarkany, I.: *Fungus Diseases and Their Treatment.* Boston, Little, Brown and Company, 1964.

Pabst, H. F., and Swanson, R.: Successful Treatment of Candidiasis with Transfer Factor. *Brit. Med. J.,* 2:442, 1972.

Vandevelde, A. G., et al.: 5-Fluorocytosine in the Treatment of Mycotic Infections. *Ann. Intern. Med.,* 77: 43, 1972.

Warts and Molluscum Contagiosum

ANDREW M. MARGILETH, M.D.

WARTS

Warts are among the most common blemishes and are not true nevi. The common wart (verruca vulgaris), flat juvenile wart (verruca plana juvenilis), filiform and plantar warts frequently disappear spontaneously. Verbal suggestion combined with monetary reimbursement for each one that disappears will hasten regression. Within one or two months about 44 per cent of common warts and 88 per cent of juvenile flat warts disappear with suggestion therapy.

If suggestion therapy is ineffective, topical application of keratolytics is advised and does not produce scarring. Application of 12 per cent salicylic acid in flexible collodion twice daily or careful application of a 40 per cent salicylic acid plaster (Duke's) cut to the exact size of the wart is effective, especially for plantar warts. The plaster is held in place for 24 to 48 hours with adhesive tape. The wart is trimmed before plaster is reapplied. If inflammation occurs, a two- or three-day waiting period is indicated. If these methods are ineffective, cryotherapy by a dermatologist is advisable.

MOLLUSCUM CONTAGIOSUM

Molluscum contagiosum is a mildly contagious viral dermatosis characterized by waxy papules of varying sizes with umbilicated centers. One application of 0.7 per cent cantharidin in collodion with a toothpick (to avoid blistering normal skin) usually suffices. After this dries (5 to 10 seconds), plastic tape is used to cover the lesion for about 12 hours. Within a day or so a blister forms, and the lesion may be scraped off. Since some children react with a large blister, it is advisable to treat only two or three lesions at the initial visit. An alternative is to remove the lesion with a sharp curet, or to freeze for 15 to 60 seconds with liquid nitrogen.

HERPESVIRUS INFECTIONS

See p. 643.

Treatment of Arthropod Bites and Stings

VINCENT J. DERBES, M.D.

For management (both prophylactic and therapeutic) of hypersensitivity reactions, see page 749.

CHIGGERS

Materials used for personal protection against chiggers function less as true repellents than as toxicants; they provide the best protection when applied to the clothing, but if inadequate clothing is worn, it may be necessary to treat the skin also. The good mosquito repellents diethyltoluamide (OFF, Meta-Delphene, Detamide), ethyl hexanediol (6–12, Rutgers 612, Octylene glycol, ethohexadiol) and dimethyl phthalate (Palatinol M, Fermine, Mipax, Avolin, DMP) are good chigger toxicants. Benzyl benzoate will withstand more wear than these and will even withstand immersion in water. Clear fingernail polish applied to the chigger bites often produces immediate relief. Antihistamines and steroids are also useful.

SCABIES

After a soaking soap-and-water bath to remove scaling and crusting detritus, an efficient scabicide is applied to the total body surface. Such agents are 1 per cent lindane (Kwell) cream or lotion; 10 per cent crotonotoluide (Eurax) cream or lotion; and 12 per cent benzyl benzoate, 2 per cent benzocaine and 1 per cent DDT (Topocide emulsion). Other trade names for benzyl benzoate preparations are Ascabin, Ascabiol, Benylate, Vanzoate and Venzonate.

LARVA MIGRANS

Classic treatment damages the skin with caustic agents (such as trichloroacetic acid) or cold (dry ice or ethyl chloride spray), so that a bleb is formed which contains the worm, thus separating it from the host. This treatment, while effective, is too traumatic for heavily infected cases. The treatment of choice is with thiabendazole (Mintezol), 50 mg. per kilogram of body weight daily for two to three days. Topical application of thiabendazole has also been reported to be beneficial.

SPIDERS

Recluse. The best treatment is administration of corticosteroids in the first 6 to 12 hours; later, antibiotic drugs are used, as well as surgery when needed. Corticosteroids should be given promptly in large doses (60 to 100 mg. of prednisone or its equivalent daily, since they may be of value in aborting or treating early systemic symptoms. Antibiotics prevent invasive infection and are essential. Antihistaminic drugs fail to prevent local necrosis. Healing cannot occur until the gangrenous tissue separates, spontaneously or by surgical débridement. Most minor bites heal with office management. Excision is not advised until necrosis appears inevitable, that is, two to five days. Excision should include all the necrotic tissue but not the widespread erythematous skin. Closure of wounds is often delayed because of indolent chronic infection which must be treated with appropriate antibiotics. Primary or secondary wound closure is feasible in some patients. Split thickness grafts are essential for large wounds or for wounds in the distal parts of the extremities where the skin is not elastic or mobile.

Black Widow. Treatment has consisted of narcotics for relief of pain and a muscle relaxant for relief of spasm. Methocarbamol (Robaxin) is thought to be of more benefit than 10 per cent calcium gluconate and produces more prolonged relief of symptoms. Methocarbamol can be administered intravenously, 10 ml. over a 5-minute period, with a second ampule in a saline solution drip. Specific treatment is the use of antivenin Lyovac (*Lactrodectus mactans*), which is available in a dried preparation with separate diluent. The preparation is stable for many years. The antivenin is administered intramuscularly after appropriate skin tests have been made, since it contains normal horse serum.

SCHISTOSOME

Since the disease is relatively brief and self-limiting, treatment is symptomatic. Antipruritic medications or lotions are usually adequate. An inexpensive, widely useful antipruritic lotion consists of 0.1 per cent betamethasone valerate cream (Valisone Cream) 15 Gm., glycerine 15 Gm. and water to 120 ml. Label it: Shake well and apply four or five times daily. If urticaria appears, antihistaminic drugs may be worthwhile.

BEES

For the most part, stings from hymenopters do not demand or receive much attention. Local applications of antipruritic shake lotions, and cool compresses or cool baths usually suffice, although antihistaminic drugs have definite value. Should there be conspicuous edema, epinephrine alone or supplemented by corticosteroids may be employed.

FLEAS

Treatment of flea bites and of papular urticaria follows the usual rules of topical and systemic anti-inflammation therapy. In the case of *Tunga penetrans,* surgical removal of the intact flea is recommended. This consists of slightly enlarging the entrance hole of the flea by means of a sterile needle, followed by gentle pressure on the sides of the aperture. The entire flea thus is forced out. The wound then is cleansed and an antiseptic dressing applied.

LICE

Benzyl benzoate and Topocide Liquid may be used for head and crab lice. To treat body lice effectively, clothing must be sterilized by boiling or by use of a hot iron, especially over seams. Clothing may be disinfected also by the use of steam under pressure. Mass delousing of troops, prisoners, refugees and civilians can be carried out successfully by simply blowing DDT powder under the clothing with a hand dust gun.

Melanin Pigmentary Disorders

ALVIN H. JACOBS, M.D.

HYPERPIGMENTATION

Café au lait spots are light tan spots of various sizes and with regular borders. They are usually of no significance and need no treatment. However, it is said that a patient with six or more such spots greater than 1.5 cm. in diameter may be assumed to have neurofibromatosis. Café au lait spots also occur commonly with Albright's disease and tuberous sclerosis.

Freckles are small, light-brown circumscribed macules which occur in response to exposure to sun. Depigmentation treatment as described below is inadvisable in the case of freckles.

Lentigines are small dark-brown macules which are not related to sun exposures and, in fact, are more common on unexposed parts of the body. Generalized lentigines in association with cardiac abnormalities have been described as the generalized lentigines syndrome. Treatment of the lentigines is not necessary, nor is it successful if attempted.

Melasma is a patchy, tan-to-brown pigmentation located predominantly on the cheeks and forehead of girls or women who are pregnant or who are taking oral contraceptives. In dark-skinned persons with much exposure to sun, melasma can be a serious cosmetic problem, and one may wish to consider depigmentation treatment (described below).

Postinflammatory hyperpigmentation may occur following subsidence of erythema due to any type of inflammation. This fades slowly over a period of months, but in dark-skinned individuals the fading is slower and depigmentation treatment as described below may be necessary.

Moles (nevus-cell nevi) are discussed under Nevi and Nevoid Tumors (page 500).

Agents to Decrease Pigmentation. Two per cent hydroquinone is an inhibitor of melanin formation. This agent, in a washable base, is rubbed thoroughly into the hyperpigmented area twice daily.* After the ointment has been applied, exposure to sunlight should be avoided.

* Manufacturer's precaution: Hydroquinone should not be used in children under 12 years of age.

It is often advisable to cover the treated area with an opaque sunscreen, such as A-Fil cream.

Hydroquinone treatment should not be used for management of freckles, but is quite useful for melasma and for larger areas of post-inflammatory hyperpigmentation.

HYPOPIGMENTATION

Albinism is a rare congenital disturbance (failure of the skin to form melanin pigment) which results from an enzymatic defect in the melanocyte. The most significant result of this absence of melanin is a strong hypersensitivity to light. There is no therapy other than prophylactic measures aimed at the light hypersensitivity. These patients must learn to avoid sunlight exposure and to use sunscreen preparations on exposed surfaces. A-Fil cream, PreSun, and Pabafilm are among the better sunscreening agents.

Vitiligo is an acquired cutaneous achromia characterized by variously sized and shaped single or multiple patches of milk-white color, usually with hyperpigmented borders and a tendency to enlarge peripherally. The skin presents no textural changes and is normal in every way except for a sensitivity to solar radiation. Some patients report some repigmentation from the border and in small perifollicular patches on exposure to sunlight in the summer, but disappearance of the repigmented areas in the winter.

Treatment of vitiligo is generally not very satisfactory. Cosmetic improvement can be achieved by staining the patches of vitiligo with Dy-O-Derm. This dye is applied to affected areas daily, after the bath, until the desired degree of staining is attained. Thereafter, one application every fourth to seventh day is sufficient. Since the dye cannot be washed off, it must be accurately applied to the lesion.

In some patients, repigmentation can be accomplished by oral administration of the psoralen compounds followed by gradually increasing exposure to the sun. The newest and apparently safest of these drugs is trimethylpsoralen (Trisoralen). The daily dosage is 10 mg., followed in 2 to 4 hours by measured periods of ultraviolet light. This treatment must be carried out daily for prolonged periods in order to maintain pigmentation. Sunlight is more effective than artificial ultraviolet irradiation, but must be taken cautiously with increasing exposures in order to avoid severe burns.

Repigmentation may begin after a few weeks; however, significant results may take as long as nine months and may require maintenance dosage to retain new pigment. If perifollicular repigmentation is not apparent after three months of daily treatment, the drug should be discontinued as a failure. To date, the manufacturer notes, the safety of Trisoralen has not been established in young persons (12 and under), and its use is therefore contraindicated.

Small, localized areas of vitiligo may be repigmented by intradermal injections of triamcinolone acetonide. The solution for injection is prepared by mixing in the syringe one part of triamcinolone acetonide (Kenalog, parenteral, 10 mg. per ml.) with three parts 1 per cent lidocaine (Xylocaine). Depending on the size of the area to be treated, 0.2 to 2 ml. of the mixture may be injected from one or several points so that the entire lesion is infiltrated. Injections should be given at two- to four-week intervals but should be terminated if no repigmentation has appeared after four treatments. Warning must be given that a temporary atrophy may supervene.

White macules exist in more than 90 per cent of patients with tuberous sclerosis when no other visible lesions typical of the disorder are evident. These hypopigmented macules are present at birth but may not be very obvious in fair-skinned infants and so must be looked for with a Wood's lamp. No treatment of the macule is necessary, but this clue should alert one to the possible future development of other manifestations of tuberous sclerosis.

Leukoderma is a patchy depigmentation usually occurring as a result of many inflammatory dermatoses and skin injuries and is frequently preceded by hyperpigmentation. These postinflammatory leukodermas are generally transient and decrease with time. Treatment should be directed only to the primary dermatosis.

An interesting type of leukoderma is the "halo nevus," or leukoderma acquisitum centrifugum. Here, a brown mole becomes surrounded by a depigmented halo that has all the earmarks of vitiligo and may be associated with vitiliginous patches in the same patient. Usually the central nevus also becomes depigmented and disappears completely. The halo nevus should not be treated, since it clears spontaneously in time.

Photodermatoses

ISAAC WILLIS, M.D.

These disorders manifest as either quantitative or qualitative abnormalities in the skin's response to sunlight or artificial light exposure. To date, nearly 40 etiologically different types of photodermatoses have been described.* For practical purposes these disorders may be classified into two groups: (1) direct photodermatoses, which are the cutaneous and sometimes systemic responses that follow overexposure to light in any normal, healthy individual, and (2) indirect photodermatoses, which require the presence of some other either endogenous or exogenous etiologic factor in combination with light exposure for clinical manifestation.

DIRECT PHOTODERMATOSES

Sunburn. The management of this disorder is essentially the same as that for a first- or second-degree burn due to other etiologic factors (e.g., thermal, electrical or chemical). For a first-degree type of sunburn, in which there is mainly erythema, tenderness and mild pain, treatment should consist of cold water or saline compresses for 20 minutes every 6 hours followed by the application of a low-strength corticosteroid cream or ointment such as 0.01 per cent Synalar, 0.025 per cent Kenalog or Aristocort, or Valisone. Aspirin in dosages of 1¼ grains every 4 hours in infants, to 5 grains every 4 hours in teenage individuals can be used to alleviate tenderness and pain. Within about 72 to 96 hours, the damaged portion of the epidermis will begin to desquamate, and at this time only a lubricating bath oil, such as Alpha-Keri or Domol, will be needed until the skin returns to normal. For treatment of a more severe sunburn in which blistering occurs, cold compresses may be applied more frequently, and the frequency of corticosteroid applications may be increased to every 3 or 4 hours until symptoms subside. In addition, either the dosage or frequency of aspirin administration may need to be increased. When severe sunburn is extensive, it may be necessary to hospitalize or closely supervise the patient in order to combat excess fluid and electrolyte loss, and constitutional signs and symptoms of systemic toxicity. In some cases it may be advantageous to administer systemic corticosteroids as soon as possible (infants, 15 to 30 mg. per day; toddlers, 30 to 40 mg. per day; children, 40 to 60 mg. per day of prednisone in three to four divided doses) and then to taper the dosage over a five- to seven-day period. Prevention and treatment of infections that may occur when bullae become denuded are important in the management of severe sunburns. Heat exhaustion due to the development of miliaria and the inability of the patient to sweat in damaged skin areas may be serious complications if the patient who has received a severe sunburn over a large surface area has not been instructed to avoid excessively hot environments for a few weeks after healing.

Chronic Actinic Damage. Except for a few normal rufous or blond individuals who receive chronic exposure to intense low-latitude sunlight, the majority of normal individuals in the pediatric age group will not show clinical signs of chronic actinic damage. However, the skin of many individuals with abnormalities that fall into the classification of heredodegenerative disorders (e.g., syndromes of Cockaynes and Rothmund-Thomson, Bloom's disease and xeroderma pigmentosum), the aminoacidurias (e.g., phenylketonuria, Hartnup disease, tryptophanuria, hydroxykynureninuria), depigmentary disturbances (e.g., albinism and vitiligo) and certain endogenously induced photosensitivity conditions will show chronic actinic damage. Early signs of damage include a change in the skin's texture with variable degrees of wrinkling, thinning and thickening, yellowing, pigmentary changes and scaling, followed by the development of premalignant keratoses and, finally, malignancies. In the early stages, several modalities of therapy, including cryosurgery with liquid nitrogen, chemosurgery using trichloroacetic acid or phenol, mechanical dermabrasion, and electrodesiccation with curettage, may be used. Chemotherapy, using 1 to 5 per cent fluorouracil (Efudex or Fluoroplex), to be applied on retiring, for 14 to 21 days is perhaps the easiest form of therapy to employ when benign and premalignant changes are present. Malignancies should be removed by surgical excision. An effective sunscreening formulation [such as PreSun or Pabanol which gives protection against short ultraviolet (UV) light] should be prescribed in the follow-up and management of these patients to minimize development of new lesions. Recent investigative findings indicate that sunscreens which protect against "photoaugmentative" long-wavelength UV (320 to 400 nanometers) should also be used in these patients. Sunscreens, such as Solbar and Uval,

* For a complete listing, one is referred to Willis, I.: Sunlight and the Skin. *J.A.M.A.*, 217:1088, 1971.

may accomplish this objective but should be applied after application of one of the short UV sunscreens listed above.

INDIRECT PHOTODERMATOSES

Phototoxic. Both the immediate type of reactions (due to such drugs as the tetracyclines, phenothiazines, thiazides, sulfonylureas, sulfonamides and griseofulvin) and the delayed reactions (due to furocoumarins such as the psoralens) clinically and pathologically resemble severe second-degree burns. Treatment is therefore similar to that outlined above for the management of severe sunburns. In addition, it is of utmost importance either to discontinue the offending drug or agent or to protect the patient from further phototoxic reactions by prescribing an appropriate long-wavelength as well as a short-wavelength UV sunscreen. Sunscreens such as Solbar, UVAL, and RVPaque (long UV sunscreens) are best applied after short UV sunscreens (PreSun or Pabanol) in order to accomplish this objective.

Photoallergy. This disorder resembles ordinary contact allergy, both clinically and histologically, and management depends on the clinical stage of the dermatitis, as follows:

Acute stage: (1) cool water or saline dressings for 20 minutes four times a day, followed by application of corticosteroid lotion (Synalar or Fluonid solutions); (2) antihistaminics (such as Benadryl elixir,† ½ teaspoon three times a day for children under 20 pounds, and 1 to 2 teaspoons three times a day for those over 20 pounds) to relieve itching; and (3) systemic prednisone (15 to 30 mg. per day for infants, to 40 to 60 mg. per day for older children) if the dermatitis is severe.

Subacute and chronic stages: (1) 0.025 per cent Synalar or comparable strength Kenalog, Valisone or Aristocort Cream four times a day; and (2) antihistaminics as outlined above. In recalcitrant cases good responses may be obtained by temporarily using high-potency corticosteroid creams such as Lidex, Synalar-HP or Aristocort-HP.

It is important to detect the photosensitizing chemical and to remove it and related chemicals from the patient's environment. Excessive light exposure should be prevented and the patient should use sunscreens as outlined above for management of phototoxicity.

Polymorphic Light Eruption. These chronic eruptions generally occur during the spring and summer and are most often caused by short UV rays. Therefore, management should include instructions to avoid exposure to sunlight, especially during the hours of 10 A.M. to 2 P.M. solar time, and to use PreSun or Pabanol sunscreens. Corticosteroid creams and antihistaminics used as outlined for the treatment of photocontact allergy may sometimes be needed to control the eruption.

Solar Urticaria. An important initial step in the management of these cases is the determination of their action spectra by means of phototesting. Then, the proper sunscreen or combination of sunscreens can be prescribed and tested for their effectiveness. Occasional benefits have been obtained with topical beta-carotene, psoralens, estrogens and quinine sulfate. The best responses have occurred with chloroquine, but its use is extremely risky in children. Therefore, the best form of management is the use of sunscreens (as outlined under phototoxicity) and antihistaminics such as Benadryl elixir.

Hydroa Aestivale. Fortunately, this vesiculobullous disorder is rare and it usually resolves either before or at puberty. Sunscreens such as Pabanol and PreSun, used alone or applied before UVAL or Solbar, will prevent or minimize its development. Topical corticosteroids are sometimes beneficial.

Xeroderma Pigmentosum. The skin of individuals with this heredodegenerative disorder eventually develop all of the changes described under Chronic Actinic Damage. Management is identical to that discussed for chronic actinic damage. Most important, one should be primarily concerned with the prevention of these changes by means of sunscreens as outlined under Phototoxicity, and by avoiding excessive and peak hour (10 A.M. to 2 P.M. solar time) exposure to sunlight.

Erythropoietic Protoporphyria. See page 370.

Lupus Erythematosus. See page 379.

Nevi and Nevoid Tumors

ANDREW M. MARGILETH, M.D.

In the following discussion a mole is defined as a localized proliferative aggregate of apparently normal melanocytes that usually appears after birth and apparently is hereditarily determined. A nevus is a localized proliferative malformation of melanocytes usually present at birth, congenitally derived and possibly hereditary. Clinically, nevi may be classified as pig-

† Manufacturer's precaution: Benadryl should not be used in premature and newborn infants.

mented, nonpigmented, vascular and nonvascular. Of the common moles and nevi in children, malignancy is rarely a consideration; therefore, excisional biopsy is indicated only in special instances.

The basic principle of management of moles and nevi is to avoid overzealous treatment so that tragic cosmetic results will not occur. One must obtain a detailed history; examine the lesion carefully with a magnifying lens, palpate and measure accurately. In cosmetically objectionable lesions a photograph is invaluable for subsequent reference. Repeat visits will facilitate deciding whether there is need for active therapy. The individual circumstances (such as appearance, location and rate of growth) in each case provide the best guidelines for continued observation or for the need for histopathologic examination or complete removal of the lesion. Consultation with a dermatologist will resolve most problems.

MELANOCYTIC TUMORS

Junctional, compound and *dermal* moles are classified by their histologic pattern in the skin. All the melanocytes are above the basement membrane in junctional moles; all the melanocytes are in the epidermis and dermis in compound moles; in a dermal mole (intradermal mole or nevus) all the melanocytes are in the dermis. These pigmented nevi may be found anywhere on the body surface. Their natural history, clinicopathologic evaluation and detailed management have been reviewed by Walton. The majority of moles require no therapy unless a sudden change occurs in growth or color, or bleeding or ulceration develops. Removal by simple or shave excision (Walton) will suffice for cosmetic reasons or for functional or anatomic reasons due to irritation, trauma and infection. Whatever method is used for removal, pathologic examination is mandatory.

Halo nevus, variously termed perinevoid vitiligo or leukoderma acquisitum centrifugum, is a pigmented mole (compound, intradermal) surrounded by a depigmented zone or halo. Single or multiple lesions are usually seen in children and located on the trunk. Treatment is rarely necessary, since eventually depigmentation will involve the central mole. The area of depigmentation also disappears gradually, but not always.

Giant hairy nevus (nevus pigmentosus et pilosus, bathing trunk nevus), present at birth, may be found anywhere on the body. The more extensive lesions involving the lower part of the trunk are commonly known as "bathing suit" nevi. Less commonly found lesions on the neck and scalp may be associated with leptomeningeal melanocytosis. Epilepsy or signs of focal neurologic abnormalities may be present. Complete excision with plastic reconstruction should be performed before puberty, since the lesions are associated with an increased incidence of melanoma or malignant degeneration in about 16 per cent of adults. Depilation alone of small, hairy, intradermal nevi may produce a cosmetically acceptable result. Shave excision (Walton) and electrodesiccation of hairy nevi in special areas (e.g., eyebrow) may be more desirable than total excision with skin grafting.

Blue nevi in children present in two forms. The common *Mongolian spot* (cellular dermal melanocytoma) is present at birth as a flat, well-defined, bluish discoloration of the lower sacral region or buttocks. Since most lesions disappear during childhood, treatment is not necessary. A few persist into adulthood.

The *dermal melanocytoma* (blue nevus) appears early in childhood as a grayish or steel-blue papule or nodule which grows slowly. If diagnosed clinically, routine follow-up is sufficient; otherwise, simple complete elliptical excision with histologic diagnosis is appropriate.

Compound melanocytoma (Spitz's benign juvenile melanoma spindle or epithelioid cell nevus) is a benign hairless papule or nodule with a smooth surface and usually pink or reddish in color. It may be present at birth and is most commonly found on the face. In many children the lesion has apparently grown rapidly during a few months prior to excisional biopsy, which is the treatment of choice. The incidence of malignant change in benign juvenile melanoma is the same as that reported for the compound mole, e.g., one in 250,000 to 500,000 children, which has been our experience over 25 years.

Malignant melanoma, very rare under the age of 15 years, occurred in 3 and 4 per cent of patients, respectively, in the 10 to 19 year age group in two clinical studies of 361 and 405 patients. Over a period of 25 years, we have observed malignant melanoma in only one child under 10 years of age. Since the risk of malignancy is so remote in the prepubertal child, regular observations in conjunction with physician and patient appreciation of danger signals are sufficient. In teenagers, especially those with lesions on the palms, soles or genitalia, any changes whatever in size, color or thickness, or ulceration or bleeding are indications to perform an elliptical excision and ascertain the histopathologic changes.

VASCULAR NEOPLASMS

Angiomas or vascular "nevi" are the most common cutaneous congenital malformations seen in children. Two major groups are seen in children: the involuting and the noninvoluting vascular lesions.

Involuting. Studies of the common involuting types (erythema nuchae, salmon patch, spider nevi or telangiectases, strawberry, cavernous, mixed strawberry-cavernous) have shown that no active therapy is necessary. A program of planned intelligent neglect is essential in order to avoid disfiguring scars. Management consists of the steps mentioned previously and the evaluation of the growth pattern of the hemangioma. The natural pattern for the strawberry or cavernous hemangioma is rapid growth (to double or triple its size) within several weeks or months during early infancy. At this time the lesion is bright red if a strawberry type, or blue if a cavernous type. When maximal size is attained, usually between 9 and 12 months of age, the color becomes a dark red.

For several months the hemangioma remains quiescent; its growth rate is the same as that of the infant. By 12 to 18 months, often earlier, spontaneous involution begins. The color gradually fades to a grayish pink; a gray-white hue appears in the center of the lesion, and this spreads until the entire area becomes white or pink. There is a decrease in tenseness as involution progresses. Although the bulk of the lesion diminishes, the area of discoloration decreases very slowly over several years.

Careful assessment of the parent's reaction and establishment of parent-physician rapport are essential before counseling and reassurance can be effected. Most parents are willing to accept watchful waiting; serial photographs showing the involution of similar lesions in other children are most convincing. The strawberry, cavernous and mixed hemangiomas spontaneously regress as follows: at age three years, 30 per cent; by four years, 60 per cent; by seven years, 76 per cent. Complications (bleeding, ulceration and infection) are uncommon (5 per cent). Ulceration or infection is treated with warm, wet compresses, surgical soap scrubs and occasionally application of bacitracin ointment, 500 units per Gm., or gentamicin cream, 0.1 per cent.

The indications for active treatment are few and must be determined individually. In rare instances in which the diagnosis is uncertain (atypical growth pattern or no evidence for a vascular lesion), excisional biopsy may be necessary. In a patient in whom a hemangioma enlarges rapidly (within a few weeks) and vital structures are compromised or tissue destruction results, the use of prednisone should be considered. If symptomatic thrombocytopenia occurs, prednisone may again be effective. Prednisone, 2 mg. per kilogram per day in two or three divided doses orally for three to four weeks, has been beneficial in 9 of our 10 patients with hemangiomas obstructing the nares, auditory canal or vision. If signs of involution occur after several weeks of daily prednisone, therapy should be continued four more weeks on alternate days in the same dose. After eight weeks, prednisone should be discontinued and the lesion watched carefully for recurrence of swelling and/or redness. Regrowth may occur (but this was not noted in nine of our patients). A second course of prednisone has been effective in other series. Plastic surgery may be necessary for redundant tissue persisting after spontaneous regression, or in a five- or six-year-old child whose lesion has not regressed.

Spider nevi (nevus araneus) are less common and occur in the older child over the neck, chest, forearms and hands. Many disappear spontaneously. If cosmetic treatment is deemed necessary, a desiccating diathermy needle applied at the center of the nevus will produce blanching. The sharp point of a pencil of carbon dioxide snow applied for 10 seconds may be equally effective.

Noninvoluting. Noninvoluting vascular neoplasms or nevi are less common in children than in adults. The therapy of a few (port-wine nevus, phlebectasia, hemangiolymphangioma, pyogenic granuloma) seen occasionally in office practice will be discussed.

Port-wine nevus or mark (nevus flammeus) is best treated by using a waterproof blemish cream (Covermark, Retouch) which adequately disguises the mark. A few of these lesions become lighter in color but rarely disappear.

Phlebectasia (venous cavernous angiectasia) and hemangiolymphangiomas are rare lesions occurring in the neck or on the extremities, or involving mucous membranes. Rarely, these involute spontaneously but slowly during the first decade. Frequent observation is necessary. Surgical removal should be done early if growth continues after the first year of age or if sudden enlargement occurs.

Pyogenic granuloma is easily diagnosed by the history of a minor wound from which a rapidly growing red granulomatous mass arose within a few weeks. These lesions bleed profusely upon the slightest trauma. The best treatment is excision or removal by electrodesiccation.

Histologic examination is recommended for all lesions because an amelanotic melanoma may be detected. Spontaneous involution may occur.

Cutaneous vascular nevi associated with systemic hemangiomatosis may be congenital or acquired, occur with one of the phakomatoses or present as a blue rubber bleb nevus or as Riley's syndrome (macrocephaly, pseudopapilledema, multiple hemangioma). These and other rare vascular tumors (hemangiectatic hypertrophy, verrucose hemangioma, angiokeratoma, racemose hemangioma) have been reviewed recently (Margileth); their management must be individualized.

Lymphangiomas are noninvoluting growths composed of vascular spaces that contain lymph. These malformations, possibly hamartomas, are pale and translucent and may exude clear fluid. Four different types have been noted, i.e., simple, cystic and diffuse lymphangiomas and lymphangioma circumscriptum. The cystic lymphangioma (cystic hygroma) commonly involves the neck axilla or inguinal areas. A few of these lesions show little or no tendency toward spontaneous involution. Surgical excision is usually necessary and should be performed electively before infiltration of deep tissues, vessels and nerves occurs. Recurrence is reported, especially if the lesion has been inadequately excised.

References

Fitzpatrick, T. B., Arndt, K. A., Clark, W. H., Jr., Eisen, A. Z., VanScott, E. J., and Vaughan, J. H.: *Dermatology in General Medicine.* New York, McGraw-Hill Book Company, 1971.

Margileth, A. M.: Developmental Vascular Abnormalities. *Pediat. Clin. N. Am.,* 18:773, 1971.

Solomon, L. M., and Esterly, N. B.: *Neonatal Dermatology,* Philadelphia, W. B. Saunders Company, 1973.

Walton, R. G.: Pigmented Nevi. *Pediat. Clin. N. Am.,* 18:897, 1971.

Other Skin Tumors

SIDNEY HURWITZ, M.D.

TUMORS OF THE EPIDERMIS

Tumors of the epidermis range in severity from benign or nevoid lesions to those which are highly malignant. Benign tumors appear frequently; malignant tumors, rare in children, are often overlooked when they do occur.

Basal Cell Epithelioma. Basal cell carcinoma (or epithelioma) generally arises from the basal layer of the epidermis. This tumor, most common in persons past middle age, has been noted upon rare occasion in children and therefore must be considered even in the young.

The majority of lesions occur on the head and neck with a predilection for the upper central part of the face. The tumor, the least aggressive neoplasm among cancers, is characterized by its capacity for local destruction. The most common type begins as a small elevated translucent nodule with telangiectatic vessels on its surface. The nodule often increases in size, undergoes central necrosis and results in an ulceration surrounded by a pearly rolled border.

No single method of therapy is applicable to all lesions. The goal, as with any skin tumor, is for permanent cure with the best functional and cosmetic result. Curettage and electrodesiccation is a simple office treatment most frequently used by dermatologists, with a cure rate of over 95 per cent. Large lesions are best treated by surgical excision with suturing or grafting when necessary. Cryosurgery with liquid nitrogen is particularly beneficial in recurrent carcinomas when other methods of therapy have been unsatisfactory. Fractional doses of radiation therapy (used for large lesions in elderly patients in whom extensive surgical procedures are difficult) should be avoided in the management of basal cell tumors in children.

Basal cell nevus syndrome is a hereditary disorder characterized by basal cell carcinomas associated with defects in other tissues, such as jaw cysts, bifid ribs and abnormalities of the vertebrae. Skin tumors in this disorder are generally multiple and occur early in life. The relatively benign course of these lesions suggests a nonradical therapeutic approach such as electrodesiccation and curettage or simple surgical excision. The use of radiotherapy should be avoided in children.

Squamous Cell Carcinoma. Squamous cell carcinoma is a malignant tumor of the epidermis rarely seen in children. Occasionally it may arise in normal skin, but generally it is seen in skin that has been injured by sunlight, trauma, thermal burn or forms of chronic irritation. In highly susceptible subjects (patients with xeroderma pigmentosum) this tumor may occur in childhood or early adult life.

The most common sites are the face (in particular the lower lip and pinna of the ear), the backs of hands and the forearms. The lesion appears as an indurated plaque-like nodule and often presents as a shallow crusted ulcer surrounded by a wide elevated border.

Because of the tendency toward deep invasion of the tissues and the possibility of metastases, treatment by electrodesiccation may not be effective. It is, however, valuable in lesions of small size (diameter under 10 mm.). Excisional surgery may be used for lesions where primary closure or simple grafting is possible. Radiation therapy is often preferred for treatment of large carcinomas, particularly on the face where surgical excision may result in objectionable scarring. When properly executed, a five-year cure rate of about 90 per cent can be obtained.

EPIDERMAL NEVI

Nevus Verrucosus. Nevus verrucosus is a benign congenital malformation of the epidermis. There are two forms of this disorder; both are present at birth or appear early in life.

In the localized type, usually only one lesion is present. It may be round or oval in shape, grayish to yellow-brown in color and warty or papillomatous in surface. The systemized type shows linear configuration and is generally limited to one side of the body. This is called *nevus unius lateralis.*

Therapy depends upon the site, the extent of the lesions and the age of the patient. Surgical excision, cryosurgery with liquid nitrogen or electrodesiccation with curettage may produce gratifying results. Dermabrasion, although initially satisfactory, may result in early recurrence.

TUMORS OF THE EPIDERMAL APPENDAGES

Nevus Sebaceus. Nevus sebaceus of Jadassohn is a solitary hairless plaque present at birth. It is yellow or yellow-brown to orange in color and has a flat, velvet-like surface. It is generally seen on the scalp but may appear on the face or neck. With puberty the lesion grows, becomes raised, thickened and nodular.

Associated tumors may develop during adolescence or in adult life. Syringocystadenoma papilliferum is commonly seen, basal cell carcinoma has been reported in 15 to 20 per cent of cases, and in rare instances a squamous cell carcinoma has arisen in the lesion.

The recognition of this lesion and its potential neoplastic change is critical. Wide local excision is mandatory, preferably before puberty. Electrodesiccation may result in recurrences; therefore, plastic surgery is recommended.

Trichoepithelioma. Trichoepithelioma (epithelioma adenoides cysticum) is a benign tumor which develops from embryonic hair structures. The tumor usually appears as multiple lesions—a dominantly inherited disorder. Occasionally it occurs as a solitary nonhereditary lesion.

Tumors generally appear during adolescence as small, firm, skin-colored nodules on the face, particularly in the nasolabial folds. Often, a few telangiectatic vessels are present over the rounded translucent surface of larger lesions.

Therapy consists of excision or electrosurgical removal of lesions. Cryosurgery with liquid nitrogen is also effective.

Benign Calcifying Epithelioma of Malherbe (Pilomatrixoma). This uncommon lesion, a benign tumor of hair structures, generally develops before the age of 21 and manifests itself clinically as a calcified deepseated nodule. The overlying skin may be normal or slightly discolored with a reddish-blue tint. The tumor usually occurs as a solitary lesion on the face or the upper extremities. Lesions may be subject to periodic inflammation or granulomatous swelling but do not become malignant.

Treatment for cosmetic purposes consists of surgical excision by a plastic surgeon. Recurrences are rarely seen.

Syringoma. Syringoma represents a benign tumor of eccrine sweat structures, predominantly seen in females, frequently appearing at adolescence. Individual lesions are small, firm, translucent, skin-colored or slightly yellow nodules. Generally 1 to 2 mm. in size, they are found primarily on the eyelids and cheeks.

For cosmetic purposes, treatment may include destruction by electrodesiccation, cryosurgery with liquid nitrogen or local surgical excision.

DERMAL TUMORS

Adenoma Sebaceum (Angiofibromas). Adenoma sebaceum, one of the cutaneous signs of tuberous sclerosis, is rarely present at birth. It occurs generally between two and five years of age, often not until puberty. Lesions appear as numerous small, firm, pink or flesh-colored dome-shaped tumors arranged in a symmetric distribution in the nasolabial folds and on the cheeks or chin.

Although its name implies sebaceous gland involvement, the term adenoma sebaceum is a misnomer. The lesions represent hamartomas composed of fibrous and vascular tissues and are more correctly termed angiofibromas.

These skin tumors require no treatment except for cosmetic reasons. Best results are seen following cryosurgery, electrodesiccation and curettage or dermabrasion. Some lesions tend to recur following superficial removal.

Keloids. Keloids represent an exaggerated connective tissue response to skin injury. Rare in infancy, their incidence increases throughout childhood, reaching a maximum between puberty and 30 years of age. Early, growing lesions are pink, smooth and rubbery, often tender, with surfaces extending beyond the area of the original wound.

Elective cosmetic procedures in persons who have a tendency to form keloids should be avoided. Keloids less than 5 cm. in diameter respond well to intralesional injections of long-acting corticosteroids (10 to 40 mg. per ml. of triamcinolone acetonide) or cryosurgery with liquid nitrogen. The use of intralesional steroid or x-ray therapy in conjunction with careful plastic surgery is helpful for larger lesions.

Lipoma. A lipoma, one of the most common benign tumors, is composed of mature fat cells. It can be seen at any age and usually occurs from puberty on. Lesions may be present on any part of the body and may be single or multiple, of variable size and with a characteristic soft, often lobulated rubbery, putty-like consistency.

Lipomas may be left untreated unless they become painful, increase in size or are large enough to be objectionable. Malignant change is very rare except in lesions of 10 cm. or more in diameter, particularly on the thighs. These should be investigated for malignancy. Surgical excision is the treatment of choice.

Dermatofibroma. Dermatofibromas are benign growths of connective tissue generally seen in adults; occasionally they are seen in children. They appear as small, well-defined dermal nodules, firmly fixed to the skin but freely movable over the subcutaneous fat. Nodules may be found on any part of the body and are common on the extremities, particularly the anterior surface of the leg. Color may vary from flesh colored to red-brown, tan or black.

Treatment is unnecessary although surgical excision may be done for cosmetic or diagnostic purposes.

Connective Tissue Nevus (Collagenoma or Juvenile Elastoma). Connective tissue nevi are localized malformations of either or both dermal collagen or elastic fibers. These benign skin lesions, often hereditary, are usually seen in young children. They appear as firm, clustered, slightly raised, pea-sized, skin-colored oval lesions which are distributed symmetrically over the abdomen, back, buttocks, arms or thighs.

Biopsy may be done for diagnostic reasons; treatment is seldom required.

The Genodermatoses

NANCY B. ESTERLY, M.D.

Most of the hereditary disorders discussed in this article are, fortunately, relatively uncommon. Since nonspecific measures and supportive care are often all that can be offered, it is important to ensure that adequate genetic counseling is provided for the families of these children.

KERATOSIS PILARIS

Keratosis pilaris, a disorder of unknown etiology, is characterized by follicular hyperkeratotic papules, which may be localized or widespread but which occur most commonly on the extensor surfaces of the upper arms and thighs. A bland emollient, such as petrolatum, Aquaphor, Eucerin or Lubriderm, applied ad libitum may be adequate to soften the lesions and alleviate dryness. If the papules are very prominent, a keratolytic agent, such as 5 per cent salicylic acid ointment or 10 to 20 per cent urea in Aquaphor or Keri Lotion, applied three times daily will be more effective.

INCONTINENTIA PIGMENTI

The cutaneous lesions of this rare, congenital and hereditary disorder exhibit three distinct stages, none of which requires specific therapy if it remains uncomplicated. Occasionally the initial vesiculobullous eruption or the second-stage verrucose lesions become pruritic and inflamed and should be treated with cool tap water compresses for 15 minutes four times a day. A corticosteroid cream, such as 1 per cent hydrocortisone, 0.1 per cent triamcinolone or 0.025 per cent fluocinolone, may be applied after the compresses. If secondary bacterial infection occurs, a topical antibiotic preparation (Polysporin, Garamycin or Bacitracin Ointment) should be used instead. Rarely, if infection is extensive, a systemically administered antibiotic may be indicated. No therapeutic measures are necessary for the third- and end-stage pigmentary phase. Dental defects are sometimes present and prosthetic dentistry may be required. Ocular manifestations, depending on the nature of the anomaly, may also necessitate ophthalmologic care.

KERATOSIS PALMARIS ET PLANTARIS

The thickening of the stratum corneum which characterizes keratosis palmaris et plantaris may be mild, severe, diffuse, focal, punctate, or striate. When the hyperkeratosis is minimal in degree, treatment may be unnecessary or restricted to simple lubrication. Petrolatum, Aquaphor or any one of a number of emollients may be used as frequently as needed to prevent dryness and fissuring, especially during the winter months. As in ichthyosis, lubrication is always enhanced by prior hydration; therefore, it is important to apply the emollient immediately after washing. If involvement of the palms and soles is severe and troublesome, a keratolytic agent should be prescribed. Five to twenty per cent salicylic acid may be incorporated into an ointment base and applied three times daily. If thickening of the stratum corneum is extreme, the concentration of salicylic acid may be increased up to 40 per cent; however, the patient must be instructed to avoid application to the less keratotic areas and to normal skin, since keratolytic agents in high concentration may cause excessive irritation, inflammation and peeling. Ten to twenty per cent urea in Aquaphor or petrolatum is another extremely useful agent which is well tolerated and preferred by many patients. Some success has been achieved with 0.1 to 0.3 per cent vitamin A acid ointment applied once daily, and again at night with an occlusive polyethylene wrap (Saran or Handi-Wrap) or disposable plastic gloves. Occlusive wraps should not be used for periods longer than 12 hours, since the moist environment and maceration of skin which result from prolonged occlusion may facilitate secondary infection. Another alternative therapeutic agent is 40 to 60 per cent (volume to volume) aqueous propylene glycol, in water, which can be applied at night and covered with an occlusive wrap. This solution of propylene glycol is stable for about four to six months. The frequency of application of any of these agents can be decreased once improvement has occurred. Painful or inflamed fissures may heal more rapidly if a protective tape (Blenderm Surgical Tape) is used to cover the fissure. Cordran Tape is occasionally useful in alleviating the discomfort associated with deep fissures.

ACRODERMATITIS ENTEROPATHICA

A vesiculobullous, eczematous skin eruption, nail dystrophy, alopecia, stomatitis, and glossitis, failure to thrive and diarrhea are characteristic features of this autosomal recessive disease of unknown etiology. An immunologic defect may coexist in some patients. Candida infection both on the skin and in the gastrointestinal tract is a frequent complication.

The oral administration of diiodohydroxyquin (Diodoquin) may bring about a dramatic remission. Infants should be started on one tablet (650 mg.) daily in two divided doses. The dosage should be adjusted as needed, depending on the response to therapy and the weight of the child. As many as 14 tablets daily have been administered to some adolescents with the disease. The patient may have to be maintained on medication indefinitely.

Although the initiation of diiodohydroxyquin therapy may ameliorate the symptoms of the disease, some infants have required additional measures. For unknown reasons the substitution of human breast milk for cow's milk combined with the administration of Diodoquin has been effective for infants refractory to Diodoquin alone. Patients with severe diarrhea and inanition may require intravenous feeding. Limited data from a few patients suggest that either cottonseed or soybean oil emulsions or casein hydrolysate (Amigen) may be of more benefit than other intravenous preparations.

Oral, paronychial and gastrointestinal candidiasis may complicate acrodermatitis enteropathica. Nystatin suspension, 100,000 units four times daily, is usually adequate for clearing intraoral lesions and suppressing Candida growth in the gastrointestinal tract. Candida infection of the skin should respond to nystatin (Mycostatin) or amphotericin B (Fungizone) cream, applied two to four times daily. Secondary bacterial infections should be treated with appropriate antibiotics.

EPIDERMOLYSIS BULLOSA

The term epidermolysis bullosa refers to a group of hereditary, chronic blistering disorders. Two of these disorders, the recessive and dominant dystrophic forms, are characterized by bullae which heal with scarring and milia formation; the remaining three types, epidermolysis bullosa simplex, Weber-Cockayne disease (epidermolysis bullosa of the hands and feet) and epidermolysis bullosa letalis, have nonscarring lesions unless resolution is complicated by secondary factors.

Since the bullous lesions are induced by trauma and friction, precautionary measures must be taken. To avoid extensive denudation of the skin, particularly in infants, gentle handling is mandatory at all times, but special care must be taken during the warmer months when the propensity to blister is increased. Soft, nonabrasive materials should be used for crib coverings and clothing, and metal closures on wearing apparel should be avoided. Paper tape is a convenient and atraumatic means of holding diapers together. Shoes should be soft and preferably made of canvas or other fabric. The use of a sheepskin pad in the crib may also be helpful. All equipment, such as cribs, strollers, infant seats and highchairs, should be adequately padded with foam-rubber or similar protective material. Only soft toys should be permitted.

Tub baths should probably be avoided in early infancy, since the amount of handling required may induce new lesions. Tepid sponge baths containing water-dispersible bath oils (Alpha-Keri, Domol, Lubath) will usually suffice until the infant is old enough to support himself in the tub. If superficial infection is present, a dilute hexachlorophene preparation may be used to wash limited areas but should be thoroughly rinsed away. Compressing for 20 minutes four times a day is an alternative to tub or sponge baths, and either normal saline, Burow's solution or 0.25 per cent silver nitrate solution may be used. Parents should be warned that silver nitrate solution will discolor the skin and fabrics with which it comes in contact.

An antibiotic ointment such as Polysporin should be applied four times a day to denuded lesions and the area covered with a nonadherent dressing (Telfa pads). Adhesive tape should never be applied to the skin, since large pieces of epidermis will be torn off on its removal. The edges of a dressing may be taped to each other or the pad held in place with a soft roller bandage such as Kerlix. Large bullous lesions should be punctured and the collapsed blister top left in place as a protective covering. Topical corticosteroid ointments (0.1 per cent triamcinolone, 0.1 per cent betamethasone or 0.025 per cent fluocinolone) may decrease the inflammatory component, but they do not prevent the formation of new lesions, and secondary infection may be promoted through their use. Prolonged application of high potency corticosteroids may result in atrophy of the skin. If severe blistering is present during the newborn period, a brief course of systemically administered corticosteroids in large doses is said to be helpful.

Oral and esophageal lesions often create severe nutritional problems, since the infant or young child may refuse his feedings. To minimize the formation of intraoral and perioral lesions in patients with the dystrophic or letalis type of the disease, infants should be fed with soft nipples, bulb syringes or devices used for patients with cleft palates. Benadryl Elixir or Xylocaine Viscous applied to the mouth just before feeding will help to alleviate pain. Cereal may have to be thinned with milk and solid foods may have to be puréed to facilitate swallowing. For the older child with moderate to severe mucous membrane lesions, a carefully selected semiliquid diet may be prescribed to provide adequate protein, iron and caloric intake. Dysphagia secondary to esophageal lesions may be palliated by brief, intensive courses of oral corticosteroids: 20 to 40 mg. per day of prednisone for children under five years of age, and up to 80 mg. per day for older children. If strictures have occurred, dilatation with bougies may be necessary in the older child.

Reconstructive surgical procedures may be required for severe strictures in the esophagus as well as for the hand and foot deformities that result from digital fusion which occurs in some forms of this disease.

Patients who have anemia resulting from blood and protein loss via the skin lesions should receive continuous oral iron therapy. A therapeutic dose of 1.5 to 2.0 mg. per kilogram body weight of elemental iron should be given three times daily (4.5 to 6.0 mg. per kilogram body weight per day) using ferrous sulfate preparations. Transfusion of packed cells may be necessary for those patients who are symptomatic from anemia and unresponsive to iron therapy because of chronic inflammation or infection.

TUBEROUS SCLEROSIS

This neurocutaneous syndrome is inherited as an autosomal dominant trait and primarily affects the skin and central nervous system, although it may also cause lesions in the bones, viscera and eyes. Hypopigmented macules, the earliest skin lesions, are simply a marker of the disease and require no treatment. The facial adenomas (adenoma sebaceum) are more cosmetically deforming and consist of smooth, pink telangiectatic nodules which may vary considerably in size and become quite numerous. These lesions can be removed by curettage and electrodesiccation, excision, surgical planing or the application of liquid nitrogen. Gingival and subungual fibromas may be treated in a similar manner. However, all of these lesions may recur, and for this reason, removal for cosmetic improvement is not indicated if patients are severely affected.

NEUROFIBROMATOSIS

Neurofibromatosis is inherited as an autosomal dominant trait and characterized by both hyperpigmented skin lesions and tumors which develop from elements of the peripheral and central nervous systems. The pigmented lesions, café au lait spots and axillary freckling, are not amenable to treatment. The neurofibromas, which can be dermal or subcutaneous, small or large, sessile, pedunculated or plexiform, may reach appreciable size, causing extreme hypertrophy of a limb or portion of an extremity. Because of the progressive nature of these tumors and the diversity in size, number and location, treatment for the most part is palliative and removal is indicated only if there is pain, severe deformity, interference with function, malignant degeneration or recurrent infection. Surgical excision is the treatment of choice; however, local recurrence is common if the lesion is not totally ablated. Surgical procedures may be especially difficult when dealing with plexiform neuromas, and the risk of postsurgical paralysis is increased. Irradiation is not effective in this disease.

ECTODERMAL DYSPLASIA

The term ectodermal dysplasia refers to a congenital and hereditary constellation of defects which involves the skin and its appendageal structures with or without associated anomalies in other organ systems. Although there are now several syndromes which can be included in this category, classically the term is used for two particular disorders: hidrotic ectodermal dysplasia and anhidrotic (hypohidrotic) ectodermal dysplasia.

In the *hidrotic form of ectodermal dysplasia* the nails are deformed, hypoplastic or absent, the hair is sparse and the palms and soles are hyperkeratotic. The nail defect cannot be treated. If the alopecia is moderate to marked, the patient should be fitted with a wig. The hyperkeratosis of the palms and soles may respond to the application of keratolytic agents (see Keratosis Palmaris et Plantaris).

In *anhidrotic ectodermal dysplasia,* absence of sweating, hypotrichosis, the peculiar facies and defective dentition are the most striking and characteristic findings, although a host of other anomalies may occur. Because of the hypoplasia or absence of eccrine sweat glands, these patients are unable to regulate their body temperature and suffer severe heat intolerance. Exposure to extreme heat should be avoided, and air conditioning is necessary if the patient is living in a warm climate. Clothing should be lightweight when the weather is warm. Older children may douse their clothing with water or undress and sit in a tub of water to cool themselves by the mechanism of evaporation.

The skin is usually thin and dry and may benefit from the routine use of a bath oil (Alpha-Keri) and a bland lubricant. Atopic dermatitis occurs with increased frequency in this disorder and should be treated with a topical corticosteroid cream. One per cent hydrocortisone applied three times daily may be adequate for the patient with mild eczema; more severe involvement may require the use of a fluorinated preparation, such as 0.1 per cent triamcinolone, 0.01 per cent fluocinolone or 0.025 per cent flurandrenolone, three times a day.

If alopecia is severe a wig should be provided. The use of a preparation such as Daragen hair-repair shampoo may make the typically unruly hair more manageable. Prosthetic dentistry is almost always required and should be provided early in life so that good nutrition can be maintained. Deficient lacrimation, when present, can be palliated by the regular use of artificial tears (1 per cent hydroxypropyl methylcellulose, one drop in each eye every 2 hours while awake). Slit-lamp examination should be performed periodically to detect corneal lesions resulting from trauma. The nasal mucosa, which is lacking in mucous glands, should be protected by saline irrigations and regular application of petrolatum. Because of the defective mucous glands in the nasal, pharyngeal and respiratory tract mucosa, these patients are more susceptible to respiratory infections. Systemic antibiotics should be prescribed depending on culture and sensitivity of the infecting organism.

If the saddle nose and protruding ears are a serious cosmetic problem in the older child, surgical reconstruction may improve the physical appearance remarkably.

ICHTHYOSIS

The ichthyosiform dermatoses can be divided into four major types: ichthyosis vulgaris, inherited as an autosomal dominant trait; X-linked ichthyosis; lamellar ichthyosis (nonbullous congenital ichthyosiform erythroderma), transmitted in an autosmal recessive fashion; and epidermolytic hyperkeratosis (bullous congenital ichthyosiform erythroderma), an autosomal dominant disorder. The ichthyoses are distinguishable not only on the basis of genetic transmission but by differences in age of onset, type and distribution of scale, involvement of fossae and palms and soles, presence or absence of blisters, histologic findings and cellular kinetics.

Treatment for the ichthyoses is restricted almost exclusively to the use of topical preparations. The most important general principle in the therapeutic approach to these patients is hydration of a dry skin and generous application of a lubricant to retard evaporative losses. Prolonged daily baths are useful not only for hydration but also because the thickened stratum corneum becomes soft and macerated and can be removed, in part, by vigorous scrubbing with a brush or rough washcloth. A water-dispersible bath oil (Alpha-Keri, Domol, Lubath, Nutra-Spa) will help soften and lubricate the skin. Immediately after bathing, while the skin is still damp, an emollient, such as petrolatum, Aquaphor or Eucerin, should be applied liberally over the entire body. Detergents and soaps with irritating additives and perfume should be avoided. Hexachlorophene-containing soaps should not be used on the infant because of the dangers of toxicity from absorption. However, older children with lamellar ichthyosis or epidermolytic hyperkeratosis frequently have an unpleasant and penetrating odor resulting from proliferation of bacteria in the macerated stratum corneum of the flexural areas; for these patients, a hexachlorophene preparation may reduce bacterial growth enough to lessen the odor.

An alternative preparation for the bath is 3 per cent sodium chloride. Ten per cent sodium chloride in petrolatum can be used as a lubricant following the bath. For patients with moderate to severe ichthyosis, 10 to 15 per cent urea in petrolatum or Aquaphor is usually more effective in removing thick scales than is a simple lubricant. A keratolytic agent, such as 3 to 10 per cent salicylic acid, may be incorporated into an ointment base for use in localized areas. Because of the hazard of absorption and systemic toxicity, salicylic acid should not be applied over extensive areas for prolonged periods. Keratolytic agents are also useful for the scalp, either in the form of an antiseborrheic shampoo (Sebulex, Sebaveen, Ionil), which should be left on the scalp for 5 to 10 minutes before rinsing, or as a liquid preparation (5 per cent salicylic acid in cottonseed or mineral oil), which can be applied to the scalp before bed and shampooed out in the morning.

Other topical preparations include vitamin A acid and propylene glycol. Vitamin A acid, 0.1 to 0.3 per cent in propylene glycol or an ointment base, is effective in the types of ichthyosis with rapid epidermal cell kinetics (lamellar ichthyosis and epidermolytic hyperkeratosis). When applied once daily, vitamin A acid reduces the quantity of scale considerably; however, this substance is extremely irritating and may cause pain and inflammation in less involved areas or in the flexures. For this reason, it must be used with care and the frequency of application reduced as the patient improves. Propylene glycol alone, in a 40 to 60 per cent (volume to volume) solution, when applied nightly with an occlusive polyethylene wrap, has apparently been effective in patients with ichthyosis vulgaris and X-linked ichthyosis.

Areas which fissure or become secondarily involved with a primary irritant contact dermatitis may be treated for a brief period with a corticosteroid cream, such as 0.1 per cent triamcinolone, 0.01 per cent fluocinolone or 0.025 per cent flurandrenolone, three times a day. Secondary bacterial and fungal infections may also occur, particularly in moist, macerated intertriginous areas, and should be treated with appropriate antibiotic or antifungal agents. Beta-hemolytic streptococcal infection commonly complicates the bullous lesions of epidermolytic hyperkeratosis. Such patients should receive a 10-day course of systemically administered penicillin.

Patients with ichthyosis tolerate extremes of temperature poorly. Decreased sweating due to blockage of the eccrine sweat duct pores may cause severe discomfort in warm weather; therefore, air conditioning may be tremendously helpful for such patients. Exposure to harsh winter weather or to extremely dry indoor heat should also be avoided. Patients with extensive disease may experience severe pruritus, particularly at night. Sedation with an oral antihistamine (Benadryl Elixir)* or a tranquilizer (Atarax or Vistaril) may be helpful in controlling this symptom.

References

Cash, R., Berger, C. K.: Acrodermatitis Enteropathica: Defective Metabolism of Unsaturated Fatty Acids, *J. Pediat.* 74:717, 1969.

Freier, S., Faber, J., Goldstein, R., and Mayer, M.: Treatment of Acrodermatitis Enteropathica by Intravenous Amino Acid Hydrolysate, *J. Pediat.*, 82:109, 1973.

* Manufacturer's precaution: Benadryl should not be used in premature or newborn infants.

Diseases of the Hair and Scalp

GEORGE F. WILGRAM, M.D.

HYPERTRICHOSIS AND HIRSUTISM

Hypertrichosis

Hypertrichosis is a state of excessive hair growth when compared with the average density of hair in men and women.

Congenital. Localized, congenital hypertrichosis can be seen as a nevoid congenital malformation and may occur with or without the presence of melanocytic nevi. Generalized hypertrichosis may occur as congenital hypertrichosis lanuginosa and is also seen in Hurler's syndrome, in congenital macrogingivae and in the Cornelia de Lange syndrome. In the latter, a profuse overgrowth of the eyebrows is particularly striking.

Symptomatic. In children, hypertrichosis can occur with erythropoietic protoporphyria as well as with porphyria cutanea tarda. It is also seen in the rare surviving case of the dystrophic type of epidermolysis bullosa and occasionally is associated with endrocrine disturbances such as hyper- and hypothyroidism. Malnutrition, dermatomyositis and, on occasion, extensive midbrain damage can be accompanied by hypertrichosis.

Hypertrichosis may be induced by drugs such as diphenylhydantoin (used in the treatment of epilepsy), streptomycin (after prolonged administration), and cortisone (after high dosages).

Patchy or localized hypertrichosis may be induced by local inflammatory changes, but this type of hair growth is temporary and usually recedes with the cessation of the inflammatory process.

Hirsutism

Hirsutism is the appearance of coarse, terminal hair in females in those areas where it is normally seen in males as a manifestation of male sexuality. The causes of hirsutism are as follows: idiopathic, adrenal, ovarian, congenital or drug-induced.

Idiopathic. In idiopathic hirsutism, no underlying disturbance is found and the excess of coarse terminal hair in young girls has to be considered a minor racial variant.

Adrenal. Among the adrenal syndromes, adrenal hyperplasia, virilizing adrenal tumors, Cushing's syndrome and adrenal dysfunction should be listed. In these adrenal syndromes the urinary 17-ketosteroids are distinctively elevated. In Cushing's syndrome the 11-hydroxy corticosteroids are also elevated. Adrenal syndromes also produce virilization.

Ovarian. Among the ovarian syndromes, tumors such as the virilizing ovarian carcinoma, arrhenoblastoma and hilus-cell tumor are known to produce hirsutism. Most of these ovarian tumors occur, however, later in life and only rarely have to be considered in childhood. The Stein-Leventhal syndrome probably is a primary biochemical defect in the production of estrogen and thus is found in girls only after their menarche. It is accompanied clinically by hirsutism, obesity and amenorrhea.

Congenital. Among congenital disorders, male pseudohermaphroditism, Turner's syndrome and precocious puberty can be recognized by hirsutism.

Drug-Induced. Iatrogenic or drug-induced hirsutism is found after prolonged administration of androgenic compounds and after the use of Cortisone.

Summary

It is important to differentiate hypertrichosis from hirsutism, since the latter is a manifestation of a severe endocrine derangement, including tumor formation which on occasion can be corrected. Therefore, a careful clinical investigation is necessary. Biochemical studies of 17-ketosteroids and 11-hydroxy corticosteroids in the urine, or of hormone levels in the blood, usually are helpful in establishing the diagnosis. Chromosome studies frequently are indicated to determine the presence or absence of a congenital abnormality such as pseudohemaphroditism or Turner's syndrome.

The treatment of hirsutism consists in the correction of the underlying endocrine defect or the removal of the hormone-producing tumor.

DIFFERENTIAL DIAGNOSIS OF HAIR LOSS

Alopecia Areata. In the United States, alopecia areata is a commonly encountered type of hair loss in pediatric practice. Characteristically, hair loss results in a smooth, whitish, shiny, bald patch. There is no erythema, edema, scaling or scarring (see page 512). On the borderline of these bald patches, plugged hair shows a so-called exclamation-point morphology upon microscopic examination; this is diagnostic for alopecia areata. After hair loss has come to a halt, fine vellus hair begins to reappear, which later is followed by normal terminal hair. Not infrequently, the regrowing hairs are vitiliginous and in some instances stay so forever. While one patch tends to fill in with regrowing hair, another patch may appear in a migratory fashion anywhere else on the scalp. Thus, alopecia areata may continue in an overlapping fashion for months and sometimes for years. It is generally agreed that the prognosis is quite good if an individual patch begins to show terminal hair within a period of approximately one year. If hair loss in any patch persists longer than one year, an eventual termination in alopecia totalis has to be considered. On occasion, alopecia totalis begins rapidly right from the onset, leading to a total loss of all scalp hair. In such instances, the prognosis for correction of the disorder is slim. While alopecia areata may occur at any age from 5 to 70 years, it is noteworthy that the sooner the onset of the disorder the more likely the development of alopecia totalis, although the overall incidence of alopecia totalis is only 2 to 5 per cent of the total number of patients with alopecia areata.

Alopecia areata can be observed in adults in hairy regions other than the scalp, such as in the axillae, on the trunk and in the pubic areas, but this would obviously not be the case in children prior to the onset of puberty. Alopecia areata of the eyebrows or eyelashes can, however, be found in both adults and children.

Frequently accompanying the hair loss are nail changes, such as extensive pitting (larger pits than in psoriasis), longitudinal ridging and irregular thickening. The cause of alopecia areata is unknown but many authors claim emotional factors to be of great importance in its induction. This author has been struck with the apparent frequency with which alopecia areata can be observed in adopted children.

Other than providing reassurance to the child and his parents, there is no true therapeutic agent available. The injection or ingestion of systemic steroids has been tried, but after cessation of steroid therapy the vellus hair temporarily induced by hypercortisonism falls out again. Excessive combing, brushing and massages should be avoided.

In cases of total alopecia, both the parents and child should be reassured that this is no reflection of the child's physical and intellectual abilities. A wig should be prescribed at an early stage and the child should be helped to adjust to the situation, if necessary with the aid of a psychiatrist.

Traumatic Hair Loss. Traumatic hair loss is the most common type of hair loss to be differentiated from alopecia areata in children. Several forms of trauma may lead to hair loss. Trichotillomania is a manifestation of anxiety or ill adjustment, leading to picking, squeezing and twisting the hair. Other types of traumatic hair loss are induced by excessive massaging, brushing and combing, as well as excessive braiding and tension. Excessive pressure on the scalp by bands may lead to temporary hair loss.

In traumatic hair loss one usually finds broken-off hair, and the pattern of hair loss is either irregular or bizarre. In no instance does one see the smooth, shiny, whitish skin of the scalp that is characteristic for alopecia areata. In traumatic hair loss, upon microscopic examination one frequently sees changes in the hair shaft resembling trichorrhexis nodosa, while in alopecia areata the exclamation-point hair can be seen at the borderline of the patches. The microscopic difference is distinctive. If trauma is applied not only to the hair but also to the scalp, one may find different degrees of scarring associated with the hair loss (see page 512).

The treatment of traumatic types of hair loss sometimes requires the ingenuity of a detective to elucidate in what manner trauma has been applied. A discussion of the problem, with gentle persuasion to desist from traumatizing the scalp again, sometimes with the aid of a psychiatrist, is all that the physician can provide.

Congenital Alopecia. Alopecia may be present at birth as a congenital abnormality. It can also coexist with progeria, ectodermal dysplasia or with disorders of amino acid metabolism. In the latter instances, other clinical manifestations or abnormal urinary amino acid excretion patterns are helpful in differentiating congenital alopecia from alopecia areata. Another congenital malformation of hair synthesis is monilethrix, in which hair under the microscope shows typical beading. Pili torti, with a typical clinical spangled appearance to the hair, can easily be diagnosed microscopically, showing twisting of the hair shaft at 180 degrees around its own axis. In most instances of congenital alopecia, hair is sparse, fine and thin rather than totally absent, and thus a differential diagnosis from alopecia areata can be made. The presence of other striking clinical features usually allows a further ready differentiation from alopecia areata, where the children are quite normal physically, except for the possible existence of anxiety.

Telogen Effluvium. Alopecia due to the so-called telogen effluvium can be seen in children after severe fever, intoxications or anemias. In less fortunate parts of the world severe malnutrition is frequently accompanied by hair loss. The telogen effluvium type of hair loss is diffuse rather than patchy and never leads to the entirely smooth, whitish, shiny appearance of the scalp typical of the bald patches of alopecia areata. Thus, a differential diagnosis is readily accomplished.

Drug-Induced Alopecia. Alopecia may be the consequence of ingestion of chemical substances, such as the inadvertent intake of thallium, which is still used as a poison against rodents; the therapeutic administration of thyroid compounds and of anticoagulants (heparin and coumarin); the intake of antimitotic agents in the treatment of malignancy; and, finally, the excessive intake of vitamin A. Among other agents which are frequently seen to produce alopecia are trimethadione employed in the control of epilepsy or chloroquine used in the treatment of systemic lupus erythematosus. Again, the chemical- or drug-induced hair loss is usually diffuse and does not lead to the same patchy baldness seen in alopecia areata, because only the hair in the most active phase of anagen would be lost by drug interference.

Alopecia Due to Endocrine Disturbances. Profuse hair loss may be observed in endocrine disorders such as hypopituitary states or hypo- and hyperthyroidism. Together with hirsutism, male pattern baldness may be seen in hyperadrenocorticism and precocious puberty. Since hair loss is just one feature among many others characteristic of the basic disorder, differentiation from alopecia areata should not prove difficult.

Alopecia Accompanied by Inflammation. Alopecia with erythema and edema with or without scaling may be seen in lupus vulgaris, leprosy, syphilis and pyogenic infections. Pediculosis should always come to mind as an important cause of pyogenic infections. Hair loss in these bacterial infections may be substantial. Virus infections such as herpes zoster, varicella and variola will likewise lead to a patchy type of hair loss which, however, shows distinct signs of inflammatory involvement.

Alopecias due to multiple insect bites and tick bites are not uncommon, but the severe inflammatory reaction usually allows ready differentiation of these disorders from alopecia areata.

Alopecia with Scaling. Alopecia with extensive scaling of the scalp and moderate inflammation should immediately raise the suspicion of a fungus infection. Fungus infections may range from the rather frequently seen infections with *Microsporon canis* or *Microsporon audouini,* to the much more rare but serious disorder of favus. Children who play in the countryside with horses or cattle may become infected with *Trichophyton verrucosum* or *Trichophyton violaceum,* leading to the kerion type of inflammatory change with scaling and alopecia of the scalp. Culture and microscopic examination of the scales and hair are diagnostic for a fungus infection. Only in those cases where alopecia areata is accompanied by seborrheic dermatitis (dandruff of the scalp) may the differentiation between alopecia areata and a fungus infection present difficulties. Some fungus infections, notably those with *Microsporon audouini* and *Microsporon canis* (40 per cent of the cases) and less so by *Trichophyton verrucosum* or *Trichophyton violaceum,* cause fluorescence of involved hair and scales, and thus a Wood's light examination is always mandatory in case of a suspected fungus infection of the scalp. The treatment of fungus infections of the scalp consists of the use of griseofulvin, ultrafine, 500 mg. two times daily for eight weeks, and of the topical application of either Tinactine or Halotex lotion two times daily.

Hair Loss with Scarring. Hair loss in children accompanied by scarring is due to traumatic factors, to preceding x-irradiation or, as is increasingly appreciated, to one of the several skin conditions that frequently affect other areas of the skin as well as the scalp. Among the latter, one has to think particularly of morphea, scleroderma, necrobiosis lipoidica, sarcoidosis and discoid lupus erythematosus. Lichen planopilaris likewise leads to hair loss and scarring. The presence of scarring with a total absence of hair follicles and an atrophic epidermis usually allows easy differentiation from alopecia areata. In case of doubt, a skin biopsy is helpful in diagnosing the disorders mentioned above.

Hair loss with scarring may also be present in congenital diseases, such as in incontinentia pigmenti, ichthyosis and congenital erythroderma, as well as in Darier's disease. In all these instances, the hair loss is just one of the many manifestations of the underlying condition, and the diagnosis should not be too difficult.

Diseases of Sweat and Sebaceous Glands

SIDNEY HURWITZ, M.D.

ACNE

Although the basic cause of acne vulgaris is as yet unknown, considerable data on its pathogenesis accumulated in recent years allow a much more rational and successful therapeutic approach to this perplexing skin disorder of the adolescent.

Acne begins at puberty, caused by an inherited keratinization process with an obstruction of the pilosebaceous unit. As a result, there is a formation of comedones; these primary lesions lead to the cutaneous manifestations seen in acne. In the open comedo (blackhead), the orifice is widely dilated and rupture of the follicular wall rarely takes place. In the closed comedo (whitehead), which is responsible for the problems in acne, breaks occur in the follicular wall, allowing sebum to escape into the surrounding dermis. Free fatty acids, the most irritating compounds in the sebum, cause inflammatory changes. These ruptured lesions appear as papules, nodules, or pustules and often form cysts, multinucleated tracts and the eventual scars associated with this disorder.

There is no single treatment for acne vulgaris. Treatment must be individualized with appropriate modifications as the activity of the disorder fluctuates. Acne should never be dismissed as being of no consequence with reassurance that the patient will outgrow it. Successful therapy depends on the cooperation of the patient and the continual interest and enthusiasm of the physician.

Relative to diet, recently carefully controlled studies refute the value of dietary restrictions imposed upon acne patients. For those few patients who attest to flares following certain foods, it is judicious to eliminate the suspicious agents until their true influence can be appropriately and individually assessed.

Local therapy may begin with various cleansing agents and topical lotions aimed at the prevention of comedo formation. These have a debatable therapeutic efficacy based upon their drying or peeling effect. The range is from mild soaps (Fostex, Acne-Aid, Acnaveen) to more abrasive skin cleansers (Acne-Dome, Brāsivol, Ionax Scrub, Pernox). The type of cleanser and the frequency of washing should be adjusted to each patient's tolerance in an effort to achieve a mild degree of skin drying without gross chapping or irritation.

Astringents such as Tyrosum or Seba-Nil may help remove lipids from the skin surface and from sebaceous gland orifices, but with limited efficacy. Sulfur, salicylic acid and resorcinol are used in various acne preparations for their reputed drying and peeling qualities. More effective topical medications appear to be the newer benzoyl peroxide preparations (Vanoxide, Loroxide, Benoxyl and Persadox lotions, or the Panoxyl gels), which offer more than just a form of epidermal irritant. They cause fine desquamation, help reduce the level of free fatty acids in sebum, and appear to be bacteriostatic for Corynebacterium acnes. A relatively low incidence of allergic contact dermatitis (1 to 2 per cent) suggests caution in the use of benzoyl peroxide preparations.

A comparatively new, still controversial, addition to the topical therapy of acne is Tretinoin, vitamin A acid (Retin-A), which seems to be particularly useful for treatment of extensive comedopapular acne. Patients should anticipate six to eight weeks of redness and peeling, necessary to unroof and extrude the impacted sebaceous material in these lesions, before a beneficial response occurs. Patients must be cautioned that this drug induces increased susceptibility to sunburn. Although it seemed advisable to avoid other topical medication when vitamin A acid is used, recent studies suggest a synergistic effect between this modality and topical benzoyl peroxide when applied at different times of the day.

The value of artificial ultraviolet light is debatable. Its major effect is to give the patient a feeling of well-being, to produce mild erythema and desquamation and a resultant tan which helps to conceal acne lesions. The risk of overexposure and conjunctival inflammation from failure to shield the eyes suggests caution and limitation as a method of home therapy.

Acne surgery, the mechanical removal of comedones, pustules and cysts, though time consuming, is extremely important for the rapid involution of individual acne lesions. This procedure is best accomplished by nicking the surface of the lesion with a sharp needle and expressing the contents with a comedo extractor. This therapy results in an immediate improvement in the patient's appearance and reduces the possibility of future scarring.

Cystic acne is benefited by intralesional injection of triamcinolone acetonide in a 2.5- to 10.0-mg. per ml. concentration; this leads to the rapid involution of nodular and cystic lesions. Extreme caution must be exercised here, since a temporary atrophy of the skin may occur when the injection is high in the dermis, particularly when higher concentrations of steroid are used. This atrophy disappears spontaneously within six months to one year.

The use of broad-spectrum antibiotics is invaluable when pustular inflammatory lesions are present. Antibiotics suppress the Corynebacterium acnes and inhibit the bacterial lipases, causing a reduction in the concentration of free fatty acids (the primary irritant of sebum). Tetracycline, effective, inexpensive and relatively free of side effects, is the antibiotic most frequently prescribed. Therapy generally begins with a dosage of 1000 mg. per day, which is gradually decreased to the lowest optimal level and usually maintained at a dosage of 250 mg. per day or every other day until clinical improvement allows its discontinuation. Long-term low dosage may be continued for many months with relatively few side effects. The possibility of tetracycline staining of teeth precludes its use for children under 12 years of age and for pregnant women after the first trimester of pregnancy. Monilial vaginitis, an occasional complication in adolescents, is more common in females who are receiving both oral contraceptives and tetracycline. Since tetracyclines, in particular demethylchlorotetracycline (Declomycin), are known photosensitizers, proper precautions and nongreasy sunscreens should be used when excessive sun exposure is anticipated. The ingestion of outdated tetracycline may cause severe toxicity. It is particularly dangerous in children who use "leftover" medication and who start and stop therapy on their own without proper medical guidance.

Penicillin appears to be of no value in the treatment of acne. Sulfa drugs have been used but their clinical results are not as favorable as those of broad-spectrum antibiotics. Cleocin and erythromycin are effective and useful when inflammatory and pustular lesions fail to respond to oral tetracycline.

Oral vitamin A, long used in acne therapy for its theoretical inhibition of keratinization, has been found ineffective (except perhaps in potentially toxic levels) and therefore has no place in the management of acne today.

Anovulatory drugs suppress the androgenic stimulation of sebum production and are beneficial in 50 to 70 per cent of females with severe, recalcitrant, pustulocystic acne. If estrogen is used, it must contain a minimum of 0.1 mg. of ethinyl estradiol or its 3-methyl ether derivative (mestranol). Side effects to be considered include nausea, weight gain, monilial vaginitis, chloasma and thromboembolic phenomena. Estrogens should never be prescribed in males, since the dose required for sebum suppression will produce feminizing side effects. These drugs should not be administered to patients under the age of 16, when possible bone growth inhibition is a consideration. Even though acne is not listed among the manufacturers' indications for use of anovulatory drugs, these preparations have been used for many years to treat acne, producing good results and a minimum of ill effects.

X-ray, once widely used in the treatment of acne, has generally been abandoned as more effective forms of therapy have developed. Superficial x-ray has been shown to reduce the size of sebaceous glands; however, problems often recur when the glands regenerate after three to four months.

Acne scars may improve to a surprising degree over a period of two to three years, but often the patient's final appearance is less than desirable. Topical chemotherapy by trichloroacetic acid and cryosurgery with liquid nitrogen have been beneficial for patients with unsightly pitting and keloidal scars. Dermabrasion, popular in the past, still offers hope for improvement in a small group of patients with residual cystic scarring and nodular lesions. It is important to note that following dermabrasion, people who pigment easily occasionally develop hyperpigmentation which appears more unattractive than the original scars. Dermabrasion therefore should be executed only in carefully selected cases by a dermatologist or plastic surgeon familiar with its techniques and potential consequences.

HYPERHIDROSIS

Hyperhidrosis is a disorder characterized by an excessive production of perspiration in response to heat or emotional stimuli. Topical and systemic therapy can be temporarily suppressive but are basically unsatisfactory. Treatment with systemic anticholinergic agents (atropine, 0.01 mg. per kilogram per dose every 4 to 6 hours, or Pro-Banthine, 1.5 mg. per kilogram per 24 hours), effective to variable degrees, is limited by side effects such as mucous membrane dryness, blurred vision and mydriasis. Sedative or tranquilizing drugs appear to be beneficial for axillary or palmar hyperhidrosis, as are aluminum salts applied locally (10 to 25 per cent aluminum chloride in distilled water).

In palmar hyperhidrosis, local astringents of value are those which inhibit the production of perspiration (Burow's soaks 1:40 or potassium permanganate 1:4000). Dusting powders, such as ZeaSORB, may be helpful. Plantar hyperhidrosis may be suppressed with a solution of 10 per cent glutaraldehyde* buffered with sodium bicarbonate to a pH of 7.5 (1.65 Gm. $NaHCO_3$ per ml.) applied topically daily or every other day. This solution causes staining and therefore is not a useful modality for treatment of the palms.

---

* Glutaraldehyde is investigational; it has not yet received approval from the Food and Drug Administration.

DYSHIDROSIS

Dyshidrosis (pompholyx) is a term applied to a condition of recurring vesiculation of the palms and soles in which hyperhidrosis and retention of sweat precedes the eruption. Although this condition may not be a disorder of the sweat glands per se, hyperhidrosis is an important accessory factor; treatment directed toward the hyperhidrosis may prove beneficial. Topical steroid creams (Aristocort 0.1 per cent, Valisone 0.1 per cent or their equivalents) and efforts to minimize excessive perspiration are helpful in controlling this disorder.

BROMIDROSIS

Bromidrosis is an embarrassing malodorous condition caused by decomposition of apocrine sweat and keratin which has been softened by excessive secretion of the feet and intertriginous areas. This disorder can be controlled by scrupulous hygiene, repeated cleansing, preferably with antibacterial soaps, frequent changes of clothing and the use of topical bacteriostatic agents and commercial deodorants. Topical aluminum salts (10 to 25 per cent aluminum chloride in distilled water) and oral anticholinergic drugs (Pro-Banthine, 1.5 mg. per kilogram per 24 hours) may help axillary eccrine hyperhidrosis, but there is little evidence to their effect upon apocrine gland secretion. Dusting powders (ZeaSORB) may absorb excessive perspiration; disagreeable odors may be reduced by soaks with Burow's solution (1:40) or potassium permanganate (1:4000).

MILIARIA

Miliaria, a common dermatosis caused by sweat retention, is characterized by a vesicular eruption secondary to prolonged exposure to perspiration, with subsequent maceration and obstruction of the eccrine ducts. There are three forms of this disorder: miliaria crystallina (sudamina), miliaria rubra (prickly heat) and miliaria profunda (a more severe form of miliaria rubra commonly seen in the tropics). Therapy is directed toward avoidance of excessive heat and humidity. Light clothing, cool baths and air conditioning are invaluable. Calamine lotion, with or without ¼ per cent menthol and ½ per cent phenol, is effective yet has a tendency to cause excessive dryness; emollient creams such as Eucerin may be helpful. Resorcinol, 3 per cent in alcohol or in Cetaphil Lotion, is therapeutically beneficial in this disorder.

ANHIDROSIS

Anhidrosis is an abnormal absence of perspiration from the surface of the skin in the presence of appropriate stimuli, often resulting in hyperthermia. This condition may be caused by a deficiency or abnormality of the sweat gland (as in anhidrotic ectodermal dysplasia) or of the nervous pathways from the peripheral or central nervous system leading to the sweat gland (as in syringomyelia, leprosy, anticholinergic drug therapy or sympathectomy). Cool baths, air conditioning, light clothing and reducing the causes of normal perspiration help to relieve symptoms.

Miscellaneous Dermatoses

ALVIN H. JACOBS, M.D.

GRANULOMA ANNULARE

The typical lesions are smooth, skin-colored firm nodules grouped in an arciform arrangement. They occur most commonly on the backs of the hands and fingers, although they often also appear about the feet and ankles.

Granuloma annulare resolves completely in two to four years. Response to treatment is erratic but the best results are from intralesional injections of triamcinolone. The technique of this type of therapy is described in the discussion of vitiligo (p. 498).

LICHEN SPINULOSUS

This is an uncommon disorder of unknown etiology. Spiny keratinous, follicular projections grouped in large patches may appear on any part of the body. They are asymptomatic. Treatment is usually unnecessary but, if desired, mild keratolytics may be helpful. For this purpose one may use 5 per cent salicylic acid in Aquaphor or Carmol Cream, which contains 20 per cent urea.

GIANOTTI-CROSTI SYNDROME

Gianotti-Crosti syndrome is a distinctive, transient and benign dermatosis of children characterized by the abrupt appearance of lichenoid papules on the extremities, face and trunk. The illness resolves in four to six weeks. No specific treatment is available. If pruritus is bothersome, calamine lotion may be applied and antihistamines administered.

17

The Eye

General Considerations of Eye Disorders

LEONARD APT, M.D.

Those eye disorders which may be recognized or treated by the pediatrician will be stressed in this section. For the most part they are the simple inflammations of the eye and its adnexa. Most other ocular diseases should be referred to an ophthalmologist. Instrumentation other than that required to remove a superficial foreign body is to be avoided by the nonophthalmologic physician.

As in other areas of medicine the key to successful therapy of eye disorders is precise diagnosis. An accurate diagnosis is derived from a careful history, a systematic inspection of the visible eye structures, ophthalmoscopy and appropriate laboratory studies. The history should include details about the symptoms and their duration, preceding illnesses or trauma, and contact with others with similar symptoms. Thorough inspection of the eye with good illumination is imperative. One must gain the child's confidence and cooperation to accomplish this. Forceful closure of the eyelids by the patient will cause the eyeball to roll up and thus conceal the cornea. Forceful separation of the eyelids by the physician with pressure on the globe may rupture a thin or perforated cornea or globe. In some instances a sedative or general anesthetic may have to be given to relax a child satisfactorily.

Since a child's medical physician is often consulted first when an eye problem arises, it is necessary that he be aware of the manifestations of a serious eye disease. Knowledge of certain danger cues is of particular importance in dealing with the "red eye," a common presenting complaint which varies in significance from benign conjunctivitis to blinding intraocular disease. A serious, or potentially serious, eye disease should be considered if any of the following signs or symptoms are present:

Visual disturbances – reduced acuity, diplopia, "spots" before the eyes, reduction in part of the field of vision.

Severe *pain* or *photophobia* suggests corneal, intraocular or orbital disease. A corneal abrasion or foreign body may be the cause.

Opacities in the cornea, lens or vitreous. A corneal opacity may be overlooked if a bright focal light aimed obliquely is not used. Opacities in the lens or vitreous can be seen as dark areas in the red ophthalmoscopic reflex.

Pupils – irregularities in size or shape are seen after trauma or with intraocular inflammation.

Persistent *discharge* or *red eye* after several days of supposedly adequate treatment.

General Remarks About Local Therapy

In young children medication in ointment form has certain advantages over liquid preparations. There is less tendency to dilution and loss of the medication with crying, and less frequent instillations are required. On the other hand, drops may be easier to instill and less messy, and do not temporarily blur the vision. In the older child it is often more convenient to use drops during the day and the ointment at bedtime.

The pediatrician should not prescribe local eye anesthetics for a painful eye for home use. Local anesthetics tend to delay corneal healing. Injury to the anesthetized eye by the parent or child may occur unintentionally.

A plea is made to avoid the indiscriminate use of local corticosteroids, or combinations of these drugs, for just any inflamed or irritated eye. Corticosteroids are effective antiallergic and antiphlogistic agents, but they may retard healing or allow the progression of serious herpes simplex or tuberculous and fungous infections of the eye. The pediatrician should make it a general rule that when an antibiotic or steroid eye preparation is given, and no definitive diagnosis has been made, the patient be referred to an ophthalmologist if no distinct improvement occurs in one to two days.

Useful Local Eye Preparations

Diagnostic Stain. Stains are used to delineate abrasions, ulcerations and foreign bodies of the cornea and conjunctiva.

FLUORESCEIN STRIPS. Strips of filter paper impregnated with fluorescein are commercially available in sterile packages. Fluorescein strips are desirable because the sterility of a fluorescein solution is difficult to maintain, particularly against contamination with *Pseudomonas pyocyanea*. The dry or slightly moistened strip is merely touched in the conjunctival fornix. No flushing of the eye is needed.

Local Anesthetics. Local anesthetics are used to alleviate pain in order to examine the eye with convenience or to anesthetize the cornea and conjunctiva prior to the removal of a foreign body (see Table 1).

The most widely used local anesthetics are tetracaine (Pontocaine), and proparacaine (Ophthaine, Ophthetic). Tetracaine has the advantages of high anesthetic potency, great stability of the aqueous solution, resistance of the solution to bacterial and fungal contamination, and low cost. The disadvantages are the moderate burning sensation with the initial instillation of the drug and the mild congestion of the conjunctival vessels that it evokes. Proparacaine causes little or no discomfort on instillation, is not toxic and has a rapid onset, but a much shorter duration of action than tetracaine. The lack of stinging and burning

TABLE 1. Local Anesthetics for Ocular Use

GENERIC NAME	TRADE NAME
Benoxinate (0.4%)	Dorsacaine
Butacaine (2%)	Butyn
Cocaine (2–4%)	–
Lidocaine (4%)	Xylocaine
Phenacaine (1%)	Holocaine
Piperocaine (2–4%)	Metycaine
Proparacaine (0.5%)	Ophthaine, Ophthetic
Tetracaine (0.5%)	Pontocaine

TABLE 2. Topical Antibiotic and Sulfonamide Eye Preparations

GENERIC NAME	TRADE NAME	CONCENTRATION OF EYE DROP	CONCENTRATION OF EYE OINTMENT
Bacitracin	Baciguent	500–1000 U./ml.*	500 U./Gm.
Chloramphenicol	Chloromycetin	0.25–0.5%	1.0%
Chlortetracycline	Aureomycin	0.5%	1.0%
Colistin	Coly-Mycin	0.1%*	0.1–0.2%
Erythromycin	Ilotycin	0.5%*	0.5%
Gentamicin	Garamycin	0.3%	0.3%
Neomycin	Myciguent	0.5%*	0.5%
Sulfacetamide	Cetamide		10%
	Bleph-10, Bleph-30	10+30%	
	Blecon		30%
	Isopto-Cetamide	10%	
	Oc-U-Med	30%	
	Op-sulfa	10+30%	
	Sodium Sulamyd	10+30%	10%
	Sulfastatin	10%	
	Sulf-30	30%	
	Vasosulf	15%	
Sulfadiazine	–		5.0%
Sulfisoxazole	Gantrisin	4.0%	4.0%
Streptomycin	–	0.25%*	0.25%*
Tetracycline	Achromycin	0.5%*	1.0%
		1.0% (oil susp.)	
Tyrothrycin	–	0.5%	0.2%*

* Not available commercially as a single drug preparation.

TABLE 3. Topical Antimicrobial Combination Eye Preparations

GENERIC NAME	TRADE NAME
Bacitracin + polymyxin B	Polysporin (oint.)
Bacitracin + neomycin + polymyxin B	Mycitracin (oint.) Neo-Polycin (oint.) Neosporin (sol.)
Chloramphenicol + polymyxin B	Chloromycetin-polymyxin (oint.)
Gramicidin + neomycin + polymyxin B	Neo-Polycin (sol.) Neosporin (oint.)
Neomycin + polymyxin B	Conjunctin (sol.) Op-Isophrin-A B (sol.) Polyspectrin (sol., oint.) Statrol (sol.)
Neomycin + sulfacetamide	Sulfacidin (sol.)
Oxytetracycline + polymyxin	Terramycin with polymyxin (oint.)

(Oint. = ointment; sol. = solution.)

TABLE 4. Topical Antimicrobial Corticosteroid Eye Preparations

GENERIC NAME	TRADE NAME
Bacitracin + cortisone	Cortone-Bacitracin (oint.)
Bacitracin + neomycin + polymyxin + hydrocortisone	Cortisporin (susp., oint.)
Chloramphenicol + hydrocortisone	Chloromycetin-hydrocortisone (susp.)
Chloramphenicol + prednisolone	Chloroptic-P (oint.)
Chloramphenicol + polymyxin + hydrocortisone	Ophthocort (oint.)
Neomycin + cortisone	Neosone (oint.)
Neomycin + hydrocortisone	Cor-Oticin (sol.) Neo-Cortef (susp., oint.) Neo-Polycin HC (oint.)
Neomycin + polymyxin + hydrocortisone	Cortisporin (susp.)
Neomycin + polymyxin + dexamethasone	Maxitrol (susp., oint.)
Neomycin + polymyxin + prednisolone	Prednefrin (susp.)
Neomycin + prednisolone	Neo-Delta-Cortef (susp., oint.) Neo-Deltef (sol.) Neo-Hydeltrasol (sol., oint.) Predmycin (sol.)
Neomycin + methylprednisolone	Neo-Medrol (oint.)
Neomycin + dexamethasone	Neo-Decadron (sol., oint.)
Oxytetracycline + hydrocortisone	Terra-Cortril (susp.)
Sulfacetamide + prednisolone	Blephamide (susp.) Cetapred (oint.) Isopto-Cetapred (susp.) Metimyd (susp., oint.) Optimyd (sol.) Sulfapred (susp.) Vasocidin (sol.)
Tetracycline + hydrocortisone	Achromycin-hydrocortisone (oint.)

(Susp. = suspension; sol. = solution; oint. = ointment; PDR = powder for suspension.)

TABLE 5. Topical Corticosteroid Eye Preparations

GENERIC NAME	TRADE NAME	CONCENTRATION
Medrysone		
Suspension	HMS	1.0%
	Medrocort	10%
Hydrocortisone		
Acetate suspension	Hydrocortone	0.5%; 2.5%
Solution	Optef	0.2%
Acetate ointment	Hydrocortone	1.5%
Fludrometholone		
Suspension	FML	0.1%
	Oxylone	0.1%
Prednisolone		
Acetate suspension	Metreton	0.2%
	Prednefrin	0.12%
	Prednefrin forte	1.0%
	Sterofrin	0.25%
	Vasopred	0.25%
Alcohol solution	Prednefrin S	0.2%
Phosphate sol. or oint.	Hydeltrasol	0.5%
sol.	Inflamase	0.125%
	Inflamase forte	1.00%
Dexamethasone		
Phosphate	Decadron	0.1% sol.; 0.05% oint.
Suspension	Maxidex	0.1%

TABLE 6. Topical Vasoconstrictor, Astringent and Antihistaminic Preparations

GENERIC NAME	TRADE NAME
Vasoconstrictors	
Epinephrine eye solution, 1:20,000	
Naphazoline, 0.1%	Albalon Privine Vasocon
Phenylephrine, 0.125% (approx.)	Degest Efricel Isopto Frin Neo-Synephrine Op-Isophrin Op-Isophrin-M Prefrin Tear-efrin

TABLE 6. *Continued*

Tetrahydrozoline, 0.05%	Visine
Astringent with vasoconstrictor	
Zinc sulfate, 0.25%, + epinephrine, 1:20,000	
Zinc sulfate, 0.25%, + phenylephrine, 0.12%	M-Z Solution
	Neozin
	Oc-U-Zin
	Op-Isophrin-Z
	Op-Isophrin-Z-M
	Phenylzin
	Prefrin-Z
	Zincfrin
Antihistamine + or — vasoconstrictor	
Antazoline, 0.5%, + naphazoline, 0.05%	Vasocon-A
Chlorpheniramine, 0.3%, + phenylephrine, 0.12%	Optihist
Chlorpheniramine, 0.1%, + phenylephrine, 0.125%	Isohist
Pyrilamine maleate, 0.1%, + phenylephrine, 0.12%	Prefrin-A

is a practical advantage in its use in infants and children.

Mydriatics and Cycloplegics. Weak mydriatics merely dilate the pupil. Strong mydriatics, in addition to dilating the pupil, paralyze accommodation by acting on the ciliary muscle. For ophthalmoscopy alone, a weak mydriatic is used, since paralysis of near vision is unnecessary. Mydriasis lasts only a few hours. Cycloplegic drugs are principally used to measure refractive errors, to immobilize the ciliary muscle in inflammatory conditions of the uveal tract and to dilate the pupil to avoid posterior synechiae in cases of iridocyclitis.

Because weak mydriatics dilate the pupil for only a few hours, cycloplegic drugs are often used when mydriasis is desired for longer periods; e.g., for daily observation of the fundus, frequent instillations of the weak mydriatics are not required. Cycloplegic drugs are also used by the ophthalmologist in the treatment of amblyopia ("lazy eye") resulting from an uncorrected refractive error in one eye, strabismus, or disuse, as in congenital cataract. The drug is instilled into the eye which has normal vision to blur the image and to prevent near vision. The patient is thus forced to use the amblyopic eye. The useful drugs for this purpose are as follows:

Mydriatics (with minimal or virtually no cycloplegic effect)
- Bis-tropamide (Mydriacyl), 0.5 per cent
- Cyclopentolate, 0.2 per cent with phenylephrine, 1 per cent (Cyclomydril)
- Eucatropine (Euphthalamine), 5 per cent
- Hydroxyamphetamine (Paredrine), 1 per cent
- Phenylephrine (Neo-Synephrine), 2.5 per cent, 10 per cent

Cycloplegics
- Atropine, 0.25–2 per cent
- Bis-tropamide (Mydriacyl), 1 per cent
- Cyclopentolate (Cyclogyl), 0.5–2 per cent
- Homatropine, 2–5 per cent
- Scopolamine, 0.2–0.5 per cent

Atropine is the most potent cycloplegic drug and is the longest acting: seven to 14 days. Mydriasis begins 40 minutes after instillation of the drug, and maximum cycloplegia occurs in about 36 hours. The lower concentrations of the drug should be used in infants and young children because toxic amounts of the drug may be absorbed. It is important to realize that absorption of toxic quantities of atropine can occur, because a 1 per cent solution provides approximately 1/120 grain of atropine powder with each drop. Pressure over the lacrimal sac when instilling the solution will help to prevent absorption of the drug through the nasal mucosa. Use of atropine in ointment form allows less chance of absorption of the drug through the lacrimal drainage system.

Scopolamine is also a potent cycloplegic. It can produce the same toxic symptoms as atropine. Mydriasis begins in 40 minutes; cycloplegia is maximal in 60 to 90 minutes, and gradually subsides in three to six days.

Homatropine is a less potent cycloplegic than atropine or scopolamine. The higher concentrations produce full mydriasis in 30 minutes and maximal cycloplegia in 60 to 90 minutes. Recovery from cycloplegia occurs in 24 to 48 hours. Toxicity from homatropine eye drops is infrequent. Instillation causes a burning sensation.

Cyclopentolate (Cyclogyl) produces rapid mydriasis and cycloplegia. Mydriasis appears in 20 minutes, and maximum cycloplegia is reached and maintained for 45 to 75 minutes after instillation of the drug. Recovery of the accommodation takes place in 6 to 12 hours, but mydriasis can persist for 24 hours. The cycloplegia, when maximal, is as profound as that obtained with atropine. Toxic effects are uncommon, but toxic hallucinatory effects and allergic reactions to the drug have been encountered in a few children.

Bis-tropamide (Mydriacyl) in the 1 per cent concentration is an ultrashort-acting cycloplegic; in the 0.5 per cent concentration the preparation is principally a mydriatic. Mydriasis and cycloplegia occur simultaneously in about 20 minutes. The duration of maximal cycloplegia is only 10 to 20 minutes. Recovery from cycloplegia is likewise rapid: 4 to 6 hours.

To achieve consistent maximal cycloplegia it is recommended that at least two instillations, about 5 minutes apart, be given. No local or systemic toxic effects from the drug have been described. It stings on instillation.

Eyelid Disorders

LEONARD APT, M.D.

BLEPHARITIS

Blepharitis is a common, chronic, recurrent inflammation of the lid margins characterized by redness, crusting ("granulated eyelids"), burning, irritation, itching, loss of eyelashes, and conjunctival irritation.

Two types are recognized by inspection. Clinical differentiation is of practical importance because knowledge of the cause aids the specific treatment. In all types, scales should be removed from the eyelid margins daily with a moistened cotton applicator or cloth. Hot moist compresses may help loosen scales.

Ulcerative Blepharitis

This is invariably caused by *Staphylococcus aureus*. Smears, cultures and sensitivity tests, however, should be obtained. The scales are hard and tenacious. Ulcers and pustules appear on the lid margins at the base of the cilia. There may be an accompanying conjunctivitis or keratitis.

Treatment. Avoid those antistaphylococcal antibiotics which later may be needed for a systemic or serious infection, because sensitization to the drug may result from its local use. The preparations most useful are bacitracin, neomycin and sulfacetamide ophthalmic ointments or liquids (Table 2, p. 517). After removal of the scales the medication is rubbed into the lid margins three or four times daily. Adrenocorticosteroids in combination with antimicrobial agents can be used to reduce the inflammation in the eye and on the eyelid caused by the staphylococcus itself or the hypersensitivity reaction that may accompany the infection.

In severe cases systemic sulfonamide or antibiotic therapy (tetracycline in low doses only in older children) may be required. Some stubborn cases have improved after the use of staphylococcus toxoid. A solution of 1000 units per ml. is given in a dose of 0.05 ml. subcutaneously, and is increased by 0.05 ml. at weekly intervals until a dose of 5 ml. has been given.

To clear the focus of infection completely in the eyelids, the ophthalmologist may find it necessary to express the meibomian glands.

General measures, such as the daily use of an antibacterial soap to control skin staphylococci, are also worthwhile.

Nonulcerative or Squamous Blepharitis

This group is subdivided into (1) seborrheic blepharitis; the scales are greasy and easily removed, seborrhea of the scalp is almost always present, and conjunctivitis or keratitis is usually absent, and (2) squamous blepharitis caused by *Hemophilus duplex* (Diplobacillus of Morax-Axenfeld), typified by minimal scaling and macerated epithelium of the eyelid margins, an angular conjunctivitis or a keratoconjunctivitis and the absence of seborrhea capitis.

Microscopic examination of eyelid margin scrapings is easily done and is of further diagnostic value. Gram-positive cocci and leukocytes are found in ulcerative blepharitis. Round or flask-shaped gram-positive budding yeasts *(Pityrosporum ovale)* are frequently found in seborrheic blepharitis; this microorganism, however, is not considered the causative agent. Large gram-negative diplobacilli with no leukocytes are seen in the second type of squamous blepharitis.

Over 90 per cent of the cases of blepharitis are staphylococcal, seborrheic or a mixture of the two. Mixed types are common. Other bacteria causing blepharitis are *Streptococcus viridans*, beta-hemolytic streptococcus, *Escherichia coli*, *Klebsiella pneumoniae* (Friedländer's bacillus) and *Pseudomonas aeruginosa*.

Treatment. SEBORRHEIC BLEPHARITIS. Sulfacetamide has antiseborrheic activity, but the commonly used antibiotics do not. Drugs that have been used for seborrheic dermatitis may also be used for the blepharitis:

- 2.5 per cent ammoniated mercury ointment applied to the lid margins twice daily
- 1 per cent yellow mercuric oxide with 1 per cent salicylic acid ointment applied twice daily
- 1 to 2 per cent sulfur ointments applied twice daily
- 1 per cent resorcinol ointment applied twice daily
- Nitrofurazone (Furacin) eye ointment applied at bedtime effective in some cases.

For the successful therapy of seborrheic blepharitis, it is imperative to treat the seborrhea that usually exists in other areas, e.g., scalp, eyebrows or ears.

Hemophilus Duplex (DIPLOBACILLUS OF MORAX–AXENFELD) BLEPHARITIS. The sulfonamides and zinc salts are the most effective drugs. Sulfacetamide ointment or zinc sulfate ophthalmic solution (0.25 per cent) or ointment (0.5

per cent) applied to the eyelid margins five or six times daily is effective.

HORDEOLUM (STY)

External Hordeolum

This is an acute, localized pyogenic infection (usually staphylococcal) of the sebaceous glands (Zeis or Moll) along the lid margin. The localized area of redness, swelling and tenderness appears on the lid margin at the base of the eyelash. A small yellow area of suppuration appears in a day or so. With rupture of the abscess, pain diminishes.

Treatment. In the early stages warm, moist compresses applied for 20 minutes four times daily hasten localization of the infection. Pressure should not be applied to hasten this process. Only when the hordeolum is entirely localized, pointing through the epidermis, should it be incised to allow the pus to drain. An antistaphylococcal ointment (bacitracin, neomycin, sulfacetamide) applied locally four to six times daily is helpful in aborting the suppuration and preventing the spread of the infection. Treatment should be continued for about one week after the sty has healed to prevent further infection in other hair follicles. For recurrent sty, treatment with staphylococcal toxoid or vaccine (see staphylococcal blepharitis) or an autogenous vaccine may be used, although these are employed rarely nowadays.

Internal Hordeolum

The acute purulent infection involves one of the meibomian glands (meibomian sty). The area of localized redness, pain, swelling or abscess appears on the conjunctival rather than the skin side corresponding to the location of the gland. Spontaneous rupture is less frequent than with the external sty. Recurrences are common.

Treatment is the same as for external hordeolum.

CHALAZION

Chalazion is a common, chronic granulomatous meibomian gland infection of unknown cause. In contrast to the acute purulent infection of this gland (internal hordeolum), there is little or no pain or tenderness unless there is a superimposed secondary pyogenic infection. Symptoms are slight. A slow-growing, hard, round mass localized in the tarsus points more commonly to the conjunctival rather than the skin side. If large enough, the mass will distort vision. The tumor may remain the same size, ulcerate through the surface and leave some remains, or be absorbed.

Treatment. If warm moist compresses and topical antibiotic-corticosteroid therapy do not significantly reduce the size of the mass in a few days, incision and evacuation of the chalazion should be performed by an ophthalmologist. For recurrent chalazia the use of an antibacterial ointment at bedtime and several times a day, and weekly massage of the meibomian glands to express secretions may be helpful.

Conjunctival Disorders

LEONARD APT, M.D.

CONJUNCTIVITIS

Conjunctivitis ranks with blepharitis as one of the most common external ocular inflammations. Inflammation of the conjunctiva may be microbial, allergic or traumatic in origin. It may be acute, subacute or chronic. In the differential diagnosis of the acutely inflamed eye, conjunctivitis can be differentiated from iritis and glaucoma by the presence of a discharge (often bilateral), normal or unaffected vision, normal pupil size and reaction to light and normal intraocular pressure.

Bacterial Conjunctivitis

Because certain bacteria cause distinct clinical features of bacterial conjunctivitis, the following classification is possible:

Purulent (Hyperacute) Conjunctivitis. Purulent discharge occurs with intense bulbar and tarsal conjunctivitis and chemosis. The gonococcus and, much less rarely, the meningococcus are the main etiologic agents. Meningococcal conjunctivitis may accompany meningitis.

Mucopurulent (Acute Catarrhal) Conjunctivitis ("Pink Eye"). The most common causative microorganisms are the *Staphylococcus aureus* pneumococcus, Koch-Weeks bacillus, and beta-hemolytic streptococcus. Intense bulbar but minimal tarsal inflammation is seen. Epithelial keratitis is rare except in the staphylococcal form. Petechial hemorrhages are most common with pneumococcal and Koch-Weeks bacillus infections. The disease is highly contagious. It may last several weeks if untreated. The eyelids seal overnight from the drying of the products of inflammation.

Subacute Catarrhal Conjunctivitis. This milder form of conjunctivitis is caused by

Hemophilus influenzae, Neisseria catarrhalis, Escherichia coli and *Bacillus proteus.*

Chronic Catarrhal Conjunctivitis. The two frequent etiologic bacteria are *Staphylococcus aureus* and Morax-Axenfeld diplobacillus, but any of the bacteria that cause the more acute forms of conjunctivitis may be found here. Typically the eye feels worse (itching, smarting, foreign body sensation) at night or in the morning. Blepharitis is common. The palpebral conjunctiva is chronically inflamed, but the bulbar conjunctiva is little affected, if at all. In the staphylococcal type frequently there are marginal infiltrates, ulcers and epithelial erosions of the cornea; loss of cilia may result. The Morax-Axenfeld bacillus characteristically produces redness most intense near the inner and outer canthi (angular conjunctivitis). The staphylococcus can also cause an angular conjunctivitis.

Treatment. The best guide for specific therapy is established by demonstrating the etiologic bacteria in smears and cultures, and then testing the sensitivity to various antimicrobial agents. From a practical standpoint this is seldom done. Often the conjunctivitis is treated empirically with a broad-spectrum antibiotic or sulfacetamide. The drug should produce few or no local sensitivities and be infrequently used in the treatment of systemic disease. Bacitracin, neomycin, polymyxin B and sulfacetamide are such drugs. If no improvement occurs in several days, cultures and antibiotic sensitivity studies are obtained and the appropriate antibiotic is used. In angular conjunctivitis due to the Morax-Axenfeld bacillus, zinc sulfate is effective in a 0.25 to 0.50 per cent solution, as well as the broad-spectrum antibiotics.

Adrenal corticosteroids have been combined with antimicrobial agents in ophthalmic preparations (Table 4, p. 518) to reduce the inflammatory and, possibly, the allergic reactions to the bacterial infection. It is best to avoid corticosteroids because of their adverse effect on latent or potential herpes simplex and mycotic infections and because of a false impression of control of the inflammatory response by the antiphlogistic action of corticosteroids.

In severe forms of bacterial conjunctivitis systemic therapy may be needed. Patients with uncomplicated conjunctivitis should not have the eyes patched. To avoid infections of other sites or other people, clean and separate cloths should be used for cleansing the eye area.

Viral Conjunctivitis

There is no specific therapy for viral conjunctivitis. The adenovirus is one of the most common agents. Therapy consists in combating secondary bacterial infections by the local use of broad-spectrum antibiotics or a sulfonamide, the relief of symptoms with the use of hot or cold compresses, and the use of local astringents or vasoconstrictors (Table 6, p. 519).

Adenovirus Conjunctivitis. The adenoviruses (adenopharyngoconjunctival or APC viruses) produce two well-organized infections: pharyngeal-conjunctival fever and epidemic keratoconjunctivitis.

Pharyngeal-conjunctival fever is seen mostly in children and is characterized by fever, malaise, sore throat, preauricular and cervical lymphadenopathy, and a follicular conjunctivitis. The palpebral conjunctiva is red, and there is a copious water discharge. The disease is usually caused by adenovirus type 3. Other types of adenovirus (except type 8) have occasionally produced the disease. It is self-limited, lasting about 10 days. Contaminated swimming pools, even those chlorinated, are frequent sources of infection. There is no specific therapy; sulfacetamide ophthalmic ointment is useful to prevent secondary bacterial infection.

Epidemic keratoconjunctivitis is highly contagious and may occur in epidemics. Type 8 adenovirus is a frequent but probably not the only viral cause. There is a sudden onset of conjunctival congestion, chemosis, profuse tearing and epithelial keratitis, but little secretion. In infants the infection may be manifested as a pseudomembranous conjunctivitis. Physicians and hospital clinics may spread the disease. The exudate contains predominantly mononuclear cells, sometimes many polymorphonuclear cells, but no inclusions. A few days later preauricular adenopathy on the affected side appears. After about 15 days subepithelial infiltrates may develop in the cornea. The corneal opacities usually clear in several months, but on occasion may never clear completely. Because the disease is highly contagious, great care should be exercised in the handling of objects used around the eye. Patients admitted to the hospital should be isolated. Topical broad-spectrum antibiotics have been used to prevent secondary infection. Topical corticosteroids have been used for the corneal opacities. Convalescent plasma, because of the antibody content, has also been used locally and intravenously. There is no evidence that any of these substances are of value.

Chlamydial Conjunctivitis

Inclusion Conjunctivitis. (See Conjunctivitis Neonatorum for discussion of the disease in the newborn.) The disease is also known as swimming pool conjunctivitis. In recent years it has been seen more frequently within the teenage hippie population. It is caused by the agent which produces inclusion blennorrhea in the newborn. It causes an acute or chronic follicular type of conjunctivitis. There is bilateral conjunctival redness and a copious exudate. The exudate contains polymorphonuclear leukocytes, plasma cells and typical cytoplasmic inclusion bodies similar to those of trachoma, but usually there is no scarring or corneal involvement. Occasionally the corneal opacities are permanent and large. The disease should be treated with oral sulfonamide or broad-spectrum antibiotic therapy for three weeks. Chlorination of swimming pools reduces the incidence of the disease.

Trachoma

This disease is one of the leading causes of blindness in some parts of the world. Contrary to general belief, it exists also in the United States. Trachoma is endemic among the Indians, in a few localities in the South and Southwest, and in certain of the alien populations. This chlamydial organism is related to the agents that cause psittacosis and lymphogranuloma venereum; it is of low infectivity. The disease occurs under conditions of poor sanitation and hygiene. The clinical picture is that of chronic bilateral conjunctival redness, mild itching, and watery discharge with scant exudate. In the early stages trachoma is indistinguishable from a mild catarrhal conjunctivitis. Cytoplasmic inclusion bodies, morphologically identical, though fewer in number, to those found in inclusion blennorrhea, are found in the conjunctival scrapings. In untreated cases inflammation of the conjunctiva continues over a period of months or years, producing papillary and then follicular hypertrophy followed by scarring. With progression of the disease the cornea becomes opacified, vascularized and scarred, thus severely impairing vision. Some of the ocular complications are due to secondary bacterial infection.

Treatment. The conjunctival inflammation in trachoma can be effectively treated with a combination of local and systemic sulfonamides or broad-spectrum antibiotics. The disease could probably be cured with local eye therapy alone, but the combination with systemic therapy hastens improvement. The preferred systemic treatment has been sufisoxazole (Gantrisin),* 100 mg. per kilogram of body weight given daily by mouth for one week, reduced to 60 mg. per kilogram of body weight for two weeks; or full tetracycline therapy in patients over 10 years of age. Local therapy is also given with tetracycline (Achromycin ophthalmic oil suspension, 1 per cent administered for six weeks, 2 drops into each eye four times daily, or tetracycline ointment into each eye four times daily for six weeks. An additional course of systemic therapy may be given after one week of no sulfonamide therapy. Corticosteroids should not be given, since they may reactivate the virus.

* Manufacturer's precaution: Sulfisoxazole is contraindicated in infants under two months of age except in the treatment of congenital toxoplasmosis as adjunctive therapy with pyrimethamine.

Exanthematous Conjunctivitis

The exanthems such as measles, chicken pox and smallpox may be accompanied by an acute catarrhal conjunctivitis. No specific treatment is given unless secondary bacterial infection occurs. If the cornea becomes involved, an ophthalmologist should be consulted for further treatment.

Vaccinial Conjunctivitis

Autoinoculation or inoculation from a contact may lead to a conjunctivitis or serious corneal involvement. Local treatment consists of idoxuridine (Herplex, Stoxil) drops (0.1 per cent solution) every hour during the day and every 2 hours during the night, or ointment (0.5 per cent), available as Stoxil ointment, used every 4 hours. Specific therapy for this complication means the use of passively administered antibodies in the form of hyperimmune gamma globulin prepared from the blood of donors who had recently been successfully vaccinated. The dose of vaccinia immune globulin is 0.6 ml. per kilogram of body weight up to a total of 20 ml. It is best not to give more than 5 ml. in one injection site. A 5-ml. vial is available from Hyland Laboratories. Vaccinia immune globulin should be used with caution if a serious keratitis accompanies eyelid lesions or a conjunctivitis. There is experimental evidence that the agent may aggravate the keratitis.

Conjunctivitis Neonatorum (Ophthalmia Neonatorum)

Any inflammation of the conjunctiva of the newborn is considered in this category. The inflammation may be due to the chemical irritant silver nitrate or to an infection acquired from an infected birth canal during parturition. The infection may be bacterial (gonococcal, staphylococcal, streptococcal, pneumococcal or other) or viral (inclusion blennorrhea).

The time of onset of the conjunctivitis is

helpful in the diagnosis. Silver nitrate conjunctivitis occurs within 24 hours after birth, bacterial conjunctivitis within two to five days, and inclusion conjunctivitis within five to 10 days. The definite diagnosis, however, is made by examining Gram- and Giemsa-stained scraping from the retrotarsal fold of the newborn showing signs of conjunctivitis and from culture studies of the material.

Silver nitrate conjunctivitis is sterile and usually clears without treatment in several days. Occasionally a secondary bacterial infection will require specific antibiotics or sulfonamide treatment.

Of the bacterial conjunctivitides, it is imperative that the diagnosis of the gonococcal type be made as soon as possible. With proper treatment the prognosis is good. The untreated or inadequately treated case results in corneal ulceration, perforation or panophthalmitis. The incidence of blindness from gonococcal conjunctivitis has been drastically reduced by prenatal treatment of the mother and by routine use of 1 per cent silver nitrate solution or an appropriate antibiotic instilled into each eye of the newborn immediately after birth. In those states of the United States in which silver nitrate need not be the only drug used for prophylaxis, erythromycin, a tetracycline, or chloramphenicol ophthalmic preparations have been used with success.

Treatment. Active treatment of gonorrheal conjunctivitis in the newborn consists in (1) topical antibiotic therapy every 1 to 2 hours—erythromycin, a tetracycline or chloramphenicol (see Table 2, p. 517); (2) systemic antibiotic therapy for four or five days—penicillin G, 30,000 units, or ampicillin, 50 mg., per kilogram of body weight injected intramuscularly every 12 hours, or erythromycin ethyl succinate, 5 mg. per kilogram of body weight given intramuscularly every 12 hours; (3) frequent irrigations of the conjunctival sac with isotonic sodium chloride solution; and (4) if the cornea is threatened, dilatation of the pupils with atropine sulfate, 0.25 per cent ophthalmic solution, 1 drop into the conjunctival sac once or twice daily.

For the nongonorrheal bacterial conjunctivitides the same local ophthalmic preparations can be used; bacitracin and neomycin are also excellent drugs for reasons previously mentioned.

Inclusion blenorrhea responds well to local sulfacetamide or to a tetracycline ophthalmic preparation.

Mucocutaneous Ocular Diseases

Treatment of the conjunctivitis associated with the mucocutaneous diseases, such as erythema multiforme, Stevens-Johnson disease and Reiter's syndrome, is mostly nonspecific, since the etiologic agent is unknown. Precipitating factors may be drugs, food allergy or infections. Mild soothing eye drops with or without astringent and vasoconstricting properties (Table 6, p. 519) may be used. Steroids used locally (Table 5, p. 518) or systemically may be helpful in controlling the allergic and inflammatory phases of the disease, but they must be used judiciously. Drugs such as the sulfonamides and antibiotics should be avoided, for they have been known to precipitate erythema multiforme and Stevens-Johnson disease. A local antibiotic should be used only when a secondary bacterial infection occurs. Choose a suitable one that the patient has not previously used, or one that unquestionably was not associated with the present episode. In severe cases visual function can be seriously impaired because of lack of tears, symblepharon, corneal ulcer, perforation and panophthalmitis in Stevens-Johnson disease, and scleritis, interstitial keratitis and hypopyon uveitis in Reiter's disease. Because of the seriousness of the eye complications it is advisable to have an ophthalmologist treat the ocular aspects of these diseases.

Allergic Forms of Conjunctivitis

Simple Allergic Conjunctivitis. The clinical manifestations of these nonspecific conjunctival inflammations are acute edema of the lids and conjunctiva, itching, photophobia, lacrimation, mild injection of the palpebral and bulbar conjunctiva, and a scanty stringy discharge. Conjunctival papillae and follicles are not present. An occasional eosinophil is present in the smear of the conjunctival scraping. There may or may not be a direct relation to an allergen such as a pollen (hay fever), cosmetic or drug.

Treatment consists in (1) removal of the offending agent if possible, (2) desensitization to the allergen, and (3) symptomatic relief with the use of local vasoconstrictors, astringents, antihistaminics and corticosteroids (Tables 5 and 6, pp. 518 and 519). Because of superior effect, the corticosteroids have replaced most of the other local preparations. It is wise to use the minimum amount of steroid needed to control the reaction and for the shortest time possible. Weak corticosteroid preparations, such as HMS or Medrocort, should be tried before using the stronger more commonly used corticosteroid eye preparations. The disadvantages of the steroids, i.e., the increase of herpes simplex, and bacterial and fungus infections, must be kept in mind. Cataracts and glaucoma have been seen in children as well as in adults who have been using corticosteroids topically for allergy. Systemic corticosteroids are rarely needed. If vasoconstrictors with or without antihistaminics (local and systemic) control the allergic reaction, steroids should not be used.

Vernal Conjunctivitis. This is a bilateral chronic conjunctivitis with symptoms which usually become worse in the spring and last throughout the warm months. The cause is thought to be allergic. The onset is between five and 15 years; symptoms become milder with the passing years. There is intense itching, lacrimation, photophobia, conjunctival injection, a stringy conjunctival discharge and, at times, a milky pseudomembrane. Giant papillary hypertrophy develops in the tarsal conjunctiva, especially the upper, to give the typical "cobblestone" appearance. The lesions may be large enough to abrade the cornea and cause corneal ulcers. Papillary hypertrophy in the limbal region appears as gray elevated lesions. Many eosinophils are seen in the smear of the conjunctival exudate.

Symptoms are relieved with topical corticosteroid drops or ointment. Vasoconstrictors and antihistaminics alone usually are insufficient. Desensitization to allergens has been disappointing. Removal to a cool climate is helpful. Beta radiation has been used to reduce the size of the hypertrophied papillae, but this is generally not necessary.

Phlyctenular Keratoconjunctivitis. The phlyctenule is a small, hard, red elevated nodule surrounded by hyperemic vessels. It appears most commonly at the limbus to involve both the bulbar conjunctiva and the cornea. The lesion is a subepithelial collection of lymphocytes; they ulcerate, but usually heal. Recurrences, especially with secondary infection, may result in corneal opacification. The outstanding clinical manifestations are intense photophobia and lacrimation. The disease has been regarded as a hypersensitivity reaction of the conjunctiva and cornea to a product of the tubercle bacillus or to other bacteria such as the staphylococcus, or to fungi.

Since malnutrition is frequently a part of the disease, general measures, such as improving the diet and hygiene, are important. A topical steroid or steroid-antibiotic combination (Tables 4 and 5, p. 518) is effective in treating the disease and the secondary infection that may be present. Investigation for a systemic disease such as tuberculosis should be made.

Nonspecific Conjunctival Hyperemia

External irritants such as smoke, smog, fumes, swimming pool or ocean water, or factors such as inadequate rest or asthenopia (eyestrain) may produce conjunctival hyperemia. Astringent eye drops with or without a vasoconstrictor (Table 6, p. 519) relieve this nonspecific inflammation. A complete eye examination should be performed if the symptoms are associated with eyestrain.

The pediatrician must consider specific diseases, such as ataxia-telangiectasia and familial dysautonomia (Riley-Day syndrome), before settling on a diagnosis of nonspecific conjunctival hyperemia.

Corneal Disorders

LEONARD APT, M.D.

In general, diseases of the cornea require early attention by an ophthalmologist. Even so-called minor affections of this portion of the eye can lead to serious ocular complications, including blindness, if they are not promptly and correctly handled by the skilled specialist. A safe rule for the nonophthalmologic physician to follow is that all diseases and injuries of the cornea (including foreign bodies) should be seen promptly by an ophthalmologist. It is important therefore for the pediatrician to learn the symptoms and signs of corneal disease to enable him to recognize this diagnostic possibility.

Patients with corneal disease may have photophobia, lacrimation, blepharospasm, pain, decreased vision, ocular discharge, hyperemia of the superficial and deep conjunctival vessels (circumlimbal flush), corneal opacity, small pupil if secondary iritis exists, and often a history of trauma. Inspection of the cornea with intense oblique focal illumination is often necessary to see a foreign body or a lesion.

The treatment of corneal diseases will not be detailed because this should be carried out by the ophthalmologist.

CORNEAL ULCERS AND INFECTIONS

Careful examination of the ocular adnexa is important because inflammation of the cornea may be secondary to other ocular diseases, e.g., blepharitis, trichiasis, trachoma, the cobblestone papillae of vernal conjunctivitis, conjunctivitis, scleritis, iritis or dacryocystitis. Systemic disease or poor general physical condition must be evaluated, for they may contribute to the development of a corneal infection.

Ulcers of the cornea can be easily seen by placing a drop or two of sterile fluorescein solution or a moistened fluorescein paper strip into the conjunctival sac and then washing out the excess with isotonic saline solution. To determine the cause of corneal ulcer, smears (Gram and Giemsa stains), cultures (bacterial and fungal) and sensitivity tests should be performed.

Simple Corneal Ulcer

This lesion may result from direct infection after a break of the epithelial barrier by trauma or by disturbances in the metabolism of the epithelium from causes such as vitamin A deficiency, corneal exposure and neurotrophic disease.

Central Corneal Ulcer

Central ulcers have an intense purulent reaction in and around the ulcer ("dirty ulcer"), with occasional extension into the deeper layers of the cornea or a reaction in the anterior chamber (hypopyon); most are bacterial. The causal bacteria in order of frequency are pneumococcus, beta-hemolytic streptococcus, *Pseudomonas aeruginosa (B. pyocyaneus),* diplobacillus of Pettit, and Friedländer's bacillus. The ulcers may develop after trauma or appear in association with a dacryocystitis (pneumococcus).

Treatment. Before antimicrobial treatment is started, smears and cultures of the ulcer material should be prepared and sensitivity studies to various antimicrobial agents pursued. Until these studies indicate the antimicrobial drug of choice, a local antibiotic mixture (Table 3, p. 518) effective against a wide range of gram-positive and gram-negative bacteria should be used at 1- to 2-hour intervals. Mixtures which contain bacitracin, neomycin and polymyxin B are available–Neosporin ophthalmic solution or ointment, Mycitracin and Neo-Polycin ophthalmic ointment (Table 3, p. 518). Gentamicin plus erythromycin or bacitracin may also be used. Local therapy alone may be all that is required in the superficial ulcers. In the more severe corneal ulcers, systemic and subconjunctival antibiotic therapy may be necessary. Cycloplegic medication is usually given because of the accompanying iridocyclitis. Local corticosteroid therapy is avoided because it interferes with tissue reparative processes and immune responses. Ulcers which progress in spite of vigorous medical therapy may benefit from covering the ulcer with a conjunctival flap, closure of the eyelids with adhesions (tarsorrhaphy) or replacement of the ulcer site by a keratoplasty.

Marginal Corneal Ulcer

Marginal ulcers are usually sterile and probably represent a toxic or hypersensitivity reaction to bacterial infection of the conjunctiva or eyelid. The acute type is seen with staphylococcal or Koch-Weeks conjunctivitis. The chronic type is secondary to staphylococcal, diplobacillus of Morax-Axenfeld, and streptococcal conjunctivitis.

Treatment. Topical corticosteroids usually cure the ulcer in three to four days. The blepharitis and conjunctivitis should be treated with bacitracin if the primary infection is due to the staphylococcus, streptococcus or Koch-Weeks bacillus. A tetracycline or sulfonamide is also effective against these bacteria as well as the diplobacillus of Morax-Axenfeld.

Phlyctenular Keratoconjunctivitis

This is discussed on page 525.

Herpes Simplex Virus Keratitis (Dendritic Keratitis)

This form of keratitis is a common corneal disease in childhood. The widespread and indiscriminate use of local steroids in recent years has significantly increased the incidence and severity of the infection and the ocular complications such as corneal perforation and loss of the eye. Dendritic keratitis is the most important corneal disease leading to loss of vision in the United States. Herpes simplex infections of the cornea tend to be chronic, leaving opaque scars that impair vision. Recurrent infections are frequent.

The patient complains of mild irritation, and has photophobia, lacrimation and blurred vision. A recent history of an infection of the respiratory tract with "cold sores" on the face is often elicited. Fever, trauma, menstruation and psychic stress may be other precipitating factors. The dendritic-shaped ulcer (seen best with fluorescein staining) and decreased corneal sensitivity characterize this type of keratitis.

Treatment. The principal treatment until recently was removal of the virus-containing epithelium, with or without chemical cauterization, by the ophthalmologist. Recently IDU (5-iodo-2′-deoxyuridine), commercially available as Herplex and Stoxil, in a 0.1 per cent solution, or in a 0.5 per cent ointment (Stoxil), has been reported to be effective against herpes simplex keratitis. Responses were best when the infection was limited to the epithelium. With stromal involvement the drug has been less effective or ineffective. IDU is incorporated into the viral DNA, resulting in the formation of defective viral particles. IDU is instilled into the eyes hourly during the day and every 2 hours during the night. Ointment is instilled into the eye every 4 hours during the day and at bedtime. Although corticosteroids are generally contraindicated in herpes simplex keratitis, in the less acute form with stromal involvement known as *disciform herpetic keratitis,* restricted use of weak local steroids, such as 0.005 dexamethasone solution, HMS or Medrocort (once or twice daily), is sometimes helpful if used along with IDU if the epithelium is healed. Disciform herpetic keratitis is possibly a hypersensitivity reaction to the superficial infection. If the keratitis is progressive in spite of medical treatment, a conjunctival flap, tarsorrhaphy or lamellar keratoplasty may be required.

Large doses of vitamins B and C, systemic administration of antihistaminics, cowpox vaccination and local administration of gamma globulin drops have been used in the treatment of herpetic keratitis, but with little consistent success.

Herpes Zoster Keratitis

The diagnosis is usually made from the characteristic skin lesions and their distribution along the ophthalmic division of the trigeminal nerve. The skin of the tip of the nose and the eye are often simultaneously involved, since the nasociliary nerve innervates both. An iridocyclitis usually accompanies the corneal involvement.

Treatment. Although steroids (without IDU) are contraindicated in herpes simplex keratitis, they frequently relieve the keratitis and iridocyclitis of herpes zoster. Severe involvement may be benefited by systemic administration of corticosteroids or ACTH (adrenocorticotropic hormone). The steroids act primarily as an antiphlogistic agent, for the disease has occurred, in some cases in a fulminating form, in patients who were receiving steroids for another disease. Cycloplegic eye drops are used for the iridocyclitis. Antibiotics to reduce secondary bacterial infection may reduce severe scarring of the cornea. Immune serum or convalescent plasma, for the passive antibody effect, has brought prompt improvement in some cases.

Vaccinia Keratitis

Vaccinia immune globulin has been used as recommended in the discussion of vaccinial conjunctivitis. Recent evidence indicates, however, that delayed immune reactions may be more common after its use. It should, therefore, be used with caution or not at all, particularly if there are no eyelid lesions or no conjunctivitis. IDU drops or ointment may be effective local therapy, since the vaccinia virus synthesizes DNA. The IDU should be used as described for herpes simplex keratitis.

Exanthematous Keratitis

Measles, chickenpox and smallpox infections of the cornea have no specific treatment. Local use of broad-spectrum antibiotics prevents secondary bacterial infections. Cycloplegics combat the secondary iridocyclitis. Steroids should be avoided.

Superficial Punctate Keratitis

This is characterized by scattered, fine punctate infiltrations in the superficial corneal layers, usually of both eyes. The lesions favor the pupillary area; they require magnification to be seen. Vision may be appreciably reduced. The lesions are nonulcerative, but most stain with fluorescein. Healing may take several years in the untreated case, but no scarring or vascularization occurs. The disease is thought to be caused by a virus. Drugs, exposure and staphylococcal infections, however, may produce the same signs and symptoms. The symptoms are photophobia, lacrimation, pain, conjunctival injection and decreased vision. Preauricular lymphadenopathy may be present.

Treatment. Topical use of corticosteroids is often beneficial. Cycloplegics are usually not needed. Local antibiotics are used only if there is a bacterial infection.

Fungal Corneal Ulcers

The incidence of keratomycosis has increased in recent years. Local antibiotic and steroid therapy seems to be an important factor in this increase. Fungi infect the cornea after a break in the epithelium from trauma or damage by inflammation. Numerous fungi, including those previously regarded as nonpathogenic, have been cultured from these indolent, slowly progressive corneal ulcers.

Treatment. Treatment should be as described for fungal conjunctivitis. Subconjunctival injections of amphotericin B (150 micrograms in 0.05 ml. of water) or nystatin (somewhat irritating) may be given in addition to topical therapy. Some control of the infection has been reported from the local use of 0.125 per cent copper sulfate given topically or by iontophoresis combined with oral potassium iodide.

Interstitial Keratitis

Most cases in children occur as a complication of congenital syphilis. Tuberculosis and leprosy are rare causes. Symptoms of intense photophobia, lacrimation, pain and gradual loss of vision, ultimately in both eyes, occur between five and 15 years of age. Inflammation and vascularization involve the deep layers of the cornea. The cornea assumes a ground-glass appearance with orange-red areas ("salmon patches") due to the vascularization. The reaction begins to subside in one to two months. Ghost vessels, seen with magnification, remain in the corneal stroma after the inflammation has subsided. An associated uveitis or choroiditis is common. Other signs of congenital syphilis may be seen, such as saddle nose, deafness and notched teeth. The serologic tests for syphilis give positive results. It is postulated that interstitial keratitis is an allergic response, since *Treponema pallidum* is not found in the cornea during the acute stage.

Treatment. There is no specific treatment for syphilitic interstitial keratitis. Systemic syphilis should be treated, but the treatment does not affect the corneal disease. Topical steroids relieve the symptoms. Systemic steroids are valuable if the local steroids do not adequately control the symptoms. The accompanying iridocyclitis is helped by the local steroids, but, in addition, a strong cycloplegic such as atropine, 1 or 2 per cent, should be instilled, 2 drops three times daily. For severe corneal scarring a corneal transplant is indicated, but only if damage to other parts of the eye does not preclude a good visual outcome. In the rare case when tuberculosis is the cause of the interstitial keratitis (usually unilateral), the systemic infection is treated.

Corneal Drying and Exposure

The following diseases are associated with the complications of corneal drying and exposure: (1) *keratitis sicca* – the result of a lacrimal gland insufficiency; (2) *exposure keratitis,* developing after facial nerve palsies, exophthalmos and prolonged periods of unconsciousness; (3) *neuroparalytic keratitis,* seen after interruption of function of the trigeminal nerve; (4) *familial dysautonomia* (Riley-Day syndrome) – corneal complications occur from the congenital absence or deficiency of tears, and corneal hypesthesia. Corneal infection may lead to intraocular infection and loss of the eye.

Treatment. The cornea should be protected with artificial tears (Bro-Lac, Lacril, Lyteers), methylcellulose solution, 0.5 to 1 per cent, 1.4% polyvinyl alcohol (Liquifilm Tears), or a bland ophthalmic ointment (Lacri-Lube). Local antibiotic ointments are used only if there is secondary bacterial infection. Flush-fitting corneoscleral contact lenses have been useful. A temporary or permanent tarsorrhaphy may be required to protect the cornea.

Scleral and Episcleral Disorders

LEONARD APT, M.D.

EPISCLERITIS

A localized inflammation of the tissue between the conjunctiva and sclera is characteristic of episcleritis. The patient has slight pain, photophobia and tenderness in the area. The localized patch of hyperemia and the absence of a discharge distinguish episcleritis from conjunctivitis. Episcleritis can occur as an isolated disease or in association with a systemic disorder, most commonly a collagen disease such as rheumatoid arthritis. About one-third of the patients have uveitis as well.

Treatment. Local vasoconstrictor drops (Table 6, p. 519) are helpful, but topical steroid medication (Table 5, p. 518) gives better relief of symptoms. A cycloplegic such as atropine, 1 per cent, 1 drop three times daily, is instilled into the eye if there is an anterior uveitis. A systemic disorder should be sought and treated.

SCLERITIS

Inflammation of the deeper scleral tissue is more severe and appears more purplish than in episcleritis. It may be localized, diffuse or nodular. Pain, photophobia and tenderness may be intense. An associated anterior uveitis is frequently present. Scleritis may be seen with systemic diseases such as the collagen diseases (particularly rheumatoid arthritis), tuberculosis, syphilis, brucellosis and gout. The severity of the scleritis is often directly related to the severity of the systemic disease.

Treatment. Topical corticosteroids are the treatment of choice. The liquid or ointment steroid (Table 5, p. 518) may be needed as often as every 2 hours during the day. Atropine, 1 per cent, is instilled into the eye three times daily if an anterior uveitis is present. The systemic disease is actively treated.

It is of interest that episcleritis or scleritis may develop in patients receiving salicylates or systemic corticosteroids for a disease such as rheumatoid arthritis. The addition of local steroid therapy is of value in such a situation.

Uveitis

LEONARD APT, M.D.

Inflammation of the uveal tract is a serious disease, for it often leads to severe visual impairment or blindness. Early diagnosis and treatment are important to prevent the ocular complications. The damaging effect of the disease is often subtle in children. There may be few or no subjective complaints or obvious signs of the disease during episodes of recurrent or chronic inflammation.

Uveitis has been popularly classified as nongranulomatous and granulomatous. *Nongranulomatous uveitis* more often involves the anterior uvea, producing the following symptoms and signs: acute onset with pain, redness, photophobia, blurred vision, circumcorneal flush, miotic or irregular pupil and, on slit lamp examination, the presence of fibrin and cells in the anterior chamber and fine white keratitic precipitates on the posterior surface of the cornea. *Granulomatous uveitis* appears more frequently as a posterior uveitis with a slow onset, minimal redness, pain or photophobia, normal or slightly miotic pupil and vision less than one would expect from the mild external manifestations of the disease. Large, yellow-gray mutton-fat keratitic precipitates are seen on the posterior surface of the cornea with the slit lamp. Iris nodules are often visible. On ophthalmoscopy single or multiple yellow or white exudative lesions are seen in the choroid with or without vitreous haze.

Uveitis presents a difficult therapeutic problem because, although numerous causes are suspected, in only relatively few cases is a specific etiologic agent detected. Nongranulomatous uveitis is thought to be a hypersensitivity reaction to bacteria (particularly the streptococcus), foods, pollens and viruses. Some studies indicate that there is a higher incidence of the disease in patients with rheumatoid arthritis. Granulomatous uveitis may result from the actual invasion of the uveal tract by any organism, but organisms are rarely isolated or demonstrated. Granulomatous uveitis may be caused by toxoplasmosis (the most frequently incriminated infection), syphilis, tuberculosis, brucellosis, leptospirosis, viruses, fungi, nematodes and sarcoid.

Treatment. The management of uveitis consists in (1) the thorough medical evaluation of the patient in search for a specific cause—the medical physician should work closely with the ophthalmologist; (2) specific treatment if the cause is found or if one is highly suspected; and (3) nonspecific ocular treatment to minimize the complications from the inflammatory process; often this is all that is or can be done.

Nonspecific treatment should include the following:

Cycloplegics to dilate the pupil to prevent posterior synechiae and to put the iris and ciliary body at rest. This reduces pain from the ciliary and pupillary spasm and decreases the inflammatory protein response in the aqueous humor. Atropine in a 1 or 2 per cent solution or ointment, instilled one to three times daily, is the preferred cycloplegic. Scopolamine, 0.25 per cent solution or ointment, may also be used, particularly if the patient is sensitive to atropine.

Mydriatics to further help the cycloplegic in obtaining wide pupillary dilatation and thus prevent or break up posterior synechiae. A drug such as 10 per cent phenylephrine (Neo-Synephrine) is a strong mydriatic and also decreases hyperemia by its vasoconstricting properties.

CORTICOSTEROIDS. Anterior uveitis may be treated with steroids applied locally or given by subconjunctival injection. The subconjunctival route is usually reserved for the more severe forms of anterior uveitis in which a higher and prolonged concentration of the drug is desired. Topical steroid drops or ointment (Table 5, p. 518) can be used every 1 to 4 hours, depending on the severity of the disease.

Posterior uveitis usually requires systemic therapy. Steroids should be given systemically in the more severe forms of anterior uveitis if local or subconjunctival medications are not beneficial. The daily dosage in children is 1 to 2 mg. per kilogram of body weight of prednisone up to a maximum of 80 mg. The equivalent dose of another corticosteroid may be used. One should use the minimum dose necessary to achieve a reasonable effect and for the shortest time needed to control the inflammation. The toxic effects and the contraindications to the corticosteroids for short- or long-time therapy must be kept in mind.

Treatment for active *ocular toxoplasmosis* deserves special mention. It consists in the combined use of pyrimethamine (Daraprim) and sulfadiazine. Corticosteroids may be given at the same time to reduce inflammation, but they should be discontinued if the inflammatory reaction in the eye worsens. Pyrimethamine is given twice daily in the total daily dosage of 4 mg. per kilogram of body weight up to 200 mg. the first day, then 1 mg. per kilogram up to 50 mg. daily. (The starting dosage is higher than that generally recommended by the manufacturer, but my young patients have tolerated it.) The sulfadiazine* dosage is a priming dose of 50 mg. per kilogram of body weight, then 100 mg. per kilogram of body weight daily up to 4 Gm. in four divided doses for one to three weeks; 50 mg. per kilogram daily is given thereafter. The average course of pyrimethamine and sulfadiazine therapy is six weeks. The drugs can be given for three months if warranted. In the acute fulminating cases clinical improvement is seen in two to three weeks.

Weekly urinalyses for sulfadiazine crystalluria or evidence of kidney irritation should be done. Since pyrimethamine is a folic acid antagonist, folinic acid, 10 mg. per day intramuscularly, should be given to prevent hematologic toxicity, e.g., bone marrow suppression, especially thrombocytopenia.

* Manufacturer's precaution: Sulfadiazine is not for use in children under two months of age.

Lacrimal Apparatus Disorders

LEONARD APT, M.D.

INFANTILE DACRYOSTENOSIS

Normally the nasolacrimal drainage system is patent throughout its length at birth. Failure of the nasolacrimal duct to canalize completely leads to persistent tearing *(epiphora)* of one eye or, rarely, both eyes in the first one to 12 weeks of life. Contrary to the statements in many pediatric textbooks, most newborn infants tear in the first week of life. Persistent tearing from dacryostenosis without dacryocystitis can be differentiated from conjunctivitis and corneal disease by the lack of conjunctival inflammation. Usually, significant dacryostenosis is followed promptly by dacryocystitis.

Treatment. Many cases of infantile dacryostenosis clear spontaneously with further canalization of the nasolacrimal duct. Massaging the contents of the lacrimal sac down through the nasolacrimal duct four to six times daily may be helpful. If this is unsuccessful, probing of the nasolacrimal duct by an ophthalmologist should be done.

INFANTILE DACRYOCYSTITIS

Obstruction of the nasolacrimal duct usually leads to infection of the lacrimal sac (dacryocystitis) by the common pyogenic bacteria. Excess tearing is then replaced by mucopurulent discharge and some conjunctival redness. There may be an acute distention of the lacrimal sac with overlying redness, pain and tenderness. Occasionally a lacrimal sac abscess will rupture and form a draining fistula. In the differential diagnosis of infantile dacryocystitis one must exclude infantile glaucoma as well as conjunctival or corneal disease.

Treatment. For the milder cases of dacryocystitis the tear sac should be massaged four to six times daily, followed by the instillation into the inner canthus of a broad-spectrum antibiotic drop (not ointment) such as bacitracin, neomycin or a tetracycline for four to seven days. Sulfacetamide is also effective if the infection is not predominantly purulent. Usually the tearing, mucopurulent discharge and conjunctival redness improve with antimicrobial therapy, but it will not be of permanent value unless the obstruction disappears or is eliminated. To avoid chronic dacryocystitis and all its troublesome complications, it is this author's policy to irrigate the lacrimal sac and to probe the nasolacrimal duct under general anesthesia if the dacryocystitis does not disappear after two separate courses of massage and antimicrobial therapy. Age is no contraindication to this procedure; it can be accomplished safely and effectively under light general anesthesia.

Severe infections of the lacrimal sac are given antibiotics systemically. An abscess of the sac requires incision and drainage.

It is advisable to obtain smears of the discharge for Gram stain study in all cases of dacryocystitis prior to antimicrobial therapy and, in addition, cultures and sensitivity studies in all cases of chronic, recurrent or severe infections.

If the patency of the nasolacrimal duct is not established by conservative measures, an external dacryocystorhinostomy should be performed. The operation is usually not done before the age of three years.

Ocular Trauma

LEONARD APT, M.D.

Prompt and appropriate care after eye injury will often save useful vision; poor management may lead to blindness. Improper initial eye care by the nonophthalmologic physician usually results from ignorance of a few fundamental rules in the correct handling of the patient with ocular trauma.

To determine the ocular structures involved and the extent of the injury, it is imperative to examine closely the external and visible structures of the eyes with good illumination and magnification, and to perform ophthalmoscopy. An accurate history is essential. Testing the patient's visual acuity before treatment is important for diagnostic, prognostic and medicolegal reasons. If an adequate examination cannot be performed by the nonophthalmologic physician, the patient should be referred to an eye physician for further care. The nonophthalmologic physician should not be the one to decide whether or not an eye injury is minor except in obvious situations such as occurs with a superficial conjunctival foreign body.

FOREIGN BODIES

Conjunctival foreign bodies can usually be safely flushed out with a stream of isotonic saline solution or removed with a sterile moistened cotton applicator. If the history suggests that a foreign body is the likely cause of the eye symptoms and none is found on the bulbar or lower palpebral conjunctiva or the cornea, then the upper eyelid should be everted for inspection. The use of a local anesthetic such as 0.5 per cent tetracaine (Pontocain) or 0.5 per cent proparacaine (Ophthaine, Ophthetic) facilitates the examination.

Corneal foreign bodies may be difficult to see unless adequate local anesthesia, oblique lighting and magnification (loupe or slit lamp biomicroscopy) are used. Fluorescein stain helps to delineate the foreign body. One drop of sterile 2 per cent fluorescein solution or a fluorescein strip is placed in the conjunctival sac and the excess washed out with isotonic saline solution. Corneal foreign bodies which are not easily removed by irrigation or with the wipe of a moistened sterile cotton applicator should be referred to an ophthalmologist for further treatment. If the foreign body is dislodged, fluorescein is again added to the eye to determine the extent of the corneal abrasion. Unless the abrasion is minute (less than a millimeter) a broad-spectrum antimicrobial agent such as sulfacetamide, neomycin or tetracycline, or a combination of bacitracin, neomycin and polymyxin B is instilled into the eye and the eye is tightly covered with a patch for 24 hours. If the abrasion is not superficial or is large (more than a few millimeters), an antibiotic is instilled and a patch is applied. The patient should be seen by an ophthalmologist. The cornea should be re-examined in 24 hours in all cases after the removal of a foreign body, for the presence of a secondary infection in the abraded area. An untreated corneal infection may lead to corneal ulceration, intraocular infection and loss of the eye.

Intraocular foreign bodies must be referred immediately to an eye physician. If there will be a delay of a few hours before the child will be seen by an ophthalmologist, the physician should test the visual acuity, instill a cycloplegic drug and a broad-spectrum antibiotic into the eye and start systemic antimicrobial therapy. Ampicillin, gentamicin or chloramphenicol in full doses has been widely used for potential or active intraocular infections because of the broad spectrum of antibacterial activity and the ability to penetrate the ocular tissues. It is important to know that small, missile-like foreign bodies may penetrate the globe and cause transient pain or no pain at all. When a history suggests the possibility of penetration of the eye by a high-velocity foreign body, the patient should be referred to an ophthalmologist for thorough evaluation.

CORNEAL ABRASIONS

Corneal abrasions are handled in the same way as described for the abrasion that remains after removal of a corneal foreign body.

LACERATIONS

Lacerations that involve the eyelid margin or the lacrimal apparatus should be treated by the ophthalmologist. Permanent notching may result from improper lid margin repair. Minor lacerations of the eyelid and brow, however, may be closed with fine sutures by the nonophthalmologic physician.

CONTUSIONS

Contusion injuries of the globe and the surrounding tissues are usually produced by blunt objects. The effects may be minor or serious, obvious or inapparent, immediate or delayed. Therefore careful study by an ophthalmologist and sufficient follow-up are necessary. A blunt injury to the eye area may result in ecchymosis of the eyelid ("black-eye"), subconjunctival hemorrhage, abrasion or rupture of the cornea, anterior chamber hemorrhage (hyphema), laceration of the iris, cataract, dislocated lens, vitreous hemorrhage, retinal edema or hemorrhage, retinal detachment, rupture of the choroid, optic nerve injury or rupture of the globe. All these complications, except for the eyelid ecchymosis, require expert eye care.

BURNS

Thermal burns of the eyelids are treated as burns of the skin elsewhere. Burns of the cornea are treated by irrigation with water or saline solution and an antibiotic ointment before sending the patient to an ophthalmologist.

Chemical burns of the conjunctiva and cornea are treated immediately by irrigation with water or isotonic saline solution. Time should not be lost in trying to neutralize the chemical. Serious damage may occur in a matter of minutes. Moreover, the heat generated by such a reaction may lead to further damage. Alkali burns of the cornea are more serious than those caused by acids because alkalis are not precipitated by the tissue proteins as are the acids.

Immediate irrigation should be carried out for at least ½ hour in the case of alkalis. The eye can be held under the water faucet stream. Local anesthetics may be used to relieve the pain. A local antibiotic ointment can be inserted into the conjunctival sac and the patient sent as soon as possible to an ophthalmologist for further care.

Retinoblastoma

LEONARD APT, M.D.

Retinoblastoma, although a relatively rare malignant tumor, is the most common intraocular tumor in infants and children. It is the most frequent cause for enucleation prior to the age of three years. The presenting symptoms are leukokoria, strabismus, dilated pupil and defective vision. Occasionally the appearance is that of uveitis, endophthalmitis or glaucoma. The disease is bilateral in about one-third of the cases. Death results from cerebral involvement by extension through the optic nerve or by metastases from the choroid by way of the blood stream. The occurrence is largely sporadic, but there is a strong hereditary potential. The chances that other siblings will have the disease are rare in the sporadic cases, but almost all the children will have the tumor if one of the parents was fortunate enough to survive the disease.

Treatment. If the disease is unilateral, enucleation is advised. The surgeon should attempt to remove at least 10 mm. of optic nerve to determine whether invasion has occurred. If the tumor has spread to the optic nerve and there is no evidence of extraocular spread, an exenteration or radiation is indicated. The remaining eye must be examined thoroughly at frequent intervals for several years.

In bilateral cases some experienced ophthalmologists are of the opinion that both eyes should be removed to ensure the best chance for survival. Others will not remove one of the two eyes if the tumor does not involve at least one-half of the globe or if the optic disc does not appear involved. Some parents refuse permission to remove both eyes.

The present recommended nonsurgical treatment of retinoblastoma is a combination of irradiation and triethylenemelamine (TEM), a potent cytotoxic antineoplastic agent. Other forms of therapy have been used, such as radon and cobalt implants, diathermy, photocoagulation and other antineoplastic drugs.

The use of TEM allows the dose of roentgen ray therapy to be reduced to safe levels. A dose of approximately 3250 r is given, and a second course may be administered. To reduce the anorexia and gastrointestinal symptoms and to increase the effectiveness of TEM, it is given intramuscularly or, better still, intra-arterially into the internal carotid artery in extensively involved eyes.*

The parenteral dose of TEM is 0.06 mg. per kilogram of body weight in infants less than six months of age, and 0.08 mg. per kilogram of body weight in older patients. The drug is given the day before irradiation therapy is started. TEM is a potent bone marrow depressant, and if an adequate dose has been given the leukocyte count will decrease to 3000 and the platelet count to 100,000 per cubic millimeter during the next three weeks. A second dose of drug is given after the blood cell count has returned to normal.

Cryotherapy has recently been used in a small number of patients, and results in certain cases have been promising.

The prognosis for survival has been dramatically improved in recent years because of earlier diagnosis, better visualization of the entire retina by the use of indirect ophthalmoscopy, and the therapy previously outlined.

---

* Manufacturer's precaution: Parenteral administration of TEM is investigational.

The prognosis is based on the number and size of the tumors, their location and evidence of spread from the retina. No longer is retinoblastoma a hopeless disease. A survival rate up to 90 per cent has been reported in those patients whose prognosis was favorable at the time that treatment was begun.

Strabismus
(Squint)

LEONARD APT, M.D.

Strabismus occurs in about 3 per cent of children. Few nonophthalmologic physicians realize that it is one of the leading causes of monocular blindness. At least 3 per cent of children have amblyopia ("lazy eye"). Approximately half of these cases are secondary to strabismus, and most of the others are due to an uncorrected refractive error in one eye. The unfortunate aspect of the problem is that in nearly every instance the blindness could be prevented if the patient were seen early by the ophthalmologist.

Normal vision and binocular function are not present at birth. These functions mature rapidly during the first years of life and become relatively fixed by the age of six years. To reach the goal of 20/20 vision with normal binocular fusion, clear images must be presented to both foveae simultaneously throughout the early years of life. Patching of the normal eye after the age of six years is not likely to effect significant improvement in the vision of an eye which has been constantly deviated.

The earlier strabismus therapy is initiated, the better is the prognosis for a functional as well as a cosmetic cure. Many pediatricians are unaware that no infant or child is too young to have an eye examination and to have treatment initiated. Parents are often misinformed by being told that it is useless to take the child to an ophthalmologist until he is older because "little can be done in the way of diagnosis or treatment and, besides he may outgrow the problem." No child outgrows a constant monocular strabismus without serious consequences – amblyopia or an abnormal sensory visual function. It is true that a child with esotropia may look improved when older because of the normal tendency for a decrease in convergence tone with time, but the functional complications remain. Most children who supposedly outgrew their "crossed eyes" never had a true deviation. They may have appeared esotropic because of the presence of epicanthal folds. Or the eyes may have looked unaligned because of a disparity between the anatomic axis and visual axis of the globe in the orbits.

Transient strabismus may be normal in the first four months of life during the period of macular development. Any transient strabismus after this time or a constant strabismus at any age demands prompt referral to an ophthalmologist so that a diagnosis can be made and the therapy started. Diseases such as retinoblastoma, intraocular infection, congenital cataract or other eye anomalies may be manifested early as a transient or constant strabismus. The pediatrician should not take the responsibility of delaying the referral of the patient unless he can absolutely rule out serious ocular disease or the presence of a true strabismus rather than pseudostrabismus.

Comitant (nonparalytic) squint is far more common than the noncomitant (paralytic) type in pediatric patients. Most cases of comitant strabismus are caused by an abnormal innervation from supranuclear sources. The nerves and the extraocular muscles are normal.

Treatment. The management of comitant strabismus includes refraction, occlusion of the nondeviating eye (if fixation is central) to prevent suppression and amblyopia in the deviating eye, orthoptic exercises and surgery. A refraction can be performed on an infant by retinoscopy, and appropriate glasses can be prescribed even in infants less than one year of age.

Convergent strabismus in children is frequently accommodative in origin. Children with hypermetropia must accommodate to get a clear image. In some children an overconvergence results. Glasses to reduce the need to accommodate may reduce or eliminate the convergent squint.

Another type of accommodative strabismus is seen in children who are not highly hyperopic, but who have an exaggerated accommodative-convergence ratio on near fixation. These patients usually respond to bifocals to reduce the need for increased accommodation with near targets, or to anticholinesterase miotics which induce "peripheral" rather than "central" accommodation by their action on the ciliary body and thus lessen convergence. The drugs most commonly used are echothiophate iodide (Phospholine Iodide) 0.03 to 0.125 per cent, and isoflurophate (DFP, Floropryl) 0.1 per cent in anhydrous peanut oil or ointment 0.025 per cent. The usual dose is 1 drop or ⅛ inch of ointment into both eyes daily. An attempt is made to reduce the frequency of instillation and the concentration of the drug to the minimum needed to control the deviation.

Toxic effects of the anticholinesterase miotics include headache, conjunctival hyperemia, abdominal pain, nausea, vomiting, diarrhea, salivation and hypotension. The effects are most severe during the first days of treatment, but subside in a few days with continued use or quickly after stopping medication. Hyperplasia of the pigment of the iris ("iris cysts") may develop after long use of the drugs. On rare occasions the cysts have become large enough to occlude the pupil. The "cysts" can be avoided or minimized by the simultaneous use of the mydriatic phenylephrine hydrochloride (Neo-Synephrine) in a 2.5 per cent solution two or three times weekly. Succinylcholine should not be used as a muscle relaxant prior to general anesthesia if the child has been receiving the Phospholine Iodide because prolonged apnea may occur.

Orthoptics are useful for fusion training. A trained technician is needed if the ophthalmologist does not perform these services. Usually the child must be at least five years old to comprehend and benefit from this training. Pleoptics is a fairly new allied field which deals mainly with the treatment of impaired vision associated with nonfoveal fixation. Frequent and intensive training sessions are required. Even with the most cooperative patient the prognosis for significant and retained improvement is guarded.

18

The Ear

Foreign Bodies in the Ear

CHARLES F. FERGUSON, M.D.

A foreign body in the external auditory canal frequently is a much more difficult problem than either the patient or the physician originally suspects. If there is any doubt as to the physician's manual dexterity, his past experience with such problems or his available equipment, he will avoid much grief by referring the patient to an otologist at once, before troublesome bleeding obscures the foreign object or trauma results in infection or irreversible damage to the delicate auditory mechanism. If the physician is experienced only with an otoscope and a wax curet, and is not adept in the use of a head mirror with external axial illumination which leaves both hands free for necessarily deft manipulation, this advice is doubly indicated. More harm is caused by inexpert attempts at removal of foreign objects in the auditory canal than would result by allowing the objects to remain indefinitely.

One point of *anatomy* essential to remember is the isthmus of the auditory canal, which is located at the junction of the outer cartilaginous and inner bony portions. If the object is inadvertently pushed medial to this narrow neck (sometimes unavoidably, if the patient makes a slight but sudden move), it will easily slip into the expanded recess of the inner bony canal, come to rest in the sulcus between the drum and the canal floor, and thereby be converted into a much more difficult problem.

Whenever *infection* is present as a result of unsuccessful foreign body removal, it must first be adequately treated. After the edema and inflammation of the wall of the canal have subsided, removal is much easier and safer. Local therapy with antibiotic drops containing cortisone (as noted under Injuries to the External Ear; e.g., Cortisporin or Coly-Mycin S otic solution) will reduce such edema and inflammation satisfactorily, although with more extensive infection, occasionally systemic administration of antibiotics may be indicated.

Unless the physician has had a great deal of experience working in the auditory canal, *general anesthesia* is heartily recommended. In many instances, even for the most experienced otologist, this is a necessity. (Adequate local anesthesia in such instances is usually not possible.) Without general anesthesia, the infant or child must be most securely mummified, with the head solidly fixed by a strong, cooperative assistant.

In the case of an *animate* object, such as an insect, it is best first to anesthetize it with chloroform or ether, and then remove it by irrigation or forceps. In the absence of such equipment, the patient might fill the canal with rubbing alcohol, mineral oil or even plain tap water which may drown the insect and allow it to float out. In the relatively common case of a tick, which has grasping, burrowing "claws," it is essential that it be anesthetized to relax its grip and that the *entire* tick (not merely the head) be removed. Otherwise the embedded legs may cause subsequent infection.

With a *hygroscopic* object, such as a pea or bean, irrigation methods should *not* be used, since such an object, unless immediately extracted, rapidly swells by absorption of water. This makes removal even more difficult. The use of alcohol or ether to dehydrate such objects is usually disappointing. Ordinarily such foreign bodies should be removed by methods other than irrigation (as discussed in the following paragraphs).

The ordinary *inanimate, nonhygroscopic* object is best removed by one of the following methods, presuming the patient is sufficiently immobilized (or anesthetized), and the operator has adequate assistance, excellent illumination, proper equipment and both hands free.

Irrigation. Use a piston-syringe and direct the stream of water, at body temperature, onto the posterior wall of the canal if the foreign body does not completely fill the canal. This is the least traumatic method and will frequently dislodge the object. Dry the canal afterward with swabs or compressed air. (Never use this method if it is suspected that the drum is perforated, or if there is, or has been, eczema or dermatitis of the canal, or other evidence of external otitis.)

Agglutination. This is a method reported from the seventeenth century. Glue, collodion or a tiny bit of adhesive attached to a small, very tightly wound cotton applicator stick may withdraw the object atraumatically. Advantages are that collodion hardens rapidly, and adhesive becomes very sticky after a strong beam of heat from a 100-watt bulb has been directed into the auditory canal.

Blunt Hook or Bent Curet. A blunt hook or bent curet frequently can be slipped between the canal wall and the foreign body, then rotated to fit behind the object to edge it outward. A thin, flexible wire curet may be less traumatic but not as strong.

Special Cup Forceps. Use a specially designed cup forceps which will firmly hold the foreign body and not force it deeper into the canal when application is made. The ordinary flat-blade tissue forceps commonly used is dangerous in this regard, since it usually *propels* rather than *retracts* the object. Its jaws are not adapted to fit about a spherical object such as a bead or a slippery piece of glass.

Surgery. When the foregoing methods fail, surgery is the safest and most conservative course. Otherwise, undue persistence may make a bad situation even worse. The canal should be opened from behind, as in the postaural mastoid operation, and the object can be removed under direct vision. This may be indicated when the foreign body has been wedged in the isthmus or pushed into the inner bony canal recess.

Complications of removal of foreign bodies from the external auditory canal are: (1) *infection,* sometimes leading to troublesome *stenosis* of the canal; (2) *chronic perforation* of the drum with or without middle ear infection; (3) *dislocation of the ossicles* with disruption of the ossicular chain, and resultant severe *hearing impairment* of up to 60 decibels; (4) forcing of the foreign body into the *middle ear* (with possible migration to the eustachian tube), where removal is more difficult, and considerable further damage is easily created.

Every conceivable object of such size and shape that either intentional or accidental introduction into the external auditory canal can be accomplished has been encountered. Every case should be treated with the utmost respect and consideration it demands, and no foreign body should be considered a simple problem until the foregoing precautions have been taken, and until it has been successfully and atraumatically extracted, leaving an intact middle ear, a normal auditory canal and an unimpaired hearing mechanism.

Otitis Externa

EDWARD A. MORTIMER, JR., M.D.

Three types of otitis externa are seen. Simple otitis externa is the most common, and is usually manifested by a malodorous discharge and slight ear pain. It is often a summertime disease related to swimming. It usually responds to gentle cleaning, keeping the ear dry and the administration of ear drops containing hydrocortisone, polymyxin B and neomycin, 4 drops four times a day. Recurrences may be prevented by the use of the same preparation once daily after swimming, or by the use of a weak acidic solution, such as 2 per cent acetic acid (Otic Domeboro solution).

More severe otitis externa may be associated with edema sufficient to occlude the canal, extreme pain and systemic symptoms. Here, systemic administration of antibiotics is required, and narcotics may be necessary for relief of pain. Removal of exudate and debris by gentle suction or other means is of paramount importance. The insertion of a wick saturated with a 2 per cent acetic acid solution may facilitate drainage.

Chronic otitis externa is usually secondary to seborrheic dermatitis and should be treated with hydrocortisone-polymyxin-neomycin ear drops, plus measures to control the seborrhea.

Otologic Infections

EDWARD A. MORTIMER, Jr., M.D.

ACUTE OTITIS MEDIA WITH INTACT DRUM

The term otitis media as used here means a purulent bacterial infection of the middle ear, manifested by bulging of the pars flaccida or whole drum with loss of mobility. Specific antibacterial therapy clearly prevents mastoiditis and has reduced the incidence of chronic perforations of the drum secondary to otitis media. It is also logical to believe that antibiotic therapy prevents secondary meningitis. The concern expressed in the past that the use of antibiotics and the discarding of myringotomies have resulted in some middle ear deafness appears to be without firm foundation on the basis of current information. Therefore, it would seem safe to rely on antibiotics as optimal therapy for otitis media. In this regard it is worth noting that almost all otitis media subsides spontaneously without complications; therefore, therapy is directed at the minority of cases that would otherwise present complications.

Because it is impractical to determine the infecting organism directly, selection of an antibiotic must depend on knowledge of the probable offending organisms. Most cases of otitis media are caused by pneumococci, a few cases by group A streptococci, and 20 to 25 per cent by *Hemophilus influenzae*. The former belief that ear infections with this latter organism are limited to children of less than five or six years appears to be incorrect. Hence, therapy must be directed against *H. influenzae* as well as pneumococci and streptococci at all ages.

Ampicillin, which is effective against both gram-positive and gram-negative bacteria, is satisfactory therapy for otitis media. The oral dose is 50 mg. per kilogram daily in four divided doses to a maximum of 2 Gm. per day. Equally acceptable is combined therapy employing sulfisoxazole (0.1 to 0.15 Gm. orally per kilogram daily),* plus one of the following penicillin regimens: a single injection of intramuscular benzathine penicillin (600,000 units to children less than 10 years and 1,200,000 units to older children); 300,000 to 600,000 units of procaine penicillin in oil with aluminum monostearate intramuscularly every third day for three doses; or oral phenoxymethyl penicillin (Pen-Vee K), 25,000 to 50,000 units per kilogram daily in three or four divided doses. Intramuscular benzathine penicillin is best *not* given to infants or children weighing less than 10 kilograms because of the smaller muscle mass and the greater risk of significant irritation (or damage to the sciatic nerve when the buttock is the injection site). In children who are allergic to penicillin, erythromycin, 40 mg. per kilogram daily to a maximum of 1 Gm. daily, plus sulfisoxazole,* is satisfactory therapy.

Therapy should be continued for a week in children seen early in the course of the illness, and longer when the process is more advanced at the time treatment is initiated.

The use of nasal vasoconstrictors in an effort to facilitate opening of the eustachian tube is warranted, though the value of this is open to question. Nevertheless, their use in patients with otitis media who are old enough to express an evaluation is often associated with symptomatic relief of pain. Phenylephrine, 0.25 per cent, 2 to 4 drops in each nostril four or five times daily, may be given. The parents should be instructed in proper positioning of the child's head so that the medication may reach the area of the eustachian orifice. Its use usually need not be continued more than four days. Many physicians prefer to use oral decongestant preparations, such as those containing pseudoephedrine (Sudafed) or other sympathomimetics. The dose of pseudoephedrine is 15 mg. for infants less than four months of age, 30 mg. for those between 4 months and 6 years, and 60 mg. for older children and adults, all given three times daily or every 6 hours. If Actifed Syrup is used, these doses can be achieved by giving ½ teaspoon to young infants, 1 teaspoon to children between 4 months and 6 years, and 2 teaspoons to the older group, inasmuch as 1 teaspoon contains 30 mg. In the case of other preparations, adherence to the manufacturer's recommendations is advised.

Usually pain subsides promptly under treatment. Salicylates may be given; rarely codeine is necessary for temporary relief of severe pain. Warm glycerin containing 5 per cent phenol may be used as eardrops, and often the application of heat in the form of a hot water bottle provides satisfactory relief of pain.

Decrease in pain occurs so promptly that myringotomy is rarely necessary in acute otitis media. The main indication for myringotomy

* Manufacturer's precaution: Sulfisoxazole is contraindicated in infants under two months of age except in the treatment of congenital toxoplasmosis as adjunctive therapy with pyrimethamine.

at present appears to be untreated otitis media of days' or weeks' duration. Such cases are seen rarely, but usually present with a history of earache in the recent past followed by deafness. Examination reveals a markedly bulging drum, often with little evidence of acute inflammation. Myringotomy is indicated for such patients to provide drainage of inspissated exudate.

Ideally, all patients with otitis media should be reexamined seven to 10 days after therapy has been initiated to be sure that the process is subsiding. Practically, only rarely do cases treated early fail to respond adequately, and in such instances prompt clinical improvement may be accepted as evidence of satisfactory progress. Pain and fever should be relieved within 24 hours; if it is not, the child should be reexamined.

ACUTE OTITIS MEDIA WITH PERFORATED DRUM

Cases of otitis media that present with ruptured drums and drainage should be treated with antibiotics and symptomatic measures as described for otitis media without perforation. Local manipulations and cleansing are unnecessary. Cultures of the exudate usually do not reveal the original offending organism because it disappears from the discharge within a few hours after rupture and is replaced by saprophytes. Drainage usually decreases promptly and disappears within three or four days; if it does not, otologic consultation should be sought.

RECURRENT OTITIS MEDIA

Prompt recurrence of otitis media within a few days of discontinuation of therapy is frequent and must be considered the result of inadequate therapy. *H. influenzae* otitis media accounts for a disproportionate number of cases of this type of recurrence. Treatment should be reinstituted; higher doses and longer duration of antibiotics should be prescribed. In addition, myringotomy may be indicated, and the possibility of mastoiditis masked by antibiotics should be considered.

A more difficult problem is that of the child who exhibits repeated otitis media, seemingly each time he contracts a respiratory infection. Occasionally a child may have six or more such episodes during the cold months. In such cases there is good evidence that low doses of a sulfonamide or ampicillin, given continuously as prophylaxis, will strikingly reduce such recurrences. Therefore, the first approach I use to such a child is the administration of sulfisoxazole, 0.25 Gm. twice daily to infants and young children less than one year of age* (approximately 10 kilograms of body weight) and 0.5 Gm. twice daily to older children. Prophylaxis should usually be continued for two years. At that time it should be discontinued in the hope that anatomic and other changes may have resulted in decreased susceptibility to otitis media. There is some evidence that adenoidectomy will reduce the incidence of recurrent otitis media for a year or two after surgery, though the response in any individual case is unpredictable, and the reduction in morbidity in otitis media is approximately counterbalanced by the morbidity resulting from the surgical procedure. If there is evidence of allergy or other underlying disturbances, either local or systemic, these should be investigated.

ACUTE MASTOIDITIS

Old-fashioned acute mastoiditis is rarely seen at present. When it occurs, it usually results from neglected otitis media. Usually, acute mastoiditis will respond to antibiotics. Because the organisms causing mastoiditis are usually pneumococci, group A streptococci, or *H. influenzae,* broad antibiotic coverage is indicated. Hospital admission is usually necessary, and ampicillin, 200 to 400 mg. per kilogram per day in four to six divided doses given intramuscularly or intravenously, is indicated. If the eardrum has perforated, cultures with appropriate antibiotic sensitivity testing may be of assistance. However, it should be remembered that the underlying offending bacterium may be difficult to identify in the presence of saprophytic overgrowth from the ear canal if more than 8 to 12 hours have elapsed since perforation. If the eardrum is bulging in the presence of acute mastoiditis, myringotomy is indicated; cultures should be obtained at this time. Simple mastoidectomy is indicated if there is evidence of perforative mastoiditis (subperiosteal abscess, Bezold's abscess or sagging of the posterosuperior canal wall) or if there is bony destruction demonstrable by x-ray.

CHRONIC OTITIS MEDIA WITH PERFORATION

Patients with chronic perforations of the drum, with or without drainage, should be managed in cooperation with an otologist. First, infection should be cleared as much as possible with systemic or topical antibiotics. Second, underlying anatomic abnormalities, such as chronic mastoiditis, granulation tissue

* Manufacturer's precaution: Sulfisoxazole is contraindicated in infants under two months of age except in the treatment of congenital toxoplasmosis as adjunctive therapy with pyrimethamine.

or cholesteatoma, should be corrected. Third, it may be necessary to attempt to repair the drum surgically.

"VACUUM" OTALGIA

Occasionally one sees afebrile, otherwise healthy children who are complaining of severe otalgia and who show retraction of the appropriate drum. Usually there is an associated feeling of fullness or deafness. This appears to be due to an obstruction of the eustachian tube with absorption of air from the middle ear, and is comparable to aerotitis. Relief may usually be obtained with nasal vasoconstrictors or oral decongestants.

BULLOUS MYRINGITIS

The main problem in bullous myringitis is that of distinguishing it from true bacterial otitis media with bulging. Only symptomatic treatment is indicated; rupture of blebs with a cotton swab or other means usually provides relief. However, in my experience, rupture of bullae often unmasks a red bulging drum which requires antibiotic therapy.

SEROUS OTITIS MEDIA

This condition is manifested by significant hearing deficit and the accumulation of uninfected serous or mucoid material in the middle ear. It is one of the most trying conditions that parents, child and physician experience. There is also considerable disagreement as to its management, largely because its origin is unclear and its natural history variable. It is probable that the basic underlying lesion is eustachian tube dysfunction. Children with respiratory allergies appear to be predisposed. Although it is said that inadequately treated or undrained otitis media is often responsible, clinical experience does not bear this out.

The critical physician finds himself in a serious dilemma in managing a child with this problem. On the one hand he is concerned that permanent hearing loss will ensue unless definitive measures are instituted. On the other hand he is reluctant to submit the family and the child to the protracted expense, inconvenience and psychic trauma associated with vigorous surgical measures, especially in the light of inadequate evidence that such measures alter the ultimate outcome of the disease.

The following would seem to be a logical plan of management at present: First, the child should be assessed from the standpoint of underlying problems, such as allergy, that might be amenable to simple measures. If there is sufficient adenoidal hypertrophy to produce significant chronic nasal obstruction, adenoidectomy should be performed. Serous otitis media by itself should not be considered an indication for tonsil and adenoid surgery, because dysfunction of the eustachian tube in this disorder is not influenced by surgery. In addition, an audiogram should be obtained from every child old enough to cooperate. This is most important as a means by which the progress of the condition may be evaluated. The child should then be followed with conservative management. Nasal vasoconstrictors, such as phenylephrine, 0.25 per cent, 2 to 4 drops four times daily, or any one of the oral decongestants containing antihistamines should be tried in dosages proportionate to age. Nasal vasoconstrictors should not be used more than three or four days without one or two days of respite.

The family should be made aware that many months may pass with no change in the condition. Often with the arrival of summer, normal hearing (both subjectively and by audiometry) returns. Relapse may occur in the autumn, however. For school children, a seat near the front of the room may be required temporarily. Periodic audiograms should be obtained, especially at times when a change in hearing is noted by the parents. Under such conservative management it is likely that most cases will subside spontaneously, even though a year or more is required. Cases that do not subside spontaneously would probably not have responded to a more vigorous regimen.

Two situations seem to warrant more active intervention after a short trial of conservative measures. The first of these is deafness which is sufficient to handicap the child in school and which cannot be adequately compensated by seating him in the front row. The second is the very young child who is learning to talk and whose speech development may be impaired by the hearing deficit. In such instances, temporary improvement in hearing may be obtained by needle aspiration of the middle ear. Unfortunately, repeated aspiration is usually required because aspiration does not affect the underlying process and consequently does not prevent reaccumulation of fluid. In some instances, repeated controlled politzerization under careful observation has appeared to shorten the course of serous otitis media. As a last resort in patients with disabling deafness, small plastic tubes may be inserted through the drums to provide constant palliative drainage. It cannot be emphasized too strongly, however, that proper management of this difficult problem requires complete cooperation between the pediatrician or generalist and the otolaryngologist.

Labyrinthitis

CHARLES F. FERGUSON, M.D.

True labyrinthitis, as the name implies, is a specific inflammatory process involving the bony or membranous labyrinth. It is almost always secondary to middle ear suppuration. In the preantibiotic era it was not an uncommon complication of otitis media or mastoiditis, but today relatively few cases are encountered.

The frequently used term "toxic labyrinthitis," which does not fall into this category, is a double misnomer. In the first place, the symptom complex to which this term refers entails a physiologic disturbance of labyrinthine function and is not actually a labyrinthitis. It is merely a temporary irritation of the stato-kinetic system. Second, there may be no true toxin involved. This term indicates merely that the real cause is not apparent. To be sure, there are transient episodes of vertigo with a gradual onset over a 24- to 48-hour period, and they may be associated with nausea or vomiting. But there is no loss of hearing, no tinnitus and no evidence of either otitis or mastoiditis. Sudden changes of position may precipitate a so-called "toxic" attack. This condition is seen in febrile diseases, such as virus infections, pneumonia and other systemic infections, and in many allergic conditions; it is also associated with certain drugs (or alcohol). In such cases, reassurance alone, with mild sedation with phenobarbital, is the only indicated treatment.

Dimenhydrinate, up to 50 mg. three or four times a day, or diphenhydramine, up to 50 mg. three or four times a day (in an older child), may raise the threshold of labyrinthine irritability and give symptomatic relief until the disturbance subsides. (Although these maximal dosages exceed those recommended by the manufacturers, I have used them successfully in my pediatric patients.) In children over 12 years of age meclizine, 25 mg. every 12 hours may be given during the acute phase.

True labyrinthitis may be circumscribed, diffuse, serous or suppurative. In *circumscribed* labyrinthitis, infection involves only a small portion of the inner ear, and the condition is usually due to an erosion of the most superficial portion of the bony labyrinth, namely, the lateral (horizontal) semicircular canal. In most cases this erosion results from pressure necrosis from an expanding cholesteatoma in a case of chronic otitis. Occasionally infection may extend directly through the oval window, or even the round window. The fistula test is usually positive in such cases; vertigo and nystagmus result from compression of the air in the auditory canal. Hearing, however, is not much more involved than in an attack of ordinary otitis media.

Treatment is that of the underlying chronic otitis. Hospitalization is frequently desirable for careful observation, and adequate prolonged treatment with full doses of antibiotics, such as penicillin, ampicillin, erythromycin or tetracycline, should be given. Later, mastoid surgery may be done to exteriorize the cholesteatoma, if it is not completely removed. Tympanoplasty to improve hearing may be associated with, or follow, this surgery if the cholesteatoma has been satisfactorily removed. Opinions still differ considerably on these points today.

Diffuse serous labyrinthitis may be secondary to a circumscribed labyrinthitis which has hitherto given no symptoms and has remained latent. In some cases it may originate primarily from an acute suppurative otitis media, with extension through the oval or round window, without necessarily producing bone necrosis, as in the circumscribed type. In such cases the fistula test is negative, because there has been no erosion. But if the *serous* labyrinthitis is secondary to a preexisting *circumscribed* labyrinthitis, the fistula test would, of course, be positive. The hearing in such cases is usually more involved than in the circumscribed type, but there is not the great loss (or complete deafness) seen in suppurative labyrinthitis. In the past this type of labyrinthitis was a complication of otitis or mastoiditis, which indicated emergency surgery to prevent the spread of infection and forestall intracranial complications.

Needless to say, hospitalization with complete bed rest is imperative in this situation, and sedation with phenobarbital should be given. Intensive antibiotic therapy (preferably parenteral to maintain maximal blood levels) must be instituted, and ampicillin or one of the sulfonamides should be used because of the possibility of intracranial extension. The middle ear must be adequately drained by a large myringotomy incision, but further surgery is not necessarily indicated unless the disease remains unchecked.

A simple mastoidectomy might be considered later if the otitis has already been of two to three weeks' duration and has not responded to intensive antibiotic therapy by complete resolution. Complete mastoidectomy with or without tympanoplasty should be done if cholesteatoma has developed in an already chronic otitis case and the fistula test is positive. Preferably, such a patient should be under the care of an experienced otologic surgeon trained to evaluate whether the underlying otitis is merely *acute* or whether it is an acute flare-up of a *chronic* infection, with or without cholesteatoma. It is important to determine whether the labyrinthitis is serous or suppurative.

Diffuse suppurative or *purulent labyrinthitis* results from gross invasion of the inner ear by bacteria, either secondary to acute or chronic otitis media or mastoiditis, or by direct extension through the oval or round window. It may follow an otologic surgical procedure. An inadequately treated serous labyrinthitis may on occasion progress to the suppurative stage. It may also result from direct extension of meningitis or a subdural abscess into the labyrinth. Complete and permanent deafness is usual, with severe whirling vertigo, tinnitus, nausea, vomiting, spontaneous nystagmus and often ataxia. The patient usually has a high fever and is acutely sick and often prostrated. Hospitalization in such cases is essential, with absolute bed rest, along with sedation as already indicated. Treatment may have to be continued for several weeks. Lumbar puncture is usually important to determine the possible presence of meningitis (or early meningeal irritation). Prolonged and intensive parenteral antibiotic and sulfonamide therapy should be given as previously noted, and if intracranial signs persist or develop, surgical drainage of the labyrinth through the mastoid may be indicated. At this time the destroyed labyrinth may have to be removed.

Injuries to the Middle Ear

CHARLES F. FERGUSON, M.D.

Trauma to the middle ear may result *indirectly* by a sudden compression of the air in the auditory canal or *directly* by a puncture wound of the tympanic membrane. Sudden air compression as occurs in a nearby or distant (though intense) explosion may rupture the drum. On occasion, however, hemorrhage may result in separation of the layers, possibly raising epithelial blebs. Such injuries may follow the inexcusable practice of boxing a child's ears with the flat palm of the hand, which produces a sudden but intense increase of pressure.

Sudden changes in middle ear pressure during airplane travel, especially if the eustachian tubes are not functioning properly at the time (because of acute nasopharyngeal infection with inflammatory edema, allergy or hypertrophied adenoids), may rupture the drum with further involvement of the middle ear. Head trauma may produce middle ear injury, and a basal skull fracture through the petrous portion of the temporal bone or the mastoid bone may cause hemorrhage from the middle ear, or drainage of cerebrospinal fluid.

A sharp blow on the head may cause dislocation of the ossicular chain with no evidence of damage to the drum, but with a severe conductive hearing loss. Symptoms of such injuries are sudden sharp ear pain, sudden fullness in the ear with impaired hearing, possibly tinnitus and even, on occasion, nystagmus.

In such injuries no manipulation is best, but a sterile cotton wick should be left in the canal until healing takes place. Even in large perforations, healing is usually complete. Ear drops and other local medications are contraindicated. If the cotton becomes wet with blood or colorless fluid (cerebrospinal fluid), the patient should be constantly and carefully observed for further intracranial injury or fractured skull, and appropriate investigative steps taken. If blood causes the tympanic membrane to bulge (hemotympanum), and there is no evidence of fractured skull or intracranial injury, sterile aspiration may be worthwhile before clotting takes place. If the contents of the tympanic cavity are already infected, myringotomy to drain the fluid and to prevent adhesions, along with systemic administration of broad-spectrum antibiotics in full doses, may be indicated for some time.

Direct injury to the tympanic membrane and middle ear frequently occurs from toothpicks, swabs, paper clips, bobby pins and pencils. On occasion, too vigorous attempts to remove wax or foreign bodies may produce such injuries. The best method of treatment is placement of a sterile cotton wick in the canal until healing has taken place, and this is usually satisfactory, even in large tears. Prophylactic antibiotic therapy may be given. An audiogram to determine possible disruption of the ossicular chain should be done, since in such instances dislocation of the incus or disruption of the incudomalleolar or incudostapedial joints may have occurred, and emergency reposition by microsurgical techniques is indicated. A hearing loss of 50 to 60 decibels by air conduction would indicate such injury. In these patients, repositioning of the incus or restoration of the continuity of the ossicular chain can be accomplished under the Zeiss operating microscope, once the injury is properly diagnosed.

Hearing Problems

ALLAN C. GOODMAN, Ph.D., *and*
WERNER D. CHASIN, M.D.

A few significant facts and concepts provide the stimulus and basis for proper management of impairment of hearing in infancy and childhood:

1. Hearing is the primary sensory input pertinent to the development of language and speech.

2. When impairment of hearing is severe with onset in the first year of life, the effects on development of language and speech are profound. Even mild and moderate hearing losses in the first few years may affect development of language.

3. Emotional, social and intellectual development are adversely affected by impairment of hearing in infancy and early childhood. For a given child, this may be true even for a mild or moderate hearing loss.

4. Failure to compensate for reduced hearing early in life by otologic, audiologic and/or educational treatment reduces the probability of adequate language and speech development; the more severe the impairment, the greater the reduction. The effects of delay on development may not be reversible. There is international consensus on the desirability of initiating treatment by the age of six months, although it is recognized that the period between the ages of 6 and 12 months may be the more practical goal in many instances.

5. Adequate methods are available for assessment of hearing early in life. The audiologist, with methods of behavioral audiometry, usually can classify an infant as having grossly normal hearing, severely impaired hearing or some intermediate degree of impairment as early as four to eight months of age. With electrophysiologic audiometry (most frequently, computer-averaged electroencephalographic changes in response to tonal stimuli), hearing threshold levels can be obtained for many infants this age and younger.

6. When hearing cannot be restored by otologic treatment (as in the infant with sensorineural hearing loss), hearing aid, auditory training, parent counseling and special educational procedures are employed to reduce the effects of the impairment on social and emotional development and to promote the development of language and speech.

IMPAIRMENT AND HANDICAP

In Table 1, categories of hearing threshold level are keyed to a scale of terms commonly used to describe hearing impairment. This is helpful in understanding the terms used in the text. The rationale for the categories of hearing level has its basis in clinical experience. Table 1 also relates numerical values of hearing levels to brief statements of the manifestations, and the probable handicap and needs for each category of impairment. More extensive discussion is provided in succeeding paragraphs. The table is a useful guide for estimating the nature and degree of difficulty most frequently imposed by a given loss of hearing. It is an oversimplification, however, and must be used with caution, because the degree of handicap imposed by a hearing loss is not determined by measurements of hearing levels alone. Other factors important for assessment of handicap and relevant to recommendations for rehabilitation and education include age at onset of hearing loss, the characteristics of the hearing loss (most significant, the reduction in ability to discriminate speech), intelligence, emotional stability, the presence of concomitant impairments and the expectations and personal needs of the child and his family.

SENSORINEURAL HEARING LOSS

The term sensorineural is used to imply that the locus of pathology is in either the cochlea or the 8th cranial nerve or both. It is the term preferred to "nerve deafness" (unjustifiably specific) and the still older "perceptive deafness" (inappropriately connotative of higher nervous system processes). Disturbances of the ability to process or make use of auditory information because of a presumed defect in the central nervous system are usually described in terms of the observed behavior; quantification in decibels is not appropriate.

Severe and Profound Bilateral Sensorineural Hearing Loss, Congenital or in Infancy

Severe congenital bilateral sensorineural hearing loss has profoundly serious effects on development of language and speech and on social and emotional development. When onset is postnatal but before development of language and speech, the consequences are little different from those of congenital hearing loss.

Many children with severe sensorineural hearing loss are also subject to recurrent otitis media. This adds to their difficulties. They should be followed for periodic treatment.

TABLE 1. Relations Between Hearing Threshold Level in dB and Probable Handicap and Needs

HEARING LEVEL dB* (*A.N.S.I. 1969 Reference*)	PROBABLE HANDICAP AND NEEDS
−10 to 26 dB†	*Normal limits. No significant handicap for most children.* Some at upper normal limits, however, have difficulty in classroom. Sustained attention may be difficult. May benefit from hearing aid.
27 to 40 dB	*Mild hearing loss. Slight handicap for some but significant handicap for many children in classroom.* Difficulty hearing faint or distant speech. Sustained attention is frequently difficult. May benefit from instruction in speech reading. May benefit from hearing aid.
41 to 55 dB	*Moderate hearing loss. Significant handicap for most children.* Will understand conversation at a distance of 3 to 5 feet but has frequent difficulty in classroom and group discussion. Sustained attention is very difficult. Speech and language may be defective. Needs hearing aid, auditory training, speech reading, speech conservation, speech and language therapy.
56 to 70 dB	*Moderately severe hearing loss. Marked handicap.* Conversation must be loud to be understood. Has great difficulty in classroom and group discussion. Speech will be defective and language skills reduced. Needs all of above-mentioned aid plus special teaching in language skills. Special tutoring in academic subjects may be necessary. Some will need special classes for the hearing impaired.
71 to 90 dB	*Severe hearing loss. Severe handicap.* May hear a loud voice about 1 foot from the ear. Understands only shouted or amplified speech. May identify environmental noises, may distinguish vowels but may not identify consonants. Speech and language will be severely defective. Needs education for deaf children in special school or classes for the deaf with emphasis on speech, auditory training and language, plus hearing aid. Some may enter regular classes after initial instruction.
More than 90 dB	*Profound hearing loss. Extreme handicap.* May hear some loud sounds. Usually cannot understand even amplified speech without visual clues. Needs are as in the preceding category. Some may enter regular schools or classes after initial instruction.

* Average of hearing levels for 500, 1000 and 2000 Hz; A.N.S.I. 1969 reference zero for pure tone audiometers is essentially the same as I.S.O. 1964.

† Many children with hearing levels within normal limits are not free of otologic abnormality, although these abnormalities are not necessarily related to handicap.

Habilitation includes use of amplification, auditory training, speech reading, special teaching and extensive counseling. Amplification with a hearing aid is of benefit even when there is little residual hearing. Although the hearing aid will not restore normal hearing, it will make audible a signal of danger or a signal that someone is talking and should be looked at. Amplification will also provide information about the temporal, stress and intonation patterns of speech. This is useful for the child in monitoring his own speech, and, when combined with visual information, can be valuable in understanding the speech of others. Special training of the child is necessary to achieve these ends. The audiologist is prepared to advise on the selection of a hearing aid, on its advantages and limitations and on the necessary special training and education. Considerable counseling and guidance of the parents are also essential. All these efforts are best accomplished at an audiology or hearing and speech center with interest and experience in pediatric problems. The earlier these efforts are begun, the better; preferably in the first year of life.

Periodic follow-up at least into adolescence is necessary for these children for several reasons: early measurements of hearing may not have been sufficiently precise, concomitant defects may not have been adequately defined or apparent at the first visits and progression of hearing loss may occur.

Initial educational treatment is directed more to the parents, and siblings if old enough, than to the affected child. The primary aim of parent education involves making the parent an effective teacher, promoting and guiding the child's language and speech development. The major points, without attempt at completeness, are these: helping the parents achieve a home environment in which the child is talked to frequently and is encouraged to communicate; showing the parents how to encourage and teach the child to associate sounds with the objects producing them (usually with his hearing aid on); showing them how to teach the child to observe the face of the talker and relate the talker's speech to the visual and auditory information the child receives; showing the parents how to contrive play-teaching situations, and how to use daily life activities (e.g., washing dishes or putting on a coat) as experiences designed to promote development of language and speech. Parental acceptance of the fact of deafness, not always attained with ease, and understanding of its implications are additional important aims. Effectiveness in this achievement influences the quality of the parents as teachers and promotes a more normal home life for all. Additional sympathetic guidance and encouragement on the part of the pediatrician is valuable. The preschool teaching and guidance may be accomplished in individual instruction, in groups of two or three, in larger nursery groups or in a combination of individual and group teaching. Opportunity for the parents to discuss problems and solutions with teachers, otologists, audiologists and with other parents is highly desirable. Following preschool, most of these children will be educated in special schools or classes for the deaf. Some may enter regular classes after initial instruction.

Indications for Referral. When parents observe that the infant is generally not responsive to loud environmental sounds (excluding fire engines and heavy trucks and other sounds which result in vibrations that can be felt) suspicion of hearing impairment is justified. Other causes for suspicion include: failure to awaken or move about in response to speech or noise when sleeping in a quiet room; by age four to five months, failure to turn his head or at least move his eyes toward the source of a sound (his name being called or other environmental sounds); by age six months, failure to turn purposefully toward the source of such sounds; by about eight months, no attempt to imitate sounds made by the parents when the parents produce sound made by the infant; at 8 to 12 months, lack of variety in melody and in sounds produced in babbling; at about 12 months, no apparent understanding of simple phrases. When any of these causes for suspicion occurs, referral for audiologic and otologic evaluation is indicated.

On the basis of experience, a number of prenatal, perinatal and postnatal circumstances have been identified that are likely to impair hearing. The most prominent high-risk conditions are as follows:

1. Any family history of hearing loss, with onset roughly under age 50, not clearly attributed to trauma, infections or ototoxic drugs.
2. Maternal rubella or other viral infections at any time during pregnancy.
3. Defects of ears, nose or throat, including malformed, low-set or absent pinnae; cleft lip or palate (including submucous cleft).
4. Birthweight less than 1500 Gm.
5. Bilirubin level greater than 20 mg. per 100 ml.
6. Prenatal treatment of the mother or postnatal treatment of the infant with ototoxic drugs.
7. Multiple congenital anomalies, any cause.

All such high-risk infants should be referred for audiologic and otologic evaluation by age four months. All should be followed regularly after the first evaluation even if hearing appears normal. The follow-up is important because not all familial impairment of hearing is evident in early infancy but may be manifested at some later time.

Application of these high-risk criteria does not detect all children with significant hearing loss since cause is unknown for many. Many, unfortunately, are not detected until age three or later because of grossly inadequate speech. One criterion which will provide earlier detection, although not as early as is desirable, is to consider as suspect children who at age two show little or no spontaneous speech. This is a more certain reason for referral if the child's speech and language development differs from that of his siblings.

Moderate and Moderately Severe Sensorineural Hearing Loss, Congenital or in Infancy

Early detection, evaluation and treatment are equally important, and for the same reasons, as in the more severely impaired children; early habilitative efforts are essentially the same. The chief differences are the better prognosis for development of good language and speech, and the greater ease with which this may be achieved. Those with the lesser degrees of hearing loss are more likely to be educated in schools for children with normal hearing, as opposed to special schools or classes for the deaf. Some of the more severely impaired children may also be educated in regular schools, most frequently after initial instruction in special schools or classes. This is highly desirable. When it occurs, special tutoring may be required in one or more subject areas, and careful monitoring of educational achievement is necessary.

Periodic follow-up at least into adolescence

is necessary. The reasons are the same as noted in the discussion of children with severe and profound hearing loss. Progression may be more likely with some of these children.

Indications for Referral. The children in this group with lesser degree of impairment may be more difficult to identify. Parents may observe that the child does not respond to sound unless it is loud and this may be more or less consistent. Most difficult to detect are those who have grossly normal hearing in lower frequencies but with marked loss at 1000 or 1500 Hz and above. The latter will hear and respond to most environmental sounds normally. They will also detect speech normally but will have considerable difficulty in understanding speech because essential acoustic information is missing. Frequent misunderstanding of conversation is a clue. When they are not discovered until school age, as occurs frequently, the primary problem may appear as "difficult" behavior because of inappropriate response to instructions and requests and "lack of attention." In some instances, parents may note that the child pays close attention to the talker's face, that he understands imperfectly and only with repetition, or that he wants the television very loud. The same high-risk conditions noted earlier should be considered. Aberrations in language and speech development may provide a sign, but this is not easy to detect accurately because of the wide range of normal at any one age early in life. It is more desirable for the pediatrician to refer such children for audiologic and otologic evaluation than to assume that the hearing is normal.

Bilateral Sensorineural Hearing Loss, Onset After Language and Speech Development

The management problems are simpler than with congenital or other early-onset impairment because language and speech have developed to some extent. The severity of the hearing loss and the age of onset are critical variables. The rehabilitative efforts include hearing aid, auditory training, speechreading, speech conservation and special teaching to foster continued development of language skills. When the hearing loss is severe and sudden, the resulting emotional upset calls for sympathetic supportive guidance and parent education.

Meningitis, measles and ototoxic drugs are frequently implicated. The etiology may also be delayed onset, hereditary, progressive hearing loss, and it may be associated with renal disease. A careful interview to elicit family history and appropriate medical evaluation are indicated. Periodic follow-up by audiology is necessary to observe for progression and to monitor social and educational accommodation to the impairment of hearing.

When the onset is sudden and the hearing loss is severe, the change in the child's responsiveness to sound will be obvious. When the hearing loss is progressive, the parents will note that the child does not respond to sound as he did previously; there is either very little response or response only to loud sound. If the child has sufficient speech and language, he will comment about his difficulty.

Severe Unilateral Sensorineural Hearing Loss

For most life situations severe or total loss of function in one ear is only a minor handicap. The ability to localize the source of a sound is impaired but in time this is usually compensated for; in this respect, however, the young man in a military combat situation is at a serious and severe disadvantage, and sportsman hunters may score less well than their colleagues. Communication in a noisy environment or in the presence of competing messages is also impaired. Obviously, a talker on the listener's "bad side" is less well heard. For some with unilateral hearing loss a special hearing aid (CROS) has helped to reduce the disadvantages. The microphone of this hearing aid is placed at the level of the impaired ear and the auditory signal is directed from there to the receiver fitted to an open earmold in the better ear.

The major concern for those with one severely impaired ear is the continued health of the better ear. Children with frequent upper respiratory infections and otitis media require especially careful control. These children, in our opinion, should not be allowed to engage in contact sports and other activities which present a high risk of head injury lest the one good ear be damaged. Periodic followup is desirable to monitor the status of the good ear.

It is frequently difficult to establish the time of onset of unilateral hearing loss in a child. Perhaps most frequently, onset is abrupt and it may be associated temporally with mumps or with other, as yet unidentified viral infections involving the cochlea. It may also be congenital, hereditary or acquired.

A progressive unilateral sensorineural hearing loss should raise the question of an acoustic neurinoma or other tumor of the cerebellopontine angle. This is fairly frequent in patients with von Recklinghausen's disease. Early diagnosis by audiologic means, vestibular evaluation and appropriate x-ray studies is essential. Such tumors, when diagnosed in their early stages, can now be removed by a translabyrinthine approach with minimal mortality and morbidity and with a good chance of preserving the integrity of the facial nerve.

Bilateral High Frequency Sensorineural Hearing Loss

There are many children with hearing loss restricted to frequencies above about 3000 Hz. In some, the condition is congenital, hereditary or other; some cases may be temporally related to infection. There is no impairment of function for communication. These hearing losses may, however, be progressive and it is prudent to follow them periodically because the progression may result in impairment at frequencies important for discrimination of speech.

FUNCTIONAL OR NONORGANIC HEARING LOSS

There are instances of impairment of hearing in which the inferred cause is motivational or emotional; there is no observable organic cause and no reasonable basis for inference of one. We refer to this as functional or nonorganic hearing impairment. In some cases there may be a functional overlay on an organic peripheral impairment. The basis for functional hearing loss, at one extreme, may represent merely a reduction of ability to do the tasks in audiologic examination, or at another extreme an emotional disturbance; the continuum may range from deliberate feigning to a psychogenic hearing loss as in a conversion hysteria. In cases of psychogenic hearing loss the impairment of function appears just as real as in organic hearing loss; the net effect is the same but the cause and treatment are different.

It is usually not difficult for an experienced clinician to identify nonorganic hearing loss. It may, however, be very difficult to distinguish between an organic component and a functional overlay or between feigning and psychogenic hearing loss.

Some children show consistent hearing loss with measurement of hearing levels for pure tones, but with changes of instruction and with measurement of hearing levels for speech, they show little or no hearing loss. Some show hearing loss with reasonable consistency with all measurements, but with electrophysiologic audiometry they show much better hearing. The latter more likely, but not necessarily, represent instances of emotional problems requiring psychiatric consultation. In both of these sets of circumstances, when we are certain that the child has hearing within normal limits and the child does not complain of difficulty in hearing, we consider that there is no significant emotional problem. When, on the other hand, the child does complain of significant difficulty in hearing in one or more listening circumstances, we believe that psychiatric evaluation is indicated.

CONDUCTIVE HEARING LOSS

In many instances conductive hearing losses are responsive to medical or surgical treatment. When hearing aids are indicated, the results are usually very satisfactory. Early treatment to bring hearing as close to normal as possible is again highly desirable. The hearing losses range from mild to moderately severe, and even with the milder losses, without very early alleviation, the probability of impairment of language and speech development is high. This is particularly true for children with bilateral congenital atresia. The adverse effects of recurrent otitis media, however, should not be taken lightly. When the latter occurs early in life, it too appears to impair language development, and during early school years it is a frequent important factor in school difficulties. Hearing aids are helpful and are often used on a part-time basis.

Congenital Deformity of External Ear

A significant hearing loss is usually associated with maldevelopment of the auricle and external auditory canal. These children should be seen for otologic and audiologic evaluation. Surgery to improve the hearing in the abnormal ear is not indicated when the deformity is unilateral. Plastic surgery is best performed at about five years of age.

When the auricles are abnormal on both sides but the external canals are patent, the hearing is not necessarily normal. For example, children with Treacher Collins syndrome usually have abnormal auricles and patent canals, but often have moderate or moderately severe hearing loss because of abnormalities of the ossicles. The hearing loss should be evaluated as early as possible. The children are then fitted with a hearing aid and operated on at age five to six years.

When the auricles are abnormal on both sides and the external canals are atretic, there is a moderately severe hearing loss. If x-ray studies demonstrate a pneumatized mastoid and audiometry reveals adequate cochlear reserve, surgery to improve the hearing can be performed. Up to age five years a bone-conduction hearing aid should be used by the child. At age five years a unilateral mastoidotympanoplasty can be performed to create an external canal and an effective tympanic sound-conducting mechanism. A mastoidotympanoplasty is not performed on the contralateral ear, although plastic surgery may be desirable for cosmetic reasons.

Unresolved Otitis Media

After treatment for acute otitis media with antibiotics and decongestants, the child should be observed at weekly intervals to see whether the eardrum returns completely to normal or continues to look slightly abnormal. The latter usually suggests a chronic serous otitis media (or "glue ear") and can be diagnosed with the pneumatic otoscope. The tympanic membrane which contains a middle ear effusion almost always flutters poorly with alternate positive and negative pressure delivered with the pneumatic otoscope. The chronically fluid-filled middle ear must be diagnosed and treated because it is a leading cause of mild to moderate hearing loss and is the most common underlying cause of recurrent acute otitis media. In addition, it is the precursor of chronic tympanomastoiditis with and without cholesteatoma.

Adenoidectomy (with or without tonsillectomy) frequently fails to reverse the chronic glue ear. The most effective treatment at the present time is a myringotomy, aspiration of middle ear fluid and insertion of a middle ear aeration tube under the surgical microscope. The tube is left in place until it is spontaneously expelled by the tympanic membrane. A new tube may have to be inserted if the fluid accumulates again. Most children outgrow the condition by age 12 years, presumably as the eustachian tube assumes normal function. Occasionally children with a chronically fluid-filled middle ear fail to respond to middle ear intubation. They need a simple mastoidectomy to exenterate cells with chronically inflamed mucosa which frequently contain cholesterol granuloma. This is most often the case in children who have a "blue eardrum" (misnamed the "idiopathic hemotympanum," which is actually a variety of the common glue ear).

In all cases of chronic glue ear upper respiratory allergy should be considered as a possible cause. Although an occasional child will respond to proper allergic management, we have, on the whole, been disappointed in the results of allergic management in this condition.

Tympanic Perforations

Persistent tympanic perforations result from overwhelming acute infection, trauma and advanced unresolved otitis media. A simple perforation causes only a slight degree of hearing loss. A moderate or moderately severe hearing loss (over 40 dB) suggests ossicular damage in addition to the more obvious perforation.

In the absence of underlying chronic infection, even large perforations may close spontaneously. The parent should be advised to prevent water from entering the diseased ear during bathing, and swimming should not be allowed. A traumatic perforation or one resulting from a resolved acute infection can be left alone to heal spontaneously for at least six months. No medications are used when there is no sign of infection.

After six months, and only if there is satisfactory eustachian tube function, as evidenced by a normal middle ear on the opposite side and ability to pass air in the affected ear by the Valsalva maneuver, a tympanoplasty may be performed. This will involve an inspection of the middle ear and repair of any ossicular damage as well as grafting of the tympanic membrane to close the perforation. When the eustachian tube is not functioning properly, surgery should be delayed for years, if necessary, since a tympanoplasty would be unsuccessful under these conditions.

Perforations resulting from advanced unresolved otitis media will usually require surgery. The indication for the latter is the eradication of chronic epitympanic and mastoid infection. Repair of the perforation is of lesser urgency, and on occasion may even be more successful if performed as a separate, subsequent procedure.

Chronic Otitis Media

It must be emphasized that in most cases of chronic otitis media there is chronic infection of both the middle ear and the mastoid air cell system, i.e., chronic tympanomastoiditis. There is either a perforation or deep retraction pocket of the tympanic membrane and signs of continued infection, either in the form of external drainage (frequently malodorous) or moisture in the ear canal without external discharge. There may be any degree of hearing loss, from minimal to marked. An advanced cholesteatoma can be present with essentially normal hearing although this is unlikely. Chronic tympanomastoiditis seldom can be cured with either systemic or topical antibiotics and usually requires surgery in the form of a mastoidotympanoplasty. Prior to surgery the infection should be at least temporarily cleared with the use of both systemic and topical antibiotics according to the culture and sensitivity test. Eardrops are effective only if debris and pus are first thoroughly cleaned from the external canal and tympanic membrane by suction or by gentle irrigation with sterile water at body temperature.

Normal-Appearing Ear

In childhood, a conductive loss with a normal-appearing tympanic membrane is due to a congenital malformation of the middle ear ossicles, traumatic dislocation or necrosis of an ossicle, postinflammatory necrosis of either the incus or stapes, congenital fixation of the stapes or, rarely, otosclerosis.

The type of loss, its degree and its significance for the child are established by audiologic evaluation. If the loss is unilateral, treatment is not urgent. If it involves both ears, either a hearing aid or surgical correction is likely to be indicated.

Surgical correction can be performed at any age, but it is preferable to wait until at least age five years or to a considerably later age if the child is prone, in addition, to recurrent middle ear infections. When the cause is otosclerosis, it is preferable to delay surgery until the patient has reached the late teens or early twenties, because the continued proliferation of bone of active juvenile otosclerosis may negate an initially good surgical result. A hearing aid is recommended in otosclerosis when the degree of hearing loss and the child's individual needs suggest its desirability.

Although most cases of conductive losses can be corrected surgically, occasionally the otologist will encounter a tympanic anomaly which is so complex that he will not attempt a reconstruction but will close the ear and recommend that the child be fitted with a hearing aid. It must be reemphasized that most cases of conductive hearing loss in children are due to a fluid-filled middle ear, and that the pneumatic otoscope should be used as part of the thorough ear, nose and throat examination of all children.

EXTERNAL OTITIS

External otitis is an occasional cause of hearing loss in children. In many cases of an apparent recurrent accumulation of excessive wax, a chronic external otitis exists. This can be recognized by inspecting the wax and noting whether it is surrounded by flakes of desquamated skin. In these patients there is a disorder of the epithelium wherein the normal self-cleaning action by migration of surface epithelium toward the external auditory meatus is absent. As a result, the canal is continuously impacted with debris. To cure this condition is difficult. Periodic gentle irrigation of the canal followed by the instillation of steroid-antibiotic ear drops is helpful in keeping the canals patent. Preventing soaps and shampoos from entering the canals and controlling allergy also help to reduce the problem.

Acute external otitis, which is much more common during the summer, is best treated by cleaning the canal with either suction or gentle irrigation with water at body temperature. Thereafter, several drops of a steroid-antibiotic ear solution are instilled three times a day. If the canal is closed by edema, a small strip of gauze (the corner of a 4- by 4-inch sponge cut off to a length of 2 inches) impregnated with Ergophene Ointment is gently inserted into the canal with an ear dressing forceps. This type of wick, if left in the ear for 24 hours, will reduce the edema so that when it is withdrawn ear drops can be instilled. Systemic antibiotics are seldom useful in the treatment of external otitis except when there is an auricular or periauricular cellulitis or lymphadenitis.

It must be emphasized that what appears to be a stubborn unilateral external otitis is often not an external otitis at all but a chronic otitis media. The perforation may be difficult to visualize, and what is apparent is only the chronic irritation of the external auditory canal which is in reality secondary to the middle ear discharge. It is obvious that such cases will not respond to a treatment regimen designed for external otitis. Such cases usually require surgery to halt the infection and prevent complications.

TRAUMA

After head injury, if blood is seen in either the external auditory canal or behind the tympanic membrane (blue eardrum), a fracture of the temporal bone is highly likely. The fracture frequently is not seen on ordinary skull films but can be demonstrated either on mastoid roentgenograms or sometimes only on mastoid laminograms. When blood is present in the canal it should be left alone and care taken to prevent secondary infection by not allowing water to enter the canal.

The Weber test indicates whether cochlear damage has occurred: if the tuning fork is heard better in the injured ear, the cochlea has been spared, but if it lateralizes to the better ear, severe cochlear damage has occurred. Immediate surgical treatment is indicated only if there is an immediate facial paralysis, evidence of spinal fluid leakage or severe labyrinthine vertigo with nystagmus toward the side of the injured ear. A facial paralysis which does not begin immediately but appears a few hours or more later can be observed, since it is probably due to edema rather than to impingement by a bony fragment. In spinal fluid otorrhea an otologist should operate, utilizing the transmastoid approach, as soon as the patient's condition permits surgery. Labryrinthine vertigo with nystagmus may be due to a dislocation of the stapes footplate and a perilymphatic fistula, and only by immediate exploratory surgery is there a chance of preserving the hearing in the ear.

All other cases of temporal bone trauma can be observed without specific therapy as long as there is no sign of infection. A hemotympanum will always resolve without any treatment. Perforations frequently will heal spontaneously. Audiologic evaluation must be performed once the ear has returned to a normal appearance, because a persistent conductive hearing loss is likely the result of a dislocated ossicle (usually the incus) and can be corrected surgically as long as cochlear function has been spared.

19

Infectious Diseases

Neonatal Sepsis, Meningitis and Pneumonia

GEORGE H. McCRACKEN, Jr., M.D.

The principal goals of therapy for neonatal sepsis and meningitis are early diagnosis and prompt institution of antimicrobial therapy. Because objective signs of infection in neonates are often lacking, therapy must be initiated before the diagnosis can be confirmed or the offending pathogen accurately identified. In most areas of the United States, *Escherichia coli* and group B beta-hemolytic streptococci account for the majority of cases of sepsis and meningitis during the newborn period. Pseudomonas species in some areas cause as many as 20 per cent, and in other areas are responsible for as little as 2 per cent of these illnesses. Other bacteria involved include *Listeria monocytogenes,* Klebsiella-Enterobacter species, rarely staphylococci, pneumococci, Salmonella and Proteus species, and on occasion other microorganisms. To choose chemotherapeutic agents intelligently, the physician must be aware of the historic and epidemiologic experience in the nursery in which the infant is housed, since initial treatment is based on the knowledge of the pathogens commonly encountered in the nursery and their antimicrobial susceptibilities.

NEONATAL SEPSIS

Once sepsis is suspected, suitable cultures should be obtained and therapy started immediately, using ampicillin and either kanamycin or gentamicin. Ampicillin is administered intravenously or intramuscularly in a dosage of 50 mg. per kilogram of body weight per day for infants under one week of age, and 150 mg. per kilogram of body weight per day for infants one to four weeks of age. The selection of the aminoglycoside antibiotic should be based on the antimicrobial susceptibilities of the enteric organisms isolated from infants in each nursery. Kanamycin is the drug of choice for the treatment of infections caused by susceptible gram-negative organisms and should be administered intramuscularly in a dosage of 7.5 mg. per kilogram of body weight every 12 hours for infants under one week of age, and 5 to 7.5 mg. per kilogram of body weight every 8 hours for infants one to four weeks of age. However, kanamycin-resistant *E. coli* have been encountered recently in some nurseries in North America. In these nurseries and when an isolate from an infant is shown to be resistant to kanamycin, gentamicin sulfate should be used in the place of kanamycin and administered in a dosage of 2.5 mg. per kilogram of body weight every 12 hours intramuscularly for infants under one week of age, and 2.5 mg. per kilogram of body weight every 8 hours for infants one to four weeks of age. Extensive studies have shown gentamicin to be effective in the treatment of neonatal sepsis, and there has been no evidence of acute renal or hematologic toxicity observed to date when gentamicin is administered in the neonatal period. In addition, ototoxicity has not been observed in infants one year following treatment with gentamicin in the neonatal period.

When the type of skin lesion or historic experience suggests the possibility of Pseudomonas infection, carbenicillin with or without gentamicin is the drug of choice. Carbenicillin is administered intravenously or intramuscularly in a "loading" dose of 100 mg. per kilogram body weight, followed by 75 mg. per kilogram every 8 hours in premature infants and every 6 hours in full-term infants under one week of age, and 100 mg. per kilogram every 6 hours in all infants one to four weeks of age. Experience has shown carbenicillin to be a safe drug when administered in this dosage to newborn infants for periods up to 10 days. If gentamicin is to be administered with carbenicillin, the drugs should not be mixed in the same solution and should be administered intravenously. Polymyxin B sulfate in a dosage of 3.5 to 5 mg. per kilogram of body weight per day intramuscularly, or colistimethate in a dosage of 5 to 8 mg. per kilogram of body weight per day, given in two or three dosages intramuscularly, is a suitable alternative.

When staphylococcal sepsis is suspected but not proved, parenteral methicillin should be substituted for penicillin, since many of the staphylococci encountered in the newborn infant are penicillin-resistant. The dosage of methicillin is 100 to 150 mg. per kilogram of body weight per day, divided into four intravenous or intramuscular injections in infants under one week of age, and 200 to 250 mg. per kilogram of body weight administered in four doses in infants one to four weeks of age. While kanamycin and gentamicin possess activity against most staphylococci, these drugs do not represent optimal therapy.

Once the pathogen is identified and its antimicrobial susceptibilities are known, the most appropriate drug or drugs should be selected. In general, kanamycin alone or in combination with ampicillin should be used for susceptible *E. coli* and Klebsiella-Enterobacter species; gentamicin alone or in combination with ampicillin for kanamycin-resistant enteric organisms; carbenicillin with or without gentamicin for Pseudomonas; ampicillin for *Proteus mirabilis,* enterococcus and *Listeria monocytogenes;* and penicillin for other gram-positive organisms, except penicillin-resistant staphylococci, for which methicillin is the drug of choice.

Guidelines for determining duration of therapy in the neonatal period are often lacking, since objective evidence of illness may be minimal. Culture of the blood should be repeated 24 to 48 hours after initiation of therapy; if the culture is positive, alteration of therapy may be necessary. In the absence of deep tissue involvement or abscess formation, treatment is usually continued five to seven days after clinical improvement. When multiple organs are involved or clinical response is slow, treatment may need to be continued for two to three weeks.

Supportive Therapy. In general, it is desirable to observe newborns with sepsis in an open or closed incubator. This permits adequate observation and stabilizes the infant's temperature.

Oxygen should be administered whenever the infant shows respiratory distress or cyanosis.

It is often not desirable to feed infants who are severely ill, and therefore maintenance of adequate fluid and electrolyte balance is essential. In general, this is best accomplished by the intravenous administration of suitable fluids. The use of nasogastric tubes for feeding in a severely sick infant is undesirable because of the possibility of vomiting and aspiration.

Many observers have reported the clinical impression that small transfusions of compatible fresh blood seem to be of benefit. There is no evidence that the administration of gamma globulin is of any value, and the use of corticosteroids is to be condemned.

The hemoglobin concentration and the urine and blood urea nitrogen concentration should be followed in patients who are receiving kanamycin, gentamicin, polymyxin or the antistaphylococcal penicillins. Albuminuria is to be expected as a consequence of sepsis during the newborn period.

NEONATAL MENINGITIS

The causative organisms are identical to those associated with sepsis in this age group. In general, therapy of meningitis is similar to that of sepsis, with the following exceptions: All infants should have a repeat spinal fluid examination and culture 24 to 36 hours after initiation of therapy. If organisms are seen on methylene blue or Gram's stain of the fluid, gentamicin is administered intrathecally* in a total daily dose of 1 to 2 mg. It is then our policy to repeat the lumbar puncture every 24 hours and administer intrathecal medication on a daily or every-other-day basis until the cerebrospinal fluid is sterile. There is a marked discrepancy in the time necessary to sterilize the cerebrospinal fluid of infants with meningitis due to gram-negative organisms compared with meningitis due to gram-positive organisms. It is not uncommon to have positive cerebrospinal fluid cultures for five to seven days or longer in infants with meningitis caused by coliform bacteria.

Parenteral antimicrobial therapy should be continued for approximately two to three weeks after sterilization of the cerebrospinal fluid. It

* Manufacturer's precaution: Intrathecal use of gentamicin is investigational.

is usually only necessary to continue therapy for a total of two weeks in patients with meningitis due to gram-positive organisms, while longer periods of therapy are necessary in infants with meningitis caused by gram-negative organisms. The patients should be carefully followed for signs of hematologic and renal toxicity.

Other principles of treatment and supportive therapy are identical to those outlined for sepsis.

Convulsions frequently occur with meningitis and are treated by the use of intravenous diazepam (Valium),† up to 10 mg. administered slowly, or with phenobarbital sodium, 4 mg. per kilogram body weight, given intramuscularly. If phenobarbital does not achieve the desired effect, an additional 2 mg. per kilogram can be injected every 45 minutes until the convulsions have ceased or until a total of 12 mg. per kilogram has been administered. If convulsions are not controlled within an hour or two after the start of sedation, diphenylhydantoin (Dilantin) in a dose of 5 to 7 mg. per kilogram body weight per day should be employed, and may be given in a single dose intravenously or intramuscularly.

NEONATAL PNEUMONIA

Congenital and Intrapartum Pneumonia

These pneumonias are found soon after birth and are usually secondary to intrauterine infection, aspiration, pulmonary hemorrhage or atelectasis. These infections are caused, in general, by the same organisms involved in sepsis and meningitis of the newborn and are treated with the same drugs. Cultures of tracheal aspirate and blood should be obtained; however, it is usually not possible to make a bacteriologic diagnosis. Penicillin and kanamycin or penicillin and gentamicin provide broad, safe and effective therapy for these pneumonias. Pseudomonas pneumonia occurs infrequently.

Pneumonias Occurring During the Later Neonatal Period

Most bacterial pneumonias occurring after the first week of life are due to coagulase-positive staphylococci, which are usually resistant to penicillin. Occasional cases of pneumococcal, streptococcal, *Hemophilus influenzae* and Klebsiella pneumonias are encountered.

Staphylococcal pneumonias usually progress very rapidly and fluid accumulates in the pleural space within hours. A diagnostic pleural tap should be performed whenever fluid is noted on x-ray or by physical examination. This permits rapid identification of the offending pathogen and the selection of the most appropriate antimicrobial therapy.

Whenever a staphylococcus is thought to be involved on the basis of epidemiology, x-ray or bacteriologic findings of the pleural fluid, methicillin in a dose of 200 to 250 mg. per kilogram body weight per day should be administered intramuscularly or intravenously. No other antimicrobial agents should be used concurrently.

If the organism is subsequently found to be penicillin-susceptible, methicillin is discontinued and penicillin G is administered in a dosage of 50,000 unts per kilogram per day intravenously or intramuscularly divided in 8-hour doses. Therapy is continued for a minimum of three weeks. Pneumococcal and streptococcal pneumonias are treated with penicillin G in a dosage of 25,000 to 50,000 units per kilogram of body weight per day intramuscularly divided into 8-hour doses. *H. influenzae* is treated with ampicillin, 150 to 200 mg. per kilogram of body weight per day intramuscularly or intravenously divided into 6-hour doses. Klebsiella is treated with gentamicin administered intramuscularly in a dosage of 7.5 mg. per kilogram of body weight per day divided into three doses.

Supportive Therapy. If fluid or air accumulates in the chest, even in relatively small amounts, either open or closed drainage should always be employed. Since pyopneumothorax as well as tension pneumothorax occurs relatively commonly, these patients should be closely observed for manifestations of these events. It is usually not necessary to leave the tubes in the chest for more than seven days.

Infants with pneumonia should receive oxygen for respiratory distress and for cyanosis. An incubator should be used to maintain their body temperature. Because of respiratory distress, oral feeding should be discontinued until the infant can tolerate them; they are replaced with intravenous administration of suitable parenteral fluids. Adequate pulmonary toilet is an important adjunct to therapy. The injection of antibiotics into the pleural cavity or the use of enzymes to "dissolve" pus is not recommended in infants, since side effects are on occasion quite severe.

† Manufacturer's precaution: The safety and efficacy of injectable diazepam (Valium) in children under 12 years of age have not been established.

Postneonatal Meningitis and Sepsis of Unknown Cause

GEORGE H. McCRACKEN, Jr., M.D.

MENINGITIS

Patients with clinical and laboratory findings of meningitis must often be treated even though the causative organism is not known. Such a situation may arise when a child has previously received inadequate or inappropriate antibacterial therapy, when the condition is diagnosed before substantial numbers of organisms appear in the spinal fluid or when the patient has a viral disease rather than a purulent bacterial infection.

Parenteral ampicillin alone is effective initial therapy of the common forms of bacterial meningitis (Hemophilus, meningococcus or pneumococcus). It is neither necessary nor desirable to add other antimicrobial agents, such as chloramphenicol or sulfonamides, to this regimen. Oral ampicillin has no place in the therapy of meningitis.

It is our practice to administer ampicillin in a dosage of 100 mg. per kilogram of body weight by rapid intravenous infusion, followed by 50 to 75 mg. per kilogram of body weight intravenously every 6 hours (200 to 300 mg. per kilogram of body weight per day)* in children past the second month of life when spinal fluid examination is suggestive or diagnostic of bacterial meningitis. Once the specific etiologic agent has been identified, ampicillin is continued for Hemophilus infection, while either ampicillin or aqueous penicillin G is effective against meningococcus and pneumococcus.

In all infants under one year of age and in any patient not showing clinical improvement within 48 hours, a second cerebrospinal fluid examination and culture should be performed. If organisms are seen on stained smear of the cerebrospinal fluid, therapy may have to be altered pending results of susceptibility studies. Parenteral therapy is continued for 7 to 10 days in patients with uncomplicated meningitis. The patient is observed without additional treatment for several days and then discharged.

If a rubelliform rash develops without signs of urticaria or serum sickness while ampicillin is being administered, it is our usual policy to continue the drug. If the infant has a history of penicillin allergy or develops urticaria or a serum sickness reaction, chloramphenicol† is substituted for ampicillin.

* This dosage of ampicillin exceeds the manufacturer's recommendation, but may be warranted here because of the seriousness of the illness.

SEPSIS

Sepsis in children past the neonatal period is caused most commonly by pneumococci, meningococci, streptococci, staphylococci and *Hemophilus influenzae,* and under certain circumstances by Salmonella, *Escherichia coli,* Klebsiella-Enterobacter species and Pseudomonas.

In general, clues to the bacteriologic diagnosis can be obtained from the clinical history. Patients with impetiginous lesions or infected wounds, a history of recent cardiac operation and similar events are likely to have staphylococcal sepsis. Multiple petechial lesions of the skin and mucous membranes suggest meningococcal infection, although Pseudomonas, pneumococci, Hemophilus, streptococci, staphylococci, rickettsiae and viruses can produce similar lesions.

Patients who have previously undergone splenectomy tend to develop overwhelming pneumococcal infections; children with diseases or undergoing therapy which suppresses immunologic responses are likely to develop Pseudomonas disease. Streptococci and staphylococci are often encountered in children with extensive lesions of the skin, such as burns, toxic epidermal necrolysis and erythema multiforme exudativum. Pseudomonas often produces disease in this latter group following therapeutic or prophylactic administration of antimicrobial agents.

When the bacteriologic diagnosis is in question in older infants and children, intravenous ampicillin, 150 to 200 mg. per kilogram of body weight per day in four doses, and intramuscular gentamicin, 5 to 7.5 mg. per kilogram of body weight per day, in three doses are administered. Kanamycin, 15 mg. per kilogram of body weight per day in two or three doses, is an acceptable alternative to gentamicin for kanamycin-susceptible enteric organisms.

In patients with shock or bleeding disorders, the aminoglycoside drugs must be given intravenously. Gentamicin or kanamycin should be given in the same dosage and administered over a 1- to 2-hour period. Major modification of dosage is required for the aminoglycoside antibiotics in patients with renal failure. In general, the usual dose is given on the first day. In moderate renal failure the dose is repeated every two or three days, while in severe

† Manufacturer's precaution: Chloramphenicol is not recommended for intravenous or intramuscular pediatric use. Chloramphenicol sodium succinate has been approved for intravenous pediatric use.

renal failure one-half the usual dose is administered every three to four days. It is advisable to obtain creatinine clearance and drug half-life values in such a patient in order to determine an accurate dosage schedule.

If the pathogen is subsequently identified as a pneumococcus, streptococcus, meningococcus or penicillin-susceptible staphylococcus, penicillin alone is used; if the organism is Salmonella or *Hemophilus influenzae,* ampicillin is used alone (chloramphenicol, 100 mg. per kg. per day divided into 4 equal doses and administered intravenously, is a satisfactory substitute).†

Suspected or proved penicillin-resistant staphylococcal infection is best treated with methicillin, 50 to 75 mg. per kilogram of body weight administered every 6 hours intramuscularly or intravenously. Methicillin is preferred to gentamicin or kanamycin, although most staphylococci are susceptible in vitro to the latter group of agents.

For Pseudomonas, carbenicillin, 100 to 150 mg. per kilogram of body weight, administered intravenously or intramuscularly every 6 hours, should be used either alone or in combination with gentamicin. The polymyxin group of drugs represents less suitable alternative agents for Pseudomonas infection in older infants and children.

Since one of the characteristics of sepsis with gram-negative organisms and staphylococci is the rapid and sudden occurrence of shock, it is essential that this be watched for. Corticosteroids in the usual dosage have no effect in either the prevention or therapy of septic shock; the use of very large doses of steroids in this condition may be warranted, but direct proof of the efficacy of this treatment is lacking in the pediatric patient.

Eosinophilic Meningitis

DONALD F. B. CHAR, M.D., *and*
LEON ROSEN, M.D.

Most cases of eosinophilic meningitis which occur on islands in the Pacific Ocean and in Southeast Asia are thought to be caused by the metastrongylid lungworm of rats, *Angiostrongylus cantonensis.* In a few instances the parasite has actually been recovered from the brain or spinal fluid of patients. It should be recognized, however, that a similar syndrome may be caused by other agents.

In older children and adults the clinical picture is characterized by headache, paresthesias and variable degrees of nuchal rigidity. Cranial nerve palsies and low-grade fever occur in a minority of cases. Younger children and infants are apt to show irritability and higher fever, and these signs can persist for several weeks. Although the prognosis generally is good, a few deaths have been recorded. The diagnosis can be established only by appropriate staining of the spinal fluid sediment to reveal the eosinophils.

Once the diagnosis has been established, little can be done except to await recovery. Treatment is largely supportive and symptomatic. The diagnostic spinal tap often relieves headache. Aspirin and other analgesic agents are useful for fever and headache. In more severe cases, in which signs of cerebral edema may be prominent, corticosteroids or the osmotic brain-dehydrating agents, such as urea or mannitol,* may be cautiously employed. Respiratory supportive measures, such as tracheostomy or artificial respiration, may be necessary if signs of brain stem compression appear. Recovery is characteristically slow, but usually complete.

Although thiabendazole, a broad-spectrum anthelmintic, affects the development of *A. cantonensis* in rats, its use against the parasite in man has not been reported and there is doubt as to the rationality of such use. It is suspected that the deleterious effects of *A. cantonensis* infection in humans are largely the result of reaction to dead or dying worms, and that not all parasites in a given patient die simultaneously. Consequently, if this view is correct, and if thiabendazole killed all the parasites at one time, treatment with the drug might do more harm than good.

Bacterial Endocarditis

CATHERINE A. NEILL, M.D.

The basic principle of therapy in endocarditis is to establish bactericidal levels of the appropriate antibiotic(s) and to maintain them long enough so that the blood is sterilized and the infecting organism destroyed.

This is a serious, debilitating, tedious, expensive and potentially lethal disease, and the difficulties in treating it show some analogies to the problems of guerrilla warfare—identifica-

† Manufacturer's precaution: Chloramphenicol is not recommended for intravenous or intramuscular pediatric use. Chloramphenicol sodium succinate has been approved for intravenous pediatric use.

* Manufacturer's precaution: Use of mannitol in pediatric patients has not been studied comprehensively.

tion of the enemy (clinical and bacterial diagnosis), defense mechanisms (drug resistance) and the limits of human tolerance (a sterile blood stream but a dead patient).

The question of *diagnosis* is of such vital import that it cannot be ignored in an article specifically devoted to therapy. Clinical diagnosis depends on a high index of suspicion in susceptible patients and on proper awareness of the protean manifestations of the disease.

Susceptible subjects include all those with congenital or rheumatic heart disease. There is some evidence that the incidence is higher in cyanotic than in acyanotic patients and in those with functioning systemic pulmonary shunts than in others. An occasional case does occur in children without a known preceding cardiac murmur or other evidence of underlying heart disease. There is some discussion as to whether these children have a bicuspid aortic valve which has not given rise to any murmurs. The age distribution is helpful, this condition being rare in children under five years of age.

Predisposing factors include dental or other oropharyngeal or genitourinary manipulations without antibiotic coverage, and occasionally oropharyngeal trauma; careful history taking and examination reveals such predisposing factors in 60 to 70 per cent of cases. A recent major predisposing factor is cardiac surgery, particularly open heart.

The classic *clinical syndrome* of fever, anemia, petechiae and splenomegaly is well known. However, atypical modes of presentation are frequent, including chest pain and pulmonary infiltrates, which may simulate pneumonia. This type of presentation is especially frequent in patients with pulmonary stenosis or functioning systemic pulmonary anastomoses. The disease may also be ushered in with symptoms of meningoencephalitis, and occasionally malaise and weight loss without other signs or symptoms apart from low-grade fever may be the chief complaint. Particularly difficult though rare modes of presentation are cardiac failure with nephrotic-like syndrome and a severe macrocytic anemia.

Iatrogenic modification of the clinical syndrome is unfortunately not infrequent. Such a patient might receive, for example, at the onset of fever a week's penicillin followed by defervescence; then recurrence and a week of chloramphenicol (defervescence, recurrence); then a week of a new antibiotic (defervescence, recurrence). After six to eight weeks of this the patient may present with severe anemia, malaise and fever and often significant weight loss. Splenomegaly is often slight and petechiae are absent. In addition to the modification of the clinical syndrome by this period of delay, the infecting organism has also been altered to an atypical form which grows out of the blood very slowly and requires a long period for exact identification.

"Changing cardiac murmurs," although repeatedly emphasized, can be characterized as a legendary rather than a useful sign. In pediatric practice a new cardiac murmur means that the patient either has mitral insufficiency from gross anemia or has developed aortic insufficiency due to valve perforation; almost certainly therapy should have been started several weeks before. In other words, to wait for changing cardiac murmurs is to wait too long. Petechiae are a special problem in cyanotic patients. A few small, frail cyanotic children get recurrent showers of petechiae on the extremities, rarely on the trunk, apparently due to some disorder of capillary fragility. So far, despite multiple venipunctures and many unhappy investigatory hours, we have not yet seen a young blue child presenting with large showers of petechiae who proved to have endocarditis.

In the postoperative patient, following cardiac surgery, differentiation of bacterial endocarditis from postpericardiotomy syndrome and postperfusion syndrome may present real difficulties. The presence of friction rubs and effusions in the former, and of leukopenia and atypical lymphocytes in the latter are frequently useful clues. Particular difficulty is now being encountered by internists in diagnosing *S. albus* endocarditis on prosthetic valves; as this type of surgery is done more frequently in the young, pediatricians will also encounter it. The only apparent symptoms are low-grade fever and general malaise appearing several months after surgery.

Bacterial diagnosis depends on adequate blood cultures and a highly competent laboratory. We have had transferred to us several patients with "negative cultures" whose first five or six consecutive cultures all grew out within 48 to 72 hours in our laboratory, and now believe that the clinician attempting to make the diagnosis must be fully and justifiably confident in the skill of the laboratory he is using. The proper laboratory techniques cannot concern us here, except to say that cultures should be both aerobic and anaerobic and kept for three weeks and then examined with a Gram stain before discarding. The clinician's role is to supply an adequate number of cultures (6 to 10) drawn over a period of 24 to 72 hours, each containing at least 1 ml. of blood for each 10 ml. of culture medium. The culture should of course be drawn with full aseptic precautions, and penicillinase should be added if the patient has recently had either penicillin or one of its analogues. Cultures of arterial blood are thought now by most authorities not to have any particular value, but bone marrow cultures have been useful in a few children who have received prior antibiotics. The time of day and the degree of fever at the time the cultures are drawn are now thought to be unimportant.

MANAGEMENT

Our present policy is to suspect the diagnosis in any patient with heart disease in whom fever persists for more than three to five days without an obvious and adequate local cause. Antibiotics are withheld, blood cultures are drawn and temperature is taken and charted every four hours. Persistent fever for five to seven days necessitates hospitalization. The younger the child, the more vital it is that a skilled pediatric house staff be available in the institution.

Following admission and the drawing of an adequate number of blood cultures, a number of decisions must be made. These include when to start therapy, the antibiotic(s) to employ, the use of other medications, the management of complications, the duration of therapy and the role of surgery. Close cooperation with a specialist in infectious disease is helpful at the beginning and throughout the course.

Starting therapy is a major decision and should, except under the very rarest circumstances, be considered an irrevocable one. In other words one should not start intravenous therapy "for a week, until we see how the blood cultures come out." In a patient who is not acutely ill and who has not received prior antibiotics, it is entirely justifiable to withhold therapy for a few days, watching the course of the fever, checking carefully several times daily for petechiae and splinter hemorrhages and awaiting the results of blood cultures, which may be positive after 72 hours. If at the end of that time the majority of the cultures taken in the first 24 hours are positive for the same organism, therapy may be confidently started.

If, after five to seven days of waiting, the clinical picture is clearly that of endocarditis and the cultures remain sterile, a decision may be made to start therapy. It is helpful at this time to make a detailed written note of the exact clinical status and the reasons for starting on this long, somewhat difficult and potentially hazardous course without bacterial diagnosis.

In a few patients therapy may be started within 24 hours of admission, immediately after six or eight blood cultures have been drawn. Indications to do this include (1) a classic clinical picture; (2) a gravely ill patient with enough clinical features to render the diagnosis probable; (3) a probable clinical diagnosis, plus evidence of aortic valve involvement or cerebral or pulmonary embolization; and (4) a prolonged preceding illness of two to three months treated with a multiple short course of antibiotics—under such circumstances the infecting organism, even with very skilled laboratory techniques, may not grow for two to three weeks and may need another week of subculture for complete identification.

Contraindications to starting therapy for endocarditis include the presence of an obvious localized focus of infection (e.g., pneumonia, tonsillitis), which should be treated appropriately, even though in some cases blood cultures may be drawn. "Positive" blood cultures, particularly with an organism likely to be a contaminant, in a child who is now afebrile should usually not be treated.

Antibiotic Therapy. For consideration of the basic approaches to antibiotic therapy, the reader is referred to the article concerning Judgment in the Use of Antimicrobial Agents. In all series the clinical course and management have been simpler and more satisfactory if the infecting organism is a penicillin-sensitive *Streptococcus viridans* (alpha strep), as it is in about 60 per cent of all cases, than if cultures reveal another organism or if no organism can be grown. The clinician can have a better and more logical understanding of available therapy if he cooperates with a group specializing in infective disease. He should be prepared for new approaches in the atypical and hazardous types of endocarditis, but in the author's opinion he should not experiment with "short cuts" or new drugs in *S. viridans* infection or in other situations in which ample experience has demonstrated a highly effective mode of therapy.

S. viridans is usually highly sensitive to penicillin, and intravenous therapy with 10 million units of penicillin G daily is used, usually without any additional antibiotic, for a minimum of two weeks. After two weeks the decision may be made to use intramuscular or oral therapy in similar doses, and this should be maintained for at least another two weeks. Because intramuscular therapy in such high doses can be painful, we prefer not to use it in children if the veins are still available.

Other organisms include the staphylococcus, the most frequent cause of endocarditis following cardiac surgery, the enterococcus and the pneumococcus. Gram-negative infections are rare but highly refractory to treatment, and fungal infections are usually, though not always, preterminal, occurring during therapy for bacterial endocarditis.

Predisposing factors may lead one to the clinical suspicion that the infection is caused by a specific organism. For example, *S. viridans* is the usual infecting organism following oropharyngeal manipulations, although the enterococcus and other relatively penicillin-insensitive streptococci may occur. Staphylococcal infections, in addition to being suspected following cardiac surgery, are also said to be the most frequent cause of endocarditis in young males without known preexisting heart disease. Gram-negative infections may follow genitourinary illness or surgical manipulation. Drug addicts characteristically develop staphylococcal or fungal endocarditis on right-sided cardiac valves. Pneumococcal endocarditis may occasionally complicate pneumococcal meningitis or pneumonia. The fact that a patient has been on preceding antirheumatic prophylaxis does not protect him from endocarditis nor does it mean that the organism is necessarily penicillin resistant.

CHOICE OF ANTIBIOTIC. The sensitivity of the organism must be determined. If it is highly sensitive to penicillin, a treatment schedule similar to that for *S. viridans* may be employed, although it is usual to add streptomycin intramuscularly for at least the first two weeks (Table 1). For enterococci, penicillin and strep-

TABLE 1. Antibiotics Used in Management of Bacterial Endocarditis

ORGANISM	DRUG OF CHOICE AND DOSE*	SECOND CHOICE*
Streptococcus viridans (penicillin-sensitive)	Penicillin G 10 million u./day I.V. 2 weeks 1 million u. b.i.d. I.M. 2 weeks	Erythromycin (max. 2 Gm.) 50 mg./kg./day I.V. 2 weeks 50 mg./kg. orally 2 weeks +Streptomycin (max. 2 Gm.) 50 mg./kg./day I.M. 1 week 25 mg./kg./day I.M. 3 weeks *or* Cephalothin (Keflin) 20 mg./kg./day I.V. q. 6 hours (max. dose 500 mg.) 20 mg./kg./day I.M. 2 weeks +Streptomycin
Enterococci, penicillin-resistant *Streptococcus viridans*	Penicillin G 20 million u./day I.V. 6 weeks +Streptomycin 25 mg./kg./day I.M.	
Pneumococci, gonococci, Group A beta streptococci	Penicillin 10 million u./day I.V. 4–6 weeks	
Staphylococci Penicillin-sensitive	Penicillin 12 million–20 million u./day I.V. 4–6 weeks	Lincomycin‡ 10 mg./kg. q. 12 hours I.V. or I.M. (Vancomycin 40 mg./kg./day I.V.)
Penicillin-resistant	Methicillin, oxacillin or cephalothin 8–12 Gm. I.V. or I.M. 6 weeks	Lincomycin‡ 10 mg./kg. q. 12 hours I.V. or I.M. (Vancomycin, bacitracin)
Coliforms, Pseudomonas	Ampicillin, streptomycin, penicillin—depending on sensitivity tests	Gentamicin, Carbenacillin } being evaluated
Bacteroides	Tetracycline† 20 mg./kg. q. 12 hours I.M. or I.V. (max. 2 Gm.) + penicillin I.M. 20 million u.	
Fungal (Candida, etc.)	Amphotericin B 1 mg./kg./day I.V.	

* The efficacy of the dose employed should be monitored by serial tube dilution studies.

† Manufacturer's note: The use of tetracyclines during tooth development (last half of pregnancy, infancy and childhood to age eight years) may cause permanent discoloration of teeth. This adverse reaction is more common during long-term use of the drugs but has been observed following repeated short-term courses.

‡ Manufacturer's precaution: Lincomycin is not indicated in the newborn (up to one month of age).

tomycin are given in combination for at least six weeks, and then, depending on progress, either penicillin is given alone or the synergistic combination is continued. Staphylococci should always be regarded as insensitive to penicillin until proved otherwise, and initial treatment should be started with large doses of a penicillinase-resistant penicillin such as methacillin or oxacillin.

NEGATIVE BLOOD CULTURES. It is usual in this situation to assume that the organism is atypical or relatively insensitive to penicillin and two antibiotics are used. Penicillin, 20 million units intravenously daily, is given together with intramuscular streptomycin for a minimum of two weeks, the therapy being changed if the cultures later become positive and indicate the use of another combination of antibiotics. In a case following cardiac surgery the high probability of a penicillin-resistant staphylococcal infection causes one to use a penicillinase-resistant penicillin as the initial treatment.

Depending on the organism and its sensitivity and on the patient's progress, other antibiotics may be used, including chloramphenicol,* polymyxin, bacitracin and vancomycin. All these drugs are toxic in various ways, and the satisfactory bactericidal levels obtained with the drugs already discussed are seldom obtainable.

Other Medical Therapy. The child is put on bed rest, usually with bathroom privileges, for the first week. If no embolization has occurred, he may be ambulated gradually, provided that good control of the intravenous management is being maintained.

Anticoagulant therapy is now rarely if ever used; it would only be considered if major pulmonary emboli continued to appear after institution of therapy. *Antipyretic drugs* should be avoided unless shaking chills and fever above 103° F. are causing great discomfort and do not respond to tepid sponging; in such cases aspirin or Tylenol in the usual pediatric doses may be used. *Sedatives* and *analgesics* should be sparingly used, because every effort is necessary to avoid complicating drug fevers. Nevertheless, occasionally a nocturnal sedative is indicated during the first week to ensure a good night's sleep, and a tranquilizer or sedative may be desirable in the young or very apprehensive patient prior to changing the site of the intravenous needle. Darvon† or morphine sulfate is very rarely necessary for pain in pulmonary emboli; if it is necessary, however, such therapy should be discontinued at the earliest possible time for obvious reasons.

Oxygen is used only if respiratory distress or severe congestive failure is present. *Anticongestive measures,* including digitalis, diuretics and a low salt diet, may be necessary if there is evidence of congestive failure.

Fluid and electrolyte intake should be carefully monitored, particularly to avoid massive overloading with sodium or potassium ions in patients on large doses of intravenous penicillin.

Probenecid‡ in doses of 250 to 500 mg. every 6 hours orally may be given to ensure higher penicillin blood levels if oral or intramuscular penicillin therapy is being used. It is not essential if satisfactory bactericidal serum levels can readily be maintained without its use.

Corticosteroids may have to be given under three special circumstances: (1) In the presence of circulatory collapse. (2) If the endocarditis is complicated by failure and the nephrotic syndrome, steroids may be helpful in the relief of edema. (3) In very rare situations, the use of penicillin together with corticosteroids allows one to continue penicillin therapy in a patient sensitive to that drug. The new penicillins, such as cephalothin (Keflin), or lincomycin§ may be used if they do not show cross-reaction. In some instances desensitization is indicated.

Complications. Anemia should be treated with small packed cell transfusions to maintain a hemoglobin of at least 10 Gm. in acyanotic patients and between 12 and 14 Gm. in those with cyanotic heart disease in whom the previous hemoglobin is known to be 15 Gm. or more. Persistent anemia after the first 10 days of therapy is a poor prognostic sign. Megaloblastic anemia, which is very rare, responds poorly to vitamin B_{12}, and again small packed cell transfusions with very careful cross matching may be needed.

In an effort to prevent *embolization,* most patients are kept at bed rest for the first week of therapy or longer if emboli are continuing. If small pulmonary emboli develop, they may be treated symptomatically and usually resolve without any residual effects. Fortunately, mas-

* Manufacturer's precaution: Chloramphenicol is not recommended for intramuscular or intravenous pediatric use. Chloramphenicol sodium succinate has been approved for intravenous pediatric use.

† Manufacturer's precaution: Safety of Darvon in children has not been established.

‡ Manufacturer's precaution: Probenecid is not recommended for children under two years of age.

§ Manufacturer's precaution: Lincomycin is not indicated in the newborn (up to one month of age).

sive emboli are rare. Systemic arterial emboli may need surgical intervention. Cerebral emboli are treated by bed rest, oxygen, respiratory supportive measures and physiotherapy.

Renal complications, including a nephrotic-like syndrome, usually respond as the congestive failure and infection come under control. Occasionally, as previously discussed, steroids may be needed for a few days or weeks.

Persistent or recurrent fever is a particularly troublesome complication. In most patients with endocarditis, defervescence occurs after three to seven days on therapy, and simultaneously a marked improvement in appetite and general well-being is noted. However, after the second week, a low-grade fever may recur; this may indicate continuing infection, thrombophlebitis, drug reaction or local inflammatory response to intramuscular injections. With careful clinical monitoring and adequate checks of bactericidal blood levels, it is usually possible to continue with the already planned course of therapy.

Assessment of Progress. Marked improvement in the clinical state, appetite, vigor and general appearance, together with defervescence, usually indicates that effective therapy has been instituted. Blood samples should be obtained after three to four days, and the serum should be bactericidal in dilutions of 1:8 in broth and preferably as high as 1:16 or more. If bactericidal levels are only obtained at high concentrations, an increase or change of antibiotics is indicated. With some enterococci or staphylococci, for example, penicillin doses of 50 million units a day or more may be needed intravenously before adequate levels are attained. An increase in hematocrit and reticulocytosis is also a favorable sign, as is the return of the sedimentation rate to normal, although continued elevation of the sedimentation rate is sometimes seen in patients who otherwise are making excellent progress.

Role of Surgery. *Noncardiac surgery,* such as removal of chronically infected teeth, is usually undertaken about one week after defervescence and establishment of satisfactory bactericidal blood levels. Clearly an abscessed tooth or an area of acute osteomyelitis may require earlier surgical intervention.

Cardiac surgery in the presence of active infection appears to be and is a heroic measure. Nevertheless, it must not be forgotten that the earliest therapeutic successes in the preantibiotic era were obtained by surgical ligation of an infected patent ductus arteriosus. Today surgical intervention is indicated as follows:

1. In endocarditis and mediastinitis following cardiac surgery, particularly in patients with a prosthetic outflow patch or a homograft. Intensive appropriate antibiotic coverage for at least a week but not more than two weeks should usually precede surgery. Removal of the infected outflow patch, direct approximation of the right ventricular myocardium, topical application of antibiotic, adequate wound drainage and postoperative maintenance of endocarditis therapy for at least another two weeks can lead and have led to cure in very ill subjects. Vacillation and reliance on medical therapy alone can lead and have led to cardiac rupture, death from massive pulmonary emboli and other disasters, all modern variations on the ancient medical maxim that infection will not be cured if a foreign body is present. The intracardiac patch used to repair a ventricular septal defect is fortunately very rarely infected, being obviously much less exposed than the mediastinum during prolonged open heart procedures. Occasionally removal of infected sutures used to repair either an atrial defect or a ventriculotomy has been necessary and successful.

2. Occasionally *progressive cardiac failure* may continue owing to aortic or tricuspid valve involvement in a case of bacterial endocarditis without prior cardiac surgery. Under heavy antibiotic coverage, removal of the infected valve and replacement by a prosthesis has been successfully undertaken, and this measure should undoubtedly be considered in a patient not responding well to adequate therapy.

3. *Aneurysm formation,* whether in the area of a ductus, a ventriculotomy site or other situations, is a clear indication for emergency cardiac surgery for two reasons: it is almost impossible to sterilize the aneurysm, and the risk of rupture is a real one.

4. *Infection on a prosthetic valve* carries a grave prognosis and repeat surgery may offer the only slim hope of cure.

Psychological Support. The best psychological support in this very trying illness is afforded by a skilled and amiable resident pediatrician capable of performing venipuncture and the maintenance of prolonged intravenous therapy with minimal trauma. Other support at consultant level is afforded by a frank discussion with the parents within 24 hours of admission concerning the necessary delay in establishing a firm diagnosis, the need for venipunctures and the minimal four-week duration of therapy.

As the days wear on, a consistent and reliable source of information to parent and child is needed (preferably one resident and one consultant), particularly in large teaching institutions where the Tower of Babel syndrome may develop, the nurse saying cultures are negative, the intern, positive, and so forth. The social worker may be valuable in exploring with the parents the implications of prolonged hospitalization, the admitting office in advising on insurance and the possibilities of financial assistance and the Child Life or similar program in supplying occupation and interest.

As soon as the child feels well enough, usually within a week of starting therapy, school contacts should be resumed and every effort made to ensure that he will graduate with the rest of his class. If therapy is successful and the staff skilled, informed and cheerful, psychologic problems are few. If it is unsuccessful, the rare and special skills needed in the management of incurable and refractory disease are called for, a subject too large for this brief article.

Discharge and Follow-up. The child is usually discharged seven to 10 days after cessation of therapy, provided that no complications are present. Activities should be moderately limited (no sports) until a return visit to the hospital is made two to four weeks later. If at that time the child is clinically well, afebrile and without evidence of recurrence of anemia or other suspicious signs, a blood culture is drawn as a precaution and the child allowed to return to his usual level of activity. Anticongestive measures are continued as appropriate, particularly in those with aortic valve involvement who warrant closer follow-up than others. Normal annual check-ups can usually be resumed.

Prophylactic antibiotics should be restarted in rheumatic subjects four to six weeks after discharge. They are not used in congenital cardiac patients after one attack of endocarditis, though we have empirically and perhaps unreasonably recommended them after two or more attacks.

Elective cardiac surgery should be postponed for at least six months after discharge to allow complete healing of myocardial and renal lesions. The desirability of surgery should then be reviewed again on its merits without undue emotional pressure because of the infective episode, because recurrences, though they do undoubtedly occur, are quite rare in less than three to five years, and because a patient who is a bad operative risk prior to endocarditis is clearly not a better one after it.

Elective cardiac catheterization should also, in the author's view, be postponed for six months or more for similar reasons and because alarming and prognostically highly inaccurate hemodynamic findings may be obtained.

PROPHYLAXIS

Suggested Treatment Schedules (American Heart Association and American Dental Association Protocol)

Day of Procedure. Give procaine penicillin, 600,000 units, supplemented by 600,000 units of crystalline penicillin intramuscularly 1 to 2 hours before the procedure.

Intramuscular penicillin is more reliable. However, because of practical considerations, some dentists and physicians rely on oral penicillin when the full cooperation of the patient is assured. If oral penicillin is to be employed, four doses (every 4 to 6 hours) of at least 0.25 Gm. of alpha-phenoxymethyl penicillin (Pen-Vee K) or 0.25 Gm. of alpha-phenoxyethyl penicillin (phenethicillin), or 500,000 units of buffered penicillin G should be given during the day of the procedure. In addition, an extra dose should be taken 1 hour before the procedure.

For Two Days After Procedure. Give procaine penicillin, 600,000 units intramuscularly each day. In selected instances, 0.25 Gm. of alpha-phenoxymethyl penicillin (Pen-Vee K) or 0.25 Gm. of alpha-phenoxyethyl penicillin (phenethicillin) or 500,000 units of buffered penicillin G, four times daily by mouth on each day, may be used for those patients in whom full cooperation is anticipated and ingestion is assured.

Contraindications to this Regimen. The main contraindication is sensitivity to penicillin. All patients should be carefully questioned for previous history suggesting penicillin sensitivity. If such a history is obtained, even if equivocal, penicillin should not be given. Under such circumstances, erythromycin should be used in a dose of 250 mg. by mouth four times daily for adults and older children. For small children, a dose of 20 mg. per pound per day divided into three or four evenly spaced doses may be used. The total dose should not exceed 1 Gm. per day.

Instrumentation of Genitourinary Tract, Surgery of the Lower Intestinal Tract and Childbirth. With these procedures, transitory bacteremia due to penicillin-resistant enterococci is apt to occur. The use of penicillin alone in the doses previously suggested cannot be expected to curtail bacteremia due to enterococci, a common cause of bacterial endocarditis.

For these reasons, it is suggested that as an empirical guide, the previously mentioned intramuscular penicillin regimen be used in combination with streptomycin, 1 or 2 Gm. intramuscularly on the day of procedure and for each of two days following the procedure. In children, streptomycin may be given in a dosage of 50 mg. per kilogram, not to exceed 1 Gm. per day. In patients who are sensitive to penicillin, a combination of erythromycin and streptomycin or a broad-spectrum antibiotic combined with streptomycin may be of some use, although it should be emphasized that very little information is available about these antibiotic combinations and their efficacy in preventing bacterial endocarditis due to enterococci.

Escherichia coli Infections

JOHN D. NELSON, M.D., *and*
KENNETH C. HALTALIN, M.D.

A variety of infections may be caused by *Escherichia coli.* Only those important because of frequency or severity are considered in this section.

SYSTEMIC INFECTION IN THE NEONATE

When systemic infection with *E. coli* occurs in the neonate, the symptomatic and antibiotic therapy is the same as that outlined under Neonatal Sepsis, Meningitis and Pneumonia (page 550).

SYSTEMIC INFECTION IN INFANTS AND CHILDREN

E. coli septicemia is uncommon after the newborn period. Generally it occurs as a complication in patients with obstructive disease of the urinary tract, in those with basic defects in host defense mechanisms or in those receiving immunosuppressive therapy. General supportive care depends on the underlying problem.

Antibiotic therapy is initiated with kanamycin or gentamicin. Kanamycin may be used in hospitals where monitoring of sensitivity testing gives assurance that 90 to 95 per cent or more strains of *E. coli* are susceptible. It is administered in a dosage of 15 mg. per kilogram per day in equally divided intramuscular doses every 8 hours. In areas such as Dallas (see Table 1), where significant numbers of strains are resistant to kanamycin, gentamicin is the preferred drug. We recommend that gentamicin be given in a dosage of 7.5 mg. per kilogram per day, administered in divided doses every 8 hours. It should be given by the intramuscular route unless the patient is in shock. For intravenous administration, the dose is diluted in sterile normal saline and infused over a 1- to 2-hour period.

If there is impairment of renal function, the dosage of either kanamycin or gentamicin must be reduced to avoid potentially toxic serum levels. Ideally, serum levels of antibiotic should be monitored under these circumstances.

Treatment is continued for five days after signs of clinical improvement; in the absence of focal complications, this usually means at least seven but not more than 10 days. When sensitivity test results are available, consideration may be given to changing to a drug with a lower toxic potential, such as ampicillin or cephalothin.

URINARY TRACT INFECTION

E. coli remains the most common single cause of urinary tract infections. In acute, uncomplicated cases, most *E. coli* are responsive to sulfa drugs. Triple Sulfas U.S.P. or sulfisoxazole* is given in a dose of 120 to 150 mg. per kilogram daily by mouth in four divided doses for seven days. In recurrent disease, the infecting *E. coli* are likely to be sulfa-resistant, and antibiotic sensitivity data must be used as guidelines for selecting alternative drugs.

It is extremely important to realize that antibiotic susceptibility results, such as those shown in Table 1, can be misleading in the case of urinary tract infections. Standards for sensitivity or resistance are established in terms of serum and tissue levels attainable with usual doses. Because far higher urinary concentrations are achieved with most drugs, *E. coli* supposedly resistant to ampicillin, for example, might actually be successfully eradicated with this drug. The best sensitivity test is the in vivo one: a repeat urine culture obtained 48 to 72 hours after start of therapy. The aim of antimicrobial therapy is to eradicate bacteriuria, not to treat fever or dysuria. The only way to ensure that this aim has been accomplished is to obtain repeat cultures, since symptoms may subside spontaneously and rapidly in the face of persisting bacteriuria.

Detailed management of urinary tract infections is presented on page 406.

---

* Manufacturer's precaution: Sulfisoxazole is contraindicated in infants under two months of age except in the treatment of congenital toxoplasmosis as adjunctive therapy with pyrimethamine.

TABLE 1. Antibiotic Susceptibilities of *E. coli* Isolated from Various Sites in Infants and Children During 1969 to 1971 at Children's Medical Center, Dallas

CULTURE SOURCE	NUMBER OF ISOLATES TESTED	PERCENTAGE SUSCEPTIBLE TO USUALLY ACHIEVABLE SERUM LEVELS OF ANTIBIOTIC						
		Ampicillin (≤ 10 mcg./ml.)	*Cephalothin* (≤ 10 mcg./ml.)	*Chloramphenicol** (≤ 10 mcg./ml.)	*Gentamicin* (≤ 5 mcg./ml.)	*Kanamycin* (≤ 10 mcg./ml.)	*Polymyxin B* (≤ 5 mcg./ml.)	*Tetracycline* (≤ 5 mcg./ml.)
Urine	962	77	78	92	97	90	97	72
Sputum or tracheal aspirate	107	78	76	94	98	85	97	76
Blood	40	98	85	100	100	88	100	88
Skin	119	76	78	95	92	79	93	79
Stool (enteropathogenic serotypes)†	264	72	75	86	94	82	92	75
Eye and ear	97	72	71	92	97	89	92	75
Miscellaneous‡	85	77	82	93	100	81	97	81
All sources	1674	76	77	92	97	87	96	74

* Manufacturer's precaution: Chloramphenicol is not recommended for intramuscular or intravenous pediatric use. Chloramphenicol sodium succinate has been approved for intravenous pediatric use.

† 99% susceptible to neomycin.

‡ Cerebrospinal fluid, peritoneal fluid, empyema, appendiceal abscess and so forth.

DIARRHEAL DISEASE

Enteropathogenic serotypes of *E. coli* seldom cause diarrheal disease in patients over a year or a year and one-half of age. Neonates, especially premature infants housed for prolonged periods in nurseries, and infants under six months of age are most vulnerable to infection. The asymptomatic carrier state occurs in about 5 per cent of infants.

General Measures. Diarrheal disease due to *E. coli* is primarily characterized by diarrhea. High fever and other manifestations of systemic toxicity are not seen in uncomplicated cases. For this reason, the severity of illness may not be appreciated until signs of gross dehydration supervene.

Patients with physical signs of dehydration must be hospitalized and managed with intravenous fluid and electrolyte therapy. In these patients it is important to determine serum electrolyte concentrations, since hyponatremia and hypernatremia occur fairly commonly. Details of fluid and electrolyte therapy are described elsewhere (page 793).

Infants who are not dehydrated are managed as outpatients. It is our practice to substitute clear liquids for formula and to discontinue solids for the first 24 hours. Recommended clear liquids include Jell-O water, glucose water, "de-fizzed" carbonated beverages, such as 7-Up and ginger ale, and clear apple juice. Homemade salt solutions should not be prescribed because of the risk of inducing hypertonic dehydration. In most patients, the formula that the child usually receives can be reinstated after the period of clear liquids. It may be given in one-half strength or in full-strength form, depending on acceptance by the child. In any event, supplementation with clear liquids should be continued. The mystique surrounding the efficacy of boiled skim milk at this stage has always escaped us and we do not advise its use because of its unacceptably high electrolyte load.

Adsorptive agents that "firm up" the stool and drugs that decrease bowel motility have no place in the treatment of infants, in our opinion. They have never been shown to shorten the course of illness and are potentially hazardous, since they mask the magnitude of fluid loss.

Antibiotic Therapy. Properly controlled studies have not been done to establish the utility of antibiotics in this disease; nevertheless, it has become standard practice to prescribe them. Neomycin sulfate oral solution is the drug of choice in areas where neomycin-resistance is infrequently encountered. It is administered in a divided dose of 100 mg. per kilogram per day, every 6 or 8 hours for five days. Continuation of therapy for longer than five days is not advised because the bacteriologic cure rate is not improved and because neomycin may induce a malabsorptive state. Colistin sulfate oral suspension is the alternate drug of choice and is given every 6 or 8 hours for five days. Dosage of colistin sulfate is currently a matter of opinion. The manufacturer's recommended dose is 3 to 5 mg. per kilogram a day orally in three divided doses, but higher doses of 10 to 15 mg. per kilogram per day have been recommended by some authorities, including The Red Book of the Committee on Infectious Diseases of the American Academy of Pediatrics.

Epidemic Diarrhea in the Premature Nursery

The Red Book recommends that infants infected with *E. coli* be removed from the nursery and exposed infants be quarantined and treated with neomycin or colistin. It also recommends that all new admissions be similarly treated until no new cases have developed and the nursery population has turned over twice.

We recommend a simpler and less disruptive method in areas where fluorescent antibody techniques are available. When an index case of *E. coli* diarrhea develops in the nursery, rectal swab specimens are obtained from all infants for rapid fluorescent antibody processing. Those infants in whom colonization has taken place are segregated and treated with oral neomycin or colistin in the dosages previously mentioned. The usual aseptic technique is followed and the remainder of the nursery functions normally. Tests are repeated on all infants after 48 hours. Using this procedure in more than a dozen outbreaks, we have never observed a new case develop once control measures were instituted. The sensitivity of fluorescent antibody technique assures that all colonized infants are identified. When culture methods alone are used, some colonized babies may be missed, and they serve to perpetuate the reservoir of infection in the nursery.

OTHER INFECTIONS

Pneumonia, peritonitis, abscesses and many other infections may on occasion be caused by *E. coli*. The information in Table 1 can be used for selection of antibiotics pending susceptibility test results. Surgery and supportive measures depend on the disease process and can be found in the appropriate chapters of this book.

Staphylococcal Infections

HARRY R. HILL, M.D., *and*
JOHN M. MATSEN, M.D.

Staphylococcal infections have continued to be a frequent and difficult clinical problem in the antibiotic era. Hospitalized patients, especially newborn infants, postoperative patients and patients with depressed host defense mechanisms, are prone to develop life-threatening staphylococcal disease. Staphylococcal pneumonia, sepsis, meningitis and endocarditis are among the most fulminating infections the clinician faces. In contrast, coagulase-negative staphylococci (*S. epidermidis*) may cause indolent but progressive disease especially in patients with indwelling vascular or cerebrospinal fluid shunts. Staphylococci alone or in association with streptococci are the most frequent pathogens isolated from cases of osteomyelitis, superficial skin lesions, minor wounds and furuncles. Thus, the physician who treats children should have a thorough knowledge of the principles of antistaphylococcal therapy.

The emergence of resistant strains of staphylococci has greatly complicated the choice of appropriate staphylococcal antibiotics. At present, 50 to 85 per cent of *S. aureus* strains isolated in hospitals are resistant to penicillin G, in contrast to a 20 to 50 per cent resistance rate in strains from outside the hospital environment. In recent years staphylococcal strains with multiple-drug resistance have been isolated. Such strains, in addition to being resistant to penicillin, may show resistance to erythromycin, chloramphenicol, tetracycline or kanamycin and, rarely, will demonstrate resistance to methicillin. An additional problem in antibiotic resistance occurs with infections due to coagulase-negative staphylococci. Two-thirds to three-quarters of these strains are resistant to penicillin and 10 to 25 per cent are also resistant to methicillin and the other penicillinase-resistant semisynthetic penicillins. The choice of an appropriate antibiotic is often difficult, therefore, and should depend on the clinical setting and the results of appropriate cultures and sensitivity patterns.

S. aureus resistant to methicillin and other penicillinase-resistant penicillins has been reported with distressing frequency in Asia and in some European centers. However, this has not been demonstrated to be a significant problem in the United States at the present time. Over the last three years we have found less than one-quarter of one per cent of *S. aureus* to be resistant to methicillin. The clinician should realize that false reports of methicillin-resistant staphylococci are not uncommon, however, since the use of methicillin discs which have chemically deteriorated can cause erroneous conclusions. Staphylococci that are resistant to methicillin are almost invariably resistant to streptomycin and tetracycline. Thus, the clinician who receives a report of methicillin-resistant staphylococci should determine if the organism is resistant to these other antibiotics. If they are not, it is likely that the report is an erroneous one.

Therapy should be initiated early in suspected staphylococcal disease to prevent abscess formation or widespread dissemination. In addition to prompt surgical drainage, high doses of a bactericidal antibiotic should be administered for a prolonged period of time in moderate to severe disease. Following initial intensive therapy of such infections, or for mild staphylococcal disease, one of a variety of new oral antibiotics may be chosen.

In assessing therapy for staphylococcal infections, a serum bactericidal titer may be determined in order to be certain that adequate antibiotic levels are being achieved. The test is performed using serial dilutions of the patient's serum taken just prior to the next dose of antibiotic. The highest dilution of this serum which completely kills all of a standard inoculum of the organism isolated from the patient is the bactericidal titer. Control of infection is usually associated with a titer of more than 1:5, but should ideally be 1:10 or greater.

Refer to Tables 1, 2 and 3 for information on parenteral antistaphylococcal preparations for penicillin-allergic and -nonallergic individuals, and on oral antistaphylococcal preparations.

Therapy for Penicillin-Susceptible Staphylococci. Penicillin continues to reign as the king of antibiotics, and there is little likelihood that it will be surpassed. As an antistaphylococcal agent, it is the drug of choice in infections due to penicillin-susceptible organisms. It should also be used in combination with one of the penicillinase-resistant drugs for initial therapy of staphylococcal disease, or of suspected staphylococcal disease when the susceptibility results are not known. Against penicillin-sensitive organisms, penicillin G is from 20 to 80 times more effective than are the semisynthetic penicillinase-resistant penicillins or most cephalosporin derivatives at similar concentrations. Aqueous penicillin G should be administered by the intravenous route in severe staphylococcal disease in doses approximating 400,000 to 500,000 units per kilogram body weight per day in six divided doses (except in neonates). It is of interest to note that one million units of penicillin, while seemingly an enormous dose, only amounts to 625 mg. of antibiotic. There is no definitive information suggesting the advantage of intravenous "push" administration of antibiotics; however, in view of the higher serum levels that are obtained, it seems wise to allow the drug to infuse over a 20-minute period.

Crystalline aqueous penicillin may also be given by the intramuscular route although the intravenous route of administration is less traumatic and more reliable serum concentrations are obtained. Procaine penicillin may also be given intramuscularly for mild to moderate disease except in neonates, in whom sterile abscesses may develop at the site of injection.

Following initial intensive therapy of moderate to severe disease, one of the oral penicillins may be utilized. Oral penicillin G is inactivated by gastric acidity, so that only one-fourth of the administered dose is absorbed. In order to obtain adequate serum concentration, four to five times the intravenous dose must be given. The phenoxyalkyl derivatives of penicillanic acid have a spectrum of activity exactly like that of penicillin G but give higher serum levels following equivalent oral doses. Phenoxymethyl penicillin (penicillin V), which is acid-resistant, is 40 per cent absorbed when given by the oral route and gives significantly higher serum levels than does oral penicillin G or equivalent doses of intramuscular procaine penicillin. The drug should be administered in doses of 25 to 50 mg. per kilogram per day in three to four divided doses. Since the presence of food in the duodenum interferes with absorption of all of the penicillins, these agents should be given 30 minutes to 1 hour prior to meals or at least 2 hours following meals.

Patients who give a history of penicillin allergy should not receive the drug unless the infection is life-threatening and there is time for appropriate skin testing and desensitization. Only 10 to 15 per cent of patients with a history of penicillin allergy will actually have positive skin tests to the major or minor penicillin determinants, suggesting true hypersensitivity to the drug. Anaphylactic reactions occur in less than 0.1 per cent of patients, but the mortality rate associated with this complication is between 10 and 25 per cent. In addition to skin rashes and serum sickness, the penicillins, and especially methicillin, may produce an interstitial nephritis. Very high serum and cerebrospinal fluid

TABLE 1. Parenteral Antibiotics Used in the Therapy of Moderate and Severe Staphylococcal Infections in the Nonallergic Individual

ANTIBIOTIC	ROUTE	DOSAGE			PERCENTAGE OF SUSCEPTIBLE STRAINS		COMMENTS
		Newborn	*Infant and Child*	*Adult or Maximum*	*Hos-pital*	*Non-hospital*	
Aqueous penicillin G	I.M. or I.V.	50,000–75,000 units/kg./day, every 12 hours	100,000–500,000 units/kg./day, every 4 hours	20–60 million units	20	60	1. Hypersensitivity (anaphylaxis $< 0.1\%$) 2. 1 million units contain 1.6 mEq. sodium or potassium
	intrathecally		1000–10,000 units	10,000 units			
Procaine penicillin	I.M. only	Contraindicated	300,000–600,000 units every 12–24 hours		20	60	1. Low serum levels 2. Contraindicated in procaine allergy
Methicillin (Staphcillin, Dimocillin)	I.M. or I.V.	100–200 mg./kg./day, every 6 hours	100–400 mg./kg./day, every 4 hours	12–15 Gm.	>99	>99	1. Acid-labile, run in over 20 minutes 2. 1 Gm. = 3 mEq. sodium 3. Nephritis may occur
	intrathecally		10–100 mg./day	100 mg.			
Nafcillin (Unipen)	I.M. or I.V.*	20–50 mg./kg./day, every 12 hours	50–100 mg./kg./day every 4–6 hours	6 Gm.	99	99	1. Phlebitis may occur 2. More active against penicillin-sensitive organisms
Oxacillin (Resistopen, Prostaphlin)	I.M. or I.V.	25–50 mg./kg./day, every 12 hours	50–100 mg./kg./day every 4–8 hours	6 Gm.	99	99	1. Lower serum concentration after I.M. administration

* Manufacturer's precaution: There is no clinical experience available on the intravenous use of nafcillin (Unipen) in neonates or infants.

TABLE 2. Parenteral Antibiotics Used in the Therapy of Moderate and Severe Staphylococcal Infections in the Penicillin-Allergic Individual

ANTIBIOTIC	ROUTE OF ADMINISTRATION	DOSAGE			PERCENTAGE OF SUSCEPTIBLE STRAINS		COMMENTS
		Newborn	*Infant and Child*	*Adult or Maximum*	*Hospital*	*Non-hospital*	
Clindamycin (Cleocin)	I.V. or I.M.	Unknown	8–40 mg./kg./day, every 6 hours	1.8 Gm./day	> 95	99	1. Few toxicities: diarrhea 2. Maculopapular rashes—10% 3. Concentration in bone
Lincomycin (Lincocin)	I.M. or I.V.	Not indicated (up to one month of age)	10–20 mg./kg./day	1.8 Gm./day	90	Most	1. Concentration in bone 2. Diarrhea
Cephalothin (Keflin)	I.M. or I.V.	30–75 mg./kg./day, every 8 hours	40–100 mg./kg./day, every 4–6 hours	12 Gm./day	99	99	1. 5% cross-reactivity in penicillin-allergic individuals 2. Crosses blood-brain barrier poorly 3. Superinfection a problem
Vancomycin (Vancocin)	I.V. only		40 mg./kg./day, over 24 hours	4 Gm./day 1st day. 2 Gm./day thereafter	Most	Most	1. Very irritating 2. Ototoxicity 3. Nephrotoxicity
Erythromycin	I.M. (Erythrocin Ethyl Succinate-I.M.) I.V. (Ilotycin Gluceptate, I.V.)	20–30 mg./kg./day in 2–4 doses	10–20 mg./kg./day, every 6–8 hours	2–4 Gm./day/ I.V.	> 90	Most	1. Bacteriostatic 2. Hepatotoxic estolate
Chloramphenicol (Chloromycetin)*	I.M. or I.V.	15–24 mg./kg./day in 3–4 doses	50–100 mg./kg./day, every 6 hours	4 Gm./day	60	80	1. Gray syndrome in neonates 2. Bone marrow depression 3. Aplastic anemia
Kanamycin (Kantrex)	I.M. or I.V.	15 mg./kg./day, every 12 hours	15 mg./kg./day, every 12 hours	1.5 Gm./day	85	95	1. Ototoxicity 2. Renal toxicity
Gentamicin (Garamycin)	I.M. or I.V.	5–7 mg./kg./day, every 8 hours	5 mg./kg./day, every 6–8 hours	Level < 10 μgm./ml.	98	98	1. Ototoxicity 2. Renal toxicity

* Manufacturer's precaution: Chloramphenicol (Chloromycetin) is not recommended for intravenous or intramuscular pediatric use. Chloramphenicol sodium succinate has been approved for intravenous pediatric use.

TABLE 3. Orally Administered Antibody for Treating Staphylococcal Infections

DRUG	DOSAGE Infant and Neonate	DOSAGE Older Child	COMMENTS
Penicillin G	100,000–200,000 units every 6–8 hours	200,000–600,000 units every 6–8 hours	1. Acid-labile 2. 20% absorbed 3. Absorption decreased by food
Phenoxymethyl penicillin (penicillin V, V-Cillin, Pen-Vee, Compocillin-V)	25–50 mg./kg./day, every 6–8 hours	125–250 mg. every 6–8 hours	1. Acid-stabile 2. 40% absorbed 3. Absorption decreased by food
Dicloxacillin (Dynapen)*	12.5–50 mg./kg./day, every 6 hours	12.5–50 mg./kg./day, every 6 hours	1. Higher blood levels than cloxacillin 2. Better activity against penicillin-resistant organisms 3. More active against pneumococci 4. 95% protein-bound
Cloxacillin (Tegopen)	25–50 mg./kg./day, every 6 hours	250–500 mg. every 4–6 hours	1. 95% protein-bound 2. Higher blood levels than oxacillin
Cephalexin (Keflex)	25–50 mg./kg./day, every 6 hours	125–250 mg. every 6 hours	1. Approx. 5% cross-reactions in penicillin-sensitive individuals 2. Excellent serum levels 3. Superinfection
Clindamycin (Cleocin)	8–20 mg./kg./day, every 6 hours	150–300 mg. every 6 hours	1. No allergic cross-reactions with penicillin 2. Well absorbed 3. Excellent bone concentration 4. Few toxicities
Lincomycin† (Lincocin)		250–500 mg. every 8 hours	1. Lower serum levels than clindamycin 2. Excellent bone concentration
Erythromycin (Pediamycin, Illosone, Ilotycin, Erythrocin)	20–40 mg./kg./day, every 6 hours	30–50 mg./kg./day, every 6 hours	1. Bacteriostatic 2. Gastrointestinal disturbances
Chloramphenicol (Chloromycetin)	25–50 mg./kg./day, every 6 hours	50–100 mg./kg./day, every 6 hours	1. Bacteriostatic 2. Excellent oral absorption 3. Excellent diffusion 4. Bone marrow depression 5. Aplastic anemia

* Manufacturer's precaution: Experience with dicloxacillin (Dynapen) in the newborn is limited; therefore, a dose for newborns is not recommended at this time.

† Manufacturer's precaution: Lincomycin is not indicated in the newborn (up to one month of age).

concentrations of penicillin, most often in patients with compromised renal function, have led to the development of seizures, owing to the direct irritative action of penicillin on neural tissue. In addition, it must be remembered that aqueous penicillin comes as a sodium or potassium salt, with one million units containing 1.6 mEq. of the electrolyte. The administration of large quantities of penicillin containing either of these electrolytes may be a factor to consider in patients with cardiac problems, uremia or cerebral edema.

Therapy for Penicillin-Resistant Organisms. Methicillin (Staphcillin) has been our initial antibiotic for use in the treatment of moderate to severe disease due to penicillin-resistant staphylococci. This was the first penicillinase-resistant antibiotic discovered, and since it first became available in 1960 it has been used extensively in the treatment of staphylococcal infections. The drug has the disadvantage of having less activity on a weight basis than penicillin against penicillin-sensitive staphylococci. The large doses required to give adequate levels to combat penicillin-resistant organisms are usually adequate, however, to provide bactericidal activity against penicillin-sensitive strains. Methicillin has the advantage of being less protein-bound than the other penicillin derivatives (35 to 60 per cent) and therefore probably gives better tissue levels. The antibiotic is administered in a dose of from 100 to 400 mg. per kilogram per day, with the latter dose being our choice in all serious infections (except in neonates). Since little drug remains 4 to 5 hours after a parenteral dose, it must be given every 4 hours. Methicillin is acid-labile, making it necessary to infuse the drug over a 30-minute period to prevent inactivation by intravenous fluids, which are normally slightly acidic. Its toxicity is similar to that of the other penicillins, with the production of skin rashes, anaphylaxis, serum sickness, reversible granulocytopenia and Coombs-positive states. There is, of course, a cross-reaction in most penicillin-allergic individuals. Methicillin may also produce a diffuse interstitial nephritis with tubular damage when given in high doses. The syndrome is characterized by the appearance, one to several weeks after the initiation of therapy, of fever, eosinophilia, rash, hematuria, proteinuria, loss of concentrating ability and azotemia. Methicillin is administered as a sodium salt with 1 Gm. containing approximately 3 mEq. of sodium. As with the penicillins, this added electrolyte load may become a problem in certain clinical states.

Nafcillin (Unipen) has greater in vitro activity than does methicillin against penicillin-sensitive and penicillin-resistant organisms. It is, however, 85 to 90 per cent protein-bound and is largely concentrated in the liver, with resultant lower serum levels. There are those who feel strongly that nafcillin should be the agent of choice over methicillin because of the large differences between the mean inhibitory concentrations and mean bactericidal concentrations observed with methicillin. Nafcillin also has greater activity against nonstaphylococcal gram-positive organisms. Further studies are needed to define the superiority of one or the other of these agents. The dosage of nafcillin in severe staphylococcal disease is 100 mg. per kilogram per day.* The toxicities are similar to those of methicillin, although nephritis has not yet been described. The drug does have irritative properties when given intravenously and phlebitis sometimes occurs. Oxacillin (Prostaphlin) may also be used but seems to offer no advantages over nafcillin or methicillin.

In the follow-up therapy of moderate to severe staphylococcal disease or in the treatment of mild disease, one of the new oral semisynthetic penicillin preparations may be used. Oxacillin (Prostaphlin) is absorbed orally but cloxacillin (Tegopen), produced by the addition of a single chloride ion to the oxacillin molecule, has slightly greater in vitro activity against penicillin-resistant staphylococci. In addition, it yields blood levels significantly higher than those produced by oxacillin after equivalent oral doses because of better oral absorption and slower hepatic excretion. Dicloxacillin (Dynapen), formed by the addition of two chloride ions to the oxacillin molecule, gives serum concentrations that are twice as great as cloxacillin and four times that of oxacillin. All three of these drugs are approximately 95 per cent protein-bound. Complications are similar to those produced by penicillin. Cloxacillin is administered in doses of 50 to 100 mg. per kilogram per day in four divided doses,† while the dose of dicloxacillin|| is 12.5 to 50 mg. per kilogram per day in four divided doses.

The cephalosporin antibiotics are closely related to the penicillins, since both contain a similar basic two-ring nucleus with a beta-lactam ring. They do not break down to form penicilloyls, however, and are less likely to show allergic cross-reactions with penicillins. The cross-reactivity or cross-sensitivity in patients allergic to penicillin has been estimated at 5 per cent. Thus, one must still be cautious in administering a cephalosporin to the penicillin-allergic individual.

Cephalothin (Keflin), which is available for parenteral administration, is effective against over 98 per cent of penicillin-sensitive and penicillin-resistant staphylococci. In doses of 40 to 100 mg. per kilogram per day, it is an effective antibiotic for treating serious staphylococcal disease parenterally. In contrast to cephalothin, which is 55 to 60 per cent protein-bound, cephaloridine has almost no protein binding. It has been associated with nephrotoxicity, however.

Cephalexin (Keflex) is an orally administered cephalosporin antibiotic which is acid-stable and is almost completely absorbed from the gastrointestinal tract. Oral administration of equivalent doses gives serum levels that are comparable to the intramuscular administration of cephalothin. In addition, the drug is only 10 to 15 per cent protein-bound. The oral dosage in children is 50 mg. per kilogram per day in four divided doses. Side effects are un-

* Manufacturer's precaution: There is no clinical experience available on the intravenous use of nafcillin in neonates or infants.

† Manufacturer's note: Pediatric capsules of sodium cloxacillin monohydrate (Tegopen) have been removed from the market. Other forms are still available.

|| Manufacturer's precaution: Experience with dicloxacillin in the newborn is limited; therefore a dose for newborns is not recommended at this time.

common and are generally related to the gastrointestinal tract, with diarrhea being mentioned most frequently. Rashes, urticaria, eosinophilia and Coombs-positive states have been reported with all of the cephalosporin derivatives. Superinfections with fungi and bacteria have also been a problem with these broad-spectrum agents.

Lincomycin and its new derivative, clindamycin, are excellent antistaphylococcal drugs that are unrelated to other antibiotics. Thus, there is no allergic cross-reactivity and little cross-resistance with other antimicrobial agents. Most strains of *S. aureus,* including most erythromycin-resistant strains and 70 per cent of methicillin-resistant strains, are inhibited by clindamycin. Recently, however, it has been reported that resistance may develop following prolonged therapy with these agents. The rapid concentration of lincomycin and clindamycin in bone within 15 minutes of an oral dose makes these drugs especially useful in treating staphylococcal osteomyelitis. Bone concentrations are approximately one-third of those found in the serum. Clindamycin appears to be superior to lincomycin in that it is 8 to 16 times more active in vitro against staphylococci, and serum levels are twofold higher after equivalent oral doses. In addition, the gastrointestinal absorption of clindamycin is delayed but not decreased significantly by food, as is that of lincomycin. Lincomycin may produce diarrhea in up to 10 per cent of patients, and occasionally this will take the form of protracted diarrheal episodes. Clindamycin may also produce gastrointestinal side effects and has been reported to cause occasional mild, maculopapular rashes. Prolonged administration of either drug has failed to produce renal, hepatic or neurologic abnormalities. Lincomycin is administered in doses of 10 to 20 mg. per kilogram per day intravenously in two to three equal doses, or 30 to 50 mg. per kilogram per day orally.‡ Clindamycin is given in doses of 8 to 20 mg. per kilogram per day in four equal doses orally, and 8 to 40 mg. per kilogram per day intramuscularly or intravenously.

Erythromycin (Erythrocin, Pediamycin, Ilosone) may be used in the oral therapy of mild to moderate staphylococcal infection. The drug is bacteriostatic, however, and resistant strains do develop. It should therefore be used only in the penicillin-allergic individual with mild disease. The dose is 40 mg. per kilogram per day given in three to four divided doses.

‡ Manufacturer's precaution: Lincomycin is not indicated in the newborn (up to one month of age).

Vancomycin (Vancocin) may also be used in the treatment of severe staphylococcal disease in penicillin-sensitive patients or when the infecting organism is methicillin-resistant. The drug is not absorbed orally but is active in the gastrointestinal tract and has been used in the treatment of staphylococcal enterocolitis. Because of its irritative properties it should not be given intramuscularly but should be reserved for intravenous use. The drug's site of action is on the cell wall and probably the cell membrane, making it a strongly bactericidal antibiotic. There appears to be no allergic cross-reaction with other drugs, since vancomycin is unlike other antibiotics. Complications of vancomycin therapy include skin rashes, anaphylaxis and phlebitis. In addition, nausea, chills, fever and a shock-like state may occur during infusion of the drug. The most serious drawbacks to vancomycin's use are ototoxicity and nephrotoxicity. With serum levels over 90 micrograms per ml., irreversible deafness has occurred. In addition, azotemia and, rarely, severe renal damage have occurred with high-dose therapy. For this reason, vancomycin should only be used for treatment of severe staphylococcal disease in a penicillin-allergic individual or when a multiple-drug–resistant strain is being treated. The dose of vancomycin is 40 to 50 mg. per kilogram per day (maximum 2 Gm. per day) by continuous intravenous drip or in four divided doses.

Bacitracin, chloramphenicol, kanamycin and gentamicin may also be used to treat staphylococcal disease. All have potential toxicities and should not be thought of as first-line antistaphylococcal agents. Chloramphenicol is occasionally useful in treating walled-off abscesses, meningitis or ventriculitis because of its ability to diffuse into tissues well.§ It is, of course, a bacteriostatic agent except in high concentrations. Kanamycin and gentamicin are effective against most strains of staphylococci and may be used in the initial therapy of suspected staphylococcal disease. Less broad-spectrum and less toxic antibiotics should be chosen, however, when staphylococci are identified as the infecting organisms.

We do not at present routinely recommend the local instillation of antibiotics into the pleural cavity, abscesses or joint fluid. Adequate concentrations of antibiotics have usually been demonstrated at the site of infection when high serum levels are obtained. Routine

§ Manufacturer's precaution: Chloramphenicol is not recommended for intravenous or intramuscular pediatric use. Chloramphenicol sodium succinate has been approved for intravenous pediatric use.

use of intrathecal antibiotics is also discouraged for staphylococcal infections. The penicillin derivatives cross the blood-brain barrier and give adequate levels when the meninges are inflamed. Recently, British investigators have advocated the intraventricular administration of methicillin in doses of 10 to 100 mg. for the treatment of ventriculitis in patients with hydrocephalus and indwelling shunts. Such therapy warrants further evaluation.

Therapy of Specific Staphylococcal Infections. NEONATAL SEPSIS AND MENINGITIS. Therapy for systemic infection due to staphylococci in the neonate must be initiated rapidly with appropriate antibiotics. The usual combination of penicillin (or ampicillin) and gentamicin (or kanamycin) used for therapy in suspected neonatal sepsis provides adequate coverage for penicillin-sensitive or penicillin-resistant staphylococci. When culture results confirm that the etiologic agent is a staphylococcus, less broad-spectrum and less toxic antibiotics should be utilized. If the staphylococcus is penicillin-sensitive, aqueous penicillin G should be administered in doses approximating 50,000 to 75,000 units per kilogram per day in two to three divided doses intravenously. If the organism is resistant to penicillin, methicillin may be administered in a dose of 100 to 200 mg. per kilogram per day in three to four divided doses. Therapy of uncomplicated sepsis should be continued parenterally for 10 to 14 days, with the latter course being preferred. Because of the high morbidity and mortality rate and the tendency for relapse to occur, high-dose parenteral therapy should be continued for three to six weeks in neonates with staphylococcal meningitis.

BREAST ABSCESS IN THE NEONATE. Breast abscesses in the neonate are almost always due to hospital-acquired penicillin-resistant staphylococci. They are best treated by adequate surgical drainage in combination with systemic antibiotics for a period of 10 days to two weeks. Strict isolation should be maintained during this period to prevent spread of infection in the nursery.

STAPHYLOCOCCAL INFECTION OF THE SKIN IN THE NEONATE. Staphylococci may produce bullous impetigo or toxic epidermal necrolysis (Ritter's disease) in the neonate. Although blood cultures are seldom positive in either disease, prompt systemic therapy with methicillin or an oral agent such as dicloxacillin should be administered. Therapy should be continued for at least 10 days. Strict isolation should be maintained.

STAPHYLOCOCCAL SEPSIS AND MENINGITIS IN THE OLDER CHILD. Therapy of staphylococcal sepsis or meningitis in the older child should include the use of both penicillin and a penicillinase-resistant penicillin derivative if sensitivities are not known. Aqueous penicillin G should be administered intravenously in a dose of 400,000 to 500,000 units per kilogram per day in four to six divided doses. Our choice for unknown or penicillin-resistant organisms is methicillin in a divided dose of 400 mg. per kilogram per day given every 4 hours. Nafcillin may also be used in a dose of 100 mg. per kilogram per day.|| Therapy should be continued parenterally for at least 10 days in uncomplicated sepsis. During this time, numerous examinations should be made for evidence of metastatic lesions in the lungs, bones, joints, viscera or central nervous system. Should such spread be detected, prolonged therapy is indicated. In the absence of evidence of seeding, oral follow-up therapy in uncomplicated sepsis is probably not necessary.

In the penicillin-allergic individual, cephalothin must be administered cautiously, since the possibility of a cross-reaction exists. The dose is 100 mg. per kilogram per day in four to six divided doses. The cephalosporin derivatives should not be considered as appropriate therapy if meningitis is a part of the clinical syndrome, owing to their unpredictable diffusion into the cerebrospinal fluid. If there is a strong indication of true penicillin allergy, our first-choice antibiotic would be clindamycin in a dose of 16 to 20 mg. per kilogram per day in four divided intravenous doses.

Staphylococcal meningitis should be treated with maximum doses of the same antibiotics used in treating staphylococcal sepsis. Most of the penicillin derivatives cross the inflamed meninges well. Again, the cephalosporins may not, and should not, be used for the treatment of central nervous system infections. Intrathecal penicillin may be administered in doses of up to 10,000 units in the older child. Methicillin has also been used intrathecally and intraventricularly in doses of 10 to 100 mg. Both drugs are somewhat irritating, however, and should not be used intrathecally unless absolutely necessary. In the treatment of coagulase-negative staphylococcal ventriculitis in patients with ventricular shunts, removal of the nidus of infection by complete shunt revision is usually necessary. Parenteral chloramphenicol (50

|| Manufacturer's precaution: There is no clinical experience available on the intravenous use of nafcillin in neonates or infants.

to 100 mg. per kilogram per day)** or methicillin (100 to 400 mg.) has been used with some success. An approach which is used successfully in such patients in our institution is to institute appropriate antibiotic therapy, bringing about a stable clinical picture. Then, under the cover of such therapy, a complete shunt revision with removal of the old shunt and insertion of a new shunt is performed and antibiotic therapy continued for 7 to 10 days.

STAPHYLOCOCCAL ENDOCARDITIS. Staphylococci have become the most common etiologic agents in postsurgical endocarditis. When coagulase-positive staphylococci are at fault, the disease is a fulminating one with rapid destruction of heart valves. Therapy should consist of prolonged high-dose administration of a penicillinase-resistant penicillin, such as methicillin or nafcillin.†† In the penicillin-allergic individual, vancomycin has been used with good results. Prolonged systemic therapy with antibiotics chosen on the basis of susceptibility testing should be administered.

STAPHYLOCOCCAL PNEUMONIA. Staphylococci produce one of the most severe pneumonic processes seen in pediatrics. The disease tends to be a fulminating one with rapid production of effusions, empyema and respiratory distress. Bullous lesions and pneumatoceles often appear and may rupture spontaneously, leading to the development of a tension pneumothorax. When such lesions are present during the acute stage of staphylococcal pneumonia, the potential for the development of a life-threatening pneumothorax must be appreciated and the means to combat it must be readily at hand. Insertion of a thoracostomy tube or even a plastic intravenous catheter may be lifesaving. When empyema develops, early surgical intervention is indicated. We do not at present instill antibiotics locally into the pleural cavity, but high-dose intravenous antibiotics are used, with methicillin being our drug of choice in a divided dose of 400 mg. per kilogram per day given every 4 hours. Parenteral therapy is continued for two to four weeks, depending on the clinical response. An additional period of oral therapy with dicloxacillin* in a dose of 25 to 50 mg. per kilogram per day for two to three weeks is then given because of the marked tendency for relapse to occur. Uncomplicated pneumatoceles are left entirely alone and usually heal without surgical intervention.

STAPHYLOCOCCAL OSTEOMYELITIS AND ARTHRITIS. Initial therapy of staphylococcal osteomyelitis and arthritis should consist of high intravenous doses of aqueous penicillin G and a penicillinase-resistant penicillin such as methicillin or nafcillin. The doses approximate those indicated for sepsis. When sensitivities are known, a single drug should be used. In the penicillin-allergic individual, lincomycin‡‡ or clindamycin is our first choice because of the tendency of these drugs to concentrate in bone. Parenteral therapy should be continued for two to six weeks depending on the amount and type of bone involvement and the clinical and laboratory responses. In the mild case with little radiologic evidence of bone involvement and a rapid clinical response with a dropping erythrocyte sedimentation rate, two weeks of parenteral therapy followed by two weeks to a month of oral therapy with cloxacillin or dicloxacillin may be adequate. In the more severe case, parenteral therapy may be indicated for longer periods of time. When oral therapy is instituted, bactericidal titers as described previously may be determined using the patient's serum. These should be repeated periodically in order to determine if the medication is being administered properly in the correct dose. Too early discontinuation of therapy may lead to the development of chronic staphylococcal osteomyelitis, which is exceedingly difficult to treat. The erythrocyte sedimentation rate, radiographic resolution, return of function and loss of point tenderness are all helpful parameters in following therapeutic progress in these patients.

Adequate surgical drainage is often required in staphylococcal osteomyelitis and arthritis. Repeated aspiration may be sufficient for peripheral joints; however, open drainage is often necessary when the hip joint is involved.

STAPHYLOCOCCAL LYMPHADENITIS. Staphylococci frequently infect the submandibular and anterior cervical lymph nodes, producing characteristically firm encapsulated nodes. These later become fluctuant and often necessitate surgical drainage. In order to hasten healing and prevent dissemination, oral cloxacillin or dicloxacillin* should be administered. At the time of surgical drainage, parenteral therapy is probably indicated.

** Manufacturer's precaution: Chloramphenicol is not recommended for intravenous or intramuscular pediatric use. Chloramphenicol sodium succinate has been approved for intravenous pediatric use.

†† Manufacturer's precaution: There is no clinical experience available on the intravenous use of nafcillin in neonates or infants.

* Manufacturer's precaution: Because of limited experience, a dose of dicloxacillin for newborns is not recommended at this time.

‡‡ Manufacturer's precaution: Lincomycin is not indicated in the newborn (up to one month of age).

STAPHYLOCOCCAL ABSCESSES, FURUNCLES AND SURGICAL WOUNDS. In local staphylococcal infections, adequate surgical drainage is the mainstay of therapy, while systemic antibiotics may be used to prevent spread. Topical agents, such as bacitracin, neosporin or gentamicin ointments, may be used for superficial skin infections. Although staphylococci may often be cultured from impetiginous lesions, they are usually secondary invaders. Penicillin aimed at the streptococcus is usually effective in eradication of these lesions.

Group A Beta-Hemolytic Streptococci Infections

HUGH C. DILLON, M.D.

Group A streptococci are among the most common causes of bacterial infections. The natural history of these infections has changed over the years, but two clinical forms of infection remain especially frequent and important: pharyngitis and pyoderma. Either may be complicated by suppurative or nonsuppurative sequela. Rheumatic fever follows only pharyngitis, but endemic and epidemic nephritis following pyoderma is common throughout many areas of the world, notably where the climate is warm and humid. Many features of pharyngitis and pyoderma differ greatly. However, similar treatment is effective for both infections.

Scarlet fever following either pyoderma or pharyngitis is less common now than in previous years. Suppurative complications vary in relation to the primary site of infection and include sinusitis, otitis media, cellulitis, lymphangitis and suppurative lymphadenitis. All are less common now than in the preantibiotic era. Serious, life-threatening infections, such as pneumonia with empyema, meningitis and infections of the bones and joints, are now relatively rare, as is erysipelas. Serious infections, with a greater likelihood of bacteremia, require more vigorous therapy.

Principles of Diagnosis and Treatment. Indications for streptococcal therapy are as follows: to prevent suppurative and nonsuppurative complications, to modify or shorten the acute infection and to minimize contagion. Therapy shortens the course of pharyngitis only minimally, but pyoderma is appreciably affected. Culture-diagnosis of streptococcal pharyngitis is essential, since clinical features resemble those caused by other agents, and vice versa. Throat cultures are simply performed and relatively inexpensive (when done in office), and treatment can be safely deferred pending results. Savings by avoiding the cost of unnecessary antibiotic therapy more than pay for the cost of a negative throat culture. Skin lesion cultures are also easily accomplished. Typical purulent lesions justify treatment without culture. Such lesions may yield streptococci *and* staphylococci; the latter are usually secondary and do not require specific antistaphylococcal therapy. Staphylococcal bullous impetigo and furuncles are clearly distinguishable from streptococcal impetigo.

When serious or life-threatening streptococcal infection is suspected, cultures of blood, cerebrospinal fluid and pus collections are obligatory. Therapy is initiated on an empirical basis with consideration given to other common bacterial agents known to cause similar disease. Culture results plus the response of the patient serve as subsequent guides to therapy.

Therapeutic Regimens. Group A streptococci are uniformly, exquisitely sensitive to penicillin. Prevention of rheumatic fever was first demonstrated by using intramuscular penicillin, given at intervals to maintain adequate daily therapeutic levels for a minimum of 10 days. Subsequent recommendations of 10-day therapy for streptococcal pharyngitis were based on these experiences, which guaranteed eradication of streptococci from a maximum percentage of patients. Single-dose preparations of intramuscular penicillin which provide the prolonged therapeutic levels needed for eradication of streptococci have supplanted preparations requiring more frequent administration. Penicillin therapy remains the standard against which agents must be compared for satisfactory treatment of streptococcal infections. It remains the drug of choice on the basis of efficacy, low incidence of toxicity and side effects, and inexpensiveness. A better perspective of relative efficacy of orally prescribed nonpenicillin agents is obtained, however, when such regimens are compared with oral rather than with intramuscular penicillin. The superiority of penicillin is less obvious in such studies.

Dose schedules for antistreptococcal agents are listed below, beginning with penicillin; alternative regimens are then listed in alphabetical order.

PENICILLIN. *Intramuscular Benzathine Penicillin G.* Patients under 90 pounds: 600,000 units; patients over 90 pounds: 1,200,000 units. Preparations containing mixtures of procaine or aqueous penicillin and benzathine penicillin G possess no material advantage over benzathine penicillin G alone. Care must be taken to ensure proper concentration of benzathine penicillin G, since it alone provides prolonged therapeutic levels needed for streptococcal eradication.

Oral Penicillin. Both phenoxymethyl penicillin (penicillin V or Pen-Vee K) and penicillin G are acceptable. The former provides more uniform absorption and is no longer more expensive than penicillin G, except in tablet form. For these reasons, Pen-Vee K is preferable. Dose schedule is 125 mg. four times a day for patients under 50 pounds, and 250 mg. four times a day for those over 50 pounds. Similar total doses, given twice daily, may be as effective as the four-times-a-day schedule.

ALTERNATIVE AGENTS. Patients allergic to penicillin may be treated with one of several effective antistreptococcal agents.

Cephalexin, a cephalosporin derivative, given in four divided doses of 30 to 40 mg. per kilogram by mouth, compares favorably with penicillin V in patients with pharyngitis and is effective against streptococcal and staphylococcal skin and soft tissue infections. The disadvantages are that it is more expensive than penicillin and cross-sensitivity with penicillins may occur.

Clindamycin, a lincomycin derivative, is now available in capsule and suspension forms and is a very effective antistreptococcal drug. Fewer gastrointestinal and other side effects have been observed with clindamycin than with lincomycin. An effective schedule is 15 mg. per kilogram per day, given in two to four doses. This agent is very effective for eradication of streptococci in patients with either pharyngitis or pyoderma. As with other antistreptococcal agents, treatment for 10 days is recommended for patients with pharyngitis; however, seven-day therapy for pyoderma appears adequate. The drug is also effective against staphylococcal pyodermas.

Erythromycin remains a safe and effective alternate agent for streptococcal infections. Suspension, chewable tablets and capsules are available for both the ethyl succinate and estolate preparations. Some evidence suggests that the estolate form allows more uniform absorption. The recommended dose range varies from 15 to 50 mg. per kilogram per day. The lower doses appear reasonably effective. Therapy given twice daily compares favorably with that given three or four times a day. Seven-day therapy for pyoderma is quite effective. Erythromycin is an exceptionally safe and well-tolerated agent, and because of its limited usefulness in more serious forms of infection, it remains an excellent alternate agent for streptococcal infections.

Streptococcal strains resistant to the above agents have been rarely encountered. Tetracyclines and sulfonamides should not be employed in the primary treatment of streptococcal infections.

Serious or life-threatening streptococcal infections should be treated with intravenous or intramuscular penicillin G. Appropriate clinical and laboratory monitoring of these infections is essential. The dose of penicillin is an empirical one and may range from one to several million units of penicillin per day, depending on the age and weight of the patient and the nature and site of infection. Limiting factors in the administration of penicillin relate primarily to the potassium content of the drug and the route of administration. The duration of therapy is dependent on the clinical response and the site of infection. In cases of well-documented penicillin allergy, clindamycin, lincomycin* or a cephalosporin should be substituted. Osteomyelitis and suppurative arthritis in particular require prolonged therapy.

Other Considerations in the Treatment and Prevention of Streptococcal Infections and Complications. STREPTOCOCCAL CARRIERS. A variable number, ranging up to 20 per cent, of healthy school children may harbor group A streptococci in the upper respiratory tract in the absence of clinical evidence of disease. The carrier state has been discussed in detail elsewhere (Dillon and Dudding). Patients with recurrent pharyngitis and positive throat cultures, in whom treatment fails to eradicate or prevent reacquisition of streptococci, should be further investigated. Small numbers of streptococci on throat culture and little or no serologic response favor the carrier state. Healthy chronic carriers appear at little risk for nonsuppurative complications.

Nongroup A beta-hemolytic streptococci, notably group C and G, are often found in the upper respiratory tract of children with or without sore throat. Such strains account for some presumed "treatment failures." Care must be taken to avoid unnecessary treatment of individuals harboring such streptococci.

RHEUMATIC FEVER PROPHYLAXIS. The American Heart Association provides definitive guidelines for primary and secondary prophylaxis. Benzathine penicillin G given as a single intramuscular injection of 1,200,000 units every

* Manufacturer's precaution: Lincomycin is not indicated in the newborn (up to one month of age).

four weeks is most effective. Alternative regimens include 125 mg. of penicillin G or V orally, given twice daily; sulfadiazine, given in a dose of 0.5 to 1.0 Gm. daily; or erythromycin, 250 mg. given twice daily. Penicillin and sulfadiazine are the preferred oral prophylactic agents. Prophylaxis following acute glomerulonephritis is not needed.

References

Dillon, Hugh C., Jr., and Dudding, Burton A.: Streptococcal Infections; in V. C. Kelly (ed.): *Brennemann's Practice of Pediatrics*. Hagerstown, Maryland, Hoeber Medical Division, Harper & Row, Publishers, 1970, Vol. II, Chapter 6, pp. 1–15.

Listeria monocytogenes Infections

HENRY G. CRAMBLETT, M.D.

Listeria monocytogenes is a short, gram-positive, nonspore-forming, motile rod which causes spontaneous infections in many species of animals. It has a worldwide distribution. Although infection with this organism in humans may cause syndromes resembling infectious mononucleosis, septicemia without localization, endocarditis and multiple focal visceral abscesses, the most commonly occurring disease in infants and children is meningoencephalitis.

Fortunately, infections due to *L. monocytogenes* are infrequent. They occur almost exclusively in the newborn and in the older child with underlying debilitating disease, and especially in those receiving steroids or immunosuppressant drugs.

Even though this organism is rare, the physician caring for children must be aware of it, because successful therapy is difficult to achieve and is predicated upon early diagnosis and energetic early and prolonged antibiotic therapy. The fatality rate with therapy is reported to be 30 to 55 per cent. Moreover, unfamiliarity with this organism may cause it to be incorrectly identified as a contaminating diphtheroid in a clinical specimen.

In vitro, many antibiotics are effective against this organism as determined by disc-sensitivity testing. However, in vivo, success is less than satisfactory. Because of the rarity of this infection, no one has been able to evaluate critically various antibiotics, either in combination or singly, in a manner suitable to permit a conclusion concerning the best therapeutic regimen. In vitro, by disc-sensitivity testing, tetracycline, streptomycin, chloramphenicol, penicillin, erythromycin, ampicillin, kanamycin and cephaloridine are all effective to varying degrees against *L. monocytogenes.*

At Columbus Children's Hospital, eight infants and children with *L. monocytogenes* meningoencephalitis have been treated in recent years. Only one patient was more than one year of age, and he was a four-year-old child with acute stem cell leukemia. Seven of the eight patients survived. All patients received penicillin in combination with at least one other antibiotic. In four patients, the second antibiotic was chloramphenicol; and in one patient each, kanamycin, erythromycin or ampicillin was the second antibiotic. In the infant who died 39 hours after admission, penicillin, kanamycin and methicillin were administered.

My personal preference for treatment of infections due to *L. monocytogenes* is a combination of penicillin and chloramphenicol administered intravenously. However, there is ample evidence from the literature that tetracycline is effective, and more recent data suggest that ampicillin alone is also effective. In short, I think that any one of these regimens may be used. The prompt institution of therapy in appropriate dosage for two to three weeks, depending on response, and intensive supportive care are factors that need to be taken into consideration if successful therapy is to be obtained in these serious, often fatal illnesses.

Penicillin G should be administered intravenously in doses of 50,000 to 100,000 units per kilogram per 24 hours. One-half of the 24-hour dose may be administered each 12 hours by continuous intravenous drip in maintenance and reparative fluids. In immature infants, chloramphenicol should be administered in a 24-hour dose of 25 mg. per kilogram. (Chloramphenicol may be administered to infants and children either orally, or, in the form of chloramphenicol sodium succinate, by the intravenous route.) Mature infants may be given 50 mg. per kilogram per 24 hours. Older children may be given 100 mg. per kilogram. The dose of tetracycline* for intravenous administration is 10 to 15 mg. per kilogram per 24 hours administered in two doses. Ampicillin should be given in a dose of 400 mg. per kilogram for the first 24 hours in four to six divided doses and subsequently reduced to 200 mg. per kilogram

* Manufacturer's note: The use of tetracyclines during tooth development (last half of pregnancy, infancy and childhood to age eight years) may cause permanent discoloration of teeth. This adverse reaction is more common during long-term use of the drug but has been observed following repeated short-term courses.

per day. (Note: The dose of 400 mg. per kilogram of ampicillin is higher than that recommended by the manufacturer. The manufacturer suggests 200 mg. per kilogram per day of ampicillin for severe infections, but adds that in some stubborn or severe cases even higher doses may be needed.)

Convulsions can be controlled with phenobarbital sodium in a dose of 4 mg. per kilogram administered intramuscularly. If seizures continue, an additional 2 mg. per kilogram may be administered every 45 minutes up to a total dose of 12 mg. per kilogram. With this regimen, diazepam (Valium) is contraindicated.

Diphtheria

LOUIS WEINSTEIN, M.D.

General Management. The patient with diphtheria should be confined to the hospital. Although this may not be absolutely necessary from the standpoint of isolation and quarantine, hospitalization is well advised because of the risk of cardiovascular and neurologic complications which may become life-threatening and require rapid and early recognition and treatment by experienced personnel. In cases in which the clinical course is benign, bed rest should be enforced for about 10 to 14 days; in complicated diphtheria the period of rest is prolonged, depending on the type and severity of the manifestations.

Good care of the skin, bladder, bowels and mouth is indicated. No special food restrictions or additions are required. Food of a consistency that can be swallowed comfortably and a diet adequate in all the nutritional elements are sufficient.

A moderate number of patients with diphtheria have considerable pharyngeal discomfort during the first few days of illness; this may be ameliorated by irrigations of the pharynx with warm physiologic saline solution and administration of codeine, 3 mg. per kilogram or 100 mg. per square meter per 24 hours, divided into six doses given either orally or subcutaneously.

Isolation. All patients must be isolated from other people. All objects such as dishes, cloth materials and bedding which the patient may contaminate must be boiled for 10 to 20 minutes in soapy water. Attendants should wash their hands with soap and water for three minutes after contact.

Although it was common hospital practice in the past to group patients with diphtheria together in large wards, such a procedure is now considered inadequate. Because antibiotic administration is effective in eliminating the carrier state, many patients may be free of organisms early in the course of the disease (one to seven days). If they are exposed to new patients brought into the same room, particularly after drug therapy has been stopped, the carrier state may recur. As a matter of fact, secondary attacks of diphtheria with faucial membrane may be observed rarely in such instances. It is best, therefore, to isolate patients with diphtheria in single cubicle or rooms in the hospital whenever possible. When such an arrangement cannot be made, the next best procedure is to move patients to "clean" wards after five or six days of antibiotic treatment and to prohibit the admission of new, untreated patients to these areas.

Isolation in the hospital is continued in uncomplicated cases until two throat and nose cultures taken 48 hours apart contain no *Corynebacterium diphtheriae*. These studies are not carried out until at least 48 hours after cessation of chemotherapy.

Antitoxin. The factors that determine the quantity of antitoxin given in the treatment of diphtheria are age and size of the patient, duration of the disease and location of the lesion. All estimations of the necessary dosage are entirely empiric, and in most instances a great excess of antibody is administered. Noteworthy is the fact that only that portion of toxin which is still free in solution in the tissue fluids, lymph and blood is capable of neutralization. Fixation of toxin to cells renders it unsusceptible to combination with antitoxin. In general, however, the older the patient, the longer disease has been present; and the more extensive the lesion, the larger is the amount of antitoxin given. If the disease has been present long enough for the pseudomembrane to disappear, little can be expected from administration of even huge quantities of antitoxin in preventing death or serious complications. Nevertheless, it is probably best in such instances to give the antiserum.

Every effort must be made to administer diphtheria antitoxin as early as possible after the diagnosis of the disease is suspected; delay beyond 48 hours must be avoided if possible, since there is evidence that the administration of even very large doses of antitoxin beyond this time may have little effect in altering the incidence or severity of complications.

The specific diagnosis can be established only on the basis of isolation and identification of the organism. In patients who have received no antimicrobial agents, this can be accomplished in 12 to 18 hours when Loeffler's medium is used. When an antibiotic has been given, however, cultures may not be positive until five to seven days after inoculation or may remain negative. In these cases it becomes important to treat patients on clinical grounds alone.

A helpful approach is to suspect diphtheria when a "typical" membrane increases in thickness and extent despite the administration of penicillin or other antibacterial drugs. If the presence of infectious mononucleosis can be ruled out, the patient exhibiting this type of lesion should be given antitoxin. A good rule to follow is to treat on the basis of strong clinical suspicion when bacteriologic studies do not quickly establish the diagnosis.

Hypersensitivity to Horse Serum. Before diphtheria antitoxin is injected, hypersensitivity to horse serum should be ruled out by appropriate examinations. The intradermal instillation of 0.1 ml. of the serum diluted 1:1000 with physiologic saline solution will give enlargement at the site of injection within 20 minutes, with urticaria, surrounding erythema and, in severe reactions, pseudopodial extensions from the central wheal in patients sensitive to horse serum. A control test using 0.1 ml. of physiologic saline solution should always be done.

The ophthalmic reaction is a more reliable indicator of clinically important hypersensitiveness, but has less value in children, in whom the significance of the reaction may be obscured by reddening of the conjunctivae due to crying. The test is carried out by putting a drop of serum diluted 1:10 with physiologic saline solution into one conjunctival sac, leaving the other as a control; it is considered positive if itching, watering and diffuse reddening of the tested eye appear within 30 minutes. *Under no circumstances should these studies be carried out without a syringe containing fresh epinephrine solution close at hand.*

Antitoxin Administration. If the skin and eye test results are negative, antitoxin may be injected without delay. In adults who show negative reactions, particularly those in whom a history of any type of allergic reactivity is present, it is best to give first 0.1 to 0.5 ml. intramuscularly and to wait 20 minutes before administering the next dose. If this is followed by no untoward effects, the quantity of serum necessary for treatment is then divided into four or six equal parts and given at 30-minute intervals until the entire amount has been administered. In nonsensitive children the total required dose may be given in a single injection.

Although intravenous instillation of antitoxin has not been thought necessary by some, it has been clearly demonstrated that the maximal serum concentration of antibody is not reached until 48 hours after intramuscular injection. Hence it is our practice to give the first half of the required dose of antitoxin by the intramuscular route, and the remaining half intravenously. The intravenous route is never used first because of the much greater possibility of producing serious hypersensitivity reactions; the initial intramuscular dose may desensitize patients who might react to antitoxin first injected into the blood.

If there are no local or systemic reactions in 30 to 60 minutes after completion of injection of the intramuscular dose, intravenous administration is accompanied by little, if any, risk. The best site for giving the serum is low in the thigh, so that, in the event of a reaction, absorption may be quickly interrupted by the application of a tourniquet above the point of inoculation.

In patients who show positive or doubtful skin and eye test results, the following procedures may be used. In those with strongly positive conjunctival reactions, serum is most dangerous and must never be given intravenously; if available, serum from another animal source should be used. If the diphtheria is severe, however, and treatment is absolutely indicated, *desensitization* must be attempted. In such instances the initial dose should be no greater than 0.1 ml. of a 1:100,000 dilution of antitoxin, administered subcutaneously. Increasing quantities, usually double the preceding one, are given every 30 minutes, if no reactions occur, until the required amount has been injected.

In some cases severe reactions may follow even the smallest dose of serum, and therapy has to be abandoned. Some clinicians advise that each injection of antitoxin be followed by epinephrine in this situation, but this has little to recommend it. Desensitization should be carried out only if the skin reaction is positive or if both tests yield doubtful results. In such patients the initial injection may be larger than 0.1 ml. of a 1:100,000 dilution, and it is usually possible to increase the quantity more rapidly. *Even the most minute amount of serum must never be given unless epinephrine solution is available for immediate use.*

Antitoxin Schedule. The schedule for diphtheria antitoxin (Table 1) recommended

TABLE 1. Amount of Antitoxin in the Treatment of Diphtheria

Mild	5000– 10,000 units	Membrane limited to a small area on one tonsil or to the nares
Moderate	20,000– 40,000 units	Both tonsils involved, or one tonsil and adjacent pillars
Severe*	40,000– 60,000 units	Extension of membrane to uvula, soft palate or nasopharynx
Malignant	60,000–100,000 units	Extensive membrane, extreme toxicity, hemorrhages in mucous membranes and skin, swelling of neck, etc.

* Instances of laryngeal and nasopharyngeal diphtheria in patients with moderately severe disease who still show activity and are seen late at the time of the first injection, and moderate diphtheria occurring as a complication of another communicable disease, should be treated as severe cases.

by the Division of Biologic Laboratories of the Department of Public Health of the Commonwealth of Massachusetts is the one we use.

A somewhat different schedule is recommended by The Committee on the Control of Infectious Diseases of the American Academy of Pediatrics. The administration of 10,000 to 20,000 units of antitoxin is recommended for lesions of the anterior nose and tonsils, 20,000 to 40,000 units for pharyngeal, uvular or laryngeal involvement, and 40,000 to 75,000 units for diphtheria involving the nasopharynx. Increase in dose is suggested "if toxicity is marked or if the patient has been ill for more than 48 hours."

SERUM REACTION. If a serum reaction occurs during or shortly after treatment, a tourniquet is applied above the site of injection in the thigh. This is followed immediately by the injection of 1:1000 solution of epinephrine hydrochloride. The dose of this agent for children is 0.01 ml. per kilogram or 0.3 ml. per square meter. The total quantity administered at one time should not exceed 0.5 ml. Injections should be given subcutaneously and, if necessary, may be repeated every 4 hours pro re nata. This drug is given if lumbar or abdominal pain or evidence of urticaria, wheezing, dyspnea, cyanosis or collapse is present. Artificial respiration may be required, and if collapse occurs, the usual methods for the treatment of shock are instituted.

Antimicrobial Drugs. Antimicrobial drugs have no effect on the clinical course of diphtheria. They are of value only in eliminating the carrier state rapidly, and they accomplish eradication of the organisms from the respiratory tract or other focus in about 10 to 12 days in more than 95 per cent of patients. Among the drugs which are useful for this purpose are penicillin and erythromycin, both having proved most effective in our experience. When crystalline benzyl penicillin G is used, a dose of 300,000 units is given intramuscularly every 4 hours. Erythromycin, 25 to 50 mg. per kilogram per day orally in four equally divided doses, is also highly effective and is the drug of choice in persons known to be sensitive to penicillin. Re-treatment a second or even a third time is indicated if bacteriologic relapse occurs. This is preferable to tonsillectomy, which may be considered a last resort if the carrier state persists despite repeated exposure to antimicrobial agents.

Management of Complications. LARYNGOTRACHEAL OBSTRUCTION. If possible, examination of the larynx and trachea by direct laryngoscopy is most desirable. In some cases it is possible to remove part or all of the laryngotracheal membrane with forceps. In others an O'Dwyer tube can be inserted under direct vision. It is not desirable, however, to tear the pseudomembrane away from the underlying mucous membrane forcefully. In most instances the presence of signs indicating occlusions of the airway should indicate immediate indirect insertion of an O'Dwyer tube.

Some clinicians prefer tracheostomy to either direct or indirect intubation. There is truly little to choose between the available methods. Tracheostomy is easier to perform with the O'Dwyer tube in place; it also offers the advantage of ease of aspiration of membrane from the tracheal lumen and makes bronchoscopy less difficult when it is necessary. Relief of the obstructed airway should *never* be delayed until cyanosis appears, because attempts at intubation at this point may produce sudden cardiac standstill.

Progressive restlessness, plus use of the accessory muscles of respiration, is the main indication for instituting measures to increase pulmonary ventilation. Oxygen should be administered after intubation or tracheostomy. In the average case the tracheal tube may be removed with safety five to six days after it has been inserted.

MYOCARDITIS. Electrocardiographic studies have revealed that in 65 per cent of patients with diphtheria, myocarditis develops at some time during the course of the disease. For those with minor changes involving the P–R or the Q–T interval or the T waves, no specific therapy is necessary or available. These patients are best kept at bed rest, however, until the electrocardiogram has again become normal.

About 10 per cent of patients who have diphtheria show physical signs of cardiac involvement. These are usually arrhythmias, varying in degree from extrasystoles to complete heart block and ventricular tachycardia; softening of the first mitral sound and various murmurs due to cardiac dilation may occur. There are no specific measures for treating the disorders of cardiac rhythm in this disease. Although quinidine has been used in some patients, especially those with ventricular tachycardia and atrial fibrillation, little beneficial effect has been noted; the process frequently progresses to ventricular fibrillation, the usual terminal event. The use of procainamide hydrochloride in this situation should be explored, particularly if ventricular tachycardia is present.

The problem of the control of cardiac failure resulting from diphtheritic myocarditis is still unsolved. Although it has been suggested that digitalis may exert a beneficial effect, the weight of evidence indicates that this drug has little or no value. Bed rest, restriction of water and sodium, and the administration of diuretics—preferably the xanthine derivatives, or in the absence of renal disease, the organic mercurial compounds—are usually sufficient. Sedation, small doses of morphine, aminophylline, oxygen and a sitting position in bed are of help when left-sided failure is prominent; in most cases, however, the failure involves mainly the right side of the circulation with pain in the abdomen because of hepatomegaly and peripheral edema, and these measures are of little help.

Peripheral Neuritis. There is no specific treatment for the average case of diphtheritic peripheral neuritis. It has been suggested that the administration of corticosteroids may be of benefit in shortening and altering the course of this type of involvement of the peripheral nerves; the studies are not validated by adequate controls, and the efficacy of this therapy remains to be proved. Rest in bed, an adequate diet and physiotherapy for weakened muscles are indicated in all cases.

Two situations that require special management are dysfunction of the swallowing mechanism and paralysis of the diaphragm and intercostal and other muscles of respiration. The inability to take food and water may be compensated for by parenteral administration of water, salt and glucose for as long as a week. After this time a thin, polyethylene nasogastric tube is passed into the stomach, where it may be allowed to remain for as long as three weeks without changing; small amounts of a fluid diet high in calories and containing added vitamins and a large quantity of protein are given every 2 to 3 hours in order to reduce the risk of vomiting and aspiration which accompanies the administration of large quantities of such a mixture. If a heavier tube is used, it is best to allow it to remain in the stomach for only about 12 to 14 hours each day and to reinsert it every morning in order to avoid pharyngeal irritation or ulceration and the possibility of aspiration. The tank respirator is the instrument of choice in the type of respiratory paralysis which occurs rarely in diphtheria.

Shock. Rarely, in the absence of either myocarditis or peripheral neuritis, severe shock may occur suddenly during the course of diphtheria. Treatment consists of the usual methods for the management of shock, such as application of heat, elevation of the foot of the bed and plasma or blood transfusion; in addition, vasoconstricting agents such as ephedrine, metaraminol bitartrate (Aramine), amphetamine sulfate (Benzedrine), levarterenol (Levophed) and mephentermine sulfate (Wyamine) may be helpful.

Questions have been raised about the efficacy of vasoconstricting agents and the possibility that they may actually impede recovery from shock. The use of fluids (blood, plasma and plasma expanders, such as the dextrans) in a quantity sufficient to restore central venous pressure to normal levels may be sufficient to eliminate the shock state in many instances; in those that fail to respond to this therapy sympathetic blocking drugs such as dibenzylene have been employed by some investigators.

It has been suggested that large doses of corticosteroids be administered when all other efforts to maintain normal tissue perfusion have failed. Although the shock that may occur in diphtheria has not been managed in this fashion, the high percentage of failures and death associated with the older methods of treatment raises the possibility of studying the value of the more recent approaches to the problem of shock of varying etiologic background.

Prophylaxis of Contacts. Persons who have been immunized actively with alum-precipitated toxoid are probably best protected against diphtheria after exposure to an active case by being given a recall or booster dose of fluid toxoid. Their respiratory tracts should be examined for the presence of *C. diphtheriae* at least twice in the first week after contact, and if organisms appear, antibiotic therapy should be instituted promptly. For adults and children not previously immunized, the administration of 2000 units of diphtheria antitoxin intramuscularly, after appropriate skin and eye tests, is usually protective against development of the disease.

Management of the Carrier State. The mere isolation of *C. diphtheriae* from the respiratory tract does not indicate a clinically significant carrier state. In all instances the organism must be studied for virulence, and treatment is applied only if toxigenic bacteria are demonstrated. The use of antibiotics, in the same quantities as in the acute phase of the clinical disease, is by far the most effective method of managing this situation. Readministration of larger doses of an antibiotic agent is usually successful in the few instances in which the first course of therapy fails to produce desired results.

Prevention. SCHICK TEST. Susceptibility to diphtheria is determined by the presence or absence of circulating antibody to exotoxin. The Schick test yields a rough estimate of the quantity of antitoxin in the circulation. The present method of carrying out this test is as follows: 0.1 ml. of highly purified diphtheria *toxin* ($1/50$ M.L.D.) dissolved in buffered human serum albumin is injected intradermally in the volar surface of the forearm; 0.1 ml. of highly purified diphtheria *toxoid* (0.01 Lf) is injected into the other arm to serve as the control. These areas are examined at 24 and 48 hours and between the fourth and seventh days. When the reaction is *positive,* the site of toxin injection begins to redden in 24 hours; this increases and reaches a maximum in about a week, at which time the lesion may be 3 cm. in diameter and moderately swollen and tender. There is usually a smaller (1 to 1.5 cm.), dark red central zone which gradually turns brown, desquamates and leaves a pigmented area. The area of *toxoid* injection shows *no reaction.* A *positive* result indicates little or no circulating antitoxin or immunity.

In a *negative* test result there is *no reaction* at the site of either *toxoid* or *toxin* instillation. This is consistent with a blood antitoxin level of $1/30$ to $1/100$ unit and immunity to ordinary exposure.

Inflammation at both sites of injection within 14 hours, which reaches a maximum in 48 to 72 hours and then fades, constitutes a *pseudoreaction.* This practically always indicates immunity plus hypersensitivity to the toxin.

The *combined reaction* begins like the pseudoreaction, but the inflammatory response at the toxin site persists for some time after that in the area of toxoid injection has faded. This type of reaction is uncommon with the use of purified Schick testing materials and indicates that the patient has delayed sensitivity to toxin. Circulating antitoxin is either absent or low in these cases. Combined reactions are uncommon in children and probably result from previous unapparent diphtheritic infection; their frequency increases with age and is highest in unimmunized groups living in areas where diphtheria is prevalent.

Antitoxic immunity is not necessarily complete. People with negative Schick test results occasionally contract diphtheria, especially if subjected to heavy exposure. On the other hand, some people with positive Schick reactions do not acquire the disease after exposure.

ACTIVE IMMUNIZATION. Diphtheria is, for the most part, a preventable disease. Immunization at the age of three months should be routine. Diphtheria toxoid is best given with tetanus toxoid and pertussis vaccine (D.P.T.) because antibody titers are higher with combined immunization than with one agent alone. Booster doses should be administered at the age of one year and again just before a child goes to school.

Although it has been suggested that Schick testing is not necessary in those who have been immunized, many physicians still carry out the tests to determine the status of antitoxic immunity. A Schick test acts as a booster. It must be reemphasized that a negative reaction does not indicate absolute protection against diphtheria; although patients with serum antitoxin levels as high as 1 unit per ml. have died of it, the disease generally is milder and much less frequently fatal when the Schick test result is negative.

Pertussis

JOHN D. NELSON, M.D.

The whooping cough syndrome may be caused by *Bordetella pertussis, B. parapertussis, B. bronchiseptica* or adenoviruses. *B. parapertussis* and *B. bronchiseptica* are uncommon causes in most areas; the proportion of cases due to adenoviruses is unknown. It is possible that viral infection accounts for some cases of whooping cough occurring in previously vaccinated children. Differentiation among the various etiologic agents cannot be made clinically and requires appropriate bacteriologic, virologic and serologic tests.

Supportive Therapy. It is a good general rule to hospitalize all babies affected under approximately one year of age, since they are at greatest risk for asphyxial death. The advantages of close observation and management of acute paroxysms outweigh the risk of hospital-acquired superinfection.

When the child with pertussis is cared for at home, the mother should be given detailed nursing care instructions. If possible the patient should be kept in a pleasant, airy room with materials for self-entertainment. Noise, dust, smoke, excitement and strenuous activity may provoke paroxysms. During a paroxysm the child should be sitting or held in the mother's lap and she can offer calm vocal reassurance to allay asphyxial anxiety. An emesis basin should be available. Adequate oral fluids and maintenance of nutrition are important facets of care. Five or six small meals daily are preferable to the usual three meals. Dry or hard foods, such as crackers, toast and meat, should not be used since they may provoke paroxysms and, more importantly, may be aspirated during a paroxysm. When the child vomits, milk or puréed foods can be offered immediately afterwards, since they are more likely to be retained at that time. Bulb suction aspiration of mucus is inadvisable in the home setting, where it is only likely to be traumatic and ineffectual in inexperienced hands.

The same general principles of rest, quiet, avoidance of unnecessary stimulation and maintenance of adequate nutrition apply to the hospitalized patient. If possible, the infant should be in a room by himself rather than in a ward with other patients. It is said that the sound of another patient's coughing may stimulate a paroxysm. The room should be near enough to the nursing station so that the infant's coughing can be heard. The whole purpose of hospitalization is defeated if the patient is allowed to go through a paroxysm without nursing attendance. The infant who loses fluid in copious mucus and vomitus requires intravenous fluid therapy. Oral liquids and soft foods are offered frequently in small amounts as tolerated. Mechanical suction equipment should be available at the bedside for emergency use, as should a supply of humidified oxygen. Routine or excessive suctioning must be avoided; it is reserved for situations in which cyanosis persists after the paroxysm. The suctioning is carried out rapidly and atraumatically immediately after a paroxysm, when the infant is somewhat refractory to stimulation of another paroxysm.

The routine use of oxygen and mist tents is to be condemned. There is no evidence that it decreases the frequency or severity of paroxysms, it is uncomfortable for the patient, it makes the patient less accessible for emergency suctioning and oxygen therapy and it increases the hazard of superinfection with Pseudomonas or other "water bugs." Oxygen and mist should be reserved for patients with complicating bronchopneumonias who are having continuous respiratory distress or symptomatology between paroxysms.

Cough suppressant medications are ineffectual.

Specific Therapy. Pertussis immune globulin (human) U.S.P. is commercially available as Hypertussis in a 1.25-ml. vial. Its effectiveness for treatment of pertussis has never been established. Nevertheless, many clinicians have used this for treating young infants, giving one vial daily for three to five doses. We personally do not recommend it.

It is not clear whether antibiotics have a significant effect on the frequency or intensity of paroxysms or on the duration of illness. It is possible that they are effective when administered early in the course of disease, but there are conflicting reports. Antibiotics are used primarily for rendering the patient noncontagious. For this purpose, chloramphenicol, tetracycline, ampicillin or erythromycin could be employed. Chloramphenicol is not recommended because safer drugs are available. Tetracycline* is useful in older children when given in a dosage of 25 to 50 mg. per kilogram per day in four equally divided doses by mouth, but ampicillin or erythromycin is preferred for infants. We have had good results with ampicillin in a dosage of 100 mg. per kilogram per day in four divided doses either orally or intramuscularly, but others have recently cast some doubt upon the effectiveness of ampicillin against *B. pertussis.* In one study, erythromycin in a dosage of 50 mg. per kilogram per day in four divided doses by mouth was found to be very effective, and our experience confirms this. If the patient vomits medication, the dose should be repeated immediately.

Antibiotic therapy should be continued for no more than five days. Pertussis organisms

* Manufacturer's note: The use of tetracyclines during tooth development (last half of pregnancy, infancy and childhood to age eight years) may cause permanent discoloration of teeth. This adverse reaction is more common during long-term use of the drug but has been observed following repeated short-term courses.

will be eliminated by that time and continuing antibiotics for an unnecessarily long period of time may predispose to secondary bacterial superinfection by prolonged alteration of normal respiratory flora.

Ampicillin is contraindicated for patients with a history of penicillin allergy. An urticarial rash occurs occasionally with ampicillin. Drug-induced diarrhea is seldom a problem when therapy is restricted to five days. Adverse reactions are rare with erythromycin.

Antibiotic therapy is indicated for complications due to bacterial superinfections (see below).

Complications. ACTIVATION OF TUBERCULOSIS. Pertussis may activate quiescent tuberculosis. Patients known to be tuberculin-positive should be treated for eight weeks with isoniazid, 8 to 10 mg. per kilogram per day in a single dose orally, if they have previously had a full course of antituberculous therapy. Those not previously treated should receive isoniazid for 12 months after pertussis.

BRONCHOPNEUMONIA. The "shaggy-heart" x-ray appearance often seen with pertussis is not indicative of secondary bronchopneumonia and is not an indication for prolonged antibiotic therapy. "Prophylactic" antibiotic treatment does not prevent superinfection; it merely ensures that superinfection will be due to bacteria resistant to that drug. In uncomplicated pertussis there are coarse rhonchi, but no respiratory distress is present between paroxysms. Development of medium or fine rales means that secondary pneumonia has supervened. In patients recently treated with ampicillin, tetracycline or erythromycin, superinfection is most commonly due to penicillin-resistant *Staphylococcus aureus.* We initiate therapy with methicillin, 300 mg. per kilogram per day in four equally divided doses intravenously or intramuscularly. This dosage is somewhat higher than that recommended in the package insert, but in our experience it is necessary for treatment of staphylococcal pneumonia. If culture of mucus coughed up during a paroxysm reveals gram-negative bacteria, treatment can be started with kanamycin (15 mg. per kilogram per day in three divided doses) or with gentamicin (5 to 7.5 mg. per kilogram per day* in three divided doses). Antibiotics are later changed to the safest appropriate antibiotic based upon in vitro sensitivity tests.

OTITIS MEDIA. Secondary bacterial infection of the middle ear occasionally complicates whooping cough. If the patient has not recently received antibiotics, the bacteria involved are generally pneumococci, *Hemophilus influenzae* or streptococci. Ampicillin is given by mouth in a dosage of 100 mg. per kilogram per day in four divided doses. If otitis develops during the course of antibiotic therapy, we recommend either myringotomy or needle aspiration of the middle ear to secure pus for direct bacterial stains and culture, with antibiotic selection based on culture and susceptibility test results.

ATELECTASIS. The most common pulmonary complication of whooping cough in our experience is atelectasis, particularly of the right upper lobe. Once the paroxysmal phase has passed, vigorous chest physiotherapy should be instituted. Spontaneous resolution usually occurs within two to three weeks. If atelectasis persists beyond this time, consideration is given to bronchoscopy. Because the right upper lobe is relatively inaccessible in small infants, we do not attempt the procedure unless atelectasis persists for at least two to three months when that lobe is involved. Reexpansion eventually occurs in virtually all patients. We have done a lobectomy on one patient whose atelectasis persisted for four months. Atelectasis is not an indication for prolonged antibiotic therapy.

OTHER COMPLICATIONS. Scleral hemorrhage, periorbital hemorrhage, epistaxis and melena are very common in pertussis. Subarachnoid hemorrhage and subdural hematomas are extremely rare. Ulcer of the frenulum may develop from irritation as the base of the tongue protrudes over the lower incisors during a paroxysm. This heals spontaneously. Hypoxic convulsions following prolonged paroxysms are managed by standard methods.

Isolation. Patients with whooping cough may be released from quarantine after completing the course of antibiotic therapy if it can be demonstrated by fluorescent antibody testing and culture that the pathogen has been eliminated. Otherwise, isolation should be maintained for four weeks after onset of illness.

Management of Exposed Individuals. Exposed susceptible individuals should be treated with antibiotics in the same dosages as indicated above for active cases. Pertussis immune globulin is no longer recommended. The antibiotic is given for five days if exposure to the active cases ceases. If the active case is being treated at home, it is wise to continue treatment of susceptible persons for 7 to 10 days. Previously vaccinated, exposed children under six years of age are given a booster dose of pertussis vaccine or of DPT (diphtheria-

* Although the dosage of 7.5 mg. per kilogram of gentamicin exceeds that recommended by the manufacturers, this dosage has worked well in our experience.

pertussis-tetanus). Although the efficacy of antibiotic treatment of exposed susceptible persons has never been subjected to critical field trials, it has now been accepted by the Committee on Infectious Diseases of the American Academy of Pediatrics as the preferred management. In following this policy for over 10 years, we have never seen a secondary household case develop in a susceptible contact treated with antibiotics. There are no asymptomatic carriers of *B. pertussis;* therefore, bacteriologic studies of exposed, asymptomatic individuals are not indicated.

Active Immunization. Refer to page 688 for discussion of active immunization for pertussis.

Bacterial Pneumonia

JEROME O. KLEIN, M.D.

Effective chemotherapy is now available for all forms of bacterial pneumonia encountered in the pediatric age group. Optimal treatment, however, requires definition of the etiologic agent. The physician must differentiate viral or mycoplasmal from bacterial pneumonia; if the agent is bacterial, he must decide on the probable species. Clinical signs and laboratory values may be of assistance but are not definitive. A major effort must be made to obtain adequate materials for bacteriologic diagnosis; these include sputum, secretions from the posterior nasopharynx and blood (bacteremia is frequent and a positive blood culture for a respiratory pathogen provides an unequivocal etiologic diagnosis). The physician should also consider the following:

1. Tracheal aspiration in young children unable to produce sputum on request.
2. Thoracocentesis when pleural fluid is present.
3. Percutaneous lung aspiration in children who are critically ill, deteriorate while on therapy or are abnormal hosts with deficient immune mechanisms (susceptible to unusual pathogens).

Therapy should be initiated promptly once bacterial pneumonia is diagnosed or strongly suspected. Initial therapy may be guided by the examination of the Gram-stained smear of sputum or tracheal aspirate. If these materials are unsatisfactory or unavailable, other criteria must be used. The relative frequency of respiratory pathogens in the various age groups may provide guidelines for initial therapy for the child with pneumonia (who has no significant underlying pulmonary or systemic illness).

Initial Choice of Antimicrobial Agents in Various Age Groups. NEONATAL PNEUMONIA. The treatment of neonatal pneumonia is similar to that of other forms of severe neonatal infection, including sepsis and meningitis: initial therapy must include coverage for gram-positive cocci, particularly group B streptococci, and gram-negative bacilli.

A penicillin is the drug of choice for the gram-positive organisms. If there is reason to suspect staphylococcal infection, a penicillinase-resistant penicillin is chosen. If there is no significant risk of staphylococcal infection, penicillin G or ampicillin is used. The latter drug may provide a theoretical advantage because of greater in vitro activity against some enterococci and some gram-negative bacilli, particularly *Escherichia coli* and *Proteus mirabilis,* when used alone or in combination with an aminoglycoside. Because high serum levels may be achieved with parenteral penicillins during the first week of life, the neonatal dosage schedule is lower than that recommended for older children (Table 1).

Choice of therapy for suspected gram-negative bacillary infection is dependent on the antibiotic susceptibility pattern for recent isolates obtained from newborn infants. The patterns vary in different hospitals or communities, and from time to time within the same institution. At the present time, a significant proportion of all gram-negative bacilli cultured from newborns at the Boston City Hospital are resistant to tetracycline, streptomycin, ampicillin and cephalothin. Strains of *Pseudomonas aeruginosa* are resistant to all antibiotics except polymyxins and gentamicin. On the basis of this information, kanamycin or gentamicin is used to initiate therapy for severe neonatal infections at this hospital.

Chloramphenicol has been used infrequently in newborn infants since the association of the gray baby syndrome with high doses of this antibiotic. Perhaps because of the now-minimal use in nurseries, chloramphenicol may be effective in vitro against gram-negative bacilli resistant to other antibiotics. Infants with neonatal sepsis due to a strain uniquely sensitive to chloramphenicol should be treated with this antibiotic in an appropriate dosage schedule (Table 1).

PNEUMONIAS IN CHILDREN ONE MONTH TO FOUR YEARS OF AGE. The vast majority of bronchopneumonias at this age are caused by respiratory viruses. Therefore, if the initial clinical findings are consistent with viral infec-

TABLE 1. Daily Dosage Schedules for Parenteral* Antibiotics of Value in Treating Bacterial Pneumonia in Newborn Infants

	DOSAGE SCHEDULE	
Antibiotic	≤ *Six Days of Age*	*One to Four Weeks of Age*
Penicillin G	50,000 units/kg./dose q12 hrs.	70,000 units/kg./dose q8 hrs.
Ampicillin, Methicillin, Nafcillin†, Oxacillin, Cephalothin	50 mg./kg./dose q12 hrs.	70 mg./kg./dose q8 hrs.
Kanamycin‡	7.5 mg./kg./dose§ q12 hrs.	7.5 mg./kg./dose q12 hrs.
Gentamicin‡	2.5 mg./kg./dose q12 hrs.	2.5 mg./kg./dose q8 hrs.
Chloramphenicol‖		
Premature	6.25 mg./kg./dose q6 hrs.	6.25 mg./kg./dose q6 hrs.
Full term	6.25 mg./kg./dose q6 hrs.	12.5 mg./kg./dose q6 hrs.

* Intramuscular or intravenous routes are satisfactory except where specifically noted.

† Manufacturer's precaution: There is no clinical experience available on the intravenous use of nafcillin in neonates or infants.

‡ Intramuscular route usually used; intravenous route preferable if shock or bleeding diathesis is present.

§ Some investigators prefer 5 mg./kg./dose every 12 hours because of decreased excretion of kanamycin in premature infants up to five days of life.

‖ Intravenous route only; inadequate absorption from intramuscular sites. Manufacturer's precaution: Chloramphenicol is not recommended for intravenous or intramuscular pediatric use. Chloramphenicol sodium succinate has been approved for intravenous pediatric use.

tion and the child can be observed closely, specific therapy should be withheld pending the results of bacterial cultures. *Diplococcus pneumoniae* and *Hemophilus influenzae* are the major bacterial agents of concern. A penicillin is the drug of choice: penicillin for pneumococcal pneumonia and ampicillin for *H. influenzae* infections. When the etiologic agent is unknown but a bacterial pneumonia seems likely, ampicillin should be used to provide coverage for both pathogens.

Staphylococcus aureus has been an uncommon cause of acute pneumonia during the past 10 years. However, if clinical signs compatible with staphylococcal disease are present (i.e., empyema, abscess formation or pneumatoceles), or if staphylococcal infections are prevalent at the time, initial therapy should include a parenteral penicillinase-resistant penicillin (methicillin, nafcillin,* or oxacillin).

PNEUMONIA IN THE CHILD FOUR YEARS OF AGE AND OLDER. *Diplococcus pneumoniae* is the major bacterial cause of pneumonia in this age group. *Hemophilus influenzae* is uncommon and need not be considered in the initial therapy.

Infection due to *Mycoplasma pneumoniae* is frequent in the school-age child, adolescent and young adult. The tetracyclines† and erythromycin are effective in reducing the duration of illness; once the diagnosis is made or strongly suspected, treatment with one of these agents is appropriate.

Chemotherapy for Specific Pathogens. PNEUMOCOCCAL PNEUMONIA. Penicillin G is the drug of choice for all children with pneumococcal pneumonia, except those considered to be allergic to that antibiotic.

For most children with mild to moderately severe disease, an oral penicillin is suitable. Phenoxymethyl penicillin (penicillin V) and phenethicillin provide significant serum antibacterial activity (approximately 40 per cent of an equivalent dose of intramuscular aqueous penicillin G). Buffered oral penicillin G is less satisfactory, since the serum antibacterial activity is approximately half that of weight equivalents of penicillin V or phenethicillin, and larger doses are therefore required.

Children who appear "toxic," who have underlying disease or who have complications such as abscesses or empyema require the higher serum and tissue antibacterial activity provided by a parenteral form. Intramuscular aqueous sodium or potassium penicillin G is rapidly absorbed, high peak levels occurring within 30 minutes; the high levels thus attained make this route optimal for treatment of severe pneumococcal disease. However, since the intramuscular preparation is painful, if therapy of any duration is anticipated the intravenous route should be used.

Procaine penicillin G administered intramuscularly attains lower peak levels (approximately 10 to 30 per cent of those achieved with the sodium or potassium salt), but activity is sustained for 6 or more hours. Since the level of antibacterial activity in the serum may be

* Manufacturer's precaution: There is no clinical experience available on the intravenous use of nafcillin in neonates or infants.

† Manufacturer's note: The use of tetracyclines during tooth development (last half of pregnancy, infancy and childhood to age eight years) may cause permanent discoloration of teeth. This adverse reaction is more common during long-term use of the drug but has been observed following repeated short-term courses.

exceeded many fold by the oral penicillins, the use of parenteral procaine penicillin G is restricted to patients who cannot tolerate the oral form (patients who vomit or who are comatose).

A single dose of benzathine penicillin G provides a low level of serum antibacterial activity for a period in excess of 14 days. Although this salt often has been effective in pneumococcal pneumonia, failures are frequent and it is not recommended.

The dosage schedule listed in Table 2 may be used to initiate therapy. The duration of therapy is dependent on the clinical response but should be continued for at least three days after defervescence and significant resolution of the radiologic and clinical signs.

STAPHYLOCOCCAL PNEUMONIA. The high incidence of penicillin G–resistant staphylococci in the hospital and in the community requires the use of a penicillinase-resistant penicillin whenever staphylococcal pneumonia is diagnosed or suspected. Later, if the culture and sensitivity data indicate that the organism is sensitive to penicillin G, it should be used instead because of its greater efficacy and lesser expense.

There are differences among the various penicillinase-resistant penicillins in oral and parenteral absorption, in vitro activity and enzyme degradation. However, clinical trials indicate that all are effective in treating staphylococcal disease when used in appropriate dosage schedules.

Since 1961 laboratories in Western Europe have reported varying proportions of strains of staphylococci resistant to methicillin and cross-resistant ˉto the other penicillinase-resistant penicillins (and some of the cephalosporins). The incidence of these resistant strains has

TABLE 2. Daily Dosage Schedules for Antibiotics of Value in Bacterial Pneumonias of Infants* and Children

ANTIBIOTIC	ROUTE	RECOMMENDED DOSE PER DAY	SCHEDULE
Penicillin G	P.O.	100,000 units/kg.	4–6 doses§
	I.M. or I.V.	100,000–200,000 units/kg.	4–6 doses
Penicillin V Phenethicillin	P.O.	50–100 mg./kg.	4–6 doses
Methicillin	I.M. or I.V.	200 mg./kg.	4–6 doses
Oxacillin Nafcillin†	P.O.	200 mg./kg.	4–6 doses§
	I.M. or I.V.	200 mg./kg.	4–6 doses
Cloxacillin Dicloxacillin	P.O.	100 mg./kg.	4–6 doses
Ampicillin	P.O.	100–200 mg./kg.	4–6 doses§
	I.M. or I.V.	200 mg./kg.	4–6 doses
Cephalothin	I.M. or I.V.	200 mg./kg.	4–6 doses
Cephalexin	P.O.	100 mg./kg.	4–6 doses§
Kanamycin	I.M.	15 mg./kg.	2–3 doses
Gentamicin	I.M. or I.V.	5 mg./kg.	3 doses
Chloramphenicol	P.O.	50–100 mg./kg.	4 doses
	I.V.‖	50–100 mg./kg.	4 doses
Lincomycin	P.O.	30–60 mg./kg.	3–4 doses§
	I.M. or I.V.	10–20 mg./kg.	2–3 doses
Clindamycin	P.O.	10–20 mg./kg.	3–4 doses
Erythromycin	P.O.	30–50 mg./kg.	4 doses
	I.V.	40–50 mg./kg.	4 doses

* One month of age and older.

† Manufacturer's precaution: There is no clinical experience available on the intravenous use of nafcillin in neonates and children.

§ Schedule at least 1 hour before meals or 2 hours after meals.

‖ Manufacturer's precaution: Chloramphenicol is not recommended for intramuscular or intravenous pediatric use. Chloramphenicol sodium succinate has been approved for intravenous pediatric use.

been low (approximately 1 per cent or less) in the United States. However, if a child with staphylococcal disease, given appropriate doses of one of these penicillins, does not respond as expected, resistance to the antibiotic must be suspected and the sensitivity of the causative organism reevaluated.

The rapid evolution of staphylococcal pneumonia and the frequent association of empyema, pneumatoceles and abscesses demand close observation and meticulous nursing care. The duration of antibiotic therapy is dependent on the initial response, the presence of pulmonary and extrapulmonary complications and the rapidity of resolution of the pneumonic process. A large parenteral dosage schedule should be used for two to three weeks followed by an oral preparation for one to three weeks.

HEMOPHILUS INFLUENZAE. This organism is susceptible to a variety of antimicrobial agents including the sulfonamides, tetracyclines, aminoglycosides and ampicillin. All have been used with success in infections due to this agent. At present, ampicillin should be considered the drug of choice in young children; it provides coverage for both *D. pneumoniae* and *H. influenzae* when there is uncertainty as to the bacteriologic diagnosis, and the high dosage schedule needed for severe forms of disease can be given without concern for dose-related toxicity (Table 2).

In mild to moderate disease, oral ampicillin should be given until the child is afebrile for at least three days. The severe disease must be treated with a regimen similar to that recommended for staphylococcal disease, namely, parenteral ampicillin for a period of at least two to three weeks.

PNEUMONIA DUE TO GRAM-NEGATIVE BACILLI. Initial therapy must be guided by the following factors: the source of infection, underlying disease process (burn, cystic fibrosis), host susceptibility (deficient immune mechanisms) and the antimicrobial susceptibility pattern for gram-negative organisms in the community and hospital. The basis for choice of antibiotic is similar to that outlined for suspected gram-negative bacillary pneumonia in the neonate. The regimen is modified if indicated by the results of the cultures and the susceptibility of the causative organism. Duration of therapy must be tailored to the clinical course and the response to therapy. Pneumonias with minimal pulmonary lesions and symptoms should be treated for at least three days after defervescence. Severe pneumonias should be treated with a regimen similar to that outlined for staphylococcal pneumonia.

Therapy for the Penicillin-Sensitive Child. If the patient has a significant history of allergic reaction to any of the penicillins, he must be considered sensitive to all of them; alternative antimicrobial agents should therefore be considered.

Cephalosporins are among the antibiotics that may be used as alternatives to penicillin. Cephalothin,‡ the parenteral form, and cephalexin, an oral preparation, are active against pneumococci and staphylococci (including penicillinase-producing strains) as well as some gram-negative organisms. The cephalosporins have been used with success in the treatment of staphylococcal and pneumococcal pneumonia.

Erythromycin and lincomycin§ are active in vitro against gram-positive cocci and are effective in the treatment of pneumococcal and staphylococcal pneumonias. Since some staphylococci may be resistant to these antibiotics, it is important to test the organism for susceptibility. Clindamycin, a chlorinated analogue of lincomycin, is well absorbed when given with meals and has greater in vitro activity and produces less gastric reaction than does lincomycin.

Vancomycin and gentamicin are effective antistaphylococcal agents and may be considered for use in the patient who is allergic to penicillin and who has severe staphylococcal disease. It may be necessary to resort to them in treating infections due to methicillin-resistant staphylococci (or the so-called heteroresistant strains).

Chloramphenicol|| should be used as an alternative to penicillin in the child with pneumonia due to *Hemophilus influenzae*.

Tetracycline should not be used in children under the age of eight years because of the frequency of tooth staining. For children over the age of eight years, it may be of value in mycoplasma pneumonia infection. The small proportion of pneumococci and the significant number (approximately 30 per cent) of strep-

‡ Cephaloridine is a derivative of cephalothin with greater activity in vitro against pneumococci, streptococci and penicillin-sensitive staphylococci; with higher and more sustained levels in serum from equivalent doses; and with less pain on injection. It is less active than cephalothin against some strains of penicillin-resistant staphylococci. The experience with cephaloridine in infants and young children is still limited, and reports of nephrotoxicity with high doses suggest caution in its use.

§ Manufacturer's precaution: Lincomycin is not indicated in the newborn (up to one month of age).

|| Manufacturer's precaution: Chloramphenicol is not recommended for intravenous or intramuscular pediatric use. Chloramphenicol sodium succinate has been approved for intravenous pediatric use.

tococci resistant to tetracyclines limit their use in infections due to these agents.

Adjuncts to Chemotherapy. Antibiotics are only part of the management of the pediatric patient with pneumonia; supportive measures, including the following, are also of the utmost importance:

1. Maintenance of fluid and electrolyte balance.
2. Humidification provided by "cool mist."
3. Oxygen for severe dyspnea or cyanosis.
4. Maintenance of mouth hygiene.
5. Antipyretics should be used sparingly, since the temperature course may provide a guideline for the therapeutic response.
6. Bronchoscopy is limited to those instances in which a foreign body, tumor or congenital anomaly is considered.
7. Tracheal intubation or tracheostomy may be considered when there is laryngeal obstruction or when the patient is having difficulty clearing the tracheal secretions and more efficient suctioning is warranted.
8. Drainage of pleural effusions may be necessary when the accumulation of fluid embarrasses respiration. Single or multiple thoracocenteses may be adequate when the volumes of fluid are small. If larger amounts are present, a closed drainage system with a chest tube under negative pressure should be placed. The tube should be removed as soon as its drainage function is completed, since delay may result in local tissue injury, secondary infection and sinus formation.
9. Intrapleural instillation of antibiotic should be considered in early cases of empyema, particularly if the fluid is loculated and the presence of fibrous adhesions is a possibility. If a chest tube is in place, antibiotics are instilled following irrigation through the tube. In susceptible infections, aqueous crystalline penicillin G, 10,000 to 50,000 units; ampicillin, 10 to 50 mg; or a penicillinase-resistant penicillin or cephalosporin, 10 to 50 mg., may be inoculated in 10 ml. of diluent (sterile water or normal saline) after the tube is clamped. The clamp is maintained for 1 hour and then released for drainage. The instillations should be repeated three to four times each day that the tube remains in place. If thoracocenteses are done, antibiotic is introduced after the pleural fluid is aspirated.
10. Because of their capacity to produce moderate or severe local irritation and febrile reactions, local instillation of intrapleural enzymes is a method sparingly used in the pediatric age group. The fibrinolytic activity of streptokinase combined with the effect of thinning of purulent exudate by streptodornase may aid the penetration of antibiotics and the process of tissue repair in the pleural space.

Meningococcal Disease

LARRY H. TABER, M.D., *and*
MARTHA D. YOW, M.D.

In 1970, 2505 cases of meningococcal disease were reported to the Center For Disease Control, with the greatest incidence (887 cases) in children under four years of age. Meningococcal infections occur most commonly in late winter or early spring. Infection is transmitted from person to person and multiple cases do occur in households, although this is uncommon.

Meningococcal disease is caused by a gram-negative diplococcus, *Neisseria meningitidis.* At the present time in the United States, most disease is caused by group B or C organisms; primarily group C. Since many of the strains are sulfonamide-resistant, penicillin G is the drug of choice in patients not allergic to penicillin (see later).

Clinical Manifestations. Meningococci characteristically infect the nasopharynx of many individuals but produce disease in only a few. This asymptomatic nasopharyngeal infection, "carrier state," occurs in approximately 2 to 25 per cent of normal infants and children.

Meningococcemia occurs in 30 to 50 per cent of patients without meningitis. Three-fourths of these patients will have a rash; petechial (most classic) purpuric, bullous and/ or morbilliform. These lesions, when present with meningitis, are highly suggestive of meningococcal disease but do not exclude other etiologic agents. Shock may appear early or late in the disease and is most frequently seen in patients with extensive purpura. Chronic meningococcemia may last for weeks with intermittent chills, fever, rash and arthralgia or arthritis. This is more common in adults than in children.

Meningitis may occur without clinical or laboratory evidence of meningococcemia. Fever, vomiting and lethargy of sudden onset are the most common symptoms in young children. Rare localization in the lungs, pleural space, pericardial sac, endocardium, myocardium and joint space may occur.

Meningococcal disease is a medical emergency; therefore, specific antimicrobial therapy should be instituted as soon as possible.

Initial Diagnostic Procedures

Complete history.

Physical examination.

Neurologic examination.

Lumbar puncture and cerebrospinal fluid studies.

Bacteriologic studies: CSF, blood, nasopharynx, skin lesions, exudates.

Ancillary laboratory studies: blood count; urinalysis, serum potassium, sodium, carbon dioxide; blood urea nitrogen; blood glucose; pH (arterial blood); prothrombin time*; partial thromboplastin time; platelet count; fibrinogen level, when indicated.

Examination of peripheral blood smear.

X-ray of chest and other x-rays, as indicated.

Electrocardiogram.

Electroencephalogram, when indicated.

Initial Therapeutic Procedures

ISOLATION. 24 to 48 hours.

SPECIFIC ANTIMICROBIAL THERAPY. Although penicillin G is the drug of choice, *ampicillin* may be used when there is any doubt about the specific etiologic agent. *Crystalline sodium penicillin G,* 100,000 to 200,000 units per kilogram per day, is given in four to six divided intravenous doses. The intramuscular route may be employed after significant clinical improvement has occurred (usually 48 to 72 hours). *Ampicillin,* 200 to 300 mg. per kilogram per day, is divided into four to six intravenous doses (the drug must be freshly prepared, diluted in sterile 0.85 normal saline and administered intravenously over a period of 5 minutes). (Note: This dosage of ampicillin is higher than that recommended by the manufacturer, but may be warranted in this instance because of the seriousness of the disease.)

Chloramphenicol† may be used in patients allergic to the penicillins. The dose employed is 100 mg. per kilogram per day, divided into three to four intravenous doses.

DURATION OF THERAPY. Meningococcemia or meningitis; until patient has been afebrile five days or a total of one week (whichever is longer).

MANAGEMENT OF CIRCULATORY FAILURE. Every patient with meningococcal disease should have initial and continuous assessment of blood pressure and urinary output. When circulatory failure is present, *rapid* intravenous therapy with normal saline, a colloid solution or whole blood is necessary to expand the intravascular fluid volume. Monitoring of the central venous pressure is necessary to assess response to therapy. An initial high venous pressure (> 12 cm.) may indicate that cardiac dysfunction is causing or contributing to the failure. (If cardiac decompensation is present, digitalization is necessary.)

With restoration of the intravascular fluid compartment, the central venous pressure usually increases and may be safely raised to 12 cm. An increase in the blood pressure and urinary output above oliguric levels (10 ml. per square meter per hour) indicates a positive response to intravenous therapy even if the central venous pressure has not been raised. If circulatory failure persists, isoproterenol, 0.2 mg. (200 micrograms) in 200 ml. of $\frac{1}{4}$ normal saline solution (1 microgram per ml.) is infused at a rate of 0.05 to 4.0 micrograms per minute. If there is no response in 15 to 30 minutes, the infusion rate is doubled. A positive response to isoproterenol is demonstrated by an increase in urinary output to more than an oliguric level (10 ml. per square meter per hour), a reduction in central venous pressure (if it is elevated) to the normal range and an increase in pulse pressure. *Infusion of isoproterenol should always be accompanied by continuous monitoring of central venous pressure, blood pressure and cardiac rhythm (cardiac arrhythmias may develop).* Correction of acidosis is mandatory. A bicarbonate solution is preferred, since the patient may have lactic acidosis.

MAINTENANCE OF OPTIMUM HYDRATION. Optimum hydration consists of correction of any deficits. Thereafter, low-maintenance fluid intake should be established in order to minimize cerebral edema.

AREATION. Maintenance of aeration and oxygenation may present problems due to (1) airway obstruction, (2) decreased respiratory effort, (3) irregular respiratory rate secondary to increased intracranial pressure or (4) seizure activity. Frequent suctioning or tracheostomy may be necessary to provide a patent airway. An artificial respirator also may be helpful, and oxygen and mist should be used if indicated.

MANAGEMENT OF INCREASED INTRACRANIAL

---

* All patients with bacterial meningitis and/or suspected bacteremia without meningitis should be observed carefully for development of disseminated intravascular coagulopathy. Prothrombin time, partial thromboplastin time, platelet count, fibrinogen level and examination of peripheral blood smear for fragmentation of red blood cells should be performed when indicated.

† Manufacturer's precaution: Chloramphenicol is not recommended for intravenous or intramuscular pediatric use. Chloramphenicol sodium succinate has been approved for intravenous pediatric use.

PRESSURE. Signs of this complication are irregular respiratory rate, increased systolic blood pressure, bradycardia and persistent seizure activity. Various methods have been employed to reduce intracranial pressure secondary to cerebral swelling. A 20 per cent solution of mannitol‡ in distilled water is employed in a dose of 1.5 to 2.0 Gm. per kilogram of body weight. In 10 to 20 minutes, a 30 to 60 per cent reduction in cerebrospinal fluid pressure lasting from 2 to 4 hours can be expected. This procedure may be repeated.

Dexamethasone has been used to reduce cerebral edema. The dosage is 0.2 to 0.4 mg. per kilogram intravenously followed by 0.1 to 0.2 mg. per kilogram intramuscularly every 6 hours.

MANAGEMENT OF DISSEMINATED INTRAVASCULAR COAGULOPATHY. See page 160.

CONTROL OF SEIZURES. Seizures can usually be effectively controlled by the parenteral use of sodium phenobarbital. An initial dose of 6 mg. per kilogram of body weight is given. If seizure activity persists, two more parenteral injections of sodium phenobarbital, 3 mg. per kilogram, are given with 30-minute intervals between each injection. Should further medication be required, paraldehyde, 0.3 ml. per kilogram in 10 ml. of vegetable oil, may be given rectally. The patient is maintained thereafter on phenobarbital, 5 mg. per kilogram per day intramuscularly in four divided doses. As soon as the child is fully responsive, this medication may be given orally in the same dosage.

PERSISTENCE OF FEVER. This may be associated with subdural effusion, development of joint effusion (usually sterile but may require aspiration), drug reaction, extensive tissue necrosis, brain abscess or patients with a marked encephalitic component to their disease, or a superimposed hospital-acquired infection such as thrombophlebitis.

Management of Exposed Persons. Penicillin may be of value in the prevention of secondary meningococcal meningitis in household contacts. Treatment with penicillin V (1 Gm. per day for four days), although it does not eliminate the organism from the pharynx, has been associated with apparent protection in high-risk individuals. Erythromycin at therapeutic levels may be substituted in the penicillin-allergic patient. Sulfonamides are no longer of any value in the *general* prophylaxis of meningococcal infection. The policy of the local hospital should be followed for management of hospital personnel exposed to the disease. Meningococcal disease has been acquired by mouth to mouth resuscitation.

‡ Manufacturer's precaution: Use of mannitol in pediatric patients has not been studied comprehensively.

References

Annual Supplement, 1970 Summary, Morbidity and Mortality Weekly Report, Center For Disease Control, Volume 19, No. 53.

Mathies, A. W., Jr., and Wehrle, P. F.: Management of Bacterial Meningitis; in B. M. Kagan (ed.): *Antimicrobial Therapy*. Philadelphia, W. B. Saunders Company, 1970, p. 226.

Infections Due to Proteus, Klebsiella, Pseudomonas and Other Gram-Negative Bacilli

JON E. ROSENBLATT, M.D., *and*
SYDNEY M. FINEGOLD, M.D.

The infections to be considered here have been divided into two groups; the first includes Proteus, Klebsiella, Pseudomonas and other gram-negative bacilli of relatively common clinical occurrence, and the second includes gram-negative bacilli of relatively uncommon clinical occurrence. Infections caused by other important gram-negative organisms, such as *Escherichia coli,* Salmonella, Shigella, *Hemophilus influenzae,* Brucella, *Franciscella (Pasteurella) tularensis, Yersinia (Pasteurella) pestis, Bordetella pertussis* and *parapertussis,* Fusobacterium, Bacteroides and *Streptobacillus moniliformis,* are covered in other articles.

GRAM-NEGATIVE BACILLI OF RELATIVELY COMMON CLINICAL OCCURRENCE

The organisms included in this group, along with suggested antimicrobial therapy, are listed in Table 1. Each of these organisms may produce a variety of clinical diseases. In addition to the susceptibility of the organisms to antimicrobial agents, factors such as the locus and severity of infection and the renal status and clinical condition of the patient may influence considerably the choice of antimicrobial drug as well as other therapy.

In treating infections caused by these gram-negative organisms, the need for in vitro drug susceptibility tests is important in view of the variability of sensitivity patterns that has been encountered. Before such data are available, choice of antimicrobial agents may be made from Table 1, but it is desirable that drug susceptibility be confirmed, particularly in the treatment of serious infections such as meningitis and endocarditis.

TABLE 1. Selection of Antimicrobial Agents for the Treatment of Gram-Negative Infections of Relatively Common Clinical Occurrence*

ORGANISM	DRUG	REMARKS
Enterobacter species (Aerobacter species)	Gentamicin† Kanamycin† Carbenicillin Nalidixic acid‡ Nitrofurantoin§	Nitrofurantoin susceptibility test may not accurately predict therapeutic efficacy in Enterobacter and Proteus urinary tract infections
Klebsiella pneumoniae	Gentamicin† Kanamycin† Polymyxin or colistin Nalidixic acid‡	Antibiotic susceptibility tests are important. Some strains may be susceptible to cephalosporins.
Proteus mirabilis	Ampicillin Penicillin G‖ Cephalothin, cephaloridine or cephalexin Kanamycin† Gentamicin† Nalidixic acid‡	
Indole-positive Proteus (*Proteus vulgaris, Proteus morganii, Proteus rettgeri*)	Kanamycin† Gentamicin† Chloramphenicol** Carbenicillin Nalidixic acid‡ Nitrofurantoin‡§	
Pseudomonas aeruginosa	Gentamicin† Polymyxin or colistin Carbenicillin‡	Combination of gentamicin and carbenicillin is usually synergistic. Both can be used in serious, life-threatening infections. Use of carbenicillin alone is associated with emergence of resistant Pseudomonas and superinfection with resistant Klebsiella
Serratia marcescens	Gentamicin† Kanamycin† Carbenicillin Nalidixic acid‡	

* In most instances, drugs are listed in order of choice.
† Manufacturer's precaution: Intrathecal use investigational.
‡ Urinary tract infection only. See Table 3.
§ Should not be given to children under one month of age.
‖ Large doses of penicillin G are required for infection other than urinary tract infection.
** Chloramphenicol is not recommended for intravenous or intramuscular pediatric use. Chloramphenicol sodium succinate has been approved for intravenous pediatric use.

Tube or plate dilution tests, if performed in a reliable laboratory, should give an accurate measure of the lowest concentration of an antimicrobial drug required to inhibit the growth of a microorganism (the MIC, or minimal inhibitory concentration). This figure then can be related to expected blood or urine levels for the dosage of drug given. Results of disc diffusion susceptibility tests are reliable only if the laboratory uses a standardized method (Kirby-Bauer method).

Urinary tract infections due to relatively resistant organisms may respond to therapy with drugs which are excreted primarily by the kidneys and which therefore achieve very high urine concentrations.

Specific information concerning routes of administration, dosage and toxicity of drugs is included in Tables 2 and 3. Footnotes indicate dosage alterations required for newborns, prematures, and patients with renal insufficiency.

Table 2 includes separate schedules of administration for each of four categories of disease: meningitis, endocarditis, other serious infections and mild to moderate infection. Table 3 includes schedules of administration for urinary tract infection.

Both polymyxin B and colistin are included, although their ranges of effectiveness and toxicity at equally effective doses are essentially identical. Both agents are now available for intravenous and intramuscular administra-

TABLE 2. Route of Administration, Daily Dosage and Toxicity of Antimicrobial Agents in Treatment of Gram-

DRUG	SERIOUS INFECTION				
	Meningitis		*Endocarditis*		*Other*
Ampicillin	I.V.	300–400 mg./kg. in 6 doses††	I.V.	200–400 mg./kg. in 6 doses	I.M. or I.V.
Carbenicillin†	I.V.	400–600 mg./kg. in 6–12 doses††	I.V.	400–600 mg./kg. in 6–12 doses	I.V.
Cephalexin		Not recommended		Not recommended‡	
Cephaloridine§		Not recommended	I.M. or I.V.	100 mg./kg. in 4 doses not to exceed 4 Gm./day	I.M. or I.V.
Cephalothin	I.V.	200–300 mg./kg. in 6 doses	I.V.	200–300 mg./kg. in 6 doses	I.M. or I.V.
Chloramphenicol‖	I.V.**	First 1–3 days, 60–90 mg./kg. in 4 doses Thereafter, 30–50 mg./kg. in 4 doses		Not recommended	I.V.**
Colistin		Not to be used	I.M.	5 mg./kg. in 4 doses	I.M.
Gentamicin	I.M. I.T.†††	5 mg./kg. in 3 doses 1–2.5 mg. (0.5 mg./ml.)	I.M.	5 mg./kg. in 3 doses	I.M.
Kanamycin	I.M. or I.V.‡‡ I.T.†††	15 mg./kg. in 2 doses 1–5 mg. (0.5 mg./ml.)	I.M.	15 mg./kg. in 3 doses	I.M.
Penicillin G	I.V.	300,000–500,000 u./kg.	I.V.	200,000–500,000 u./kg.	I.V.
Polymyxin B	I.T.††† I.M. or I.V.	< 2 yr. 2 mg. > 2 yr. 5 mg. 2.5 mg./kg. in 3 doses	I.M. or I.V.	2.5 mg./kg. in 3 doses	I.M. or I.V.
Streptomycin†	I.T.†††	1–5 mg. (0.5 mg./ml.)	I.M.	15 mg./kg. in 2 doses (30 mg./kg. may be used for first few days if indicated)	I.M.
Sulfadiazine§§	I.V.	120 mg./kg. in 4 doses‖‖	I.V.	120 mg./kg. in 4 doses‖‖	I.V.
Tetracycline*** (including oxytetracyline and chlortetra-cycline)	I.V.	First 1–3 days, 15–20 mg./kg. Thereafter, 15 mg./kg. (by continuous drip)		Not recommended	I.V.

* Between-meal administration to avoid food in stomach.

† Not to be used as sole therapy.

‡ May be used as follow-up treatment in certain serious infections after initial therapy with a parenteral cephalosporin.

§ Not to be used in patients with impairment of renal function. Also, safety of cephaloridine in premature infants and infants under one month of age has not been established.

‖ Chloramphenicol dosage should not exceed 25 mg./kg./day in premature infants and newborns up to the age of two weeks. An initial dose of 25 mg./kg. may be given to seriously ill patients in this age group. Despite the absence of specific instances of drug toxicity related to renal insufficiency, because of theoretical considerations the manufacturer recommends that the dose be adjusted downward in patients with impairment of renal function.

** I.V. administration by intermittent, not continuous, infusion. *Manufacturer's precaution:* Chloramphenicol is not recommended for intravenous or intramuscular pediatric use. Chloramphenicol sodium succinate has been approved for intravenous pediatric use.

†† Authors' dosage higher than that recommended by manufacturer; severity of illness and low toxicity, however, may warrant high dose.

Negative Infection for Patients with Normal Renal Function

Serious Infections		MILD TO MODERATE INFECTION (OTHER THAN URINARY TRACT)	TOXICITY AND SIDE EFFECTS
100–200 mg./kg. in 6 doses	P.O.*	75 mg./kg. in 4 doses	Hypersensitivity reactions
400–600 mg./kg. in 6–12 doses	I.M. or I.V.	200 mg./kg. in 6 doses	Hypersensitivity reactions
Not recommended‡	P.O.	50 mg./kg. in 4 doses	Hypersensitivity reactions; neutropenia; eosinophilia
100 mg./kg. in 4 doses not to exceed 4 Gm./day	I.M.	30–50 mg./kg. in 4 doses	Nephrotoxicity
100–200 mg./kg. in 6 doses	I.M.	60 mg./kg. in 4 doses	Hypersensitivity reactions; neutropenia;
First 1–2 days, 30–60 mg./kg. Thereafter, 30 mg./kg. in 4 doses	P.O., I.V.**	30 mg./kg. in 4 doses	Gray baby syndrome in neonates; dose-related reversible anemia; aplastic anemia
5 mg./kg. in 4 doses	I.M.	5 mg./kg. in 4 doses	Neurotoxicity (paresthesias, respiratory arrest at high doses); nephrotoxicity
5 mg./kg. in 3 doses	I.M.	2.4–3.0 mg./kg. in 3 doses	Eighth nerve damage (mainly vestibular); nephrotoxicity
15 mg./kg. in 2 doses	I.M.	15 mg./kg. in 2 doses	Eighth nerve damage (mainly auditory); nephrotoxicity; respiratory arrest at high dosage
100,000–500,000 u./kg.	I.M. I.V.	20,000–30,000 u./kg. 100,000–400,000 u./kg.	Hypersensitivity reactions
2.5 mg./kg. in 3 doses	I.M. or I.V.	2.5 mg./kg. in 3 doses	Neurotoxicity (paresthesias, respiratory arrest at high doses); nephrotoxicity
15 mg./kg. in 2 doses (30 mg./kg. may be used for first few days if indicated)	I.M.	15 mg./kg. in 2 doses	Eighth nerve damage; respiratory arrest at high doses
120 mg./kg. in 4 doses‖‖	P.O.	60–120 mg./kg. in 4 doses‖‖	Crystalluria; hypersensitivity reactions
First 1–3 days, 15–20 mg./kg. Thereafter, 15 mg./kg. (by continuous drip)	I.M. P.O.	6 mg./kg. in 2 doses 30 mg./kg. in 4 doses	Staining of teeth; nausea, vomiting and diarrhea; liver damage; negative nitrogen balance; Fanconi-type renal damage from outdated tetracyclines

††† Intrathecal administration: total dose to be administered over a 10-minute period daily for the first three days and every second day thereafter until no longer required. Braces indicate concurrent administration. *Manufacturer's precaution:* Intrathecal use of *gentamicin* and and *kanamycin* is investigational.

‡‡ I.V. administration only when I.M. administration is not possible.

§§ Use is hazardous in newborn patients.

‖‖ Peak serum levels should be maintained between 8 and 15 mg./100 ml. Adequate urine output should be maintained and urine should be alkalinized.

*** Desirable not to use these agents in children under eight years of age. *Manufacturer's note:* The use of tetracyclines during tooth development (last half of pregnancy, infancy and childhood to age eight years) may cause permanent discoloration of teeth. This adverse reaction is more common during long-term use of the drugs but has been observed following repeated short-term courses.

TABLE 3. Route of Administration and Daily Dosage of Antimicrobial Agents in Treatment of Gram-Negative Urinary Tract Infection for Patients with Normal Renal Function

DRUG	ROUTE	DAILY DOSAGE
Ampicillin	P.O.*	40–60 mg./kg. in 4 doses
Carbenicillin	I.M. or I.V.	100 mg./kg. in 4 doses
Cephalexin	P.O.	25–50 mg./kg. in 4 doses
Cephaloridine§	I.M.	30–50 mg./kg. in 4 doses
Cephalothin	I.M.	30–50 mg./kg. in 4 doses
Chloramphenicol†‡	P.O.	30 mg./kg. in 4 doses
Colistin	I.M. or I.V.	5 mg./kg. in 4 doses
Gentamicin‡	I.M.	2.4 mg./kg. in 3 doses
Kanamycin‡	I.M.	15 mg./kg. in 2 doses
Nalidixic acid‖	P.O.	First 2 weeks, 50 mg./kg. in 4 doses If treated longer, then 25 mg./kg. in 4 doses
Nitrofurantoin‖	P.O.	6 mg./kg. in 4 doses (oral preparation not to be used in patients under one month of age)
Penicillin G	P.O.* or I.M.	25,000 u./kg. in 4 doses
Polymyxin B	I.M. or I.V.	2.5 mg./kg. in 3 doses
Streptomycin**	I.M.	15 mg./kg. in 2 doses
Sulfadiazine‖	P.O.	60 mg./kg. in 4 doses
Tetracyclines†† (including oxytetracycline and chlortetracycline)	P.O.	15–30 mg./kg. in 4 doses

* Between-meal administration to avoid food in stomach.

§ Safety of cephaloridine in premature infants and infants under one month of age has not been established.

† Chloramphenicol dosage should not exceed 25 mg./kg./day in premature infants and newborns up to the age of two weeks. An initial dose of 25 mg./kg. may be given to seriously ill patients in this age group.

‡ Should be used only in serious urinary tract infections.

‖ Use is hazardous in patients under three months of age.

** Not to be used as sole agent.

†† Desirable not to use these agents in children under eight years of age. *Manufacturer's note:* The use of tetracyclines during tooth development (last half of pregnancy, infancy and childhood to eight years) may cause permanent discoloration of teeth. This adverse reaction is more common during long-term use of the drugs but has been observed following repeated short-term courses.

tion. Polymyxin B has been administered intrathecally in meningitis due to gram-negative bacilli.

Carbenicillin is a relatively new penicillin derivative chemically closely related to ampicillin. Its antibacterial activity is similar to that of ampicillin, except that it is also active against Pseudomonas. Although the minimal inhibitory concentrations are high (25 to 150 micrograms per ml.), large doses can be safely given and produce serum concentrations in excess of these levels.

There have been a number of new tetracycline derivatives introduced in recent years (doxycycline, minocycline and methacycline). However, they have approximately the same activity against gram-negative bacilli as does tetracycline; the only differences are pharmacologic. Primarily, they persist longer in the blood than does tetracycline and can therefore be given at longer intervals and lower dosage. However, they are also more expensive. Minocycline may be particularly useful in prophylaxis against meningococcal infection. Doxycycline does not accumulate in the blood in the presence of renal failure and might be especially useful in azotemic patients. However, since doxycycline does have a low renal clearance, it is probably not useful in the treatment of urinary tract infections in these patients. The new derivatives are not included in the tables, since in most circumstances they appear to have no real therapeutic advantage over tetracycline in these infections.

Cephalexin is a new orally absorbed cephalosporin derivative which has an antibacterial spectrum similar to that of the other cephalosporins. It may be useful in certain gram-negative infections of the soft tissues, respiratory tract and urinary tract, and as follow-up therapy for patients with serious infections initially treated with a parenteral cephalosporin.

Initial treatment of meningitis due to gram-negative bacilli should include intrathecal as well as parenteral administration of antibiotics. Gentamicin is probably the best agent with which to start therapy until culture and antibiotic susceptibility results are available. Dosage recommendations are found in Table 2.

Several of the antimicrobial agents suggested are potentially toxic. Cephaloridine should not be used in patients with impaired renal function. With the drugs colistin, gentamicin, kanamycin, polymyxin B, streptomycin, tetracycline, sulfadiazine, nitrofurantoin, nalidixic acid and possibly chloramphenicol, the hazard of toxic reaction is increased with impairment of renal function, because these drugs are excreted by the kidney. At any dosage level, reduction in excretion leads to increase in serum level. Therefore, with renal impairment, dosage should be reduced and the patient observed for evidences of toxicity. The hazard of chloramphenicol and sulfonamide toxicity is increased when there is impaired liver function; thus premature and newborn infants are at greater risk when treated with these drugs.

Table 4 includes recommendations for altered dosage schedules of antimicrobial agents in the presence of renal failure. Although formulas for the calculation of gentamicin and kanamycin dosage in the presence of renal failure exist, these are not entirely reliable. The availability of simple and rapid methods for the assay of aminoglycoside antibiotics dictates the measurement of serum levels in azotemic patients and other complicated cases whenever possible.

The choice of antimicrobial agents may also be influenced by the prospect of the complication of superinfection, which is more likely to occur when the drug is effective against a broad-spectrum of microorganisms and is used with a higher dosage. This is related to the suppres-

TABLE 4. Alteration in Dosage Schedules in Presence of Renal Failure*
(Unit dose given at intervals indicated)

		SEVERITY OF RENAL FAILURE			
DRUG	UNIT DOSE	*Mild (1.2–2.5 mg./100 ml.)†*	*Moderate (2.0–5.0 mg./100 ml.)*	*Severe (5.0 mg./100 ml.)*	SIGNIFICANT DIALYSIS EFFECT
Ampicillin		No change from normal dosage			Yes (H)‡
Carbenicillin	25–100 mg./kg.	q2–4h	q4–12h	q12–24h	Yes (H, P)‡
Penicillin		No change from normal dosage but avoid large doses in severe renal failure			No (H, P)
Cephalexin	25–50 mg./kg.	q8–12h	q24h	q48h	Yes (H, P)
Cephaloridine		Not to be used in renal failure			
Cephalothin	15–65 mg./kg.	q4–6h	q6h	q8–12h	Yes (H, P)
Chloramphenicol		No change from normal dosage§			No (H, P)
Colistin	1.2 mg./kg.	q24h	q36–60h	q60–90h	No (H, P)‖
Gentamicin**	1–1.7 mg./kg.	q8–12h	q12–24h	q48–96h or longer††	Yes (H, P)
Kanamycin‡‡	7.5 mg./kg.	q12–24h	q24–60h	q60–96h or longer	Yes (H, P)
Polymyxin B	0.8 mg./kg.	q24h	q36–60h	q60–90h	No (H, P)
Streptomycin	7.5 mg./kg.	q24h	q24–72h	q72–96h	Yes (H, P)
Sulfadiazine	15–30 mg./kg.	q6h§§	Do not use		Yes (P)
Tetracycline‖‖	7.5 mg./kg. (give p.o. only)	q12h	q24–48h	q72–96h	Yes (H, P) Peritoneal dialysis may be variable

* Note: These dosage schedules should be viewed only as rough guides. Changing renal function and other factors influence serum levels. Assays should be used whenever possible, especially with the more toxic antibiotics. In addition, hepatic dysfunction further limits the dosages of ampicillin, carbenicillin, chloramphenicol and tetracycline.

† Serum creatinine levels.

‡ H = hemodialysis; P = peritoneal dialysis.

§ Manufacturer's precaution: Chloramphenicol is not recommended for intravenous or intramuscular pediatric use. Chloramphenicol sodium succinate has been approved for intravenous pediatric use.

‖ Small amounts may be removed by peritoneal dialysis.

** Can give unit dose each third half-life; half-life = 3.5 times the serum creatinine (in hours).

†† Can give unit dose q8h for two doses on first day in severe infections.

‡‡ Can give unit dose each third half-life; half-life = 3 times the serum creatinine (in hours).

§§ Maintain good urine output and keep serum levels between 8 and 15 mg./100 ml.

‖‖ Manufacturer's note: The use of tetracyclines during tooth development (last half of pregnancy, infancy and childhood to eight years) may cause permanent discoloration of teeth. This adverse reaction is more common during long-term use of the drugs but has been observed following repeated short-term courses.

sion of normal flora which otherwise might prevent establishment of potential pathogens. Therefore, whenever possible a "narrow spectrum" antibiotic, specifically active against the infecting organism, should be used rather than a "broad-spectrum" agent.

In addition to the judicious use of antimicrobial agents, the treatment of patients seriously ill with gram-negative infection demands attention to many other factors. Fluid and electrolyte balance must be maintained. Proper oxygenation must be ensured, and airway obstruction should be relieved. Urinary obstruction should be relieved, and when continuous catheter drainage is required, attention should be given to the use of a suitable closed drainage collection system to avoid infection or superinfection of the urinary tract. In many instances, continuous drainage with an indwelling catheter can be avoided by repeated intermittent catheterizations. Intermittent catheterization carries a much lower risk of urinary infection than does continuous drainage with an indwelling catheter. Abscesses, empyemas and other collections of purulent material should be aspirated and, if necessary, drained surgically. Accessible infected areas should be debrided of necrotic material. Patients with endocarditis should be observed for evidence of congestive cardiac failure; when indicated, treatment with digitalis preparations and diuretic drugs should be given.

When endotoxin shock is encountered in gram-negative infection, measures for the correction of the circulatory disturbances associated with this complication should be instituted. As a guide to this therapy, the introduction of a catheter for the measurement of central venous pressure is frequently invaluable. In addition to fluid administration to combat hypovolemia, drug therapy should be instituted to increase cardiac output and peripheral perfusion. On the basis of currently available information, isoproterenol appears to be the drug of choice for this purpose. When isoproterenol is used, central venous pressure measurement is mandatory to ensure the maintenance of an adequate circulating blood volume. The drug should be infused intravenously in an aqueous 5 per cent dextrose solution containing 10 micrograms of isoproterenol per ml. at an initial rate of 1 to 2.5 micrograms per minute. The rate may then be adjusted to obtain maximal therapeutic effect consistent with safe cardiac rate and absence of ventricular arrhythmias.

Therapy should be evaluated by the improvement in perfusion of vital organs rather than by the maintenance of any given blood pressure level. If perfusion of vital organs is not increased by the previously mentioned treatment, as judged by criteria such as failure to increase urine flow and to improve mental status, intravenous metaraminol or norepinephrine should be added to the treatment. The use of steroid therapy in endotoxin shock has been recommended by some authors, but improvement of survival rate has not been demonstrated, and the hazards attending such therapy must be considered.

The disseminated intravascular coagulation syndrome (consumption coagulopathy) is also a frequent accompaniment of endotoxin shock. The presence of ecchymoses, decreased platelets and a prolonged partial thromboplastin time is usually enough justification for the institution of heparin therapy.

Finally, consideration should be given to the prevention of gram-negative infection. Urinary tract catheterization should be avoided when possible and particularly the use of an indwelling urethral catheter. A well-designed closed urinary drainage collection system should be used with the indwelling urethral catheter to minimize the likelihood of introduction of infection into the urinary tract. In addition to urinary catheters, intravenous catheters and cannulas have been shown to be possible sources of systemic infection. Such devices should not be used longer than necessary, and when they are used for more than one day, the puncture or cutdown site should be redressed and inspected daily. Ideally, intravenous sites should be changed every 48 hours and scalp-vein needles are preferable to the larger intravenous catheters.

GRAM-NEGATIVE BACILLI OF RELATIVELY UNCOMMON CLINICAL OCCURRENCE

The organisms in this group, with suggested choices of antimicrobial drugs, are listed in Table 5. This group contains a number of organisms described previously under different generic and species designations (given in parentheses). The suggested choices of antimicrobial agents are culled largely from the literature and in many cases reflect extremely limited experience. They therefore must be regarded as guides to therapy and should be augmented by in vitro drug suspectibility tests and clinical observation. In the case of cholera, it is most likely that proper fluid and electrolyte management of patients contributes more to recovery than do antimicrobial drugs. Methods of administration and dosages of drugs are listed in Table 2.

TABLE 5. Selection of Antimicrobial Agents for the Treatment of Gram-Negative Infection of Relatively Uncommon Clinical Occurrence*

ORGANISM	DRUG	REMARKS
Acinetobacter anitratus *(Herellea vaginicola,* *Achromobacter anitratus)*	Kanamycin† Gentamicin† Polymyxin or colistin Nalidixic acid‡	
Acinetobacter lwoffi *(Mima polymorphia*—oxidase neg., *Achromobacter lwoffi*	Gentamicin† Kanamycin† Polymyxin or colistin Chloramphenicol§ Tetracycline‖ Nalidixic acid‡	
Actinobacillus actinomycetem- *comitans*	Tetracycline‖ Streptomycin Chloramphenicol§ ? Ampicillin ? Gentamicin† ? Kanamycin†	
Actinobacillus lignieresii	Kanamycin† ? Polymyxin or colistin	
Aeromonas hydrophila *Aeromonas shigelloides*	Gentamicin or kanamycin† Chloramphenicol§ Tetracycline‖ Polymixin or colistin	
Alcaligenes species	Chloramphenicol§ Cephalothin Ampicillin Gentamicin† Kanamycin† Carbenicillin Polymyxin or colistin Nalidixic acid‡	
Arizona	Chloramphenicol§ Kanamycin† ? Ampicillin ? Cephalothin ? Tetracycline	Available data inadequate—drug susceptibility tests important
Bartonella bacilliformis	Penicillin G Chloramphenicol§ Streptomycin Tetracycline‖	
Bordetella bronchiseptica	Tetracycline‖ Polymyxin or colistin Chloramphenicol§	
Calymmatobacterium granulomatis *(Donovonia granulomatis)*	Tetracycline‖ Streptomycin Chloramphenicol§	
Chromobacterium	Kanamycin or gentamicin† Tetracycline‖ Chloramphenicol§	
Citrobacter *(Escherichia freundii,* Bethesda-Ballerup)	Gentamicin† Polymyxin Kanamycin† Chloramphenicol§ Tetracycline‖ Carbenicillin Nalidixic acid‡ Nitrofurantoin‡**	

TABLE 5. Selection of Antimicrobial Agents for the Treatment of Gram-Negative Infection of Relatively Uncommon Clinical Occurrence*—Continued

ORGANISM	DRUG	REMARKS
Comamonas terrigena (*Pseudomonas terrigena*, *Lophomonas alcaligenes*)	Chloramphenicol§ Tetracycline‖	Available data inadequate—drug susceptibility tests important
Edwardsiella tarda	Chloramphenicol§ Tetracycline‖ Kanamycin† Ampicillin	
Enterobacter hafniae	Gentamicin† Kanamycin† Carbenicillin Tetracycline‖ Nalidixic acid‡	
Enterobacter liquefaciens	Gentamicin† Carbenicillin Kanamycin† Nalidixic acid‡	
Erwinia	Gentamicin† Chloramphenicol§ Colistin Kanamycin† Nalidixic acid‡	
Flavobacterium	Erythromycin Chloramphenicol§ ? Gentamicin† ? Carbenicillin Nalidixic acid‡	Much strain variation — drug susceptibility tests important
Hemophilus aphrophilus	Penicillin G Gentamicin† Cephalothin Chloramphenicol§ Tetracycline‖	
Klebsiella rhinoscleromatis	Streptomycin Tetracycline‖ Chloramphenicol§ Penicillin	Available data inadequate—drug susceptibility tests important
Moraxella kingii	Penicillin	Available data inadequate—drug susceptibility tests important
Moraxella lacunata (*Moraxella liquefaciens*)	Penicillin Ampicillin Chloramphenicol§ Tetracycline‖	
Moraxella nonliquefaciens, *Moraxella osloensis*, *Moraxella phenylpyrouvica* (*Mima polymorpha* var. *oxidans*)	Penicillin Ampicillin Cephalothin Chloramphenicol§ Gentamicin† Kanamycin† Nitrofurantoin‡** Nalidixic acid‡	
Pasteurella multocida (*Pasteurella septica*)	Penicillin B Kanamycin† Cephalothin Tetracycline‖ Chloramphenicol§	
Providence (*Proteus inconstans*)	Kanamycin† Carbenicillin Gentamicin† Nalidixic acid‡	

TABLE 5. Selection of Antimicrobial Agents for the Treatment of Gram-Negative Infection of Relatively Uncommon Clinical Occurrence*—Continued

ORGANISM	DRUG	REMARKS
Pseudomonas alcaligenes	Tetracycline‖ Gentamicin† Kanamycin† Polymyxin	
Pseudomonas cepacia *(Pseudomonas multivorans)* *(Pseudomonas kingii)*	Chloramphenicol§ Kanamycin† Nalidixic acid‡ Sulfonamides‡	
Pseudomonas fluorescens	Gentamicin† Kanamycin† Tetracycline‖ Polymyxin or colistin	
Pseudomonas maltophilia	Chloramphenicol§ Polymyxin or colistin Gentamicin† Kanamycin† Nalidixic acid‡	
Pseudomonas pseudomallei	Tetracycline‖†† Chloramphenicol§ Kanamycin† Sulfonamides Novobiocin ? Ampicillin ? Gentamicin†	Doxycycline and methacycline may be more active than tetracycline
Pseudomonas putida	Gentamicin† Kanamycin† Polymyxin or colistin Tetracycline‖	
Pseudomonas stutzeri	Gentamicin† Kanamycin† Polymyxin or colistin Ampicillin Carbenicillin Tetracycline‖ Nalidixic acid‡	
Vibrio cholerae	Tetracycline‖ Chloramphenicol§	Fluid and electrolyte management more important than specific antimicrobial therapy
Vibrio fetus	Tetracycline‖ Chloramphenicol§ Ampicillin Streptomycin Kanamycin† Erythromycin	
Vibrio parahaemolyticus	Gentamicin† Tetracycline‖ Erythromycin Ampicillin Cephalothin Chloramphenicol§ Kanamycin†	
Yersinia enterocolitica	Tetracycline‖ Chloramphenicol§ Streptomycin Kanamycin† Sulfonamides	

TABLE 5. Selection of Antimicrobial Agents for the Treatment of Gram-Negative Infection of Relatively Uncommon Clinical Occurrence*—Continued

ORGANISM	DRUG	REMARKS
Yersinia pseudotuberculosis (*Pasteurella pseudotuberculosis*)	Tetracycline‖ Streptomycin Chloramphenicol§ Kanamycin† Ampicillin Cephalothin	

* In most instances, drugs are listed in order of choice.

† Manufacturer's precaution: Intrathecal use is investigational.

‡ Urinary tract infection only.

§ Manufacturer's precaution: Chloramphenicol is not recommended for intravenous or intramuscular pediatric use. Chloramphenicol sodium succinate has been approved for intravenous pediatric use.

‖ Manufacturer's note: The use of tetracyclines during tooth development (last half of pregnancy, infancy and childhood to age eight years) may cause permanent discoloration of teeth. This adverse reaction is more common during long-term use of the drugs but has been observed following repeated short-term courses.

? Indicates strain variability or inadequate data.

** Manufacturer's precaution: Should not be given to infants under one month of age.

†† Single drug therapy is probably adequate for the pnemonic form of the disease. Combination therapy is recommended for the septicemic form of the disease but adequate data are not available to permit evaluation of this therapy.

Infections Due to Anaerobic Cocci and Gram-Negative Anaerobic Bacilli

SYDNEY M. FINEGOLD, M.D.

Special Bacteriologic Problems in Anaerobic Infection. In general, in anaerobic infections the bacteriologic results will not be available as quickly as in other bacterial diseases, particularly if the infection is mixed (as it is in two-thirds of cases). There are several other bacteriologic problems with regard to anaerobic infections which are of considerable importance to the clinician who is concerned with administering proper therapy. Some laboratories may fail to recover certain or all of the anaerobes present in a specimen. This is particularly true if the specimen is not put under anaerobic conditions very promptly (for transport to the laboratory). If care is not taken to avoid "contamination" of the specimen with normal flora, anaerobes may be recovered which have nothing to do with the patient's illness. For example, coughed sputum should not be submitted for anaerobic culture; a percutaneous transtracheal aspirate or lung puncture specimen must be obtained (unless an empyema is present). Not all laboratories are equipped to identify accurately anaerobes, and presumptive results may be very misleading. Finally, standardized disc susceptibility tests are not yet available for all anaerobic bacteria. Some laboratories have used a disc test without measurement of zones of inhibition or by applying the Kirby-Bauer-Sherris standards (which were developed for aerobic and facultative organisms); results obtained with these techniques are completely undependable. Conventional tube or plate dilution tests, with incubation in an anaerobic jar are satisfactory.

The Importance of *Bacteroides fragilis.* It is most important to note when *Bacteroides fragilis* may be involved in infection (this organism is recovered from infections more often than any other anaerobe) because it is more resistant to antimicrobials than is any other anaerobe and is the only commonly encountered anaerobe resistant to penicillin. *B. fragilis* is a predominant member of the normal bowel flora and is found in the female genital tract as well. It has been said that infections below the diaphragm should not be treated with penicillin because of the frequent involvement of *B. fragilis* in such infections, and that infections above the diaphragm may be treated effectively with penicillin. These guidelines are not always helpful in the individual case, particularly when the patient is quite ill and it is important that the antimicrobial therapy be appropriate from the beginning. *B. fragilis* is encountered frequently enough in pulmonary and in central nervous system infections that one should provide coverage for it unless the bacteriology is already well defined or the infection is not of great severity.

Specific Antimicrobial Agents for Anaerobic Infections. Table 1 lists the most useful drugs and their activity against various anaerobic bacteria; this should serve as a reliable guide when susceptibility results are not available. In seriously ill patients with suspected anaerobic infection but with inadequate bacteriologic data, chloramphenicol is presently the drug of choice. As indicated earlier, penicillin G is excellent except for *B. fragilis.* However, occasional strains of anaerobic cocci (Peptococcus) or streptococci (Peptostreptococcus) require as much as 8 units per ml. for inhibition. Other penicillins and cephalosporins are often less active against anaerobes than is penicillin G. In general, ampicillin and cephaloridine are roughly comparable to penicillin G in activity against these organisms. Tetracycline, once the drug of choice for anaerobic infections, is no longer satisfactory for use without prior susceptibility testing because many different anaerobes have become resistant. Two-thirds of *B. fragilis* isolates in many institutions are resistant currently. Preliminary data indicate that doxycycline and minocycline are much more active against *B. fragilis* and other anaerobes than is tetracycline. Three other agents are effective for treatment of anaerobic infection: lincomycin, clindamycin and metronidazole. Clindamycin is better than lincomycin in this regard; the anaerobes most commonly resistant to clindamycin are *Fusobacterium (Sphaerophorus) varium* (and strains of certain species of clostridia other than *C. perfringens*). Metronidazole is also very active against most anaerobes (the major exception being certain of the cocci, particularly those that are microaerophilic), but there is much less clinical experience with this compound in systemic anaerobic infections than with clindamycin. Rifampin is also very active against most anaerobes in vitro but has not been studied clinically; development of resistance would most likely be a problem. Metronidazole, lincomycin, erythromycin, vancomycin and rifampin are not yet approved by the Food and Drug Administration for anaerobic infections.

When the infecting organism is susceptible and the patient is not hypersensitive, penicillin G is the drug of choice for these infections, particularly when bactericidal activity may be important, as in subacute bacterial endocarditis. Daily intramuscular or intravenous dosage of 30,000 to 60,000 units per kilogram given in four to six doses is adequate for most suscep-

TABLE 1. Susceptibility of Nonsporulating Anaerobes to Antimicrobial Agents

	MICROAEROPHILIC AND ANAEROBIC COCCI	*BACTEROIDES FRAGILIS*	*BACTEROIDES MELANINOGENICUS*	*FUSOBACTERIUM VARIUM*	*OTHER FUSOBACTERIUM SPECIES*	*EUBACTERIUM AND ACTINOMYCES*
Penicillin G	++++	+	++++	+++*	++++	++++
Lincomycin§‖	+++	+ to ++	+++	++	+++	++ to +++
Clindamycin	+++	+++	+++	++	+++	+++*
Metronidazole§	++	+++	+++	+++	+++	?
Tetracycline**	++	+ to ++	+++	++	++ to +++	++
Chloramphenicol	+++	+++	+++	+++	+++	+++
Erythromycin§	++ to +++	+ to ++	++	+	+	++ to +++
Vancomycin§	++ to +++	+	+	+	+	?+++

++++ Drug of choice
+++ Good activity
++ Moderate activity
+ Poor or inconsistent activity

* Few strains resistant.
§ Use in anaerobic infections not yet approved by F.D.A.
‖ Not indicated in the newborn up to one month of age.
** Manufacturer's note: The use of tetracyclines during tooth development (last half of pregnancy, infancy and childhood to age eight years) may cause permanent discoloration of teeth. This adverse reaction is more common during long-term use of the drug but has been observed following repeated short-term courses.

tible infections, but certain strains of anaerobic cocci in particular and certain types of infection (brain abscess, endocarditis) may require 150,000 to 300,000 units or more per kilogram per day intravenously.

Chloramphenicol is given in a dosage of 25 to 50 mg. per kilogram per day orally at 6-hour intervals. Intravenously, the succinate salt is used as a 10 per cent solution in a small volume of isotonic saline or 5 per cent dextrose, so that each dose (given at 6- or 8-hour intervals) may be run in over a 30-minute period. Smaller doses may be indicated for premature and neonatal patients because of the hazard of the "gray syndrome." Chloramphenicol should not be used intramuscularly. Patients should also be observed carefully for possible bone marrow depression; complete blood cell counts should be obtained once or twice weekly, and periodic serum iron and reticulocyte counts may be useful in indicating toxicity early.

Lincomycin may be given to children over one month of age orally in doses of 30 to 60 mg. per kilogram per day, divided into three or four equal doses, and intramuscularly or intravenously in a dosage of 10 to 80 mg. per kilogram per day in two or three doses. For intravenous administration, lincomycin should be added to 250 ml. or more of 5 per cent dextrose in water or normal saline and given as a slow infusion. The most common side effects of lincomycin therapy are diarrhea and other gastrointestinal symptoms, and rash or urticaria. Neutropenia and abnormalities in liver function tests are seen rarely. Because lincomycin has a profound effect on anaerobes in the normal intestinal flora, one must be alert to the possibility of enterocolitis due to lincomycin-resistant *Staphylococcus aureus.*

Clindamycin is preferable to lincomycin because of distinctly greater activity against anaerobes and fewer side effects. Dosage is 8 to 20 mg. per kilogram per day, divided into three or four equal doses. Parenterally, clindamycin may be given either intramuscularly or intravenously in a dosage of 10 to 40 mg. per kilogram per day in three to four equal doses.

Tetracycline, intravenously, should be administered in a dosage of 20 mg. per kilogram per day, divided into two or three doses given every 8 to 12 hours (or by continuous drip throughout the day).* Each dose of the drug should be diluted to at least 100 ml. and administered by slow drip over all or most of the 8- or 12-hour periods; do not administer tetracycline with blood or with solutions containing calcium. When feasible, switch to oral therapy, using a daily dose of 25 to 30 mg. per kilogram divided into four doses given every 6 hours. Do not use milk or antacids containing calcium or aluminum to minimize intestinal side effects of tetracycline therapy, because calcium, aluminum and magnesium inactivate the antibiotic. Tetracycline should not be given, particularly by the intravenous route, to patients with impaired renal or hepatic function if other suitable drugs are available.

Erythromycin may be given orally or intravenously in a daily dosage of 30 to 40 mg. per kilogram divided into four doses. The most common side effect is diarrhea; nausea and vomiting occur less frequently. Intrahepatic cholestasis is seen occasionally with the estolate derivative of erythromycin.

Other Factors Influencing Choice of Chemotherapy. As in the therapy of other types of infections, other factors will influence the choice of drugs: the toxicity of chloramphenicol, whether the patient is allergic to penicillin, the poor spinal fluid levels achieved with clindamycin, the excellent bactericidal activity of metronidazole against *B. fragilis,* the lack of a parenteral preparation of metronidazole, the renal and hepatic functional status of the patient and so forth. Certain antimicrobial agents, such as the aminoglycosides, are so inactive against anaerobes that they predispose the patient to superinfection with these organisms.

The nature of other organisms in a mixed infection will also influence the choice of drugs. In general, antimicrobial therapy for anaerobic infections requires high dosage and prolonged treatment because of the prominent tissue necrosis and the marked tendency for relapse.

Adjunctive Therapy. Adjunctive therapy is extremely important in the proper management of infections due to anaerobes. Drainage of collections of pus and excision of necrotic tissue are often necessary and in minor infections are all that is required. Septic phlebitis occurs in some patients, and if pulmonary emboli result, anticoagulant therapy or venous ligation may be indicated.

Local use of hydrogen peroxide or zinc peroxide is occasionally helpful. In rare situations, notably when débridement is not feasible, hyperbaric oxygen therapy might prove beneficial.

---

* Manufacturer's note: The use of tetracycline during tooth development (last half of pregnancy, infancy and childhood to age eight years) may cause permanent discoloration of teeth. This adverse reaction is more common during long-term use of the drug but has been observed following repeated short-term courses.

Hemophilus Influenzae Infections

PAUL F. WEHRLE, M.D.

Hemophilus influenzae organisms occur most frequently as silent unrecognized infections of the upper respiratory tract of normal children and adults. They are found in a rough unencapsulated untypeable form and as one of six recognized smooth encapsulated serotypes. These serotypes include type B, which is responsible for virtually all cases of meningitis and the majority of the invasive forms of the disease. *H. influenzae* type B is the most common cause of acute bacterial meningitis in childhood, and is responsible for many episodes of acute bacterial sepsis involving other organs. Although it may produce a primary nasopharyngitis in susceptible children, it is likely that most of these episodes reflect preceding or concomitant viral infections. Direct extension of the infection may involve the paranasal sinuses, middle ear, epiglottis and lower respiratory tract. From many of these areas, hematogenous spread may occur and involve meninges, joints, subcutaneous tissues and, rarely, bones or pericardium.

Since virtually all invasive disease due to *H. influenzae* is caused by type B organisms, and since these are almost invariably susceptible to ampicillin, chloramphenicol and tetracycline, one of these agents is the preferred method of antimicrobial therapy. Due to the effectiveness and lack of toxicity, ampicillin is the preferred drug. Patients allergic to the penicillins and under eight years of age should be treated with chloramphenicol. Tetracycline should be administered only to individuals over eight years of age, since dental enamel hypoplasia and discoloration are clearly associated with the use of this antibiotic in infancy and early childhood.

ACUTE BACTERIAL MENINGITIS

As noted, *H. influenzae* is the most common cause of acute bacterial meningitis in childhood. Although occasional cases are seen during the neonatal period, the peak incidence is at one year of age. The frequency declines rapidly with increasing age, and only about 5 per cent of the cases occur among children over 10 years of age and among adults.

Meningeal infections should be regarded as true medical emergencies. In older infants and children the symptoms and signs can usually be recognized without difficulty. Fever, headache and vomiting, together with the customary signs of meningeal irritation, are usually the presenting complaints. If meningitis is suspected, examination of spinal fluid should be performed promptly. If organisms consistent with *H. influenzae* are seen on the Gram stain, or if this infection is suspected in the absence of such organisms, antimicrobial therapy should be promptly initiated. An initial intravenous dose of 50 mg. per kilogram of ampicillin should be administered. This should be followed by at least 150 mg. of ampicillin per kilogram per day given in six divided doses by intermittent intravenous infusion at 4-hour intervals. The use of the intravenous route ensures that the drug is actually being absorbed and that inactivation within the intravenous administration system is avoided. In addition, large doses of the penicillins given intramuscularly are at times followed by subcutaneous fat atrophy, even when the injection has been intended to be deep in the muscular tissue.

When there is strong reason to believe that penicillin cannot be tolerated, chloramphenicol* is an acceptable substitute for the treatment of *H. influenzae* meningitis. This should be administered in doses of 100 mg. per kilogram per day, with reduction of the dose to 50 mg. per kilogram per day after response has been assured. In newborn infants, chloramphenicol dosage should not exceed 25 mg. per kilogram per day given in four divided doses at equal intervals. If chloramphenicol is used, careful monitoring for signs of toxicity should be carried out.

Intrathecal administration of antibiotics is unnecessary for the management of *H. influenzae* meningeal infections.

Supportive therapy is an essential feature of treatment, since death can occur before antimicrobial therapy can produce its desired effect. The problems that require the greatest attention are shock, acute cerebral edema and maintenance of the airway.

Blood pressure must be monitored carefully. If difficulty is encountered in maintenance of blood pressure after proper hydration, an indwelling central venous catheter should be inserted. With such monitoring, the rapid infusion of fluids (saline, albumin or blood) will usually restore the effective arterial circulation. If central venous pressure increases without concomitant improvement of circula-

* Manufacturer's precaution: Chloramphenicol is not recommended for intravenous or intramuscular pediatric use. Chloramphenicol sodium succinate has been approved for intravenous pediatric use.

tion, isoproterenol may be used to improve circulatory status.

Pharmacologic doses of hydrocortisone or other glucocorticoids have been advocated by some, and data are available indicating their effect in restoring arterial circulation. As yet, however, data indicating increased survival after administering these drugs are not available. The frequent occurrence of stress ulcers of the gastrointestinal tract and superinfection suggests caution in their use. Disseminated intravascular coagulation occurs both in meningoccemia and in pneumococcal sepsis but is seldom seen in *H. influenzae* forms of meningitis. Heparin will reduce the clotting defect, but has not yet been shown to improve the frequency of survival.

Acute cerebral edema of severe degree can be expected to occur in approximately 2 per cent of *H. influenzae* meningitis patients and usually accompanies the fulminant form of the disease. Mannitol† or urea given by relatively rapid infusion in full therapeutic doses for diuresis has been helpful, although attention should be given to possible electrolyte imbalance following the diuresis.

Tracheostomy or assisted ventilation (or both) may be required in those patients with respiratory depression. The irregular "meningitic" form of breathing can be expected in some patients but is not in itself an indication for assisted respiration.

Monitoring the Effects of Therapy. Patients with severe disease present special problems in management and may require additional diagnostic measurements for effective monitoring.

It is helpful to examine the spinal fluid between 24 to 36 hours after initiation of antimicrobial therapy. The spinal fluid sediment at this time should not yield demonstrable microorganisms, and culture should be negative. Although the white cell count and protein levels may be increased over the initial values, the spinal fluid glucose concentration should be greater than that observed initially, provided effective therapy has been given and the organisms are susceptible to the antibiotic selected. Should fever recur during the course of therapy or should there be signs of delayed resolution or exacerbation of the meningeal symptoms, the clinician should not hesitate to repeat the spinal fluid examination.

With the exception of early infancy, when therapy is continued for a minimum of three weeks, treatment is continued until the patient has been afebrile for at least five days. At that time, a final spinal fluid examination should be performed. If the cell count is found to be less than 30 cells, if the glucose levels are normal (approximately two-thirds of blood sugar levels), if the protein concentration is approaching normal and if no microorganisms are seen, therapy may be discontinued. It is appropriate to observe the patient for an additional two days after therapy has been stopped, since relapses are occasionally seen in *H. influenzae* meningitis.

When the criteria for discontinuance of therapy are not met, the patient should be carefully reevaluated, since there may be mastoiditis, subdural effusion, brain abscess or other sites of continued infection. Approximately 10 per cent of infants with *H. influenzae* meningitis can be expected to develop subdural effusions. If subdural effusion is present, daily subdural taps should be instituted, removing up to 25 ml. of fluid daily from each side and permitting the fluid to drip into a tube. Syringe aspiration should not be done. Surgical intervention is indicated for those patients in whom fluid continues to form over a period of three weeks of daily taps and observation. These individuals represent less than 1 per cent of the total cases seen.

Fever persisting after the first three or four days of treatment is often associated with subdural effusion. Other causes include improper or inadequate antimicrobial therapy; phlebitis occurring at the site of intravenous infusions; local or cerebral abscesses; localized infections associated with urethral catheters, tracheostomy tubes or other foreign objects; mastoiditis or sinusitis; and drug fevers. When fever does persist, the patient should be carefully evaluated with these possibilities in mind.

Rehabilitation. During convalescence, careful evaluation must be made of motor, sensory and intellectual function. Despite effective therapy, deafness or other sensory organ deficits and motor or intellectual impairment may follow meningitis. These sequelae are often readily demonstrable during convalescence, although if relatively mild in degree, careful evaluation during subsequent months may be required to identify the defect. Proper corrective measures for such defects must be instituted and are part of the total care of the patient.

Prophylaxis for Household Contacts. Second cases of *H. influenzae* meningitis in fami-

---

† Manufacturer's precaution: Use of mannitol in pediatric patients has not been studied comprehensively.

lies occasionally occur, and parents should be asked to watch other children for signs of fever and listlessness. When identified, the patient should be evaluated and treated promptly. Since second cases of *H. influenzae* in family associates are extremely infrequent, there is no need for prophylactic antimicrobial therapy among household associates, even young children.

Prevention. Although a vaccine is currently under evaluation for the prevention of *H. influenzae* type B infections, it is not likely to be available for use in the near future.

ACUTE EPIGLOTTITIS (SUPRAGLOTTITIS)

Epiglottitis is an acute life-threatening emergency occurring most frequently between the ages of two and seven years. It should be suspected in any febrile, acutely ill child with upper airway obstruction. Audible stridor may be absent. If this condition is suspected, preparation should be made for an emergency tracheostomy prior to examination of the pharynx. If the epiglottis is found to be inflamed and edematous, a tracheostomy is recommended, and blood and pharyngeal cultures should be obtained. Therapy should be instituted with either ampicillin, chloramphenicol or tetracycline. Ampicillin therapy is preferred.

OTITIS MEDIA

Among the bacterial causes of otitis media occurring among infants and young children, *H. influenzae* ranks second in frequency to the pneumococcus. The inflammation tends to be less intense than that seen with pneumococcal infection. Otitis media may be treated with oral ampicillin in doses of at least 100 mg. per kilogram per day given in four divided doses.

OTHER CONDITIONS

Osteomyelitis and *septic arthritis* are sometimes due to *H. influenzae*. These require orthopedic consultation and, sometimes, surgical drainage. Antimicrobial therapy is identical to that for acute meningitis and should be continued for a minimum of three weeks.

Cellulitis, pneumonitis and *sinusitis* due to *H. influenzae* can be expected to respond promptly to ampicillin. In sinusitis, appropriate drainage should be assured if the infection is to be eradicated.

Alternative antibiotics to ampicillin which are effective against *H. influenzae* in diseases other than meningitis and osteomyelitis include chloramphenicol, tetracycline and erythromycin. Chloramphenicol is well absorbed and reaches adequate tissue levels. It should be used only in serious situations when the other drugs cannot be employed with equal effect.

Tetanus

GEORGE H. McCRACKEN, Jr., M.D., *and*
FLORENCE N. MARSHALL, M.D.

Tetanus in the United States is a disease of slowly declining incidence; approximately 100 cases are reported annually for an incidence rate of 0.13 per 100,000 population. Peak incidence occurs in newborn infants and in the elderly, and the case-fatality ratios are maximal also at the extremes of age. On the other hand, tetanus is a common disease in certain areas of the world, particularly in underdeveloped countries where the disease accounts for considerable morbidity and mortality in neonates and young children. The social, economic and medical problems operative in these countries are unique and so different from those in the United States that consideration of therapy in this section will be limited to the disease as encountered in the United States only.

Treatment. Since tetanus is encountered infrequently in the United States, very few physicians or medical center personnel have extensive experience with the disease. The main clinical findings which should lead to the suspicion of tetanus are trismus, generalized rigidity and intermittent seizures. There is no loss of consciousness. Other conditions to be ruled out are meningitis, intracranial hemorrhage, tetany, bizarre forms of epilepsy, oropharyngeal abscess or tumor, rabies, strychnine poisoning and phenothiazine reactions. A detailed history should be obtained in order to determine the possible mode of infection, the approximate incubation period and the duration of symptoms. These data have epidemiologic and prognostic implications.

Once the diagnosis is suspected or proved, the patient should be transferred to a medical center equipped with intensive care facilities. The optimal care of tetanus, particularly in the newborn infant, requires a coordinated effort by medical, nursing and anesthesiology personnel.

Airway and Ventilation. Recurrent laryngospasms or accumulation of excessive secretions in the oro- and hypopharynx may require special attention to maintaining a patent airway. In the older child, excessive secretions may be controlled by gentle, repeated oral and nasopharyngeal suctioning and elevation of the foot of the bed.

In neonates and young children it is frequently necessary to maintain the airway by nasotracheal intubation. Employment of such a tube requires fastidious nursing care: i.e., saline, 1 ml., suctioning, and sighing (hyperinflation) every hour and as necessary to prevent obstruction with secretions. Care must be taken to humidify totally the inspired gases. Generally such tubes are changed on a routine basis every week so that alternate nostrils are used. The size of tube employed should be approximately 0.5 mm. smaller in diameter than can be maximally placed. The neonate should be placed in either an open or closed incubator in order to maintain a constant environmental temperature and supply of oxygen, if necessary. Vital signs should be monitored and determination of blood gas values is frequently helpful in evaluating the respiratory status.

In patients requiring heavy sedation or neuromuscular blockade, nasotracheal intubation or tracheostomy is necessary to supply assisted ventilation by means of a positive pressure apparatus. Because of the stimulatory effects of the nasotracheal tube, its use should be carefully considered. Tracheostomy carries hazards in the neonate and small child and it should never be a routine procedure.

CARE OF LOCAL WOUND. The umbilicus is the usual site of infection in neonates, and puncture wounds and lacerations account for the majority of infected lesions in older infants and children. Wounds suspected of infection should be cultured for *Clostridium tetani* and other pathogens. Omphalitis is frequently observed in neonates and may be due to streptococci, staphylococci or enteric bacteria.

The infected umbilical stump is treated by débridement and cleansing with an antibacterial soap suspension, such as 3 per cent hexachlorophene, followed by a dilute solution of hydrogen peroxide. This should be repeated several times during the first 48 hours.

Puncture wounds or deep infected lacerations should be exposed and debrided. Washing and cleansing as specified above are helpful in removing debris. The wound should be kept open and dry.

The local instillation of tetanus antitoxin around suspected wounds has never been proved effective and should not be employed. Parenteral penicillin therapy is usually effective in eradicating the vegetative phase of the tetanus bacillus and is used as a supplement to local therapy. Omphalitis or cellulitis around infected wounds should be treated as indicated by the culture and susceptibility studies of the offending pathogen.

ANTITOXIN THERAPY. The primary goal of antitoxin therapy is to neutralize toxin not yet bound to nervous tissue. It has no immediate curative action. The efficacy of antitoxin therapy in tetanus has been questioned, particularly in mild cases of the disease. However, until evidence clearly indicates otherwise, antitoxin should be administered to all patients with tetanus.

There are two antitoxin materials commercially available: homologous tetanus antitoxin (human tetanus immune globulin) and heterologous tetanus antitoxin (equine or bovine). Although the equine material has been used more extensively, the human immune globulin is clearly the preferred therapeutic agent because it is not associated with serum sickness and anaphylactic reactions and because it has greater persistence in serum.

Recent studies at the Hôpital Albert Schweitzer in the Artibonite Valley of central Haiti have demonstrated the comparative efficacy of 500 units of tetanus immune globulin (human) and 10,000 units of equine antitoxin in the treatment of tetanus neonatorum. Additional studies have shown that 500 and 1500 units of tetanus immune globulin are equally efficacious in the neonatal form of the disease.

Based on these data, we currently recommend 500 units of tetanus immune globulin (human) administered intramuscularly for the treatment of tetanus neonatorum. The proper dosage of tetanus immune globulin in older infants and children is unknown, but approximately 200 units per kilogram of body weight (to a total of 2000 to 6000 units) appear adequate. The intravenous route should not be used and it is not necessary to skin test the patient prior to administration.

In those areas outside the United States where it is not feasible to use this preparation because of cost and lack of availability, 10,000 units of tetanus antitoxin of equine origin is adequate. Larger doses are unnecessary and may be associated with increased morbidity. This preparation may be administered intravenously or intramuscularly. Patients beyond the neonatal period should be tested for dermal hypersensitivity to the preparation and closely observed after administration for signs of systemic reactions.

Several points deserve reemphasis: (1) There is no reason to use the more toxic and shorter-lived equine preparation in the treatment of tetanus in the United States. (2) Local instillation of antitoxin around the site of infection is unnecessary. (3) Antitoxin does not reverse the effects of toxin already bound in the central nervous system.

SEDATIVE-RELAXANT THERAPY. The primary purposes of sedative and relaxant therapy are to prevent convulsions and to minimize muscle spasm. While receiving therapy, the patient should remain responsive to ordinary stimuli without developing convulsions or significant clonus, and respiration should not be depressed. The success of any specific therapeutic regimen is dependent in part on the experience of the physician and anesthesiologist, adequacy and number of nursing personnel and the ready availability of proper, functioning emergency equipment. Treatment in a well-equipped and staffed intensive care unit, the availability of an experienced anesthesiologist and constant observation cannot be overemphasized in the management of tetanus in pediatric patients, particularly in neonates.

A number of sedatives and tranquilizers have been used alone and in combination in the treatment of tetanus. These include the various barbiturates, particularly phenobarbital and pentobarbital, the phenothiazines, diazepam, chloral hydrate and paraldehyde. In general, phenobarbital alone is a safe and effective sedative for the control of spasms and convulsions in mild and some cases of moderately severe tetanus. The dose of phenobarbital is 2 to 7 mg. per kilogram of body weight administered every 4 to 6 hours according to individual needs. It is preferable to administer this drug orally if possible; otherwise, the intravenous route is preferred over repeated intramuscular doses. If severe seizures occur during phenobarbital therapy, 10 to 15 mg. of pentobarbital for neonates and 20 to 30 mg. for older infants and children may be administered intravenously or orally, as indicated. As the frequency and severity of seizures diminish, the dose of phenobarbital is decreased.

Chlorpromazine,* a phenothiazine, has been used alone and, more frequently, in combination with phenobarbital to control muscle spasms and seizure activity in patients with tetanus. The drug is employed in a dosage of 0.2 to 0.5 mg. per kilogram of body weight administered every 6 hours, preferably by the oral route. The combined use of chlorpromazine and phenobarbital is particularly useful in patients with moderate to severe tetanus.

Diazepam (Valium) has been used successfully in the management of some patients with tetanus. When used alone in mild tetanus, the drug has a sedative and muscle relaxant effect. Doses of 2 to 10 mg. may be used, and the drug can be administered orally, intramuscularly or intravenously.† When combined with phenobarbital or chlorpromazine, seizure activity and muscle spasm of patients with moderate to severe tetanus may be controlled. The dose of phenobarbital should be reduced when used in combination with diazepam.

Mephenesin (Tolserol) and methocarbamol (Robaxin) have been used with variable success in patients with tetanus. They are thought to achieve muscle relaxation by central depression of external stimuli. Triple therapy with phenobarbital, a phenothiazine and a muscle relaxant has been used successfully in tetanus neonatorum.

Patients with severe tetanus and those not responding to the above regimens may require neuromuscular blockade with curare-like agents. If tubocurarine is used, a dosage of 0.2 to 0.3 mg. per kilogram, administered intravenously, may be repeated as often as every 1 to 2 hours when muscle spasms interfere with adequate ventilation. When this routine is followed closely, the course of the disease can be assessed by the curare requirements. Therapy with these drugs requires intermittent positive pressure respiration by way of nasotracheal intubation of tracheostomy, and constant supervision by trained personnel. Patients treated by neuromuscular blocking agents should be cared for in intensive care units under the direct supervision of an anesthesiologist. Sedation with phenobarbital or intermittent doses of diazepam are usually required to control seizure activity during the early phase of therapy.

Although a darkened, quiet area has been stressed in the management of tetanus patients, this appears to be far less important in controlling muscle spasms and seizure activity than the regulation of vibratory stimuli and excessive handling of patients. Indeed, a well-illuminated area allows better observation and care.

ANTIBIOTIC THERAPY. The primary aim of antimicrobial therapy is the eradication of tetanus bacilli from the focus of infection. Penicillin G is effective against the vegetative form

* Manufacturer's precaution: Chlorpromazine is not recommended for children under six months of age except when lifesaving.

† Injectable diazepam (valium) in studies in vitro has been shown to be capable of displacing bilirubin from albumin as a result of the action of its sodium benzoate preservative. Thus, injectable preparations of diazepam should probably be avoided in the neonate, and used with caution in other infants and children who have elevated serum bilirubin levels. *Note:* Manufacturer's precaution: safety and efficacy of injectable Valium in children under 12 years of age have not been established. Oral Valium is not for use in children under six months of age.

of the organism and is therefore the drug of choice in the newborn and young infants. The tetracyclines are a suitable alternative but should not be given in infancy and early childhood (up to eight years of age) because of their adverse effects on dentition and bone growth. Buffered penicillin G is administered intravenously to neonates and young infants in a daily dosage of 50,000 units per kilogram of body weight. Intramuscular injections of procaine penicillin G once daily are satisfactory when there is no reason for an intravenous infusion, but may stimulate the patient to have a seizure. Therapy should be continued five to seven days.

MANAGEMENT OF FLUID AND CALORIC INTAKE. The maintenance of fluid, electrolyte and pH balance, and caloric intake are very important in patients with tetanus. In general, oral or nasogastric feeding should be attempted whenever possible. This is usually feasible in patients with mild to moderately severe tetanus. The advantages of these feedings are as follows: (1) provision of adequate calories, (2) provision of a route of administering sedatives and relaxant drugs and (3) minimization of the chance of peptic ulceration, which can complicate the course in some tetanus patients. Nasogastric feedings are particularly useful in tetanus neonatorum. Oral and nasogastric feedings must be carried out with extreme care by experienced nursing personnel to avoid aspiration of the feeding mixtures or stomach contents and precipitation of seizures and/or muscle spasms. The nasogastric tube should be removed and changed daily.

Patients with severe tetanus or with recurrent laryngospasms should not be fed orally or by way of nasogastric tube until properly controlled with medication. Intravenous fluids containing maintenance electrolytes and 5 per cent glucose are satisfactory for several days. Intravenous alimentation may be indicated in patients with evidence of undernutrition and in those unable to tolerate nasogastric or oral feedings. This form of alimentation must be under the supervision of trained personnel and an experienced dietitian. Gastrostomy has proved useful in older children and is not a complicated procedure.

COMPLICATIONS. The most common complications of tetanus in neonates and young children are pulmonary problems; skin infections such as omphalitis, cellulitis or abscess formation around wounds; gastrointestinal bleeding from peptic ulceration; and septicemia. Pulmonary complications may result from mucous plugs which partially block a bronchus, resulting in atelectasis and infection distally; problems related to intubation or tracheostomy; aspiration of oral or nasogastric feedings; or laryngospasm, which may precipitate or be aggravated by the other pulmonary problems. Adequate humidification, gentle suctioning of secretions, sighing the patient, routine changing of the nasotracheal tube, proper aseptic technique in the use of the respiratory equipment, care in feeding and handling patients and judicious use of antimicrobial therapy will minimize these complications.

TETANUS PROPHYLAXIS

Active Prophylaxis Against Tetanus. Complete primary immunization with tetanus toxoid provides long-lasting protective antitoxin levels. Augmentation of immunity is rapid following a booster dose in persons who have previously received at least two doses of tetanus toxoid. The preferred form of toxoid is the adsorbed or alum-precipitated preparation.

The Committee on Infectious Diseases, the American Academy of Pediatrics and the Public Health Service Advisory Committee on Immunization Practices currently recommend the following immunization schedule for tetanus prophylaxis: Primary immunization in infants and children up to six years of age consists of four doses of combined vaccine (diphtheria and tetanus toxoids and pertussis bacterial vaccine), administered intramuscularly at four- to six-week intervals for the first three doses, and with a one-year interval between the third and fourth doses. Ideally, immunization should be initiated at two to three months of age. Older children and adults should receive three doses of tetanus and diphtheria toxoid, adult type, given intramuscularly with a four- to six-week interval between the first and second doses, and a 6- to 12-month interval between the second and third doses. Immunization of women in the child-bearing years is the only sure way of preventing tetanus in newborn infants in areas where good obstetric or midwifery care is not available.

Booster doses of diphtheria-pertussis-tetanus vaccine should be given to children four to six years of age (usually at the time of entrance into school). Thereafter, and for all other persons, a booster of diphtheria and tetanus toxoid (adult type) should be given at 10-year intervals, unless tetanus toxoid alone is administered as part of wound management (see below). There is no need to administer booster doses of toxoid every three to five years as has been the routine, or prophylactically prior to camping trips and the like. Indeed, there is evidence that overimmunization may be associated with an increased incidence and severity of reactions.

Passive Prophylaxis. Passive prophylaxis with tetanus antitoxin should be considered in a patient who has had less than two previous immunizations with toxoid, and whose wound is considered "tetanus-prone" and has been unattended for more than 24 hours. The value of passive immunity is the immediate but transient conferral of protection.

Tetanus immune globulin (human) should be the only antitoxin used in prophylaxis because of its longer half-life in serum and freedom from adverse reactions. The currently recommended prophylactic dose of tetanus immune globulin is 5 to 10 units per kilogram of body weight, up to a maximum dose of 250 mg., for wounds of mild to moderate severity. Should the human preparation be unavailable, equine antitoxin may be used in a dose of 3000 to 5000 units; doses of over 10,000 units are excessive and unwarranted. Careful screening for sensitivity must precede administration of the equine antitoxin and the patient should be followed carefully for development of serious adverse reactions.

Wound Management. The primary purpose of wound management is to prevent tissue necrosis and secondary infection which provide a milieu for growth of *Clostridium tetani.* Thorough cleansing and surgical débridement should be carried out. Disinfection with topical antibiotics should not be relied upon. Procaine penicillin or tetracycline may be used for contaminated wounds and administered for five days.

The following table is a guide to tetanus prophylaxis in wound management.§ Combined tetanus-diphtheria toxoid (Td) is used for active immunization, and tetanus immune globulin (TIG) is used for passive immunization.

HISTORY OF TETANUS IMMUNIZATION	CLEAN, MINOR WOUNDS		ALL OTHER WOUNDS	
(Doses)	*Td*	*TIG*	*Td*	*TIG*
Uncertain	Yes	No	Yes	Yes
0–1	Yes	No	Yes	Yes
2	Yes	No	Yes	No*
3 or more	No†	No	No‡	No

* Unless wound more than 24 hours old.
† Unless more than 10 years since last dose.
‡ Unless more than five years since last dose.

§ Recommendations of the United States Public Health Service Advisory Committee on Immunization Practices. *Morbidity and Mortality Weekly Report,* Vol. 21, No. 25, 1972.

The concurrent administration of toxoid and antitoxin at separate sites provides adequate immediate protection and initiation of active immunity. The adsorbed or alum-precipitated toxoid (not fluid toxoid) should always be used. Additional doses of toxoid should be given to patients with histories of inadequate previous immunization.

Shigellosis

KENNETH C. HALTALIN, M.D.

Shigellosis occurs acutely in three clinical forms: simple diarrhea, dysentery and a toxic form in which central nervous system symptoms predominate. The approach to treatment varies with the clinical expression of disease.

Fluid and Electrolyte Therapy. Replacement of water and electrolyte losses and subsequent maintenance of optimal hydration are the most important aspects of treatment. Details of fluid and electrolyte therapy are described elsewhere. Patients with diarrhea but without dehydration or systemic toxicity can be managed as outpatients with oral alimentation. Clear liquids may be used for this purpose: plain water, glucose water, ginger ale or 7-Up, and clear apple juice are well accepted by younger infants. Carbonated beverages should be "defizzed" by shaking the bottle. Older infants and children may prefer clear soups and weak tea solutions with added sugar. The practice of prescribing homemade salt solutions is to be condemned because the chance of inducing hypertonicity through error in preparation is too great. After 12 to 24 hours, a more substantial oral intake can usually be permitted. One-half strength formula is suitable, plus bland solids, such as apple sauce, rice cereal and bananas.

Patients with clinical signs of dehydration require intravenous fluid and electrolyte therapy. It is essential to keep pace with the continuing bowel losses in patients with dysentery, since fluid and electrolyte deficits may be massive. Oral intake should be resumed as promptly as possible. It is unwise to prolong intravenous fluid therapy unduly at the expense of an adequate oral intake. Oral feedings of clear liquids can usually be started in 24 hours, and half-strength formula and bland solid foods can be started in 48 hours. Shock is usually due to fluid loss, but it is seen rarely in the absence of apparently significant dehydration. If patients do not respond promptly to the usual intravenous infusions, transfusions of whole blood, plasma or plasma expanders should be used.

Antimicrobial Therapy. To be effective against shigellosis, an antimicrobial agent must satisfy two criteria: the organism must be susceptible in vitro and therapeutic concentrations of drug must be attained in the serum and bowel wall. Ampicillin has been shown to be effective for severe shigellosis and also for milder disease provided that the infecting strain is susceptible. In some areas, notably those where shigellosis is usually due to *S. sonnei,* the incidence of ampicillin-resistance is so high that ampicillin is of limited value. It should be stressed that organisms resistant to ampicillin are often also resistant to other agents of proved efficacy. For this reason it is wise to determine the in vitro susceptibility of each patient's strain and to be aware of the current antibiotic susceptibility patterns in a given area.

The dose of ampicillin is 100 mg. per kilogram per day divided into 6-hour doses for five days (a total of 20 doses). It is effective by the oral, intravenous and intramuscular routes of administration.

The intravenous route is preferred for initiation of therapy in patients who are excessively toxic or who are not able to take and retain oral medication. Ampicillin should be added to the calibrated chamber of the infusion set every 6 hours rather than directly to the bottle of fluid. Many patients can be treated orally from the outset.

Ampicillin is the drug of choice for patients with shigellosis who have been in Central America, where infection with *S. dysenteriae* type 1 has been epidemic. This strain is resistant to sulfonamides, tetracycline and chloramphenicol.

Previously, sulfonamides, tetracyclines and chloramphenicol were widely used, but the high percentage of resistant strains precludes their routine use for the initiation of therapy. In addition, tetracycline and chloramphenicol have well-known adverse effects that make their use in pediatric patients undesirable.

Orally nonabsorbable antibiotics, such as neomycin, kanamycin, colistin and polymyxin B, are frequently recommended for treatment of shigellosis. These agents are ineffectual in eliminating shigellae from the stools and do not shorten the course of illness. Furazolidone is ineffective for shigellosis and nalidixic acid has little effect on the natural course of illness. Iodochlorhydroxyquin, paromomycin and cephalexin have also been recommended, but there is insufficient evidence upon which to judge their effectiveness.

Other Measures. Absorptive agents and drugs that reduce bowel motility may occasionally be useful in older children in whom abdominal cramping is severe, but their use should be avoided in infants because they tend to mask the magnitude of the fluid loss.

Hyperpyrexia should be treated vigorously to avoid convulsions. Anticonvulsant agents should be used when indicated. Specifically treatable causes of convulsions, such as hyponatremia, hypocalcemia and hypoglycemia, must not be overlooked. Hypernatremia rarely occurs in shigellosis.

Because multiple cases of shigellosis within a household are the rule, it is advisable to identify and treat other cases in an effort to eradicate disease from the family unit. Attention should also be paid to traditional public health measures and the education of the family in matters of personal and interpersonal hygiene.

Typhoid Fever

HENRY G. CRAMBLETT, M.D.

Typhoid fever continues to occur in children, although with much less frequency than in the past. A total of 407 cases in children and adults in the United States was reported to the Center for Disease Control in 1971. Sources of infection for children include chronic carriers, of which there are many in each metropolitan area, or by environmental fecal contamination during natural disasters such as floods, where the usual means of sanitation are interrupted. Because of its relative rarity, typhoid fever is often not considered in the differential diagnosis of children with fever of unknown origin. The clinical picture in children may vary considerably, but the most consistent finding is fever. In our experience, fever may be present for as short a period as five days or as long as 30 days before the diagnosis is established. Other clinical manifestations include vomiting, diarrhea, abdominal pain, splenomegaly, anorexia and weight loss, lethargy, cough, headache, hepatomegaly, rose spots and meningismus.

In considering the diagnosis of typhoid fever in children, it is important to remember that blood cultures are more often positive early in the course of the disease than are stool cultures.

Specific Treatment. Chloramphenicol is the drug of choice for treatment of typhoid fever in children, providing the causative strain is sensitive. I recommend a course of chloramphenicol sodium succinate in a dose of 75 to 100 mg. per kilogram per 24 hours in four divided doses administered intravenously for a minimum of 14 days. In children who are extremely toxic and who respond to therapy slowly, I occasionally administer chloramphenicol for as long as three weeks. In patients receiving prolonged therapy, chloramphenicol may be administered orally as chloramphenicol palmitate, in the same 24-hour dosage and at 6-hour intervals, during the latter part of the therapeutic course.

Therapeutic response to chloramphenicol is often less than dramatic. The majority of children will become afebrile within 72 hours, but it is not uncommon for an occasional patient to continue to have spiking fever for several days beyond this. It also is disconcerting to have positive blood cultures during chloramphenicol therapy. This, however, should not be a deterrent to continuing chloramphenicol.

Even though chloramphenicol is the drug of choice for treatment of typhoid fever due to a sensitive organism, this does not relieve the physician from the responsibility of monitoring the patient carefully for possible adverse reactions. As a matter of routine procedure, when chloramphenicol is used it is mandatory that the physician ascertain whether the child has ever had a previous course of chloramphenicol. If so, this should be recorded carefully in the chart. It should be explained to the parents that occasionally an idiosyncratic reaction to chloramphenicol occurs, especially in those who have had short, interrupted courses of the drug in the past. In the event that the child has not had a previous course of chloramphenicol toxicity, this, too, should be included in the official record of the patient. While it is less likely that an idiosyncratic reaction resulting in total aplastic anemia will occur in this situation, it has been reported. It is more common, however, to see a gradual depression of the bone marrow, which can easily be detected by appropriate hematologic monitoring, in which case the chloramphenicol can be discontinued. I customarily discontinue chloramphenicol if the total white blood cell count falls below 5000 per cubic millimeter or if the percentage of polymorphonuclear cells in the peripheral blood falls below 30 per cent.

Recently, cases of typhoid fever occurring in Mexico and in American tourists returning from Mexico have been studied; the causative strain, *Salmonella typhi,* has been resistant to chloramphenicol. In such a situation, antibiotic sensitivities should be obtained and the antibiotic regimen selected accordingly.

Ampicillin in large doses has been recommended as being an efficacious alternate drug to chloramphenicol when the patient has received short interrupted courses of chloramphenicol in the past (in which case the danger of idiosyncratic total bone marrow depression is more likely to occur) or when the patient manifests bone marrow depression during chloramphenicol therapy. While I have had no personal experience with this therapeutic regimen, it is my recommendation that if ampicillin is used it should be given intravenously in doses of 200 mg. per kilogram per day in four divided doses for a period of two weeks.

Treatment of Relapse. In a review of 42 patients treated at Columbus Children's Hospital, only one patient had a relapse of disease after treatment with chloramphenicol, and this occurred 90 days after completion of antibiotic therapy. The organism remained sensitive to chloramphenicol, and the patient subsequently was cured with re-treatment with chloramphenicol.

General Measures. Most deaths occur because of inadequate supportive care or failure to recognize and treat important complications early. During the early part of hospitalization, therefore, much attention must be given to supportive measures. Often the patient is extremely toxic, semistuporous and accordingly needs close attention to eye care and oral hygiene to prevent corneal ulcerations and suppurative parotitis. Even though the patient rarely has diarrhea, he may become dehydrated owing to poor oral intake and/or persistent high fever. When the patient is able to take oral fluids, these should be encouraged. A bland, high-caloric diet should be started as early as possible. Enemas may be used to relieve constipation, but cathartics should be avoided. Urinary output should be monitored and palpation of the bladder performed as indicated to detect urinary retention. Antipyretics should not be used for fever because of the possibility of an adverse reaction with cardiovascular collapse. Excessively high temperatures should be treated with tepid sponge baths. Paralytic ileus is treated with nasogastric suction and appropriate intravenous fluids.

Isolation of Patient. The patient should be isolated and excreta should be very carefully disposed of after decontamination. While *Salmonella typhi* is often absent from the stool during the early course of illness, it may be excreted later in the course of the disease. Health authorities may require three consecutive negative stool and urine cultures taken at least 24 hours apart, not earlier than one month after onset of disease, in order to declare the patient free of the carrier state.

Complications. Complications include intestinal perforation, septic foci outside the gastrointestinal tract, encephalopathy with convulsions and intestinal hemorrhage.

Control Measures. A heat-killed, phenol-preserved or acetone-derived typhoid vaccine is available which may be administered to children at high risk. Indications for the use of this vaccine include travel to foreign countries where typhoid fever is endemic, or travel to areas of natural disaster, especially where there has been flooding. Administration of vaccine after exposure is of little value in preventing typhoid fever. Immunization may be performed by administering two doses of 0.5 ml. vaccine subcutaneously to children 10 years of age and over, four or more weeks apart, or three doses at weekly intervals. Children six months to 10 years should receive two doses of 0.25 ml. subcutaneously four or more weeks apart, or three doses at weekly intervals. Repeat injections are recommended every one to three years if there is continued exposure. Recall injections may be administered intradermally, 0.1 ml., into the flexor surface of the forearm; or subcutaneously, 0.5 ml. for those 10 years old and over and 0.25 ml. for infants and children under 10 years of age.

Salmonellosis

HENRY G. CRAMBLETT, M.D.

Over 1200 serotypes of salmonella have been identified in the laboratory. Potentially, under appropriate circumstances, any one may cause disease in the human host. Certain types of salmonella, other than *Salmonella typhi*, can cause enteric fever or a typhoid-like syndrome. The treatment is the same as for typhoid fever. The most common clinical manifestation of salmonella infection is gastroenteritis. Localized infections due to salmonella can occur in any organ of the body. The other group of patients from whom positive stool cultures are obtained are those who have asymptomatic infections or who are chronic carriers of the organism.

GASTROENTERITIS

The true incidence of salmonella gastroenteritis in infants and children is unknown. Undoubtedly, many children with this disease are not diagnosed and countless others are unreported. There has been, however, no decrease in reported human isolations by the Center for Disease Control, as has been the case with typhoid fever. Salmonella surveillance charts show that these infections occur perennially, but there is an obvious peaking during the summer months. During the period of time when all infants and young children with gastroenteritis were admitted to one diarrhea ward at Columbus Children's Hospital, salmonella infections accounted for approximately 2 to 3 per cent of all admissions to that service.

After an incubation period as short as 4 hours and as long as seven days, the patient characteristically has fever, nausea, vomiting, diarrhea and abdominal cramps. Stool cultures are consistently positive and, by definition, blood cultures are negative.

Antibiotic Therapy. Antibiotics are not indicated for otherwise healthy patients with salmonella gastroenteritis. It has been demonstrated that antibiotics tend to prolong the carrier state and there is no convincing evidence that the duration of disease in patients with negative blood cultures is diminished by such therapy.

Circumstances under which one would consider the use of antibiotics include patients with unusual susceptibility to localized infection with salmonella—that is, patients with hemoglobinopathies or patients in whom the gastrointestinal disease tends to be protracted and severe—and neonates.

My practice is to withhold antibiotics in the usual patient with salmonella gastroenteritis. However, if the results of a positive stool culture are reported and the patient is still symptomatic (especially febrile), or if he falls into the category of being a patient at increased risk of salmonella complications, I prescribe ampicillin in a dose of 100 mg. per kilogram divided into four doses orally per day for a period of seven days. I do not recommend routine follow-up stool cultures following antibiotic therapy because invariably such cultures will be sporadically positive, especially in the infant.

It is important that the physician explain to the parents that great care must be taken in the months following salmonella infection to handle the child's excreta in a sanitary manner and to prevent the child from fecally contaminating objects in the environment, especially foodstuffs, which might be consumed by other siblings or young children.

General Measures. If fluid and electrolyte losses as a result of vomiting and/or diarrhea are severe enough to warrant hospitalization, appropriate fluid and electrolyte replacement should be instituted. As in other cases of severe diarrhea, it is my practice to put the infant on intravenous fluids and withhold oral feedings for 36 to 48 hours. Following this period, the usual regimen for reinstitution and orderly increase in oral feedings may be undertaken. In infants, one may start with glucose water and proceed to skim milk and bland soft low residue foods. In older children, clear liquids and broth soups may be used. I do not use anything specifically designed to decrease vomiting or stooling.

FOCAL INFECTIONS

The most serious localized infection is meningitis. This is most common in neonates and very young infants, and may prove to be a very difficult infection to eradicate. Accordingly, aggressive and prolonged antibiotic therapy is indicated.

I recommend chloramphenicol* as the drug of choice unless the infant is immature. The dose to be used ranges from 25 to 100 mg. per kilogram per day, depending on the age and maturity of the patient. Frequent repeat examinations of the cerebrospinal fluid should be performed to assess the progress of therapy. In the event that the cerebrospinal fluid and/or clinical condition does not improve within three to five days, ventricular taps may be indicated. If there is evidence of localized ventriculitis, I recommend intraventricular instillation† of chloramphenicol in a dose of 25 mg. Antibiotic therapy should be continued for at least three weeks or longer if response to therapy has been slow.

If ampicillin is chosen for primary therapy, I recommend parenteral administration of 400 mg. per kilogram per day in four divided doses for 24 to 48 hours. The dose can then be decreased to 200 mg. per kilogram per day for the remainder of the course of therapy (three weeks or longer).

Infections involving other organs are treated in much the same way. Antibiotic therapy should be prolonged and surgical drainage of pus is mandatory.

VACCINATION

Because of the large number of serotypes of salmonella and because of the difficulty in preparing an efficacious immunogenic antigen against the most common types, there is no satisfactory vaccine available for prevention of these infections.

* Manufacturer's precaution: Chloramphenicol is not recommended for intravenous or intramuscular pediatric use. Chloramphenicol sodium succinate has been approved for intravenous pediatric use.

† Intraventricular use of chloramphenicol is investigational.

Brucellosis

SAMUEL P. GOTOFF, M.D.

The manifestations of brucellosis are quite variable, and spontaneous remissions may occur. Specific antibiotic therapy is usually effective, but relapses may ensue following the recommended course of therapy.

A tetracycline‡ should be given in a total dose of 30 to 40 mg. per kilogram per day divided into four doses given every 6 hours by mouth. The maximal dose is 500 mg. every 6 hours. Oral administration is preferred, but tetracycline, 12 to 20 mg. per kilogram per day, may be given intravenously or intramuscularly every 12 hours. The tetracycline should be continued for 21 days.

In severe cases of acute brucellosis streptomycin is given in addition to tetracycline. The total dose is 30 mg. per kilogram per day divided into two doses given intramuscularly for two weeks. The maximal pediatric dose rarely exceeds 1 Gm. daily. Streptomycin should not be used alone. Erythromycin, chloramphenicol§ or kanamycin may be employed in patients who cannot take tetracycline. Ampicillin does not appear to be effective in the treatment of brucellosis. Clinical or bacteriologic relapses should be re-treated with tetracycline for three weeks and streptomycin for two weeks in the dosages just recommended.

In the unusual case in which marked toxicity is present, prednisone, 5 to 10 mg. four times a day, may be given by mouth for three or four days. Excision and drainage are required for brucellar osteomyelitis and arthritis. General supportive measures, such as limitation of activity and maintenance intravenous fluids, are employed depending on the severity of the disease. Acetylsalicylic acid, 10 mg. per kilogram every 4 hours, may be given as needed for relief of pain. Splinting or traction may be helpful in cases of arthritis. Isolation of the patient is not required.

Prevention of brucellosis depends on ulti-

‡ Manufacturer's note: The use of tetracyclines during tooth development (last half of pregnancy, infancy and childhood to age eight years) may cause permanent discoloration of teeth. This adverse reaction is more common during long-term use of the drugs but has been observed following repeated short-term courses.

§ Manufacturer's precaution: Chloramphenicol is not recommended for intravenous or intramuscular use. Chloramphenicol sodium succinate has been approved for intravenous pediatric use.

mate eradication of the disease in animals. Contact with infected animal tissue and the use of unpasteurized dairy products must be avoided until that time. Brucellar vaccines are not indicated for man.

Tularemia

SAMUEL P. GOTOFF, M.D.

The different clinical forms of tularemia generally respond quite well to specific antimicrobial agents. Streptomycin, 30 mg. per kilogram per day in two divided doses intramuscularly for one week, is the treatment of choice. The maximal dose should rarely exceed 1 Gm. daily for a child. Less effective but adequate alternative forms of therapy are either a tetracycline* in a dose of 30 to 40 mg. per kilogram per day orally, or 12 to 20 mg. per kilogram per day intravenously or intramuscularly for 10 days. Relapses may be treated with another course of the original drug, but, again, streptomycin is preferable.

Acetylsalicylic acid, 10 mg. per kilogram, may be given every 4 hours for relief of pain. Isolation of the patient is not required, but exudative lesions should be covered with dressings and handled with rubber gloves. Draining lymph nodes should be treated with saline soaks daily. A fluctuant abscess should be excised and drained after antibacterial therapy has been initiated. Ocular lesions should be treated with saline soaks. Extension of conjunctival ulcers into the cornea is an indication for topical atropine.

Tularemia is prevented by keeping children away from the infected animal reservoir. Wild game (rabbits) should be thoroughly cooked. Children should be protected against the bites of infected flies and ticks by the use of proper clothing and insect repellents. Vaccination is indicated for the rare child at high risk.

* Manufacturer's note: The use of tetracyclines during tooth development (last half of pregnancy, infancy and childhood to age eight years) may cause permanent discoloration of teeth. This adverse reaction is more common during long-term use of the drugs but has been observed following repeated short-term courses.

Plague

K. F. MEYER, M.D.

Bubonic plague is accounted for by association with wild rodents (sylvatic or campestral plague) and is widespread. Many plague foci exist and perpetuate themselves throughout the western United States, to be discovered only when human and rodent deaths indicate their presence. Before 1965, the yearly total of cases was three; in 1970 it increased to 13, but returned to two in 1971. The increase possibly reflects a larger number of persons being exposed to wild rodent activity, either by their style of living or during summer and fall outdoor recreational activities. Every human case is a warning of the rather unusual, unsuspected and accidental transmission of the plague bacillus from a rodent reservoir to man. Statistics for the period 1950 to 1971, dealing with 54 patients, show that children under 15 years of age are the primary group affected (28 or 52 per cent of cases).

A presumptive clinical diagnosis of plague is unfortunately beset with difficulties. In areas where medical workers are unfamiliar with plague, it is imperative to regard all cases of inguinal, axillary and sometimes cervical lymphadenopathy with a high index of suspicion, especially when the history suggests exposure to wild rodents. A delay in administration of specific chemotherapy is costly. Bacteriologic diagnosis can be obtained within a few minutes during the earliest stages of infection by puncture of the edematous area surrounding an involved lymph node and examination of the exudate film stained with Giemsa or Wayson dye mixture or by fluorescent antibody technique. A stained blood cell count may reveal plague bacilli and leukocytosis (20,000 to 25,000 cells), with a shift to the left. In every suspected case, the physician should obtain blood for culture.

Serodiagnostic procedures using the hemagglutination or complement fixation test with fraction I may establish the diagnosis in retrospect. Refer serum specimens to Ecological Investigations Program, C.D.C., P. O. Box 551, Fort Collins, Colorado 80521.

Treatment. Streptomycin is the antimicrobial drug of choice; penicillin is ineffective. Intramuscular administration of 20 to 40 mg. per kilogram in four divided doses for three to five days is followed by drugs such as tetracycline, chloramphenicol or sulfonamides. The total daily dose of streptomycin for a child should be less than maximal dosage, owing to the danger of a severe Herxheimer reaction. To avoid liberation of plague toxins capable of causing severe shock by the bacteriolytic streptomycin, ultimate sterilization of the tissues is accomplished with bacteriostatic drugs.

It has been reported that plague meningitis may successfully be cured with aqueous penicillin, sulfadiazine† and chloramphenicol sodium succinate administered intravenously every 6 hours (Martin et al.). Moderate amounts of streptomycin combined with chloramphenicol or tetracycline seem to be reasonable initial therapy for plague meningitis.

Clinical response is rapid, even dramatic, provided prompt therapy follows onset of the illness. The disease becomes rapidly refractory to specific treatment as it progresses. Therefore, when specific therapy is not instituted within the first 15 hours of overt illness, antimicrobial drugs seldom favorably alter the outcome of the disease, particularly if blood-stained sputum is present in primary pneumonic plague or if microscopically countable bacilli appear in the blood smear in severe septicemic plague.

Symptomatic Management and Isolation. In the treatment of patients having received specific chemotherapy at a stage at which the infection has already induced extensive toxic damage, great difficulties in maintaining the fluid and electrolyte balance may be encountered.

Bubonic plague uncomplicated by pulmonary manifestations is not directly contagious, and isolation is unnecessary. Hospitalization is recommended in view of superior facilities for efficient treatment and adequate nursing care. Manipulation of buboes and surgery should be avoided. Exudates from ulcers or pus from draining lymph nodes should be handled with rubber gloves.

Care of patients suffering from primary pneumonic plague requires different methods. To reduce the chances for spread of infection during the transport of a patient to the hospital, tetracycline, 12 to 15 mg. per kilogram (0.5 Gm. for patients 12 years of age and older), should be administered intramuscularly or intravenously before the patient leaves home. Isolation in a separate room is essential. All contacts should be placed promptly on oral prophylactic chemotherapy, adult contacts receiving oral tetracycline in a daily dose of 1 Gm., or 2 to 5 Gm. of sulfonamides, for six days. The deplorable incidence of pneumonic plague infections among hospital personnel working with isolation patients shows that precautions are essential. Use of a proper mask, goggles and a cloth hood with a frontal mica window is indispensable.

Only under unusual circumstances is immunoprophylaxis with formalin-killed plague vaccine recommended. This vaccine is partially effective, but protection is not achieved until completion of basic and booster inoculations two or three months after the first inoculation.

† Manufacturer's precaution: Sulfadiazine should not be used in infants under two months of age.

References

Martin, A. R., et al.: Plague Meningitis. A Report of Three Cases in Children and Review of the Problem. *Pediatrics,* 40:610, 1967.

Meyer, K. F.: Pasteurella and Franciscella; *in* R. J. Dubos and J. G. Hirsch: *Bacterial and Mycotic Infections of Man.* 4th ed. Philadelphia, J. B. Lippincott Company, 1965, pp. 659–697.

Pollitzer, R.: *Plague.* World Health Organization Monograph Series 22, 1954.

Reed, W. P., et al.: Bubonic Plague in the Southwestern United States—A Review of Recent Experiences. *Medicine,* 49:465–486, 1970.

Tuberculosis

EDWIN L. KENDIG, JR., M.D.

Early diagnosis of tuberculosis is essential for an optimal therapeutic result.

Preventive Therapy. Results from the United States Public Health Service Isoniazid Prophylaxis Study among household contacts indicate that isoniazid is effective in reducing the incidence of tuberculous disease in this group. However, for infants born of tuberculous mothers, it is advised that BCG vaccine be administered as soon after birth as is practicable.

General Therapy. Whenever a child is found to be tuberculin-positive, the tuberculous contact must be removed as soon as possible. This entails a chest x-ray of all adult contacts, including grandparents, baby sitters, household servants and any others who may have been in contact with the child.

An adequate, high protein diet and the usual vitamin supplement for a growing child are indicated, but the question of bed rest varies with the type of disease. In most instances, bed rest is not required.

The need for protecting the child from intercurrent infection should be stressed, since not only measles but also any acute infection may lower resistance. The tuberculin-positive child who has not had rubeola should be protected against this disease by the use of measles vaccine, but the vaccine should be administered only when he is receiving antituberculosis chemotherapy (including isoniazid). Protection of the child from a source of tuberculous infection in the home must also not be overlooked.

Chest x-rays at appropriate intervals are necessary.

Antimicrobial Therapy. Isoniazid (INH), streptomycin (SM), para-aminosalicylic acid (PAS) and ethambutol are the four antimicrobial agents of greatest efficacy in the treatment of tuberculosis in childhood. However, other drugs, including pyrazinamide, viomycin, cycloserine, ethionamide and kanamycin, may have limited value; rifampin is particularly promising.

ISONIAZID (INH). Isoniazid is the most effective antituberculosis agent known, and it is the only drug which tends to prevent the complications of tuberculosis. Accordingly, it must be included in every therapeutic regimen unless contraindicated because of the patient's hypersensitivity to the drug or because the causative organism is isoniazid-resistant.

Resistance to isoniazid has not been of serious clinical significance in the treatment of children. As a consequence, the drug can be used alone in the treatment of uncomplicated primary tuberculosis. In progressive primary tuberculosis, isoniazid is used in conjunction with para-aminosalicylic acid (PAS). In severe forms of tuberculosis, such as miliary tuberculosis and tuberculous meningitis, a triple drug regimen, with isoniazid, streptomycin and PAS, is utilized. Whenever the patient does not show satisfactory improvement, another drug (usually ethambutol or rifampin) is substituted for streptomycin or PAS, but INH is always included.

When isoniazid is administered orally, a plasma concentration 20 to 80 times the usual inhibiting concentration of the drug (which is 0.05 microgram per ml.) may be attained within a few hours; effective high concentrations persist for 6 to 8 hours. Isoniazid penetrates freely into the cerebrospinal fluid and into caseous tissue. It is excreted mainly in the urine. The principal side effect of the drug, neurotoxic in manifestation, either as convulsions or as peripheral neuritis, results from competitive inhibition of pyridoxine metabolism. Such a side effect has been described mainly in adults, however, and pyridoxine deficiency does not appear to be a problem in children, although precautions must be exercised during adolescence. Pyridoxine, 25 to 50 mg. daily (10 mg. for each 100 mg. of isoniazid), should be added to the treatment schedule during this period. Other side effects include gastrointestinal dysfunction and allergic reactions. Rarely, isoniazid may be hepatotoxic. Since hepatic dysfunction is now reported more frequently in adults than was the case in previous years, the parent of the patient for whom INH is prescribed should be questioned carefully at monthly intervals for any symptoms or signs of isoniazid toxicity.

The problem of adequate isoniazid dosage may be approached in one of two ways. Since children tolerate isoniazid much better than do adults, the dosage may be as much as 20 mg. per kilogram of body weight per day, with a maximal daily dosage of 500 mg. On the other hand, combined therapy with PAS may be utilized. The PAS apparently competes with isoniazid for acetylation in the liver, and this competitive effect results in a high blood level of isoniazid. The present trend in the treatment of tuberculosis is the simultaneous use of isoniazid and PAS or another antimicrobial agent (streptomycin or ethambutol). In the treatment of pulmonary tuberculosis in adults, ethambutol has largely replaced PAS. Triple drug therapy has no statistical advantage over treatment with two drugs (if one of the drugs is isoniazid), but it is nevertheless preferred by many investigators in the treatment of serious forms, such as tuberculous meningitis and miliary tuberculosis.

Isoniazid is available for oral administration as tablets of 50, 100 and 300 mg. and as a flavored syrup containing 10 mg. per ml. A preparation for parenteral administration (intramuscular or intrathecal) is also available.

STREPTOMYCIN (SM). Streptomycin in a concentration of 1.6 micrograms per ml. inhibits growth of the tubercle bacillus. After parenteral administration it rapidly appears in the blood, reaching a peak value in 2 hours. The drug diffuses into the pleural fluid but does not pass the cerebrospinal fluid barrier to any appreciable extent unless there is inflammation of the meninges. Streptomycin is largely excreted in the urine, with an 80 per cent recovery within 24 hours after administration.

The principal toxic effect of streptomycin is involvement of the 8th cranial nerve. Although loss of vestibular function may be permanent, children usually adjust to this defect without symptoms. Involvement of the auditory branch constitutes a real danger, but this effect is much less frequent now than in the days of prolonged streptomycin therapy. Allergic manifestations, such as fever and dermatitis, may occur, and agranulocytosis has been reported.

Streptomycin is administered by intramuscular injection in a suggested dosage of 20 to 40 mg. per kilogram of body weight per day, with a maximal daily dosage of 1 Gm. Dosage is at the lower level (20 mg.) except in meningitis and other fulminating forms of tuberculosis. Although a single daily injection of the drug is usually given, the daily dose may be divided into two injections for a small or emaciated patient.

Streptomycin is never used as the sole therapeutic agent because of the rapid development of drug resistance. It is routinely given with at least one other tuberculostatic agent.

Experience has not proved the value of intrathecal administration of streptomycin, and use of the drug in this manner has been largely discontinued.

Streptomycin is supplied in crystalline form, usually as a sulfate, in vials containing 1 and 5 Gm.

PARA-AMINOSALICYLIC ACID (PAS). This drug has bacteriostatic activity against the tubercle bacillus, and also can delay the emergence of microbial resistance to streptomycin. Thus, it was of great value when streptomycin was the most effective antimicrobial agent. It also delays bacterial resistance to isoniazid, but such resistance has not been of serious clinical significance in children.

As previously mentioned, the chief value of PAS is that it apparently competes with isoniazid for acetylation in the liver, thereby increasing the amount of free isoniazid in the blood.

When administered orally, PAS is readily absorbed and diffuses into serous surfaces and reaches the cerebrospinal fluid in small amounts. It has no intracellular activity and is rapidly excreted in the urine.

Gastrointestinal disturbances constitute the principal toxicity, but hypokalemia, leukopenia, hepatitis and a goitrogenic effect have been described. The drug may also be the cause of severe allergic reactions, including dermatosis and an otherwise unexplained fever.

Children usually have a much better tolerance for all forms of PAS than do adults. The drug should be prescribed in a dosage of 200 mg. per kilogram of body weight per day in three or four divided doses (maximal daily dosage of 12 Gm.). When salts of PAS (sodium, potassium, calcium) are used, the dosage should be correspondingly larger: 250 to 300 mg. per kilogram of body weight per day. The drug is supplied as 0.5-Gm. tablets, as a powder and as a solution of the sodium salt. The solution is stable for only 24 hours, and then only if kept in the dark and refrigerated.

ETHAMBUTOL.* This drug is a very effective antimicrobial agent. As with PAS, when it is given in combination with other antimicrobial agents, it delays the onset of microbial resistance. It is also better tolerated and has less tendency to produce toxicity than does PAS. So far the drug has been used largely in adults, where it appears to be gradually replacing PAS, but the dosage I have found to be satisfactory in children is 20 mg. per kilogram of body weight per day orally for four to six weeks, and 15 mg. per kilogram of body weight per day thereafter. With larger dosage, a few instances of retrobulbar neuritis with resultant loss of vision have been noted in adults. At the recommended dosage and with precautions that include monthly studies of visual acuity, visual fields and tests for green color vision, there appears to be much less danger of this complication. The drug should be discontinued if there is a two-line loss of visual acuity as measured on a Snellen eye chart, if there is contraction of visual fields or if there is loss of green color vision. Ethambutol is supplied in 100-mg. and 400-mg. tablets and is administered in a single daily oral dose.

RIFAMPIN. Rifampin is the newest and one of the most promising of the antituberculosis chemotherapeutic agents. It is a semisynthetic, orally administered derivative of rifamycin SV, and thus far appears to be relatively nontoxic, although occasional liver toxicity has been noted. Gastrointestinal disturbances, dermatoses and reversible leukopenia may occur. It is recommended for use in combination with at least one other antituberculosis drug. Suggested dosage is 10 to 20 mg. per kilogram of body weight per day (maximum daily dose of 600 mg.). Rifampin is administered in a single daily dose and is supplied in 300-mg. capsules.

ETHIONAMIDE. This agent is also available for use in combination with one or more antituberculosis agents when bacterial resistance to isoniazid and streptomycin exists. The dosage I have used for children is 10 to 20 mg. per kilogram of body weight per day in two or three divided doses (maximum of 750 mg.), although manufacturers' pediatric recommen-

* Manufacturer's precaution: Ethambutol is not recommended for children under 13 years of age, since conditions for safe use have not been established.

dations are as yet unavailable. The drug may be hepatotoxic and also may cause severe gastrointestinal dysfunction. Ethionamide is administered orally and is supplied as 250-mg. tablets. The drug may also be given rectally.

PYRAZINAMIDE. This drug is effective only for a short time; however, its ensuing ineffectiveness cannot be correlated with the emergence of pyrazinamide-resistant tubercle bacilli. There has also been much evidence of hepatic toxicity. The Committee on Therapy of the American Trudeau Society (now the American Thoracic Society) concluded that when used alone, pyrazinamide has only a limited effect, and that its serious hepatotoxic action tends to outweigh its therapeutic value. The drug is administered orally in a dosage of 20 to 30 mg. per kilogram of body weight per day (maximum of 2 Gm.) in three divided doses. It is supplied in 0.5-Gm. tablets.

VIOMYCIN.† This drug has tuberculostatic properties, but it is less potent than streptomycin and is not devoid of toxicity. Toxic manifestations include depletion of plasma electrolytes, increased blood urea nitrogen level, the appearance of albumin, casts, white and red blood cells in the urine, acoustic nerve damage, unexplained fever, eosinophilia and urticaria. The drug is rarely used in children, therefore, and is indicated only when other therapy is not effective. It is administered intramuscularly twice weekly in a dosage of 30 mg. per kilogram of body weight (maximal dose of 4 Gm. per week) and should always be utilized in combination with another antituberculosis agent. It is supplied as a sulfate in vials containing 1 and 5 Gm.

CYCLOSERINE.‡ This drug is not as effective as isoniazid or streptomycin. It also has a number of toxic effects, the tendency toward convulsions being the most important. Cycloserine is given orally in a dosage of 5 to 15 mg. per kilogram of body weight per day in two or three divided doses (less in renal tuberculosis). Maximal daily dosage is 500 mg. It is supplied in 250-mg. capsules.

KANAMYCIN. Kanamycin is a streptomycin type of drug, which may have all the toxic effects of streptomycin and, in addition, may show renal toxicity. It is rarely used in the treatment of tuberculosis in children. Dosage is 10 to 15 mg. per kilogram of body weight per day.

ADRENOCORTICOSTEROIDS. Cortisone apparently suppresses the usual inflammatory response of the body, with impairment of granulation tissue formation, macrophage activity and fibroblastic repair. From this mechanism, it appears likely that cortisone promotes progression of tuberculous disease in the lung. This deleterious effect can be overcome, however, by specific, effective antimicrobial treatment. Indications for the use of adrenocorticosteroids in specific forms of tuberculosis will be presented subsequently under individual headings.

POSITIVE TUBERCULIN REACTION

Treatment of a child with a positive tuberculin reaction and no other evidence of disease is aimed at the prevention of complications (Table 1).

If the patient is less than 6 years of age, he should be given isoniazid in a dosage of 10 to 15 mg. per kilogram of body weight per day for one year. The drug may be administered in a single daily dose or in two divided doses. Such a child is not considered infectious, and activity is not curtailed. Follow-up roentgenograms are suggested one to three months after diagnosis and again at the completion of one year of therapy. Naturally, if there is symptomatic evidence of worsening of the disease process during that period, such a routine must be correspondingly altered. After the

† Manufacturer's precaution: Safety of viomycin in children has not been established.

‡ Manufacturer's precaution: Safety of cycloserine in children has not been established.

TABLE 1. Treatment of Patient with Positive Tuberculin Reaction

PATIENT	DRUG	DOSAGE	MAXIMUM DAILY DOSAGE	NUMBER OF DAILY DOSES	DURATION OF THERAPY
< Six years of age	Isoniazid	10–15 mg./kg.	300 mg.	1 or 2	12 months
> Six years of age	Individualize	See text			
Recent converter (within 12 months)	Isoniazid	10–15 mg./kg.	300 mg.	1 or 2	12 months

first year, an annual chest x-ray is indicated. The tuberculous adult is, of course, removed from contact with the patient as soon as possible.

Studies indicate that the first year after tuberculous infection is the most dangerous period, and it is recommended that any child who converts from a negative to a positive tuberculin reaction within a one-year period be given the treatment already outlined. This, of course, accentuates the value of the routine annual tuberculin test.

Although it is not nearly as certain that a child over the age of six years with no physical or roentgenographic evidence of tuberculous disease benefits from isoniazid therapy, there is a growing belief that any child with a positive tuberculin reaction and no other evidence of disease should receive isoniazid for one year. If such a child does not receive antimicrobial therapy, and most of them do, he should have a careful follow-up with routine monthly examinations, an occasional roentgenogram throughout the ensuing year and an annual chest roentgenogram thereafter. All children, particularly girls, with a positive tuberculin reaction merit special attention during puberty and adolescence. At present it is our policy to institute a one-year course of isoniazid therapy in adolescents who have a positive tuberculin reaction and who have not received a previous course of isoniazid therapy.

ASYMPTOMATIC PRIMARY TUBERCULOSIS

Although, strictly speaking, the child with a positive tuberculin reaction and no other evidence of disease belongs in the category of asymptomatic primary tuberculosis, only those with roentgenographic evidence of active tuberculosis as well as a positive tuberculin reaction will be considered here.

It is recommended that the patient with asymptomatic primary tuberculosis be given isoniazid in a dosage of 10 to 20 mg. per kilogram of body weight per day for one year (Table 2). Administration of the drug, follow-up examinations and roentgenograms are the same as outlined under Positive Tuberculin Reaction. Activity of the child with primary tuberculosis is not restricted. Search for and removal of the tuberculous adult are, of course, indicated.

PROGRESSIVE PRIMARY PULMONARY TUBERCULOSIS

Pulmonary progression of primary tuberculosis and chronic pulmonary tuberculosis require a more intensive therapeutic approach. Antimicrobial treatment consists of isoniazid, 15 to 20 mg. per kilogram of body weight, with a maximal daily dosage of 500 mg., and PAS, 200 mg. per kilogram of body weight, with a maximal daily dosage of 12 Gm. (Table 3). Isoniazid is given in one or two daily divided

TABLE 2. Treatment of Asymptomatic Primary Tuberculosis

DRUG	DAILY DOSAGE	MAXIMAL DAILY DOSAGE	NUMBER OF DAILY DOSES	DURATION OF THERAPY
Isoniazid	10–20 mg./kg.	400 mg.	1 or 2	12 months

TABLE 3. Treatment of Progressive Primary Pulmonary Tuberculosis

DRUG	DAILY DOSAGE	MAXIMAL DAILY DOSAGE	NUMBER OF DAILY DOSES	DURATION OF THERAPY
Isoniazid	15–20 mg./kg.	500 mg.	1 or 2	12 months or longer
PAS	200 mg./kg.	12 Gm.	3 or 4	12 months or longer
If response is unsatisfactory, add streptomycin	20 mg./kg.	1 Gm.	1 (in some cases, 2)	One month after satisfactory clinical response
For endobronchial disease, add prednisone	1 mg./kg.	60 mg.	4	6–12 weeks

doses, and PAS in three or four divided doses. If the child does not respond satisfactorily to this treatment, substitute ethambutol (see manufacturer's precaution, p. 615), 15 mg. per kilogram of body weight, for PAS; or add streptomycin, 20 mg. per kilogram of body weight per day, with a maximal daily dosage of 1 Gm. Streptomycin is given once each day intramuscularly, although for a small or emaciated patient the daily dose may be divided into two injections. Streptomycin therapy is continued for one month after satisfactory clinical response, but isoniazid and PAS (or ethambutol) therapy should be carried out for at least one year, and sometimes longer.

Atelectasis is an important pulmonary complication. Since this may be either extrabronchial (impingement of a mass of lymph nodes upon the bronchus causing occlusion of the lumen) or endobronchial (penetration of the wall of a bronchus by a caseous lymph node), bronchoscopic examination is desirable. Incomplete obstruction of the lumen due to a check-valve mechanism may also occur and result in hyperaeration (so-called obstructive emphysema). Treatment of endobronchial tuberculosis has not been satisfactory, and there is good evidence that the use of adrenocorticosteroids, in conjunction with antimicrobial therapy, may be of value in early cases. Prednisone in a dosage of 1 mg. per kilogram of body weight per day should be continued for 6 to 12 weeks.

TUBERCULOSIS IN THE NEWBORN

Congenital tuberculosis is a rarity, and tuberculosis in the newborn period is relatively uncommon. When the mother is known to have pulmonary tuberculosis, the newborn infant should be isolated from her at delivery. It is suggested that BCG vaccine be promptly administered to the newborn infant; if the vaccine is administered when the infant is two weeks of age or more, a tuberculin test and chest roentgenogram must be performed prior to vaccination. A negative result should be obtained in both studies before the infant is vaccinated. After BCG vaccination the infant should continue to be isolated from the mother for at least six weeks, and until the mother's tuberculous disease is so controlled that contact with the infant is deemed advisable.

If the mother has evidence of hematogenous tuberculosis or far-advanced pulmonary disease with sputum positive for tubercle bacilli, the infant should be isolated from the mother and isoniazid (15 to 20 mg. per kilogram of body weight per day) should be given to the infant for three months; the infant should have a tuberculin test and chest roentgenogram at the end of that period; if both are negative, BCG vaccination is performed. The infant should, of course, be isolated from the mother for an additional six-week period and until the mother is no longer considered infectious.

Isoniazid prophylaxis for a one-year period in children born of tuberculous mothers has also been recommended.

If the infant has already acquired tuberculous infection, isoniazid (15 to 20 mg. per kilogram of body weight per day) should be administered for at least one year; if there has been progressive tuberculous involvement, a more radical therapeutic approach is required.

TUBERCULOUS PLEURISY WITH EFFUSION

Isoniazid and PAS are given for a 12-month period. Prednisone, 1 mg. per kilogram of body weight per day orally in four divided doses, is given only until pleurisy with effusion seems to be controlled (Table 4).

Although studies indicate that subsequent pulmonary function is not improved by the use of adrenocorticosteroids, it does appear that they exert an immediately favorable effect on

TABLE 4. Treatment of Tuberculous Pleurisy with Effusion

DRUG	DAILY DOSAGE	MAXIMAL DAILY DOSAGE	NUMBER OF DAILY DOSES	DURATION OF THERAPY
Isoniazid	15–20 mg./kg.	500 mg.	1 or 2	12 months or longer
PAS	200 mg./kg.	12 Gm.	3 or 4	12 months or longer
Prednisone	1 mg./kg.	60 mg.	4	Until pleurisy with effusion is controlled

the pleurisy with effusion, promoting a rapid control of fever and the disappearance of the fluid.

Diagnostic aspiration should always be carried out, but subsequent aspirations are necessary only when there is respiratory embarrassment.

MILIARY TUBERCULOSIS

Miliary tuberculosis is an extremely serious form of the disease, and therapy consists of a triple drug regimen with isoniazid, 20 mg. per kilogram of body weight per day; PAS, 200 mg. per kilogram per day; and streptomycin, 20 to 40 mg. per kilogram per day (Table 5). If the patient does not show satisfactory improvement, ethambutol (see manufacturer's precaution, p. 615) or rifampin may be substituted for streptomycin or PAS. Isoniazid and PAS are continued for at least one year, but streptomycin is given for one month after satisfactory clinical response. Prednisone has been recommended for extreme dsypnea, but it is used only for the period necessary to control the dyspnea.

It is desirable that cerebrospinal fluid examinations be performed at regular intervals in order to make an early diagnosis if meningitis occurs. These procedures are indicated at weekly intervals during the early stages of treatment and less often thereafter.

CHRONIC PULMONARY TUBERCULOSIS

Since the lesions of chronic pulmonary tuberculosis in children are extremely unstable, prompt therapy should be instituted (Table 6). Isoniazid, 10 mg. per kilogram (maximum daily dose of 300 mg.) and either para-aminosalicylic acid, 200 mg. per kilogram of body weight (maximum daily dose 12 Gm.) per day, or ethambutol (see manufacturer's precaution,

TABLE 5. Treatment of Miliary Tuberculosis

DRUG	DAILY DOSAGE	MAXIMAL DAILY DOSAGE	NUMBER OF DAILY DOSES	DURATION OF THERAPY
Isoniazid	20 mg./kg.	500 mg.	1 or 2	12 months or longer
PAS	200 mg./kg.	12 Gm.	3 or 4	12 months or longer
Streptomycin	20–40 mg./kg.	1 Gm.	1 (in some cases, 2)	1 month after satisfactory clinical response
Prednisone	1 mg./kg.	60 mg.	4	Use only during period of extreme dyspnea

TABLE 6. Treatment of Chronic Pulmonary Tuberculosis

DRUG	DAILY DOSAGE	MAXIMAL DAILY DOSAGE	NUMBER OF DAILY DOSES	DURATION OF THERAPY
Isoniazid	10 mg./kg.	300 mg.	1 or 2	2 years after sputum is negative
PAS	200 mg./kg.	12 Gm.	3 or 4	2 years after sputum is negative
or				
Ethambutol*	15 mg./kg.	–	1	2 years after sputum is negative

* Ethambutol is not recommended for children under 13 years of age, since conditions for safe use have not been established.

Table 6), 15 mg. per kilogram, should be given for two years after the sputum has become negative for tubercle bacilli.

TUBERCULOSIS OF THE SUPERFICIAL LYMPH NODES

Tuberculosis of the lymph nodes most commonly involves the superficial cervical glands.

Whenever there is a positive tuberculin reaction and lymph nodes measure 2 cm. or more in diameter and are increasing in size or showing early signs of suppuration, treatment by excision and, of course, isoniazid and PAS therapy for a full year are indicated (Table 7). If the mass of nodes is too great, or if complete liquefaction of the node has already occurred and excision cannot be carried out, aspiration of the node (when liquefied) and the oral use of isoniazid and PAS may be effective. Isoniazid and PAS are administered for one year. Tonsillectomy is advised only if there are indications for it.

TUBERCULOUS MENINGITIS

Before the discovery of streptomycin, tuberculous meningitis was presumably 100 per cent fatal. At present, with the use of isoniazid, PAS and streptomycin, approximately 85 per cent of the few such patients admitted to the Medical College of Virginia Hospitals are salvaged.

The treatment consists of a triple drug regimen: isoniazid in daily dosage of 20 mg. per kilogram of body weight (maximum of 500 mg.), PAS in daily dosage of 200 mg. per kilogram of body weight (maximum of 12 Gm.) and streptomycin in daily dosage of 20 to 40 mg. per kilogram of body weight (maximum of 1 Gm.) (Table 8). The first two drugs are given for at least one year, and streptomycin is given for one month after satisfactory clinical response, as determined by the general condition of the patient, disappearance of fever and improvement in the cerebrospinal fluid picture. Although it may sometimes be necessary to substitute rifampin or ethambutol in the therapeutic regimen, antimicrobial agents appear to be reasonably effective in the treatment of tuberculous meningitis *if* they can reach the organism.

Use of prednisone may decrease the likelihood of cerebrospinal fluid block, and, in addition, reduction of the inflammatory process may lessen the danger of irreversible thrombotic phenomena. Use of prednisone after cerebrospinal obstruction has occurred often results in dissolution. Obviously, however, pre-

TABLE 7. Treatment of Tuberculosis of the Superficial Lymph Nodes

	DRUG	DAILY DOSAGE	MAXIMAL DAILY DOSAGE	DURATION OF THERAPY
Excision or aspiration and:	Isoniazid	15–20 mg./kg.	500 mg.	12 months or longer
	PAS	200 mg./kg.	12 Gm.	12 months or longer

TABLE 8. Treatment of Tuberculous Meningitis

DRUG	DAILY DOSAGE	MAXIMAL DAILY DOSAGE	NUMBER OF DAILY DOSES	DURATION OF THERAPY
Isoniazid	20 mg./kg.	500 mg.	1 or 2	12 months or longer
PAS	200 mg./kg.	12 Gm.	3 or 4	12 months or longer
Streptomycin	20–40 mg./kg.	1 Gm.	1 (in some cases, 2)	1 month after satisfactory clinical response
Prednisone	1 mg./kg.	60 mg.	4	6–12 weeks

vention of such block is more desirable. The drug is usually administered for a 6- to 12-week period.

Promptness of response to antimicrobial therapy varies considerably. In general, the earlier the diagnosis, the more prompt the response. An affected child may lie in a stuporous, semicomatose or even comatose state for months and finally effect an almost complete recovery or even a complete recovery.

TUBERCULOSIS OF BONES AND JOINTS

The bones most frequently involved are the head of the femur (hip), the vertebrae and the fingers and toes. The American Thoracic Society recommends that tuberculosis of the bones and joints be treated with isoniazid and PAS for 18 to 24 months. Dosage of these drugs is the same as that outlined under therapy of progressive primary tuberculosis (Table 9).

All superficial and accessible abscesses should be drained. Immobilization is not necessary in the nonweight-bearing structures; however, if weight-bearing structures (such as vertebrae and the hip) are involved, whatever means are necessary to prevent weight-bearing are carried out. For example, treatment of tuberculosis of the spine (Pott's disease) may vary widely. Some utilize only a hard mattress and the aforementioned drug therapy; others feel that a plaster cast is advisable. Fusion is advised by some orthopedists, and others use fusion only when there appear to be special indications for it.

RENAL TUBERCULOSIS

For renal tuberculosis, treatment should be carried out for a two-year period. Triple drug therapy with isoniazid, PAS and streptomycin has been advocated for this period, but in cases in which the urogram shows no abnormality, streptomycin may be discontinued after six months. One authority gives isoniazid, PAS and one other drug—oral cycloserine, ethionamide or ethambutol—for two years, usually in a single daily dose. Dosage of isoniazid is 15 to 20 mg. per kilogram of body weight per day; PAS, 200 mg. per kilogram per day; and streptomycin (when used), 20 mg. per kilogram three times weekly. For cycloserine, dosage is 4 to 5 mg. per kilogram of body weight per day; for ethionamide, 10 mg. per kilogram per day; and for ethambutol, 15 mg. per kilogram per day (maximal dosages and manufacturer's precautions as indicated in Table 10). Since there is a possibility that ureteral stricture may appear during therapy, an intravenous pyelogram and ureteral calibration every four months during treatment and annually thereafter for a 10-year period seems advisable.

INTRA-ABDOMINAL TUBERCULOSIS

Intra-abdominal tuberculosis has been a rarity on the pediatric service of the Medical College of Virginia in recent years. Treatment of tuberculous enteritis requires the same antimicrobial therapy routine as is outlined in Table 3, as well as the usual general measures for tuberculosis. A low residue diet of adequate caloric and vitamin content is also helpful. Therapy is otherwise symptomatic.

Tuberculosis of the mesenteric and retroperitoneal lymph nodes usually does not require local treatment. Rarely, excision of enlarged or calcified abdominal lymph nodes may be necessary for relief of pain.

Tuberculous peritonitis is treated in the same manner as tuberculosis in general (Table 3). If there is an associated enteritis, a low residue diet provides some symptomatic relief. The addition of adrenocorticosteroid therapy may also be helpful.

TUBERCULOSIS OF THE SKIN

Treatment of tuberculosis of the skin is the same as for tuberculosis in general (Table 3). Local treatment is symptomatic.

TABLE 9. Treatment of Tuberculosis of Bones and Joints*

DRUG	DAILY DOSAGE	MAXIMAL DAILY DOSAGE	DURATION OF THERAPY
Isoniazid	15–20 mg./kg.	500 mg.	18–24 months
PAS	200 mg./kg.	12 Gm.	18–24 months

* Drain all superficial and accessible abscesses. Immobilize involved weight-bearing structures.

TABLE 10. Treatment of Renal Tuberculosis

DRUG	DAILY DOSAGE	MAXIMAL DAILY DOSAGE	DURATION OF THERAPY
Isoniazid	15–20 mg./kg./day	500 mg.	2 years
PAS	200 mg./kg./day	12 Gm.	2 years
Streptomycin or	20 mg./kg. 3 times weekly	1 Gm.	2 years (6 months in very mild cases)
Cycloserine* or	4–5 mg./kg./day	500 mg.	2 years
Ethionamide† or	10 mg./kg./day	750 mg.	2 years
Ethambutol‡	15 mg./kg./day		2 years

* Manufacturer's precaution: Safety of cycloserine in children has not been established.

† Manufacturer's precaution: Optimum dosage of ethionamide has not been established. However, this does not preclude its use if crucial to therapy.

‡ Manufacturer's precaution: Ethambutol is not recommended for children under 13 years of age, since conditions for safe use have not been established.

OTHER INDICATIONS FOR ANTIMICROBIAL THERAPY

Any tuberculin-positive child who receives adrenocorticosteroid therapy for another disease should be given concurrent isoniazid therapy (10 to 20 mg. per kilogram).

Since measles causes deterioration of tuberculous disease, and since isoniazid is effective in preventing that deterioration, isoniazid, 10 to 20 mg. per kilogram of body weight, should be given for a minimum of four weeks in any tuberculin-positive child who contracts measles. The same therapy should be used in the tuberculin-positive child with pertussis.

PREVENTION OF TUBERCULOSIS

Three methods are reasonably effective in preventing tuberculous infection: isolation of adults with infectious tuberculosis, the use of BCG vaccine and the administration of isoniazid to household contacts of tuberculous patients.

Results from the United States Public Health Service Isoniazid Prophylaxis Studies among tuberculin-positive household contacts indicate that isoniazid is effective in reducing the incidence of tuberculous disease in this group of children. Further studies by the United States Public Health Service have shown that extending the use of isoniazid to all household contacts results in less tuberculous disease during the year of prophylactic therapy and continuing good effect lasting at least through the 10 years following discontinuation of isoniazid therapy.

BCG vaccine increases resistance to exogenous tuberculous infection, and is mainly used in this country for children living in a home in which there is an adult with infectious tuberculous disease, or one with potentially infectious disease, such as a mother who has been discharged from a sanatorium with apparently arrested tuberculosis. It is recommended for children born of tuberculous mothers. It is also useful in population groups in which there is a high incidence of tuberculous infection. The BCG vaccination may be effected by the multiple puncture technique or by the intracutaneous route.

In order to be eligible for BCG vaccination, the patient should have a negative tuberculin reaction (PPD, 0.0001 mg.; or OT, 0.1 mg.) and a negative chest roentgenogram within the previous two weeks. Eight to 12 weeks after vaccination, the same procedures should be carried out. This time the tuberculin reaction should be positive, and if this is not the case, the vaccination is repeated.

The multiple puncture disc method, as described by Rosenthal, is the preferable procedure. The vaccination is performed over the deltoid region, and the area should be cleansed with acetone and allowed to dry thoroughly. There should be no constriction of the arm. Three drops of BCG vaccine are placed on the skin of the deltoid area, using a syringe and a 22-gauge needle. The disc is picked up by a sterile magnet-type holder, allowing the wide margin of the disc to extend beyond the magnet and away from the operator. The operator holds the disc at a 30-degree angle and distributes the vaccine over an area of about 2.5 square cm., tapping with the wide margin of the disc. The points of the disc are dipped into the vaccine, and the disc is rotated slightly so that all points become moistened with BCG vaccine. The disc is placed in the center of the vaccine site, with the long axis of the holder at a right angle to the arm, and the magnet is moved to the center of the disc. This will avoid bending the disc.

The arm under the vaccine site is grasped with the operator's other hand, thereby tensing the skin over the vaccination area. With the butt of the magnet in the curve of the index finger, downward pressure is applied so that the points of the disc are well buried in the skin. Enough pressure is applied so that penetration of the points is readily felt by the hand. With pressure still exerted, the disc is rocked forward and backward and from side to side twice. The grasp underneath the arm is then released. The operator slides the magnet toward himself and off the disc, maintaining a slight downward pressure.

After a successful procedure, the disc remains flat on the arm, with the points still in the skin. If the points are on top of the skin, the procedure must be repeated. The disc is again picked up with the magnet, allowing the wide margin to extend beyond the magnet. By utilizing the wide margin of the disc, the vaccine is gently tapped so that each perforation of the skin is covered with vaccine. If too much pressure is exerted, the vaccine will be pressed out of the perforations. The vaccine is allowed to dry on the arm without a dressing. The vaccinated area should not be washed for 24 hours.

Infants and children from tuberculous households (and all adults) should receive the two-site method of BCG vaccination. This procedure differs from the foregoing only in that a larger area of the deltoid region is cleansed; one vaccination site is in the upper portion, and a second in the lower portion. Materials for use in BCG vaccination may be obtained from the Research Foundation, 70 West Hubbard Street, Chicago, Illinois 60610. BCG vaccine is also commercially available from the Eli Lilly Company, 740 South Alabama Street, Indianapolis, Indiana 46206.

References

Avery, M. E., and Wolfsdorf, J.: Diagnosis and Treatment: Infants of Tuberculous Mothers. *Pediatrics,* 42:519, 1968.

Committee on Drugs, American Academy of Pediatrics: Infants of Tuberculous Mothers: Further Thoughts. *Pediatrics,* 42:393, 1968.

Committee on Therapy, American Thoracic Society, the National Tuberculosis and Respiratory Disease Association and the Center for Disease Control: Joint Statement on the Preventive Treatment of Tuberculosis. *Am. Rev. Resp. Dis.,* 104:460, 1971.

Kendig, E. L., Jr.: Management of Infants Born of Tuberculous Mothers. *New England J. Med.,* 281:520, 1969.

Mitchell, R. S.: Control of Tuberculosis. *New England J. Med.,* 276:842, 1967.

Nemir, R. L., et al.: Prednisone as an Adjunct in the Chemotherapy of Lymph Node–Bronchial Tuberculosis in Childhood. *Am. Rev. Resp. Dis.,* 95:402, 1967.

Rosenthal, S. R.: *BCG Vaccination Against Tuberculosis.* Boston, Little, Brown and Company, 1957.

Starr, S., and Berkovich, S.: Effects of Measles, Gamma Globulin Modified Measles and Vaccine Measles on the Tuberculin Test. *New England J. Med.,* 270:386, 1964.

Leprosy

CALVIN C. J. SIA, M.D.

The therapy of choice for all varieties of leprosy is sulfone therapy. The parent drug, dapsone (4,4′-diaminodiphenylsulfone, DDS, DADPS, "parent sulfone"), is the drug of choice based on therapeutic efficacy, cost and ease of administration. Dapsone is given initially in small doses, with the effective dosage reached only after a suitable period of time and increments made cautiously in borderline disease. In giving this drug one is cautioned to be aware of possible sulfone sensitivity and drug resistance with long-term therapy. Blood cell counts and urinalysis should be performed periodically. For the child, the following dosage is recommended:

First month	10 mg. twice a week
Second month	20 mg. twice a week
Third month	25 mg. twice a week
Fourth month	50 mg. twice a week
Thereafter	100 mg. twice a week

In indeterminate or tuberculoid leprosy (closed), treatment should be given for at least two years, or at least one year after all clinical signs of activity have disappeared. In lepromatous and borderline leprosy (open), treatment is continued for at least four years, or at least two years after all clinical signs of activity have ceased, and the acid-fast bacillary material is no longer seen on skin smears. The term clinical activity refers to any extension of existing lesions or the appearance of new lesions, the persistence of redness or elevation of the lesions or an increase in signs of peripheral nerve damage.

In attempting to reach optimal dosage, sulfone blood levels may be obtained monthly. A good therapeutic level has been about 0.5 mg. per milliliter.

Other sulfones which are more costly than dapsone (DDS) are derivatives of the "parent sulfone." These include sulfoxone (Diasone), solapsone (Sulphetrone), sodium acetosulfone (Promacetin) and thiazolsulfone (Promizole).

In lepra reactions, a complete study should be done at that time and active therapy withheld. The treatment should be symptomatic and conservative, using analgesics, antihistamines and ephedrine hydrochloride. Cortisone, systemically and locally, has also been used in severe exacerbations.

Physical rehabilitation plays a larger role in the total care of the child with developing deformities and contractures. Physical therapy, early orthopedic care and plastic surgery may be necessary in the total care.

References

Browne, S. G.: Leprosy. *Brit. Med. J.*, 3:725, 1968.
Chung-Hoon, E.: Personal communications.
Cochrane, R. G.: Chemotherapy of Leprosy. *Practitioner*, 188:67, 1962.
Doull, J. A.: Current Status of the Therapy of Leprosy. *J.A.M.A.*, 173:363, 1960.
Trowell, H. C., and Jelliffe, D. B.: *Disease of Children in the Subtropics and Tropics*. London, Edward Arnold Ltd., 1958.

Infections with the Unclassified Mycobacteria

EDWIN L. KENDIG, Jr., M.D.

In recent years it has been established that human disease can be caused by mycobacteria previously considered to be harmless. These organisms, called unclassified (atypical, anonymous) mycobacteria, may be the cause of a disease process simulating tuberculosis.

Chronic suppurative lymphadenitis is the usual form of this disease in children, but other systems (such as bone and skin) may be involved.

The usual antituberculosis drugs are utilized in treatment, but these agents are not always effective; they are more effective in group I and much less effective in group II, III and IV infections. In the treatment of group III infections, authorities have advised the use of drug combinations, often four drugs: one injectable and three oral, In fact, all treatment usually consists of at least two drugs used concomitantly. Ethambutol* and ethionamide† are probably the most effective drugs for oral administration, and next to streptomycin, kanamycin is the most effective injectable drug.

Isoniazid should be given orally in a dosage of 20 mg. per kilogram of body weight per day in a single dose or in two divided doses (maximal daily dosage of 500 mg.) and para-aminosalicylic acid (PAS) in a dosage of 200 mg. per kilogram of body weight per day orally in three or four divided doses (maximal daily dosage of 12 Gm.). If the organism is even partially sensitive, medication should be continued for one year. Streptomycin in a single intramuscular daily dose of 20 to 40 mg. per kilogram of body weight (maximal daily dose of 1 Gm.) is continued until clinical improvement is noted, and the drug may then be administered three times each week. The duration of treatment with this drug depends on the course of the disease, but if such treatment is prolonged, the patient should be carefully watched for possible damage to the 8th cranial nerve.

Ethambutol is given orally in a suggested dosage of 20 mg. per kilogram of body weight per day for four to six weeks and 15 mg. per kilogram of body weight per day thereafter. It is given in a single daily dose. The drug appears to be an effective and relatively safe agent, although use in pediatric patients under 13 years of age is experimental. It is well tolerated, and there have been few reports of allergic reactions. So far, the drug has been used mainly in adults, and with large dosage a few instances of retrobulbar neuritis with resultant loss of vision have been noted. At the recommended dose and with precautions that include monthly studies of visual acuity, visual fields and tests for green color vision, there appears to be much less danger of this side effect. The drug should be discontinued if there is more than a two-line loss of visual acuity as measured on a Snellen eye chart, if there is contraction of the visual field or if there is loss of green color vision.

Ethionamide, also available for use in combination with one or more drugs, is administered orally in a suggested dosage of 10 to 20 mg. per kilogram of body weight. (Dosage in children has not been established.) It is given

* Manufacturer's precaution: Ethambutol is not recommended for children under 13 years of age, since conditions for safe use have not been established.

† Manufacturer's precaution: Optimum dosage of ethionamide has not been established. However, this does not preclude its use if crucial to therapy.

in two or three divided doses. The drug may be hepatotoxic.

Kanamycin, given intramuscularly in a dosage of 10 to 15 mg. per kilogram, is similar to streptomycin and may have all the toxic effects of streptomycin plus renal toxicity.

Early reports suggest that rifampin possesses significant activity against certain strains of atypical mycobacteria. Suggested dosage is 10 to 20 mg. per kilogram of body weight (maximum daily dose of 600 mg.).

Prompt excision of suppurative lymph nodes is the most important part of the therapeutic approach. Since there is a tendency toward early and complete liquefaction of affected lymph nodes, these nodes should be completely removed as soon as possible. In adults with pulmonary disease who have localized lesions which have not responded to chemotherapy and are in satisfactory general condition, pulmonary resection is the treatment of choice. They should continue to receive the same antimicrobial therapy as previously outlined. There have been a few reports of pulmonary disease in children, but such involvement in this age group must be very rare.

Skin lesions caused by *Mycobacterium balnei (marinum)* must often be excised and the patient is always given the same antimicrobial therapy.

Patients with clinical disease caused by the unclassified mycobacteria should not be treated in a tuberculosis sanatorium.

References

Bialkin, G., Pollak, A., and Weil, A. J.: Pulmonary Infection with *Mycobacterium kansasii. J. Dis. Child.,* 101:739, 1961.

Black, B. G., and Chapman, J. S.: Cervical Adenitis in Children Due to Human and Unclassified Mycobacteria. *Pediatrics,* 33:887, 1964.

Committee on Diagnostic Skin Testing, American Thoracic Society: Current Indications for the Use of Atypical Mycobacterial Skin Test Antigens. *Am. Rev. Resp. Dis.,* 102:468, 1970.

Krieger, I., Hahne, O. H., and Whitten, C. F.: Atypical Mycobacteria as a Probable Cause of Chronic Bone Disease. *J. Pediat.,* 65:340, 1964.

Mollohan, C. S., and Romer, M. S.: Public Health Significance of Swimming Pool Granuloma. *Am. J. Public Health,* 51:883, 1961.

Reid, J. D., and Wolinsky, E.: Histopathology of Lymphadenitis Caused by Atypical Mycobacteria. *Am. Rev. Resp. Dis.,* 99:8, 1969.

Rynearson, T. K., Shronts, J. S., and Wolinsky, E.: Rifampin: In Vitro Effect in Atypical Mycobacteria. *Am. Rev. Resp. Dis.,* 104:272, 1971.

Syphilis

PAUL J. WIESNER, M.D.

In the United States, the reported incidence of congenital syphilis in patients under one year of age has increased from 277 cases in 1969 to 422 cases in 1972. This represents an increased rate per 10,000 live births from 0.8 to 1.3 during the same period and closely parallels the reported incidence of early infectious syphilis in the general population.

Several critical periods in the course of congenital syphilis may be identified as important in treatment aimed at preventing complications of the disease. The first period begins with acquisition of infection by a female of childbearing age and extends approximately to the fourth month of pregnancy. Syphilitic infection in the mother rarely, if ever, involves the fetus prior to the fifth month of pregnancy. The greatest effort should therefore be expended to identify and treat the infection in the mother prior to this time, thereby preventing infection of the fetus.

With the onset of the fifth month, *Treponema pallidum* crosses the placenta in a high percentage of women with early syphilis. Syphilitic infection of the fetus is less common in women with longstanding infection. The infection in the fetus and neonate is, in many respects, analogous to early syphilis in the adult, except that it is less benign and may on occasion lead to stillbirth or neonatal death. In addition, involvement of developing structures, such as cartilage, bones and teeth, results in deformities not seen following adult-onset syphilis. Treatment of the mother during late pregnancy, or of the neonate, arrests the infection. Completeness of recovery varies with the severity and location of pathology established at the time of treatment, and with associated factors such as secondary infection and nutritional status.

For those children not developing early signs and symptoms, the prognosis is excellent if treatment is administered prior to two years of age. In older children, pathology may be irreversible, and in the particular instances of the poorly understood inflammatory lesions of interstitial keratitis and 8th nerve deafness, the disease may actually progress in spite of therapy.

As in adult syphilis, penicillin is the drug of choice. Dose-interval schedules were established in vitro in animals, and then in adult patients during the early penicillin era of the late 1940s and early 1950s. The high incidence of syphilis made large clinical trials possible. This work revealed the exquisite sensitivity of *T. pallidum* in vitro to as little as 0.005 microgram per ml. of penicillin. It is eliminated from rabbit testis when serum levels of 0.005 to 0.01 mg. per ml. are achieved. These data, in conjunction with the clinical trials, lead to the general formulation that all forms of uncomplicated syphilis require exposure of the organism to a serum level of 0.03 to 0.2 units per ml. over an eight- to 14-day period for cure.

Unfortunately, little information is available describing the serum and other pertinent body fluid levels after administration of the various dosages and preparations of penicillin in children in different age groups. Treatment studies of large numbers of patients with congenital syphilis have been conducted only with aqueous penicillin G. On the basis of these studies, it is recommended that small infants be treated with aqueous penicillin G given in equally divided intramuscular doses every 3 to 6 hours, over a 10-day period, for a total dose of at least 100,000 units per kilogram body weight.

The above regimen would, in most cases, require hospitalization of the infant or child. The advent of repository forms of penicillin in the early 1950s obviated this need in many clinical settings. However, the precipitous decrease in incidence of syphilis in the 1950s made it difficult to conduct appropriate clinical trials with these newer penicillin preparations. As a result, treatment studies of congenital syphilis with repository forms of penicillin involve only small numbers of patients. However, over the years, various treatment schedules have become established.

Small infants may be treated with aqueous procaine penicillin G given intramuscularly in two equally divided daily doses for a total of 100,000 to 200,000 units per kilogram of body weight. For larger infants under two years of age, in whom more muscle mass is available for injection, possible alternative schedules are 100,000 to 200,000 units of aqueous procaine penicillin G per kilogram of body weight, divided into three doses at two- to three-day intervals, or 100,000 units per kilogram of body weight of benzathine penicillin G either in a single intramuscular injection or in two doses one week apart. The volume required for such a single injection serves as a contraindication for use in smaller infants.

For children between the ages of two and 11, or for children who weigh less than 70 pounds, either a total of 100,000 to 200,000 units per kilogram of body weight of aqueous procaine penicillin G divided into 10 daily intramuscular doses, or a total of 100,000 units per kilogram of body weight of benzathine penicillin G given intramuscularly at one visit may be used.

Children 12 years of age or older may be treated with one of the following schedules: a total of 6 million to 9 million units of procaine penicillin G with aluminum monostearate given intramuscularly in doses of 1,200,000 units at three-day intervals, or 600,000 to 1 million units of aqueous procaine penicillin G, given in daily intramuscular doses for 10 days.

While there are some data available for the efficacy of penicillin regimens, there are only a very limited number of reports reflecting use of other antimicrobial agents when penicillin is contraindicated. Tetracycline and erythromycin have been employed. In children under age eight, 6 to 8 Gm. of erythromycin per kilogram of body weight is used, to be given orally every 6 hours for 10 days. Tetracycline is contraindicated in this age group because of staining of teeth and possible toxicity to bone. Older children require either 20 to 30 Gm. of erythromycin, given in four daily doses of 500 mg. each for 10 to 15 days, or 30 to 40 Gm. of tetracycline over 10 to 15 days. Unfortunately, these dosages are in the ranges that may cause gastrointestinal side effects.

Recommended follow-up for congenital syphilis should begin with repeat clinical examinations to document resolution of active lesions. A pretreatment quantitative Venereal Disease Research Laboratory (VDRL) slide test establishes a base line titer. Following treatment, the quantitative VDRLs should be repeated to document a fall in titer. At least one spinal tap should be performed to document the absence or resolution of central nervous system involvement. A cerebrospinal fluid (CSF) VDRL, protein determination and cell count are the important parameters.

For children under age two, the quantitative VDRL on serum is recommended at monthly intervals for six months, then at three-month intervals for one year. If only one spinal fluid examination is done, the preferred time is 12 months after treatment. For children older than age two, if the spinal fluid VDRL is nonreactive, a quantitative VDRL should be done at six-month intervals for two years. If spinal fluid is reactive, a VDRL serologic test and a spinal fluid examination should be done quarterly for one year and semiannually for a second year.

Generally, in children under age two, lesions heal rapidly and the serologic and spinal fluid VDRLs revert rather rapidly to nonreactive. The CSF protein and cell count should return to normal. In older children titers of blood may descend very slowly or remain static. Therefore, serofastness does not indicate that previous therapy has been inadequate or that additional treatment is needed. In some cases, the CSF VDRL may not become nonreactive but the cell count and the protein should return to normal. A rising serum VDRL or the failure of CSF cell counts and protein to fall steadily to normal indicates continued activity of the disease and dictates re-treatment.

Adequate follow-up is of increasing importance as one shifts from the better studied aqueous penicillin G to other forms of penicillin for which there are fewer data, or to nonpenicillin drugs, for which data are confined to individual case reports.

The management of late complications of congenital syphilis often requires individualized specialized care. With interstitial keratitis and nerve deafness, the advice of an appropriate specialist should be sought, since these complications often progress in spite of penicillin therapy alone. For interstitial keratitis, topical steroids may be used in addition to penicillin, usually with good results. Systemic corticosteroids as an adjunct to penicillin, have been reported to be of value in the treatment of nerve deafness.

Generally, the therapy for acquired syphilis in children is similar to that for congenital syphilis.

Leptospirosis

ROBERT E. KOEHLER, M.D.

The clinical course of leptospirosis is often biphasic. The initial or leptospiremic phase, characterized by fever, vomiting, headache, muscle aches and prostration, subsides in four to eight days. Fever then may return a few days later as the second phase of the illness begins; meningitis and ocular complications are more likely to occur during this second period. The onsets of hepatic, renal and hemorrhagic manifestations correlate poorly with phase of illness; these complications may begin at any time in the course of the disease.

General Measures. Hospitalization is recommended for all patients with leptospirosis early in their illness. This is advisable particularly from the standpoint of permitting a careful watch to be kept for renal, hepatic, hemorrhagic and other potentially serious complications.

Since specific antibiotic therapy is often started late and is of relatively little benefit, general supportive measures are particularly important. Nursing care should include monitoring of fluid intake and output. The staff should be encouraged to report promptly the occurrence of dyspnea, oliguria or hemorrhage into the skin, gastrointestinal tract or other areas. Severely ill patients should be turned frequently to lessen the risk of secondary pulmonary complications. Severe protracted vomiting is best managed by discontinuing oral intake and instituting intravenous fluid and electrolyte replacement. Aspirin and codeine help lessen fever, headache and muscle aches, but salicylates should be used with caution if gastrointestinal bleeding occurs. Strong cathartic agents that may predispose to gastrointestinal bleeding should not be used.

The patient's blood and cerebrospinal fluid may contain viable leptospires early in the course of the disease, and the organism has been isolated from urine of convalescent patients as late as several weeks after symptoms abate. Hospital personnel should be instructed to exercise care in the disposal and laboratory analysis of such fluids, keeping them away from mucosal surfaces and broken or abraded skin. Isolation of the patient is not necessary.

Antibiotic Treatment. Many workers have demonstrated in vitro the leptospirostatic effects of penicillin and many of the commonly used broad-spectrum antibiotics. The question of the efficacy of antibiotic therapy in human leptospirosis has been much more difficult to answer because of the great variability in the clinical severity and complication rate in the untreated illness. Two clinical studies failed to demonstrate any difference in the severity of illness in patients treated with penicillin or broad-spectrum antibiotics as opposed to untreated controls. On the other hand, two controlled studies and many uncontrolled observations support the claim that there is a reduction in the duration and severity of fever when antibiotic therapy is begun within four days of onset of symptoms. There is no clear evidence of beneficial effects of antibiotic therapy begun later in the course of the disease. Antibiotics do not appear to lessen the frequency of renal, hepatic or other complications. The use of antibiotic therapy is advised until the question of its effectiveness is settled.

Since the lower dose levels of penicillin used in treatment of hospitalized patients

(10,000 to 15,000 units per kilogram every 6 hours) have not shown clear evidence of effectiveness, penicillin, if used, should probably be given in dosages comparable to those used for treatment of bacteremias due to penicillin-sensitive organisms (100,000 units per kilogram per day, intravenously), even though proof of efficacy at this higher level is also lacking. Therapy should probably be continued for at least five days. As an alternative regimen, tetracycline* can be given orally every 6 hours in a dose of 25 mg. per kilogram per day for five days.

Undesirable effects of penicillin treatment which have occurred in some patients, particularly those receiving the initial dose early in the course of the disease, include a sharp rise in temperature and transient worsening of the other signs and symptoms of the disease within 24 hours after the initial dose of penicillin (Herxheimer reaction). Occasionally this reaction includes a drop in blood pressure requiring treatment with pressor amines.

Management of Complications. The presence or absence of protein, cells and casts in the urine is not a good indicator of the extent of renal involvement, and monitoring of renal function should include daily assessment of urinary output and periodic measurement of blood urea nitrogen and serum creatinine. When azotemia and oliguria are noted, a determination must be made as to whether these abnormalities are due to salt and water depletion or to actual renal involvement with acute tubular dysfunction. Jugular venous distention, orthostatic changes in blood pressure and condition of skin and mucous membranes should be evaluated. Measurement of central venous pressure and the ratio of urine osmolality to plasma osmolality (U_{osm}/P_{osm}) may also be helpful in making this distinction. Diuresis can usually be induced in patients with prerenal azotemia by the intravenous administration of physiologic saline, 20 ml. per kilogram. Patients with serum creatinine greater than 2 mg. per 100 ml. and U_{osm}/P_{osm} less than 2 usually do not respond to the administration of a fluid load and should be treated in accordance with the accepted principles of management of acute tubular necrosis. Since the long-term prognosis after recovery from severe renal involvement with leptospirosis is good, there should be no hesitation in the use of peritoneal dialysis or hemodialysis when these measures are required.

Hemorrhage may occur as purpura, epistaxis, hemoptysis or gastrointestinal bleeding and appears to be due to capillary injury although hypoprothrombinemia and a low platelet count are sometimes noted as well. Transfusions may be required.

No additional therapeutic measures are known to be helpful in the management of hepatic or meningeal involvement with leptospirosis.

Iridocyclitis occasionally occurs as a complication, usually appearing late in the clinical course or as much as several weeks after recovery. An ophthalmologist should be consulted regarding management of ocular complications.

* Manufacturer's note: The use of tetracyclines during tooth development (last half of pregnancy, infancy and childhood to age eight years) may cause permanent discoloration of teeth. This adverse reaction is more common during long-term use of the drugs but has been observed following repeated short-term courses.

Rat Bite and Rat-Bite Fever

JAY P. SANFORD, M.D.

Rat-bite fever occurs throughout the world, with a higher incidence in urban areas where sanitation is poor and the rat population is great. In the United States, approximately one-half of the reported cases have occurred among children under 12 years of age. Rat-bite fever is said to follow about 10 per cent of rat bites; however, with an estimated 14,000 persons bitten by rats annually in the United States, this frequency appears excessively high.

RAT BITES

The primary wounds are incurred on the face or extremities during sleep; they may vary from a simple puncture wound to lacerations. Initial wound management should consist of prompt cleansing with soap and water, although it has been stated by some clinicians that immediate wound cleansing does not prevent rat-bite fever. The wounds should then be debrided adequately to remove devitalized tissue. As with all contaminated traumatic wounds, tight primary closure should not be performed except to cover tendons. Additional primary wound management should include appropriate tetanus prophylaxis, although I am unaware of tetanus occurring following a rat bite. A child who has previously received at least two doses of tetanus toxoid should receive the recommended dose (check the manufacturer's package insert) of tetanus-diphtheroid toxoid intramuscularly. However, even in wound management it is unnecessary to use booster injection more than every five years. If passive immunization is to be used, i.e., when the child has had less than two previous injections of tetanus toxoid or when the wound has been untended for more than 24 hours, tetanus immune globulin (human) (TIG) should be used. The recommended adult prophylactic dosage of TIG is 250 units and should be given concurrently with tetanus toxoid; however, each should be given with separate syringes and at separate sites. Children's dosage of TIG should be calculated by body weight (4 units per kilogram). Larger doses may be used when the injury is severe or the risk of tetanus infection is high. Antirabies prophylaxis is seldom, if ever, required. Specifically, among more than 5000 laboratory-confirmed instances of wildlife rabies in the United States between 1970 and mid-1972, there was only one instance of rabies in a rat.

RAT-BITE FEVER

In addition to the usual (group A streptococcal and staphylococcal) pyogenic infections, two clinically similar but etiologically distinct diseases may follow rat bites, and both are designated rat-bite fever.

Streptobacillary rat-bite fever is caused by the pleomorphic gram-negative bacillus *Streptobacillus moniliformis,* while spirillary rat-bite fever is caused by *Spirillum minus.* In the United States, streptobacillary rat-bite fever is more common. *S. moniliformis* is found in the oropharynx of healthy rats. Though several epidemics have apparently been associated with the ingestion of raw milk (Haverhill fever), the portal of entry is usually an animal bite.

Following a bite, the primary wound usually heals promptly, and after an incubation period of 1 to 22 (usually less than 10) days the patient abruptly develops severe chills, fever, vomiting, headache and pains in the back and joints. The fever tends to remit in two to five days. About the third day, a morbiliform, petechial rash appears on the feet and hands in over 90 per cent of patients. After remitting briefly, the fever recurs and is characteristically (70 per cent of patients) associated with arthralgia and arthritis.

Spirillum minus is a cause of ocular infection in rats, with the organism apparently reaching the rat's mouth via the nasolacrimal ducts. Following a bite, the initial wound usually heals promptly. After an incubation period of 4 to 28 (usually greater than 10) days, inflammation recurs at the primary wound site, with associated fever and regional lymphadenitis. A roseolar-urticarial rash may be present, but it is less evident than that which occurs in streptobacillary rat-bite fever. Arthritis is rare. The fever is typically relapsing in character. Laboratory findings include a white blood cell count of 5000 to 30,000 and false-positive VDRL tests in about one-half of patients.

Both streptobacillary and spirillary rat-bite fever are optimally treated with penicillin (penicillin V, 50,000 units per kilogram per day orally, divided into three or four doses; or procaine penicillin G, 50,000 units per kilogram per day intramuscularly, divided into two doses) for 10 days. In children with penicillin hypersensitivity, tetracycline* (50 mg. per kilogram per day orally, divided into three or four doses) for 10 days represents an effective alternative antimicrobial agent.

Pneumocystis carinii Pneumonitis

WALTER T. HUGHES, M.D.

Pneumocystis carinii pneumonitis occurs almost exclusively in patients with a serious underlying disease which has compromised the host's resistance to infection. The infection remains limited to the lung even in fatal cases. Pathologically, the disease is primarily an alveolitis, with interstitial edema causing a diffuse alveolar-capillary blockade.

Successful management requires early diagnosis, specific antimicrobial therapy and intensive supportive management. The procedure required to obtain material for diagnostic studies is needle aspiration of the lung, lung biopsy or endotracheal brush catheter technique. Pneumothorax is a complication of these procedures, and management demands attention to this hazard. Also, optimum treatment of the primary disease should be maintained.

Specific Therapy. Pentamidine isethionate, an aromatic diamidine, is the drug of choice. Manufactured under the name Lomidine by May and Baker Ltd., Dagenham, England, the drug is investigational and available in the United States only through the Center for Disease Control, Atlanta, Georgia. Physicians may obtain the drug to treat specific cases by calling the Parasitic Disease Drug Service (day: (404) 633-3311, ext. 3672; and night: (404) 633-2176).

Pentamidine is administered as a single daily dose of 4 mg. per kilogram, intramuscularly. Therapy is continued for 10 to 14

* Manufacturer's note: The use of tetracyclines during tooth development (last half of pregnancy, infancy and childhood to age eight years) may cause permanent discoloration of teeth. This adverse reaction is more common during long-term use of the drugs but has been observed following repeated short-term courses.

days. If improvement is apparent after five days of treatment, the dosage may be reduced to 3 mg. per kilogram per day. The total dosage should not exceed 56 mg. per kilogram. Intramuscular injections should be given deeply into the anterolateral aspect of the thigh. Each 100 mg. of the drug should be dissolved in 1 ml. of sterile distilled water. Filtration of the drug in solution through a Millipore filter (0.22-micron pore size) immediately before injection is advisable to ensure sterility for the immunosuppressed host.

Adverse effects of pentamidine include the following: (1) induration, abscess formation and necrosis at injection sites; (2) nephrotoxicity; (3) hypoglycemia or, rarely, hyperglycemia; (4) hypotension; (5) alteration in liver function; (6) tachycardia; (7) hypocalcemia; (8) nausea and vomiting; (9) skin rash; (10) anemia; (11) hyperkalemia; and (12) thrombocytopenia.

A combination of pyrimethamine and sulfonamides has been shown to have some therapeutic effect in animals (Frenkel et al.) and prophylactically in nursery epidemics (Post et al.). However, its efficacy in active *P. carinii* pneumonitis has not been determined.

Strict Isolation. Since the mode of transmission of *P. carinii* is unknown, it is advisable at this time to isolate the patient from other individuals at high risk for infection.

Supportive Measures. OXYGEN. All patients are placed in an oxygen tent with Fi–O_2 of 40 to 50 volumes per cent. The flow rate should exceed the minute volume of the patient (12 to 14 liters per minute).

VENTILATORY THERAPY. Assisted or controlled ventilation is indicated in patients with arterial blood pH of less than 7.25, arterial oxygen tension less than 60 mm. Hg and arterial blood CO_2 tension greater than 60 mm. Hg. Patients with acutely elevated pCO_2, without pH changes, and with or without hypoxemia should be considered candidates for ventilatory therapy.

WITHHOLD IMMUNOSUPPRESSIVE CHEMOTHERAPY. Patients receiving immunosuppressive drugs should have these discontinued if the status of the primary disease permits. Corticosteroids are of no benefit, and may be deleterious to the course of the pneumonitis (Hughes et al.).

INTRAVENOUS FLUIDS. Fluid and electrolyte quantities are calculated by the patient's needs but should contain 5 or 10 per cent glucose to prevent hypoglycemia during pentamidine therapy. Metabolic acidosis must be corrected.

ANTIBIOTICS. Bacterial pneumonia or sepsis may occur in association with *P. carinii* pneumonitis. In the seriously ill patient with marked neutropenia (absolute neutrophil count less than 1000 per cubic millimeter) or evidence of bacterial infection, antibiotics should be given. Cephalothin, 100 mg. per kilogram per day, and gentamicin, 5 mg. per kilogram per day, are administered intravenously until the results of cultures are known.

NUTRITION. Efforts should be made to improve the nutritional status of the patient by dietary means even during the acute stage of the disease. Multivitamins should be given empirically. The value of intravenous alimentation has not been determined.

ANEMIA. Give blood transfusion if hemoglobin level is less than 9 Gm. per 100 ml. The hemoglobin content must be sufficient to result in an arterial oxygen content of 15 to 20 ml. per 100 ml. of blood at an arterial oxygen tension of 100 mm. Hg.

PNEUMOTHORAX. Pneumothorax may be a complication to diagnostic procedures. If the pneumothorax is small with no adverse effect on respiration, close observation is adequate. If the pneumothorax is more extensive, insertion of a thoracotomy tube with a water seal drainage system is necessary.

Parameters to Monitor. The following measurements should be made to recognize adverse events because of the infection, the primary disease or the therapy:

1. *Serum immunoglobulins* at the onset of the illness. Administer immune serum globulin (165 mg. per ml.) 1.5 ml. per kilogram, if the immunoglobulin G level is below 300 mg. per 100 ml.

2. *Blood urea nitrogen (BUN) and urinalysis* every three days. If the BUN exceeds 40 mg. per 100 ml., withhold pentamidine for one or two days.

3. *Roentgenograms of chest* daily until clinical evidence of improvement. If needle aspiration of the lung, lung biopsy or endotracheal brush catheter technique has been used as a diagnostic procedure, chest roentgenograms should be made at 30-minute, 4-hour and 12-hour intervals after the procedure to detect pneumothorax.

4. *Blood glucose* 4 to 6 hours after each injection of pentamidine. Administer glucose if value of blood glucose is less than 40 mg. per 100 ml.

5. *Serum calcium and phosphorus* every three days. If the serum inorganic phosphate level becomes increased and the calcium level becomes decreased from normal values on the

basis of renal insufficiency, give calcium lactate, 15 to 20 Gm. per day, or calcium carbonate, 5 to 8 Gm. per day orally. The diet should be low in phosphate and 25,000 to 50,000 units of vitamin D is given orally.

6. *Blood pressure, pulse and respiratory rate* every 6 hours or more frequently if the condition is critical.

7. *Serum glutamic oxaloacetic transaminase (SGOT)* every three days; withhold pentamidine for one to two days if evidence of hepatic toxicity exists.

8. *Hemoglobin, WBC count and differential, and platelet estimate.*

9. *Body weight, intake and output* daily.

10. *Arterial blood gases:* measure pH, pCO_2, pO_2 and base excess or deficit initially and as often as necessary, based on severity of clinical course.

11. *Serum electrolytes:* measure sodium, chloride, potassium and carbon dioxide content every three days or more frequently if indicated.

Expected Course. Fever, tachypnea and pulmonary infiltrates usually persist with little change for four to six days. If no improvement is apparent after one week of therapy, concomitant or secondary infection most likely exists. These infections have included bacterial pneumonia or sepsis, systemic candidiasis, aspergillosis, cryptococcosis, histoplasmosis and cytomegalovirus inclusion disease as well as other viral infections.

Recurrent *P. carinii* pneumonitis may occur several months after apparent recovery in 10 to 15 per cent of cases.

Prevention. No effective means for prevention of *P. carinii* infection are known for the compromised host. Since protein-calorie deprivation is a factor in host susceptibility to *P. carinii* pneumonitis, maintenance of proper nutritional status is probably important in prevention of this disease.

References

Frenkel, J. K., Good, J. T., and Schultz, V. A.: Latent Pneumocystis Infection of Rats: Relapse and Chemotherapy. *Lab. Invest.*, 15:1559, 1966.

Hughes, W., Price, R., Kim, H. K., Coburn, T., Grigsby, D., and Feldman, S.: *Pneumocystis carinii* Pneumonitis in Children with Malignancies. *J. Pediat.*, 82:404, 1973.

Post, C., Fakowhi, T., Dutz, W., Bandarizadeh, B., and Kohout, E. E.: Prophylaxis of Epidemic Infantile Pneumocystosis with a 20:1 Sulfadoxine and Pyrimethamine Combination. *Curr. Ther. Res.*, 113:273, 1971.

Western, K. A., Perera, D. R., and Schultz, M. G.: Pentamidine Isethionate in the Treatment of *Pneumocystis carinii* Pneumonia. *Am. Int. Med.*, 73:695, 1970.

Measles
(Rubeola)

HARRIS D. RILEY, JR., M.D.

The ideal approach to the "treatment" of measles is prevention by immunization.

All susceptible persons – those who have not had natural measles or who have not received measles vaccine–should be immunized.

Unless protected by vaccine, virtually all children will at some time have clinically evident measles. It is particularly important to immunize children who are still susceptible before they enter nursery school, kindergarten or elementary school, because otherwise they may be responsible for transmission of measles to other children in the community.

PREVENTION

Active Immunization

Live Attenuated Measles Virus Vaccine (Edmonston, Schwarz and Moraten Strains). Measles virus vaccine, live, attenuated, prepared from the Edmonston or Schwarz and Moraten (further attenuated) measles virus strains is widely used in the United States. The Edmonston strain is propagated in either chick embryos or canine renal cell cultures; it may be given alone or simultaneously with measles immune globulin, according to the manufacturers' directions. The Schwarz and Moraten strains are prepared only in chick embryo cell cultures; they are suitable for administration without the concurrent administration of measles immune globulin.

The live attenuated measles virus vaccines produce a mild or inapparent noncommunicable infection. Fifteen per cent of those patients receiving either the Edmonston strain with measles immune globulin, or the further attenuated strains, experience fever, with temperatures of 103° F. (39.4° C.) (rectal) or higher, beginning about the sixth day after vaccination and lasting no longer than five days. About twice as many (30 per cent) of those receiving the Edmonston strain vaccine without measles immune globulin have similar responses. The majority of children responding with high fever experience relatively little discomfort and minimal toxicity.

An antibody response develops in virtually all susceptible children who are given live attenuated measles virus vaccines. The antibody titers following Edmonston strain vaccine administered with measles immune globulin, or from the further attenuated strains alone, are slightly lower. However, all three of these vaccine schedules appear to confer lasting protection against naturally occurring measles, and live attenuated measles virus vaccines are among the safest immunizing agents available. To date, serious reactions associated with their use have been very rare.

Inactivated Measles Virus Vaccine. Inactivated vaccines derived from Edmonston strain measles virus and prepared either in chick embryo or monkey cell cultures are available (Measles Virus Vaccine, Inactivated). These vaccines should be administered in a three-dose schedule, at monthly intervals, with a booster six months later. Following primary immunization with inactivated measles virus vaccine, the protection achieved in normal children has been satisfactory for the first few months, but has been shown to decline rapidly thereafter. Inactivated measles virus vaccine should not be used for immunizing normal children (see Previous Immunization with Inactivated Measles Vaccine). It should be restricted for use in children in whom live attenuated measles virus vaccine may be contraindicated, such as those with leukemia, lymphomas or other generalized malignancies, and in those receiving corticosteroids, alkylating agents, antimetabolites or irradiation therapy. Reactions to inactivated measles virus vaccine are infrequent and mild and resemble those observed after administration of other alum-precipitated products (e.g., diphtheria and tetanus toxoids).

Recommendations for Use. AGE. For maximum efficacy, live attenuated measles virus vaccine should be administered when children are at least 12 months old. It can be given to infants at 9 to 12 months of age, with the realization that the proportion of vaccine responses may be slightly reduced. This proportion is further decreased if measles immune globulin is administered with the vaccine. At the present time, vaccination of adults is rarely necessary because nearly all persons are immune by age 15. Limited data indicate that reactions to vaccine are no more common in adults than in children.

HIGH-RISK GROUPS. Immunization against measles is particularly important for children with chronic illnesses, such as heart disease, cystic fibrosis and chronic pulmonary diseases, as well as for malnourished children and those living in institutions.

PREVENTION OF NATURAL MEASLES FOLLOWING EXPOSURE. Live attenuated measles virus vaccine usually can prevent disease if administered before or on the day of exposure to natural measles. Limited studies reported to date indicate that adverse effects are not induced by measles immunization following exposure.

Precautions in the Use of Live Attenuated Measles Virus Vaccine. SEVERE FEBRILE ILLNESSES. Vaccination should be postponed until recovery is complete.

TUBERCULOSIS. The exacerbations of tuberculosis that have been related to natural measles infection, by analogy, might accompany infection with live attenuated measles virus. Therefore, any individual with known active tuberculosis should be under active treatment when given measles vaccine. Although tuberculin skin testing is desirable as a part of ideal health care, it need not be a routine prerequisite in community measles immunization programs. The value of protection against natural measles outweighs the theoretical hazard of possible exacerbation of tuberculosis infection by the administration of the vaccine.

MARKED HYPERSENSITIVITY TO VACCINE COMPONENTS. Measles vaccine produced in chick embryo cell cultures should not be given to children who are hypersensitive to ingested egg proteins. Similarly, vaccine produced in canine cell cultures should not be administered to children who are highly sensitive to dog hair or dog dander. To date, no reactions of the anaphylactic type following the administration of measles vaccine have been reported in the United States.

Contraindications to Use of Live Attenuated Measles Virus Vaccine. LEUKEMIA, LYMPHOMAS AND OTHER GENERALIZED MALIGNANCIES. Administration of live attenuated measles virus vaccine to children with leukemia has occasionally been followed by severe complications, such as fatal giant cell pneumonia. Theoretically, attenuated measles virus infection might be potentiated by other severe underlying diseases, such as lymphomas and generalized malignancies.

ALTERED RESISTANCE FROM THERAPY. Steroids, alkylating drugs, antimetabolites and radiation may predispose patients to untoward complications because of altered resistance.

PREGNANCY. Purely on speculative grounds, physicians are reluctant to risk causing fetal damage that theoretically might be related to attenuated virus infection. Immunization with inactivated vaccine is not contraindicated during pregnancy.

MANAGEMENT OF PATIENTS WITH CONTRAINDICATIONS TO LIVE ATTENUATED MEASLES VIRUS VACCINE. If immediate protection against measles is required for persons in whom use of live attenuated measles virus vaccine is contraindicated, passive immunization with measles immune globulin (dose, 0.25 ml. per kilogram) should be given as soon as possible after a known exposure. It is important to note, however, that the preventive dose of measles immune globulin which is effective in normal children may not be equally so in children with acute leukemia. Inactivated measles virus vaccines may induce longer lasting protection than that provided by measles immune globulin, but many children with leukemia and those receiving immunosuppressive drugs respond poorly.

Previous Immunization with Inactivated Measles Vaccine. Atypical measles, sometimes severe, following exposure to natural measles has occasionally been observed in children previously immunized with inactivated measles virus vaccines. Untoward local reactions, such as induration and edema, have, at times, been observed when the live measles virus vaccine was administered to persons who had previously received inactivated vaccine.

Despite these reported instances of unusual association, children who have been given inactivated measles vaccine should also be given the live vaccine for full and lasting protection against natural infection.

Simultaneous Administration of Live Virus Vaccines and of Combined Vaccines. In the past, it was recommended that there be an interval of one month between administration of live virus vaccines. The rationale for the recommendation was the theory that superimposed reactions and diminished antibody responses might result if two or more live virus vaccines are given simultaneously. The only exception to this practice has been the use of live poliovirus vaccine when administered as a trivalent mixture. However, interference of one vaccine with the antibody response to another has posed the only significant problem. For example, instances of partial interference have been noted between live measles and yellow fever vaccines given simultaneously, and between those two vaccines and smallpox vaccine.

Combined or simultaneous administration of various live virus vaccines offers obvious advantages, particularly when the child will be inaccessible for further immunization or when there is a threat of concomitant exposure. Several new vaccines are now available which contain two or three of the live attenuated viruses already in wide use as single agents. These include measles and rubella vaccine, as well as measles, mumps and rubella vaccine. Experience to date indicates that these products are both safe and effective when used as directed. Data indicate that antibody response to each component of these combination vaccines is comparable with antibody response to the individual vaccine given separately. There is no evidence that adverse reaction to the combined product occurs more frequently or more severely than known reactions to the individual vaccine. The obvious convenience of giving already selected antigens in combined form should encourage consideration of using these products when appropriate. They can, therefore, be recommended, with obvious advantage in reduction in the number of injections for any given child and a concomitant decrease in the required visits to a physician's office or clinic. Which combination to administer will vary with the past immunization, experience and needs of any particular child, as well as the choice and priorities of any physician or health planning group. Past restrictions on the simultaneous administration of live virus vaccines have been modified with the experience of a new antigen. If one chooses on a single occasion to administer multiple separate injections for the monovalent measles, rubella and/or mumps vaccines, only those same specific virus strains incorporated in the combination product can be used with certainty; until further data are available, further strains cannot be recommended with such simultaneous administration.

Now that specific combined preparations have been carefully evaluated in field studies and subsequently licensed for general use, the restriction on giving these particular antigens simultaneously is no longer relevant.

Passive Immunization

Live attenuated measles virus vaccine will usually prevent the disease if administered before or on the day of exposure to natural measles. Since this is a rare situation, measles should be prevented or modified in exposed susceptibles by the administration of immune human serum globulin (ISG). A preventive dose of 0.25 ml. per kilogram of body weight should be given intramuscularly as soon as possible after exposure. When ISG is given after the fourth or fifth day of exposure, the disease is rarely prevented but it is modified. Although a modified attack of measles confers permanent immunity in most persons, this does not usually occur when the disease has been completely prevented. Therefore, active immunization should be carried out approximately two months later.

If the exposed susceptible child is known

to have leukemia, disseminated malignant disease, or "Swiss" type of agammaglobulinemia or has been on immunosuppressive drugs, 20 or 30 ml. of ISG intramuscularly should be given.

TREATMENT

The treatment of uncomplicated measles is supportive. Patients should usually remain in bed and are frequently more comfortable in a dimly lighted room because of the photophobia which accompanies the disease. During the active phase of the disease children usually do not desire solid foods; fluid requirements should be met by the use of soft drinks and ices. Fever may be controlled by the use of aspirin, 60 mg. per year of age every 4 to 6 hours to a maximum of 3.6 Gm. (60 grains) per day. The harassing cough is frequently resistant to the common antitussives, but the use of these agents is not contraindicated. Humidification of the room usually makes the patient more comfortable. As the fever disappears and the anorexia and malaise subside, normal diet and activity may be resumed.

The measles virus produces a generalized inflammatory reaction throughout the respiratory tree. The most frequent complications are respiratory in nature, particularly otitis media and pneumonia. Neurologic complications are more common in measles than in any of the other exanthems. Persistent fever beyond the third day of rash is usually the result of a complication.

Otitis media is the most frequent complication. It is usually due to one or a combination of the following organisms: pneumococci, *Hemophilus influenzae* and beta-hemolytic streptococci. Treatment can be accomplished by the use of the following:

1. Benzathine penicillin G, 600,000 units intramuscularly for patients weighing less than 50 pounds, and 1,200,000 units for patients weighing over 50 pounds; plus oral sulfisoxazole (Gantrisin),* 60 mg. per kilogram of body weight initially, followed by 180 mg. per kilogram of body weight per day divided into three or four doses for at least 14 days. (Sulfisoxazole may be omitted in patients older than five years.)

2. Ampicillin, 50 to 100 mg. per kilogram of body weight per day orally in four doses for a minimum of 14 days. Depending on the response, it may be desirable to continue chemotherapy for a longer period of time.

Pulmonary complications are second to otitis media in frequency but rank first as a cause of death. *Pneumonia* may result from an extension of the viral infection, from a superimposed bacterial infection or from a combination of both. When it is caused by the measles virus itself, it is interstitial in distribution. More commonly, it is due to secondary bacterial infection by the pneumococcus, streptococcus, staphylococcus or *H. influenzae.* Differentiation of a bacterial from a viral agent is frequently very difficult. Treatment of bacterial pneumonia in a child may be successfully carried out in a variety of ways, but treatment should be continued for a minimum of 10 days: (1) cephalothin, 40 to 80 mg. per kilogram per 24 hours intramuscularly, or cephaloridine, 30 to 100 mg. per kilogram per 24 hours;† (2) ampicillin, 50 to 100 mg. per kilogram per day; or (3) procaine penicillin, 30,000 units per kilogram per day in two doses.

Because of the frequency and severity of staphylococcal pneumonia, it is our practice to include specific antistaphylococcal drugs in the therapeutic regimen of young children with clinically severe pneumonia. These drugs include cepalothin or cephaloridine, or one of the antistaphylococcal penicillins (oxacillin, cloxacillin, methicillin); they are given until the particular cause of the pneumonia can be eliminated.

Croup, although usually mild, is common and may be severe. The management should be the same as for other patients with this disorder, particularly as it relates to the relief of upper airway obstruction.

Encephalitis is a serious, potentially crippling or fatal complication that occurs in a clinically overt form in an incidence of 1 to 1.5 per 1000 cases of measles. There appears to be no correlation between the severity of measles and that of neurologic involvement, or between the severity of the initial encephalitic process and the prognosis. It rarely occurs in association with modified measles. In a few instances it becomes manifest in the preeruptive period, but more often the onset is two to five days after the appearance of the rash; it is probably due to the measles virus itself. Encephalitis is characterized by fever, headache, drowsiness and, frequently, signs of meningeal irritation. Convulsions and coma are common. The cerebrospinal fluid usually shows a lymphocytic pleocytosis with some elevation of the protein. Occasionally the fluid may be

* Manufacturer's precaution: Sulfisoxazole (Gantrisin) is contraindicated in infants under two months of age.

† Manufacturer's precaution: Safety of cephaloridine in premature infants and infants under one month of age has not been established.

normal. The course is unpredictable, and the treatment is symptomatic and supportive. Attentive nursing care is essential, and attention to fluid and electrolyte needs by the intravenous route is usually indicated. For long-term care, nutrition by nasogastric tube or gastrostomy may be necessary. Phenobarbital, 6 mg. per kilogram of body weight per day in three or four divided doses, diphenylhydantoin (Dilantin), 6 to 8 mg. per kilogram of body weight per day in two or three doses, or diazepam (Valium),‡ given by slow intravenous injection in a dose of 1 to 5 mg., may be used for seizure control. There is no convincing evidence that corticosteroids are efficacious. In severe encephalitis other supportive measures may be needed. The use of intravenous mannitol§ and hypothermia in the management of cerebral edema has been useful in our hands. If shock is present, the use of blood, plasma and isotonic solutions along with careful monitoring of cardiovascular and respiratory status may be lifesaving. If respirators, intravenous catheters or urinary catheters are used, the possibility of secondary infection is greatly enhanced and appropriate measures to detect and treat this complication should be taken. In hemorrhagic measles, if disseminated intravascular coagulopathy ensues, the use of heparin is necessary.

Rubella
(German Measles)

SAUL KRUGMAN, M.D.

Rubella in children is generally a mild, asymptomatic and self-limited disease which requires no treatment. Although complications are rare, encephalitis and thrombocytopenic purpura may occur. The disease in adolescents and adults is more apt to be associated with constitutional symptoms such as fever, malaise, painful lymph nodes and, occasionally, arthralgia and arthritis.

Joint manifestations associated with rubella are transient, generally subsiding in one to two weeks. The symptoms respond to aspirin therapy; corticosteroids are not indicated. Neither have corticosteroids been shown to be useful for the treatment of other complications of rubella, such as thrombocytopenic purpura and encephalitis.

CONGENITAL NEONATAL RUBELLA

Rubella acquired during the first trimester of pregnancy is associated with an increased incidence of congenital malformations, stillbirths and abortions. Infants with congenital rubella have exhibited the following clinical manifestations, either singly or in combination: (1) low birth weight; (2) congenital lesions of the eyes, such as cataract, glaucoma, retinitis and coloboma; (3) deafness; (4) microcephaly, meningoencephalitis or mental retardation; (5) congenital heart disease, particularly patent ductus arteriosus and ventricular septal defects; (6) thrombocytopenic purpura; (7) hepatomegaly; (8) splenomegaly; (9) jaundice (hepatitis); and (10) bone lesions. Infants with congenital rubella infection have been shown to excrete virus from the pharynx and urine for several months after birth. These virus-shedding infants are contagious. These findings highlight the importance of isolating these infants from presumably susceptible women early in their pregnancy.

Infants with congenital rubella should be considered contagious for at least three months after birth. The period of contagion may be assessed more accurately if virus isolation facilities are available. Under these circumstances it may be possible to shorten the period of isolation. In rare instances an infant with congenital rubella may shed virus for more than one year.

EFFICACY OF GAMMA GLOBULIN

The available evidence indicates that human immune serum globulin may modify or suppress the clinical manifestations of rubella without preventing viremia. During the 1964 epidemic there were many well-documented reports of congenital rubella in infants whose mothers received human immune serum globulin after exposure.

At present it is difficult to justify the *routine* use of gamma globulin for prophylaxis of rubella in the first trimester of pregnancy. In situations in which a therapeutic abortion would be performed if infection occurred, the administration of gamma globulin would be unwise because of its potential to mask the disease without preventing viremia. On the other hand, if a therapeutic abortion would not be considered because of religious or other contraindications, human immune serum globulin should be given promptly after exposure. The recommended dose is 20 ml. intramuscularly.

‡ Manufacturer's precaution: Safety and efficacy of injectable diazepam in children under 12 years of age have not been established.

§ Manufacturer's precaution: The use of mannitol in pediatric patients has not been studied comprehensively.

Recent studies with human immune serum globulin containing a high titer of rubella antibody have been very encouraging. Inoculation of this rubella immune globulin preparation after exposure has been followed by no clinical illness, no detectable viremia, decreased shedding of virus from the pharynx and modification of the antibody response.

LIVE ATTENUATED RUBELLA VIRUS VACCINE

Two live attenuated rubella virus vaccines have been licensed for use in the United States.* In general, these vaccines have been well tolerated. Inoculation of rubella vaccine has been followed by an antibody response in approximately 95 per cent of susceptible persons. Rubella antibody levels have been lower than those observed after natural infection, but they have persisted for the seven-year period of observation of groups of children who received the experimental vaccines.

Live rubella vaccine is recommended for children 1 to 12 years of age. The highest priority should be given to kindergarten and elementary school children because they are the major source of rubella virus dissemination in the community. A past history of rubella is not reliable enough to exclude children from immunization.

Routine immunization of adolescent and adult women of child-bearing age may be hazardous because of the danger of inadvertently administering vaccine before pregnancy is evident. However, susceptible women of child-bearing age should be immunized if the possibility of pregnancy is essentially nil. Each case must be individualized. When vaccination is contemplated, the following steps are indicated: (1) One should determine rubella susceptibility by the hemagglutination inhibition test. (2) Immune women should be reassured. (3) Susceptible women who are vaccinated must be advised strongly against becoming pregnant for the next two months. In addition, they should be advised that transient arthralgia and possible arthritis may occur two to four weeks after vaccination.

As stated previously, live rubella vaccine is contraindicated for pregnant women. It is not recommended for children with altered immune states caused by leukemia, lymphoma, generalized malignancy or therapy with corticosteroids, alkylating drugs, antimetabolites or radiation. Vaccination should be postponed during severe febrile illnesses.

* 1. HPV-77 strain in duck embryo cell culture (Meruvax, Merck Sharp and Dohme, West Point, Pennsylvania).
2. Cendehill strain in rabbit kidney cell culture (Cendevax, Smith, Kline and French Laboratories, Philadelphia, Pennsylvania).

Reference

Proceedings of the International Conference on Rubella Immunization. *Am. J. Dis. Child.*, July and August issues, 1969.

Varicella and Herpes Zoster

SIDNEY KIBRICK, M.D., PH.D.

Varicella and herpes zoster are different clinical manifestions of infection with the same viral agent, varicella-zoster or V-Z virus. Varicella is the result of primary infection with this agent. Zoster represents reactivation of a latent varicella infection in an individual whose immunity has waned. Occasionally it may result from an exogenously acquired reinfection in such patients. There is no specific therapy for these disorders but supportive measures are of value.

VARICELLA (CHICKENPOX)

In its uncomplicated form, this is a benign, self-limited disease of childhood. Treatment is symptomatic. Constitutional reactions, such as malaise, high fever and headache, may be treated with aspirin or similar antipyretics and analgesics. Pruritus may be relieved by calamine lotion (more effective with 0.25 per cent menthol added) and tepid starch or sodium bicarbonate baths. Oral antihistaminics, phenothiazine derivatives or sedation may also be helpful, especially at bedtime.

Scratching should be prevented to reduce the possibility of secondary infection and scarring from premature removal of crusts. Fingernails should be kept short and clean; for infants, mittens or restraints may be necessary. Careful bathing with soap and water and use of clean underclothes will diminish the risk of bacterial superinfection. In patients with painful oral or pharyngeal mucous membrane lesions, warm saline or dilute Karo syrup gargles are often soothing. Bed rest is advisable as long as new lesions continue to appear, especially in more severe cases.

Complications. BACTERIAL INFECTION. The most common complication of varicella is secondary bacterial infection of the lesions on the scalp and skin. The organisms most frequently responsible are hemolytic *Staphylococcus aureus* and streptococci. When involvement is limited, warm saline soaks generally suffice. With more widespread infection, especially when associated with fever or leukocytosis, antibiotics specific for the infecting organisms should be given. Prompt recognition and adequate antibiotic treatment of secondary bacterial infection are important, since such infections may give rise to subcutaneous abscesses, bacteremia and metastatic sepsis.

Bacterial infections of the respiratory tract may also occur, usually after the acute stage of the rash. In the child under five years, laryngotracheitis and suppurative bronchitis are the most common manifestations, with *Hemophilus influenzae* as the chief offender and, less frequently, with hemolytic streptococci or pneumococci. Treatment consists of cool humidified air and antibiotics specific for the etiologic agent. Bacterial pneumonias may also occur. They are generally associated with a leukocytosis and secondary rise in fever. Here also, specific antibiotic therapy should be instituted. Occasionally, supportive measures are required, e.g., oxygen and, for impending cardiac failure, digitalization.

Varicella Pneumonia. Primary varicella pneumonia (pneumonia due to varicella virus) is rare and generally mild in children; it is common and frequently severe in adults. In the more severe cases the association of persistent respiratory distress with rapid shallow respirations may lead to exhaustion and death. Antibiotics are of no value in this complication and should be given only to provide specific therapy for superimposed bacterial infections or for broad-spectrum coverage pending results of cultures when the diagnosis is in question. Treatment is otherwise supportive, consisting of measures such as oxygen for cyanosis, digitalization for signs of cardiac failure and direct resuscitative rebreathing techniques if respiration becomes severely compromised. The value of adrenal steroids in this complication is unproved. A short-term trial of steroids (three or four days) may be warranted in a severely ill patient with a high degree of diffusion block who is doing poorly.

Although primary viral pneumonia is rare in children, *croup* due to this agent is occasionally encountered. Treatment consists of cool, humidified air and other supportive measures, as required.

Encephalitis. This is a relatively uncommon complication, with an incidence of about 1:10,000 and a 5 per cent fatality rate. In the patient with coma, good nursing care and supportive measures are especially important. Hydration and nutrition must be maintained by either parenteral fluid therapy or tube feeding, and aspiration must be prevented. Superimposed pulmonary infection may occur and requires specific antibiotic therapy. Although corticosteroids have been used, their efficacy has not been established.

Thrombocytopenia. This is uncommon, usually mild or subclinical and transitory. Occasionally it may be severe and associated with petechiae, bleeding from various orifices and internal hemorrhage. Hemorrhage should be treated with transfusions of fresh whole blood. When thrombocytopenia is severe and endangers life, steroid therapy often quickly controls or decreases bleeding and may cause a rapid increase in platelets. It is therefore worthy of trial even though the effects may be only temporary.

Ocular Lesions. Rarely, vesicles may appear on the cornea and conjunctiva in varicella. They are usually superficial and heal without scarring. In herpes zoster ophthalmicus and occasionally in varicella, the keratitis may be more severe with resultant scarring and impairment of vision. It is important, therefore, that treatment of ocular involvement in these disorders be carried out by or in conjunction with an ophthalmologist.

Superimposed bacterial infections may also occur, especially in ophthalmic zoster. Antibiotics may be given, either systemically or topically, depending on the severity of the infection, but the choice of antibiotic should be determined by results of culture and sensitivity tests.

Ophthalmic preparations containing steroids are sometimes employed to relieve the keratitis and iridocyclitis of herpes zoster. The use of such preparations is not without risk and should be under the direction of an ophthalmologist.

Topical iododeoxyuridine (IDU) has occasionally been used to treat the ocular manifestations of varicella and zoster. The value of such treatment is uncertain. Its use should be supervised by an ophthalmologist.

Miscellaneous Complications. Hepatitis, orchitis, hypoglycemia with convulsions, and myocarditis have all been observed as complications of varicella. Treatment is symptomatic and supportive.

Reye's syndrome, an acute cerebral edema and fatty infiltration of the liver, occasionally occurs in association with varicella. Therapeutic measures are directed primarily toward correction of the acute hepatic failure. This syndrome has been successfully treated in a few cases by peritoneal dialysis or, alternatively, by the administration of insulin and glucose to inhibit lipolysis (Riley).

Varicella and Steroids. Susceptibile patients exposed to varicella shortly after completing a course of steroids or during steroid treatment for some other disorder may acquire a severe infection with diffuse involvement of internal organs, frequently with fatal termination. In some but not all such cases the underlying disorder may have contributed to the fatal outcome. The risk is greatest if the patient is receiving steroids at the time infection is acquired. If such patients are exposed to varicella, therefore, steroid dosage should be reduced to 1 to 1½ times physiologic levels (0.7 to 1.0 mg. of cortisone per kilogram per day) as rapidly as is consistent with safety. Such patients should also receive gamma globulin immediately after exposure; preferably, they should receive zoster immune globulin (ZIG) if it is available (see below).

Gamma Globulin. Pooled gamma globulin given intramuscularly *within three days* of exposure to varicella results in modification, but not prevention, of the disease. Such attempts at modification should be made in susceptible persons who are in the following high-risk groups: patients receiving or recently completing high level steroid therapy or under treatment with antimetabolites or other depressants of antibody response, patients with blood dyscrasias or other severe underlying disease and infants under three months of age whose mothers did not have varicella before delivery. A dose of 0.6 ml. of gamma globulin per kilogram of body weight up to a total of 30 ml. is suggested.

ZOSTER IMMUNE GLOBULIN (ZIG). This is a gamma globulin fraction of plasma with a high titer of V-Z antibody, obtained from patients convalescing from V-Z infection. It prevents varicella in normal children when given in a 2-ml. dose within 72 hours following household exposure. In a larger dose (5 ml. given intramuscularly) it will also prevent varicella in susceptible high-risk individuals who have had a household or other close exposure to V-Z. Since ZIG is in short supply, it is presently available only for the following susceptible high-risk groups: (1) patients with leukemia or other malignancies, (2) patients with immune deficiencies or disorders and (3) patients receiving medications that depress the immune response (e.g., corticosteroids, antimetabolites). Consultants to be contacted with requests for ZIG are listed in Judelsohn's report from the Center for Disease Control.

Antimetabolites, Cytotoxic Drugs. Despite the in vitro efficacy of IDU, cytosine arabinoside (Ara–C) and adenine arabinoside (Ara–A) against V-Z virus, the value of these agents for systemic treatment of varicella and disseminated zoster in immunosuppressed patients has not yet been substantiated in controlled clinical trials. Since these drugs may be associated with marrow toxicity or further immunosuppression, consideration of their use should be delayed pending outcome of such trials.

HERPES ZOSTER (SHINGLES)

This is relatively uncommon in the pediatric age range. When it occurs, the associated pain, which is often severe and persistent in older persons, is generally mild and of short duration. Discomfort can usually be relieved by analgesics such as aspirin and, if necessary, codeine. Neither steroids nor gamma globulin is of value for this purpose.

As in varicella, the lesions in the vesicular stage may be treated with calamine or a similar drying lotion. During the crusted stage a bland ointment may expedite softening and disappearance of crusts.

Ocular manifestations may be severe. They have already been discussed (see p. 637).

Bacterial infection of the ruptured vesicles occasionally occurs. It may be treated either topically or systemically, but the choice of antibiotic should be guided by results of culture and sensitivity tests.

Since exposure to zoster may occasionally result in varicella, patients with zoster should not be admitted to open wards and should be kept from contact with high-risk varicella groups. The infectivity of zoster, however, appears to be considerably less than that of varicella.

References

Judelsohn, R. G.: Prevention and Control of Varicella-Zoster Infections. *J. Infect. Dis.*, 125:82, 1972.

Riley, H. D., Jr.: Reye's Syndrome. *J. Infect. Dis.*, 125:77, 1972.

Smallpox

C. HENRY KEMPE, M.D.

There is no specific therapy for smallpox at present. Penicillin and the broad-spectrum antibiotics, however, are highly effective in preventing the secondary bacterial complications that frequently occur during and after the pustular phase of the disease. Procaine penicillin, 400,000 units a day intramuscularly, or any one of the tetracycline preparations* in dosage ranging from 10 to 20 mg. per kilogram per day is indicated.

The drug N-methylisatin beta-thiosemicarbazone (Marboran) is under trial as a therapeutic agent in early treatment. Vaccinia immune gamma globulin has a place in the prevention or modification of smallpox in persons known to have been exposed, if it is given in the incubation period or in the preeruptive phase of the disease.

The N-methylisatin beta-thiosemicarbazone decreases the incidence of smallpox after exposure regardless of vaccination status. In more than 1100 household contacts given the drug by mouth, three mild cases of smallpox occurred. In a comparable group of contacts who did not receive the drug there were 78 cases of smallpox and 12 deaths. The drug was effective even when given more than six days after contact. Further trials with different dosage schedules are in progress.

A related compound, 4-bromo-3-methylisothiozole-5-carboxaldehyde-thiosemicarbazone, has been tested in therapeutic trials in hospital patients. There is slight indication that the drug may reduce the mortality rate in the severe types of smallpox in vaccinated patients, but have little effect in severe cases in unvaccinated patients. These trials are continuing with an increased dose of the drug.

Other preparations, such as 5-iodo-2-deoxyuridine, 6-aza-uracyl-riboside and sulfone derivatives, are being studied, but none has yet been tested against smallpox.

The mild or discrete case of smallpox requires little except strict attention to oral and skin hygiene, fluid intake and routine analgesia. Fingernails should be cut short to prevent scratching, and antipruritic colloid baths in the scabbing period after the 12th day of the disease tend to minimize discomfort.

Severe discrete or confluent cases should be treated like serious thermal burns (see elsewhere in text). In most cases of severe smallpox, severe dehydration results because of the pain associated with swallowing. Intravenous fluid therapy may be difficult in the face of massive skin involvement. Fluid requirements increase as with any febrile illness, and fluid loss from the skin may be considerable. Oliguria and eventual renal insufficiency may further interfere with the patient's recovery.

The use of intensive parenteral fluid therapy or the early institution of feeding through a polyethylene stomach tube holds promise. Boiled skimmed milk with added carbohydrate (10 per cent) supplies calories and fluids through the critical 10 days of the early eruptive period. With the use of intensive fluid therapy and prophylactic use of antibiotics, mortality rates in the pediatric age group can be reduced to between 10 and 30 per cent.

All local applications to the skin and baths are to be discouraged. It is important, however, to attempt to clean the eyes with warm normal saline solution to prevent matting and to decrease the chances of permanent involvement of the sclera. There is no evidence that corticosteroids are of value in the treatment of this condition.

Penicillin and tetracycline are of value if started in the pustular phase, approximately on the sixth or seventh day of the disease, and reduce the bacterial complications involving lungs, bones and skin. Other supportive care is as noted previously.

Hemorrhagic smallpox is virtually universally fatal, and no treatment has been successful to date. Specific clotting deficiencies, particularly factor V and platelets, suggest intravascular clotting and the possible therapeutic employment of heparin. Currently under study are early use of N-methylisatin beta-thiosemicarbazone and the intravenous use of heparin or dextran. Oxygen and, when indicated, digitalis are of value.

Complications and Prognosis. Bacterial complications include sepsis, pneumonitis, osteomyelitis and septic arthritis. Iritis, corneal ulceration and severe conjunctivitis may lead to decrease in visual acuity, depending on their severity.

The prognosis of hemorrhagic smallpox is virtually hopeless. The prognosis for survival in children suffering from confluent smallpox is also extremely grave. Children suffering from modified smallpox or discrete smallpox due to previous successful vaccination have a good prognosis, especially if they receive optimal supportive therapy.

Control Measures. ISOLATION. Strict hospital isolation in screened wards is required until all scabs have disappeared.

CONCURRENT DISINFECTION. All articles associated with a smallpox patient must be sterilized in high pressure steam or, alternately, by boiling them before removing from the patient's room.

---

* Manufacturer's note: The use of tetracyclines during tooth development (last half of pregnancy, infancy and childhood to age eight years) may cause permanent discoloration of teeth. This adverse reaction is more common during long-term use of the drugs but has been observed following repeated short-term courses.

TERMINAL DISINFECTION. Thorough disinfection of the patient's room is required, and the walls and ceiling should be painted.

VACCINATION. All contacts should be promptly vaccinated or revaccinated and observed for 16 days from the last day of exposure. Vaccination *after* contact usually does not protect against smallpox unless accompanied by vaccinia immune gamma globulin. Vaccination, to ensure protection, must be done *before* exposure to smallpox. It is important to ignore a history of recent vaccination if exposure has occurred unless there is definite evidence of the formation of a recent scar to show that vaccination has, indeed, been successful.

N-METHYLISATIN BETA-THIOSEMICARBAZONE. This investigational drug, 1.5 to 3 Gm. orally twice a day for two days, decreases smallpox after known intimate exposure regardless of vaccination status. The material frequently causes emesis, and it is desirable to administer antiemetics prophylactically. Further toxicity has not been noted in the dosage used, but potential damage to liver and bone marrow should be watched for.

VACCINIA IMMUNE GAMMA GLOBULIN. Early evidence indicates that vaccinia immune gamma globulin given to close contacts of patients with smallpox may prevent or modify the disease in the contact. The intramuscular administration of vaccinia immune gamma globulin should follow revaccination by 12 to 24 hours. Dosage is a single intramuscular injection of 0.12 to 0.24 ml. per kilogram of body weight.

Vaccinia immune gamma globulin has been prepared and distributed through the financial cooperation of the Blood Program of the American Red Cross and is available commercially from Hyland Laboratories, Los Angeles, California.

References

Bauer, D. J., St. Vincent, L., Kempe, C. H., and Downie, A. W.: Smallpox Prophylaxis. *Lancet,* 2:501, 1963.

Bauer, D. J., et al.: Prophylaxis of Smallpox with Methisazone. *Am. J. Epidemiol.,* 90:130, 1969.

WHO Expert Committee on Smallpox: *World Health Organization Technical Report Series* No. 283, 1964, p. 23.

Vaccinia

Smallpox Vaccination

C. HENRY KEMPE, M.D.

Indications for Vaccination. Children should no longer be vaccinated routinely. Selective vaccination is advised for travelers to areas where smallpox is endemic, for health personnel, and in the presence of an epidemic. For certain travelers, WHO requires revaccination every three years. In areas of the world where smallpox is endemic, *yearly* successful vaccination is required to give solid protection.

Contraindications to Vaccination. Childhood eczema is an absolute contraindication to vaccination. The presence of a sibling with eczema in the family of the child to be vaccinated also is an absolute contraindication to vaccination because serious secondary vaccinia infections are likely to occur. If vaccination is desired in this situation, the sibling with eczema must be placed in a separate household and must have no contact with the vaccinated child for at least 15 days.

Infants and children who have had many repeated bacterial infections or who have failed to thrive should not be vaccinated. Children suffering from dysgammaglobulinemia have a high mortality rate after smallpox vaccination.

Further contraindications include all forms of leukemia, lymphoma and malignancy as well as other blood dyscrasias, as well as patients who are receiving corticosteroids or antimetabolites for x-ray therapy.

Method of Vaccination and Care of Lesion. To minimize the risk of unnecessary complications, the following practices are recommended.

AGE FOR PRIMARY VACCINATION. In nonendemic areas, primary vaccination need not be done. Otherwise, there are no conclusive data indicating the exact period when complication rates are minimal. The presence of some transplacental maternal immunity, provided the mother has been vaccinated, may be desirable in modifying the primary vaccination reaction, and therefore vaccination may be carried out in the first months of life. Vaccination of newborn infants has been carried out without complications. In such cases in endemic areas, revaccination should be carried out after an interval of six months. If primary vaccination is delayed for several months, children who are at increased risk, such as those suffering from the Swiss type of agammaglobulinemia, will have been readily identified by their clinical course and will, therefore, not become a casualty of smallpox vaccination.

SITE FOR VACCINATION. Primary vaccination and revaccination are best performed on the outer aspects of the upper arm, over the insertion of the deltoid muscle or behind the midline. Reactions are less likely to be severe on the upper arm than on the lower extremity or other parts of the body. With proper technique, resultant scars are small and unobtrusive.

PREPARATION OF THE VACCINATION SITE. With clean skin, the best preparation is none at all. The use of chemical skin cleaners may leave a residue that contains virus-inactivating material, whereas vigorous physical cleansing of the site may create minute abrasions, which then can become the site of secondary vaccinia eruptions, with resultant involvement of a comparatively large skin area.

VACCINATION TECHNIQUE. Regardless of age, routine primary vaccination should be carried out with no more than three pressures made with the side of a needle. These pressure points should be as close as possible, and carried out at only one site. With the highly potent vaccines currently in use, numerous pressures are not necessary and should not be utilized in a nonimmune person. When children and adults are to be revaccinated after a lapse of more than five years, the same small number of pressures should be used. For revaccination within a five-year period, in persons known to have had a major reaction, the full complement of 30 strokes can safely be used.

VACCINATION REACTION. The terminology for the reactions after vaccination or revaccination should follow that recommended by the Expert Committee on Smallpox of the World Health Organization. A successful primary vaccination is one that on examination after seven to 10 days presents a typical jennerian vesicle. If this is not present, vaccination must be repeated with fresh vaccine, applying a few more strokes of the needle. The successful revaccination is one that on examination one week (six to eight days) later shows vesicular or pustular lesions, *or* an area of definite palpable induration and congestion surrounding a central lesion; this lesion may be a scab or an ulcer. These reactions are termed *major reactions;* all others should be called *equivocal reactions.* A major reaction indicates virus multiplication with consequent development of immunity. An equivocal reaction may merely represent an allergic response, which could be elicited by inactive vaccine or poor technique in someone who had been sensitized by earlier vaccination, or the equivocal reaction may result from sufficient immunity to prevent virus multiplication.

Because the allergic response cannot be readily differentiated from the one due to true immunity, another vaccination should be performed using a different lot of vaccine if there is a possibility that it is of weak potency, and the procedure should be completed with an additional number of pressures. The site should be examined one week later; if the result is again equivocal, revaccination is repeated, using a full 30 pressures. For the sake of expediency, an equivocal reaction to revaccination with a minimal insertion may be followed by vaccination at two sites, not less than 2 inches apart, using known potent vaccine. This method makes a third return unnecessary in most instances.

In summary, successful smallpox vaccination consists in the production of a major reaction. When potent vaccine and good technique are used, the repeated inability to produce a major reaction can be assumed to be due to solid immunity from previous immunization.

Complications of Smallpox Vaccination. ERYTHEMA MULTIFORME. A generalized maculopapular eruption may occur at the height of the vaccinia reaction. There is no systemic reaction in addition to those of an uncomplicated vaccination. Lesions are usually not pruritic, although the reaction is an allergy to the vaccinia virus. Treatment is reassurance and any oral antihistiminic. The rash disappears in two to four days.

ECZEMA VACCINATUM. Infants suffering from eczema are peculiarly susceptible to infection with vaccinia virus, and this complication accounts for the largest number of childhood deaths from serious complications of smallpox vaccination. Such children should, therefore, never be vaccinated, even though their lesions appear to be dry, unless they are likely to be exposed to smallpox. They must also be carefully guarded against exposure to siblings and other children who have been vaccinated and who may, in turn, infect them.

Lesions first occur in the area of eczema three to four days after exposure. Soon new crops arise in areas of the skin previously uninvolved. Patients are febrile and toxic for five to 15 days.

Affected children should be treated as if they were suffering from severe thermal burns. The use of oxygen, blood, plasma and electrolytes, as well as penicillin, is indicated (see the discussion under Burns).

Evidence suggests that there is a primary defect in the production of specific antibodies against the vaccinia virus. The use of passively administered antibodies in the form of vaccinia immune gamma globulin has proved to be a valuable adjunct in the specific therapy of this complication. The dose of vaccinia immune gamma globulin is 0.6 to 1 ml. per kilogram of body weight, and it is given once or twice intramuscularly. In serious cases N-methylisatin beta-thiosemicarbazone (Marboran)* should be used in doses of 200 mg. per kilogram orally at once, followed by 50 mg. per kilogram every 6 hours for no more than three days.

GENERALIZED VACCINIA. Generalized vaccinia in children not suffering from skin disorders is seen when viremia happens to occur during primary vaccination, giving rise, in turn, to a generalized skin eruption, each lesion simulating a primary vaccination.

Lesions usually continue to appear in crops over a four- to six-day period after the onset of the disease, which frequently coincides with the height of the primary vaccination reaction (8 to 14 days after vaccination).

The mortality rate of generalized vaccinia in the absence of eczema is much lower, because this complication occurs more frequently in children over two years of age.

The *treatment* is identical to that for eczema vaccinatum.

PROGRESSIVE VACCINIA (VACCINIA NECROSUM; PROLONGED VACCINIA). This extremely rare complication of vaccination is characterized by a complete inability to make specific antibodies against the vaccinia virus. This results in progressive spreading of the primary vaccination take, and eventually most of the arm as well as the rest of the body becomes involved with necrotizing lesions. The systemic reaction is usually mild during the first six weeks of the disease, but progressively increases in the subsequent weeks and eventually leads to death four to six months after onset.

This complication is certainly very frequent in children suffering from either the Bruton or the Swiss type of agammaglobulinemia. But in four instances the quantitative gamma globulin levels were normal even though a qualitative effect (dysgammaglobulinemia) existed.

The logical course of treatment is the provision of large amounts of antivaccina antibodies in the form of vaccinia immune gamma globulin, given in doses of 0.6 to 1 ml. per kilogram of body weight intramuscularly every 8 to 10 days until lesions are entirely healed. Large amounts of high titer serum from adults recently successfully vaccinated or repeated exchange transfusions from such donors have been successful in the Bruton type capable of delayed hypersensitivity response. But even a single blood transfusion can cause a fatal graft-versus-host reaction in the athymic lymphopenic patient, and blood must never be used in such patients.

If antibody therapy does not result in immediate improvement, therapy with N-methylisatin beta-thiosemicarbazone should be instituted. (Such therapy can be carried out at the center for treatment of vaccinia gangrenosis at the University of Colorado School of Medicine, provided the patient is transferred to Denver.) The oral dose is 200 mg. per kilogram at once, followed by 50 mg. per kilogram every 6 hours for three days. After a rest of three to four days, an additional three-day course should be given. The disease has been promptly arrested in approximately half the patients treated to date.

POSTVACCINATION ENCEPHALITIS. This is a rare complication of smallpox vaccination with an incidence of less than one per 100,000 vaccinations.

Encephalitic symptoms usually develop at the height of the primary vaccination reaction and not later than the 15th day after vaccination.

The mortality rate is 25 per cent, but there is usually eventual physical recovery of those who survive. Behavioral disorders are frequent. It is thought by many that this complication occurs more commonly after the age of three, and because it is almost exclusively associated with primary vaccination, most physicians prefer early vaccination. The mortality rate, on the other hand, appears to be much higher in the younger child. The complication can be markedly decreased by simultaneous administration of 2 ml. of vaccinia immune gamma globulin intramuscularly into the thigh at the time of primary vaccination.

Vaccinia Immune Gamma Globulin. Vaccinia immune gamma globulin has been prepared and distributed through the Quarantine Services of the United States Public Health Service, and is also available commercially from Hyland Laboratories, Los Angeles, California.

References

Kempe, C. H.: The End of Routine Smallpox Vaccination in the United States. *Pediatrics,* 49:1489, 1972.

Neff, J. M., et al.: Complications of Smallpox Vaccination, I. National Survey in the United States, 1963. *New England J. Med.,* 276:125, 1967.

* Marboran is an investigational drug.

Herpes Simplex Infections

A. J. NAHMIAS, M.D.

Herpes simplex virus (HSV) infections in children can be either primary or recurrent and are most commonly caused by HSV type 1. On the other hand, the majority of neonatal infections are caused by HSV-2. In view of the potential life-threatening and debilitating sequelae, major problems in herpes simplex virus infections are neonatal herpes, encephalitis, eczema herpeticum and infection in the immunodeficient, immunosuppressed or severely malnourished hosts. Less severe, but occasionally with complications, are herpetic infections of the eye, mouth (gingivostomatitis), lips, skin and genitalia.

General Considerations. It is particularly difficult to evaluate the true effectiveness of most therapeutic measures, in view of the unpredictable prognosis of the more severe forms of HSV infection. In case of recurrent infections, it is also usually difficult to determine that a particular regimen is effective, since the frequency of recurrences varies so greatly within any one individual. General aspects of approaches that are under evaluation are presented first and their potential use in various types of HSV infection discussed later.

ANTIVIRAL AGENTS. Several antiviral drugs are under investigation. Of these, topical 5-iodo-2′-deoxyuridine (IDU) has been most widely used in human therapy, particularly for disease of the eye. Systemic administration of IDU or other inhibitors of viral DNA synthesis—cytosine arabinoside (ara-C) and adenine arabinoside (ara-A)—have been employed in patients with severe forms of herpetic disease. Controlled studies are currently being done to evaluate their effectiveness (see below).

GAMMA GLOBULIN. Although this material contains herpes simplex virus antibodies, its main use might be in preventing viral dissemination via the blood, assuming virus is not present in peripheral leukocytes. Gamma globulin does not appear to affect cell-to-cell spread once infection is established. The possibility of direct transmission of virus via neuropathic pathways from skin, eye or nasopharynx to central nervous system would also curtail effectiveness of this substance. Transplacentally transmitted antibodies in some newborn cases may also be ineffective for similar reasons.

TRANSFER FACTOR. Preparations of dialyzable substances from lymphocytes of individuals with prior HSV infection have been used in a limited way in cases of the Wiskott-Aldrich syndrome with severe herpetic infections. The use of such preparations for the alleviation of the frequency of recurrences of infection with HSV are currently under investigation.

PHOTOINACTIVATION. It has been recently proposed that the application of dye solutions of neutral red or proflavine to herpetic lesions followed by exposure to light would reduce the duration of lesions and the frequency of herpetic recurrences. The effectiveness of this approach requires confirmatory studies, particularly in its application to herpetic infections in children.

VACCINES AND CORTICOSTEROIDS. Experimental herpes simplex virus vaccines have had limited use for recurrent, debilitating infection. A type 1 herpes simplex virus vaccine appears to benefit patients with severe, frequent, recurrent HSV type 1 infections (eyes, skin above waist, lips). Use of smallpox vaccine for treatment of recurrent herpes has too many potentially severe consequences and too few truly demonstrable advantages to be warranted. Effectiveness of adjunct drugs, such as topical corticosteroids, has not been well evaluated (except in combination with IDU for disciform herpetic keratitis), and systemic steroids may be potentially harmful.

NEONATAL HERPES

Recent evidence supports the concept that most cases of neonatal herpes are acquired by passage of the infant through an infected maternal genital tract. The minimal risk of an infant developing neonatal herpes from a mother with genital herpes detected after the thirty-second week of gestation is approximately 10 per cent. If the virus is present at the time of delivery, the minimal risk is 40 per cent. At least one third of infected infants develop a severe disease resulting in death or in serious neurological or ocular sequelae. Although there is a higher risk to infants whose mothers had primary infections, transplacental antibodies are not fully protective, and infants born to mothers with recurrent infections also risk developing severe herpetic disease. The possible prevention of neonatal herpes by performing a cesarean section on the mother prior to rupture of membranes has become an important consideration.

Decision for abdominal delivery requires

close collaboration between obstetrician and pediatrician. Cytologic and virologic confirmation of a genital herpetic infection in a woman close to delivery should be obtained when possible. Amniocentesis may be performed and if the amniotic fluid contains virus, it is doubtful that a cesarean section would be helpful. If a cesarean section is to be performed, it should be done before membrane rupture or as soon as possible thereafter (within 4 hours of rupture).

Every case should be individualized, balancing maternal risk from abdominal delivery against risk to the newborn. Infants born to mothers with concurrent genital or nongenital infections are isolated and observed carefully for clinical or laboratory evidence of herpetic infection, and topical IDU drugs are administered to both eyes every 2 hours or IDU ointment is applied every 4 hours.

The effectiveness of systemic antiviral drugs in infections of the newborn is not well established. This form of therapy should be used only after approval of the clinical trials committee of the institution, the parents and the Food and Drug Administration. Two controlled studies to evaluate the possible usefulness and potential toxic side effects of these drugs are currently under way. It must be realized that occasionally infants with generalized herpes or herpetic encephalitis survive without drugs.

One study is to evaluate responses to systemic cytosine arabinoside, as compared to a placebo. Any physician can participate in this study by contacting Dr. G. Royer, Upjohn Company, Kalamazoo, Michigan. Cytosine arabinoside or the placebo is administered intravenously as a push dose of 20 mg. per square meter, followed by 180 mg. per square meter given over the next 2 hours. This regimen is followed daily for five days. Close monitoring of hematopoietic, liver and kidney function is necessary. Criteria for inclusion in the study have been developed by a group of 15 experts. It is obvious that one needs first to ascertain the diagnosis of herpes simplex virus infection by laboratory means.

In another study, under the direction of Dr. L. Chien and Dr. C. Alford of the University of Alabama, a comparison of systemically administered adenine arabinoside and a placebo is being evaluated in cases of herpes simplex virus infection in the neonate. Adenine arabinoside is administered intravenously as a continuous drip over 12 hours at a dose of 15 mg. per kilogram per day for a period of 7 to 10 days. Close monitoring of hematopoietic, liver and kidney function is also necessary when using this drug.

HERPETIC MENINGOENCEPHALITIS OUTSIDE THE NEWBORN AGE GROUP

Current data suggest that the encephalitic form of herpetic infection is caused by HSV-1. On the other hand, HSV-2 infections, which are infrequent in children outside the newborn age group, may cause a benign form of meningitis. Patients with the encephalitic form of herpetic infection may survive, although neurologic sequelae are often severe. Evaluation of the effectiveness of systemic antiviral therapy is therefore difficult. Diagnosis in the patient outside the newborn age group is more difficult to establish, because skin and other herpetic lesions are uncommon and when present, may be coincidental to the encephalitis. Since the virus is infrequently recoverable from the cerebrospinal fluid outside the newborn age group, diagnosis must be established, whenever possible, by brain biopsy and demonstration of the virus, preferably by culture techniques. (Electron microscopy and immunofluorescent tests might also be helpful.)

A collaborative interhospital study, under the direction of Dr. L. Chien and Dr. C. Alford of the University of Alabama, is comparing systemically administered adenine arabinoside, iododeoxyuridine and placebo. Adenine arabinoside is administered intravenously as a continuous drip over 12 hours at a dose of 15 mg. per kilogram per day for a period of 10 days. Iododeoxyuridine is administered intravenously at a dose of 100 mg. per kilogram per day for a period of 5 days. The drug is infused over a 45 minute to 1 hour period. Close monitoring of hematopoietic, liver and kidney function is required.

Other standard forms of management of encephalitis include close monitoring and appropriate therapy for convulsions, shock or possible bacterial or mycotic superinfection. Decompression of the brain appears to be important in the management of this condition. The benefit of systemic corticosteroids for this purpose, as contrasted to their potential risk, has not been well evaluated.

HERPES INFECTION IN IMMUNOSUPPRESSED HOSTS

Patients with certain forms of cancer such as leukemias or lymphomas, and those on immunosuppressive therapy such as that following renal transplantation, may develop severe herpes simplex virus infections. Local infections, as of the skin, in such patients may occasionally become extensive and chronic; less commonly, they may involve the esophagus or the lungs or may disseminate to internal organs. The effectiveness of adenine arabinoside is also currently being evaluated in such patients in the collaborative study directed by Dr. Chien and Dr. Alford.

Local infection must be persistent for 7 days before the patient is entered in the study. The patient receives either placebo or adenine arabinoside for 7 days. The drug is administered intravenously as a continuous drip over 12 hours at a dose of 10 mg. per kilogram per day. Close monitoring of clinical and virological responses, as well as of hematopoietic, liver and kidney function, is necessary.

HERPES OF THE SKIN AND ECZEMA HERPETICUM

The use of IDU ointment for skin infections is not particularly effective. Bland ointments are usually sufficient, although topical antibiotic ointment, such as Neosporin (polymyxin B, neomycin and bacitracin) may be helpful in preventing or treating skin bacterial superinfection.

Eczema herpeticum is a more serious herpetic complication of atopic children and particularly patients with the Wiskott-Aldrich syndrome. It is very difficult to prevent children with atopic eczema from having contact with herpes-infected persons, since subclinical infections are so common. An attempt should be made to prevent contact with persons who have overt herpetic lesions. It is also important to keep atopic patients from being placed in hospital rooms recently occupied by patients with eczema herpeticum (or eczema vaccinatum).

In the treatment of patients with eczema herpeticum, fluids and occasionally blood transfusions are given to correct electrolyte losses and anemia (particularly in the Wiskott-Aldrich syndrome with thrombocytopenia and bleeding in the skin lesions). Gamma globulin in doses of 20 to 40 ml. is given intramuscularly to prevent further blood-borne viral dissemination. Topical IDU drops are administered to both eyes to prevent ocular herpetic involvement. We give systemic antibiotics, usually nafcillin* or oxacillin (200 mg. per kilogram per day intravenously), unless appropriate cultures reveal organisms not susceptible to these drugs. If there is suspicion of pseudomonas infection, we do not hesitate to add gentamicin (5 mg. per kilogram per day intravenously).

If evidence of generalized herpetic disease or encephalitis develops in such patients, particularly those with the Wiskott-Aldrich syndrome, use of systemic antiviral drugs might be considered (as outlined in the previous section). The potential value of transfer factor in cases of the Wiskott-Aldrich syndrome with severe HSV infections is currently under study.

HERPETIC GINGIVOSTOMATITIS AND LABIALIS

Therapeutic measures are required for only the more severe form of gingivostomatitis, with fever, vesicles and ulcers over the tongue and many parts of the mouth, gingival inflammation, oral pain and cervical lymphadenopathy. Major considerations are prevention of dehydration and relief of pain. Use of a topical anesthetic, such as lidocaine (2 per cent) in a viscous base, a few minutes before feeding allows the child to take in fluids and bland foods. Sedatives, such as elixir of phenobarbital, may be added. Oral hygiene may be maintained with hydrogen peroxide (3 per cent, diluted 1:1) or mouthwashes, such as Cēpacol. In general, these measures are needed for a short period, because the mouth lesions recede within a few days. In rare instances, lack of oral intake and vomiting may require hospitalization for parenteral fluid therapy to restore fluid and electrolyte balance.

Recurrences of herpetic lesions in the mouth are infrequent. Therefore, recurrences of vesicles or ulcers in the mouth are almost always due to canker sores and not herpesvirus. Recurrences of herpes are usually localized to the mucocutaneous junction of the lip (cold sores) and adjacent skin. Since certain conditions, such as sunlight and emotional stress, might precipitate the recurrences, avoidance of these factors may be helpful.

There have been several forms of treatment of recurrent herpes simplex infections in recent years. We avoid use of corticosteroids or of smallpox vaccinations. Topical iododeoxyuridine (0.5 per cent in a petrolatum-base ointment) may be helpful, if applied locally every 1 or 2 hours. Idoxuridine in a higher concentration (5 per cent in 100 per cent dimethyl sulfoxide) has been found by British workers to

* Manufacturer's precaution: Intravenous use of nafcillin is investigational.

be beneficial; however, this form of the drug is not approved for use in the United States. More recently, photodynamic inactivation has been claimed to be beneficial in curtailing not only the duration of lesions, but also the frequency of recurrences. This regimen involves rupturing early vesicular lesions, applying a 0.1 per cent aqueous neutral red solution and exposing the lesion to an ordinary, cool, white, 15-watt fluorescent lamp for 15 minutes at a distance of 6 inches. New lesions developing over the next 24 to 72 hours are treated in a similar manner. We have no direct experience with this form of therapy, which awaits confirmatory studies, particularly in children. When herpetic lesions occur at great frequency (every one to two months), particularly if facial lesions are associated with ocular involvement, the inactivated herpes simplex 1 vaccine (Eli Lilly and Company), still in the experimental stage, may prove beneficial.

RECURRENT APHTHOUS STOMATITIS (CANKER SORES)

Like recurrent herpes labialis, recurrent canker sores might be distressing to a few patients. Canker sores may be painful, may occur in one or more sites inside the mouth or on the tongue and may be accompanied by malaise and low-grade fever. Less frequently, such lesions may occur on the genitalia or be associated with joint or systemic manifestations (Behçet's syndrome).

It has recently been suggested that aphthous stomatitis may be an autoimmune disease or may be related to oral alpha-hemolytic streptococci. On this basis, treatment with a tetracycline suspension (Achromycin), held in the mouth for two minutes and then swallowed, may be helpful. Treatment, to be reserved for children over five years of age, is seldom necessary for longer than five days (four times a day). Milder cases are handled by an oral rinse of topical anesthetic, such as lidocaine (2 per cent in a viscous base), three times daily before meals. On occasion, application of a topical corticosteroid (Kenalog in Orabase) to the lesions four times daily may help relieve the symptoms. In very severe cases, systemic corticosteroid therapy may be indicated.

HERPANGINA AND ORAL LESIONS OF HAND-FOOT-AND-MOUTH SYNDROME

Certain enteroviral infections occurring mostly in the summer and fall may cause papular, vesicular and ulcerative lesions in the posterior part of the mouth (herpangina). Other enteroviruses, particularly Coxsackie virus A16, may produce such lesions in the anterior part of the mouth and thereby be confused with herpetic infection. However, such patients have vesicles or papules primarily on the hands and feet. Although these patients may have sore throat and fever, no therapy is indicated, and antibiotics should be avoided.

THRUSH (ORAL CANDIDIASIS)

Treatment of oral candidiasis is limited to infants with visible lesions, particularly when these affect food intake. One course of nystatin (Mycostatin) is usually sufficient for treatment. This consists of dropping 1 ml. (100,000 units) of the suspension in the mouth, swabbing over involved areas and repeating four times daily until lesions have cleared and for about three days thereafter. Application of a 1 per cent aqueous gentian violet solution in a similar fashion may be useful, although rather messy.

Recurrence of oral candidiasis, if treatment has been given properly the first time, should make one suspect an underlying problem, such as a rare case of thymic aplasia. In older infants and children, oral candidiasis is usually a complication of antibiotic therapy. Less frequently, it might result from other forms of therapy, such as antimetabolites. Recurrent oral candidiasis, occasionally combined with skin involvement, should make one suspect a hormonal defect, malignancy or immunologic disorder, particularly one associated with defective cellular immune mechanisms. Therapy with nystatin in children with associated underlying conditions is usually only temporarily effective. Repeated courses are usually needed unless the underlying condition is treated.

TRAUMATIC APHTHAE

These ulcerative lesions result from trauma to the oral mucosa, such as from the edges of carious teeth, hard toothbrushes and inadvertent bites. Therapy consists simply of recognizing and removing the irritant.

VINCENT'S ANGINA

This condition is rare in children, and most cases diagnosed as Vincent's angina are really of herpetic etiology. Vincent's angina is probably a result of lowered resistance to organisms present in the mouth, particularly fusiform bacilli and spirochetes. It is most commonly found in children with poor oral hygiene or debilitating conditions. Therapy should include, therefore, correction of predisposing factors, such as poor dentition. Local rinses with hydrogen peroxide (3 per cent, diluted 1:1) are used four times a day. In addition, penicillin V, 125 to 250 mg. given every 6 hours orally for five days, appears to be helpful.

Reference

Nahmias, A. J., Alford, C. A., and Korones, S. B.: Infection of the Newborn with *Herpesvirus hominis*. *Adv. Pediat.*, 17:185, 1970.

Mumps

SYDNEY S. GELLIS, M.D.

Bed rest is voluntarily sought by children who feel ill; most do not, and bed rest need not be enforced. Even in adolescent males, ordinary activity or bed rest appears to bear no relationship to the development of orchitis. Strenuous physical work or exercise should be prohibited, however, in the patient old enough to develop orchitis. For parotid or other salivary gland swelling, acetylsalicylic acid, 65 mg. per kilogram of body weight per 24 hours divided into six doses, is usually helpful. Some patients feel greater relief with the use of an ice collar, whereas in others, heat gives more comfort. Diet may be given as tolerated; children may not have increased pain from ingestion of citrus fluids as do adults.

Complications. Mumps may produce thyroiditis, hepatitis and myocarditis. These require special treatment, and corticosteroids may be very useful. Little can be done to diminish damage from neuritis, transverse myelitis, deafness or postinfectious encephalitis. Fortunately, these are rare complications.

MENINGOENCEPHALITIS. Usually symptomatic treatment is sufficient. In patients with intense headache that does not abate with salicylates, lumbar puncture may be followed by great improvement.

PANCREATITIS. Symptomatic treatment is undertaken; intravenous fluids are given if vomiting occurs.

ORCHITIS. Bed rest should be insisted upon until pain and swelling have subsided. A suspensory or adhesive tape cradle between the thighs protects the testes from sudden movement of the legs. An ice bag propped beneath the testes but not upon them gives additional comfort. Narcotics may be needed for adults with orchitis but are rarely necessary for the adolescent boy.

Although controlled studies indicate that there is little to be gained by corticosteroids, they may in individual cases give relief of pain. In patients with severe pain and swelling, a three- or four-day course consisting of 300 mg. of cortisone daily divided into four doses may prove helpful to the patient who is miserable with fever and pain. Surgical incision of the tunica albuginea testis for relief of swelling, a procedure that had a modicum of popularity in an earlier era, seems to have been discarded.

In addition to medication, the patient with orchitis benefits from reassurance; most adults fear that they will be left sterile by the complication, but the incidence of sterility is very low.

Prevention. LIVE ATTENUATED MUMPS VACCINE. This vaccine is administered subcutaneously as a single dose. The vaccine is lyophilized and comes with diluent, which is added just prior to use. Children under one year of age should not receive the vaccine because of possible interference by maternal neutralizing antibodies. It should not be given to pregnant women, to patients known to be sensitive to eggs, to people with leukemia, lymphoma or other malignancies, to patients receiving immunosuppressive agents or to those having diseases with defective immune response. There is no consensus as to the administration of the vaccine to all children, because there is little information about the duration of immunity conveyed by the vaccine. If the vaccine should prove to give life-long immunity, there could be little argument against its administration routinely to all children. Until more is known about the duration of protection, it probably should be reserved for prepubertal males with no history of mumps.

Administration to fathers of young children known to have been exposed to the infection is unlikely to be effective because it takes about four weeks following immunization for antibodies to develop and because children are infectious for several days before swelling of salivary glands is apparent. However, because the majority of adult males without a history of mumps have had subclinical infection and are immune, the vaccine will have a considerable effect on morale.

INACTIVATED VACCINE. The live attenuated vaccine is so much more effective than the old inactivated vaccine that there should be little use for the latter.

HYPERIMMUNE GAMMA GLOBULIN. This

preparation has limited use as a means of producing passive immunity because of its cost, the large dose required (10 to 20 ml., which exceeds that recommended by the manufacturer) and its questionable effectiveness.

Influenza

JOHN M. ADAMS, M.D.

Epidemic influenza and other commonly recognized viral infections of the respiratory passages are not affected by any known specific antimicrobial agents. Treatment should consist primarily of general measures designed to ease the discomfort and general aches. There is no readily available method for the accurate diagnosis of influenza early in the patient's illness. Epidemiologic features and clinical signs and symptoms are still the most valuable diagnostic aids. Influenza occurs in epidemics which appear suddenly in a community, and it is frequently first recognized by high absenteeism in the schools. The epidemic in any one community is short-lived; a period from 10 days to two weeks may represent the height of the attack.

There are three immunologic types of influenza. The A form tends to occur in epidemics every two to three years; epidemics of influenza B appear at longer intervals, usually from four to six years; influenza C occurs sporadically, but has not been found to occur in epidemics. Although the diagnosis of "the flu" is frequently made throughout the respiratory season, the actual incidence of influenza is nearly zero in nonepidemic periods. During an epidemic the diagnosis of an acute respiratory disease as influenza has a high probability of being correct.

Wise management depends on a reasonably accurate diagnosis. The incubation period is short, one to two days with a rather abrupt onset of fever and chills, sore throat and general aches and pain. The illness lasts about two to four days unless complications occur. Differentiation of any single case of influenza from other acute respiratory illnesses may be difficult; but as pointed out previously, when groups of cases occur, influenza may be recognized readily by its distinct clinical features. In military installations, symptomatology in seasoned personnel as well as in recruits is considered highly characteristic of epidemic influenza. A well-established epidemic of Asian or A2 influenza occurred at the National Boy Scout Jamboree in Valley Forge, Pennsylvania. The most common complaints among the boys were fever, headache, cough and sore throat. Many also complained of general discomfort and prostration. Muscle aches and abdominal pain were important clinical features. Inflammation of the eyes and running noses as well as red throats were recorded in three quarters of the boys. About one-fifth had signs of inflammation in the chest, which was confirmed by x-ray findings on several occasions.

Final diagnosis depends either on the isolation of the virus or detection of specific antibodies in the convalescent serum as compared to a specimen obtained early in the acute phase of illness. These procedures are not practical for the individual case but are carried out by many city, county and state diagnostic laboratories.

Prevention. At the present time, vaccination would appear to be the most hopeful method for the control of influenza. Until recently, the search for effective drugs against the influenza virus has failed to control the disease. An antiviral drug known as amantadine has proved useful in prevention but *not in treatment* of the Asian type of influenza. Amantadine hydrochloride taken by mouth has been approved by the Food and Drug Administration for the prevention of influenza. It was designed to prevent illness caused by the A2 strain of influenza virus, but must be taken continuously to have a preventive effect. The drug appears to act by interfering with the virus's ability to penetrate the host's cells rather than by stimulating the production of antibodies. It should be reemphasized that the drug does not have therapeutic value, and that its effectiveness is limited to prevention. The dose has not been clearly defined and the recommended dose has been considered by some to be too close to the toxic level. Its widespread use at the time of epidemics has been criticized on the basis that further clinical trials are needed to establish its safety and effectiveness.

The main method of prevention employed in the United States today is the inoculation of killed vaccines. When properly constituted, these have been shown to be highly effective in prevention. A leading authority in the field of influenza immunization has strongly urged wider application of the vaccine, particularly among school children where its effectiveness should be comparable to that which has been demonstrated in military situations. A widespread vaccination program of school children and their families would not only benefit the recipients but would also provide a shield against dissemination to the rest of the community.

Influenza vaccines have not been widely accepted because of concern over febrile reactions. These reactions may be readily controlled with salicylates. Vaccines produced in egg cultures should not be given to sensitive individuals. A highly purified vaccine which does not produce febrile reactions but which does induce high antibody levels may be available in the near future. Ruben and Jackson reported recently on a new influenza vaccine, called TNBP vaccine, which has the advantage of purity and a broad range of dosage. Larger doses produced a better antibody response with less local reaction.

Murphy and associates reported on new recombinant viruses administered intranasally and found one which was attenuated to a degree desirable for a vaccine. The men who received the live virus did not develop symptoms, but they did develop antibodies which induced complete resistance to influenza when challenged with a virulent wild-type virus.

The Influenza Commission lists several indications for vaccination. It should be given to those with chronic debilitating diseases and to pregnant women, particularly during the last trimester when the risk is highest. People involved in community functions concerned with health services, public safety, public utility and transportation should be vaccinated. A vaccine dosage schedule suggested for infants and children is shown in Table 1.

The latest formulation of the vaccine differs from that of 1971–1972 as follows: The potency of the type A strain has been increased from 400 to 700 chick cell agglutinating (CCA) units. The type B strain for 1972–1973 contains 300 CCA units. Doses for children are specified in the manufacturers' package labeling. Vaccines from all producers are highly purified and should be less often associated with adverse reactions than were the previous vaccines.

The preferred route is under the skin or subcutaneously, but on occasion the intradermal route has been employed for a booster response following previous immunization. It is recommended that vaccination be carried out as soon as possible after September 1 and completed by mid-December. It is important that immunization be performed before influenza occurs in a particular community. It takes approximately two weeks following vaccination for one to develop immunity. In the face of an impending epidemic, even a single dose will afford some protection, and it may be followed by a booster injection in two weeks in order to increase its effectiveness.

Treatment of Uncomplicated Influenza. Bed rest is considered most important. For the protection of the patient as well as others, visiting should be rigidly limited. Infants and young children should be encouraged to take fluids in order to prevent dehydration. Moderate degrees of fever are to be expected, and these are usually well tolerated by children. An antiviral substance, known as *interferon,* made by cells in response to acute infection is more effective at elevated temperature levels, and unless fever is excessively high, methods such as administering salicylates to reduce it are not indicated. When cough is interfering with rest, humidity and syrups containing codeine may be helpful. This type of medication will also help relieve the aches and pains of acute influenza.

The fever of influenza runs a limited course and often disappears rapidly. When fever persists, complications should be suspected. If indicated, antibiotics may be employed for the common complications. The common ones are otitis media, sinusitis and pneumonia. Rarely, the central nervous system may be involved. Symptoms of irritability, increased fever and convulsions may indicate the onset of meningoencephalitis. A lumbar punc-

TABLE 1. Schedule for Bivalent Influenza Vaccine, 1972–1973

AGE GROUP	IMMUNIZED PREVIOUSLY	NO PRIOR INFLUENZA VACCINE
3 months–5 years	0.1–0.2 ml. given once	0.1–0.2 ml. given 3 times at intervals of 0, 2 weeks and 2 months
6–12 years	0.5 ml. given once	0.5 ml. given twice at 2-month intervals

ture should be done in order to substantiate the diagnosis and to rule out complicating bacterial meningitis. Supportive therapy is indicated and, rarely, a tracheostomy will be necessary. Steroids have no place in therapy but should be continued if the patient is on this medication for other reasons prior to the onset of influenza. The management of the specific complications is dealt with in other sections of this book.

References

Murphy, B. R., Chalhub, E. G., Nasinoff, S. R., and Chanock, R. M.: Temperature-Sensitive Mutants of Influenza Virus, II. Attenuation of *ts* Recombinants for Man. *J. Infect. Dis.*, 126:170–178, 1972.

Ruben, F. L., and Jackson, G. G.: A New Subunit Influenza Vaccine: Acceptability Compared with Standard Vaccines and Effect of Dose on Antigenicity. *J. Infect. Dis.*, 125:656–664, 1972.

Rabies

JAMES J. CEREGHINO, M.D.

Human rabies appears no longer to be uniformly fatal. Nevertheless, prophylaxis following animal bites remains the treatment of choice. Treatment is dependent on the circumstances of the biting incident, the extent and location of the wound, the vaccination status of the patient and of the biting animal, and the relative risk of infection in the involved species for that area (available through local or State Health Departments).

Prophylaxis Following Animal Bite. FIRST AID. Immediate copious flushing of the wound with water and soap or detergent should be done before medical care is obtained.

LOCAL TREATMENT. Local treatment attempts to reduce to below an infective level the amount of rabies virus implanted in the wound. Animal studies indicate that the virus is not highly virulent when inoculated into muscles. The virus level may be reduced by vigorous swabbing of the wound with a quaternary ammonium virucidal agent [benzalkonium chloride (Zephiran) or benzethonium chloride (Phemerol)]. Quaternary ammonium compounds should not be used on mucous membranes, about the eyes or in combination with anionic soaps (hexachlorophene), because the large organic ions of opposite charges attract one another and destroy the virucidal action. Wounds in which rabies is suspected should not be sutured.

Animal studies indicate that infiltration of antirabies serum under the wound is effective in preventing infection. Presumably this is also true for humans. The dose (preferably not less than 5 ml.) is determined by the site of the wound. A careful history for sensitivity to horse serum and tests for hypersensitivity need to be done.

SYSTEMIC TREATMENT. The exposure of intact skin to the saliva of a rabid animal does not warrant systemic antirabies treatment, since all evidence indicates that the virus must reach nerve tissue to be infective.

The World Health Organization Expert Committee on Rabies, and the Public Health Service Advisory Committee on Immunization Practices recommend the systemic use of antirabies serum in severe exposure wounds when the biting animal is a healthy dog or cat. The combined use of serum and vaccine is recommended in mild or severe exposure wounds caused by a dog or cat known to be rabid at the time of attack or by an unprovoked attack from a skunk, fox, raccoon, coyote or bat, or in severe exposure wounds caused by a dog or cat when the biting animal cannot be located or has signs suggestive of rabies at the time of attack. Vaccine alone is recommended in mild exposure wounds caused by a dog or cat which cannot be located, and in the initial treatment of mild exposure wounds caused by a dog or cat with signs suggestive of rabies at the time of attack. In the latter case, the vaccine is stopped if the animal is healthy five days after exposure or if acceptable laboratory negativity has been demonstrated in the animal.

Tetanus prophylaxis or antibiotic treatment may also be indicated.

While serum alone has some effectiveness, combined use of serum and vaccine is the most effective treatment. Serum provides passive antibodies during the 10 or more days required to produce active antibody from the vaccine. Serum is most effective if given in the first 72 hours after the bite. A single dose of serum is recommended in order to avoid interference phenomena between the passive serum antibodies and the antigenic vaccine response.

Antirabies Serum. Antirabies serum is a purified and concentrated horse serum product (Lederle Laboratories). When used systemically, about 15 per cent of recipients develop serum sickness. A human rabies immune globulin (Cutter Laboratories) is currently being investigated by the Center for Disease Control in Atlanta, Georgia.

Antirabies Vaccine. It is difficult to document the value of a vaccine. In India, 465 people were identified who had been bitten by animals proved capable of transmitting rabies. A complete treatment with Semple vaccine was given to 316 while 106 received no treatment. In the treated group 8.86 per cent died, while in the untreated group 48.11 per cent died.

The most commonly used vaccine is the duck embryo vaccine (DEV) (Eli Lilly and Company), consisting of virus grown in duck embryo and inactivated by beta-propiolactone. Another available product is Semple vaccine (National Drug Country), consisting of virus-infected rabbit brain and cord, inactivated by phenol. Rabies deaths in treated individuals have occurred with both vaccines. DEV stimulates earlier production of antibodies. With the Semple vaccine, neurologic complications occurred once in every 4000 to 8000 patients in the United States. The fatality rate has ranged from 25 to 40 per cent, with up to one-third of the survivors having neurologic sequelae. With DEV, only six instances of neurologic reaction have been seen in over 200,000 people immunized.

The minimal course of DEV treatment consists of one subcutaneous dose administered under the abdominal skin, using alternate sides, each day for 14 days. Each dose should be given in a previously unused site. The dose is the same for adults and children. Desensitization may be required. Administration of DEV is accompanied by immediate stinging or burning at the site of injection. Local erythema and induration of earlier inoculation sites are common, especially from days six to 10. Fever and regional lymphadenopathy may be seen. The manufacturer reports three cases of anaphylactic shock, all occurring within 15 minutes after the first dose. Gastrointestinal reactions, urticaria and dyspnea may occur immediately after vaccination. Supplemental doses of vaccine are recommended 10 and 20 days after completion of the series, particularly if antirabies serum was used.

In persons bitten by wild animals, administration of two doses of vaccine daily for the first seven days is recommended, followed by one dose daily for another seven days for a total of 21 doses of vaccine.

If antibody is not present after the course of immunization, additional booster doses may be given. Antibody titers may be obtained from the Center for Disease Control in Atlanta, Georgia, through a State Board of Health laboratory.

A single dose of rabies vaccine given to individuals who have demonstrated an antigenic response to a potent vaccine administered as long as 15 to 25 years previously will result in a rise in antibody titer in four to eight days.

Preexposure Immunization. Physicians may wish to consider preexposure immunization for children who will be living in areas outside the United States where rabies is endemic and the child will be contacting native animals. The preexposure course used in high occupational risk persons has been two to three doses of 1 ml. of DEV administered deep subcutaneously in the upper arm at one-month intervals, followed by a booster dose six months later.

Management of Human Rabies. Rabies no longer appears to be uniformly fatal once manifestations appear. A six-year-old boy is the first documented case of recovery from rabies. Recovery was attributed to aggressive treatment to prevent hypoxia, increased intracranial pressure, cardiac arrhythmias, seizures and superimposed infections.

Diagnosis of human cases is usually established at postmortem examination, thus giving the erroneous impression that rabies is uniformly fatal. Despite a proliferation of diagnostic laboratory tests, it remains difficult to establish a premortem diagnosis. Assistance in diagnosis and treatment can be obtained from the Center for Disease Control in Atlanta, Georgia, through a local or State Health Department.

References

Cereghino, J. J., et al.: Diagnosis and Treatment. Rabies: A Rare Disease but a Serious Pediatric Problem. *Pediatrics,* 45:839–844, 1970.

Hattwick, M. A. W., et al.: Recovery from Rabies. A Case Report. *Ann Int. Med.,* 76:931–942, 1972.

Recommendation of the Public Health Service Advisory Committee on Immunization Practices: Rabies Prophylaxis. Center for Disease Control: Zoonoses Surveillance, May, 1972. Issued August, 1972.

World Health Organization Expert Committee on Rabies, Fifth Report. World Health Organization Technical Report Series No. 321. Geneva, World Health Organization, pp. 33–35, 1966.

Lymphogranuloma Venereum

NICHOLAS J. FIUMARA, M.D., M.P.H.

Lymphogranuloma venereum (LGV) is an acute and a chronic minor venereal disease caused by an organism related to the psittacosis group and occupying a place intermediate between the rickettsiae and the true viruses. It has been classified as being in the genus Bedsonia.

The disease manifests itself by an evanescent papule, pustule or herpetiform ulcer on the genitals and, less often, in the mouth (fellatio). It is then followed by a moderately tender lymphadenopathy, most often of the inguinals in the male; in the female, the deep pelvic and perianal nodes may be involved. Occasionally there is a generalized lymphadenopathy with enlargement of the spleen and, less often, of the liver. The nodes are moderately tender; they characteristically enlarge by elongation, with their long axis parallel and on either side of the groin fold. Alternate areas of softening and induration can be palpated. The periadenitis causes the overlying skin to adhere to the node. As rupture of the fluctuant areas occurs, multiple draining fistulas result. Often the adenitis is accompanied by "fever of unknown origin," with chills and generalized arthralgia.

The diagnosis can be confirmed as follows:

Frei Skin Test. It should be read at 72 hours. It usually becomes positive a week or so after the appearance of the lymphadenopathy. However, a negative Frei test in a patient who has had lesions for three or more weeks speaks strongly against the diagnosis of lymphogranuloma venereum.

Complement Fixation Test. If positive in a dilution of 1:80 or higher, it is significant. Two samples taken a week or more apart and showing a significant rise in titer are diagnostic.

The earlier the treatment is given in the course of this disease, the better the results. Lymphogranuloma venereum responds favorably to a number of wide-spectrum antibiotics as well as to the sulfonamides. The drug of choice is tetracycline,* 500 mg. four times a day for seven days, followed by 250 mg. four times daily for the next 14 days.

Sulfadiazine, 1 Gm. four times daily for three weeks, may be used in early cases.†

Complications of lymphogranuloma venereum, such as rectal strictures, polypoid masses and elephantiasis, require surgical treatment.

Infectious Mononucleosis

JAMES C. NIEDERMAN, M.D.

Infectious mononucleosis is an acute disease caused by the Epstein-Barr virus, a member of the herpes group. It is prevalent among children and young adults, especially in the 15- to 25-year age group. Characteristic clinical features include (1) fever, sore throat and adenopathy, (2) an increase in lymphocytes and monocytes (usually greater than 50 per cent and including more than 10 per cent atypical lymphocytes, (3) the transient appearance of heterophil antibody and beef cell hemolysins, (4) the development of persistent antibody against Epstein-Barr virus and (5) abnormalities of liver function.

Most cases of infectious mononucleosis are mild or moderate in severity. An irregular fever is present for one to two weeks and subjective symptoms usually persist for two to three weeks. During the febrile period, rest in bed with bathroom privileges is advisable as long as the patient experiences sore throat, headache, excess malaise and anorexia. Isolation techniques are not necessary. Most patients recover uneventfully in two to three weeks, with gradual increase to normal activities.

Gargling and irrigation of the throat with warm saline solutions are useful for pharyngitis and membranous tonsillitis. Aspirin, 1 grain or 60 mg. per dose per year of age, up to 10 grains or 0.60 Gm. every 4 hours, usually controls pharyngeal discomfort and headache. Occasionally, codeine may be necessary for relief of these symptoms. In toxic patients, who have severe exudative pharyngotonsillitis which makes airway obstruction a potential hazard, corticosteroid therapy is employed and a tracheostomy set should be readily available. Prednisone or its equivalent in other steroid preparations may be utilized. An initial prednisone dose of 10 to 15 mg. four times daily is decreased gradually and usually discontinued after a period of seven to 10 days. Corticosteroids in full doses have been used in treating other severe complications, which include central nervous system involvement, thrombocytopenic purpura, hemolytic anemia, myocarditis and pericarditis.

Antibiotics have no effect on uncomplicated cases of this disease; and gamma globulin does not prevent or modify illness. If the throat culture is positive for hemolytic streptococci, a full course of oral penicillin (200,000 to 400,000 units four times daily) or an equivalent amount of erythromycin or parenteral penicillin should be administered over a 10-day period.

Splenomegaly develops in approximately one-half of infectious mononucleosis cases; these patients should be cautioned about heavy lifting, abdominal trauma and vigorous athletics until splenomegaly has subsided. Although extremely rare, splenic rupture is one of the few potentially fatal complications of this disease.

* Manufacturer's note: The use of tetracyclines during tooth development (last half of pregnancy, infancy and childhood to age eight years) may cause permanent discoloration of teeth. This adverse reaction is more common during long-term use of the drugs but has been observed following repeated short-term courses.

† Manufacturer's precaution: Sulfadiazine is contraindicated in infants under two months of age.

Severe abdominal pain is unusual in infectious mononucleosis except in the presence of splenic rupture, which necessitates immediate splenectomy.

Although hepatic enlargement is detectable in only about 10 per cent of patients, serum transaminase, cephalin flocculation and thymol turbidity values are elevated in many cases for several weeks. Jaundice develops in approximately 4 or 5 per cent of patients, and requires only rest in bed until the serum bilirubin returns to a normal level. No special diet is indicated.

In rare instances, patients may experience symptoms for several months, and their laboratory abnormalities are slow to resolve. In these cases, atypical lymphocytes persist and heterophil antibody titers may remain elevated for months after onset of acute illness. During this time, only symptomatic therapy is indicated.

Acute Infectious Lymphocytosis

SAMUEL KARELITZ, M.D.

Acute infectious lymphocytosis is most likely a viral infection. It occurs most commonly in children under 10 years of age but may occur in young adults, and lasts two to four weeks or longer. The revealing diagnostic finding is a white blood cell count ranging from about 40,000 to 100,000 and more. Seventy-five to 95 per cent of the cells are mature lymphocytes, and the eosinophils may be slightly increased.

The disease is self-limiting, usually without sequelae. Since the condition has occurred among siblings and in institutions, it must be regarded as contagious. Yet the patient need not be isolated, nor should the contact be quarantined.

There is no serum to treat the disease or vaccine to prevent it. Thus, the treatment has to be symptomatic. Antibiotics are not indicated except for complications ordinarily requiring antibiotic therapy. The child may be ambulant. He may have the diet to which he is accustomed. His clothes may be laundered with the family clothes. No private toilet facilities are required.

Other diseases which may have lymphocyte counts as high as those in infectious lymphocytosis are pertussis, leukemia and infectious mononucleosis. These entities are easily excluded by clinical observation and laboratory data.

Cat-Scratch Disease

SIDNEY KIBRICK, M.D., PH.D.

In almost all instances this disease is self-limiting and benign. There is no specific treatment. Antibiotics have no effect and the value of steroids is unproved. Constitutional symptoms, such as pain, fever and malaise lasting from days to several weeks, are common and may be treated with aspirin or other analgesics.

The adenopathy characteristic of this disorder usually subsides within one or two months but may persist much longer. Adenitis which has not progressed to suppuration by six weeks generally tends to subside without abscess formation. Warm, moist compresses may hasten this regression.

The suppurating fluctuant node is most simply and effectively treated by closed aspiration, using 18- or 19-gauge needle and local anesthesia. When pus is thick, instillation of saline may facilitate this process. Generally, only one or a few aspirations are necessary. This procedure not only relieves painful adenopathy but also provides material for preparation of skin test antigen.

Treatment by incision and drainage is not recommended, since it is more frequently followed by the development of sinus tracts and chronic drainage than is closed aspiration. Incision for biopsy may also be followed by this complication.

Under certain circumstances, surgical excision of the involved nodes may be indicated. This procedure should be reserved for the following cases: (1) those failing to respond to repeated closed aspirations, (2) patients with persistent draining sinuses, (3) patients with persistent adenopathy of sufficient severity and pain to interfere with their normal activities and (4) those equivocal cases in which a biopsy is needed to rule out the possibility of malignancy or some other serious disease.

There is no evidence that cat-scratch disease is spread from man to man. Accordingly, it is not necessary to isolate or quarantine patients with this disease.

Cytomegalovirus Infections

JAMES B. HANSHAW, M.D.

CONGENITAL INFECTION

Approximately 90 per cent of congenital cytomegalovirus infections are asymptomatic; the remaining 10 per cent may have mild to severe, even fatal, cytomegalic inclusion disease. Although several drugs such as prednisone, cytosine arabinoside, 5-iododeoxyuridine (IUDR), 5-fluorodeoxyuridine (FUDR) and interferon inducers have been used experimentally in patients, there is no evidence that these drugs have any lasting effect on the progression of the disease. Both cytosine arabinoside and IUDR can induce a diminution in virus excretion in some patients. However, in view of the possible toxicity of these compounds and their unproved efficacy, they cannot be recommended. They should never be used in hospitals that do not have ready access to platelet transfusions.

Most infants with symptomatic infection do not require therapy. Exchange transfusion is rarely necessary for indirect hyperbilirubinemia. Neonatal sepsis, an unusual complication of cytomegalic inclusion disease, is due to enteric organisms or a streptococcal infection. Thus, the therapy would not be different from that used in other newborns with sepsis (p. 550). Since congenital cytomegalic inclusion disease may be a cause of spastic quadriplegia, mental retardation and obstructive hydrocephalus, long-range measures dealing with these chronic problems must be planned on an individual basis.

ACQUIRED INFECTION

Until recently, clinically apparent disease due to cytomegalovirus infection had not been recognized except in patients with primary or iatrogenic immune deficiency. It is now known that infections in previously healthy individuals may result in a variety of abnormalities, including an infectious mononucleosis-like illness (cytomegalovirus mononucleosis), infectious polyneuritis, hepatomegaly with abnormal liver function tests and pneumonitis. The latter manifestation is more often associated with a deficiency of cellular immunity such as that induced by corticosteroid therapy in homotransplantation. In such instances the pneumonitis may be benefited by a temporary reduction of immunosuppressive therapy. Although leukemic patients with cytomegalovirus pneumonitis have apparently responded clinically to FUDR, more data on virus excretion during therapy are needed before the efficacy of this compound can be adequately evaluated.

Prevention. Cytomegalovirus mononucleosis may occur in previously healthy young adults or following the transfusion of fresh blood. The greater the number of transfusion units, the higher the probability of cytomegalovirus transmission. Because of the lability of cytomegalovirus, this complication of transfusion can be diminished significantly by using citrated blood that has been stored for more than 72 hours.

There is no available vaccine for the prevention of cytomegalovirus infection.

Viral Respiratory Disease

EDWARD A. MORTIMER, JR., M.D.

Viral respiratory disease comprises many different syndromes, including the common cold, pharyngitis, bronchiolitis, nonbacterial croup, bronchopneumonia and the influenza syndrome (la grippe). Etiologically almost any respiratory virus may be responsible for any one of these syndromes, although there is a tendency for some specific agents to be associated more frequently with one or another symptom complex, such as the respiratory syncytial viruses with bronchiolitis, or the parainfluenza viruses with croup. Specific therapy of these syndromes is discussed elsewhere.

General management should include keeping the patient comfortable by symptomatic therapy of specific manifestations and the avoidance of unnecessary treatment, such as the use of antibiotics. In influenza or the influenza-like syndrome, defined as a febrile viral illness with moderate to severe systemic symptoms but few respiratory complaints, fluids, bed rest and aspirin or acetaminophen (Tempra, Tenlap or Tylenol) represent the best means of relief. The doses are 60 mg. of aspirin or acetaminophen per year of age, given no more often than four times in 24 hours. Care must be taken to avoid salicylism.

In viral respiratory diseases with moderate coughing, any one of various expectorant cough preparations, given according to the manufacturer's directions, may be employed. Narcotic suppressives such as codeine may sometimes be required when cough interferes significantly with sleep, but these are usually not needed.

A mild non-narcotic preparation containing glyceryl guaiacolate is Robitussin; the dose is 1 teaspoon every 4 hours to children three years and older; younger children should receive half this dose. Robitussin A-C contains 10 mg. of codeine per teaspoon; the dose is the same.

Mycoplasma Pneumoniae Infections

SIDNEY J. SUSSMAN, M.D.

The literature indicates that *Mycoplasma pneumoniae infections* usually involve the lower lobes (Denny et al.), and that the white blood cell and differential counts are relatively normal. However, one can never be confident of the diagnosis on initial examination, because the symptoms, signs, x-ray findings and blood counts are often strikingly similar to those found in other types of bacterial and viral pneumonias. *Mycoplasma pneumoniae* infection in a patient with sickle cell anemia may be the one exception to this observation. Here the pneumonia may be fulminant and perhaps more severe than that produced by other respiratory organisms. The clinician must institute therapy after initial evaluation of the patient, with the knowledge that confirmation of a mycoplasma infection requires two to three weeks.

In the absence of a firm bacteriologic diagnosis, the physician usually begins with penicillin in routine pneumonias. Failure of response is the best clue that the patient may be infected with *Mycoplasma pneumoniae* (Shulman et al). This is usually apparent by the fifth day, at which time one should seriously consider *Mycoplasma pneumoniae* as the causative agent and switch to erythromycin, 50 mg. per kilogram per day, or tetracycline,* 50 mg. per kilogram per day. This rule is especially applicable to pneumonias in children 5 to 19 years of age, where one finds the highest incidence of *Mycoplasma pneumoniae* infections. Despite the fact that neither drug has antimicrobial effect in vivo against *Mycoplasma pneumonia* (Slotkin et al.), there is adequate clinical experience to support their effectiveness (Kingston et al.). Therapeutic response is usually not dramatic, but the clinical course is abbreviated under the influence of these drugs. Adequate antibody response is not diminished by either drug even if therapy is instituted early.

* Manufacturer's note: The use of tetracyclines during tooth development (last half of pregnancy, infancy and childhood to age eight years) may cause permanent discoloration of teeth. This adverse reaction is more common during long-term use of the drugs but has been observed following repeated short-term courses.

Mycoplasma pneumoniae infections in children are usually mild (Denny et al.), and other treatment beyond antibiotics is generally unnecessary. However, in the severely ill patient, oxygen, fluids, mist and decongestants are indicated. Extension of the organisms to other organs is rare, and therefore other forms of treatment directed to those parts of the body are usually unnecessary.

Spread within families has been well documented. On occasion, the organism causes epidemics. Individual recurrences occur but are very rare. The physician must be aware of these situations and use erythromycin or tetracycline when clinically indicated.

References

Denny, F. W., Clyde, W. A., Jr., and Glezen, W. P.: *Mycoplasma pneumoniae* Disease: Clinical Spectrum, Pathophysiology, Epidemiology, and Control. *J. Infect. Dis.,* 123:74–92, 1971.

Kingston, J. R., Chanock, R. M., Mufson, M. A., Hellman, M. A., James, H. H., Fox, B. S., Manko, M. A., and Boyers, J.: Eaton Agent Pneumonia. *J.A.M.A.,* 176:118–123, 1961.

Shulman, S. T., Bartlett, J., Clyde, W. A., Jr., and Ayoub, E. M.: The Unusual Severity of Mycoplasmal Pneumonia in Children with Sickle Cell Disease. *New England J. Med.,* 287:164, 1972.

Slotkin, R. I., Clyde, W. A., Jr., and Denny, F. W.: The Effect of Antibiotics on *Mycoplasma pneumoniae* In Vitro and In Vivo. *Am. J. Epidemiol.,* 86:225–237, 1967.

Viral Hepatitis

SAUL KRUGMAN, M.D.

Viral hepatitis is one of the most important unsolved problems in preventive medicine today. The control of this disease will depend in great part on the isolation, identification and attenuation of the viruses which cause this infection. This important objective has not been achieved. However, during the past 25 years, studies on the natural history, epidemiology and prevention of viral hepatitis have provided data needed for the formulation of rational procedures for the control of the disease.

Viral hepatitis is caused by at least two viruses: virus A (infectious hepatitis) and virus B (serum hepatitis). The two types of hepatitis have the following distinctive clinical, epidemiologic and immunologic features: the *incubation period* for viral hepatitis, type A is 15 to 50 days, and for type B, 50 to 160 days; regarding *age incidence,* type A usually occurs in children and young adults, and type B occurs at any age but predominantly in adolescents and adults; *transmissibility* of hepatitis A virus is chiefly by close contact, but also by parenteral exposure, and of hepatitis B virus chiefly by inoculation of contaminated blood or blood products, and also by close contact; *Australia* or hepatitis B antigen (HB Ag) is not present in type A hepatitis, but usually is present in type B during the incubation period and the acute phase of the disease: HB Ag may persist for years in chronic carriers; *immunity* is homologous following infectious and serum hepatitis, but neither confers immunity against the other.

Prevention of Viral Hepatitis, Type A. Since the infection is spread chiefly via the fecal-oral route, procedures designed to block intestinal oral pathways should be used for control. These measures include scrupulous handwashing, proper sterilization of food utensils, fly abatement and exclusion of potentially infected food handlers. Although close contact is the most common mode of transmission of infectious hepatitis, common source epidemics stemming from contaminated food, milk and water supplies may also occur.

The efficacy of human immune serum globulin for the prevention or modification of viral hepatitis type A has been well established. It is recommended for children and adults who have had an intimate exposure to a person with the disease. It is also indicated for persons living in the same household because they are likely to have direct or indirect contact with the infectious virus. On the other hand, the routine use of immune serum globulin for children and adults in schools, offices and factories is not warranted; spread of the disease is unlikely under the conditions in these open facilities. However, in institutions for mentally retarded children and in other closed areas where hepatitis is endemic, immune serum globulin is indicated for new admissions and new employees. The dose is dependent upon the type of exposure; a proposed schedule is shown in Table 1.

Prevention of Viral Hepatitis, Type B. Contaminated blood, blood products and needles are the most common sources of hepatitis B virus infection. The most common mode of transmission is the parenteral route, but the virus can infect via the oral route. Blood obtained from commercial donors carries a ten- to fifteen-fold greater risk of causing hepatitis than blood obtained from volunteer donors. The indications for administering blood or blood products should be carefully assessed to be sure that the potential advantages of the transfusion warrant the potential risk of transmitting hepatitis.

The following precautions are indicated for the screening of blood donors: (1) Reject persons whose blood contains HB Ag; (2) reject persons who are suspected of being addicted to narcotics; (3) reject those who have received blood or had contact with a patient with hepatitis within the past six months; (4) reject donors who have had hepatitis in the past; and (5) reject donors whose blood was previously suspected of causing hepatitis.

The use of disposable equipment is indicated if feasible. Equipment which cannot be discarded should be thoroughly cleaned and sterilized. The virus can be inactivated by boiling for at least 10 minutes, autoclaving at 15 pounds pressure or being subjected to dry heat at 338° F. (170° C) for 30 minutes.

The use of immune serum globulin for the prevention of viral hepatitis type B has not proved as effective as its use for viral hepatitis type A. There have been conflicting reports, ranging from no protection to minimal protection. Consequently, the routine use of immune serum globulin for prevention of serum hepatitis is not warranted.

Treatment. There is no specific treatment

TABLE 1. Recommended Dose of Immune Serum Globulin for Prevention of Viral Hepatitis Type A

TYPE OF EXPOSURE	DOSE (*ml./lb.*)	TOTAL DOSE* (*ml.*)	
Single or short-term	0.01–0.02	0.5	(up to 50 lb.)
		1.0	(50 to 100 lb.)
		2.0–3.0	(over 100 lb.)
Prolonged or continuous	0.03–0.06	1.0–2.0	(up to 50 lb.)
		2.0–3.0	(50 to 100 lb.)
		5.0	(over 100 lb.)

* Repeat once after five months if exposure is continuous.

for children with type A or type B viral hepatitis. The disease is generally so mild that bed rest is unnecessary after the acute stage. The return to activity is usually gauged by the child's desire. The diet is also determined by the patient. When anorexia is present, food is rejected; liquids, such as broth and fruit juices, should be offered. A normal diet is recommended when the appetite returns. Corticosteroids and other drugs are not indicated for children with uncomplicated hepatitis.

FULMINANT HEPATITIS. Sudden onset of mental confusion, emotional instability, restlessness, coma and hemorrhagic manifestations may progress to a fatal outcome within 10 days. Under these extraordinary conditions the following measures should be considered: (1) corticosteroid therapy; (2) withdrawal of protein from the diet; (3) oral neomycin, 25 mg per kilogram of body weight every 6 hours, to suppress bacterial flora of the intestinal tract; (4) laxatives and cleansing enemas; and (5) exchange transfusion.

Enterovirus Infections

HARRY T. WRIGHT, JR., M.D.

The group of enteroviruses (Coxsackie viruses group A, Coxsackie viruses group B, ECHO viruses and polioviruses) consists of over 60 serologically distinct viruses that inhabit the gastrointestinal tract and possess similar physical and chemical properties. Most enteroviral infections are asymptomatic or result in mild illnesses with clinical manifestations referred to the central nervous system, the gastrointestinal tract, the heart, the respiratory tract and the skin. Some distinctive clinical diseases may be associated with infection with certain enteroviruses. These include paralytic poliomyelitis, herpangina, human hand, foot and mouth disease, pleurodynia and generalized disease of the newborn with encephalitis and myocarditis.

No specific therapy is known which directly affects the enteroviruses or influences the course of diseases caused by them. Currently available antiviral agents are not applicable to the treatment of enteroviral infections in man, and once signs of illness have appeared, the administration of gamma globulin will not alter the course of the disease. Because of the large number of viruses involved, it would appear impractical to consider a vaccine other than the poliovirus vaccines. Various nonspecific measures, such as aspirin and fluid therapy, relieve symptoms caused by these infections.

Occasionally, supportive treatment may be lifesaving when designed to control the life-threatening manifestations that occur, such as airway obstruction and hypoventilation.

ACUTE RESPIRATORY DISEASE AND BRONCHOPNEUMONIA

Acute respiratory disease (upper respiratory infections) can be caused by Coxsackie viruses group A, Coxsackie viruses group B and, rarely, ECHO viruses. Bronchopneumonia can be caused by Coxsackie viruses group A and Coxsackie viruses group B, but this etiology is probably unusual. Treatment is symptomatic and includes aspirin, cough syrup, bed rest and adequate fluid intake. Secondary bacterial infection is not usually a problem; therefore, antibiotics are not indicated.

GASTROINTESTINAL DISEASE

There is little firm evidence to implicate the enteroviruses in gastroenteritis except in a few epidemics in which ECHO viruses have been isolated; therefore, the most important therapeutic principle is to exclude treatable causes of gastroenteritis. Treatment is symptomatic and most children can be managed with oral fluids; intravenous therapy is rarely necessary.

HERPANGINA (VESICULAR OR ULCERATIVE TONSILLOPHARYNGITIS) AND ACUTE LYMPHONODULAR PHARYNGITIS

Herpangina is caused by a number of the Coxsackie viruses group A, and acute lymphonodular pharyngitis is apparently caused specifically by Coxsackie viruses group A, type 10. Children with these lesions are treated symptomatically with aspirin and with a liquid or soft diet. Citrus juices may irritate the mouth lesions; however, clear liquids such as apple juice, tea and Jell-O water are tolerated well. Local anesthetics such as lidocaine (Xylocaine) viscous may relieve the pain caused by the mouth lesions.

HAND-FOOT-AND-MOUTH DISEASE

Hand-foot-and-mouth disease is caused by Coxsackie viruses group A, types 5 and 16. This disease is characteristically benign and self-limited, although a fatality associated with Coxsackie virus group A, type 16 infection has been reported. Treatment is entirely symptomatic and is similar to that suggested for herpangina and acute lymphonodular pharyngitis.

NONSPECIFIC FEBRILE ILLNESS, WITH OR WITHOUT RASH

The nonspecific febrile illnesses, with or without rash, have been reported with certain of the Coxsackie viruses group A, Coxsackie viruses group B, ECHO viruses and polioviruses. Patients usually experience mild illnesses, and symptomatic therapy is all that is necessary. Since the rash associated with ECHO 9 virus infections can resemble the rash of meningococcemia, it is important to perform appropriate studies to differentiate between the two diseases so that antimicrobial therapy will not be withheld if it is indicated.

PLEURODYNIA (BORNHOLM'S DISEASE, EPIDEMIC MYALGIA)

Pleurodynia is almost always caused by Coxsackie viruses group B, although ECHO viruses have rarely been implicated. In adults the characteristic onset is with sudden, severe chest pain (devil's grip), whereas in children, abdominal pain is the more frequent presenting symptom. With severe pain, codeine may be required. Intractable coughing among children, devoid of any abnormality in the respiratory tract, may occur. The severe paroxysms are sometimes refractory to any type of cough medication; however, a beneficial effect can often be derived from rock candy.

ENCEPHALOMYOCARDITIS IN NEWBORNS; MYOCARDITIS AND PERICARDITIS IN OLDER CHILDREN AND ADULTS

The myocarditis of newborns and the myocarditis and pericarditis of older children and adults caused by enteroviruses is almost always due to one of the Coxsackie viruses group B; however, ECHO viruses and Coxsackie viruses group A have rarely been isolated.

Precaution should be taken to protect newborn infants from exposure to and infection with Coxsackie viruses group B. Because of the potential danger when Coxsackie viruses group B are introduced on an obstetric service, the woman who at the time of delivery has fever and other evidence of an acute viral infection is suspect and should be isolated. Newborn infants with myocarditis due to these agents may require oxygen and digitalis. The use of digitalis in myocarditis is discussed on page 136.

ENCEPHALITIS

Encephalitis can be caused by certain Coxsackie viruses group A, Coxsackie viruses group B, ECHO viruses and polioviruses. Therapy is nonspecific but is designed to preserve vital functions through support measures. Phenobarbital sodium, paraldehyde and diphenylhydantoin sodium (Dilantin) appear to be equally effective as anticonvulsive drugs. If frequent or sustained convulsions appear, it may be necessary to give diazepam (Valium)* intravenously. The smallest amount of diazepam necessary to stop a convulsion is indicated (usually 0.1 to 0.2 mg. per kilogram). Anticonvulsive drugs should be used with caution, since they may augment any respiratory irregularities or depression already present.

Dexamethazone intramuscularly, urea intravenously and mannitol† intravenously have been used with variable results in these patients to reduce cerebral edema. Cooling measures, including aspirin, an ice blanket and, occasionally, thorazine,‡ may be necessary with hyperpyrexia, and respiratory aid may be necessary for inadequate respiratory exchange.

ASEPTIC MENINGITIS

Aseptic meningitis may be caused by a variety of enteroviruses, including Coxsackie viruses group A, Coxsackie viruses group B, ECHO viruses and polioviruses. This is a benign and self-limited disease and treatment is entirely symptomatic. A more extensive discussion of management of this syndrome appears on page 660.

POLIOMYELITIS (PARALYTIC DISEASE)

Although the vast majority of poliomyelitis is caused by the polioviruses, paralytic disease has also been associated with several Coxsackie viruses group A, Coxsackie viruses group B and ECHO viruses.

Prevention and Control. Although the methods of the spread of poliomyelitis are not clearly understood, there is no definite evidence that isolation of individuals or communities for a prolonged period of time affects the course of an epidemic. Immunization procedures, however, do prevent poliomyelitis.

Active Immunization. Two kinds of vaccines are available for active immunization; a formalin-inactivated vaccine (Salk) given by injection, and an oral vaccine containing live attenuated poliovirus strains (Sabin). Both vaccines produce adequate immunity in infants,

---

* Manufacturer's precaution: The safety and efficacy of injectable Valium in children under 12 years of age have not been established.

† Manufacturer's precaution: Use of mannitol in pediatric patients has not been studied comprehensively.

‡ Manufacturer's precaution: Thorazine is not recommended for children under six months of age except when lifesaving.

children and adults. Currently, the vaccine of choice is the oral trivalent material, although monovalent vaccines, each containing one of the three attenuated poliovirus types, are available. Infants should receive their first dose at two to three months of age, a second dose eight weeks later and a third dose eight weeks after the second. A fourth dose is given at 15 to 18 months of age and a fifth dose is given before starting to school. The oral trivalent vaccine is easy to administer, has an adequate immunogenic effect and results in a prolonged persistence of antibody. At present, whether booster doses of vaccine are needed after the initial series (five doses) is unknown.

PASSIVE IMMUNIZATION. Pooled human gamma globulin has been administered intramuscularly in a dosage of 0.14 ml. per pound to reduce infection by polioviruses and to lessen the severity of paralysis in children. It must be injected prior to exposure or very early in the incubation period to have beneficial effects. Protection lasts about five weeks.

The emergence of vaccines for the production of active immunity has resulted in far less need for passive protection against this disease, and poliomyelitis immune serum globulin (human) is now infrequently used.

Management. Management of the patient with poliomyelitis varies with the type of clinical disease encountered as well as with the stage of disease.

There is no specific treatment for paralytic poliomyelitis. Convalescent serum or gamma globulin does not alter the course of events once signs of illness have appeared. Although mild and suspect cases of abortive and nonparalytic forms of poliomyelitis may be managed at home, all patients with acute paralytic poliomyelitis should be hospitalized. Complete bed rest during the febrile period and early convalescence is vital for all patients with this disease. There appears to be a close correlation between the amount of physical activity early in the major illness and the incidence and severity of subsequent paralysis. Constant clearing of the throat is an early sign of swallowing dysfunction; weakness of the arms may be followed by weakness of the muscles of respiration; the inability to void may precede more serious disease, such as weakness or paralysis of the legs.

PARALYTIC POLIOMYELITIS. A firm, hard mattress should be provided, and the bed should be equipped with a foot board to prevent footdrop. A blanket roll under the knees may reduce extensor muscle spasms of the legs and back, and small changes in position often relieve pain. The patient's posture should be changed from side to side periodically for the relief of pain due to muscle spasm.

Hot moist packs (the Sister Kenny method) applied over the painful areas usually bring relief of pain and relaxation to tight muscles. Hot baths may be more efficient than hot packs for smaller children. Aspirin offers useful analgesia. Intravenous feedings may be necessary but oral feedings are usually sufficient. Neostigmine methylsulfate (Prostigmin) hypodermically, 0.04 mg. per kilogram, may be used to treat abdominal distention and constipation. Bethanechol chloride (Urecholine Chloride; for dosage see discussion of Acute Aseptic Meningitis Syndrome) may be useful in relieving urinary retention. However, urinary retention may be transitory and bladder function may return to normal within two or three days. If this is the case, intermittent catheterization with a straight French catheter may be all that is necessary. Some patients need catheters (Foley) continuously for a period of time. These patients should be observed closely for urinary tract infections, which frequently follow the insertion or prolonged use of a catheter.

All patients with acute paralytic poliomyelitis should be observed carefully for evidence of respiratory paralysis. The signs of hypoxia include restlessness, anxiety, insomnia, lethargy, muscle twitchings, cyanosis and dilatation of the pupils; stupor and death may follow. Because the patient with weakness of the respiratory muscles tends to retain carbon dioxide, oxygen tents are contraindicated. In order to rest the involved muscles, it is advisable to place the patient in a mechanical respirator (preferably the Drinker or tank respirator) before the latter stages of hypoxia are reached. The vital capacity should be measured frequently. If it is reduced one-half to two-thirds the predicted value, the respirator should be used for "rest periods" of at least 1 hour of every three or four while the patient is awake, and continuously while the patient is sleeping. If the vital capacity is one-third to one-half the predicted value, continuous respirator care is indicated. Optimal ventilation is best attained by adjusting the respiratory rate and depth, depending on the results of frequent monitoring of blood gases by determinations of the pH, pCO_2 and pO_2.

During this stage the patient needs much reassurance. He should be encouraged to move as much as possible the muscles that are partially paralyzed, although exercise to the point of fatigue is inappropriate. Attempts at passive movement and muscle reeducation should be initiated by physiotherapists soon after the pain subsides.

BULBAR POLIOMYELITIS. Patients with cranial nerve involvement may develop a nasal twang, swallowing difficulties and pooling of secretions. These patients are placed in the Trendelenburg position (15 degrees) on the side to encourage the pooling of secretions from the oropharynx and mouth. Frequent aspiration of the patient's mouth and oropharynx to remove secretions is of prime importance. Patients with mild cases of disease frequently learn to use the mechanical aspirator upon themselves. Intravenous feedings are usually indicated until a soft diet may be taken by the patient.

Patients with severe disease, with an obstructed airway as manifested by laryngeal stridor and with vocal cord paralysis and cyanosis, and patients needing a mechanical respirator should have tracheostomies performed. Strict aseptic technique in the care of the tracheostomy is necessary to prevent bacterial infections at the tracheostomy site and in the lungs. A different, sterile catheter should be used each time the tracheostomy is aspirated.

Patients with severe bulbar spinal disease may progress from lethargy to stupor and coma, and may need a tracheostomy and a tank respirator. These patients should be tested for hypoxia or hypercapnia by determining the blood gases (pH, pCO_2 and pO_2), since hypoxia may disappear in some patients when proper ventilation is achieved.

Anticonvulsant drugs for convulsions in patients with encephalitic involvement should be used with caution, since they may potentiate any respiratory depression that may be present. Phenobarbital sodium, paraldehyde, diazepam (Valium),§ and diphenylhydantoin sodium (Dilantin) have all been used effectively.

With extensive medullary or brainstem involvement, high fever and hypotension, frank shock may appear as a terminal event. Shock is a very grave complication, and although the usual therapy may be tried (vasoconstrictors and blood volume expanders), it is usually unsuccessful.

CONVALESCENCE. The patient is usually afebrile within two weeks after the onset of disease. Measures to reduce pain and spasm and to prepare the muscles for reeducation and use include aspirin, hot packs for 20 to 30 minutes every 2 to 3 hours and hydrotherapy in a Hubbard tank. Passive exercises to the extremities through the range of motion of all joints should be performed after the use of hot packs.

Within six weeks after the onset of disease, muscle pain and spasm have diminished and a careful program of muscle strengthening and reeducation may be planned by the physical therapist and the orthopedist. The process of weaning the patient from the respirator should be quite gradual, with the time out of the respirator increased in small increments, never allowing the patient to become fatigued. Periods of unassisted breathing may be attempted when the patient can maintain a normal respiratory rate without the use of accessory muscles and without anxiety.

When the patient no longer has upper airway obstruction or lower respiratory disease and is able to clear his own airway with a cough, the tracheostomy tube may be removed.

The child with paralytic disease should be under the long-term supervision of an orthopedist, since undetected, untreated, minimal skeletomuscle imbalances may result in permanent deformities in the child who is growing rapidly.

§ Manufacturer's precaution: Safety and efficacy of injectable diazepam in children under 12 years of age have not been established. Oral diazepam is not for use in children under six months of age.

References

Curnen, E. C.: The Coxsackieviruses. *Pediat. Clin. N. Am.*, 7:903, 1960.

Horstmann, D. M.: Enterovirus Infections: Etiologic, Epidemiologic and Clinical Aspects. *California Med.*, 103:1, 1965.

McAllister, R. M.: Echovirus Infections. *Pediat. Clin. N. Amer.*, 7:927, 1960.

Portnoy, B.: Pediatric Virology. *California Med.*, 102:431, 1965.

Ward, R.: Poliomyelitis. *Pediat. Clin. N. Amer.*, 7:947, 1960.

Wright, H. T., Jr., Landing, B. H., Lennette, E. H., and McAllister, R. M.: Fatal Infection in an Infant Associated with Coxsackie A16 Virus. *New England J. Med.*, 268:1041, 1963.

Acute Aseptic Meningitis Syndrome

HARRY T. WRIGHT, JR., M.D.

Aseptic meningitis is a clinical syndrome which is usually considered benign and self-limited. The principal features are as follows: acute onset of fever, signs of meningeal irritation and alteration of cerebrospinal fluid to include pleocytosis, increased protein, normal sugar and an absence of bacteria. The initial lumbar puncture may reveal a polymorphonuclear leukocyte response; later in the disease, lymphocytes predominate in the cerebrospinal fluid.

Mumps virus is perhaps the most common single cause of the aseptic meningitis syndrome; however, enteroviruses (Echo viruses, Coxsackie viruses and polioviruses) can also cause extensive epidemics of aseptic meningitis. Although the aseptic meningitis syndrome is usually a benign viral infection requiring no special diagnostic or therapeutic measures, it must be remembered that some patients may have serious or potentially fatal diseases and initially present with signs and symptoms similar to those of aseptic meningitis.

Management. The most important principle of therapy consists of making an accurate and appropriate diagnosis. If aseptic meningitis is known to be prevalent in the community and if the patient is alert and active, although manifesting some signs of meningeal irritation, and if examination of the cerebrospinal fluid reveals pleocytosis, no microorganisms and a normal concentration of glucose, then the diagnosis of aseptic meningitis is most likely, and observation rather than the initiation of antibiotic therapy is the recommended course of action. If the initial lumbar puncture reveals a predominance of polymorphonuclear leukocytes and a borderline-low cerebrospinal fluid sugar, if the patient has been treated with antibiotics prior to admission or if the clinical condition of the patient worsens after hospitalization, it is my policy to repeat the lumbar puncture in 4 to 6 hours to confirm the diagnosis of aseptic meningitis.

Treatment of aseptic meningitis is symptomatic and no specific therapy is available. Bed rest, using a firm mattress if possible, analgesics and antipyretics will bring symptomatic relief. If spasms of the extensor muscles of the legs and back occur, then a blanket roll under the knees may help. Rarely, vomiting may be severe enough to necessitate intravenous fluid therapy; however, oral feedings usually suffice.

Patients with aseptic meningitis are usually hospitalized for observation for two or three days. This period of observation is usually adequate to rule out any treatable diseases. If patients become toxic or have an illness that is characterized by progressive deterioration, if the patient acquires a petechial rash with evidence of meningeal irritation, if the patient demonstrates evidence of skeletomuscular weakness or swallowing difficulties or if the patient cannot be adequately cared for at home during his acute and convalescent illness, then hospitalization is required and essential. If the patient is hospitalized, he should be isolated, since some of the viral agents that cause this syndrome are readily communicable.

Aspirin has been useful for headache and muscle pain. Bethanechol chloride (Urecholine Chloride) given orally (0.6 mg. per kilogram per day with a maximum single adult dose of 30 mg.) in three divided doses, or subcutaneously (0.15 to 0.2 mg per kilogram per day with a maximum single adult dose of 5 mg.), has been of benefit in some patients with urinary retention.

Although clinical manifestations are usually gone within two weeks, convalescence may be delayed even in patients with relatively mild disease. The generalized malaise apparently persists more frequently in older children and young adults than it does in infants and young children.

Because a certain number of patients with aseptic meningitis may have mild myelitis without the development of the more obvious paralysis, an important part of the management of these patients is careful evaluation by a physical therapist about 48 to 72 hours after the patient becomes afebrile, and this examination should be repeated six weeks to 60 days after the onset of the illness. Functional muscle impairment may not necessarily show up during the early days of convalescence but may be apparent later. If any deficits are found, appropriate physical and orthopedic therapy should be instituted. Several enteroviruses, other than polioviruses, have occasionally caused significant and severe muscle function impairment lasting up to two years following the acute illness.

References

Adair, C. V., Gauld, R. L., and Smadel, J. E.: Aseptic Meningitis, A Disease of Diverse Etiology. *Ann. Int. Med.*, 39:675–704, 1953.

Lepow, M. L., Carver, D. H., Wright, H. T., Jr., Coyne, N., Thompson, L. B., Woods, W. A., and Robbins, F. C.: A Clinical, Epidemiologic and Laboratory Investigation of Aseptic Meningitis During the Four-Year Period, 1955–1958. *New England J. Med.*, 266: 1181–1193, 1962.

Wehrle, P. F., and Leedom, J. M.: Management of the Aseptic Meningitis Syndrome. *Pediat. Portfolio 1*, April 12, 1971.

Encephalitis Infections—Postinfectious and Postvaccinal

HORACE L. HODES, M.D.

Encephalitis is considered to be primary if it occurs during the acute state of an infection. "Primary infectious encephalitis" refers to cases caused by the direct action of a virus upon nerve tissues of the brain. Primary infectious encephalitis may be caused by a large number of viruses, including herpes, mumps, enteroviruses and arthropod-borne (ARBO) viruses, such as St. Louis virus, Western equine encephalitis virus, Eastern equine encephalitis virus, Japanese encephalitis virus and others. Coxsackie and ECHO viruses also cause encephalitis, with symptoms of meningeal involvement often being prominent in such cases. In a very small percentage of cases, infectious mononucleosis may cause primary encephalitis.

We shall not discuss here subacute sclerosing panencephalitis (SSPE), which appears to be encephalitis caused by measles virus acting as a "slow" virus.

Postinfectious encephalitis refers to cases of encephalitis in which neurologic symptoms appear when signs of a generalized viral infection are waning or as long as three or four weeks after all symptoms of the generalized disease have disappeared. Measles, varicella, rubella and smallpox may be followed by encephalitis. In general, postmeasles and postsmallpox encephalitis are more severe than those following varicella and rubella.

In postinfectious encephalitis the causative virus is not recoverable, at least in its complete infectious form, so that some indirect mechanism appears to be responsible for the injury to the brain. One such mechanism which has some supporting evidence is that the virus brings about some change in nerve tissue and that antibody against the altered tissue reacts with nerve tissues and injures them.

The term *postvaccinal encephalitis* is applied to encephalitis which occurs after injection of a vaccine. The injury to the nervous system is almost certainly not due to infectious virus particles or to living bacteria, although it should be noted that the incidence of postvaccinal encephalitis is lower with killed rabies vaccine than it is with rabies vaccines which contain a small number of infectious rabies virus particles. It is certain that vaccines for yellow fever and for pertussis and antirabies vaccines may be followed by postvaccinal encephalitis. The same is true for vaccinia virus which is used for vaccination against smallpox. The incidence of postvaccinal encephalitis has varied greatly from one country to another. In the United States the vaccination of approximately 4 million people in New York City was followed by 45 cases of postvaccinal encephalitis, an incidence of 1 per 100,000 vaccinations. Vaccination of 53,000 soldiers of the Royal Netherlands Army resulted in 13 cases of postvaccinal encephalitis, an incidence of 24 per 100,000 vaccinations. The reasons for the variation in the incidence of postvaccinal encephalitis are not known.

In England several years ago the Beckenham strain of attenuated measles virus vaccine apparently caused a number of cases of encephalitis, and the use of this vaccine strain was discontinued. In the United States there have been no proved cases of encephalitis due to any type of measles vaccine and the further attenuated chick embryo cultivated measles virus vaccines which are now in use have not caused encephalitis in any instance.

Treatment. Treatment for encephalitis (with the possible exception of herpes virus encephalitis) is entirely symptomatic. Convulsions are controlled with the drugs usually employed for this purpose. Dexamethasone in a dose of 0.25 to 0.50 mg. per kilogram per day, given intramuscularly, is very effective for decreasing cerebral edema. Respiratory failure, usually due to injury to the nerve cells which control respiration, is treated with any one of a number of mechanical respirators. Difficulty in swallowing is dealt with by intermittent or continuous aspiration of the pharynx. If these measures do not keep the airway open and prevent aspiration, an artificial airway must be provided by a tracheostomy tube or by placing a plastic tube through the larynx into the trachea.

Several years ago Dr. B. E. Juel-Jensen reported that cytosine arabinoside (cytarabine) had brought about a "dramatic recovery" in five patients with several forms of generalized herpes virus hominis infection and that a very similar result was obtained in the treatment of a man with early simian virus encephalitis. These patients were given cytarabine intravenously once daily for five days in doses ranging from 0.3 to 2.0 mg. per kilogram per day. Since this report, a number of patients with herpes virus encephalitis have been treated with cytarabine. In one such case a dose of 20 mg. per square meter per day given intravenously once daily for five days was used together with intrathecal application of 10 mg. of cytarabine. This treatment was unsuccessful. At the present time it must be concluded that the value of cytarabine for herpes virus encephalitis has not yet been established. Also, it should be kept in mind that the drug is quite toxic, causing severe bone marrow suppression. The author believes that at present cytarabine should be used only in patients with severe herpes virus encephalitis. The same is true for adenine arabinoside, a drug which acts in a manner similar to cytarabine but is said to be less toxic. Again, the experience with adenine arabinoside in the treatment of generalized herpes virus disease and herpes virus encephalitis is not large enough to establish its value.

The prognosis in patients with encephalitis varies greatly, depending on the etiologic agent. In general the outcome is best in postvaccinal encephalitis and poorest in primary encephalitis. For primary encephalitis, prognosis is certainly worst with rabies, which has very nearly a 100 per cent fatality rate. Among the ARBO virus diseases which occur in the United States, Eastern equine encephalitis is the most severe. Measles encephalitis is the most severe of the common postinfectious encephalitides.

Ornithosis
(Psittacosis)

JOSEPH W. ST. GEME, JR., M.D.

The relationship between parrots and pneumonia in humans was first suggested near the turn of the century. In 1929 to 1930, a world-wide pandemic resulted in official restrictions on the importation of psittacine birds into the United States. Over the next 20 years it was learned that chickens, pigeons, ducks, turkeys, pheasants and hawks carry the organism responsible for this "viral" pneumonia. Healthy birds as well as sick birds may carry the organism and infect the human host.

The spectrum of psittacosis ranges from very mild flulike illness to an abrupt onset of high fever, severe headache and nonproductive cough, which may progress to delirium and death. Fever may reach 103 to 105° F., last seven to 10 days and lyse by the second or third week of illness. Malaise, anorexia, nausea, vomiting, abdominal pain, joint discomfort and myalgia may accompany the illness. Bradycardia relative to fever occurs occasionally.

Some patients present with shaking chills, rales and the physical and radiographic findings of typical lobar pneumonia. The more classic pattern of psittacosis is lobular, interstitial pneumonitis with scant physical findings at the outset, inconspicuous cough, gradual evolution of pulmonary radiographic changes and thin sputum becoming more mucoid but nonpurulent as infection progresses. Hepatomegaly and splenomegaly may occur. As anticipated, some episodes of psittacosis are asymptomatic and most infections are mild, ambulatory illnesses. Fatal illness is rare. Overwhelming systemic infection can develop with diffuse involvement of the reticuloendothelial organs, hepatitis, toxic nephrosis, pericarditis and multifocal aseptic meningitis.

Man acquires this infection by inhalation of dried avian excreta, contact with infected tissues and rare bites. Transmission between humans has been very unusual. Fatal cases have been from such a source. Psittacosis is infrequent in children under 10 years of age. The incubation period is usually seven to 15 days but can be as long as 30 to 39 days.

Treatment. The tetracyclines are optimal antimicrobial therapy and should be administered in the usual dose for age.* Oral pediatric therapy is 25 mg. per kilogram daily in four divided doses. For older children the adult dose of 1 Gm. per day may be administered. Oral tetracycline should be given at least 1 hour before and 2 hours after meals. Larger doses may be used for severe infection. The total daily intravenous dosage is 12 mg. per kilogram in two divided doses.

Although a rapid response may occur, more often the response to treatment is too slow to make a therapeutic diagnosis. Because the antimicrobial effect is suppressive rather than bactericidal, and infection can be persistent in humans as well as birds, therapy should be sustained for two to three weeks. Significant tracheitis and bronchitis can accompany more extensive psittacosis, producing thick, bloody, gelatinous and viscid mucous plugs. These plugs may require nebulized, warm mist therapy and expectorants to liquefy and eliminate them. Stubborn plugs and atelectasis should respond to positive pressure aerosol therapy, vigorous percussion and postural drainage. Ample fluids, antipyretics and rest should suffice for supportive therapy.

Rickettsial Infections

HENRY G. CRAMBLETT, M.D.

The most common rickettsial infection in the United States is Rocky Mountain spotted fever. In the year 1971, 432 cases were reported to the Center for Disease Control. Other rickettsial infections, and their frequency, reported to the Center for Disease Control include the following: Rickettsialpox (1), typhus fever (flea-borne, murine) (23), and Q fever (25).

* Manufacturer's note: The use of tetracyclines during tooth development (last half of pregnancy, infancy and childhood to age eight years) may cause permanent discoloration of teeth. This adverse reaction is more common during long-term use of the drugs but has been observed following repeated short-term courses.

Since general therapy and management of patients with rickettsial infections are similar, only Rocky Mountain spotted fever will be discussed in detail.

Specific Therapy. Both tetracycline and chloramphenicol are effective in the therapy of rickettsial infection, although the response to therapy may not be dramatic, especially in the latter stages of the disease.

Generally, in patients who are only mildly or moderately ill, I prescribe tetracycline* orally in a dose of 50 mg. per kilogram per day in four divided doses. The total daily dose should not exceed 2 Gm. The duration of therapy should be seven to 10 days.

In the more severely ill patients who are hospitalized, I customarily use chloramphenicol. To the severely ill patient, chloramphenicol succinate should be administered intravenously in a dose of 50 to 100 mg. per kilogram per 24 hours given in four divided doses. The total daily dose should not exceed 2 Gm. and the total course of drug should be seven to 10 days. If one chooses to use chloramphenicol, it is mandatory that one ascertain whether the patient has had chloramphenicol in the past. If this is the case, the danger of an idiosyncratic bone marrow depression must be considered if chloramphenicol is used. If the patient has not had chloramphenicol in the past, there is less likelihood of this severe complication of antibiotic therapy. For monitoring purposes, complete blood counts should be performed every other day, and if the total peripheral white count drops below 5000 per cubic millimeter or if the per cent of peripheral polymorphonuclear cells drops to 30 per cent or below, chloramphenicol should be stopped. In all circumstances the parents must be informed of the potential danger of chloramphenicol and the reason for choosing it in terms of efficacy versus toxicity. Occasionally, after cessation of therapy, there may be a recurrence of signs and symptoms. In this case, retreatment for a subsequent seven-day period is indicated. If there is hepatomegaly and impairment of liver function, it is probably wise to choose chloramphenicol rather than tetracycline.

There is suggestive evidence that sulfonamides are harmful in Rocky Mountain spotted fever and therefore should not be given.

Supportive Therapy. Fever and headache are common symptoms of the disease. It is worthwhile to attempt to control both of the symptoms with the use of acetylsalicylic acid but, not uncommonly, this drug fails to relieve the pain. In those patients who are distinctly uncomfortable, codeine phosphate, 0.8 to 1.5 mg. per kilogram of body weight orally, or 0.8 mg. per kilogram subcutaneously, may be used.

In patients who are moderately to severely ill and who are likely to be hospitalized, careful attention must be given to maintaining adequate fluid and electrolyte equilibrium. Hypoelectrolytemia may occur as a complication of the disease. The reason for this is not clear but may be the result of inappropriate antidiuretic hormone effect. Therapy of this complication with concentrated electrolyte solutions is rarely successful and may be contraindicated.

Recognition and Treatment of Complications. All patients have vasculitis to a varying degree. The more severely ill patients may have edema involving the periorbital area, face and extremities. It may be necessary to use plasma expanders in order to maintain a satisfactory circulating blood volume.

Intravascular coagulation may occur in patients with Rocky Mountain spotted fever. One must be especially judicious in deciding whether therapy is indicated once the diagnosis of disseminated intravascular coagulation has been made. It is our opinion that heparin therapy in such patients may be deleterious.

Patients may manifest varying degrees of involvement of the central nervous system, including delirium, semicoma, confusion, coma and convulsions. Examination of cerebrospinal fluid may reveal a pleocytosis and increase in protein content. Convulsions can be controlled with phenobarbital sodium in a dose of 4 mg. per kilogram administered intramuscularly. If seizures continue, an additional 2 mg. per kilogram may be administered every 45 minutes up to a total dose of 12 mg. per kilogram. With this regimen, diazepam (Valium) is contraindicated. If there is evidence of increased intracranial pressure, the use of intravenously administered mannitol† should be considered.

Myocarditis and heart failure may occur in the severely ill patient. Observation for and therapy of this complication must be a part of the careful monitoring of the patient. Careful records should be maintained of fluid intake and output along with daily weights to prevent congestive failure.

Avascular necrosis is seen most often in the digits (fingers and toes), ear lobes and scrotum. The local care of lesions should be such that

---

* Manufacturer's note: The use of tetracyclines during tooth development (last half of pregnancy, infancy and childhood to age eight years) may cause permanent discoloration of teeth. This adverse reaction is more common during long-term use of the drugs but has been observed following repeated short-term courses.

† Manufacturer's precaution: Use of mannitol in pediatric patients has not been studied comprehensively.

the added deleterious factor of pressure necrosis is not operative. Antibacterial ointments may be used for prevention of secondary bacterial infection of these open wounds.

Thrombocytopenia may be treated by platelet transfusions or transfusion of fresh whole blood.

Prevention. The disease is spread by the bite of a tick. *Dermacentor andersoni,* the wood tick, is the vector most commonly responsible for adult infections, while the dog tick, *Dermacentor variabilis,* is the most important vector in childhood infections. In endemic areas where children will be exposed to wooded areas and/or have dogs as pets, parents must exercise a careful vigilance for ticks on their children. While it is recommended that children playing in wooded areas with pets wear tight-fitting clothing and be completely covered, this is not practical in the endemic areas in the hot summer months. Twice daily inspection of children with prompt removal of ticks may be helpful in preventing the disease. If the ticks can be removed before they have had the opportunity to become attached and engorged, with subsequent regurgitation of rickettsiae into the blood of the victim, this is of obvious practical significance.

Another practical suggestion is to be very certain that dogs, particularly those that are household pets, be de-ticked daily during the tick season.

It is the opinion of many practicing physicians in endemic areas that the incidence of Rocky Mountain spotted fever has decreased because of the use of antibiotics early in the prodromal stage of the disease. Ill children in endemic areas with definite tick exposure in whom tetracyclines are administered may in fact have abortive disease. Although there is no evidence to support such a practice, I personally feel that a therapeutic trial with tetracycline may be indicated in this circumstance, particularly in the child with severe headache and fever and who, upon careful physical examination, does not have any detectable cause for such symptoms.

A killed rickettsial vaccine is available for prevention of Rocky Mountain spotted fever. This vaccine must be administered in three subcutaneous injections of 1 ml. each at weekly intervals. Its protection is of short duration and a booster must be given annually. Moreover, the efficacy of this vaccine has not been fully established. Accordingly, I do not recommend its use.

Systemic Mycotic Infections

JOHN P. UTZ, M.D., *and*
WILLIAM E. LAUPUS, M.D.

The systemic mycotic infections encountered in the United States may be considered primary (histoplasmosis, blastomycosis, coccidioidomycosis, actinomycosis and sporotrichosis) or opportunists (candidosis, aspergillosis, cryptococcosis and mucormycosis [phycomycosis]). The latter infections are seen with striking frequency in various conditions such as diabetic acidosis, lymphoma (especially Hodgkin's disease), leukemia, immunosuppressive (azathioprine) or corticoid therapy, sarcoidosis and especially the hereditary, immune-deficiency states (hypogammaglobulinemia, Wiskott-Aldrich or Swiss type disease). Under these conditions not only do the clinical manifestations reflect the underlying predisposing condition, but also therapy directed toward correction of the underlying condition sometimes solves or ameliorates the complicating fungal infection.

Although in many areas most fungal in-

TABLE 1. Chemotherapeutic Agents in the Systemic Mycoses

DISEASE	DRUG: *First Choice*	DRUG: *Second Choice*
Actinomycosis	Penicillin	Lincomycin*
Nocardiosis	Sulfonamide	Ampicillin
Histoplasmosis	Amphotericin B	Sulfonamide
Blastomycosis	Amphotericin B	2-Hydroxystilbamidine
Sporotrichosis	Potassium iodide	Amphotericin B
Candidosis	Amphotericin B	Flucytosine
Cryptococcosis	Amphotericin B	Flucytosine
Coccidioidomycosis	Amphotericin B	No other drug
Aspergillosis	Amphotericin B	No other drug
Mucormycosis	Amphotericin B	No other drug

* Manufacturer's precaution: Lincomycin is not indicated in the newborn (up to one month of age).

fections may be entirely subclinical, most patients with mycoses who come to the physician are seriously ill with symptoms such as fever, chills, anorexia, weight loss, sweating at night and lassitude. The first major mode of therapy is general care for such children: the dehydration and electrolyte derangements require proper rehydration and replacement. An attractive high protein, high caloric, vitamin-rich diet is reasonable. Other symptoms, such as sleep-disturbing cough, shortness of breath, pleuritic pain, airway obstruction and respiratory acidosis, similarly require appropriate treatment.

In addition to its diagnostic value in obtaining biopsy material, surgery is often essential in these infections. Abscesses must usually be drained, and cavitary or fungous ball lesions, which produce hemoptysis, and irreversibly damaged (necrotic, fibrotic and avascular) lesions (e.g., actinomycosis) must be resected.

However, the third, essential, and most important mode of treatment is chemotherapy.

Sulfonamides. Sulfadiazine has been the drug usually employed in patients who have nocardiosis. A daily dosage (0.065 to 0.1 Gm. per kilogram per day) sufficient to achieve a serum level of approximately 10 mg. per 100 ml. should be given.* Primarily because of the frequency of metastatic abscesses, notably in the brain, such treatment has been disappointing, and it has been a common practice to supplement sulfonamides with either streptomycin (15 mg. per kilogram per day) or ampicillin (150 mg. per kilogram per day). Therapy should be prolonged for at least 12 weeks or until lesions have cleared or stabilized.

Penicillin. Actinomycosis of the cervicofacial, thoracic or abdominal form is best treated with benzyl-penicillin (G), 10 million units intravenously for two to four weeks. After that and especially if the patient is able to go home, it has seemed reasonable to continue treatment orally with phenoxymethyl penicillin in a dosage of 500 mg. four times daily. Therapy must be continued for eight weeks or until the lesion has cleared or remained stabilized for four weeks.

2-Hydroxystilbamidine. This drug is chemotherapeutically active and relatively less toxic than alternative agents in rare children who develop blastomycosis. We have not had occasion to use this drug in children,† but *in adults* the dosage we have employed without problems has been 225 mg. in 500 ml. of 5 per cent glucose in water given daily. It has been customary to treat the patient for approximately four weeks (or 8 Gm. total dosage) as a course of therapy. Because some of the stilbamidines are not stable and fluoresce on exposure to light, it is customary to protect the dissolved solution and the infusion bottle from light.

Potassium Iodide. Use of this drug is limited to patients who have cutaneous lymphatic sporotrichosis. The usual dose is 9 to 12 ml. given daily in three doses. Such side effects as acneiform skin eruptions, lacrimation, parotid swelling, nausea and vomiting can usually be controlled by stopping the drug for a few days and resuming therapy at a slightly lower dosage. Although the duration of therapy has not been established and probably differs from patient to patient, the drug should be continued for approximately four weeks after lesions have healed completely or stabilized.

Amphotericin B. For the remaining mycoses, aspergillosis, histoplasmosis, blastomycosis, candidosis, cryptococcosis, coccidioidomycosis, mucormycosis (phycomycosis), and more resistant forms of sporotrichosis, amphotericin B is the standard chemotherapeutic agent. It is given intravenously in 5 per cent glucose in water over a 2- to 6-hour period. The initial day's dose should not be more than 1 mg., but the dose can be increased thereafter by daily increments of 5 or 10 mg. until an optimal dose of 1 mg. per kilogram (not exceeding 50 mg.) per day has been achieved. The maximal concentration given should not be greater than 10 mg. per 100 ml. The total dose and the duration of therapy are not established, and, indeed, vary from infection to infection, but at least four weeks' therapy should be given for every mycosis (except for mucormycosis, in which the disease usually resolves, fatally or otherwise, in three to four days).

Administration of this drug is accompanied by unpleasant side effects, such as chills, fever, nausea, vomiting, anorexia, headaches and general malaise. When such symptoms occur frequently enough to warrant attention, 25 to 50 mg. of hydrocortisone may be given intravenously at the beginning of the infusion. An even more serious side effect, however, is nephrotoxicity, with rising blood urea nitrogen and serum creatinine levels and decreasing concentrating ability and clearances. It is virtually impossible to avoid all renal toxicity, and a serum creatinine level of 3.0 (1.5 for children under 10) or a blood urea nitrogen concentration of 50 mg. per 100 ml. can serve as a reason-

* Manufacturer's precaution: Sulfadiazine is not recommended for infants under two months of age.

† Manufacturer's note: Children's dosage of 2-hydroxystilbamidine has not been established.

able limit beyond which treatment must be altered. A few days without treatment, administration of the drug on only alternate days or resumption at a slightly lower dosage is usually sufficient to maintain renal function within acceptable limits. Anemia is frequently encountered, in part due to decreased red cell survival resulting from the infection and in part due to decreased red cell production stemming from probable bone marrow suppression by the drug. This anemia is generally mild and tends to stabilize as the infection is brought under control. Iron is of no value, and transfusions are rarely necessary. Hypokalemia, often symptomatic, is another complication and can be prevented by administration of potassium salts orally.

Flucytosine (5-Fluorocytosine). In selected cases of cryptococcosis and systemic Candida infections, this agent is an alternative to amphotericin B. Before starting therapy it is critical that the laboratory do tube dilution studies to determine the sensitivity of the fungus to the drug. With minimum inhibitory concentrations of 12.5 micrograms per ml. or less and if the patient can swallow, the drug should be given orally in a dosage of 150 mg. per kilograms per day in four divided doses. At present there is no liquid preparation. The duration of therapy has been arbitrary but is usually six weeks. The drug is well tolerated, and it has been difficult in the patients so far treated to distinguish side effects from manifestations of the other underlying disease, or of the treatment for it or of the infection. However, the following determinations should be regularly obtained during therapy: serum creatinine or blood urea nitrogen, serum glutamic oxaloacetic transaminase, alkaline phosphatase, hemoglobin and leukocyte count.

Histoplasmosis

AMOS CHRISTIE, M.D.

Unfortunately, a truly effective agent has not been found for the treatment of histoplasmosis. A variety of drugs and antibiotics have been tried by us and by others without uniformly favorable results.

At Vanderbilt the current method of choice for treatment of the primary lesions only is the use of triple sulfonamide suspension.* This is based on the in vitro evidence that it is impossible to grow the fungus when levels of 12 to 15 mg per 100 ml. are placed in the media. Therefore, we give the suspension in doses which produce levels of 6 to 8 mg. per 100 ml. in the blood. This dose varies with age, weight or surface area and with excretory capability. At least 150 mg. per kilogram per day orally in divided doses is required to attain the level indicated. This is well tolerated by the patient; it can be accurately regulated by laboratory methods available to all pediatricians; and we believe it to be the method of choice for all primary varieties of histoplasmosis at this time.

Amphotericin B (Fungizone) has been used in the progressive disseminated forms of the disease, and favorable results have been reported. In its present form, however, the drug is pyrogenic, producing chills and high fever. It is poorly absorbed from the gastrointestinal tract, and nephrotoxicity is well documented. Methods for determining blood levels have been developed and are helpful. This drug should never be given outside a hospital. Since it must be given for weeks, economic implications are apparent.

* Manufacturer's precaution: Triple sulfonamide suspension is not for use in infants under two months of age.

References

Christie, A.: The Disease Spectrum of Human Histoplasmosis. *Ann. Int. Med.,* 49:544, 1958.

Little, J. A., Bruce, J., Andrews, H. A., Crawford, K., and McKinney, G.: Treatment of Disseminated Infantile Histoplasmosis with Amphotericin B. *Pediatrics,* 24:1, 1959.

Coccidioidomycosis

H. E. EINSTEIN, M.D.

PRIMARY PNEUMONITIS

Simple bed rest is all that is needed for the majority of patients, with early return to normal activity when symptoms subside and x-rays stabilize. Most children can be expected to be back in school or at play within a period of two to four weeks. The occasional pulmonary cavitary residual may require surgical removal if it bleeds or becomes secondarily infected, or when rupture into the pleural cavity with empyema formation occurs. Cavities that persist for over a year, if more than 2 cm. in size or if enlarging, are usually resected electively to prevent the above-mentioned problems.

PROGRESSIVE PRIMARY PNEUMONITIS

This form of disease, which still is nondisseminated, is characterized by delayed clearing of the infiltrate or effusion, or persistent hilar adenopathy; this is usually accompanied by a complement fixation antibody titer of 1:64 dilution or above. It is seen particularly in infants and non-Caucasians. A course of amphotericin B, usually 0.5 to 1 Gm. total dose, is indicated to hasten recovery and prevent dissemination.

DISSEMINATED DISEASE

Metapulmonary lesions must be treated with amphotericin B systemically and, whenever feasible, locally. This includes skin, bone and joints, lymph nodes and serous membranes, and the affected structures in visceral and meningeal disease. The total dosage varies from 0.5 Gm. to a total dose of 3 Gm., depending on the extent of involvement and the age of the child. The drug is given intravenously daily or every other day in a concentration of 0.1 mg. per ml. in 5 per cent dextrose in water. The initial dose is 0.25 mg. per kilogram of body weight and is increased to the usual daily dose of 1 mg. per kilogram within one week.

Renal damage is invariably present and dose related. Weekly creatinine clearance values are the most reliable monitors of this complication. Hypokalemia is a usual concomitant and potassium supplementation is mandatory. Nausea, vomiting, chills and general malaise are seen in varying degrees in all patients and are treated symptomatically. Hypochromic anemia is frequently present but rarely requires treatment. Occasionally, corticosteroids are required to suppress the toxicity of the disease or drug.

Local Treatment. Amphotericin is very active locally and should be used in conjunction with systemic therapy whenever possible. This includes injection into serous cavities, joints and draining sinuses, and skin application in lotion or ointment form. Coccidioidal osteomyelitis is treated by surgical débridement, followed by drip infusion and drainage of the involved bone or joint. (Injection into serous cavities, joints, and draining sinuses is considered investigational.)

Meningitis presents a special difficult case. The patient initially requires local therapy, given every other day, along with intravenous therapy. This is given intrathecally (investigational), preferably in the cisterna magna. Dosage usually ranges from 0.1 to 0.5 mg. of amphotericin per injection. Long-acting corticoids, such as Depo-Medrol, are usually administered in the same injection to decrease the reaction. This treatment is continued until cell count diminishes, at which time the treatment interval can be lengthened; however, long-term suppressive treatment must be continued in this disease, which is frequently marked by relapse. An intraventricular silicone reservoir (Ommaya) may be implanted in one of the lateral ventricles, or preferably into the cisterna magna, as a secondary form of treatment if intracisternal punctures are not feasible.

PREVENTION

Prevention of coccidioidal infection is impossible in the endemic area. Attempts at environmental control to avoid unnecessary exposure to dust, and soil treatment against dust have been attempted with varying degrees of success. An active vaccination program, hopefully, will be available soon; an effective vaccine has been developed and is awaiting clearance for field trials.

Reference

Einstein, H. E.: Coccidioidomycosis; in H. A. Buechner (ed.): Management of Fungus Diseases of the Lungs. Springfield, Illinois, Charles C Thomas, Publisher, 1971.

Visceral Larva Migrans

C. H. MOK, M.B.B.S., D.C.H.

Visceral larva migrans, occurring mainly in young children, is characterized not only by chronic eosinophilia, hepatomegaly and hyperglobulinemia, but at times also by involvement of the eye and other organs. It is the result of larval migration in the tissues. The most common roundworms of dogs and cats, *Toxocara canis* and *Toxocara cati,* distributed widely throughout the world, appear to be the most frequent cause. Puppies and nursing bitches are the most infectious. Generally the course is benign but prolonged, although a few affected children have died.

There is no effective specific treatment. Mild cases require no therapy. Moderately severe ones may need supportive measures. In very severe cases, particularly patients with extensive pneumonitis, myocarditis or encephalitis, the anti-inflammatory effect of adrenocorticosteroid may prove lifesaving.

Diethylcarbamazine (12 mg. per kilogram of body weight per day orally in divided doses for 21 days), though not demonstrably affecting the eosinophilia, may improve other manifestations, such as fever, malaise, anemia, cough and hepatomegaly.

Thiabendazole (25 mg. per kilogram body weight twice daily orally for two days), a broad-spectrum anthelminthic with larvicidal effect, gives satisfactory and prompt symptomatic relief. It is usually well tolerated in children.

Side effects—anorexia, nausea, vomiting and dizziness—if they occur, are usually transitory and mild.

Preventive measures are of great importance. Regular deworming with piperazine is recommended for puppies, nursing bitches, all other dogs, kittens and cats. Children should be discouraged from handling any animal which might be carrying Toxocara eggs, and hands must be washed after handling. Puppies that are not house-trained and nursing bitches should not be allowed indoors because of the possibility of contaminating furnishings. Careful collection and disposal of excreta from suspected animals may prevent contamination of soil, lawns and gardens.

Attempts should be made to stop a child's pica habit, which is often associated with helminthic infection and at times with behavior problems, anemia and lead poisoning. The mother's cooperation is essential.

Trichuriasis

Whipworm

FRANK E. SMITH, M.D.

Heavily infected or hospitalized patients can be treated with hexylresorcinol. The agent is given orally as a single dose following an overnight fast. The drug should be swallowed promptly in order to minimize mucosal irritation, in the amount of 0.1 Gm. per year of age, the total dose not to exceed 1 Gm. for larger children or adults. A concomitant enema of 500 ml. of a 0.1 to 0.2 per cent solution of hexylresorcinol retained for 1 hour will supplement the oral program. A cleansing enema may be given in 4 hours. Repeat courses may be undertaken in four days. Systemic toxicity occurs infrequently, the major side effects of hexylresorcinol being local irritation of mucosal surfaces.

A secondary drug which "cures" one-third of patients treated is thiabendazole. This drug can be used for ambulatory patients in a dose of 25 mg. per kilogram orally, given after meals twice daily for two days. The toxic effects of thiabendazole are described elsewhere in this text.

Schistosomiasis

ALFRED W. SENFT, M.D., M.P.H.

Schistosomiasis is a general term which refers to infection by one of several species of flatworm intravascular parasites. Although nontransmissible in the United States, the disease is occasionally diagnosed in returning tourists, veterans or international agency personnel (or their families) who have had imprudent or accidental exposure to fresh waters harboring infected snails. On a worldwide basis, schistosomiasis probably accounts for the most widespread and persistent morbidity of any single disease known to man; about 8 per cent of the total world's population is currently affected. The disease is most often acquired in early childhood during wading, swimming or outdoor washing activities.

The therapy of schistosomiasis is presently not entirely satisfactory. There is considerable variation in drug response by the three common species *(S. mansoni, S. hematobium* and *S. japonicum),* with *S. japonicum* generally requiring more intensive or more prolonged drug administration. The classic method of treatment consists of intravascular or intramuscular injection of one of several kinds of trivalent antimony preparations. Although many formula variations are known, the most common drugs used are antimony potassium tartrate (tartar emetic) or antimony sodium gluconate (Triostam)* for intravenous use, and dimercaptosuccinate (Astiban) or the catechol disulfonate (Fuadin) forms of antimony for intramuscular treatment. Antimony has the capacity to bind to phosphofructokinase enzyme (PFK), thus compromising the ability of the worm to use glucose in the Embden-Meyerhof pathway. However, antimony toxicity in humans is severe in 1 to 5 per cent of cases treated. Nausea and vomiting are common, and dangerous myocardial fibrillation occurs periodically. In spite of its low chemotherapeutic–toxic ratio, antimony compounds are still widely used in Africa, Egypt and South America, since single or multiple courses of treatment are effective, even though dangerous. These antischistosome preparations, whether given intravenously or intramuscularly, have similar cumulative toxic manifestations which reflect the total quantity of antimony ion administered. Generally, a total adult therapeutic regimen given by any route and in various configurations consists of

* Triostam is not available in the United States.

about 400 to 800 mg. of antimony base. Intramuscular antimony is administered on alternate days until a total of 10 to 15 mg. of base per kilogram have been given.

Three newer drugs have had recent widespread trials. These are lucanthone, hycanthone and niridazole. Niridazole (Ambilhar) interferes with worm vitelline metabolism and ovarian function. In addition, it deranges the worm's glycogen storage and mobilization. The action of lucanthone and its hydroxylated analog, hycanthone, is thought to be primarily against the worm's gut and reproductive organs.

Niridazole is given orally (25 mg. per kilogram for seven days).† There follows a conversion into albumin-bound metabolites, which are slowly released in the urine and feces. During this phase the urine becomes dark in color and is unpleasantly malodorous. Niridazole administration is sometimes accompanied by electrocardiographic and electroencephalographic changes; occasionally mental confusion, schizophrenic behavior and convulsions occur. These seem to be related to the ability of the patient's liver to metabolize the parent compound. Therefore, although these toxic manifestations appear reversible, these hazards have limited the use of an otherwise fairly effective schistosomacidal agent.

Lucanthone (investigational) is also given orally (15 mg. per kilogram for seven days). It is bitter and causes some transient yellowish pigmentation of the skin and sclera. Its chief disadvantage is that it is quite toxic, with numerous symptoms: nausea, vomiting, vertigo, tremors and headache.

Hycanthone (Etrenol) is given intramuscularly in a dose of 3 ± 0.5 mg. per kilogram. There are many reports of cure following a single injection. However, sequential treatment of residual egg-positive cases may be required as a three- or six-month follow-up. Hycanthone dosage is often followed by headache, vertigo, anorexia and diarrhea. Generally these symptoms are mild. The most common adverse reaction is vomiting (up to 50 per cent of those treated). This reaction is usually moderately severe and of short duration and has, in general, not been a major deterrent in treatment. Hepatic toxicity has been reported in treated patients, principally those who have had severe liver deficiency or other concomitant hepatic disorders. Thus, hycanthone ought not to be used in a patient with a history of recent jaundice or known liver malfunction. Adverse reactions have recently been calculated to appear at a rate of about 1:20,000.

Hycanthone is currently under considerable scrutiny because of the appearance, in a schistosome laboratory strain, of drug fastness. In addition, selective bacteria and some mammalian cell lines have shown mutations in the presence of hycanthone. Thus, there has been hesitance to certify this drug for use in the United States. The available evidence, based on continuing in vitro studies and the experience with about 450,000 patients treated throughout the world, suggests that this drug is quite effective and acceptably safe for use in humans. One disadvantage of this drug is that it is not useful against *S. japonicum* infections.

Schistosome therapy is presently in a state of considerable ferment; it is likely that therapeutic procedures will be radically revised in the next two or three years. In view of the fact that these parasites have been found to salvage purines rather than synthesize the base, it appears that a number of purine analogs may be used to poison the parasite's nucleotide or proteosynthetic pathways. Therefore, certain analogs of adenosine which are customarily used for tumor therapy may be found to be useful antischistosome agents in the future.

† Niridazole (Ambilhar) is investigational in the United States. It is available from the Parasitic Disease Drug Service, Center for Disease Control, Atlanta, Georgia.

Filariasis

P. E. C. MANSON-BAHR

Diethylcarbamazine (Banocide, Hetrazan, Notezine) acts on microfilariae and is used when pathology is caused by microfilariae in onchocerciasis and tropical eosinophilia. Toxic effects are nil except in reactions caused by death of the parasites. Suramin* (Bayer 205, Moranyl) is used when filariasis is caused by the adult worms *Wuchereria bancrofti* (Bancroftian filariasis) and *Onchocerca volvulus* (onchocerciasis). It is, however, a particularly toxic drug in its effects on the kidney and has consequently fallen out of favor; if albumin appears in the urine during treatment, the drug must be stopped. Diethylcarbamazine also acts on adult *Loa loa* (loiasis), in which both microfilariae and adult worms are present.

BANCROFTIAN FILARIASIS

The ill effects of Bancroftian filariasis are caused by lymphatic obstruction and take many years to appear. They are very rare in children except in the Malayan form of filariasis. Microfilaria carriers do not need treatment if there

* Suramin is not commercially available in the United States. It may be obtained from the Parasitic Disease Drug Service, Atlanta, Georgia.

are no other symptoms. Diethylcarbamazine is given in doses of 6 mg. per kilogram in three divided doses daily for three weeks. This will cause the microfilariae to vanish from the blood, only to reappear six to nine months later. Repeated courses of the drug may have some effect on the adult worm. In developed cases of lymphedema with recurrent lymphangitis and filarial fever, there is some evidence that a course of Banocide will prevent the attacks. The affected limb must be elevated and bandaged to reduce the edema which must then be controlled by a permanent elastic stocking; this will also prevent further attacks. The adult worms are usually dead in the late stages of filariasis and therefore no antiadult treatment is necessary.

LOIASIS

Diethylcarbamazine acts on both the adult and larval forms of *loa loa.* The dosage is 6 mg. per kilogram daily in three divided doses for three weeks. If there is a heavy microfilaremia, a severe reaction may be expected with headache and encephalopathy. This can be prevented by starting with small doses, 12.5 to 25 mg. daily, and building up to the maximum dose. Repeated courses of therapy are not necessary.

ONCHOCERCIASIS

Onchocerciasis can affect children, though the later effects, such as blindness, take time to develop and do not occur during childhood. Diethylcarbamazine is given as 6 mg. per kilogram per day in three divided doses for three weeks. However, to avoid severe skin reactions caused by death of the microfilariae, this dosage should be reached in stages starting with a small daily dose of 25 mg., and increasing gradually over one week to the maximum dose. Skin reactions must be treated with antihistamines and, if severe, with steroids. If the eyes are involved, steroid drops should be placed in the eyes before starting treatment with diethylcarbamazine. Eye involvement is an indication for macrofilaricidal drugs, and suramin* may be given intravenously in doses of 1 Gm. weekly for five weeks. The dose should be reduced to the correct amount on a weight-for-age basis. The urine must be tested for albumin before each injection; if albuminuria occurs, the drug must be stopped. The skin should be cleared of microfilariae with a preliminary course of diethylcarbamazine.

If diethylcarbamazine is the only drug used, repeated courses will have to be given every nine months, up to eight or even nine in number. Signs of relapse to be looked for are a return of pruritus, and the reappearance of microfilariae in a skin snip. A good test for the presence of microfilariae in the skin is the Mazzotti reaction. Diethylcarbamazine is given in a single dose of 50 or 100 mg. and the patient is observed for 8 hours. If pruritus or a skin rash appears during this time, this is evidence that microfilariae are present in the skin. A negative test means that there are no microfilariae in the skin.

* See footnote, p. 670.

TROPICAL EOSINOPHILIA

Diethylcarbamazine has a curative effect in doses of 6 mg. per kilogram body weight in three divided doses daily for three weeks. The symptoms of asthma and the eosinophilia rapidly disappear, but there may be a recurrence six to nine months later when more microfilariae develop; however, this is uncommon. If there is a relapse, the course of diethylcarbamazine must be repeated.

DRACUNCULOSIS (GUINEA WORM)

A guinea worm may be extracted without breaking if a dose of metronidazole, 400 to 800 mg., is given 2 hours before extraction. The anti-inflammatory effect of the drug allows the worm to be wound up on a match stick and extracted painlessly. A dose of steroid has the same effect.

Leishmaniasis

P. E. C. MANSON-BAHR, M.D.

Pentavalent antimony† diamidine drugs and amphotericin B (Fungizone) are used in the treatment of all forms of leishmaniasis. Kala-azar is treated primarily with pentavalent antimony or urea stibamine, and with diamidine drugs or amphotericin B only if these drugs fail. Cutaneous leishmaniasis may be treated with pentavalent antimony, pyrimethamine (Daraprim) or cycloguanil pamoate (Camolar). Mucocutaneous leishmaniasis should be treated with amphotericin B if it fails to respond to treatment with antimony.

Children withstand *pentavalent antimony*† very well. Dosage for patients 5 to 15 years of age is 400 mg. per 4 ml. daily intramuscularly. Below the age of five, use 200 mg. per 2 ml. daily – never less than 200 mg. For Indian kala-azar give six daily injections for a total of 2.4 Gm. for children five to 15, and 1.2 Gm. for those below five. For kala-azar in all other parts of the world give 30 daily injections for a total of 12 Gm. for children five to 15, and 6 Gm. for those below five. The dosage for

† Pentavalent antimony is investigational in the United States.

patients above the age of 15 is 600 mg. per 6 ml. daily intramuscularly. For Indian kala-azar give six daily injections for a total of 3.6 Gm. For kala-azar in all other parts of the world give 30 daily injections for a total of 18 Gm. This regimen should cure 98 per cent of cases.

*Urea stibamine** (para-aminophenylstibinic acid) is given in a dosage of 125 mg. daily intravenously for children five to 15 years of age, and 65 mg. for those below five. Patients above the age of 15 should be given a dosage of 250 mg. Six doses are given for Indian kala-azar. In other parts of the world urea stibamine should be given in courses of 10 daily intravenous injections to a total of 2.5 Gm. for adults, 1.25 Gm. for the older children and 0.65 Gm. for those under five, which may be repeated twice.

The toxic effects of pentavalent antimony are much milder than for other forms of antimony. Very large doses (as much as 1.8 Gm. a day) have to be given. Nausea, abdominal pain and colic, anorexia and headache are the main toxic effects. These subside immediately on cessation of the drug, which is excreted quickly.

With respect to *diamidine drugs,* hydroxystilbamidine isethionate† is given when pentavalent antimony has failed. The dosage is 250 mg. daily intravenously for 10 days followed by 10 days of rest and repetition of the course up to a total of three courses or 30 injections totaling 7.5 Gm. Children under 15 should receive 125 mg. daily, and under five years, 65 mg. daily.

Hydroxystilbamidine isethionate causes a release of histamine and produces a decrease in blood pressure. This should be counteracted in all cases by the simultaneous administration of an antihistaminic: promethazine hydrochloride (Phenergan), 12 mg. orally three times a day. Children under 15 should receive half-doses, and under five, quarter doses.

Amphotericin B, initially 0.25 mg. per kilogram of body weight, is given daily, gradually increasing to 1 mg. per kilogram dissolved in 5 per cent dextrose to give a concentration not in excess of 0.1 mg. per milliliter of solution. This solution is infused intravenously over 3 to 6 hours every other day for three to eight weeks according to the reaction of the patient. Toxic and potentially dangerous reactions are frequent and include anorexia, headache, chills and fever. Antipyretics, such as aspirin, 650 mg. three times a day, or promethazine hydrochloride, 12 mg. three times a day orally, are given in conjunction with the medication. If these do not control the reactions, a steroid preparation, such as prednisone, 5 to 10 mg. three times a day, should be given orally. Albuminuria necessitates halting the drug.

Pyrimethamine, 25 mg. three times a day by mouth, may be given for seven days, and repeated twice if necessary. For children under 15, the dose should be 12.5 mg., and under five, 6.25 mg. Cycloguanil pamoate‡ may also be used as a repository drug in a single intramuscular injection of a suspension containing 140 mg. per ml. of dosage. For children under one year, give 1 ml.; for children between one and five years, give 2 ml.

* Urea stibamine is not available in the United States.

† Manufacturer's precaution: Children's dosage of 2-hydroxystilbamidine has not been established.

Malaria

RODNEY C. JUNG, M.D., PH.D.

The treatment of malaria may have one or more objectives: (1) termination of an attack (therapy in the narrow sense), (2) prevention of an attack without prevention of infection (suppression), (3) prevention of infection (prophylaxis), (4) prevention of relapse (radical cure) and (5) termination of the carrier state in falciparum malaria.

Therapy: Termination of an Attack. This requires a drug which will destroy the parasites infecting the erythrocytes. The two most effective drugs are amodiaquine (Camoquin) and chloroquine (Aralen). For nonimmune patients the manufacturer recommends a total dose of 25 mg. of base per kilogram of body weight administered in three days as follows: First dose: 10 mg. per kilogram (maximum, 600 mg. base). Second dose: 5 mg. per kilogram (maximum 300 mg. base) 6 hours after first dose. Third dose: 5 mg. per kilogram 18 hours after second dose. Fourth dose: 5 mg. per kilogram 24 hours after third dose. All doses are in terms of base. Amodiaquine is given in a dose of 100 mg. to children up to two years of age, 200 mg. for those two to five years old and 400 mg. for those five to 15 years old. The dose may be repeated daily on the two following days.

Persons with partial immunity require much smaller dosages.

If the patient is not able to take oral medication because of vomiting, a 5 per cent chloroquine solution is available for intramuscular

‡ Cycloguanil pamoate is not available in the United States.

administration. A single dose of this preparation should not exceed 5 mg. of base per kilogram of body weight, and the total dose over 24 hours should not exceed 10 mg. per kilogram of body weight (maximum of 800 mg.). Parenteral administration should be stopped and oral therapy instituted as soon as possible.

Chloroguanide (Paludrine) and pyrimethamine (Daraprim) are not recommended for treatment, especially in falciparum malaria, because their action is delayed. In the case of resistant malaria, quinine must be used.

Suppression: Prevention of Attack. As in therapy, the point of activity of the drug is against the blood stages of the parasites.

Amodiaquine and chloroquine are both effective. Chloroquine is given once weekly in accordance with the following schedule:

WEIGHT (*lb.*)	CHLOROQUINE *Base (mg.)*	PRIMAQUINE* *Base (mg.)*
10–15	20	3
16–25	40	6
26–35	60	9
36–45	80	12
46–55	100	15
56–100	150	22.5
over 100	300	45

Chloroguanide and pyrimethamine are preferred in some parts of the world, but there is a greater tendency for occurrence of strains of malaria resistant to these two drugs. Suppressive medication should be continued for one month after leaving the endemic zone.

Prophylaxis: Prevention of Infection. A prophylactic drug destroys exoerythrocytic parasites.

In falciparum malaria which is not resistant to chloroquine, suppression by the above method during residence in and continued for a month after departure from the endemic area prevents the blood infection.

If there is exposure to chloroquine-resistant falciparum malaria, some authorities believe that risk of infection may be partially reduced by ingestion once weekly of amodiaquine or chloroquine combined with primaquine. For dosage, see schedule above. Chloroquine, 300 mg. of base, combined with primaquine, 45 mg., in a single tablet is commercially available. Caution: Primaquine may cause hemolytic reactions in persons, especially Negroes, who have a glucose-6-phosphodehydrogenase defect. When exposure is in an area where chloroquine-resistant malaria does not occur, suppression may be expected to be effective and chemoprophylaxis is not necessary provided that therapy directed at *radical cure* is carried out after departure from the endemic area.

Radical Cure: Prevention of Relapse. To produce radical cure, not only must the blood infection be terminated but the exoerythrocytic parasites also must be eliminated. In the case of falciparum malaria, cure of the attack is the same as radical cure provided that there has been no exposure subsequent to the inoculation of the patent infection.

In other types of malaria it is necessary not only to treat the blood infection or attack in the manner previously described, but also to eliminate the exoerythrocytic forms by administration of primaquine. This is given in a dose of about 0.2 mg. *of base* per kilogram of body weight per day (maximum of 15 mg.) for 14 days.

Destruction of Gametocytes to Terminate the Carrier State. This is indicated only in falciparum malaria. Gametocytes in the other types of malaria perish with the other erythrocytic forms during treatment of the attack. Falciparum gametocytes may be destroyed by administration of primaquine in a single dose of 0.2 to 0.4 mg. of base per kilogram of body weight (maximal dose, 15 mg. in Negroes, 30 mg. in Caucasians). If falciparum gametocytes are the *only* form of parasites detectable, the patient does not have clinical malaria and the indication of treatment is public health rather than clinical.

Treatment of Resistant Falciparum Malaria. Patients who have falciparum malaria which has not responded to treatment with chloroquine or amodiaquine as previously described, who are from an area of chloroquine-resistant malaria or who have recrudescence following such treatment should be treated with quinine. If the patient is severely ill and there is no knowledge regarding the susceptibility of the strain to chloroquine, quinine should be administered as quinine sulfate. The daily dosage of quinine for children is approximately 25 mg. per kilogram of body weight divided into two or three equal parts administered at equal intervals for seven to 10 days.

Patients should be kept at bed rest during treatment. If oliguria occurs, the drug should be temporarily discontinued.

If the patient is unable to receive oral medication because he is comatose or vomiting, quinine may be given intravenously. This is definitely hazardous and should be done only if no other method of treatment is feasible. It is given as quinine dihydrochloride in 0.1 per cent solution in normal saline by slow intra-

* Manufacturer's precaution: Children's dose for primaquine has not been established.

venous drip, with continuous observation of blood pressure and pulse to detect adverse cardiovascular reaction. The dose is 10 mg. per kilogram over 2 hours and may be repeated in 8 hours if absolutely necessary. The total in 24 hours should not exceed 20 mg. per kilogram.

If the infection responds to quinine therapy but subsequently recrudesces, re-treatment with quinine is indicated with prolongation of the course to 21 days.

If asexual parasites persist in the blood during quinine therapy even though there may be a favorable clinical response, the patient should receive pyrimethamine for three days plus sulfadiazine concurrently with the quinine. Pyrimethamine may be given in a daily dose of 6 mg. for children less than one year old, 12.5 mg. for those one to seven and 25 mg. (adult dose) for those over seven.

Adequate hydration must be maintained during this treatment.

Chagas' Disease

RODNEY C. JUNG, M.D., PH.D.

No fully satisfactory treatment for Chagas' disease (infection with the American trypanosome *Trypanosoma cruzi*) has been developed.

Acute Chagas' disease is treated symptomatically. Heart failure due to Chagas' myocarditis is treated with diuretics and digitalis preparations as in other types of myocarditis. Digitalis is not highly effective.

To date no drug has been found to be active against the intracellular forms of the parasite, though several compounds destroy the blood forms. The presently available drugs therefore may be expected to be helpful only during the acute phase, if at all, when parasitemia is evident, and not in the chronic phase when circulating trypanosomes are very scarce.

The 8-aminoquinoline drugs, for example, including primaquine and isopentaquine, appear to ameliorate the course of acute Chagas' disease, but do not eradicate the infection.

Primaquine, the only one of these drugs which is commercially available in the United States, is given in a dosage of about 0.2 mg. of base per kilogram of body weight daily for 14 days. The maximal daily dose is 15 mg.* The most important untoward effect is hemolysis. This is particularly prone to occur in Negroes, in whom the drug therefore should not be used unless definitely indicated.

* Manufacturer's precaution: Children's dose of primaquine has not been established.

Bayer 2502, an investigational drug which appears to be more effective, and more toxic, is available under certain conditions from the Parasitic Disease Drug Service, National Center for Disease Control, Atlanta, Georgia.

In endemic areas, the most commonly seen forms of Chagas' disease are the chronic forms. These are mostly cases of chronic heart disease with conduction disturbances and are seen primarily in adults. Treatment is symptomatic.

In the case of other disorders due to destruction of autonomic ganglia seen in adults late in the course of the disease, the treatment, if any, may be surgical, as for correction of cardiac achalasia (megaesophagus) and acquired aganglionic megacolon. The muscular dysfunction in cardiac achalasia may be ameliorated by administration of nitrites such as those used for angina pectoris. Belladonna preparations may decrease discomfort but increase dilation.

Amebiasis

RODNEY C. JUNG, M.D., PH.D.

With regard to treatment, intestinal amebiasis must be regarded as two distinct diseases: nondysenteric amebiasis and dysenteric amebiasis.

A large number of drugs may be used effectively in the treatment of *nondysenteric* amebiasis. The most important of these are metronidazole (Flagyl), arsenicals, broad-spectrum antibiotics and iodized oxyquinolines.

Metronidazole appears to be the most effective amebicidal drug available. It is efficacious and safe with doses to adults of 500 to 750 mg. three times daily for five days. Dosage for children is 35 to 50 mg. per kilogram of body weight daily divided into three doses orally for 10 days.

Diiodohydroxyquinoline is usually effective in a dosage of about 30 mg. per kilogram daily for two to three weeks. Maximal dosage is 650 mg. three times daily.

Certain broad-spectrum antibiotics are also effective. With large doses or prolonged administration, these drugs cause gastrointestinal side effects, including diarrhea, often mistakenly thought to be due to the parasitic infection. Before accepting the routine use of broad-spectrum antibiotics, the physician should seriously consider the possibility that he may thereby encourage the development of antibiotic-resistant pathogenic bacteria in his community or institution.

Oxytetracycline, chlortetracycline and tetracycline, though relatively effective, tend to cause staining of the teeth in young children (to eight years of age) and hence are less desirable. The dosage is 20 to 30 mg. per kilogram of body weight per day divided into four equal doses. Maximal dosage is 250 mg. four times daily.

In *amebic dysentery* the physician's first objective is to relieve the dysentery. Eradication of the infection can come later. In severe cases supportive treatment, including bed rest and a bland diet, may be needed. Demulcent preparations are not particularly helpful, but opiates are valuable in relieving both pain and tenesmus. If fluid and blood losses have been great, these must be replaced.

Three types of drugs are highly effective in checking amebic dysentery: the broad-spectrum antibiotics, metronidazole and emetine. The dosage of metronidazole has already been given. Antibiotics may sometimes be effective in checking dysentery even when they do not eradicate the parasites. Tetracyclines, though effective, have the disadvantage previously mentioned. We have successfully terminated dysentery with erythromycin stearate in a dosage of 30 to 50 mg. per kilogram of body weight a day for five to seven days. Maximal daily dosage is 1 Gm.

Emetine hydrochloride is given hypodermically for three to five days in a dose of 1 mg. per kilogram of body weight per day, up to a maximal daily dosage of 60 mg. in older pediatric patients. Children over eight years of age should receive not more than 20 mg. daily, and those under eight should receive not more than 10 mg. daily. Usually it provides dramatic relief of dysentery, although it is not likely to eradicate the infection. Because of its toxic effects on the heart, it is advisable to keep the patient in bed during emetine therapy and for a day or two afterward. After dysentery has ceased, the remaining amebic infection may be treated as nondysenteric amebiasis.

Dehydroemetine (investigational), which is somewhat less toxic than emetine, though equally effective, is given in a dose of 1 to 1.5 mg. per kilogram of body weight daily for a similar period.

Amebic abscess of the liver may be treated with metronidazole or emetine hydrochloride or dehydroemetine (investigational) for 10 days in the dosages previously mentioned. Because of its high absorbability, metronidazole may be effective against hepatic amebiasis in a lower dosage than that necessary for intestinal amebiasis. With emetine, precautions must be observed because of toxicity to the heart. A safer but somewhat less effective drug than emetine is chloroquine diphosphate (Aralen). Although the pediatric dosage of chloroquine for treatment of amebic abscess has not been established in the United States, I have had success with a dosage of about 10 mg. per kilogram of body weight per day in two or three divided doses for two weeks. Since this drug is relatively more toxic to children than to adults, the daily dose should not exceed 500 mg., and the single dose should not exceed 250 mg.

Any of these drugs will fail at times. Cure rates may be improved by concurrent utilization of two or more of the agents. It has been reported that the concurrent administration of tetracycline with metronidazole will further improve response to treatment.

Reference

Rubidge, C. J., Scragg, J. N., and Powell, S. J.: Treatment of Children with Acute Amoebic Dysentery. Comparative Trial of Metronidazole Against a Combination of Dehydroemetine, Tetracycline, and Diloxanide furoate. *Arch. Dis. Child.*, 45:196, 1970.

Amebic Meningoencephalitis

D. H. H. PULLON, M.B., M.R.C.P., F.R.C.P.E., F.R.A.C.P., D.C.H.

At the time of writing, only three cases of amebic meningoencephalitis have been reported in the literature to have survived: one with *Acanthamoeba astronyxis* infection, and two given amphotericin B to kill amebae of the Naegleria group.

Should headache, vomiting and neck stiffness occur subsequent to bathing in a warm pool during the previous two weeks in an endemic area, no more than two or three ml. of cerebrospinal fluid is taken initially by the lumbar route. Because cerebral edema often develops rapidly in amebic meningoencephalitis, the specimen is taken slowly with a needle no larger than 21 gauge.

If convulsions or coma are present, cerebral edema is presumed if amebae are found, and a continuous intravenous drip infusion is started. Mannitol, 2 Gm. per kilogram as a 25 per cent solution is given with 10 per cent dextrose over 15 to 30 minutes.* This dose is repeated every 6 hours for six doses in the first instance, provided the blood urea is below 70 mg. per 100 ml. Besides attention to acid-base

* Manufacturer's precaution: Use of mannitol in pediatric patients has not been studied comprehensively.

balance and fluid intake, sodium and potassium supplements are necessary to keep pace with urinary output and electrolyte loss. Blood sugar and serum calcium and magnesium checks are performed.

Hypothermia to 30° C. is employed and the preservation of a clear airway and adequate respiratory function are required. Dexamethasone is not given, since it may combine with amphotericin B and so decrease the effectiveness of this drug in the tissues.

Diazepam† is given to control epileptiform convulsions. It is administered intravenously 1 mg. per minute, up to a total dose of 0.5 mg. per kilogram. The total daily dose is 0.8 mg. per kilogram divided into six equal doses. Phenobarbital is given concurrently in a parenteral dose of 4 mg. per kilogram up to a total of 8 mg. per kilogram for the first 24 hours, divided into four to six doses; thereafter, a total daily dose of 3 to 5 mg. per kilogram is given. As an alternative to diazepam, paraldehyde may be given intramuscularly, 0.15 ml. per kilogram per dose, repeated every 4 to 6 hours. Diphenylhydantoin sodium, (Dilantin) 5 mg. per kilogram per 24 hours intravenously every 6 hours, may be added to the anticonvulsant regimen. Chlorpromazine, 1 to 2 mg. per kilogram per 24 hours, given every 6 hours, may also be used to control restlessness and vomiting, but the patient should be kept normotensive. For patients over 40 kilograms, dosage is calculated on a surface area basis.

Amphotericin B is given intravenously in a dose of 1 mg. per kilogram per day. No work-up from a smaller dose is carried out, since many of the troublesome side effects are not seen because the patient is usually unconscious and because of the lethal nature of the condition. Instructions supplied with the drug are carefully followed. Daily infusions stabilized to a pH of 5.5 with buffer are given over a 6-hour period from a burette different from that used for other intravenous preparations. Renal toxicity is probably reversible with the modest total dose required.

Amphotericin B is given intrathecally (investigational) in a dose of 0.5 mg. twice weekly. Freshly made dilutions using sterile distilled water, with 0.25 mg. per ml., are used. Two ml. of this solution are diluted slowly repeatedly with 10 ml. of cerebrospinal fluid, and by injection of small volumes, the whole dose is given.

Amphotericin B is also given intraventricularly (investigational) in a dose of 0.1 mg. three times weekly and may be gradually increased to 0.5 mg. three times weekly. Premedication with an antiemetic, such as chlorpromazine in a dose of 1 to 2 mg. per kilogram intramuscularly, is given before each insertion.

Sulfadiazine in a dose of 150 mg. per kilogram per day as a continuous intravenous infusion is also given to kill Hartmannellid types of amebae.

The use of an Ommaya indwelling reservoir may be indicated in the future if intraventricular amphotericin B is required over several weeks, if there is difficulty in entering the cerebral ventricles or if intrathecal injections of amphotericin B are not tolerated. The use of surgical decompression for unresponsive cerebral edema is in the investigational stage.

In conclusion, amebic meningoencephalitis is so fulminant a condition that speed in applying therapy is essential for any chance of success.

† Manufacturer's precaution: Safety and efficacy of injectable diazepam in children have not been established.

References

Anderson, K.: Institute of Medical and Veterinary Science, Adelaide, Australia. Personal communication.

Carter, R. F.: Primary meningo-encephalitis. An appraisal of present knowledge. *Trans. Roy. Soc. Trop. Med. Hyg.*, 66:193, 1972.

Mandal, B. N., et al.: Acute Meningo-encephalitis due to amoebae of the order myxomycetale. *New Zeal. Med. J.*, 71:16, 1970.

Meyer, J. S., et al.: Treatment with glycerol of cerebral oedema due to acute cerebral infarction. *Lancet*, 2:993, 1971.

Balantidiasis

FRANK E. SMITH, M.D.

The decision for treatment of balantidiasis may be based on clinical grounds including: (1) dysenteric balantidiasis, (2) chronic balantidiasis associated with intermittent diarrhea, (3) balantidiasis associated with malnutrition or other serious disease and (4) proctoscopic visualization of mucosal ulcerations harboring the organism.

The treatment of choice is oxytetracycline* (Terramycin), 15 to 20 mg. per kilogram per day administered orally. The total daily dose is divided into four equal doses, and the regimen is continued over a course of seven to 10 days.

* Manufacturer's note: The use of tetracyclines during tooth development (last half of pregnancy, infancy and childhood to age eight years) may cause permanent discoloration of teeth. This adverse reaction is more common during long-term use of the drugs but has been observed following repeated short-term courses.

Hemorrhage, dehydration and shock may complicate the dysenteric form of balantidiasis and necessitate active measures of support, including fluid, electrolyte and blood replacement as individual situations dictate. Coincident infection with other bowel pathogens, e.g., Shigella organisms, not infrequently complicates balantidiasis and necessitates specific therapy as outlined elsewhere in this book.

Stools should be reexamined at the end of a course of treatment, and in older patients proctoscopic examination will verify healing of the characteristic ulcerations of the disease.

Giardiasis

FRANK E. SMITH, M.D.

Patients with symptomatic giardiasis, coincident malabsorption with or without diarrhea, hypogammaglobulinemia and simultaneous infection with other enteric pathogens are candidates for chemotherapy. In most instances a three-day course of quinacrine (Atabrine) eliminates the parasite from the stools. The drug is administered orally, three times a day, the total dose not to exceed 7 mg. per kilogram. For larger children and adults, a single dose should not exceed 100 mg. Stools may be checked for the parasite two weeks after treatment. Occasionally stools become negative after treatment, but symptomatic disease continues. In such situations, duodenal aspirates may affirm continued presence of *Giardia lamblia* and indicate re-treatment.

Complications of treatment with quinacrine include nausea, vomiting, abdominal cramps, drug fever and yellowing of the skin. The gastrointestinal symptoms may be minimized by giving the drug after meals with a glass of fruit juice.

An alternative treatment program preferred by many employs metronidazole (Flagyl).* The drug is administered orally in a dose of 250 mg. three times a day for 10 days in larger children and adults. For smaller children, 125 mg. three times a day for 10 days are taken. Side effects occur much less frequently compared to Atabrine, and most commonly are gastrointestinal with nausea being the most frequent. Occasionally, diarrhea, anorexia, abdominal cramps or epigastric distress may be seen. Dizziness, ataxia and vertigo occur extremely rarely and serious hematologic toxicity has not been appreciated, even though this compound is a nitroimidazole. The drug is contraindicated in patients with active neurologic disease or a history of blood dyscrasia. The former contraindication is based on experimental data from animals when the drug is given in substantial dosage and from limited information from human subjects suffering from overdoses much above the therapeutic range. The neurologic findings have been transient in observed patients.

* Manufacturer's precaution: Flagyl is considered investigational for the treatment of giardiasis.

Ascariasis

FRANK E. SMITH, M.D.

A two-day course of piperazine (Antepar) eliminates roundworms in 95 per cent of patients. Piperazine as tablet, syrup or wafer is given orally as a single dose of 75 mg. per kilogram per day for two days. Pretreatment purging is not necessary. Stools should be reexamined two to three weeks following treatment.

Piperazine is a well-tolerated and safe drug in therapeutic dosage, but transient side effects occur; they include nausea, vomiting, headache and abdominal cramps. Urticaria has been reported rarely, and when large doses are administered transient neurologic findings have been seen.

Mixed infections of ascaris, strongyloides and trichuris have been treated successfully with the broad-spectrum anthelmintic thiabendazole (Mintezol), although trichuris is less sensitive to this drug than are the other worms mentioned.

Enterobiasis

FRANK E. SMITH, M.D.

When the decision is made to treat infection caused by this ubiquitous organism, it is appropriate to include the family members of the patient in a simultaneous course of therapy to minimize reinfection.

Piperazine is administered orally in a single dose of 50 to 60 mg. per kilogram per day for five to seven days. This program eliminates the parasite in more than 90 per cent of subjects so treated. The side effects of piperazine are discussed under Ascariasis.

Pyrvinium pamoate (Povan) is a useful alternative agent in the treatment of enterobiasis. A single oral dose of 5 mg. per kilogram clears the stools of the organism in most cases, but a second dose given seven days later eliminates residual worms. Nausea, vomiting and staining of the teeth and undergarments by this red dye are not infrequent complications of treatment. Patients should be instructed not to chew the tablets and that the bright red stools are not cause for alarm.

A cellophane tape test seven days following treatment checks the efficacy of therapy.

Hookworm

HARRY MOST, M.D.

Hookworm infections in the United States are almost all due to *Necator americanus.* Occasionally an infection acquired abroad may be due to *Ancylostoma duodenale.*

Although the susceptibility of these species varies to some extent with the drug used, it is possible to reduce the intensity of infection or to eradicate hookworms and often other concomitant parasites, such as Ascaris, Strongyloides and pinworms, by the use of agents which affect more than one type. For Necator infections, tetrachloroethylene is preferred. The demand for this drug is so slight that it is not generally available for human use. Clinics which treat significant numbers of patients who have hookworm infections frequently have the drug put up in gelatin capsules which are then made available to the patients; otherwise it may be necessary to prescribe a veterinary preparation, which is perfectly satisfactory and safe since it contains U.S.P. tetrachloroethylene.

The drug is administered in the fasting state without prior dietary preparation and without purgation. The dose is 0.10 to 0.12 ml. per kilogram of body weight (maximum dose 5 ml.). The drug is usually available in 0.5- and 1-ml. soft gelatin capsules. For children too young to take capsules, the requisite amount of drug may be removed from the capsule by syringe and given by mouth with any appropriate diluent. Tetrachloroethylene may produce central nervous system stimulation or depression, and it is desirable to keep the patient in bed for several hours during and after treatment. A light breakfast may be given within 2 hours after the drug has been administered, but should not be followed by purgation.

Although treatment may not be curative following a single course of drug, the chances for cure are enhanced if tetrachloroethylene is given together with bephenium (Alcopara) on three successive mornings. The usual dose of bephenium is 5 Gm. for a 12-year-old child, to which 2 ml. of tetrachloroethylene may be added.

In multiple infections or when tetrachloroethylene is not readily available, thiabendazole is preferred. It also rids the host of most of the Ascaris worms and all the Strongyloides and pinworms if they too are present.

Angiostrongyliasis

DONALD F. B. CHAR, M.D. *and*
LEON ROSEN, M.D.

Two species of the metastrongylid genus Angiostrongylus are known to cause disease in man. The first to be recognized as a human pathogen, *Angiostrongylus cantonensis,* is responsible for cerebral angiostrongyliasis (also known as eosinophilic meningitis or meningoencephalitis); the second, *Angiostrongylus costaricensis,* is responsible for abdominal angiostrongyliasis.

It is generally accepted that most cases of eosinophilic meningitis are caused by *A. cantonensis,* a lungworm of rats, although the parasite has only rarely been recovered from the brain or spinal fluid of patients. It should be recognized, however, that a similar syndrome may be caused by other agents. In older children and adults the clinical picture of cerebral angiostrongyliasis is characterized by headache, paresthesias and variable degrees of nuchal rigidity. Cranial nerve palsies and low-grade fever occur in a minority of cases. Younger children and infants are apt to show irritability and higher fever, and these signs can persist for several weeks. Although the prognosis generally is good, a few deaths have been recorded. The diagnosis can be established only by appropriate staining of the spinal fluid sediment to reveal the eosinophils.

Once the diagnosis has been established, little can be done except to await recovery. Treatment is largely supportive and symptomatic. The diagnostic spinal tap often relieves headache. Aspirin and other analgesic agents are useful for fever and headache. In more severe cases, in which signs of cerebral edema may be prominent, corticosteroids, or the osmotic brain-dehydrating agents, such as urea or mannitol,* may be cautiously employed. Respiratory supportive measures, such as tracheostomy or artificial respiration, may be necessary if signs of brainstem compression ap-

* Manufacturer's precaution: Use of mannitol in pediatric patients has not been studied comprehensively.

pear. Recovery is characteristically slow, but usually complete.

Although thiabendazole, a broad-spectrum anthelmintic, affects the development of *A. cantonensis* in rats, its use against the parasite in man has not been reported and there is doubt as to the rationality of such use. It is suspected that the deleterious effects of *A. cantonensis* infection in humans are largely the result of reaction to dead or dying worms, and that not all parasites in a given patient die simultaneously. Consequently, if this view is correct, and if thiabendazole killed all the parasites at one time, treatment with the drug might do more harm than good.

A. costaricensis has an entirely different habitat from that of *A. cantonensis,* both in its normal rodent hosts and in man. In the latter, it produces pathologic lesions in the appendix and adjacent intestine and lymph nodes, consisting of granulomatous inflammation with intense eosinophil infiltration. Clinically, the human disease is characterized by pain in the right iliac fossa, or occasionally elsewhere in the abdomen, prolonged fever, anorexia and vomiting. Physical examination reveals the presence of an intra-abdominal mass which can be confused with malignant tumors or bacterial abscesses. Leukocytosis and eosinophilia (usually more than 10 per cent) are present, as well as radiologic evidence of intestinal pathology such as difficulty in filling, spasticity and irritability. Diagnosis can be established only by the examination of surgical specimens, since larvae of the parasites have not been found in the feces of patients. Treatment also is surgical.

Tapeworm

HARRY MOST, M.D.

The three most common tapeworms in the United States in order of their frequency in children are *Hymenolepis nana* (the dwarf tapeworm), *Taenia saginata* (the beef tapeworm) and *Diphyllobothrium latum* (the fish tapeworm). The beef tapeworm is usually detected when segments have been passed in the stool. Segments may also be passed and identified in infections with the other tapeworms, but in addition the diagnosis can be made by stool examination.

The drug of choice for all three intestinal tapeworms of man is quinacrine hydrochloride (Atabrine). The proper use of this drug requires adherence to a very low residue or preferably liquid diet on the day before treatment. A mild laxative such as milk of magnesia is prescribed in the evening, and later a soapsuds enema may be given to clean out the large intestine and to facilitate the search for the tapeworm scolex. The drug is administered in a fasting state in three divided doses at 20- to 30-minute intervals. The total dose for children is 0.4 Gm. for those weighing 18 to 34 kilograms, 0.6 Gm. for those weighing 35 to 45 kilograms, and 0.8 Gm. for those weighing more than 46 kilograms.

The drug may produce nausea and vomiting. If there is a history of emotional disturbance, Atabrine should not be used because instances of psychosis in such patients have been observed following its use. Nausea and vomiting may be prevented or minimized by the administration of each dose with an ounce of orange juice and with the administration of an antiemetic such as chlorpromazine† 30 minutes before treatment is initiated. If severe vomiting occurs in spite of these measures, treatment may subsequently be given successfully by the administration of the full amount of Atabrine in solution given through a duodenal tube. A saline purgative is usually given 2 hours after oral treatment, and in the case of duodenal treatment it may be administered with the Atabrine at the same time through the tube.

If the scolex is not found after treatment, re-treatment should not be considered for six to 12 weeks, during which segments or positive stool findings would indicate failure.

Yomesan, if approved by the Food and Drug Administration, is the preferred drug for all tapeworms. It is currently available only through the Center for Disease Control, U.S. Public Health Service, Atlanta, Georgia.

Alternative Drugs for Selected Parasitic Infections

SHIRLEY L. FANNIN, M.D.

The following table is presented for two reasons: (1) to list drugs which could be used if the treatment of a disease discussed in the text (indicated by*) is not desirable for a given patient and (2) to add treatments for conditions not described in the text.

† Manufacturer's precaution: Chlorpromazine is not recommended for children under six months of age except when lifesaving.

TABLE 1. Alternative Drugs for Parasitic Infections

ORGANISM	DRUG AND STRENGTHS	UNDER 15 LB.	15 TO 30 LB.	30 TO 60 LB.	60 LB. AND OVER
PROTOZOA					
**Giardia lambia*	Metronidazole (Flagyl)[13]—tablets: 250 mg.	25 mg. t.i.d. for 10 days	50 mg. t.i.d. for 10 days	125 mg. t.i.d. for 10 days	250 mg. t.i.d. for 10 days
**Balantidium coli*	Diiodohydroxyquin (Diodoquin, Moebiquin)—tablets: 210, 650 mg.	Not recommended	162 mg. t.i.d. for 20 days	325 mg. t.i.d. for 20 days	650 mg. t.i.d. for 20 days
AMOEBA					
**Entamoeba histolytica*	Carbarsone (*p*-carbamidobenzine arsonic acid)—tablets: 250 mg.	Not recommended	Not recommended	250 mg. b.i.d. for 7 days	250 mg. t.i.d. for 3 weeks
	Bismuth glycolyl arsanilate[8]—tablets: 500 mg.	Not recommended	Not recommended	250 mg. t.i.d. orally before meals for 8 days	500 mg. t.i.d. orally for 8 days before meals
	Paromomycin (Humatin)—capsules: 250 mg.; syrup: 25 mg./ml.	25 mg./kg. orally daily for 5 days	25 mg./kg. orally daily for 5 days	25 mg./kg. orally daily for 5 days	25 mg./kg. orally daily for 5 days
	Dehydroemetine[1]—ampules: 30 mg./ml.	Not recommended	1.5 mg./kg. I.M. daily for 6–10 days	1.5 mg./kg. I.M. daily for 6–10 days	1.5 mg./kg. I.M. daily for 6–10 days
NEMATODES, ROUNDWORMS					
**Ascaris lumbricoides* (roundworm)	Hexylresorcinol[2] (Crystoids)—capsules: 100 and 200 mg.	Not recommended	200 mg. single dose	500 mg. single dose	1 Gm. single dose
**Trichuris trichiura*	Hexylresorcinol (S.T.-37)—0.1%	62.5 ml. of 0.1% solution by rectal retention for 1 hr.	125 ml. of 0.1% solution by rectal retention for 1 hr.	250 ml. of 0.1% solution by rectal retention for 1 hr.	500 ml. of 0.1% solution by rectal retention for 1 hr.
	Stilbazium (Monopar)	Not recommended	Not recommended	50 mg./kg. single dose for 3 days	50 mg./kg. single dose for 3 days
	Thiabendazole (Mintezol)—suspension: 100 mg./ml.	25 mg./kg./day for 2–4 weeks	25 mg./kg./day for 2–4 weeks	25 mg./kg./day for 2–4 weeks	25 mg./kg./day for 2–4 weeks
Strongyloides stercoralis (threadworm)	Thiabendazole (Mintezol)—suspension: 100 mg./ml.	25 mg./kg. b.i.d. for 2 days	25 mg./kg. b.i.d. for 2 days	25 mg./kg. b.i.d. for 2 days	25 mg./kg. b.i.d. for 2 days
	Pyrvinium pamoate[3] (Povan)—syrup: 100 mg./ml.; tablets: 50 mg.	A daily dose of 5 mg./kg. (maximum of 31 mg.) for 4 days	A daily dose of 5 mg./kg. (maximum 62.5 mg.) for 4 days	A daily dose of 5 mg./kg. (maximum 125 mg.) for 4 days	A daily dose of 5 mg./kg. (maximum 250 mg.) for 4 days
	Stilbazium (Monopar)	Not recommended	Not recommended	500 mg. oral single dose	1 Gm. oral single dose

TABLE 1. Alternative Drugs for Parasitic Infections—*Continued*

ORGANISM	DRUG AND STRENGTHS	UNDER 15 LB.	15 TO 30 LB.	30 TO 60 LB.	60 LB. AND OVER
Necator americanus (hookworm)	Hexylresorcinol (Crystoids) —capsules: 100 and 200 mg.	Not recommended	200 mg. single dose	500 mg. single dose	1 Gm. single dose
Ancylostoma duodenale (hookworm)	Triclofenol piperazine 5% solution in polyethylene glycol	Not recommended	Not recommended	25 mg./kg. b.i.d. for 2 days	25 mg./kg. b.i.d. for 2 days
Enterobius vermicularis (pinworm)	Stilbazium (Monopar)	Not recommended	Not recommended	10 mg./kg. in single dose orally	10 mg./kg. in single dose orally
CESTODES, TAPEWORMS **Taenia saginata, Taenia solium, Diphyllobothrium latum*	Niclosamide[1] (Yomesan) — tablets: 500 mg.	A single dose of 250 mg. after a light breakfast	A single dose of 500 mg. after a light breakfast	A single dose of 1 Gm. after a light breakfast	A single dose of 2 Gm. after a light breakfast
	Dichlorophen[1] (anthiphen)— tablets: 500 mg.	Not recommended	Not recommended	70 mg./kg. divided in 3 doses in 24 hours	70 mg./kg. divided in 3 doses in 24 hours
Hymenolepis nana	Hexylresorcinol[2] (Crystoids) —capsules: 100 and 200 mg.	Not recommended	200 mg. single dose	500 mg. single dose	1 Gm. single dose
	Niclosamide[1] (Yomesan) — tablets: 500 mg.	A single dose of 250 mg. after a light breakfast	A single dose of 500 mg. after a light breakfast	A single dose of 1 Gm. after a light breakfast	A single dose of 2 Gm. after a light breakfast
FLUKES					
**Schistosoma mansoni*	Stibophen[4] (Fuadin) — ampules: 5 ml.	Not recommended	1 ml. daily I.M. 5 days per week for 4 weeks, to total of 20 ml.	2 ml. daily I.M. 5 days per week for 4 weeks, to total of 40 ml.	4 ml. daily I.M. 5 days per week for 4 weeks, to total of 80 ml.
	Sodium antimony dimercaptosuccinate (Astiban)[1,4] —vial, powder: 500 mg.	Not recommended	Total dose of 34 mg./kg. (maximum 500 mg.) given I.M. in divided doses in 5–7 days	Total dose of 34 mg./kg. (maximum 1 Gm.) given I.M. in divided doses in 5–7 days	Total dose of 34 mg./kg. (maximum 2 Gm.) given I.M. in divided doses in 5–7 days
	Niridazole[1,5] (Ambilhar) — tablets: 500 mg.	Not recommended	25 mg./kg./day orally for 5–10 days	25 mg./kg./day orally for 5–10 days	25 mg./kg./day orally for 5–10 days
**Schistosoma japonicum, Schistosoma hematobium*	Potassium antimony tartrate[6]	Not recommended	I.V. doses of 2, 3, 4, 5, 6 and 7 ml. on alternate days, continuing at 7 ml. on alternate days for 10 doses (total of 90 ml.)	I.V. doses of 4, 6, 8, 10, 12 and 14 ml. on alternate days, continuing at 14 ml. on alternate days for 10 doses (total of 180 ml.)	I.V. doses of 8, 12, 16, 20, 24 and 28 ml. on alternate days, continuing at 28 ml. on alternate days for 10 doses (total of 360 ml.)

TABLE 1. Alternative Drugs for Parasitic Infections—*Continued*

ORGANISM	DRUG AND STRENGTHS	UNDER 15 LB.	15 TO 30 LB.	30 TO 60 LB.	60 LB. AND OVER
	Stibophen[4] (Fuadin) — ampules: 5 ml.	Not recommended	1 ml. daily I.M. 5 days per week for 4 weeks, to total of 20 ml.	2 ml. daily I.M. 5 days per week for 4 weeks, to total of 40 ml.	4 ml. daily I.M. 5 days per week for 4 weeks, to total of 80 ml.
Clonorchis sinensis (liver fluke)	Chloroquine phosphate[7] (Aralen)—tablets: 125 and 250 mg.	Not recommended	Not recommended	125 mg. t.i.d. for 6 weeks	250 mg. t.i.d. for 6 weeks
Paragonimus westermani (lung fluke), *Fasciola hepatica* (sheep liver fluke)	Bithionol[8]	Not recommended	Not recommended	50 mg./kg. on alternate days for 15 days	50 mg./kg. on alternate days for 15 days
FILARIA					
Wucheria bancrofti	Suramin sodium[1, 9] (Antrypol)—ampules: 1.5 Gm.	25 mg. (test dose) I.V., then 125 mg. weekly for 5–10 doses	50 mg. (test dose) I.V., then 250 mg. weekly for 5–10 doses	100 mg. (test dose) I.V., then 500 mg. weekly for 5–10 doses	200 mg. (test dose) I.V., then 1 Gm. weekly for 5–10 doses
	Mel W (Trimelarsen)[8]	Not recommended	37.5 mg. I.M. daily for 4 days	75 mg. I.M. daily for 4 days	150 mg. I.M. daily for 4 days
	M Sb B (Sb analog of Melarsen)	Not recommended	75 mg. t.i.d. for 7 days	150 mg. t.i.d. for 7 days	300 mg. t.i.d. for 7 days
*LEISHMANIA *Leishmania braziliensis* *Leishmania tropica* (cutaneous leishmaniasis)	Glucantime (*N*-methylglucamine antimonate)	Not recommended	100 mg./kg./day for 15–20 days	100 mg./kg./day for 15–20 days	100 mg./kg./day for 15–20 doses
	Ethylstibamine (Neostibosan)—ampules: 50, 100 and 300 mg.	25 mg. I.V., then 37.5 mg. I.V. daily or every 2 days for 16 doses	50 mg. I.V., then 75 mg. I.V. daily or every 2 days for 16 doses	100 mg. I.V., then 150 mg. I.V. daily or every 2 days for 16 doses	200 mg. I.V., then 300 mg. I.V. daily or every 2 days for 16 doses
Leishmania donovani	Ethylstibamine (Neostibosan)—ampules: 50, 100 and 300 mg.	25 mg. I.V., then 37.5 mg. I.V. daily or every 2 days for 16 doses	50 mg. I.V., then 75 mg. I.V. daily or every 2 days for 16 doses	100 mg. I.V., then 150 mg. I.V. daily or every 2 days for 16 doses	200 mg. I.V., then 300 mg. I.V. daily or every 2 days for 16 doses
TRYPANOSOMES African trypanosomiasis[10] (early)	Pentamidine[1] (Lomidine)—ampules (3 ml.): 40 mg./ml.	4 mg./kg. I.M. every 1 to 2 days for 10 doses	4 mg./kg. I.M. every 1 to 2 days for 10 doses	4 mg./kg. I.M. every 1 to 2 days for 10 doses	4 mg./kg. I.M. every 1 to 2 days for 10 doses
	Suramin sodium[1, 9] (Antrypol)—ampules: 1.5 Gm.	25 mg. (test dose) I.V., then 125 mg. weekly for 5 to 10 doses	50 mg. (test dose) I.V., then 250 mg. weekly for 5 to 10 doses	100 mg. (test dose) I.V., then 500 mg. weekly for 5 to 10 doses	200 mg. (test dose) I.V., then 1 Gm. weekly for 5 to 10 doses

ORGANISM	DRUG AND STRENGTHS	UNDER 15 LB.	15 TO 30 LB.	30 TO 60 LB.	60 LB. AND OVER
(late disease with CNS involvement)	Melarsoprol[1, 11] (Arsobal)	10 mg. I.V. daily for 3 doses; after 1-week interval, 3 doses, increasing to 20 mg.; after 1-week interval, 20 mg. daily for 3 doses	20 mg. I.V. daily for 3 doses; after 1-week interval, 3 doses, increasing to 40 mg.; after 1-week interval, 40 mg. daily for 3 doses	45 mg. I.V. daily for 3 doses; after 1-week interval, 3 doses, increasing to 90 mg.; after 1-week interval, 90 mg. daily for 3 doses	90 mg. I.V. daily for 3 doses; after 1-week interval, 3 doses, increasing to 180 mg.; after 1-week interval, 180 mg. for 3 doses
	Suramin sodium[1, 9] (Antrypol—ampules: 1.5 Gm.	25 mg. (test dose) I.V., then 125 mg. weekly for 5 to 10 doses	50 mg. (test dose) I.V., then 250 mg. weekly for 5 to 10 doses	100 mg. (test dose) I.V., then 500 mg. weekly for 5 to 10 doses	200 mg. (test dose) I.V., then 1 Gm. weekly for 5 to 10 doses
	followed by Tryparsamide[12]	250 mg. I.V. every 5 to 7 days for 10 to 20 doses as required	500 mg. I.V. every 5 to 7 days for 10 to 20 doses as required	1 Gm. I.V. every 5 to 7 days for 10 to 20 doses as required	2 Gm. I.V. every 5 to 7 days 10 to 20 doses as required
(chemoprophylaxis)	Pentamidine[1] (Lomidine)—ampules (3 ml.): 40 mg./ml.	3 mg./kg. I.M. every 3 to 6 months	3 mg./kg. I.M. every 3 to 6 months	3 mg./kg. I.M. every 3 to 6 months	3 mg./kg. I.M. every 3 to 6 months
	Suramin sodium[1, 9] (Antrypol)—ampule: 1.5 Gm.	37 to 87 mg. I.V. or I.M. every 2 to 3 months	75 to 175 mg. I.V. or I.M. every 2 to 3 months	150 to 350 mg. I.V. or I.M. every 2 to 3 months	300 to 700 mg. I.V. or I.M. every 2 to 3 months

* See text for treatment of choice.

[1] Not available for clinical use in the United States. Must be obtained as an investigational drug from Parasitic Disease, Service, Center For Disease Control, United States Public Health Service, Atlanta, Georgia 30333.

[2] Hexylresorcinol should be given on an empty stomach and should be followed in 2 to 4 hours with a purge of magnesium sulfate. Hexylresorcinol is contraindicated in patients with peptic ulcer. The drug should not be chewed because it is caustic and may produce burns in the mucous membranes of the mouth.

[3] Pyrvinium pamoate may cause nausea and vomiting; it turns the stool red.

[4] Stibophen and sodium antimony dimercaptosuccinate are contraindicated in renal and cardiac disease, and in hepatic disease not caused by schistosomiasis (but note that Schistosoma infections usually cause hepatic disease). Either drug should be stopped in the event of recurrent vomiting, progressive albuminuria (urine tested weekly), severe persistent joint pain, purpura or intercurrent febrile infection. Sodium antimony dimercaptosuccinate may cause a toxic dermatitis, usually not severe enough to compel discontinuance.

[5] Niridazole is available through Ciba in Switzerland.

[6] Potassium antimony tartrate should be given slowly intravenously, since it may produce a hacking cough, vomiting and severe or fatal reactions if given rapidly.

[7] Chloroquine usually does not cure, but produces temporary suppression of ova. Chloroquine may cause nausea and vomiting, nervousness, insomnia, headache, and blurring of vision, but evidently not irreversible eye changes such as occur in long-term use. It rarely causes leukopenia and other blood dyscrasias.

[8] Investigational in the United States.

[9] Suramin sodium may cause renal irritation and agranulocytosis.

[10] Rhodesian trypanosomiasis should be treated with both suramin sodium and melarsoprol, since CNS invasion occurs very rapidly. This is the standard procedure recommended by the East African Trypanosomiasis Research Unit for every case except when infection is known to have occurred within the past three to four weeks.

[11] Melarsoprol may cause myocardial damage, albuminuria, hypertension, neuritis and colic. Fatalities have been reported. In frail patients, begin with as little as 1/5 of the recommended dose and increase the dose progressively.

[12] Tryparsamide should be used under investigational conditions. It may cause impaired vision (usually temporary if the drug is stopped) and optic atrophy. Careful observation of the eyes, especially the visual fields, is indicated.

[13] Metronidazole (Flagyl) is considered investigational for the treatment of giardiasis.

Toxoplasmosis

B. H. KEAN, M.D.

Toxoplasmosis is now recognized as one of the most prevalent diseases; approximately one-half billion humans are infected. One of every thousand infants in the United States is born with a congenital infection, and one-third of these are damaged. In almost any age group the percentage of infection is numerically related to age. At 5 years, the prevalence is somewhat less than 5 per cent; at age 20, the prevalence is 20 per cent; of 5000 women with a mean age of 27, 33 per cent were infected (Kimball et al.).

Although it has been known that many infections are acquired by the ingestion of raw or poorly cooked meat, the recent discovery that *Toxoplasma gondii* is a coccidian with its definitive cycle in the cat has eliminated much of the mystery about the acquisition of the parasite (Hutchison and Dunachie, Frenkel). The precise role played by the cat and cat feces in the dissemination of the infection to humans remains to be elucidated.

No drug or combination of drugs cures toxoplasmosis; but, in certain stages, the course of the disease can be modified by therapy.

CONGENITAL TOXOPLASMOSIS

A mother infected *before* pregnancy does not transmit the disease. Only if the infection is acquired by the mother during pregnancy is congenital toxoplasmosis possible.

Asymptomatic. The child is born with the mother's titer or higher. The titer does not fall rapidly, but no clinical abnormalities can be detected. IgM antibodies are an indicator of infection (Remington et al.). These infants probably should be treated. Asymptomatic toxoplasmosis must be distinguished from *"serologic" toxoplasmosis.* The infant is born with the same titer as that of the mother, but he is not infected. The infant's titer drops relatively rapidly at gradients of one half per month, and usually is negative in four months. Obviously, no treatment is needed.

Systemic Toxoplasmosis. Encephalitis with microcephalus or macrocephalus, cerebral calcification, retinochoroiditis, hepatitis, carditis, dermatitis and so forth, in various combinations and degrees, require vigorous repeated treatment even with dangerous drug regimens. Unfortunately, there has been little evidence that therapy of the severely damaged infant alters the prognosis.

Delayed (Latent) Toxoplasmosis. Unrecognized in infancy, evidence of the disease appears in early or late childhood. Treatment is probably useless but may be attempted in an effort to avoid further damage.

Retinochoroiditic Toxoplasmosis. Retinochoroiditic toxoplasmosis as the only evidence of the disease can appear or be recognized at any time from birth to middle adulthood. If the disease is inactive, the patient should be watched at regular intervals. Every exacerbation should be treated vigorously with specific antitoxoplasmic drugs and corticosteroids. Prophylactic treatment at regular intervals, e.g., once yearly, may be considered.

ACQUIRED TOXOPLASMOSIS

Acquired toxoplasmosis is generally less serious than the congenital form and usually requires no treatment.

Asymptomatic. Asymptomatic toxoplasmosis is recognized only by the presence of a positive titer. No treatment is needed.

Lymphadenitic Toxoplasmosis. Enlarged lymph nodes, especially the posterior cervical chain, fever, lassitude and rising titers characterize this type. The syndrome is often confused clinically with infectious mononucleosis. No controlled study data of the efficacy of drug therapy are available. In most of these children treatment is not needed since they recover spontaneously, albeit, on occasion, slowly (Kean).

Typhus-like Toxoplasmosis. This is a systemic infection with involvement of the central nervous system, lungs, heart, liver, skin and other organs. It may be caused by an especially virulent strain or represent some inability of the patient to handle a usually benign disease. Therapy must be vigorous and prompt.

Toxoplasmosis in the Immunodeficient Patient. This type occurs in patients with Hodgkin's disease, leukemia or disseminated malignancy under treatment with immunodepressant drugs. It may be reactivation of prior acquired or congenital disease, or it may represent a new infection. Despite the ultimate poor prognosis, these patients respond surprisingly well to treatment.

SPECIFIC THERAPY

Two drugs, pyrimethamine and sulfadiazine, used synergistically, are recommended for the treatment of toxoplasmosis (Eyles).

Pyrimethamine (Daraprim). A folic acid antagonist, this drug is an excellent antimalarial; in experimental toxoplasmosis in animals it prolongs life and may cure. Its use demands frequent, e.g., biweekly, monitoring of the peripheral blood, since its major toxic effects are bone-marrow suppression with thrombocytopenia, leukopenia and anemia. Folinic acid (Leucovorin) or yeast, or both, should be administered simultaneously. Folinic acid does not interfere with the antitoxoplasmic effect of pyrimethamine as may folic acid.

Sulfadiazine. Sulfadiazine (or triple sulfonamide) also has specific antitoxoplasmic effects and, incidentally, anti-malarial qualities.

Its capacity to suppress the proliferative phase of toxoplasmosis approximates that of pyrimethamine, but both have little or no effect on the chronic or cyst stage of the parasite.

The toxicity of the sulfonamides is too well known to require description here.

DRUG SYNERGISM. The simultaneous use of pyrimethamine and sulfadiazine is synergistic to a five- to ten-fold level, whereas toxicity is only modestly additive. For this reason, the two drugs are almost always given jointly.

Corticosteroids. In active toxoplasmic retinochoroiditis, corticosteroids are used with pyrimethamine and sulfadiazine. They may be useful also in the rare, acute typhus-like syndrome. In large doses, corticosteroids theoretically could exacerbate the disease.

Spiromycin (Rovamycine). An antibiotic, not available in the United States, Spiromycin is recommended by some French workers (2 Gm. daily in divided doses for six weeks). If patients exhibit hypersensitivity to pyrimethamine and sulfadiazine, an effort may be made to obtain the preparation.

Dose Schedules. *Pyrimethamine:* 1 mg. per kilogram daily for 21 to 30 days, administered once daily (maximum 25 mg. per day). If pyrimethamine cannot be administered orally, an intravenous form of pyrimethamine (isethionate)* may be obtained from Dr. George Hitchings, Burroughs Wellcome & Co. (telephone (919) 549-8371).

Sulfadiazine (or triple sulfonamide): 100 mg. per kilogram per day for 21 to 30 days administered as 25 mg. per kilogram four times daily (maximum 4 Gm. per day).

Folinic Acid (Leucovorin, citrovorum factor; also available as Calcium Leucovorin): 2 to 5 mg. intramuscularly three times weekly for three to six weeks. Five Gm. of baker's yeast daily should be given for a similar period.

The dose of all drugs is usually doubled for the first two days of treatment. In severe cases, when sight or life is threatened, drug dosage may be doubled and extended to six weeks.

* Manufacturer's precaution: The intravenous form of pyrimethamine is investigational.

References

Eyles, D. E.: An Evaluation of the Curative Effects of Pyrimethamine and Sulfadiazine, Alone and in Combination, on Experimental Mouse Toxoplasmosis. *Antibiot. and Chemother.*, 5:529–539, 1955.

Frenkel, J. K., Dubey, J. P., and Miller, N. L.: *Toxoplasma gondii* in Cats: Fecal Stages Identified as Coccidian Oocysts. *Science*, 167:893–896, 1970.

Hutchison, W. M., and Dunachie, J. F.: The Life Cycle of the Coccidian Parasite, *Toxoplasma gondii*, in the Domestic Cat. *Trans. Roy. Soc. Trop. Med. Hyg.*, 65:380–399, 1971.

Kean, B. H.: Clinical Toxoplasmosis—50 years. *Trans. Roy. Soc. Trop. Med. Hyg.*, 66:549–571, 1972.

Kimball, A. C., Kean, B. H., Fuchs, F.: Congenital Toxoplasmosis: A Prospective Study of 4048 Obstetric Patients. *Am. J. Obstet. Gynec.*, 111:211–218, 1971.

Remington, J. S., Miller, M. J., and Brownlee, I.: IgM Antibodies in Acute Toxoplasmosis: I. Diagnostic Significance in Congenital Cases and a Method for Their Rapid Demonstration. *Pediatrics*, 41:1082–1091, 1968.

Cholera

LAWRENCE S. C. GRIFFITH, M.D.

Therapeutic management of childhood cholera depends on recognition of the critical differences between pediatric and adult patients with this disease. The child with cholera excretes a diarrheal stool that differs chemically from that of an adult. Fecal losses of sodium, chloride and bicarbonate are less and potassium losses are greater than in the adult (Table 1). Administration of excess sodium and failure to provide sufficient "free" water to the child unable to drink are among the major problems in the therapy of childhood cholera.

TABLE 1. Mean Electrolyte Composition (mEq./liter) of Cholera Diarrhea*

	Na^+	Cl^-	K^+	HCO_3^-
Pediatric	97	74	23	32
Adult	134	97	17	46

* Pediatric and adult concentrations are significantly different ($P < 0.05$).

Treatment. The therapy of cholera consists of the careful parenteral replacement of the fecal electrolyte and water losses. On admission the child is obtunded, thirsty and markedly dehydrated (average 7 to 8 per cent of body weight). The blood composition of the average child with cholera at the time of hospitalization and in convalescence is listed in Table 2. On admission the child has a high plasma protein and low bicarbonate concentration, but the serum sodium concentration is normal. With correction of the metabolic acidosis the serum potassium level can fall significantly.

TABLE 2. Blood Composition in Pediatric Cholera Patients*

	ADMISSION	CONVALESCENT
Plasma specific gravity	1.0345	1.0240
Plasma protein concentration (Gm./100 ml.)	10.2	6.3
Osmolality (mOsm./liter)	269	267
BUN (mg./100 ml.)	24	11
Hematocrit (%)	49	34
$[Na^+]$ Wp (mEq./liter)†	143	143
$[Cl^-]$ Wp (mEq./liter)†	110	107
$[K^+]$ Wp (mEq./liter)†	4.9	3.9
$[HCO_3^-]$ Wp (mEq./liter)†	10	25
pH	7.162	7.415

* Average values from 42 children.
† Corrected for plasma water.

Because the first hours of therapy are of critical importance, the child with cholera should be admitted to a pediatric ward where special care can be rendered. After 12 to 24 hours, if the child is awake, taking water by mouth and generally stable, he can be transferred to an open ward. An adult "watcher," often a relative, is assigned to stay with the child throughout hospitalization.

The child is initially weighed, examined and placed on a cholera cot to facilitate complete stool collection. This cot has a 6- to 8-inch hole over which the child is positioned while the diarrheal stools are collected in a standard-size bucket. The volume of stool should be measured every 4 hours, using a graduated dipstick. A blood specimen should be drawn by an 18 to 20 gauge needle placed in a brachial, jugular, scalp or femoral vein. A stool culture for *Vibrio cholerae* as well as other pathogens is obtained on admission, and then daily until negative for three consecutive days. A rectal temperature should be taken every 6 hours. The child with cholera who is in water and electrolyte balance is afebrile. Fever (greater than 100.8° F.) is uniformly present whenever significant hypernatremia exists and is often the first abnormal sign brought to the physician's attention.

FLUID REPLACEMENT. The volume and electrolyte deficits initially present must be rapidly corrected intravenously during the first 2 to 4 hours after admission (rehydration phase). Continuing stool losses should be replaced on a volume-for-volume basis (maintenance phase). Oral administration of plain water must begin as soon as the child can safely drink. A child should drink 60 to 80 ml. per kilogram of "free" water per day. An intake-output record is kept at the patient's bedside and should be checked every 4 hours.

A plasma specific gravity (or protein concentration) should be determined on admission, after initial rehydration is complete and then twice daily until diarrhea has stopped. Determination of plasma specific gravity by the copper sulfate method is easy and accurate under field conditions. Plasma protein concentration can be measured even more simply with a hand refractometer. Using either the plasma specific gravity or protein concentration and the patient's admission weight (in kilograms), the volume deficit present at the time of hospitalization or during therapy can be satisfactorily corrected by administration of the volume shown in Table 3 and described in the following paragraphs.

TABLE 3. Parenteral Solutions for Pediatric Cholera Therapy*

	NAMRU-2 PEDIATRIC CHOLERA SOLUTION	NAMRU-2 PEDIATRIC CHOLERA REPLACEMENT–HYDRATION SOLUTION†
Composition		
Na^+ (mEq./liter)	90	70
Cl^- (mEq./liter)	64	49
HCO_3^- (mM./liter)‡	45	35
K^+ (mEq./liter)	15	12
Ca^{++} (mEq./liter)	2	1
Mg^{++} (mEq./liter)	2	1
Glucose (%)	5	5
Initial Rehydration		
Serum specific gravity (ml./kg. each 0.001 > 1.025)	6	7
Serum protein concentration (ml./kg. each 0.1 > 6.6 Gm./100 ml.)	1.6	1.8
Maintenance replacement	100% replacement of fecal volume	150% replacement of fecal volume

* See text for explanation of therapeutic regimens.
† 150% intravenous replacement of stool losses provides: Na^+ = 105, Cl^- = 74, K^+ = 18, HCO_3^- = 53, Ca^{++} = 1.5 and Mg^{++} = 1.5 mEq. per liter stool.
‡ As acetate.

Either of two therapeutic solutions is recommended for the treatment of cholera in childhood (Table 3). The electrolyte compositions of both solutions are designed to replace fecal losses in the pediatric patient and have been adjusted to correct the larger than expected bicarbonate deficit present at the time of admission.

The *U.S. Naval Medical Research Unit No. 2 (NAMRU-2) pediatric cholera solution* is administered on a volume-for-volume replacement of continuing stool losses. The amount given initially on admission is calculated as 6 ml. per kilogram per each 0.001 greater than 1.025, or using plasma protein concentration, 1.6 ml. per kilogram per each 0.1 greater than 6.6 Gm. per 100 ml. Supplemental dextrose (5 per cent) in water should be given intravenously to any child who is unable to drink adequate amounts of "free" water (60 to 80 ml. per kilogram per 24 hours) or who begins to exhibit signs of hypernatremia.

The *NAMRU-2 pediatric cholera replacement-hydration solution* is a more dilute solution, and a volume equal to 150 per cent of stool output should be given. The initial volume given on admission is calculated as 7 ml. per kilogram per each 0.001 greater than 1.025, or 1.8 ml. per kilogram per each 0.1 greater than 6.6 Gm. per 100 ml. Use of this solution in this manner has the advantage of providing adequate amounts of "free" water parenterally to all children with cholera.

ANTIBIOTICS. Each child should receive tetracycline* by mouth, 100 mg. four times a day until the stool culture is negative for *V. cholerae* on three consecutive days. Tetracycline is usually required for a total of seven days. If tetracycline is not available, furazolidone† by mouth, 15 mg. four times a day, has proved to be almost as effective as tetracycline. This therapy will reduce by two-thirds the volume and duration of diarrhea.

POTASSIUM. Replacement of fecal potassium losses should be by the intravenous rather than the oral route.

ORAL REPLACEMENT. Present clinical evidence does not support the routine use of oral glucose–electrolyte solutions in both the rehydration and maintenance phases of pediatric cholera therapy. No treatment center should, by choice, rely solely on oral replacement therapy in children with cholera.

COMMENTS. The treatment of cholera is the intravenous replacement of fecal losses. There is no justification for the administration of cardiotonic, antiperistaltic or anti-inflammatory drugs, such as epinephrine, nikethamide, atropine, bismuth, kaolin, paregoric or steroids.

Complications. HYPERNATREMIA. Hypernatremia has been a major complication in the treatment of children with cholera. The mean fecal sodium concentration in childhood cholera is 97 mEq. per liter. The sodium concentrations of lactated Ringer's solution, Dacca 5:4:1 and isotonic 2NaCl:1$NaHCO_3$ solutions are, respectively, 130, 133 and 154 mEq. per liter. Use of these solutions on a volume-for-volume replacement basis in the pediatric patient provides at least 34 per cent more sodium than is lost in the child's stool. Because large replacement volumes are required, a significant net positive sodium balance can develop.

This problem is worsened if a child is unable to drink his maintenance "free" water. Nearly 25 per cent of pediatric cholera patients are unable to drink for periods of 2 to 12 hours. This most commonly happens immediately after admission and emphasizes the importance of close observation during this initial therapeutic period.

The progression of clinical findings that follow excess sodium and insufficient "free" water administration includes fever, thirst, tachycardia, tachypnea, vomiting, oliguria or anuria, increased muscle tone, convulsions, delirium, coma, shock and death. These complications are similar to the syndrome described as hypernatremia or hypertonic dehydration. Such a child may appear to be quite dehydrated and the physician or nurse will often increase the rate of intravenous fluids, believing that the child has lost stool into his intestinal lumen that has not passed per rectum. Additional isotonic fluid at this time will aggravate his condition.

Treatment of a child with hypernatremia is the cautious intravenous administration of dextrose (5 per cent) in water, 30 to 50 ml. per kilogram over a 2- to 3-hour period. If "free" water is given too rapidly to the hypertonic child, neurologic findings similar to those of hypernatremia can be seen.

VOLUME OVERLOAD. Despite the large amount of diarrhea excreted by the pediatric patient, overzealous fluid administration is more common than insufficient volume replacement.

OTHER COMPLICATIONS. The prolonged oliguria or anuria that accompanies hypernatremia should not be mistaken for renal shutdown; it responds to intravenous "free" water administration. Hypoglycemia has been rarely seen in the malnourished child with cholera, but it is not a significant factor in the large number of children whose neurologic problems

---

* Manufacturer's note: The use of tetracyclines during tooth development (last half of pregnancy, infancy and childhood to age eight years) may cause permanent discoloration of teeth. This adverse reaction is more common during long-term use of the drugs but has been observed following repeated short-term courses.

† Manufacturer's precaution: Furazolidone is not recommended for infants under one month of age because of the possibility of producing hemolytic anemia.

are related to hypernatremia. Low serum magnesium and calcium levels have not been found in pediatric cholera patients.

Preventive Measures. There is not commercially available at the present time a single intravenous solution that is suitable for treatment of pediatric cholera. It is recommended that arrangements be made for commercial preparation of recommended solutions by any treatment center that is, or that anticipates, treating children with cholera.

Cholera vaccine should be administered to all children (and adults) who might become exposed to *V. cholerae.* Stool cultures should be taken on all contacts of a cholera patient and any asymptomatic cholera carrier should be treated with tetracycline. Improved sanitation facilities offer the greatest hope of cholera eradication in a given geographic area.

References

Griffith, L. S. C., et al.: Electrolyte Replacement in Pediatric Cholera. *Lancet,* 1:1197, 1967.

Griffith, L. S. C., et al.: Pediatric Cholera: Evaluation and Therapy, in R. S. Gordon (ed.): *Symposium on Cholera, Palo Alto, July 1967,* Bethesda, Maryland, Office of International Research, 1967, p. 201.

Active and Passive Immunization

ALEX J. STEIGMAN, M.D.

ACTIVE IMMUNIZATION

Recovery from an illness or from infection with the many hundreds of microbial agents with no resulting illness results in extensive *natural* active immunity. We are here discussing *artificial* active immunity.

A product employed for inducing artificial active immunity should be safe, effective and technically easy to use, and should be under regular review for effectiveness, for undesirable side effects and for whether need for its use continues to exist. Individual judgments are often necessary; the tendency to use a routine calendar for everyone regardless of circumstances is not desirable. Rigid legislative requirements, whether recently imposed or outmoded but still followed, are not always wise.

There is biologic variation among individuals. Response to an immunization procedure (as well as to an illness) may be influenced by age, pregnancy, concurrent illness, medications, nutritional status and unidentified environmental and genetic factors. *It is very important to observe the instructions printed on the package inserts of all preparations used.*

For those naturally acquired infectious diseases which result in enduring active immunity, the patient develops humoral antibody, and in many infections there also develops local antibody (IgA) along the path of entry of the infection. Additionally, cell-mediated immunity results with certain infectious agents. Subsequent exposure results in a sharply accelerated cellular and antibody response which tends to abruptly arrest the process.

Antibacterial Vaccines for Specific Active Immunization

Diphtheria and tetanus immunizations are accomplished by injecting toxoids which engender antitoxin. The basic pathology in these two disorders is due to their respective exotoxins. Immunization against these two diseases, therefore, has a very high rate of success with few side effects and with durable immunity. Vaccines comprised of killed bacteria, such as those for pertussis, typhoid, cholera and plague, are more likely to result in side effects and result in less durable immunity. (See Tables 1 and 2.)

Antibacterial Vaccines Used Regularly

TETANUS: toxoid; reactions rare; superbly effective with lasting immunity; overuse should be avoided.

DIPHTHERIA: toxoid; reactions very uncommon; good protection; carrier state and/or cutaneous diphtheria may exist despite circulating antibody (i.e., negative Schick test).

PERTUSSIS: extract of whole organism; local reactions not rare, general and neurologic reactions not frequent; protection from pertussis in early infancy depends on avoiding household contact with infected siblings.

Antibacterial Vaccines for Special Situations

BCG: used when exposure to active tuberculosis is likely and when other means of prevention, including chemoprophylaxis, cannot be assured.

TYPHOID: recommended only if considerable risk of exposure is anticipated; effectiveness limited.

CHOLERA: used only when required by international travel restrictions; effectiveness very limited.

PLAGUE: used only where very intense exposure can be reasonably expected; not very effective.

Antiviral Vaccines for Specific Active Immunization

Attenuated live virus vaccines are a relatively recent development. Best results are expected when the virus concerned exists in

TABLE 1. Active Immunization: Proposal for Healthy Normal Infants

AGE*	VACCINE	COMMENT
2 months	DTP, TOPV†	A minimum of 6- to 8-week intervals between these three injections is desirable for maximum effect.
4 months	DTP, TOPV	
6 months	DTP, TOPV	
1 year	Measles, rubella, mumps	May be given separately or combined, e.g. measles-rubella (M-R) or measles-mumps-rubella (M-M-R).
1½ years	DTP, TOPV	
4–6 years	DTP or Td, TOPV	
14–16 years	Td†	Repeated ± every 10 years; wound boosters for tetanus given if 5 years since last dose.

* Age chosen for convenience; may be altered, especially if child febrile or ill at time, or if reaction to previous DTP has occurred, which is most likely due to the pertussis component.

† *Abbreviations:* DTP = diphtheria and tetanus toxoid combined with pertussis vaccine in alum adjuvant.
TOPV = trivalent oral poliovaccine.
Td = adult type combined tetanus and diphtheria toxoids containing less diphtheria component than DT.

TABLE 2. Active Immunization: For Children Failing to be Immunized in First Year of Life

	AGES 1 THROUGH 5	AGE 6 AND OVER
Initial Visit*	DTP, TOPV†	Td,† TOPV
1 month later	Measles, rubella, mumps	Measles, rubella, mumps
2 months later	DTP, TOPV	Td, TOPV
4–6 months later	DTP, TOPV	Td, TOPV
1 year later	DTP, TOPV	Td, TOPV

* Local conditions influence decisions of sequence to follow; e.g., one may wish to give measles vaccine first if measles has been occurring, postponing DTP and TOPV for a month.

† *Abbreviations:* See Table 1.

one or only a few subtypes. Effective combinations are available. Duration of resulting immunity is probably less than that which results from natural infection. Influenza and rabies vaccines are made of killed viruses.

Antiviral Vaccines Used Regularly

POLIOMYELITIS: attenuated viruses; trivalent oral poliovaccine (TOPV) is highly effective; reactions *in children* unknown or negligible; recipients may excrete vaccine virus to close contacts.

MEASLES: attenuated virus; single injection effective; reactions mild; those who received killed measles vaccine in the past (no longer available) may suffer unusual local reactions when injected with live vaccine, or systemic illness and unusual rash when exposed to wild measles long afterward; vaccine virus not communicable to contacts of recipients.

RUBELLA: attenuated virus; reactions mild except for arthropathy, incidence of which is higher in females and increases with age; small risk of communicability to nonimmune close contacts; does not entirely prevent asymptomatic re-infection. (See special precaution in the package insert for girls of childbearing age.)

MUMPS: attenuated virus; negligible reactions, not communicable to contacts of recipients.

Antiviral Vaccines for Special Situations

SMALLPOX: a closely related live virus (vaccinia) used; formerly recommended routinely but now used in special situations, including health personnel and in compliance with legal and travel regulations.

INFLUENZA: killed viruses; zonal centrifuged now resulting in fewer reactions than previously; effectiveness variable but improving; usually recommended for children with chronic pulmonary, cardiac or metabolic disorders.

YELLOW FEVER: attenuated virus; required for travelers in specified countries.

RABIES: killed virus; most often used after exposure, unlike other vaccines; reactions frequent, especially locally; close judgment required in selecting recipients; duck-embryo vaccine preferred.

PASSIVE IMMUNIZATION

Every newborn benefits from passive immunization by receiving maternal immunoglobulins (essentially IgG class) via cord blood. This lasts for a variable but relatively short period of time, until the normal half-life decay of the IgG results in waning protection.

The immunoglobulins of human plasma can be concentrated (Cohn fraction II), resulting in a 16.5 per cent viscous solution referred to as immune serum globulin–human (ISG). Because many adult blood donors have significant levels of antibody to measles and to infectious hepatitis, ISG may be used for exposed susceptible persons. Humans can also be deliberately hyperimmunized against a single microbe, e.g., that for tetanus, pertussis, mumps or vaccinia, and their plasma concentrated as gamma globulin. All human globulin solutions must be injected only intramuscularly.

Animals can be artificially hyperimmunized against a specific agent and their serum fractionated into gamma globulin. There is a risk of anaphylactic reactions and serum sickness; antisera of animal origin are used only when no other protective means is available. Their use should be preceded by a scratch test (a drop of 1:100 serum dilution) or a conjunctival test (a drop of 1:10 serum dilution), either of which is preferred to an intradermal test by many physicians.

Passive immunization, whether with serums of human or animal source, is generally used as prophylaxis *after exposure* to an infectious agent. An exception is the use of ISG for persons anticipating a high degree of exposure to infectious hepatitis (IH).

Bacterial Infections

Botulism: horse serum antitoxin; specific types A, B, E or F, or polyvalent; used on suspicion or confirmation of previous case; consult local or state health department or Center for Disease Control, Atlanta, Georgia (telephone (404) 633-3311).

Diphtheria: horse serum antitoxin; usual dose for household exposure of a susceptible child is 10,000 units intramuscularly; for therapeutic doses see Diphtheria, p. 575.

Pertussis: human gamma globulin; value uncertain; used for very small unimmunized exposed infants; 1.5 ml. daily for several days or 5 ml. in one dose intramuscularly.

Tetanus: human or horse antitoxin; for passive prophylaxis, human serum is very much preferred, using 250 to 500 units intramuscularly, infiltrating some into the wound; is not necessary if active immunization has been accomplished; if horse serum must be used, give 3000 to 6000 units intramuscularly; these are prophylactic doses; for therapeutic use see p. 603.

Virus Infections

Infectious hepatitis: (IH, HAV; not useful for serum hepatitis SH, HBV): ISG; for household contacts give 0.02 to 0.04 ml. per kilogram of body weight intramuscularly as soon as possible after exposure; effective for five to six weeks. For continuous intense exposure, give 0.06 ml. per kilogram and repeat in five to six months.

Measles: ISG; a *preventive dose* following exposure is 0.25 ml. per kilogram soon after exposure; if unimmunized children with leukemia, immunodeficiency or other high risk situation are exposed, give 20 to 30 ml. intramuscularly; for most unimmunized children in good health who are exposed, one may give the live attenuated measles vaccine and in a separate site inject 0.04 ml. per kilogram of ISG, which is the *modifying dose.*

Vaccinia and Smallpox: Vaccinia immune globulin–human (VIG). This is used as therapy for eczema vaccinatum, accidental vaccinia in vulnerable sites especially around the eyes and generalized vaccinia; it is used prophylactically for a child with extensive skin lesions, such as eczema, who is exposed to a recently vaccinated person, and prophylactically for someone exposed to smallpox; eczematous children who must travel to areas with a genuine threat of smallpox may be vaccinated followed by VIG (0.3 ml. per kilogram) intramuscularly; VIG is available through the American Red Cross and Hyland Laboratories, Costa Mesa, California.

Rabies: a horse serum (from Lederle) is available for persons exposed to rabies; serum reactions occur in 15 to 20 per cent of subjects; is used in conjunction with rabies vaccine.

Passive Immunization for Other Infections

The value of *standard* ISG for nonimmune persons exposed to varicella, rubella and serum hepatitis (SH; HBV) is very questionable, even with large doses. Efforts are underway to develop *special* human serum globulins for these infections. A small supply of ZIG (zoster immune globulin)* is available for very special situations in nonimmune children exposed to chickenpox.

* Use of ZIG (zoster immune globulin) is investigational. It is available from the Center for Disease Control, Atlanta, Georgia.

20

Allergy

Atopic Dermatitis

SHELDON C. SIEGEL, M.D.

Atopic dermatitis is a common skin disorder of childhood. Because knowledge of its etiology and pathogenesis remains obscure, the treatment is often nonspecific and challenging. Successful management usually requires a diversified therapeutic program encompassing a number of different approaches and modalities of treatment. These include (1) prophylactic measures, (2) environmental control, (3) control of infection, (4) topical therapy, (5) systemic corticosteroids, (6) antipruritic measures, (7) dietary restrictions and (8) psychologic management.

Prophylactic Measures. DIETARY. Based on suggestive evidence that the incidence of atopic dermatitis may be reduced by feeding infants human breast milk in contrast to cow's milk formulas, it would seem advantageous to advise mothers of potentially allergic infants to breast feed their infants. Although more controversial, it has also been advocated that infants predisposed to allergic disease by heredity be given a soybean milk substitute (Neo-Mull-Soy, ProSobee, Isomil) from birth until several months of age to avoid sensitization to milk and, in turn, the development of atopic dermatitis. For similar reasons, withholding the introduction of strong sensitizing foods, such as egg white and citrus juices, during the first few months of life when the gastrointestinal tract is more permeable to intact proteins would seem desirable.

IMMUNIZATIONS. Since many children with atopic eczema are sensitive to eggs, caution should be exercised in administering vaccines prepared from viruses harvested from embryonated chicken eggs, e.g., influenza virus vaccine. Fortunately, live measles vaccine and live mumps vaccines, because they are grown on chicken embryo tissue cultures, are tolerated by most egg-sensitive children. If a child cannot ingest eggs, preliminary scratch skin testing with undiluted vaccine should be performed. If the scratch test is negative, an intradermal skin testing with 1:100 dilution of the vaccine should be carried out before administering the vaccine. Preliminary skin testing is usually not necessary for the administration of other routine immunization agents, such as diphtheria, pertussis and tetanus (DPT).

Environmental Control. The principal purpose of carrying out environmental control measures is to reduce the number of pruritic stimuli and allergens to which the patient is exposed. Although opinion varies as to the role inhalant allergens play in the etiology of atopic eczema, there is general agreement that they are important factors in the genesis of allergic respiratory disease (allergic rhinitis and asthma). Since up to 80 per cent of children with atopic eczema later develop allergic rhinitis or asthma, or usually both, it is important that potential dander be removed from the child's environment.

The control of irritating and sensitizing contacts should be an essential part of this approach to treatment. This can be accomplished by washing sheets and clothing with mild soaps, without bleaching, followed by thorough rinsing. Fabrics that come in contact with the child's skin should not contain wool. Cotton and other smooth-textured fabrics are usually best tolerated.

For bathing and cleansing the infant, colloid baths prepared with powdered oatmeal (Aveeno) or cornstarch—one half cup to a bathtub of water—and the use of soap substitutes, such as Lowila Cake, Aveeno Bar or Neutrogena, are preferable during the acute stages of the atopic eczema. Because of recent reports of its toxicity, hexachlorophene should be avoided, especially when the lesions are extensive.

Extremes of either temperature and humidity should also be avoided since they tend to exacerbate atopic eczema. To control these aggravating factors, air conditioners and humidifiers can be helpful. Sweating, which usually will bring on intense itching, can be minimized by avoiding excessive exercise or too much clothing.

Control of Infection. Patients with atopic eczema are unusually susceptible to a number of viral infections—vaccinia, herpes simplex and molluscum contagiosum viruses. Since this susceptibility exists even when the eczema may be mild or quiescent, it is important to withhold smallpox vaccination and to prevent contact with other vaccinated individuals or those infected with herpes simplex viruses. When the complication of eczema vaccinatum does arise, it can be effectively treated with intramuscularly administered vaccinia immune globulin (0.6 to 1 mg. per kilogram of body weight), and in serious cases, methisazone (Marboran)* may be useful in doses of 200 mg. per kilogram as a starting dose, followed by 50 mg. per kilogram every 6 hours for no more than three days.

Secondary bacterial infections of the lesions are also common. Extensive pyogenic lesions are best cultured and treated with appropriate systemic antibiotics. When the infections are localized to small areas of the skin, topical antibiotics, such as neomycin and bacitracin, which are not normally administered systemically, may be useful.

Topical Therapy. The type of topical therapy selected will depend on the stage of the presenting cutaneous lesions; the more weepy, oozing and crusted the skin lesions are, the wetter the treatment should be. Such lesions are best treated with wet compresses of saline or Burow's solution (which can be easily prepared by dissolving one Domeboro tablet or packet of powder to a pint of cool water). Although any type of soft fabric may be used for applying the compresses, porous materials, such as cheesecloth or surgical gauze containing at least 12 layers, are particularly suitable for wet compress treatments. The packs should be applied for at least 15 minutes of each hour. After each application the packs are removed, rinsed in the prescribed solution and then reapplied.

For the subacute stages, lotions, creams and pastes are the most useful. By far the most effective topical agents that are beneficial in this stage of the dermatitis are the corticosteroid preparations. There are now over 200 different topical corticosteroid preparations on the market. These are available in varying concentrations of different corticosteroids and in different types of vehicles, such as sprays, lotions, creams and ointments. Although often combined with many other active dermatologic agents, including tars, antibacterial, antifungal, antiseborrheic and antihistaminic preparations, they are best administered by themselves. The choice of the appropriate preparation is made on the basis of good dermatologic therapy. Some of the newer synthetic preparations have an advantage in that they possess greater anti-inflammatory activity than hydrocortisone in doses less than their equivalent potencies. Table 1 lists some of these synthetic topical preparations, their trade names, the manufacturers, the type of vehicles and their concentrations.

Some of these preparations contain a paraben preservative which can lead to contact sensitization. When sensitivity to this agent is suspected or known, a paraben-free preparation such as Valisone can be used. The physician should become familiar with a few of the agents listed in Table 1, the type of compound selected often based on the type of vehicle in which it is contained, and its cost. As a general rule, creams are better tolerated than ointments. When the lesions are extensive and large amounts of topical corticosteroids are required, the possible complications related to their percutaneous absorption should be kept in mind. For similar reasons, other potentially toxic topical preparations, such as boric acid, should be completely avoided.

Although less effective than topical corticosteroids, other preparations can be used quite effectively for the subacute stages of eczema. One such preparation which has proved useful for the author is Rosen's ointment, also known as 1-2-3 preparation because of the proportions of its composition:

Burow's solution	10.0
Aquaphor	20.0
Lassar's paste	30.0

Mild coal tar preparations may also be effective at this stage of dermatitis and can reduce the need for corticosteroids.

* Use of methisazone (Marboran) is investigational.

TABLE 1. Topical Preparations

STEROID	TRADE NAME	MANUFACTURER	VEHICLE	CONCENTRATION, %
Betamethasone	Celestone	Schering	Cream	0.2
Betamethasone valerate	Valisone	Schering	Cream	0.1
			Ointment	
			Aerosol	0.15
Desonide	Tridesilon	Dome	Cream	0.05
Dexamethasone	Decadron	Merck, Sharp & Dohme	Cream	0.1
			Spray	
	Hexadrol	Organon	Cream	0.04
Dichlorisone	Diloderm	Schering	Cream	0.25
			Aerosol	
Fludrocortisone	Alflorone	Merck, Sharp & Dohme	Ointment	0.1
			Lotion	0.1
	F-Cortef	Upjohn	Ointment	0.1
Flumethasone pivalate	Locorten	Ciba	Cream	0.03
Fluocinolone	Synalar	Syntex	Cream	0.025, 0.1
			Ointment	0.025, 0.1
	Fluonid	Derm Arts	Solution	0.01
Fluocinonide	Lidex	Syntex	Cream	0.05
			Ointment	0.05
Fluorometholone	Oxylone	Upjohn	Cream	0.025
Flurandrenolide	Cordran	Lilly	Ointment	0.025, 0.05
			Cream	0.025, 0.05
			Lotion	0.05
			Tape	
Hydrocortamate	Ulcort	Ulmer	Ointment	0.05
Methylprednisolone	Medrol	Upjohn	Ointment	0.25, 1.0
Prednisolone	Meti-Derm	Schering	Cream	0.5
			Aerosol	
Triamcinolone acetonide	Kenalog	Squibb	Ointment	0.025, 0.1
			Cream	0.025, 0.1
			Lotion	0.025, 0.1
			Spray	
	Aristocort	Lederle	Ointment	0.1
	Aristoderm Foam	Lederle	Foam	0.1

For the more chronic stages of the skin, tars and quinolone preparations may prove helpful. There are only a limited number of tar preparations available which contain solely tar derivatives. These include carbonis detergens, Tar Doak lotion and paste, Tarbonis cream and Supertah. These preparations should not be used on patients sensitive to tars or on acutely inflamed skin, and should be discontinued if photosensitization, folliculitis or furunculosis develops. The quinolone derivative iodochlorhydroxyquin (Vioform) is useful because of its bactericidal and fungicidal properties.

An occlusive dressing using corticosteroid preparations may be useful in treating small lichenified patches of eczema. Since this type of dressing enhances secondary infection, precautions should be taken to avoid this complication.

Thickened, lichenified lesions may only require the application of lubricating preparations such as Aquaphor, Lubriderm, Polysorb or Cetaphil Lotion.

Systemic Corticosteroids. Systemic corticosteroid therapy is usually best avoided for this condition because exacerbations are frequently noted upon its discontinuance and because, once used, the patient will prefer this routine of administration over the safer topical therapy. However, as a temporary expedient, systemic corticosteroid may be helpful when the lesions are extensive and unresponsive to other therapy. Usually a short three-day course of prednisone, 2 mg. per kilogram per day in three divided doses, followed by topical corticosteroid and other ancillary therapy will suffice.

Antipruritic Measures. Measures which prevent or reduce severe pruritus and in turn minimize exacerbations produced by scratching and rubbing are important in the management of atopic eczema. Topical therapy, especially the corticosteroids, are helpful in this regard. However, incorporation of topical antipruritic agents such as phenol or menthol are rarely helpful and usually poorly tolerated.

Colloid baths, as described above, if tolerated, are beneficial in controlling itching during the acute stages; tar baths (e.g., Alma-Tar Bath, Zetar, Balnetar) may also be useful after the acute inflammation has subsided. The use of topical anesthetic preparations, including the antihistamines, is contraindicated not only because they are usually ineffective but also because of their strong sensitizing properties.

Sedatives including the antihistamines may help to reduce scratching and irritability, especially during the night. Hydroxyzine (Atarax, Vistaril), 0.5 mg. per kilogram per dose four times a day; elixir diphenhydramine (Benadryl),* 1 mg. per kilogram per dose twice a day; phenobarbital, 2 mg. per kilogram per dose three times a day; or chloral hydrate, 20 mg. per kilogram per dose on retiring, is particularly useful in infants and small children. Some temporary relief of the itching can also be obtained by the use of cold or hot packs and with aspirin. At times all of the above measures will fail to control the pruritus, and restraints or covering of the lesions may become necessary to prevent undue scratching; cotton gloves or socks placed over the hands can be very helpful in this regard. Keeping the fingernails short will also minimize the extent of self-inflicted excoriations.

Dietary Restrictions. During infancy and early childhood, dietary restrictions may be of some help in the management of recalcitrant cases. The diet should exclude cow's milk, beef, pork, fish, citrus fruits, eggs, wheat, chocolate and any other foods suspected of exacerbating the skin lesions. The basic elimination diet (e.g., soybean milk substitute, rice, applesauce, pears, carrots, string beans, lamb and a synthetic A, D and C vitamin supplement) should be strictly followed for a period of at least two weeks. If the dermatitis improves, other foods are reintroduced into the diet every three to four days. With prolonged dietary restrictions, care should be taken to ensure that the diet is nutritionally adequate.

Immunotherapy. This approach to therapy is not indicated in patients who have no associated respiratory allergic manifestations. Although allergy injections are thought by some allergists to be helpful in older patients with inhalant sensitivities, insufficient evidence is available to permit firm conclusions as to its effectiveness in the treatment of atopic dermatitis. Since patients with this skin disorder also often poorly tolerate high doses of antigens, caution should be exercised when administering immunotherapy injections to patients with asthma or allergic rhinitis who have concomitant eczema.

Psychological Management. Tension and emotional stresses may trigger itching with consequent aggravation of the dermatitis. Furthermore, as is the case with any chronic or disfiguring disease, emotional and financial problems may arise as a result of the illness. The constant attention and energies required for care of a child with atopic dermatitis usually have a wearing and adverse psychologic effect on the entire family. If financially feasible, the simple recommendation of engaging someone to help with the care of the child and family chores can be of great benefit. A sympathetic and understanding physician can do much to alleviate the anxiety associated with this disease, and reassurance, explanation of the disease process and encouragement should also be an integral part of the physician's therapeutic approach to this disease. In rare instances, outside psychologic counseling may be necessary.

* Manufacturer's precaution: Elixir diphenhydramine (Benadryl) is not for use in premature or newborn infants.

Allergic Rhinitis

HEINZ J. WITTIG, M.D., *and*
DONALD M. MacQUEEN, M.D.

With the total prevalence of allergic disease being estimated somewhere between 10 and 20 per cent in the general population, the upper respiratory tract, particularly the nasal mucosa, is the most frequently affected shock organ in human atopy. Because of a wide range of morbidity from this type of atopic illness which often does not require medical care, precise assessment of this prevalence is difficult to establish. Cases of allergic rhinitis are less often referred to specialists than are patients with bronchial asthma or allergic dermatitis. A recent survey of the patient material in a referral-type university allergy clinic indicated that 61 per cent of patients could be diagnosed as having allergic rhinitis, most often in combination with bronchial asthma.

CLASSIFICATION

Allergic rhinitis is commonly classified as seasonal and nonseasonal, the seasonal variety being referred to as hayfever or pollinosis and the nonseasonal as perennial allergic rhinitis (PAR). Patients with hayfever have demonstrable hypersensitivity to grass, tree or weed pollens. Seasonal variations of symptomatology are fairly well correlated with the atmospheric prevalence of specific pollen species of the windborne (anemophilous) type. Skin test–reactivity with antigens prepared from such pollens is uniformly demonstrable. However, large-scale cross reactivity with insect-borne pollens on skin testing may obscure the picture, although the latter type of pollens have very little clinical significance. Diagnostic and therapeutic considerations must, therefore, be based on a thorough understanding of the aerobiology of pollens and mold-spores of a particular geographic region. Fungal spores may have periods of seasonal prevalence similar to pollens, and clinical hypersensitivity to molds may therefore be confused with pollinosis. Most patients can be identified as being either pollen- or mold-sensitive, although both conditions may coexist and require a combined therapeutic approach.

Perennial allergic rhinitis may be due either to sensitization of the nasal mucosa to one or more perennially present antigens (house dust, animal dander, foods and so forth) or multiple seasonal sensitivities with overlapping prevalence. Its etiologic diagnosis requires much more expertise and effort than that of hayfever. PAR is sometimes difficult to differentiate from nonallergic problems of the nasal and paranasal tissues, such as chronic sinusitis, vasomotor rhinitis and rhinitis medicamentosa, which is often the result of overuse of nose drops. The establishment of nasal eosinophilia, a positive family history of allergy and some evidence of atopic sensitization, either by skin testing or by demonstrable increase of symptomatology upon antigenic exposure, are helpful in this differentiation.

CLINICAL PICTURE

Allergic rhinitis is characterized by sneezing, rhinorrhea, nasal itching, swelling of the mucosa and, often, associated conjunctivitis. This picture may be obscured by superinfection with purulent exudate, erythema and a change of the nasal cytology toward neutrophil cells. Polypoid degeneration of the mucosa is rare in young children and mostly limited to the perennial form of allergic rhinitis with frequent infection.

TREATMENT

Most patients with allergic rhinitis respond reasonably well to oral antihistaminic and sympathomimetic therapy, if coupled with a conscientious effort on the patient's part to exercise environmental control. Only if these measures fail, or if involvement of the lower respiratory tract becomes apparent, will it be necessary to consider additional antiallergic therapy, such as hyposensitization or corticosteroid therapy.

Environmental Control. EPIDERMOIDS. This constitutes sensitizing exposure to animal hair and feathers. Elimination of the responsible antigens in this type of allergy can be readily accomplished after their identification. Even though positive skin tests to dog hair, cat hair or feathers do not invariably coincide with clinical sensitization, and even though clinical sensitivity to epidermoids may not yet be demonstrable in a young child, patients with allergic rhinitis should not have hairy pets in the house and should not have feather pillows. Casual exposure to outdoor pets is not usually significant. The problem with indoor pets arises from animal dander being incorporated into the house dust and carried from room to room by hot-air heating systems and air-conditioning.

HOUSE DUST. This is the most important single sensitizing environmental factor. In the authors' clinic, 58 per cent of all patients have exhibited a 3+ or 4+ skin test reaction to house dust antigen. The nature of the house dust antigen or antigens has been the subject of considerable investigative effort over the last decades. The ubiquity of this material in all parts of the world has invited the suspicion of a specific chemical entity as "the" house dust antigen, although its origin must vary with different cultural settings. Experience has shown that the presence of house dust requires the availability of decaying organic material, such as cotton fibers, human or animal skin particles and debris from clothing and furniture, plus warmth and humidity. Patients with house dust sensitivity therefore benefit from meticulous cleanliness and a cool and dry environment. Some years ago, fungal antigens were suspected to constitute "the" dust antigen, but subsequent studies have failed to show identity of the immunologic reaction of dust sensitive sera with reactivity to mold extracts. The abundance of gram-negative saprophytic bacteria in house dust has persistently raised the suspicion of endotoxin being an important factor in house dust allergy. Recently, some mite species (particularly *Dermatophagoides pteronyssinus* and *D. farinae*) have been shown to contribute a major portion of the antigenic material to house dust. Worldwide studies have confirmed this. However, not all patients with dust-sensitivity are mite-sensitive, and individual atopic factors vary from case to case. Be this as it may, the dust-sensitive patient must use frequent vacuuming and wet-mopping in his environment and attempt to maintain a relatively low humidity. But even under optimal conditions, total avoidance of dust is only possible in an operating room type of setting, and hyposensitization therapy is often attempted.

Electrostatic precipitating filters have been employed with some success as a means of controlling house dust. These are fairly expensive devices which are most effectively installed into the home-heating and air-conditioning systems. They must not be confused with widely advertised mechanical filter-type air-cleaning machines, which are often coupled with ozone-producing ultraviolet light fixtures with irritating qualities.

MOLDS. Fungal spores require a relative humidity in excess of 40 per cent for optimal growth. Nutritional requirements of many fungal species are minimal, colony growth being observed on plastic, metal, wood and plaster, as well as organic materials. Cleaning mold-infested surfaces with Lysol or Zephiran is effective. Porous walls can be sprayed with fungus-inhibiting paint additives. Mold-infested rooms or cellars can be effectively treated with formaldehyde by allowing this material to evaporate from empty coffee cans over a period of a few days every few months, while the respective rooms are kept closed and sealed for this time. Air-conditioning is the most effective single factor in mold control. In areas with high outside (atmospheric) mold-spore counts, avoidance is practically impossible and immunotherapy (treatment by hyposensitizing injections) is often indicated.

POLLENS. Theoretically, some pollen species (particularly ragweed) could be avoided by having the patient travel to pollen-free areas during the height of the pollen seasons. Practically, this is rarely feasible for most individuals, particularly since the height of the ragweed season coincides with the start of the school year and the end of summer vacation. Air-conditioned houses are relatively pollen-free, but children cannot be kept inside during summer months. Moving from one section of the country to another may temporarily solve the problem of regional pollinosis. However, susceptible patients are prone to acquire clinical hypersensitivity to locally prevalent pollens after a few years. For example, foreign students from ragweed-free countries who were enrolled at the University of Michigan were observed to develop ragweed allergy within about three years at the same prevalence rate as local students. For most pollen-sensitive patients, the greatest promise lies in judicious use of symptomatic medication and in immunotherapy.

MISCELLANEOUS. Aside from pollens, molds, dust and epidermoids, there are innumerable air-borne substances with potentially sensitizing qualities. Most important among these are kapok (in cushions and in furniture), silk, wool, insecticides, food particles, gums, the dust from the wings of insects and tobacco smoke. Once identified, all of these items should be avoided. If occupational exposure is necessary, patients will have to be instructed in the use of air-filters and face masks. Hyposensitization should not be necessary.

Hyposensitization Therapy

Immunotherapy by hyposensitizing injections with the sensitizing antigens should be limited to severely allergic patients with sensitivity to unavoidable antigens. Best results can be expected when this type of treatment is used with specific antigens, rather than with broad-range mixtures. Ideally, injected antigen choices should be made subsequent to provocative testing, by which only those allergens are identified which cause clinical symptoms, rather than those which cause positive skin tests only.

The mechanisms by which immunotherapy is thought to be effective in vivo have recently found laboratory confirmation. Three such mechanisms are described: (1) the production of IgG type blocking antibodies which develop within a few months of injection therapy; (2) a gradual decrease of IgE type skin-sensitizing antibodies over several months or years of treatment; and (3) an as yet poorly understood development of "tolerance," characterized by a loss of the histamine-releasing qualities of tissue mast cells and blood basophils. Since patients for whom this type of therapy has been elected will be committed to years of injection therapy with considerable expense and some potential hazards, physicians who direct the administration of this treatment should have appropriate experience and expertise.

Hazards of hyposensitization therapy include (1) anaphylactic reactions from erroneous overdoses in highly sensitive patients; (2) continuous worsening of the clinical course by chronic overdosage; and (3) the gradual development of delayed (Arthus type) reactions from long-term injections with certain antigens, particularly house dust and molds. The decision-making and long-term guidance of immunotherapy is therefore best left to physicians with special training in this field, while the actual weekly giving of injections can be executed in any practitioner's office.

Properly directed immunotherapy is generally rewarding when carried out over a period of years, although complete "desensitization" is rarely accomplished. Whether immunotherapy in patients with allergic rhinitis will prevent the development of bronchial asthma is still a disputed subject.

Pharmacologic Therapy

Antihistamines (Table 1). Since the acute symptomatology of allergic rhinitis, particularly in its seasonal form, appears to be mediated by histamine, antihistaminic therapy has been the time-honored choice of treatment in this disease. Receptor sites on shock organ cells for histamine appear to be occupied by these drugs in a competitive fashion.

The 1972 *Physician's Desk Reference* lists 103 antihistaminic preparations, to be given either alone or in combination. On the grounds of their chemical structures, several groups of antihistamines have been identified which are considered separately in Table 1. Some patients may respond more favorably to representative drugs from one group than from another.

Practical use of antihistamines in allergic rhinitis depends on achieving a balance between the desired histamine antagonism and undesirable side effects, of which sedation and an atropine-like drying effect are the most notable. Susceptibility to these side effects varies among patients and from group to group, with a general correlation between effectiveness and sedative action. However, a recent study conducted in the authors' laboratory has demonstrated that this correlation is not uniformly applicable, a representative of the ethanolamine group (diphenhydramine HCl) giving a relatively high side-effect score, with the lowest effectiveness measured in terms of suppression of wheal and flare reactions from allergy skin testing.

Previous warnings against the use of antihistamines in cases of coexisting allergic rhinitis and bronchial asthma have probably been exaggerated. While the drying effect of antihistamines may present some hazard in the severe acute asthmatic attack, asthmatic patients may otherwise actually benefit from histamine antagonism and may make use of this therapy in the prevention of attacks.

Antihistamines are readily absorbed from the gastrointestinal tract, and oral administration brings about a detectable therapeutic effect within 30 minutes. The duration of this effect is short (3 to 6 hours), but a prolonged effect (8 to 12 hours) can be obtained from a number of commercially available sustained-release preparations. The recommended dosages indicated on the package inserts should be considered only as broad guidelines and may require considerable adjustments for individual patients in regard to side effects and effective range. Some patients appear to metabolize antihistamines poorly and have a prolonged and significant therapeutic effect from low dosages, with associated sedative symptoms, while others tolerate and need much higher quantities. Furthermore, the side effects from a given antihistamine may subside with continued use, while effectiveness persists. On the other hand, some patients will benefit from alternating use of different groups of antihistamines from week to week.

Sympathomimetics (Table 2). Marked swelling of the nasal mucous membranes often fails to respond to antihistamines, but does respond to sympathomimetic drugs such as ephedrine, phenylpropanolamine hydrochloride or pseudoephedrine hydrochloride. Numerous commercial preparations contain these drugs in combination with antihistamines (Table 3). Anticholinergic additives (e.g., isopropamide in Ornade) are found in some combination drugs which attempt to inhibit rhinorrhea by their specific drying effects.

Sympathomimetic amines with alpha-adrenergic action are often used topically as nasal sprays or nose drops. In this application, vasoconstriction and relief of swelling is much more dramatic and rapid than in the systemic use of these amines. However, there is often a rebound vasodilation occurring an hour or so after the use of such topical agents, and long-term use should be avoided because of the hazard of resulting atrophy of mucosal tissues. Generally, there is very little justification for the use of sympathomimetic nose drops and sprays in children.

Corticosteroids. The topical use of corticosteroids (e.g., Decadron Turbinaire, containing water-soluble dexamethasone in an aerosol with Freon as the inert propellant) has received favorable acceptance in some cases of severe nasal obstruction from chronic allergic rhinitis. These units deliver about 0.08 mg. of dexamethasone with each whiff. The usual starting dose is two whiffs in each nostril three times daily. After the initial effect is obtained, some patients can be maintained on continued in-

TABLE 1. Antihistamines Used in Allergic Rhinitis

GROUP	TRADE NAME	GENERIC NAME	MANUFACTURER	PREPARATIONS AVAILABLE	DOSAGE
ETHANOLAMINES (marked sedation, low G.I. side effects)	Benadryl*	Diphenhydramine HCl	Parke, Davis	Capsules: 25 mg. Kapseals: 50 mg. Elixir: 10 mg./4 ml. Injection: 10 mg./ml.	Children over 20 lb.: 12.5 to 25 mg. t.i.d.–q.i.d. Children under 20 lb.: 5 to 10 mg. t.i.d.–q.i.d. (½ tsp. Elixir)
ETHYLENEDIAMINE DERIVATIVES (moderate sedation, higher incidence of G.I. side effects)	Pyribenzamine	Tripelennamine	Ciba	Tablets: 50 and 25 mg. Lontabs: 50 and 100 mg. Elixir: 20 mg./5 ml.	Children: 25 to 50 mg. t.i.d.–q.i.d. Infants: 10 to 20 mg. t.i.d.–q.i.d. Lontabs: 50 mg. b.i.d. for children over 5 yr.
ALKYLAMINES (less sedation, CNS stimulation more common)	Chlor-Trimeton	Chlorpheniramine	Schering	Tablets: 4 mg. Repetabs: 8 and 12 mg. Syrup: 2 mg./5 ml.	Children over 12 yr.: 4 mg. t.i.d.–q.i.d. Children under 12 yr.: 2 mg. t.i.d.–q.i.d. Infants: 1 mg. t.i.d.–q.i.d. Repetabs: 12 mg. b.i.d. over 12 yr.; 8 mg. b.i.d. 6–12 yr.
	Teldrin	Chlorpheniramine	Smith, Kline & French	Spansules: 8 and 12 mg.	Children over 12 yr.: 12 mg. b.i.d. Children 6–12: 8 mg. b.i.d.
	Over-the-counter medications: Alleroid, Contac, Coricidin, Dristan and Novahistine; all contain chlorpheniramine in various amounts and combinations				
	Actidil	Triprolidine HCl	Burroughs Wellcome	Tablets: 2.5 mg. Syrup: 1.25 mg./5 ml.	Children over 12 yr.: 2.5 mg. b.i.d.–t.i.d. Children under 12 yr.: 1.25 mg. b.i.d.–t.i.d. Infants: 0.6 mg. b.i.d.–t.i.d.
	Polaramine	Dexchlorpheniramine maleate	Schering	Repetabs: 4 mg. and 6 mg. Syrup: 2 mg./5 ml.	Children over 12 yr.: 6 mg. Repetab b.i.d. Children 6–12 yr.: 4 mg. b.i.d. Children under 6 yr.: syrup 2 mg. q.i.d.
	Dimetane	Brompheniramine maleate	Robins	Tablets: 4 mg. Extentabs:† 8 mg. and 12 mg. Elixir: 2 mg./5 ml.	Children over 12 yr.: 4–8 mg. t.i.d.–q.i.d. or Extentab 12 mg. b.i.d. Children 6–12 yr.: 4 mg. t.i.d.–q.i.d. or Extentab 8 mg. b.i.d. Children under 6 yr.: 0.2

	Disomer	Dexbrompheniramine maleate	Schering	Tablets: 2 mg. Chronotabs: 4 mg. and 6 mg. Syrup: 2 mg./5 ml.	Children over 12 yr.: 2–4 mg. t.i.d.–q.i.d. or Chronotab 6 mg. b.i.d. Children 6–12 yr.: 1–2 mg. t.i.d.–q.i.d. or Chronotab 4 mg. b.i.d. Children under 6 yr.: ½–1 mg. t.i.d.–q.i.d.
PHENOTHIAZINES (marked sedation)	Phenergan	Promethazine	Wyeth		Not usually used in treatment of allergic rhinitis.
PIPERAZINES (marked sedation but most powerful antihistaminic action)	Atarax	Hydroxyzine HCl	Roerig	Tablets: 10, 25, 50 and 100 mg. Syrup: 10 mg./5 ml.	Children over 12 yr.: 25 mg. b.i.d.–q.i.d. Children 6–12 yr.: 10 mg. b.i.d.–q.i.d. Children under 6 yr.: 5–10 mg. b.i.d.–q.i.d.
	Vistaril	Hydroxyzine pamoate	Pfizer	Capsules: 25, 50 and 100 mg. Suspension: 25 mg./5 ml.	Same as Atarax
PIPERIDINES (moderate sedation, increases appetite)	Periactin	Cyproheptadine	Merck, Sharp & Dohme		Not usually used in treatment of allergic rhinitis

* Manufacturer's precaution: Benadryl is not for use in premature or newborn infants.
† Manufacturer's precaution: Dimetane Extentabs are contraindicated in children under 12 years of age.

TABLE 2. Sympathomimetics ("Decongestants") Used in Allergic Rhinitis

GROUP	TRADE NAME	GENERIC NAME	MANUFACTURER	PREPARATIONS AVAILABLE	DOSAGE
CATECHOLAMINES	Neo-Synephrine	Phenylephrine	Winthrop	Elixir: 5 mg./5 ml.	Children over 12 yr.: 10 mg. t.i.d. Children under 12 yr.: 5 mg. t.i.d.
				Nasal solution or spray: 0.125, 0.25 and 0.5%	Children over 12 yr., nasally: 0.5% Children under 12 yr., nasally: 0.25% Infants, nasally: 0.125%
PHENYLISOPROPYLAMINES	Sudafed	Pseudoephedrine	Burroughs Wellcome	Tablets: 30 and 60 mg. Syrup: 30 mg./5 ml.	Children over 12 yr.: 60 mg. t.i.d.–q.i.d. Children under 12 yr.: 30 mg. t.i.d.–q.i.d.
		Phenylpropanolamine (used only in combinations)			
		d-Isoephedrine (used only in combinations)			

TABLE 3. Combinations Used in Allergic Rhinitis

PREPARATION	CONTENTS	DOSAGE
Actifed (Burroughs Wellcome)	Tablets: Triprolidine HCl 2.5 mg. Pseudoephedrine HCl 60 mg.	Children over 6 yr.: 1 t.i.d. Children 1–6 yr.: ½ t.i.d.
	Syrup: Triprolidine HCl 1.25 mg./5 ml. Pseudoephedrine HCl 30 mg./5 ml.	Children over 6 yr.: 10 ml. t.i.d. Children 1–6 yr.: 5 ml. t.i.d. Infants: 2.5 ml. t.i.d.
Dimetapp (Robins)	Extentabs: Brompheniramine maleate 12 mg. Phenylephrine HCl 15 mg. Phenylpropanolamine HCl 15 mg.	Children over 12 yr.: 1 b.i.d.
	Elixir: (per 5 ml.): Brompheniramine maleate 4 mg. Phenylephrine HCl 5 mg. Phenylpropanolamine HCl 5 mg.	Children over 12 yr.: 10 ml. t.i.d.–q.i.d. Children 6–12 yr.: 5 ml. t.i.d.–q.i.d. Children under 6 yr.: 2.5 ml. t.i.d.–q.i.d.
Triaminic (Dorsey)	Timed-Release Tablets: Phenylpropanolamine HCl 50 mg. Pheniramine maleate 25 mg. Pyrilamine maleate 25 mg.	Children over 12 yr.: 1 t.i.d.
	Timed-Release Juvelets: Phenylpropanolamine HCl 25 mg. Pheniramine maleate 12.5 mg. Pyrilamine maleate 12.5 mg.	Children 6–12 yr.: 1 t.i.d.
	Syrup (per 5 ml.): Phenylpropanolamine HCl 12.5 mg. Pheniramine maleate 6.25 mg. Pyrilamine maleate 6.25 mg.	Children over 12 yr.: 10 ml. q4h Children 6–12 yr.: 5 ml. q4h Children 1–6 yr.: 2.5 ml. q4h
	Concentrate oral drops (per ml.): Phenylpropanolamine HCl 20 mg. Pheniramine maleate 10 mg. Pyrilamine maleate 10 mg.	One drop/kg. q.i.d.
Ornade (Smith, Kline & French)	Spansules: Chlorpheniramine maleate 8 mg. Phenylpropanolamine HCl 50 mg. Isopropamide iodide 2.5 mg.	Children over 6 yr.: 1 q12h
Drixoral (Schering)	Sustained Action Tablets: Dexbrompheniramine maleate 6 mg. *d*-Isoephedrine sulfate 120 mg.	Children over 12 yr.: 1 b.i.d.–t.i.d.
Disophrol (Schering)	Chronotabs: Same as Drixoral	Same as Drixoral
	Tablets: *d*-Isoephedrine sulfate 60 mg. Dexbrompheniramine maleate 2 mg.	Children over 12 yr.: 1 b.i.d.–t.i.d. Children 6–12 yr.: ½ b.i.d.–t.i.d.
Rondec (Ross)	Chewable Tablets: Carbinoxamine maleate 2.5 mg. Pseudoephedrine HCl 60 mg.	Children over 6 yr.: 1 q.i.d. Children under 6 yr.: ½ q.i.d.
	Syrup (per 5 ml.): Carbinoxamine maleate 2.5 mg. Pseudoephedrine HCl 60 mg.	Children over 6 yr.: 5 ml. q.i.d. Children under 6 yr.: 2.5 ml. q.i.d. Infants: ½–1 ml. q.i.d.

frequent use of the Turbinaire. Systemic absorption of the corticosteroid by this method is demonstrable (0.3 to 0.5 mg. per day) but not sufficient to warrant fear of significant adrenal suppression.

In some instances, severe seasonal allergic rhinitis may warrant the consideration of short term systemic corticosteroid treatment. Since the effect of hyposensitization therapy is far from approaching ideal goals, and since some patients do not attain sufficient benefits from antihistaminic and sympathomimetic treatment to be restored to an acceptable state of health, some patients are best managed by the administration of 15 to 25 mg. of prednisone daily for a few weeks, until the peak of their allergy season has subsided and treatment can be discontinued. However, chronic corticosteroid therapy for perennial allergic rhinitis should be avoided because of the well-known disadvantages of adrenal suppression and so forth.

Disodium Cromoglycate. Favorable reports have appeared in the literature from England on the intrabronchial as well as the intranasal use of disodium cromoglycate in IgE-related respiratory disease. The principle of the pharmacologic action in this treatment is not established, but disodium cromoglycate does not appear to be an antihistamine, steroid or sympathomimetic drug. It is reported to modify mediator release from tissue mast cells by a heretofore undetermined mechanism. Disodium cromoglycate is used by insufflation as a powder (20 mg. per dose in bronchial use and 10 mg. per dose in intranasal use) on a continual basis to prevent symptoms. It does not modify symptoms once they have become apparent.

Bronchial Asthma

BERNARD A. BERMAN, M.D.

Bronchial asthma is a reversible obstructive bronchitis of apparent allergic origin. It is characterized by paroxysmal spasms of dyspnea and cough with audible wheezing, which in large part can be relieved by sympathomimetic drugs. The precise pathophysiology of this disorder has yet to be defined. The disease is characterized by spasm of smooth muscle of the bronchial tree, increased mucus gland secretion, edema and local and tissue fluid eosinophilia. Inheritance is presumably dominant with incomplete penetrance. The precipitating factors are legion and include pollens, dust, molds, animal dander, foods and a variety of noxious agents, as well as emotional factors.

Once the physician has excluded those diseases with which asthma can be mistaken, a plan of therapy should be undertaken. It is important to recognize that the signs and symptoms of asthma are subject to so many variations that an orderly approach to therapy is often difficult.

Three major groups of medicaments provide the foundation for treatment of bronchial asthma: the catecholamines, the xanthines and the corticosteroid hormones. The catecholamines include epinephrine, isoproterenol, and ethylnorepinephrine; ephedrine, not a true catecholamine, exerts a similar effect. The xanthines are usually available in pure form or as soluble double salts. Corticosteroid hormones provide anti-inflammatory action suitable for most atopic hypersensitivity states, but one must balance their advantages against the known deleterious reactions. A variety of synthetic preparations followed the development of cortisone and hydrocortisone, and most were designed to provide a potent response and minimize side effects.

Theophylline, caffeine and theobromine are methylated xanthines with diverse pharmacologic actions. Our interest will focus on the theophyllines because they relax bronchial smooth muscle. Theophyllines can be administered orally, intravenously and rectally. Modifications of theophylline—for example, the addition of ethylenediamine, forming aminophylline—enhance beneficial effects by providing greater solubility and higher blood levels, and they minimize gastrointestinal upset. Aminophylline contains 81 per cent anhydrous theophylline, dyphylline (available as Lufyllin) contains 71 per cent theophylline and choline theophyllinate (Choledyl) contains 64 per cent theophylline. The physician should be familiar with the theophylline preparations that he prescribes, and he must realize that calculations of dosages may have to be modified depending on the percentage, by weight, of theophylline available.

Theophyllines in combination with catecholamines or their derivatives produce a synergistic response, because both groups of drugs stimulate the accumulation of cyclic adenosine monophosphate, which induces bronchial muscle relaxation. The biochemical routes to achieve accumulation of cyclic adenosine monophosphate are different for each group of drugs.

Side effects of theophylline are multiple, and range from nausea, vomiting, hematemesis and excitability, to coma, convulsions and death.

During the past few years the theophyllines have acquired a new respectability. For example, aminophylline has been found to be both safe and effective when it is administered intravenously in a dose of 3 to 4 mg. per kilogram over a 20-minute period. However, to avoid many of the pitfalls of aminophylline toxicity, and this is particularly applicable to hospitalized patients, it is important to assess the patient as follows:

1. The dehydrated and vomiting patient should be rehydrated before receiving the drug.

2. Patients should be questioned as to the amount of theophylline given just prior to hospitalization and when the last dose was given. It takes 6 to 8 hours for blood levels of theophylline to drop below a therapeutic effect.

3. Check the previous modality of administration before giving theophylline. For example, prior rectal infusion provides higher blood levels than does oral administration.

4. Be familiar with the side effects of theophylline. Some of the early signs and symptoms associated with bronchial asthma mimic the side effects of theophylline overdose—for example, vomiting.

5. Do not write fixed 6- to 8-hour orders for intravenous aminophylline. The patient should be monitored carefully for signs of toxicity and in some instances more than 6 to 8 hours may have to elapse before the next dose.

There has been a surge of interest in the oral use of theophylline. High doses of theophylline, from 6 to 10 mg. per kilogram per dose, have been used successfully during the past few years, with side effects occurring in no more than 5 to 10 per cent of the patients. Titrate the dosage and start at 6 to 7 mg. per kilogram. Gradually increase the dose to clinical response or tolerance, whichever comes first, but do not administer more than 10 mg. per kilogram for any one single dose.

Adrenergic agents activate two broadly defined receptor sites—alpha and beta—stimulation of which results in a fairly predictable response. Alpha stimulation causes vasoconstriction of mucosal blood vessels, while beta activity relaxes bronchial smooth muscles and stimulates the heart. All of the adrenergic drugs induce both alpha and beta activity, but their responses can be graded as preeminently alpha, beta or both. Furthermore, there are now subgroupings of beta activity—$beta_1$, myocardial stimulant; $beta_2$, smooth muscle relaxation. Isoproterenol has profound $beta_1$ and $beta_2$ activity, inducing both cardiac and bronchial effect. Epinephrine has a similar beta response, but induces, simultaneously, alpha stimulation. Ethylnorepinephrine is primarily a $beta_2$ agent, producing bronchial smooth muscle relaxation. The beta receptor site is probably the locale of adenyl cyclase, stimulation of which results in accumulation of cyclic adenosine monophosphate.

Epinephrine, a potent bronchodilator with many disagreeable side reactions, including pallor, palpitation, trembling, anxiety, nausea, vomiting and pressor effect, is still very useful. The most common mistakes in administering epinephrine are (1) unnecessary delay when it is needed, and (2) giving initially too large a dose. For a child 6 to 12 years of age, it is best to inject 0.10 ml. subcutaneously and repeat, if necessary, every 15 to 20 minutes until relief of symptoms or tolerance, whichever comes first, occurs; do not exceed a dose of 0.50 ml. Because ethylnorepinephrine, a $beta_2$ agent (distributed as Bronkephrine), has a far greater safety margin than both epinephrine and isoproterenol (Isuprel), and because it is effective without the many side reactions of epinephrine and isoproterenol, it is the drug of choice for home administration for bronchial asthma, and in many cases, for hospital use. For a child 6 to 12 years old, the initial dose is 0.40 ml. subcutaneously; directions for repeating the dose are the same as those for epinephrine. The maximal total dose of ethylnorepinephrine should not exceed 1.25 ml. The short action of epinephrine and ethylnorepinephrine can be prolonged by using Sus-Phrine, 0.10 ml. subcutaneously for children between 6 to 12 years, and 0.15 to 0.20 ml. subcutaneously for those older than 12 years.

For inhalational therapy, isoproterenol (Isuprel), isoetharine (Bronkosol, primarily $beta_2$) and epinephrine are available in packaged metered aerosols. Bronkosol is preferred because it is longer acting than both isoproterenol and epinephrine and, further, has less cardiotonic and pressor response. All aerosolized medicaments with bronchodilator activity are effective in suitable situations, but one must be cognizant of the harmful side reactions that can occur, particularly when these drugs are overused and abused. Continued use, in many instances, causes rebound phenomena with concomitant worsening of the asthma. Continued inappropriate use, when combined with injections of epinephrine can produce sudden death. Metered aerosol adrenergic agents, although rarely prescribed, are useful for nocturnal spasms, exercise-induced wheezing and acute attacks unresponsive to oral preparations.

Ephedrine, the most popular oral adrenergic agent, has marked analeptic activities. Even though it is claimed to be effective, from a pharmacologic point of view it is a rather weak agent. When combined with theophylline, as well as sedative agents, it is available as Tedral, Marax, Duovent and Verequad. These combinations usually contain 24 mg. of ephedrine and approximately 130 mg. of theophylline. The precise oral dosage of ephedrine is not well defined; however, the average dose is 20 to 25 mg. of ephedrine every 4 hours for older children (this dose is contained in tablets of Tedral, Marax, Duovent and Verequad) and one-half this dose for the younger child. Ephedrine Syrup N.F. contains 0.4 Gm. per 100 ml. Timed-release capsules of ephedrine are also available—Ectasule Minus Sr. and Jr. are timed-action pellet capsules for an 8- to 12-hour effect. The senior preparation contains 60 mg. of ephedrine, while the junior is available in 30 mg. per capsule. Similar preparations are Slo-Fedrin A 30 (30 mg. ephedrine) and Slo-Fedrin A 60 (60 mg. ephedrine). For milder episodes of wheezing, Tedral, Marax and other such combinations are satisfactory. For more profound and serious episodes of bronchospasm, whether acute or chronic, ephedrine and theophylline can be prescribed separately, in order to maximize their therapeutic benefits, or additional theophylline can be added to the patient's baseline medication.

EXAMPLE CASES

Let us consider specific examples of asthma and develop treatment programs for each.

Case I

An eight-year-old had intermittent episodes of wheezing occurring with or without infection for 1½ years. Symptoms were worse in the morning, at bedtime and during sleep. He had daily episodes of exertional cough and wheezing.

A. *History.* Complete history, including previous signs and symptoms of allergic disease.

B. *Profile of the environment.*
   1. Pets in the home or at grandparents or friends. Pets include feather- or fur-bearing animals.
   2. Emphasis on bedroom, playroom and parents' room. Look for furniture with feathers or kapok. Rugging in playroom may have ozite pad, composed of cattle and hog hair.
   3. Basement—damp basement means mold, and unused attic implies excessive amounts of dust. Father performing house improvements, such as scraping the floors, increases dust content. Painting aggravates symptoms.
   4. Kindergarten—collection of pets and plants.
   5. Family home in country visited on weekends—dust and molds. Hand-me-down furniture stuffed with feathers. Barn with grain dust and excessive mold content. Contact with various farm animals.

C. *Physical Examination.* Chest clear on auscultation; forced expiration produces scattered bilateral wheezes. Other findings include the various stigmata of allergic disease: allergic salute, shiner eyes, nasal crinkle and pale boggy turbinates.

D. *Laboratory.*
   1. CBC.
   2. Nasal smear for eosinophils.
   3. Spirometry.
   4. Chest x-ray.
   5. Tuberculin test.
   6. Blood test.
   7. Alpha-1-antitrypsin.
   8. Sweat test and immunoelectrophoresis if indicated.
   9. Scratch and intradermal allergic skin tests.

E. *Discussion with parents.*
   1. Allergic cleanliness.
   2. Humidification, preferably with cool mist vaporizer.
   3. Coordination by the physician of the child with his environment to effect the best possible clinical results. This may require letters and personal phone calls to school teacher, gym teacher, family physician and school nurse. All activities must be designed for the personal needs of the child.

F. *Therapy.*
   1. Child previously on Marax,* ½ tablet q.i.d. and only as needed. By history, there are indications that the child is having day-to-day obstructive disease (exertional wheezing). Therefore, medication should be administered on a continuous basis, t.i.d. or q.i.d.; if child is sleeping, do not disturb. Continue Marax, ½ tablet t.i.d.
   2. Add Slo-phyllin,† 125 mg. every 8 hours. The child weighs 28 kilograms; calculate the theophylline doses on the basis of 7 mg. per kilogram per dose. On this basis, the child should tolerate approximately 200 mg. of theophylline every 6 to 8 hours. With Marax, ½ tablet, he is receiving only 65 mg. q.i.d. With the addition of Slo-phyllin t.i.d. (capsules contain 125 and 250 mg. of anhydrous theophylline—if capsule cannot be swallowed, empty pellets into a suitable vehicle) to the Marax t.i.d., the child will have 190 mg. of theophylline available with each dose.
   3. Hydration. The most effective expectorant is adequate fluid intake; therefore, give the patient with acute bronchospasm ½ to 1 glass of water or fruit juice every hour on the hour. Iodides and glyceryl guaiacolate are said to liquefy viscid mucus, but we have not been impressed with the effect of guaiacolates. Iodides may be helpful. Whether iodides are used for short or longer periods of time, the patient should be monitored for adverse reactions—nausea, swelling of salivary glands, goiter and acne (occurring in adolescents or adults). Saturated solution of potassium iodide is available for administration. The dose is usually expressed as drops per age and administered t.i.d. For example, for

---

* Manufacturer's precaution: Marax is not recommended for children under two years of age.

† Manufacturer's precaution: Slo-phyllin should not be administered within 12 hours of receipt of another theophylline preparation by any route.

our eight-year-old child, administer 8 drops of saturated solution of potassium iodide t.i.d. in a vehicle such as milk or water.

Case II

A nine-year-old boy had been sick for three weeks with sneezing, rhinorrhea, itchy eyes and sudden onset of wheezing. Wheezing became intense and was unrelieved by ½ to 1 tablet of Verequad q.i.d. The child was seen in the physician's office during September. Past history indicated that during August and September of the previous two years the child had had signs and symptoms of ragweed hayfever. Physical examination revealed an acutely ill dyspneic nine-year-old white male with rapid respirations and audible wheezing. The temperature was normal. The child weighed 35 kilograms. There were no objective signs of infection.

A. *Therapy.* Bronkephrine (ethylnorepinephrine), 0.40 ml. subcutaneously or intramuscularly. Some improvement noted. Child was still wheezing 20 minutes later. Bronkephrine was repeated twice over the next 40 minutes. At the end of 1 hour, the child had improved but wheezes were still heard with and without forced expiration.

B. *Instructions to parents.*
1. Force fluids every hour on the hour.
2. Allergy-free environment.
3. Verequad, 1 tablet q.i.d.
4. Slo-phyllin,* 125 mg. every 8 hours.
5. Prednisone (generic), 5-mg. tablets. Administer 15 mg. t.i.d. for four days.
6. Return in 48 hours for reevaluation.
7. Skin tests to be performed at a later date.
8. Chest x-ray if indicated.

Comment. This child weighed 35 kilograms. The theophylline dosage was calculated on the basis of 7 mg. per kilogram for each dose. Verequad contains 130 mg. of theophylline, and when combined with 125 mg. of Slo-phyllin,* the total theophylline dosage was 255 mg.

Delta-1 steroids, preferably prednisone, are the steroids of choice for acute and chronic severe allergic conditions unresponsive to optimal traditional therapy. In this case, the use of prednisone was designed for a self-limited episode of moderately severe pollen asthma. The recommended dose is 2 mg. per kilogram for 24 hours. From a practical standpoint, provide a minimum of 30 mg. to a maximum of 75 mg. per day, depending on the severity of the problem.

This patient received and responded promptly to short-burst, four-day prednisone treatment, which was stopped abruptly. For more severe cases, short-burst, initial high-dose prednisone may have to be followed by single-dose, alternate-day therapy, administered every other day after breakfast, for short or longer periods of time, but certainly for no longer than needed. Never administer an alternate-day program without first initiating short-burst, high-dose prednisone for three to four days. For alternate-day treatment, which is far more suitable and effective for children than for adults, always resort to the smallest dose of prednisone, e.g., 10 to 15 mg., which, when administered with adjunctive decongestants and/or bronchodilators, suppresses the major manifestations of the allergic reaction. In children up to 12 years, linear growth is generally undisturbed when doses as high as 40 mg. are offered every other day. When prednisone is ineffective, one or more of the following factors are responsible: (1) an incorrect diagnosis, (2) an insufficient dosage, (3) an associated infection or (4) an unusually severe allergic reaction. If contemplating long-term, alternate-day therapy, perform a tuberculin test. For those requiring corticosteroid hormones, always conduct an allergic survey.

* See manufacturer's precaution, p. 703, footnote.

Case III

A four-year-old child had repeated colds and wheezing during the fall, winter and spring months. The patient was known to have a constant stuffy, nose, allergic salute and occasional fits of nocturnal coughing. The current episode, similar to many previous episodes, began with rhinorrhea and minimal cough. Within 24 hours the patient developed a tight cough; by the second day he had a wheeze; and on the third day he had a temperature of 102° F. Physical examination revealed a well-developed, well-nourished child with some respiratory distress: harsh cough and audible wheeze, and minimal retraction. The findings were those of an upper respiratory tract infection: noisy chest with wheezing and rhonchi. Laboratory procedures included CBC, nasal smear for eosinophils, throat culture, chest x-ray and tuberculin test. Arrangements were made for a sweat test and immunoelectrophoresis at a later date.

The following program was to be administered by the parents:

(1) Expectorant cough mixture containing codeine, 4 grains; ephedrine, 6 grains; glycerine, 2 drams; syrup of hydriotic acid and Robitussin, enough to make 4 ounces. Give ½ to 1 teaspoonful q.i.d.

2. Force fluids.

3. Elixir of Dimetapp, 1 teaspoonful t.i.d. If wheezing develops, discontinue Dimetapp, and substitute Slo-phyllin Syrup, 1 to 2 teaspoonfuls q.i.d.

4. Cool mist vaporizer during sleeping hours.

5. Antibiotics—Erythrocin granules, 1 teaspoonful three to four times a day.

6. Allergic cleanliness.

7. Return to office periodically for reevaluation, allergic work up and allergic therapy (hyposensitization may be included if warranted).

Comment. This case is illustrative of a child with a diagnosis of recurrent upper respiratory tract disorder of allergic origin, perennial allergic rhinitis and bronchial asthma. Children who are afflicted with recurrent upper respiratory tract disorder of allergic origin often have a predictable and rhythmical pattern to their syndrome. That is, parents can often describe with a fair degree of accuracy those signs and symptoms which herald an attack. It has been our experience that when treating such a child, the parents should be instructed to administer, simultaneously, a series of medications, all of which should be given at the very first signs of an impending episode, which in this case were nasal congestion and cough. The purpose of giving these medications is to abort or at least to limit the more severe features of the attack. Thus, in this case the child was started immediately on an expectorant cough mixture, decongestant/antihistaminic, forced fluids and bed rest. When it was evident that the process had evolved to a full-blown picture, including elevation of temperature, despite the use of the aforementioned medications, the child was started on, simultaneously, an antibiotic.

Because recurrent upper respiratory tract disorder of allergic origin is a frequent precursor of noninfectious bronchial asthma, it is recommended that all such children have a complete allergic survey as well as allergic treatment. The decision to implement hyposensitization is often clear-cut, but at other times it is less well defined. It has been our policy that if after evaluation, including appropriate skin tests, there is a correlation between history and skin tests, and if allergens cannot be removed or avoided, then a trial program of immunotherapy should be considered.

Case IV

A 10-year-old boy had day-to-day wheezing for at least three years. All competitive activities were limited because of severe asthma. Previous management included hyposensitization and the use of appropriate bronchodilators on an as-necessary basis. The patient was previously tested and had clinical sensitivity to a variety of pollens as well as to dust, molds and animal dander. The family maintained very strict allergic cleanliness. On many occasions during the past three years, and for periods longer than two to three weeks at a time, the patient had received corticosteroid hormones—dexamethasone (Decadron), sometimes as alternate-day therapy and at other times by inhalation of dexamethasone (Decadron Respihaler). Physical examination revealed a tired-appearing chronic asthmatic with distorted chest—increased anteroposterior diameter—and noisy breathing due to wheezing. He weighed 45 kilograms and his height was well below the third percentile. He had a cushingoid appearance.

The patient underwent the following laboratory procedures: CBC, throat culture, alpha-1-antitrypsin evaluation, sweat test, immunoelectrophoresis, chest x-ray, sinus x-ray, spirometry and allergic evaluation.

The following therapy was initiated:

1. Discontinuance of hyposensitization program.
2. High-dose theophylline—Slo-phyllin, 375 mg. (capsules of 125 and 250 mg. taken together) every 6 to 8 hours, to be administered along with ephedrine given as Ectasule Minus Sr. (time-pellet capsule containing 60 mg. of ephedrine) every 8 to 12 hours, if tolerated.
3. Pulmonary rehabilitation, including postural drainage, breathing exercises, cupping and specialized program of exercise at the local YMCA, including swimming, parallel bars, rope climbing and ball throwing. The specialized program was administered to the limits of the patient's capabilities.

Because the patient had poor response to theophylline and ephedrine, he was also started on alternate-day steroids, using prednisone. Because the dose was governed by the severity of the illness, the initial dose was 60 mg. a day for four days, followed by 25 mg. as a single dose every other day after breakfast. After a two-month period of observation, he was no better and was a pulmonary and emotional cripple. Arrangements were therefore made for the patient to be admitted to a residential inpatient home for asthmatic children.

Comment. It is important to reemphasize that the delta-1 steroids, preferably prednisone, are recommended because they lend themselves to alternate-day therapy. Methyl-prednisolone and prednisolone are also suitable for this method of treatment. However, dexamethasone, betamethasone and triamcinolone, although potent corticosteroid hormones, are never to be used for alternate-day administration, since these steroid preparations if administered every other day will cause adrenal suppression within one week because of the manner in which they are excreted. Because dexamethasone and triamcinolone are available in liquid form, they may be used in young children, but only as short-burst therapy—for example, no longer than three to four days, and only in those acute or severe allergic states unresponsive to traditional treatment. Frequent inhalations of dexamethasone (Decadron Respihaler) are dangerous because 40 to 50 per cent of the active aerosolized material is absorbed, and signs and symptoms of adrenal suppression will develop quickly.

In this case, the patient had previously been treated with intermittent bronchodilators, administered only when symptoms of asthma were profound. Hypoxemia, a fairly consistent finding in children with intractable asthma, induces bronchospasm, and this process, once established, can become self-perpetuating. Therefore, chronic obstructive disease requires continuous therapy three or four times a day to aim for a wheeze-free chest.

This child had intractable asthma. More than 90 per cent of all children afflicted with bronchial asthma and treated appropriately respond favorably to modern allergic therapy. That is, they can eventually function fairly well in a competitive society. On the other hand, the child with intractable asthma, often steroid-dependent, is a pulmonary and, at times, an emotional cripple. For these patients a trial of cromalyn sodium is desirable. The application for this drug has been approved by the Food and Drug Administration. Its release, however, although imminent, is still pending because of problems relating to the package insert. Cromalyn sodium, first synthesized in England in 1965, has generated significant interest in treating severe childhood asthma, particularly those patients who are steroid-dependent. The drug, available in capsules each containing 20 mg. of the active agent, is administered four times a day by a device suitable only for inhalation (cromalyn is poorly absorbed from the gastrointestinal tract).

Cromalyn has no specific antihistaminic, anti-inflammatory or bronchodilator activity. It does not prevent the antigen and cell-bound antibody reaction, but it does apparently prevent the mast cell from releasing chemical mediators—histamine and slowly-reacting substance of anaphylaxis—both responsible in part for the asthmatic attack. Thus, this drug offers a unique method of interrupting the chain of events leading to the asthmatic spasm, events which are usually inevitable once the child is exposed to known sensitizing or precipitating factors. Therefore, cromalyn is effective only if administered prior to the challenge, having no useful action after the event. Given this information, the drug should be prescribed solely as a prophylactic agent, prior to the asthma attack. Once asthma develops, cromalyn offers no beneficial action and should be temporarily discontinued. The physician must then rely on traditional methods of treatment. To repeat: cromalyn is not the drug to use once moderate to severe asthma is in progress.

As far as patient selection is concerned, the patient's ability to use the device properly is clearly one factor, although children as young as five years have been successfully instructed to do this. Also, children with severe asthma are worthwhile candidates. In our study, where treatment was initiated in children with intractable as well as steroid-dependent asthma, 40 per cent derived significant benefits, especially from long-term administration and only when adjunctive measures—chronic bronchodilator therapy, adherence to environmental controls, hyposensitization therapy and so forth—were also used.

Although side effects are minimal and consist chiefly of local irritative reactions (dry throat, cough, occasional nausea), the physician must consider the advantages of the drug versus the potential risk resulting from long-term administration of an inhaled powder. Thus, from time to time wean the patient from the drug if there has been a satisfactory response. Afterward, if it is still needed, re-introduce the drug. In most instances improvement can be anticipated within a few days to several weeks. Do not expect miracles when you prescribe cromalyn. Even if the criteria for its use are fulfilled, it is still not possible to predict the child's response.

If cromalyn therapy is ineffective, referral of the child with intractable asthma to a residential home should be considered. It must, however, be recognized that residential facilities for the massive population of intractable asthmatics are limited.

Case V

An eight-year-old child with severe bronchospasm was examined in the emergency room. The episode occurred at the height of the grass season and was unresponsive to Tedral, forced fluids and insertion of a 125-mg. aminophylline suppository. Physical examination revealed a moderately dyspneic child with wheezing over both lung fields. The chest x-ray was within normal limits. The CBC indicated moderate eosinophilia. The patient received 0.4 ml. of ethylnorepinephrine and showed moderate improvement. The dose was repeated twice, with injections spaced 20 minutes apart. His air exchange was good, but considerable wheezing was still present. He was then placed on an intermittent positive pressure breathing (IPPB) machine using Bronkosol (isotharine), 8 drops in 2 ml. of saline; later, the child had a clear chest. He was observed in the accident room for another 4 hours and then discharged, wheeze-free, on supportive medication.

Comment. What is available for a child with acute bronchospasm if there is an unsatisfactory response to orally administered bronchodilators? (1) Injection of epinephrine, Bronkephrine or Sus-Phrine. For home administration, a responsible adult is taught to inject ethylnorepinephrine. (2) Aerosolized medications administered by metered appliances or, if there is severe obstruction, by IPPB apparatus, the latter usually in a hospital setting. (3) Rectal administration of theophylline.

Although we have resorted to rectal aminophylline for acute bronchospasm and although often the results are satisfactory, it is not the preferred method of treatment by our group. Suppositories are available as 125-, 250- and 500-mg. strength solutions of aminophylline (Aminet), or as Fleet Theophylline, 30 ml.-volume in 250-mg. and 500-mg. strength. When dealing with preparations that are available only in fixed dosage, care must be taken not to exceed the recommended 7 mg. per kilogram rectal dose. It is also unwise and dangerous to order ½ suppository to achieve recommended dosage. Suppositories are so manufactured that there is an uneven dispersion of theophylline. Also, when suppositories are used on a day-to-day basis, rectal irritation of the mucosa can occur.

Case VI

A nine-year-old with severe asthma of three days' duration, not responding to three injections of epinephrine, was admitted to the hospital. The traditional definition of status asthmaticus—failure to respond to three subcutaneous injections of epinephrine—has been embraced by some, but others have modified this definition to include those unresponsive not only to epinephrine but also to intravenous aminophylline and IPPB. Status asthmaticus is a medical emergency, and the care of such a patient warrants a team approach involving an anesthetist, allergist, pediatrician and pulmonary specialist, as well as competent skilled nursing personnel and physical therapists. Scaling the severity of status asthmaticus cannot be achieved unless both the clinical assessment of the patient and serial blood gases are monitored. The nine-year-old status patient had the following laboratory procedures: CBC, chest x-ray, blood gases determinations, urinalysis, and electrolyte determinations. His state of hydration was then estimated, using previous fluid intake, history of vomiting, presence of fever and duration of asthma. When first examined, this child, not unlike other status patients, had hypoxemia (arterial pO_2 = 64 mm. Hg), but the pCO_2 and pH were near normal. Ketonemia in children is often present and its magnitude is proportionately greater in a child five years of age or younger. The following orders were written for this patient:

1. Nothing by mouth.

2. Intravenous fluids, 80 to 160 mg. per kilogram per 24 hours.

3. Corticosteroid hormones–Solu-Medrol, 1 to 2 mg. per kilogram for an individual dose by intravenous push, repeated every 4 hours.

4. Oxygen to be administered by nasal prongs and/or mask. For nasal prongs: 3 to 4 liters per minute; for mask: 5 to 6 liters per minute. If the patient is intolerant to prongs or mask, an oxygen tent should be used with a flow rate of 10 to 13 liters per minute. Oxygen tents are unreliable because even with a high flow rate of oxygen, the concentration in the tent is often as low as 25 per cent. Although oxygen, no matter how administered, is to be moisturized, ultrasonic nebulization should be avoided. Ultrasonic nebulizers merely increase the workload of the patient. The particles which are deposited high in the respiratory tract are irritants. Because of the high density of the inhaled particles, there is an added workload for a child already burdened by severe obstructive disease. For children, excessive oxygen intake does not diminish the central nervous system's response to accumulated carbon dioxide. Once the patient is stabilized and improved and has an adequate air exchange, the mask and/or prongs can be discontinued and an oxygen tent substituted.

5. IPPB therapy. We prefer to use Bronkosol because it is a $beta_2$ agent with minimal cardiac effect; furthermore, its action is more prolonged than that of isoproterenol. Isoproterenol should be used with extreme caution in children who present with a significantly lowered arterial pO_2, because this drug further increases perfusion defects, thus lowering the oxygen concentration even more. IPPB with any agent should be avoided if the patient has been exposed to undue and excessive amounts of aerosolized adrenergic agents prior to hospitalization. In such patients, use of intermittent positive pressure can further diminish the air exchange as well as cause cardiac arrythmias. When Bronkosol is used, the dose is 5 to 10 drops diluted in 2 ml. of saline. It should be repeated every 2 to 4 hours if needed. If there is marked dyspnea and apprehension during the interval between Bronkosol administration, IPPB therapy with saline (without Bronkosol) can be helpful.

6. Sedation. The best form of sedation is reassurance and comfort by qualified nursing or resident personnel at the bedside. If further sedation is required, use chloral hydrate, 20 to 25 mg. per kilogram per dose by mouth or rectum; no single dose should exceed 1 Gm.

7. Frequent arterial blood gas determinations are necessary. For this, use the brachial or radial arteries. If acidosis is present, give sodium bicarbonate, 2 mEq. per kilogram of body weight. One-half of the total dose can be infused quickly over a 15-minute period, and the remainder during the next 30 minutes. After sodium bicarbonate administration, blood gases should continue to be monitored frequently, and if the base excess is a deficit value of 5 or more, or if the pH is 7.3 or less, the bicarbonate treatment should be repeated, rarely up to three to four times in 24 hours.

8. Expectorants. Adequate hydration is the most effective expectorant available. On occasion, sodium iodide, 250 mg. for the younger child and 500 mg. for the older child, may be added to the intravenous fluids and run in over a 24-hour period. Its clinical effect is difficult to measure.

9. Sympathomimetic agents. Do not use epinephrine or other adrenergic preparations until the patient's condition is improved, as determined by blood gases and clinical appearance.

10. Aminophylline. Give 3 to 4 mg. per kilogram intravenously over a 20- to 30-minute period. Refer to the prior discussion regarding the pitfalls of theophylline administration.

11. Antibiotics. Since infection is a frequent complication of status asthmaticus, antibiotics in suitable doses are recommended.

12. Physical therapy. Postural drainage, breathing exercises and cupping may be introduced when the condition is stabilized.

13. Assisted ventilation. If the patient's condition deteriorates and respiratory failure is impending, assisted ventilation can be a lifesaving procedure. The anesthesia and/or pulmonary staff will now manage the patient. The following criteria are necessary to confirm incipient respiratory failure: (*a*) cyanosis, (*b*) severe retractions and dyspnea, (*c*) depression in level of consciousness, (*d*) lessened response to painful stimuli, (*e*) hyperinflated chest with poor air exchange–diminution of wheezing and rhonchi by auscultation, (*f*) rising arterial pCO_2, usually above 60, often associated with lowered pO_2 and a pH below 7.25.

Serum Sickness

SHELDON C. SIEGEL, M.D.

Serum sickness is a generalized acute inflammatory disease resulting from deposition of circulatory antigen-antibody complexes in vascular structures. The term serum sickness originally pertained to the symptoms and signs that developed in certain people after being injected with therapeutic antisera (usually of horse or rabbit origin). However, reactions to several drugs, especially penicillin, may simulate serum sickness very closely in their clinical manifestations and probably have a similar pathogenesis.

The symptoms usually appear 7 to 12 days after exposure to the antigen. Patients previously sensitized to the offending agent may produce antibodies more rapidly and consequently develop an earlier onset of symptoms, usually within one to five days (an accelerated serum reaction).

Treatment. The treatment of serum sickness is largely symptomatic. Since the disease can be variable in its clinical manifestations, the choice of therapeutic agents should be governed by the severity of the reaction as well as by the organ systems predominantly involved.

When an acute anaphylactic reaction develops, therapeutic measures as outlined under Anaphylaxis should be promptly initiated.

Urticaria and angioedema are most effectively relieved by the antihistaminic and antiserotonin drugs. A wide variety of antihistamines is available. One antihistamine that is effective and has a low incidence of side effects is chlorpheniramine (Chlor-Trimeton, Teldrin). It is administered orally in a dose of 0.35 mg. per kilogram of body weight per 24 hours in four divided doses (not to exceed 4 mg. per dose). For more prolonged effects and when sedation is desirable, promethazine (Phenergan), 0.5 mg. per kilogram per dose, not to exceed 25 mg. per dose, may be used. Because of individual variation in drug response and differences in the incidence of side effects, other antihistamines may be more suitable for a specific patient. When switching antihistamines, it is best to select a drug with a different chemical structure.

Hydroxyzine (Atarax, Vistaril), 2 mg. per kilogram per 24 hours in three divided doses orally, and cyproheptadine (Periactin), 0.25 mg. per kilogram per 24 hours in four divided doses orally, which also has antiserotonin as well as antihistamine properties, are especially useful as antipruritic agents. Local applications of lotions containing phenol or menthol (e.g., calamine lotion) and starch baths (1 cupful of starch to a tubful of water) may also be helpful in relieving pruritus.

For severe angioedema and urticarial lesions that remain uncontrolled by the antihistamines, epinephrine 1:1000 may be of benefit when administered in a dose of 0.1 ml. per kilogram (maximum dose of 0.5 ml.). A more sustained action can be obtained by using a suspension of epinephrine in thioglycolate (Sus-Phrine) in a dose of 0.1 ml. for young children and 0.15 ml. for older children. The dose may be repeated every 6 hours.

Acetylsalicylic acid, 65 mg. per kilogram per day or 65 mg. (1 grain) per year of age every 4 hours, may be prescribed for the fever and symptoms in the joints. The dose should not exceed 3.6 Gm. per 24 hours.

When the patient fails to respond to these measures and in the absence of specific contraindications, corticosteroids should be administered. Prednisone or prednisolone is the steroid of choice. The dose must be individualized, depending upon the severity of the reaction and the size of the patient. A suggested dosage schedule is 2 mg. per kilogram per 24 hours in divided doses; the dose should generally not be less than 20 mg. a day for infants, nor usually exceed 60 mg. a day in older children. Once the desired effects have been achieved, the dose should be gradually tapered to the minimal amount that will suppress the reaction. Since serum sickness reactions are self-limited, it is rarely necessary to continue the hormones for more than a couple of weeks.

Prevention and Precautions. 1. Foremost in the measures to prevent serum sickness is the avoidance of the use of foreign sera and unnecessary drugs whenever possible. Their use can be greatly curtailed by: (*a*) mass primary immunization (especially to tetanus, pertussis and diphtheria) with periodic boosters of the appropriate antigens and (*b*) substitution of human hyperimmune globulins (Cutter, Breon, Savage, Flint or Hyland Laboratories) for foreign sera when passive immunization becomes necessary.

2. Before any therapeutic or diagnostic agents are administered, a detailed history should be obtained regarding: (*a*) possible previous adverse reactions, especially to the agent in question—a drug, biologic product or foreign serum should never be administered when a history of a possible reaction has been elicited, except under extenuating circumstances when one of them might be necessary to save the patient's life; (*b*) presence of atopic background (allergic rhinitis, bronchial asthma or atopic dermatitis) in the patient—persons who are sensitive to proteins of the species from which the sera are derived are more apt to have serious, immediate reactions, and extreme caution and conservatism are warranted in these subjects; (*c*) previous injection of serum—special precautions should be taken for these patients, because a history of previous administration of serum greatly increases the likelihood of a serum sickness reaction. Anaphylactic reactions

and accelerated reactions are also more likely to occur.

3. Skin or ophthalmic testing for sensitivity to the serum is imperative prior to the administration of serum irrespective of whether the patient has previously received serum or experienced a reaction to the serum in question. Usually the initial intracutaneous or ophthalmic test may be performed with a 1:100 saline dilution of the serum. In persons with a history of atopy of a previous reaction, the initial dilution should be 1:1000, and preferably a scratch test should be done first. A positive skin or ophthalmic test strongly suggests sensitivity; on the other hand, a negative test in no way assures against a reaction occurring.

Desensitization. When the patient exhibits a positive skin or ophthalmic reaction or is known to be sensitive to a foreign serum, substitution of an antitoxin from another species is advisable. On rare occasions when this is not possible and a foreign serum is required as a lifesaving measure (e.g., antitoxin for snakebite), rapid desensitization may be carried out. The technique is basically the same as other desensitization procedures. The procedure is extremely hazardous and should always be performed in a hospital by a physician prepared to treat anaphylaxis. Although coverage with the antianaphylactic drugs (antihistamines, Adrenalin, corticosteroids) might be helpful in preventing minor systemic reactions, they will not prevent a severe reaction, and reliance on these agents alone could lead to disastrous results. The following schedule for desensitization to foreign sera is presented as a rough guide.

1. The initial dose is determined by scratch and intradermal testing (dilutions are made with normal saline). First, perform the scratch test with a 1:1000 dilution. If the result is negative perform an intradermal test with the same solution (1:1000); if the result is positive, begin treatment with 1:1000 as the initial concentration. If the result of the intradermal test is still negative, perform the same test with a 1:100 dilution. Unless a large reaction is observed, this concentration may be used for the first dose.

2. Start an intravenous infusion with 100 mg. of cortisol succinate (Solu-Cortef) and 25 mg. of diphenhydramine (Benadryl), or their equivalents, in 500 ml. of 5 per cent glucose and saline. One-tenth to 0.15 ml. of Sus-Phrine, a suspension of epinephrine in thioglycollate and glycerin, is administered subcutaneously.

3. The first dose of diluted serum is then injected subcutaneously at a site in an extremity where a tourniquet could be placed proximally if a reaction should occur. Subsequent injections are given every 30 minutes, approximately doubling the dose each time until the full dose is administered.

NUMBER OF DOSE	AMOUNT OF SERUM IN ML.	DILUTION
1	0.1	1:1000
2	0.2	1:1000
3	0.4	1:1000
4	0.7	1:1000
5	0.1	1:100
6	0.2	1:100
7	0.4	1:100
8	0.7	1:100
9	0.1	1:10
10	0.2	1:10
11	0.4	1:10
12	0.7	1:10
13	0.1	Undiluted
14	0.2	Undiluted
15	0.4	Undiluted
16	0.7	Undiluted
17	1.0	Undiluted

4. When a dose of 1 ml. of undiluted serum has been reached, additional injections are best administered intramuscularly, particularly when large doses of antitoxin are necessary as in the treatment of diphtheria. As with the subcutaneous route, the dose is doubled every 30 minutes until the desired amount of antiserum has been administered. Use of the intravenous route for administering serum is best avoided unless massive amounts of antiserum are required in critically ill patients. For this purpose the serum should be diluted one hundredfold in saline and given slowly.

Angioneurotic Edema

FRED S. ROSEN, M.D., *and*
HARVEY R. COLTEN, M.D.

Angioneurotic edema is a symptom which consists of circumscribed areas of swelling of the subcutaneous areas of tissue. The swelling is never discolored or red, is never painful and usually does not itch. The symptom may arise from a hereditary defect or on an allergic basis.

HEREDITARY ANGIONEUROTIC EDEMA

Hereditary angioneurotic edema results from a genetically determined deficiency in the C1 inhibitor, an alpha-2 globulin of the blood which inhibits the enzymatic activity of the first component of complement (C1). The life span of patients with hereditary angioneurotic edema is frequently shortened by asphyxiation consequent to laryngeal edema.

Diagnosis. Affected individuals are prone to sudden, unheralded attacks of circumscribed subcutaneous edema. The swelling, which may be severe enough to cause remarkable disfigurement of the affected part, evolves very quickly and usually subsides within 72 hours. There is no discoloration, redness, pain or itching associated with the edema. Despite the undistinguished appearance of the edema, involvement of the mucous membranes of the hypopharynx and larynx may result in untimely death from asphyxiation.

A rash, reminiscent of erythema marginatum, is recognized by some affected patients, particularly children, and it may occur without associated swelling. All affected individuals have recurrent attacks of abdominal pain due to collections of edema fluid in the intestinal wall. The colic may be severe and spasmodic. Bilious vomiting or copious, watery diarrhea ensues; the hemoconcentration due to fluid loss is reflected in the rising hematocrit as the attack progresses. Abdominal attacks often are not accompanied by cutaneous swelling and thus may be confused with peptic ulcer, biliary colic, appendicitis or some other cause of the acute abdomen.

Although trauma is clearly related to attacks of angioedema, more frequently the cause of any individual bout of swelling is obscure. Patients have frequently associated menses, violent exercise, extremes of temperature and psychic trauma with the onset of attacks of angioedema. The earliest symptoms usually occur sometime in the first decade of life. Colic is frequently noted in affected infants. The frequency and severity of attacks typically exacerbate at adolescence and subside in the fifth decade of life (Donaldson and Rosen, 1966; Landerman, 1962).

Treatment. Daily administration of methyl testosterone linguets has prevented attacks of angioedema in approximately one-third to one-half of the patients. It must be taken daily in a single dose of 10 to 25 mg. The mechanism of its effect is not known. Methyl testosterone therapy is not recommended for children.

Epsilon-aminocaproic acid has been successful in halting attacks of angioedema. However, the side effects with chronic administration of this agent are so annoying that its usage has been very limited. An analogue, tranexamic acid, has been found to have fewer side effects, causing only occasional minor gastrointestinal distress. In doses of 1 to 3 Gm. orally per day, it has proved effective in aborting attacks of angioedema. The drug has not yet been released by the Food and Drug Administration.

Infusions of plasma have been recommended in the therapy of attacks of angioedema. However, this approach is not recommended by us for several reasons: it has been of questionable value and is not innocuous in the view of several observers who have attempted to use it. It is not possible to raise the level of C1 inhibitor above 7 mg. per 100 ml., a level under which attacks of angioedema occur, except by infusing very large amounts of plasma. For instance, 100 ml. of plasma would raise the inhibitor level by 1 mg. per 100 ml. in a 40-kilogram child. Fresh plasma contains more substrate for C1 than does inhibitor; consequently, its administration early in the course of an attack, prior to the onset of tachyphylaxis, might in fact exacerbate the symptoms. Such an event has been observed.

Epinephrine is useful in controlling swelling in very few patients. Hydrocortisone also provides benefit very rarely in patients. Antihistamines are of no use. Intravenous administration of diuretics, such as Mercuhydrin or ethacrynic acid,* is helpful in halting the progression of life-threatening angioedema.

Tracheostomy should be performed without hesitation in patients with laryngeal obstruction. It is frequently life-saving.

A large number of compounds, including several phosphonate esters, are known to inhibit C1 and C1 activation in vitro. The likelihood of finding a nontoxic analogue remains promising for future therapy of hereditary angioneurotic edema.

NONHEREDITARY ANGIONEUROTIC EDEMA

Nonhereditary angioneurotic edema is generally a benign clinical condition of diverse etiology. Food ingestion, drugs and insect stings in appropriately sensitive individuals, and psychic or physical factors may precipitate attacks of angioedema. The clinical consequences of angioedema are a function of the site involved; angioedema of the larynx may be fatal if prompt therapy is not instituted. Angioedema secondary to acute infection or to connective tissue disorders must be differentiated, since the diagnostic and therapeutic efforts must be specific for these primary diseases.

In the case of angioedema due to an

* Manufacturer's precaution: Until further experience is accumulated in infants, therapy with the oral and parenteral forms of ethacrynic acid is contraindicated.

obvious precipitating event (e.g., insect sting), an etiologic diagnosis by means of history and skin testing is not difficult. Avoidance of exposure, hyposensitization and the availability of an emergency kit consisting of sublingual Isuprel or an oral ephedrine preparation and antihistamine (e.g., Benadryl) are generally successful in preventing subsequent episodes of angioedema. The emergency kit should be carried by the patient at all times during periods when exposure to stinging insects is likely.

In contrast, in the case of other causes of angioedema, identification of the specific etiologic agent is often more difficult. For example, in angioedema due to food ingestion, skin testing is of doubtful value; and if the onset of clinical symptoms is delayed for several hours following ingestion of the offending agent, the history may not be helpful. In fact, it is estimated that in nearly 50 per cent of all cases of nonhereditary angioedema, an etiologic diagnosis is not made.

Accordingly, although elimination of the offending agent is the most successful therapy, symptomatic therapy may be the only available measure. Aqueous epinephrine is of value, particularly in the more severe cases. Parenteral or oral antihistamines and/or oral sympathomimetics (ephedrine) are also indicated. Maintenance of adequate ventilation in instances of laryngeal edema may require intubation or tracheostomy if the response to epinephrine is not prompt. The role of corticosteroids in the treatment of angioedema has not been rigorously studied, though those agents are frequently employed. In no instance should corticosteroids be considered a substitute for epinephrine in the emergency treatment of severe cases of angioedema.

Allergic Gastrointestinal Disease

HAROLD I. LECKS, M.D.

The successful treatment of allergic gastrointestinal disease requires identification and removal of the offending allergen. In many instances detection is extremely difficult and marked by many uncertainties. In part this arises from the wide range of symptoms and syndromes usually considered those of gastrointestinal allergy, and in part from the lack of methodology for establishing the causal allergen and from the fact that other target organ systems (viz., respiratory) may be affected concurrently.

Gluten enteropathy, protein-losing gastroenteropathy, ulcerative colitis, regional enteritis, Heiner's syndrome and lactose intolerance have all been related causally to food hypersensitivity, although the relationship has not always been clear-cut. Of even more uncertain allergic origin are aphthous ulcers, infantile colic, cyclic vomiting, constipation or diarrhea, excessive flatus, tension fatigue syndrome and recurrent abdominal pain. Recent observations have also documented symptoms of food hypersensitivity (such as banana and melon) affecting the upper gastrointestinal tract during episodes of seasonal rhinitis (pollenosis). These findings lend support to earlier concepts suggesting an alteration in allergic tolerance to the same or unrelated antigen in one organ system (viz., the gastrointestinal tract) when another is affected (viz., the respiratory system).

Identification of Offending Allergen. Of the techniques used to establish the causal allergen, detailed interrogation of the parents and possibly the child remains the most satisfactory. Questioning should encompass not only suspected and previous food intolerances (particularly in infancy) but also intense food dislikes, food excesses, family food disagreements, frequency of feeding of foods under question and daily diet schedules.

When the clinical history fails to uncover a potential offender, either of two courses may be followed: arbitrary feeding of a diet selected because of low allergenicity (hypoallergenic diet, or the utilizing of one or two foods (e.g., rice, lamb) initially for 24 to 48 hours with gradual reintroduction of other foods at varying intervals (usually two to three days), noting whether or not the symptoms are provoked. Obviously the former plan is most applicable to children with suspected gastrointestinal allergy.

The author has listed in Table 1 the most frequently used menu in his practice for the infant or child under a year or two of age. In the older patients Rowe's diets (cereal-, wheat-, milk-, egg-free) or modifications are also useful. More complex dietary programs have been suggested by Rinkel, with the added diagnostic innovation of attempting to reproduce the gastrointestinal complaint by injection of the suspected food—a time-consuming and potentially hazardous technique which has not yet been widely evaluated.

With all types of dietary manipulation, assessment of obscure symptoms may be difficult unless carried out under controlled periods of observation. This is best done with the patient institutionalized and offered at least two challenge feedings. In the older child, masked or disguised feedings may be necessary.

TABLE 1. Hypoallergenic Diet for Infants and Young Children

Milk substitute—Mull-Soy and Neo-Mull-Soy (Borden Co.), Sobee and ProSobee (Mead Johnson), Isomil (Ross), Soyalac (Loma Linda)

Cereals—rice (also oat, corn, poi, rye, etc.); bread—Rye-Krisp Baltic rye (1011 Marlborough Street, Philadelphia, Pa. 19125)

Vegetables—beets, white and sweet potato, carrots, broccoli (also legumes, asparagus, etc.); soups made from these vegetables

Fruits—apple, pear, plum, banana (also apricot, grape, etc.); juices of these fruits

Meats—lamb (also capon or rooster, pork, etc.)

Desserts—fruits listed and their gelatin products

Spreads—oleomargarine (kosher, jellies of the listed fruits)

Vitamins—synthetic (Tri-Vi-Sol, Poly-Vi-Sol, Decca-Vi-Sol—Mead Johnson)

Comment: Amounts fed to the patient are dependent on age, and known specific disagreements are excluded.

Concurrent roentgenologic survey of the gastrointestinal tract may be helpful. Gastric dilatation, increased small bowel motility, intestinal puddling of barium and segmentation of the intestinal wall have been reported as characteristic albeit not diagnostic findings. Proctoscopic examination with or without intraluminal suction biopsies from the distal duodenum or proximal jejunum with light and electron microscopy may be required when the distinction must be made between a malabsorption state of allergic origin and gluten-induced enteropathy.

Although the value of skin testing in the detection of food allergens is controversial, in some instances it may facilitate diagnosis by narrowing the spectrum of suspected allergens. Positive tests elicited by the prick method have greater clinical significance, especially if large reactions occur, than do those elicited by intradermal or Prausnitz-Küstner testing. Such reactions contradict further identification testing with these allergens. Rarely, however, does a generalized reaction occur from a prick test with a food previously known to cause anaphylactic symptoms. These findings may indicate a past and, less frequently, a future sensitivity and must be interpreted with such qualifications in mind. The reliability of testing in infants is less than in the older child, probably because of the peculiar physiologic state of the infant's integument (vascularity, nature of collagen, electrolyte and water content, enzyme composition and so forth) and the relative immunologic incompetence of the infant's lymphoid system, rather than because of testing techniques or the potency and nature of the extract used. Skin irritability and dermographism are common.

Serologic determinations for a variety of antibodies to food proteins have also been used as a measure of correlating the suspected allergen with the gastrointestinal complaint. Coproantibodies (precipitins) have also been detected for antigens such as milk and wheat in patients with gluten enteropathy and with milk protein hypersensitivity. Its specificity, however, has been challenged, since this immunologic response has occurred in patients with a diarrheal stool and in the normal stool. Milk precipitins have also been found in the serum of a heterogeneous group of patients, some of whom do not have evidence of malabsorption. The significance of these findings is uncertain. Except for the passive cutaneous anaphylaxis antibody, little relationship exists. It is possible that with further modifications the recently devised radioimmunoassay method for the measurement of serum antibodies of the IgE variety may provide an in vitro test for the detection of food allergens.

A number of other measures have also been suggested as diagnostic procedures for defining the gastrointestinal allergen, including serial leukocyte and eosinophil counts, and pulse rate determinations made before and after challenge of the patient with the causal allergen, usually a food. There is some question as to their value in childhood allergy. Even the presence of an eosinophilia in the blood, tissue or secretions of the gastrointestinal tract as an indicator of an allergic illness is controversial, because this may occur in the neonate or infant until three or more months and is present in a number of nonatopic gastrointestinal illnesses (e.g., ulcerative colitis). However, a provocative eosinophilia following challenge with the specific allergen may be more meaningful diagnostically. Recently, in a group of infants with milk intolerance, varying abnormalities of intestinal absorption (D-xylose absorption and excretion, fat malabsorption), quantitative disturbances in disaccharide enzyme estimation, histologic changes in the jejunal mucosa as well as eosinophilic cell infiltration in biopsies obtained from the rectal submucosa following topical (enema) application of the antigen have been reported.

Treatment. When an elimination diet is selected for a child, it is necessary that food fillers and additives be excluded. Many of the currently prepared foods, particularly fruits and vegetables, have added cereals to increase their bulk, homogeneity and ease of preparation. Parents must therefore be instructed to read

TABLE 2. Cereal-Milk-Egg Elimination Diet for Child over Two Years*

The following foods are permitted:

Vegetables
White potato
Sweet potato or yam
Lettuce
Spinach and chard
Carrots
Artichokes
Tomato and squash
Asparagus
Peas and string beans
Lima beans

Fruit
As desired

Meat, Fish, Poultry
As desired, except that hens and hen turkeys must be avoided

Soups
All clear soups

Fats
Soy bean oil
Bacon fat
Lard

Desserts
Gelatin or tapioca with fruit juice
Cakes or cookies made from arrowroot, soy bean flour or potato starch

Beverages
Tea, coffee, carbonated beverages (except for cola drinks), fruit juices, nectars, soy bean formulas, vegetable base liquids (Coffee Rich, etc.)

Sweets
Maple or cane sugar syrup
Sugar
Honey
Molasses
Jam
Jelly

Seasonings
Salt
Vinegar (white)
Vanilla

Breads
Only those made from arrowroot, soybean flour or potato starch

Vitamins
Synthetic preparation (Tri-Vi-Sol, etc.)

Note: Avoid foods with "concealed" cereal grains, e.g., meat loaves, canned-meat dishes, frankfurters, beer and ale, commercial salad dressings, food prepared with bread and cracker crumbs and baking powder. Use water-pack or dietetic canned fruits.

Comment: More detailed menus with additional recipes and directions for the preparation and use of these diets are published elsewhere: Department of Dietetics, University of Michigan; Dietary Department of Massachusetts General Hospital, Nutrition Division, Department of National Health and Welfare, Ottawa, Ontario, Canada.

Absolute adherence to the diet is imperative. If undesirable weight loss occurs, more of the prescribed carbohydrates, sugar, fats and oils must be taken.

* Modified from Rowe.

labels. If "pure" foods are unobtainable commercially, parents should be taught how to prepare these foods at home. Various mechanical grinders and blenders are now available for this purpose.

In the newborn or in early infancy, cow's milk protein (especially β-lactoglobulin) is by far the most common food allergen. The most suitable substitute is breast milk; if this is not available, one of the soy bean formulas may be used. Though a few patients are able to tolerate heat-modified cow's milk (evaporated or powdered), the majority of infants do best when a complete milk substitute is used. Presumably these patients are intolerant to the heat-stable protein fractions, of which casein is the most notable. Unfortunately, gallons of soy bean milk have been fed infants without critically appraising the need for this type of feeding. Many of these patients have nonatopic gastrointestinal symptoms, usually of functional origin (spitting, regurgitation, colic, irritability).

Prior to the formula revision of the currently available soy bean substitute feedings, a variety of complications had been reported to occur with their prolonged feeding, including gastrointestinal upset with napkin contact and monilial dermatitis (disturbances of intestinal bacterial flora? superinfection?), avitaminosis (vitamin A), hypoproteinemia, iodide-deficient goiter and pseudotumor cerebri. Fortunately the newer preparations are now more elegantly prepared and resemble milk not only in its quantitative distribution of carbohydrate, fat, protein, vitamins and minerals, but in color as well.

In the older child presenting the malabsorption syndrome presumed to be of allergic origin, cow's milk and wheat appear to be frequent offenders. One or the other or both may be implicated as causal allergens. Immunologic data suggest a possible antigenicity between these two proteins, and it is possible that initial sensitization with cow's milk may potentiate gluten hypersensitivity and lead to a pattern of absorptive disorders (D-xylose, fat and so forth). Usually rigorous dietary exclusion is required and may extend over a prolonged period of time. If the child refuses or is unable to take a cow's milk substitute, a daily calcium and mineral supplement should be prescribed.

Following the elimination of a food allergen from the diet of an infant or child, a period of time must elapse before tolerance to this particular food is established. Usually these intervals are variable, extending from a few weeks in some instances to several years in other patients. How tolerance is brought about is uncertain and cannot be identified with any immunologic phenomenon. Occasionally in the older patient the shock organ may change; for example, respiratory symptoms may appear instead of gastrointestinal complaints after ingestion of the offending food or allergen. In a few children, particularly those with exquisite sensitivity to egg, peanut, fish or buckwheat, tolerance rarely occurs. Efforts have been made to desensitize such patients, using a graduated feeding program whereby the offending food is initially introduced in an extremely dilute mixture and eventually fed to the child in its natural state after cautious increases in its concentration. Many programs have been designed for this purpose. Other approaches to desensitization have included the use of propeptans (specific digestive products of the causal foods, based upon the phenomenon of antianaphylaxis); and hyposensitization with extracts of the food allergen, either by injection or sublingual feeding. These latter measures not only appear to have little clinical value but may even lead to untoward reactions.

Drug therapy of allergic gastrointestinal disease is usually employed for symptomatic relief or as a supportive measure until an etiologic diagnosis is made. Antihistamines, antispasmodics, sedatives, opiates and corticosteroids have all been used at one time or another, depending upon the symptomatic needs of the patient. In the child with the allergic malabsorption syndrome, the sulfonamides may be extremely useful when bowel control (diarrhea) is lost as a consequence of respiratory infection, perhaps because they stabilize intestinal bacterial flora. In a few patients with ulcerative colitis or protein-losing enteropathy, presumably of allergic origin, the corticosteroids have also been used for prolonged periods until the causative allergens have been found. With eczematous and contact dermatitis of the lips, oral mucosa, anus and rectum, topical steroids prepared in an adherent base have proved most beneficial (Kenalog in Orobase). Disodium cromoglycate, one of the newer antiasthmatic drugs, has also been used in infants intolerant to milk protein, and if substantiated by further trials may provide a new chemotherapeutic tool in the management of gastrointestinal allergy.

Prophylaxis must also be considered in the treatment of allergic gastrointestinal disease. From the studies of Glaser and of Johnstone, evidence suggests that the exclusion of cow's milk, egg and wheat-containing foods from the diet of infants with an allergic family background for the first six to nine months of life will significantly lessen the incidence of asthma, perennial allergic rhinitis and other allergic diatheses in later childhood.

References

Anderson, L. B., et al.: Melon and Banana Sensitivity Coincident with Ragweed Pollenosis. *J. Allergy,* 45:310, 1970.

Goldstein, G. B., and Heiner, D. C.: Clinical and Immunological Prospectives in Food Hypersensitivity. *J. Allergy,* 46:270, 1970.

Contact Dermatitis

DOUGLAS E. JOHNSTONE, M.D.

The method of treatment of contact dermatitis in children depends on whether the eruption is due to a *primary irritant,* such as detergents, soap, foods, wool, urine, chemicals or a mechanical abrasion, or whether it is due to a *delayed type cellular hypersensitivity* following repeated contact with plant oleoresins (poison ivy, poison oak, poison sumac, ragweed, tomato plant, goldenrod or other garden weeds), rubber constituents, nickel, dyes, formaldehyde, mercury compounds or other chemicals. Success in treatment may also depend upon recognition of the mode of transmission of the contactant. It may come in obvious direct contact, or it may be delivered indirectly by wind-borne smoke or the fur of a favorite pet to a bed- or chair-bound patient. A careful history is mandatory. Intense itching and vesiculation suggest a diagnosis of the hypersensitivity type of dermatitis rather than a primary irritant rash.

Primary irritant dermatitis usually responds to the removal of the irritant and rest of the skin involved. Expose the area of rash to the air as often as practical. If the lesions are weeping, it is helpful to use baths of Aveeno or Linit starch (1 to 2 cupfuls added to a half tub of water after dissolving in a pan of water). If sedation seems indicated, give diphenhydramine hydrochloride (Benadryl), 4 to 5 mg. per kilogram of body weight per day orally in three or four doses. In the subacute phase use local applications of Desitin ointment (a mixture of Lassar's paste and cod liver oil) three times a day. If the eruption persists, one should consider the possibility of a secondary infection with bacteria or *Candida albicans.* (See Bacterial Infections of the Skin and Fungous Infections.)

Treatment of the hypersensitivity type of contact dermatitis requires more individual care according to the stage of dermatitis present.

Individualize treatment and maintain good communication with the patient's parent by phone and repeat personal reevaluations of the patient's progress until the lesions have completely healed. Be sure that the patient and parent know exactly what is expected of them. Give explicit directions in writing.

Protect areas of dermatitis from excessive heat, cold, wind, moisture, sunlight and abrasion.

Relieve itching to prevent scratching and subsequent scarring or secondary infection. Choose drugs with a large margin of safety such as diphenhydramine (Benadryl) and hydroxyzine (Atarax). For diphenhydramine hydrochloride the dosage is 4 to 6 mg. per kilogram of body weight per day orally in three or four divided doses. (Maximal daily dose is 100 mg.) For hydroxyzine hydrochloride the dosage is 1 to 3 mg. per kilogram of body weight per day orally in three divided doses.

In cases of extreme discomfort and intense itching, the dose of either of these drugs may be gradually increased up to twice the previously mentioned doses or to the point of drowsiness, whichever dose is smaller. Also, aspirin (65 mg. or 1 grain per year of age every 4 to 6 hours, as needed) is antipruritic. (Maximal dose is 10 grains.)

Promptly treat secondary infection with systemic antibiotics. Secondary infection usually manifests itself by an increase in local tenderness with or without a purulent exudate. Early recognition and treatment is mandatory to prevent sepsis, pyarthrosis and acute glomerulonephritis. Antibiotics should be chosen by the results of culture and sensitivity determinations. They should be given systemically rather than applied locally. When laboratory facilities are not available, prescribe dicloxacillin, 12.5 mg. per kilogram of body weight per day by mouth in four doses. For children suspected of penicillin sensitivity, give erythromycin, 40 mg. per kilogram of body weight per day by mouth in four doses.

Local treatment in the acute phase should include cooling of the skin and removal of crusts and scales as well as residuals of previous medication. Cooling and drying of the skin can be accomplished by evaporation of wet dressings. Thoroughly moisten two or three layers of loosely applied gauze with one of the following:

Burow's solution: Dissolve one Domeboro tablet or packet in 1 quart of cool water.

Potassium permanganate: Dissolve one crushed 65-mg. tablet in one quart of cool water.

Saline: Add one level teaspoonful of table salt to 1 pint of water.

Additional methods of cooling and soothing include use of oatmeal baths (add one cupful of Aveeno to half a tub of tepid water; let the solution dry on the patient's skin after soaking).

In the subacute phase of contact dermatitis, drying is no longer desirable. Liquid emulsions, such as Lubriderm Lotion, are helpful. Local application of a cream containing triamcinolone or fluocinolone, such as Aristocort; Synalar or Cordran, is very useful. Apply it thinly at least four times a day until lesions are nearly healed.

In patients with severe manifestations of contact dermatitis, systemic corticosteroid therapy may be used when the measures mentioned do not control the symptoms satisfactorily. For the first two to three days prescribe 20 to 30 mg. of prednisone per day by mouth divided into three doses given at meal time. As soon as the itching and inflammation begin to subside, the dose is gradually reduced over a period of 10 to 15 days. Other local measures described may be continued during the steroid withdrawal period. Be sure to keep the patient under close observation and warn the parents of the dangers of steroid medications.

What you *do not do* may be as important as what you do to treat patients with contact dermatitis.

Do not irritate the skin. During the acute phase of the eruption, avoid irritating medications. Ointments macerate acutely inflamed skin and intertriginous or hairy areas. Wool and soap must be avoided. Before applying a cream or an ointment to a large affected area, one should first perform a "use test," i.e., apply the medication to an area the size of a dime and watch for several hours for signs of primary irritation, before using it on a larger area.

Do not use local agents capable of sensitizing the skin. Dermatologic preparations of sulfonamides, penicillin, thimerosol (Merthiolate), dyes, neomycin, local anesthetics and antihistamines can sensitize the patient so that he may never again be able to take these agents.

Do not permit swimming, body contact sports or contact with persons infected with bacterial infections or viruses such as herpes simplex or cowpox.

Hospitalization is occasionally required if the dermatitis is widespread. All persons who may come in contact with the infant hospitalized for contact dermatitis (medical personnel, housekeeping persons and visitors) should be screened for obvious signs of contagious bacterial or viral infections before being permitted to enter the patient's room.

Drug Allergy

BERNARD A. BERMAN, M.D.

Adverse reactions to drugs may occur on an immunologic as well as on a nonimmune basis. The incidence of such reactions is increasing for a variety of reasons, but mostly because of increased awareness of, and a proliferation of, newer and more complex pharmacologic agents, and an indiscriminate use of drugs. Nonimmune reactions, which are often difficult to distinguish from allergic responses, include intolerance, overdose, side effects, idiosyncrasy and secondary effects.

Allergic reactions to drugs result from sensitization to the drug or, more often, from one or more of its degradation products. This explains why with few exceptions, scratch and intradermal tests with a suspect drug are unreliable: the precise degradation or breakdown products responsible for sensitization are usually unavailable for testing.

Not only are the clinical expressions of drug allergies diverse, but the immune response is also heterogeneous. A specific drug, with multiple antigenic determinants, can incite a variety of immune phenomena, involving complement, many classes of immunoglobulins, chemical mediators and so forth. To bring some order to what appears to be a broad but unrelated spectrum of immune and clinical response, Gell and Coombs designed a classification that makes clear how a single drug can induce, under appropriate circumstances, one or multiple dissimilar clinical and immune reactions.

Type I. Type I involves humoral antibodies and is IgE-dependent. Symptoms occur as a consequence of antigen-antibody reactions releasing pharmacologically active substances, including histamine. Urticaria, angioedema, rhinorrhea, asthma and anaphylaxis are included in type I reactions. The cutaneous expression of drug allergy—urticaria—occurs far more often than do respiratory symptoms. Both scratch and intradermal skin tests are available, chiefly for type I reactions.

Type II. This is a cytotoxic response. The antibody (IgG and/or IgM) combines with an antigen on the surface of the red blood cell and, in the presence of complement, hemolysis occurs. This reaction is noted with penicillin or with any drug having an affinity for red blood cells.

Type III. When a precipitating antibody (IgG), with complement available, combines with an antigen and forms microprecipitates, (toxic complexes) surrounding and in the walls of small blood vessels, as well as in the basement membrane, tissue-damaging enzymes are released. The Arthus phenomenon, an example of type III reaction, is manifested clinically by some aspects of serum sickness. Hypersensitivity pneumonitis is another expression of type III reaction.

Type IV. Type IV delayed reactions, of which the tuberculin tests and contact dermatitis are classic examples, occur frequently. Unlike type I reactions, which result from humoral antibodies, type IV reactions are cell-mediated. The antigen combines with sensitized lymphoid cells, releasing active substances responsible for tissue injury to the host.

Aphorisms Relating to Drug Allergy

1. Patients who react to one drug are more likely to react to others.
2. Before prescribing any drug, obtain as precise a history as possible of the patient's prior experience with the drug.
3. If a choice is available between an oral or systemically administered drug, always choose the oral route.
4. Always check the exact composition of the drug, particularly if the prescription is a combination of drugs. The *Physician's Desk Reference* is an excellent source of reference; e.g., a patient known to be aspirin-sensitive had an explosive episode of urticaria after receiving Percodan-Demi (contains aspirin).
5. The incidence of drug allergy is greater in adults than children.
6. Always stop a drug at the first sign of an adverse reaction. Patients and/or parents should be given such instructions before prescribing the medication. For example, a patient with atopic dermatitis, treated with Mycolog, had a flare-up of rash. Despite worsening of eruption, topical medicament was applied more frequently and vigorously. Four days later, the drug was stopped. Patch testing revealed sensitivity to a specific perfume used in the manufacture of Mycolog.
7. Intermittent administration of drugs is more likely to result in an allergic reaction.

8. Reactions generally do not occur on initial exposure. Usually a latent period exists prior to reaction. An exception to this is illustrated by reactions provoked by chemically related drugs. For example, a patient with known sensitivity to procaine received a sulfa preparation, which is biologically related to procaine, and promptly developed an urticarial reaction.

9. A thorough history and sound clinical judgment still remain the most important methods for diagnosis of penicillin allergy. Major and minor determinants, degradation byproducts of penicillin, both suitable and necessary for testing, are as yet not commercially available.

10. Patch testing, useful for type IV reactions, and expressed clinically as contact dermatitis, is a common procedure which is useful and safe, only if it is performed and interpreted correctly.

11. Patients with proved drug sensitivity should wear a bracelet or other conspicuous emblem detailing their specific sensitivities. Medic-Alert Foundation, P. O. Box 1009, Turlock, California, provides this type of emblem.

12. Aspirin is probably the most widely used and abused medication in the United States. Aspirin sensitivity, probably not mediated by immune mechanisms, is a source of concern because it is seen with increasing frequency. Acetaminophen, available as Dularin, Tylenol and Valadol, is a suitable substitute and should be used in preference to aspirin, unless the latter is clearly needed. The dose is the same as for aspirin. Allergic reactions to acetaminophen are rarely encountered, gastric irritation is minimal or absent and the unusual bleeding tendencies seen with aspirin have not been described when acetaminophen is given in recommended dosage.

13. Corticosteroid hormones are not useful for immediate effect in severe drug allergic reactions (type I). Epinephrine and antihistaminics are needed for immediate effect, and corticosteroid hormones should be included only if it is anticipated that a beneficial response is required 4 to 24 hours later.

Treatment. Obviously, in the presence of any untoward or unanticipated response, any drug should be stopped immediately. For specific treatment, only those therapeutic agents, useful in managing type I mediate reactions, will be discussed.

For the itching of urticaria, resort to antihistaminics. It is impossible to anticipate reactions to antihistamines, because each patient varies considerably in side effects and clinical response. Excitability is often encountered and is a reason for discontinuing these agents. Soporific effects need not dictate abandonment of the drug, because this effect is useful at bedtime to provide a restful sleep in an otherwise unhappy, pruritic child. The choice of the best antihistaminic for a particular patient is often made after several have been tried. Therefore, any of the following can be used as directed, but the dosage may have to be lowered or increased, according to the requirements of the patient: Benadryl and Phenergan are excellent choices for night-time use, since they produce not only an antipruritic response but also a fairly strong sedative and, at times, a soporific effect. For a child two to five years of age, give 2 to 4 teaspoonfuls of Benadryl or, alternatively, ½ to 1 teaspoonful of Phenergan Fortis. For older children, 50-mg. doses of Benadryl are available. For day-time, any one of the following can be used in a dose of ½ (1 teaspoonful) or one tablet for morning and midafternoon, saving Benadryl and/or Phenergan for bedtime: Chlor-Trimeton, Dimetane, Triaminic and Periactin.

Acetaminophen (Dularin, Tylenol or Valadol), in usual doses for children, is another antipruritic drug which can be administered with an antihistaminic to control itching.

Ataractic agents are occasionally beneficial in the treatment of itching disorders because of their additional antihistaminic effect. Atarax, 1 teaspoonful three times a day for younger children, or a 10- to 25-mg. tablet three times a day for older children, can be helpful.

As a night-time substitute for antihistamines and particularly when sedation is desirable, use chloral hydrate (Noctec), 1 to 2 teaspoonfuls. Phenobarbital more often than not stimulates the child.

Ephedrine, 12 to 24 mg. orally, is often useful when combined with an antihistaminic agent.

Epinephrine, with vasoconstrictive as well as bronchodilator activity, is the recommended drug of choice for acute type I conditions, the initial dose varying according to the severity of the reaction. For those with milder symptoms, start with 0.1 to 0.15 ml. subcutaneously and repeat as frequently as needed, up to tolerance. For others with more severe involvement, 0.20 ml. given subcutaneously is the initial dose; this is repeated usually once or twice at 15-minute intervals.

Refer to Bronchial Asthma for the choice and dose of delta-1 corticosteroid hormones.

For the management of anaphylaxis, see page 718.

Hypersensitivity to Physical Factors

ALAN A. WANDERER, M.D.

Various physical factors such as cold, heat, pressure and light can induce hypersensitivity-like reactions, such as urticaria and angioedema. Physical allergy is the commonly accepted medical nomenclature used to describe this group of reactions, but the term is considered somewhat inaccurate since immunologic mechanisms have been suggested in only a few of the disorders, i.e., acquired cold urticaria and dermographism.

The most common clinical entities included in this classification are (1) acquired cold urticaria: nonfamilial cold sensitivity is manifested in all age groups and is characterized by the development of local or generalized urticaria after cold exposure; (2) heat (cholinergic) urticaria: development of hives after activities that increase body temperature, i.e., emotional stress or exercise; and (3) dermographism: unique pressure sensitivity that can induce urtication. Acquired cold urticaria is the least benign of the group, since 40 to 50 per cent of these patients will experience systemic symptoms, such as nausea, vomiting, tachycardia, angioedema and syncope. The life-threatening aspects of cold urticaria are obvious for the patient who may develop systemic symptoms while swimming.

Avoidance of Physical Factors Inducing Symptoms. It is very important for the patient with a physical allergy to be made aware of his diagnosis so that he may attempt to avoid the circumstances which induce symptoms. In particular, patients with acquired cold urticaria should be forewarned of the dangers of swimming. The very sensitive cold urticaria patient may have to move from cold climates if his symptoms are severe and frequent. Individuals with light urticaria may also develop systemic symptoms, and thus should try to avoid prolonged exposure to sunlight and other light sources which emit wavelengths (2800 to 5000 Å) of light that can induce their symptoms. Cholinergic (heat) urticaria is often induced after increased body heat production, such as after exercise. Patients can often reduce the intensity of their symptoms by minimizing these physical activities.

Pharmacologic Therapy. Recent clinical studies indicate that acquired cold urticaria can be effectively suppressed with cyproheptadine hydrochloride (Periactin). This compound can suppress the induction of urticaria and angioedema after prolonged exposure to cold. The dosage should be titrated according to the patient's weight, the side effects of the drug (appetite stimulation and occasional mild sedation) and the degree of cold sensitivity. The amount recommended may vary between 2 to 4 mg. orally four times a day. The individual daily dose of Periactin should, not exceed 0.5 mg. per kilogram per day. Hydroxyzine hydrochloride (Vistaril, Atarax) is another drug which may be effective in the treatment of cold, light or heat sensitivity. Dosages of 10 to 25 mg. orally four times a day may be recommended. The usual children's dose (under six years) is 50 mg. daily in divided doses. For the patient with cholinergic urticaria which develops after vigorous exercise, a single dose of hydroxyzine hydrochloride taken 2 to 3 hours before the planned physical activity may be all that is required to suppress the symptoms. Other antihistamine drugs, such as diphenhydramine hydrochloride (Benadryl), 1.5 mg. per kilogram of body weight orally every 6 hours, and chlorpheniramine maleate (Chlor-Trimeton), 0.1 mg. per kilogram orally every 6 hours, may be used in the treatment of physical allergies, but their effectiveness is frequently unsatisfactory. Corticosteroids appear to be ineffective in the management of these disorders. Patients with severe light sensitivity may find it impractical to avoid all light sources that might induce their symptoms. Light screening preparations are available for topical application. Two preparations are recommended for protection against light energy sources: Pabafilm for light wavelengths below 3200 Å, and Uval for wavelengths above 3200 Å.

Since life-threatening angioedema and systemic reactions can occur in patients with physical allergies, the treatment is the same as in other similar medical emergencies. Aqueous epinephrine 1:1000 (0.1 to 0.4 ml.) should be administered subcutaneously or intramuscularly for these situations. If appropriate, further efforts should be made to establish an airway and maintain adequate blood pressure.

Anaphylaxis

SHELDON C. SIEGEL, M.D.

Anaphylaxis is a hypersensitivity reaction induced in man by the administration of an antigen to which the individual is specifically hypersensitive. Fundamentally, the pathophysiology consists in increased capillary permeability and smooth muscle contraction, which in man results in a variable clinical picture. Usually the onset is unexpected and occurs within seconds to minutes after exposure to the offending agent. Generally anaphylactic reactions which occur abruptly and precipitously are the most severe and often end fatally. In those reactions which are not immediately fatal, the severity of the anaphylaxis may vary from nausea and mild urticaria to severe respiratory embarrassment and shock.

Management. The key to successful management of anaphylactic reactions is the speed with which the physician is prepared to institute appropriate therapy. Since seconds may count, the necessary drugs and equipment must be accessible at a moment's notice in an emergency kit. The following drugs and equipment are suggested for the contents of such a kit:

I. Drugs
   A. Epinephrine hydrochloride solution 1:1000, 1-ml. ampules or 30-ml. vials
   B. Injectable antihistamine—e.g.:
      1. Diphenhydramine (Benadryl), 10-ml. vials (10 mg. per ml.) or 1-ml. ampule (50 mg. per ml.)
      2. Chlorpheniramine maleate (Chlor-Trimeton), 1-ml. ampule or 10-ml. vial (10 mg. per ml.)
   C. Injectable aminophylline, 250 mg. in 10-ml. ampules
   D. Water-soluble corticosteroid esters—e.g.:
      1. Hydrocortisone sodium succinate (Solu-Cortef), 100 mg. per vial
      2. Hydrocortisone phosphate injectable (Hydrocortone), 2- and 10-ml. vials (50 mg. per ml.)
      3. Dexamethasone sodium phosphate, 1- and 5-ml. vials (4 mg. per ml.)
   E. Injectable adrenergic agents
      1. Metaraminol bitartrate (Aramine), ampules or vials (10 mg. per ml. or 10-ml.)
      2. Levarterenol bitartrate (Levophed), 4-ml. ampules (2 mg. per ml.)
      3. Isoproterenol HCl, 1- and 5-ml. ampules (1:5000 solution, 0.2 mg. per ml.)
   F. Parenteral fluids
      1. Five per cent dextrose in normal saline
      2. Five per cent dextrose
      3. Normal salt-poor serum albumin, 20-ml. vials
   G. Injectable anticonvulsant drugs—e.g.:
      1. Amobarbital sodium (Amytal), 65-mg. ampules
      2. Diazepam (Valium), 2- and 10-ml. ampules (5 mg. per ml.)
   H. Sodium bicarbonate 50-ml. ampules (0.9 mEq. per ml.)

II. Equipment
   A. Tourniquets
   B. Intravenous infusion tubing
   C. Assorted sterile syringes and needles
   D. Several sizes of airways and endotracheal tubes for children
   E. Lifesaving tube
   F. Ambu bag
   G. Aspirator or suction bulb
   H. Surgical instruments for venesection
      1. Scalpel
      2. Hemostats
      3. Suture material

In addition to the kit, oxygen should be available in the immediate vicinity. Ideally, a suction machine and positive pressure resuscitation apparatus should also be nearby.

At the first sign of an impending anaphylactic reaction, the following drugs should be promptly administered and the described additional measures taken as indicated:

Epinephrine 1:1000, 0.3 to 0.5 ml., should be administered either subcutaneously or intramuscularly. If no response is noted within 5 minutes, the dose may be repeated. In the event of severe shock with vascular collapse, 1 ml. of 1:1000 epinephrine diluted in 10 ml. of saline solution should be administered by slow intravenous injection. An intravenous infusion should be started at the same time so that subsequent medications can be rapidly administered by the intravenous route.

If the anaphylaxis has been caused by a therapeutic agent injected into an extremity, a tourniquet should be placed proximal to the site to delay absorption, and an additional 0.25 ml. of epinephrine injected directly into the previous injection site.

The administration of epinephrine should be followed immediately by an intramuscular or intravenous injection of an antihistaminic such as diphenhydramine (Benadryl). The dose for an older child should be comparable to that for an adult, 50 mg.; for an infant or younger child, use 1 mg. per kilogram, not exceeding 50 mg. per dose or 150 mg. per day.

When bronchospasm develops despite the administration of epinephrine, aminophylline should be slowly administered intravenously in a dose of 4 mg. per kilogram of body weight.

Oxygen administered promptly will minimize the development of hypoxia, which may in itself contribute to vascular collapse and cerebral edema. Vigilance must be kept at all times to make certain the patient has adequate ventilation. Excess secretions should be removed by suction. If the airway becomes completely obstructed by angioedema, intubation or tracheostomy may be necessary.

If cardiovascular collapse ensues, measures

to support blood pressure and circulation are mandatory. Priority should be given to restoration of blood volume, especially when massive urticaria and angioedema have developed. This can be best accomplished by the intravenous administration of a colloid such as 5 per cent serum albumin. In any prolonged episode of anaphylactic shock, measurement of central venous pressure becomes virtually a necessity to evaluate properly the adequacy of volume replacement. When the central venous pressure is low (less than 5 cm. water) additional crystalloid and colloid fluids are required. Central venous pressure greater than 10 cm. of water suggests myocardial insufficiency. These patients may be helped by the intravenous administration of isoproterenol hydrochloride (Isuprel), 1 mg. diluted in 500 ml. of 5 per cent dextrose infused at a rate of 1 to 2 ml. per minute (1 to 4 micrograms per minute), depending on response. Persistence of hypotension and low central venous pressure (despite adequate fluid replacement) may necessitate the use of a vasopressor agent such as metaraminol, 0.4 mg. per kilogram, diluted in 500 ml. of crystalloid fluid and administered slowly intravenously by drip. In the event of cardiorespiratory arrest, cardiac massage and artificial respiration are the only recourse.

Because of their slow onset of action, the corticosteroids should be administered only after the "front line" therapy has been instituted. Although these agents have profound beneficial effects on most hypersensitivity reactions, reliance on them in the acute phase of anaphylactic and bronchospastic reactions to the exclusion of the rapidly acting drugs could be disastrous. When utilized for these acute reactions, the water-soluble steroid esters (100 to 200 mg. of hydrocortisone phosphate [Hydrocortone] or its equivalent) injected intravenously are preferable. Since the development of angioedema may be delayed for several hours, it is important to continue corticosteroids for at least two days after the onset of the reaction. When the acute reaction has subsided, prednisone, 2 mg. per kilogram, should be given in divided doses; the dose should generally not be less than 20 mg. a day for infants, nor usually exceed 60 mg. a day in older children.

Prevention. Anaphylactic reactions are to a great extent iatrogenic and in many instances can be prevented by adhering to the following principles of prophylaxis.

Foremost in the measures to prevent anaphylactic (and other drug) reactions is the scrupulous avoidance of unnecessary drugs. Antibiotics, especially penicillin, are the most common causes of these reactions. They deserve special scrutiny, since it has been estimated that 95 per cent of these drugs are administered without appropriate indications.

Foreign serum antitoxins are also frequent offenders. Their administration can be greatly curtailed by (1) mass primary immunization (especially to tetanus, pertussis and diphtheria) with periodic booster doses of the appropriate antigens; (2) substitution of foreign serums with human hyperimmune globulins (Cutter or Hyland Laboratories) when passive immunization becomes mandatory.

Of prime importance is the simple measure of obtaining a detailed history from patients before the administration of any proposed therapeutic or diagnostic agents. Special emphasis should be placed on (1) possible previous adverse reactions, especially to the agents in question, and (2) presence of atopic allergies (allergic rhinitis, atopic dermatitis or bronchial asthma) in the patient or his family. Since there are suggestive data that anaphylactic reactions occur 3 to 10 times more often in atopic persons than in "normals," extreme caution and conservatism are warranted in these subjects. A drug, biologic product or foreign serum should never be administered when a history of possible reaction has been elicited, except under extenuating circumstances when they might be necessary to save the patient's life. Attempts to corroborate a positive history or to "prove" an allergic reaction by a small test dose are extremely dangerous and are to be condemned.

Preliminary testing with potential anaphylactic agents is in general unreliable, though in certain specific cases, such as biologic products, penicillin and foreign serums, it may provide valuable information. Nevertheless, a negative scratch, intradermal or conjunctival test result in no way assures against an anaphylactic reaction. A positive result, on the other hand, strongly suggests its likelihood. Caution should be taken in performing any of these procedures, since the tests themselves may produce anaphylactic reactions. A scratch test should usually be performed and interpreted as negative before doing intradermal testing. Appropriate dilutions of antigens should also be used. These will vary with the type of preparation being tested (e.g., foreign serums should be diluted to at least 1:100, and bee antigen should be diluted to 1:1,000,000,000 as the initial test dose).

As yet, an accurate, easily performed screening test to detect individual reactions to drugs has not been developed. Nevertheless, skin testing with degradation products of penicillin has been shown to have predictive value in sorting out potential anaphylactic reactors to penicillin. Both the major haptenic group [P.P.L. (benzylopenicilloyl combined with polymers of lycine—penicilloyl-polylysine)] and mixtures of the minor haptenic groups [M.D.M. (benzylpenicillin, sodium benzylpenicilloate and sodium benzylpenilloate)] should be used in testing. Positive reactions to the M.D.M. are more likely to predict anaphylactic sensitivity. Although neither of these penicillin antigens is available commercially, dilution of benzylpenicillin to 1000 units with 0.1 normal concentration of sodium hydroxide or alkaline-buffered saline and kept at room temperature for two weeks before use is thought by some authorities to produce the minor determinant antigens. It should be kept in mind that skin tests with either the "major" or "minor" antigens of penicillin will *not* predict other late allergic reactions, including the morbilliform rashes, serum sickness, hemolytic anemias and agranulocytosis.

Other in vitro screening procedures for detecting anaphylactic sensitivities, such as hemagglutination, basophil degranulation tests, histamine release of leukocytes, lymphocyte transformation tests and macrophage migration inhibition tests, are technically difficult to perform and impractical for clinical use. Because the results of these latter tests are also not completely dependable, they should be considered in the same light as skin test results, i.e., a negative test does not rule out a potential reaction, but a positive one suggests its likelihood.

Since reactions following the oral administration of drugs are usually less frequent and less severe than those following parenteral administration, it is best to use the oral route whenever possible. Remember, however, that in highly sensitive persons even the oral administration of drugs may result in severe reactions.

On rare occasions, when a foreign serum, biologic product or drug is mandatory for saving a patient's life, and another suitable preparation cannot be substituted, rapid desensitization may be warranted. The technique is basically the same as other desensitization procedures. The procedure is extremely hazardous, and should always be performed in a hospital by a physician prepared to treat anaphylaxis. Although "coverage" with the previously described antianaphylactic drugs might be helpful in preventing minor systemic reactions, they will not prevent a severe reaction, and reliance on these agents alone could lead to disastrous results. Because the details of the technique of desensitization might vary with the therapeutic agent in question and the degree of sensitivity of the patient, the following schedules for desensitization to penicillin are presented only as rough guides.

A. Penicillin desensitization

1. The patient is "covered" with the antianaphylactic drugs: cortisol antihistaminics and epinephrine as described for serum desensitization.
2. Increasing quantities of the desired crystalline penicillin are then administered intramuscularly in an extremity (at a site where a tourniquet could be placed proximally in the event of a systemic reaction) every 30 minutes as indicated in the following schedule:

DOSE NUMBER	AMOUNT OF PENICILLIN IN UNITS
1	10
2	100
3	1000
4	10,000
5	100,000
6	1,000,000

In order to prevent death from anaphylaxis, it is important that a physician be in attendance at the time of the reaction. For this reason, all patients receiving medications parenterally should remain under observation in the physician's office or clinic at least 15 to 20 minutes after the injection. Since most anaphylactic reactions have their onset within this period, this measure will ensure prompt institution of appropriate therapy.

21

Accidents and Emergencies

Food Poisoning

ALLEN W. MATHIES, Jr., M.D., Ph.D.

Food poisoning is caused by the ingestion of preformed toxins of microorganisms occurring in food or food products. The most common types are as follows:

STAPHYLOCOCCAL FOOD POISONING

Common sources—meat, milk, bakery products
Onset of symptoms—within 6 hours
Usual symptoms—salivation, nausea, vomiting, abdominal cramps

CLOSTRIDIUM PERFRINGENS FOOD POISONING

Common sources—beef, poultry
Onset of symptoms—about 12 hours
Usual symptoms—nausea, diarrhea

BOTULISM

Common sources—home-processed string beans, meat, olives, chili peppers (types A and B), canned seafood (type E)
Onset of symptoms—20 to 36 hours
Usual symptoms—diplopia, difficulty swallowing, weakness, dizziness, paralysis

Management. General. Most cases of staphylococcal and clostridial food poisoning are mild and self-limited. The vomiting and diarrhea are actually useful in eliminating the ingested toxin. Food and milk should be withheld while nausea and vomiting are present; however, weak tea, broth and carbonated beverages may be tolerated. In more severe cases, parenteral fluid and electrolyte therapy may be needed to replace losses. Nausea and vomiting may be controlled by the use of trimethobenzamide (Tigan) rectal suppositories, 100 mg. for a patient 15 kilograms or less, and 200 mg. for a patient 15 to 40 kilograms; or by the use of prochlorperazine (Compazine)* rectal suppositories, 2.5 to 5 mg. (Prochlorperazine is not recommended in children under 10 kilograms; in such children, parenteral therapy is almost always necessary.) If parenteral medication is needed, prochlorperazine, 0.12 mg. per kilogram intramuscularly, usually controls the symptoms. These medications can be repeated every 4 hours if necessary. Prochlorperazine occasionally causes alarming extrapyramidal signs and symptoms. This appears to be an idiosyncratic reaction and is not dose-related. Intravenous diphenhydramine (Benadryl), 50 mg., rapidly relieves the symptomatology.

Attempts to control diarrhea should be withheld until the nausea and vomiting have disappeared. Abdominal cramps occasionally may be severe enough to warrant the use of narcotics. Sedation may be accomplished with codeine sulfate, 5 mg. per kilogram orally or subcutaneously every 6 hours; meperidine hydrochloride, 1.5 mg. per kilogram orally or intramuscularly every 4 to 6 hours; or morphine sulfate, 0.1 to 0.2 mg. per kilogram orally or subcutaneously. Antibiotics are not indicated.

Specific. Specific antisera are available for treatment of botulism and may be particularly helpful if given within a few hours after onset of symptomatology. Bivalent botulinus antitoxin for types A and B is available from Lederle Laboratories. Type E monovalent an-

* Manufacturer's precaution: Prochlorperazine (Compazine) is not recommended for children under 20 pounds or under two years of age.

titoxin is available through the Center for Disease Control in Atlanta, Georgia. The antitoxin is of equine origin, and appropriate skin tests to determine sensitivity to horse serum must be carried out prior to administration. The usual dose of antitoxin varies between 10,000 and 50,000 units given intravenously.

Supportive measures are of tremendous importance in the care of the patient with botulism. Parenteral fluids must be administered and particular attention must be paid to the maintenance of an adequate airway. Tracheostomy is indicated if the respiratory muscles and pharyngeal muscles are so involved that they cause pooling of secretions. Assisted ventilation, either in a tank respirator or with a positive pressure machine, may be necessary during the period of maximal muscle involvement.

Acute Poisoning

FREDERICK H. LOVEJOY, Jr., M.D., *and* JOEL J. ALPERT, M.D.

In spite of significant reductions in mortality from many diseases, deaths among children from accidental as well as intentional ingestion of poisonous substances persist. Further, nonfatal ingestions are extremely common, accounting for an estimated 750 to 1000 times the number of total fatal cases, since the majority of accidental childhood poisonings remain symptom-free and unreported. In view of this extraordinarily high attack rate with a low morbidity and even lower mortality, any proposed therapy must be reasonable, and its indications clearly thought through. With this in mind, the principles of management of acute poisoning are as follows:

1. Identification
2. Removal
   a. Mechanical
   b. Chemical
   c. Enhanced excretion
   d. Dialysis
3. Dilution and cathartics
4. Supportive measures
5. General and specific antidotes
6. Treatment for specific and known poisoning
7. Prevention

IDENTIFICATION

Ingestions in children involve those substances commonly available in the home, such as aspirin, tranquilizers, sedatives and common household products (polishes, detergents, bleaches). Low income families are especially vulnerable because of the increased prevalence of lead, narcotic drugs and kerosene in these homes. In most instances the child will be seen or the parent will call for help prior to the onset of symptoms. Generally the ingested product is known. In some cases the nature of the product ingested is not clear or in fact unknown. The physician needs to rapidly ascertain what has been taken, how much has been taken (one swallow in a two- or three-year-old is equal to approximately 4 to 5 ml.) and when the possibly poisonous substance was taken. It is important that the largest estimated amount be used in determining therapy. Further, when more than one child is involved in an ingestion, it should be assumed that each child consumed the total amount ingested and both should be treated. Knowing what the ingestion is not is also helpful. Specifically knowing that a hydrocarbon or a caustic has not been taken and that the child is not comatose or convulsing allows one to then proceed, even in an uncertain situation, to removal.

The physical status of the child is rapidly ascertained over the telephone or by direct physical examination. Useful information includes knowing that the child is alert, and is not comatose, not having seizures and not exhibiting unusual behavior. Important history, indicating a recent ingestion, includes gastrointestinal and neurologic symptoms. Especially valuable in the physical examination are vital signs, eyes, odor of the breath, color of the urine and color of the vomitus. Lacking a specific history of the substance ingested, these parameters can provide clues as to the identity of the ingested substance.

Preserving any vomitus or urine may be helpful in instances of unknown ingestions. Further, it is most important to save the container or bottle from which the ingested material came. Unfortunately, many materials ingested have not been stored in their original containers.

REMOVAL

Removal is the most important aspect of management. If an error is made, it is better to err in the direction of inducing unnecessary emesis, as long as the emetic used is safe and effective.

Mechanical Removal. Mechanical methods include the use of blunt objects to provoke vomiting, and gastric lavage. Spoons, sticks or fingers placed in the posterior pharynx are almost always unsuccessful, although they may be worth a try if no other means are available.

Gastric lavage is effective but has certain disadvantages. It is a traumatic procedure. The patient must come to the hospital prior to removal of the ingested material; this results in a significant loss of time during which removal could have been instituted. Gastric lavage is not useful for removing tablets when the tablets are bigger than the tube. Further, as shown by the failure of complete removal of barium following gastric lavage, liquids are less effectively removed as well. Finally, dilution during the process of lavage may in fact enhance absorption.

Gastric lavage may be reserved for the lethargic patient. The technique is to use the largest tube possible (number 8 to 12 French for a child). The exception to this would be for the removal of hydrocarbons in an obtunded or unconscious patient. In these instances a smaller tube is indicated. All tubes should be well lubricated and should be cooled to ease passage. The patient should be turned on his left side with his head lower than his hips. If the patient is obtunded or comatose, respiratory paralysis with succinylcholine and endotracheal intubation with a cuffed endotracheal tube will protect the trachea during lavage. The passage of the tube via the nares is preferred in the older child. The oral passage is preferred in the younger child. Lavage is performed with half isotonic or isotonic saline (150 to 1500 ml.) until clear. At the time of removal of the tube, an antidote such as charcoal may be left in the stomach. The tube should be pinched during the process of removal to avoid spillage and aspiration of gastric contents.

Chemical Removal. Chemical removal may be accomplished with copper sulfate, apomorphine or ipecac syrup. Copper sulfate is used in Europe as a chemical emetic, but is not used in the United States because (1) it is not usually available and (2) it is toxic if emesis does not occur.

Apomorphine is a safe, fast, effective means of inducing emesis. Its disadvantages include the necessity of coming to the doctor or hospital for therapy, as well as its instability when left unused for an extended period of time. When not in use it should be kept in the dark, and tightly stoppered. It should be checked for discoloration every three to four weeks. It is remarkably effective, however, causing emesis within 2 to 3 minutes in 100 per cent of cases. The dosage for a child is 0.1 mg. per kilogram per dose subcutaneously given once only. Levallorphan (Lorfan),* 0.02 mg. per kilogram per dose, or nalorphine (Nalline), 0.1 mg. per kilogram per dose, may be used to counteract the drug's possible central nervous system depressant effects. Apomorphine's most appropriate use is in those cases in which more rapid emesis is indicated than can be provided by ipecac syrup.

The most effective and safest way of inducing emesis in the home is ipecac syrup (it is the emetic of choice even in the office or the hospital). It will be taken easily by a child and directions for its use can be easily given over the telephone. It may be inexpensively purchased over the counter; no prescription is required. The product has a remarkably long shelf life. When given properly, emesis occurs in 80 to 99 per cent of cases within 20 minutes of administration. Return of the ingested material is estimated to be 90 to 100 per cent. The fluid extract, which is 14 times as concentrated as ipecac syrup, should never be used for emesis. Fortunately, the fluid extract has been removed from the *United States Pharmacopeia*. The dose of ipecac syrup in the child above one year is 15 to 20 ml. (1 tablespoon). This should be followed by 200 ml. of fluid, preferably water, to facilitate examination of the vomited contents. Finally, it is essential that the child be kept active to assure full effectiveness of the drug. Vomiting will occur within 15 to 20 minutes. If it does not, the 15-ml. dosage may be repeated. If the child has not vomited in 30 minutes, no further ipecac should be administered and gastric lavage should be instituted. The ingestion of phenothiazines is not a contraindication to the use of ipecac syrup. In fact, ipecac syrup will be as effective in the face of such an ingestion as in any other situation. In the child over one year of age, 30 ml. or less of ipecac syrup is not cardiotoxic. Further, the present availability of ipecac syrup in 30-ml. amounts will prevent the use of an excessive dose. In the child less than one year of age a dose of 5 to 10 ml. should be used; this dosage may be repeated once.

Charcoal, which is not an emetic, has been recommended widely for use in acute ingestions. It is discussed on page 727. It should never be given if the plan is to give ipecac

* Manufacturer's precaution: Levallorphan tartrate (Lorfan) is for use in treatment of significant narcotic-induced respiratory depression. Lorfan is *ineffective* against respiratory depression due to barbiturates, anesthetics and other non-narcotic agents or pathologic causes, and may increase respiratory depression in these instances.

syrup subsequently, since it binds the ipecac syrup as well as the ingested poison.

Removal by Enhanced Excretion. In some instances, removal by emesis is either unsuccessful or is performed sufficiently long after the ingestion for absorption to have occurred. In the majority of cases symptoms will be mild, and simply allowing the body to excrete the drug (via kidneys, liver or lungs) is the preferred method of therapy. Occasionally, symptomatology will be sufficiently severe to necessitate more rapid removal. All methods of removal that enhance excretion carry some risk. Thus, the physician must be certain that the risks from enhanced removal are less than those from the ingested drug. If absorption has occurred and is of potential danger, the physician may proceed to one of the following methods of removal.

Fluid diuresis is the most common method of enhancing excretion. The mechanism involved includes a shorter time for exposure of the drug to reabsorptive sites in the distal tubules, increased glomerular filtration and dilution of the drug in the kidney relative to the blood, thus resulting in a higher drug gradient from blood to urine. Fluid diuresis is most effective for those drugs excreted by the kidneys. During diuresis, input and output are carefully monitored and care is exerted to prevent fluid overload. Renal shutdown or congestive heart failure is a contraindication to this form of therapy.

Ionized diuresis is a less commonly used method of removal. Its mechanism of action is based on the fact that diuresis is favored when the drug is maintained in its ionized form. Since the ionized form in the tubule will not cross back into the blood, decreased tubular reabsorption and thus increased excretion of the absorbed drug is the result. Alkalinization of acidic compounds (for example, aspirin and barbiturates) may be accomplished through the use of bases [sodium bicarbonate, sodium lactate, THAM (trihydroxymethylaminomethane) or Diamox]. As electrolytes are lost in the urine, both serum and urinary sodium and potassium are carefully monitored. The more acidic the drug ingested, the more effective will be alkalinization; the more neutral the drug, the less effective ionized diuresis and the more effective fluid diuresis. Acidification of the urine may be used for basic compounds (for example, amphetamines and strychnine). Ascorbic acid and ammonium chloride have been used in these instances.

When the pH of the ingested drug is neutral, ionized diuresis will be less effective. Osmotic diuresis in these situations can be effective and is a relatively safe method of removal. The mechanism of action of osmotic diuresis is that the osmotic load prevents reabsorption of the drug in the proximal tubules, loop of Henle and distal tubules. The method should not be used if decreased renal function, hypotension, cardiac disease, or pulmonary edema is present. During the procedure, frequent weights and careful monitoring of serum and urine electrolytes and central venous pressure are indicated. Adequate sodium and potassium must be supplied during therapy. The physician should aim for a sustained urine excretion rate of 0.1 ml. per kilogram per minute, or, in rough figures, an excretion rate of three to five times normal. Osmotic agents include urea and mannitol. Mannitol† may be used as a 25 per cent solution at a dose of 0.5 Gm. per kilogram per dose given every 4 to 6 hours or when the urine specific gravity falls below 1.025. In adults the dose for 50 per cent urea is 1 ml. per kilogram per hour given over a 4-hour period of time, then followed by a rate of 0.25 ml. per kilogram per hour.

Finally, diuretics may be used to increase urine excretion rates. Both ethacrynic acid‡ (1 mg. per kilogram per dose) and furosemide§ (1 to 3 mg. per kilogram per dose) have been used. The precautions and desired excretion rates previously noted for osmotic agents and ionized diuresis also apply to these two drugs.

Removal by Dialysis. Dialysis is an extreme form of therapy and should be used infrequently and in situations in which there is no less dangerous alternative. Methods include peritoneal dialysis, hemodialysis, exchange transfusion and lipid dialysis. There is less experience with the use of these methods in the pediatric patient than in the adult. Before these methods are attempted, it must be clearly evident that conservative modalities of therapy are inadequate to handle the emergency. Clinically, dialysis should be considered for a dialyzable drug, with existing oliguria and anuria, hypotension and respiratory depression.

Peritoneal dialysis is a slower method of removal than is hemodialysis. It is ineffective for drugs that have poor peritoneal clearance

---

† Manufacturer's precaution: Use of mannitol in pediatric patients has not been studied comprehensively.

‡ Manufacturer's precaution: Until further experience is accumulated, therapy with oral and parenteral forms of ethacrynic acid is contraindicated in infants.

§ Manufacturer's precaution: Furosemide should not be given to children until further experience is accumulated.

as well as for drugs that are tissue-bound. It is contraindicated in cases where the peritoneal cavity is infected. Extensive abdominal surgery is considered a relative contraindication. Peritoneal dialysis is relatively easily performed (as compared to hemodialysis) and is particularly effective for the drugs listed in Table 1. It can be effective for the correction of electrolyte and acid-base disturbances.

Hemodialysis is particularly useful when plasma levels are elevated. Tissue-bound drugs are poorly dialyzed, as are plasma protein-bound drugs. Protein may be added to the dialysate fluid to increase the gradient in instances of protein-bound drugs. In addition, "ion trapping," created by increasing the pH gradient between the blood and the dialysate, will result in increased removal of the ionized fraction in the dialysate. The drugs for which hemodialysis is effective are also included in Table 1. At the moment, hemodialysis is less commonly used for children than is peritoneal dialysis or exchange transfusion.

Exchange transfusion is particularly useful for the small child and for drugs which are highly protein-bound and remain in the circulation for prolonged periods of time. The drugs for which exchange transfusion is used are also listed in Table 1.

Lipid dialysis is still largely a research

TABLE 1. Currently Known Dialyzable Poisons*

BARBITURATES†
Barbital–1, 2
Phenobarbital–1, 2
Amobarbital–1, 2
Pentobarbital–1, 2
Butabarbital–1, 2
Secobarbital–1, 2
Cyclobarbital–1, 2

GLUTETHIMIDE†–1, 2

DEPRESSANTS, SEDATIVES AND TRANQUILIZERS
Diphenylhydantoin–1, 2
Primidone–2
Meprobamate–1, 2
Ethchlorvynol†–1, 2, 3
Ethynylcyclohexyl carbamate–1
Methyprylon–1, 2
Diphenylhydramine–1, 3
Methaqualone–1, 2
Heroin–1
Gallamine triethiodide–1
Paraldehyde–1, 2
Chloral hydrate–1
Chlordiazpoxide–1

ANTIDEPRESSANTS
Amphetamine–1, 2
Methamphetamine–1, 2
Tricyclic secondary amines–1
Tricyclic tertiary amines–1
Monoamine oxidase inhibitors–1
Tranylcypromine–1
Pargyline–1
Phenelzine–1
Isocarboxazide–1
Imipramine–1

ALCOHOLS
Ethanol†–1, 2
Methanol†–1, 2, 3
Isopropanol–1
Ethylene glycol–1, 2

ANALGESICS
Acetylsalicylic acid†–1, 2, 3
Methylsalicylate†–1, 2, 3
Acetophenetidin–1
Dextropropoxyphene–1, 2
Paracetamol–1, 3

ANTIBIOTICS
Isoniazid–1, 2
Carbenicillin–1, 2
Streptomycin–1
Kanamycin–1, 2
Neomycin–1, 2
Vancomycin–1
Penicillin–1
Ampicillin–1
Sulfonamides–1
Cephaloridine–1
Chloramphenicol–1
Tetracycline–1
Nitrofurantoin–1
Polymyxin–1
Cycloserine–2
Quinine–1, 2

METALS
Arsenic–1, 2
Calcium–1, 2
Iron–1, 4
Lead–1
Lithium–1
Magnesium–1
Mercury–1, 4
Potassium–1, 2
Sodium–1, 2
Strontium–1

HALIDES
Bromide–1
Chloride–1
Iodide–1
Fluoride–1

ENDOGENOUS TOXINS
Ammonia–1, 2, 3
Uric acid†–1
Bilirubin–1, 2, 3
Lactic acid–1, 2
Myasthenia gravis–1
Porphyria–1
Cystine–1
Endotoxin–1
Hyperosmolar state†–1, 2
Water intoxication–1, 2

MISCELLANEOUS
Thiocyanate†–1
Aniline–1, 2, 3
Sodium chlorate–1, 2, 3
Potassium chlorate–1, 2, 3
Eucalyptus oil–1, 2
Boric acid–2
Potassium dichromate–1, 4
Chromic anhydride–1
Digoxin–1, 2
Sodium citrate–1
Dinitro-ortho-cresol–1
Amanita phalloides–1
Carbon tetrachloride–1
Ergotamine–2
Cyclophosphamide–1
5-Fluorouracil–1
Methotrexate–1
Camphor–1
Trichloroethylene–1, 2
Carbon monoxide–1

* Adapted from Schreiner, G. E.: Dialysis of Poisons and Drugs—Annual Review. *Trans. Am. Soc. Artif. Int. Organs,* Vol. 16, 1970.

† Kinetics of dialysis thoroughly studied and/or clinical experience extensive.

1 = hemodialysis.
2 = peritoneal dialysis.
3 = exchange transfusion.
4 = chelation and dialysis.

procedure. It is used for drugs that are highly lipid-soluble, the mechanism for removal being based on a gradient effect between the tissues, blood and the dialysate fluid.

DILUTION AND ENEMAS

Though dilution and enemas are relatively ineffective, there will be occasional specific indications for their use. Dilution in particular is relatively ineffective. Its main action seems to be one of calming the parent and the older child. It does, however, have the deleterious side effect of hastening transit of the ingested poison into the lower gastrointestinal tract, from which removal is difficult. Laxatives hasten transit through the bowel, thus decreasing absorption of the poison. Laxatives, however, have the additional effect of irritating the mucosa. As many poisons are in themselves irritating, laxatives are unnecessary and may compound the problem. Enemas are infrequently used but are indicated for drugs that have been given per rectum and from which symptoms may result.

SUPPORTIVE MEASURES

When significant absorption has occurred, various body organs and their functions must be supported. The organs most commonly affected by poisoning include those of the cardiac, pulmonary, hepatic, renal and central nervous systems. Immediate supportive therapy is directed toward the respiratory and cardiac systems.

The establishment of effective respiratory exchange is critical and is accomplished by the clearing of secretions, the use of oral airways and the use of endotracheal intubation with mechanical support. A nasogastric tube is indicated for removal of the ingested poison as well as for emptying stomach contents in an effort to prevent subsequent aspiration pneumonia. Shock should be treated with volume expanders (blood, plasma, albumin) and pressors (Aramine, levarterenol, Isuprel). Maintenance of fluid homeostasis and correction of losses by intravenous fluids is needed. Intake and output should be carefully monitored. Frequent vital signs, the avoidance of central nervous system stimulants, and diligence not to overtreat with large doses of antidotes are necessary. Cardiac therapy may include the use of digoxin for myocardial failure and appropriate therapy for arrhythmias. Atropine is used in instances of bradycardia secondary to excessive vagal effect. The therapy of convulsions includes the use of barbiturates (phenobarbital and pentobarbital), paraldehyde, Dilantin, Valium,|| oxygen, effective suction and care to prevent self-injury. The therapy for respiratory failure includes the use of Nalline, Lorfan** or Narcan.†† Renal failure treatment regimens may be necessary when glomerular or tubular injury has occurred. Occasionally, dialysis will be needed. Analgesics for pain may include aspirin, Demerol or morphine. Prophylactic antibiotics are not indicated. Antibiotic therapy may be needed in the rare case in which superinfection occurs.

GENERAL AND SPECIFIC ANTIDOTES

Local antidotes may be used to decrease or to prevent absorption of an ingested drug. Systemic antidotes may be used once a drug has been absorbed to counteract its deleterious effects. Antidotes that effect absorption in addition to the local antidote include the universal antidote (not recommended) and activated charcoal.

The following compounds may be treated by the use of local antidotes which act as neutralizers:

1. *For acid ingestion* – neutralization by weak alkalis (magnesium hydroxide, milk of magnesia).
2. *For alkali ingestion* – neutralization by weak acids (vinegar diluted 1:4, 1 per cent acidic acid or lemon juice).
3. *For fluoride ingestion* – calcium (milk or calcium lactate) to precipitate the fluoride as calcium fluoride.
4. *For iron ingestion* – the use of sodium bicarbonate (through the formation of ferrous carbonate) to relieve abdominal discomfort, decrease absorption and prevent intestinal erosion and ulceration.

Activated charcoal is the best available local antidote that works by absorption, and its contribution to management has been recently emphasized. It is a tasteless, fine black powder which is the residue of the distillation of wood pulp. Its effectiveness depends on its small particle size and large surface area. Indiscriminate use of activated charcoal is discouraged, particularly when effective means of removing the poison are present. It should be used only for drugs against which it is known to be effective (Table 2). It is not effective for cyanide, ethyl

---

|| Manufacturer's precaution: The safety and efficacy of injectable Valium in children under 12 years of age have not been established. Oral Valium is not for use in children under six months of age.

** See manufacturer's precaution, p. 724, footnote.

†† Manufacturer's precaution: Narcan is not recommended in neonates; its safety in children has not been established.

TABLE 2. Drugs Absorbed by Activated Charcoal*

Amphetamines	Diphenylhydantoin	Penicillin
Antipyrene	Glutethimide	Phenol
Aspirin	Iodine	Phenolphthalein
Atropine	Ipecac	Primaquine
Barbiturates	Methylene blue	Propoxyphene
Camphor	Morphine	Quinine
Cantharides	Muscarine	Salicylates
Chlorpheniramine	Nicotine	Sulfonamides
Cocaine	Opium	Stramonium
Colchicine	Oxalates	Strychnine
Digitalis	Parathion	

* Adapted from Corby, D. G., Fiser, R. H., and Decker, W. J.: *Pediat. Clin. N. Am.*, 17:545–556, 1970.

and methyl alcohol and alkali and acid ingestions. Once a complex has been formed, disassociation of that complex usually does not occur. Repeated dosages are not more effective than one dose, except in the rare instance when a drug is reexcreted into the gastrointestinal tract (e.g., imipramine). The amount of charcoal needed by weight is generally five to ten times greater than the ingested drug. The suggested dose is 1 Gm. per kilogram per dose, or 1 to 2 tablespoons in 8 ounces of water. Certainly, the earlier the drug is given the more effective it will be. It should never be used prior to administration of Ipecac Syrup.

The universal antidote contains charcoal (used to absorb chemicals), magnesium hydroxide (to neutralize ingested acids) and tannic acid (to precipitate heavy metals and alkaloids as well as to neutralize bases). The use of the universal antidote is to be condemned because it is ineffective, the tannic acid is hepatotoxic and the ingredients actually neutralize each other.

Systemic antidotes are used when a drug has been absorbed, symptoms exist and inactivation of the drug is indicated. Approximately 14 specific antidotes exist. The specific antidotes preceded by an asterisk are effective immediately and may be required in order to save the victim's life.

1. *BAL* (dimercaprol), given either intramuscularly or intravenously at a dosage of 2.5 to 4 mg. per kilogram per dose every 4 hours, is effective in heavy metal poisoning because of its greater affinity for the heavy metal than that exerted by the sulfhydral radicals of the body. BAL is particularly effective in the treatment of gold, arsenic, bismuth, chromium, copper and nickel poisonings. Early therapy is desirable.

2. *EDTA* (calcium disodium edetate), given intramuscularly or intravenously for heavy metal poisoning at a dosage of 30 to 50 mg. per kilogram per day in four divided doses, has a greater affinity for the ingested metal than the affinity exerted by the sulfhydral radicals of the body. It is particularly effective for lead, uranium, magnesium, chromium, cobalt, copper, radium and selenium ingestions.

3. *Penicillamine,* given orally in a dose of 25 mg. per kilogram per dose, works by the same mechanism as BAL and EDTA. It is, however, less potent than these two drugs. Its use is better saved for the chronic and less acute ingestion.

4. **Nitrates and thiosulfate* are used in the therapy of cyanide poisoning. Cyanide has a particularly strong affinity for ferric iron, found in the body's oxidizing enzymes, and thus causes an irreversible inhibition of these critical functions. The principle of therapy is to supply iron in its ferric form (as found in methemoglobin) to bind cyanide, thus protecting the iron contained in the cellular oxidizing systems. Amyl nitrite ampules are broken in a gauze sponge and held over the nose for 15 to 30 seconds of each minute until intravenous sodium nitrite can be prepared. For children greater than 25 kilograms, 10 ml. of sodium nitrite is then given intravenously as a 3 per cent solution at a rate of 2.5 to 5 ml. per minute. For children less than 25 kilograms, the dose is 10 mg. per kilogram per dose. The drug may then be repeated once at 5 mg. per kilogram per dose. This results in the conversion of hemoglobin ferrous radicals to ferric, thus creating available ferric iron to bind and inactivate the ingested cyanide. Then, sodium thiosulfate is given intravenously as a 25 per cent solution in a dosage of 50 ml. at a rate of 2.5 to 5 ml. per minute. This results in the formation of thiocyanate, which is then excreted from the body.

5. **Nalline, Lorfan and Narcan* are used in the therapy of narcotic ingestions. Narcotics exert their effect by depressing the respiratory and central nervous systems. These drugs work to counteract this effect. Nalline, at a dose of

0.1 mg. per kilogram per dose, Lorfan,** at a dose of 0.02 mg. per kilogram per dose, or Narcan,‡‡ at a dose of 0.01 mg. per kilogram per dose, are all effective. Narcan is preferable in that it causes no respiratory depression if the diagnosis is in error and a narcotic agent has not been ingested. These drugs, given intravenously, are effective in 2 minutes, and last up to 4 hours. Given intramuscularly, they act in 5 to 10 minutes. To achieve an effect similar to the intravenous route, the intramuscular dose should be increased by 50 per cent.

6. *Vitamin K_1* is used in the therapy of warfarin and Dicumarol ingestions. These latter drugs exert their deleterious effect by inhibiting prothrombin formation. Vitamin K_1, given in a dose of 5 to 10 mg. orally; reverses this inhibitory effect on prothrombin synthesis.

7. *Deferoxamine* is the specific agent used in the therapy of iron ingestion. It competes effectively with the protein-carrying globulin transferrin, and in combination with iron results in excretion of the drug. Recommended therapy is now limited to intramuscular or intravenous usage, since oral use is associated with increased absorption. The recommended dose is 1 Gm. or 20 mg. per kilogram given every 4 to 12 hours, depending on the clinical response. The total dose should not exceed 6 Gm. per 24 hours. Given intravenously it may induce hypotension. Thus, the intramuscular route is preferable provided there will be adequate absorption of the drug from the tissues. If the intravenous route is necessary, the dose used is 0.5 Gm. to 1 Gm. every 4 to 12 hours by slow infusion (depending on the clinical response), not to exceed 15 mg. per kilogram per hour.

8. **Ethanol* is used in the therapy of methanol ingestions. Methanol is toxic owing to its conversion by the dehydrogenase enzyme to formaldehyde and formic acid. Ethanol has a greater affinity for the dehydrogenase enzyme than methanol does and thus blocks the conversion of methanol to its toxic products. The recommended dose of ethanol, given either intravenously or by mouth, is 0.75 to 1.0 ml. per kilogram per dose, followed by 0.5 ml. per kilogram per dose every 4 hours for four days.

9. **Atropine sulfate and PAM* are used in the therapy of insecticide ingestions, specifically the cholinesterase-inhibitor insecticides. Insecticides act by combining with and inactivating acetylcholinesterase. The accumulation of acetylcholine causes the symptoms. Atropine sulfate, in a dose of 1 mg. intravenously for a child and 2 to 3 mg. for an adult, with additional doses at 15- to 30-minute intervals until muscarinic effects disappear and full atropinization is accomplished, is the indicated treatment. PAM (2-pyridine aldoxime methiodide), in a dose of 0.25 Gm. (may be repeated twice within a 24-hour period), is an alternative form of therapy.

10. **Methylene blue and ascorbic acid* are used in the therapy of methemoglobinemia. A number of compounds, including nitrates, aniline, chlorates, phenacetin, nitrobenzene, sulfonamides, quinones and dyes, are responsible for the conversion of hemoglobin ferrous iron to its ferric state, thus producing methemoglobinemia. This results in a shift of the oxygen saturation curve to the left, poor oxygen-carrying capacity and decreased delivery of oxygen to the tissues. Reduction of ferric iron to its ferrous form is accomplished through the use of methylene blue. A dosage of 1 to 2 mg. per kilogram per dose of methylene blue given intravenously as a 1 per cent solution is used. This dose may be repeated in 3 to 4 hours. Oxygen is given as well. Since methylene blue is toxic, its use should be determined by the concentration of methemoglobin (40 per cent or greater is accepted as severe) and by clinical symptoms.

11. *Calcium* is used in the therapy of fluoride ingestions. Fluoride is toxic owing to its corrosive effect on the gastrointestinal mucosa. Calcium (calcium chloride, calcium lactate, calcium gluconate), binds with the ingested fluoride and is the specific antidote.

12. *Chlorpromazine*§§ may be used in the therapy of amphetamine ingestion. The hyperactivity induced by the amphetamines may be decreased through the oral or intramuscular use of chlorpromazine in a dose of 1 mg. per kilogram per dose. Reduction of this dose to 0.5 mg. per kilogram per dose is indicated when a barbiturate has been ingested along with the amphetamine.

13. *Benadryl* is used in the therapy of the extrapyramidal reactions induced by the phenothiazines. Benadryl, given at a dosage of 1 to 2 mg. per kilogram per dose intravenously, results in immediate relaxation. Generally, a maintenance dosage of Benadryl will be necessary over the next 24 hours to prevent recurrence of symptoms.

14. **Oxygen* is used in the therapy of carbon monoxide poisoning. The high affinity

** See manufacturer's precaution, p. 724, footnote.

‡‡ See manufacturer's precaution, p. 727, footnote.

§§ Manufacturer's precaution: Chlorpromazine is not recommended for children under six months of age except when lifesaving.

of hemoglobin for carbon monoxide may be reversed through use of high concentrations of oxygen. The individual poisoned by carbon monoxide may be effectively treated through the inhalation of 100 per cent oxygen over a 30-minute period of time.

TREATMENT FOR THE SPECIFIC AND KNOWN POISONING

Table 3 lists certain common substances of low toxicity which require either no treatment at all or, in the case of ingestions of large quantities, only emesis. There are many substances that, although theoretically poisonous, usually do not produce symptoms because of the small amounts taken. Table 4 lists in alphabetical order the most common poisons, their symptoms and an outline for their therapy. This table emphasizes emergency treatment, and the reader is urged to use definitive references or to contact the manufacturer or the nearest poison control center for more detailed aspects of therapy.

PREVENTION

Finally, no therapy for a poisoning is complete until the reasons for the poisoning have been fully explored and advice as to future preventive measures has been completely outlined and explained to the parent.

References

With these resources, the majority of serious ingestions can be managed satisfactorily.

Alpert, J. J., and Lovejoy, F. H., Jr.: Management of Childhood Poisoning. *Current Problems in Pediatrics,* March, 1971.

Arena, J.: *Poisonings: Chemistry—Symptoms—Treatments.* Springfield, Illinois, Charles C Thomas, Publisher, 1970.

Coleman, A. B., and Alpert, J. J.: Poisoning in Children. *Pediat. Clin. N. Am.,* 17:471–758, 1970.

Dreisbach, R. H.: *Handbook of Poisoning: Diagnosis and Treatment.* 6th Ed. Los Angeles, Lange Medical Publications, 1969.

Gleason, M., Gosselin, R., and Hodge, H.: *Clinical Toxicology of Commercial Products.* 3rd ed. Baltimore, The Williams & Wilkins Co., 1970.

Goodman, L., and Gilman, A.: *The Pharmacological Basis of Therapeutics.* 4th ed. New York, The Macmillan Company, 1970.

Kingsburg, J. M.: *Poisonous Plants of the United States and Canada.* Englewood Cliffs, New Jersey, Prentice-Hall, Inc., 1964.

TABLE 3. Common Ingestions of Low Toxicity

NO TREATMENT REQUIRED	REMOVAL NECESSARY ONLY IF LARGE AMOUNTS INGESTED
Ball-point inks	After-shave lotion
Bar soap	Body conditioners
Bathtub floating toys	Colognes
Battery (dry cell)	Deodorants
Bubble bath soap	Fabric softeners
Candles	Hair dyes
Chalk	Hair sprays
Clay (modeling)	Hair tonic
Crayons with A.P., C.P. or C.S. 130-46 designation	Indelible markers
Dehumidifying packets	Matches (greater than 20 wooden matches or 2 books of paper matches)
Detergents (anionic)	No Doz
Eye make-up	Oral contraceptives
Fish bowl additives	Perfumes
Golf balls	Suntan preparations
Hand lotion and cream	Toilet water
Ink (blue, black, red)	
Lipstick	
Newspaper	
Pencils (lead and coloring)	
Putty and Silly Putty	
Sachets	
Shampoo	
Shaving cream and shaving lotions	
Shoe polish (occasionally aniline dyes present)	
Striking surface materials of matchboxes	
Sweetening agents (saccharin, cyclamate)	
Teething rings	
Thermometers	
Toothpaste	

DRUG	TOXICITY	SYMPTOMS	TREATMENT
Acids (Lysol)	Toxicity related to concentration and duration of exposure and less to amount	1. Corrosive burns of mucous membranes of mouth, esophagus and stomach with possible stricture 2. Pain in area of burns 3. Circulatory collapse and shock	1. Emetics and lavage are contraindicated 2. Immediate neutralization with milk of magnesia, magnesium oxide, milk, magnesium hydroxide 3. Opiates for pain 4. Intravenous therapy for shock 5. For further therapy see under *Alkali*
Alkali (Lye, Drano, Saniflush, Clinitest)	Toxicity related to concentration and duration of exposure and less to amount	1. Corrosive burns of mucous membranes of mouth, esophagus and stomach 2. Pain in area of burns 3. Circulatory collapse and shock 4. Complications include esophageal and gastric perforation, glottic edema, pulmonary edema, pneumonia, stricture formation of esophagus	1. Emetics and lavage are contraindicated 2. Immediate neutralization with vinegar diluted 1:4, 1% acetic acid, lemon juice 3. Opiates for pain 4. Intravenous therapy for shock 5. With evidence of esophageal or gastric burn (clinically or by esophagoscopy), prednisone 2–3 mg./kg./24 hr. for 2 weeks and then tapered for 2 weeks 6. Broad-spectrum antibiotic coverage while on steroids 7. Following therapy, upper gastrointestinal series for evidence of stricture 8. Dilation of stricture if present
Aminophylline	Symptoms when therapeutic dose exceeded	1. Agitation, restlessness 2. Vomiting 3. Fever 4. Tachycardia and cardiac arrhythmias 5. Convulsions 6. Vasomotor collapse 7. Respiratory failure	1. Ipecac syrup for oral ingestions 2. Enemas for rectally administered overdose 3. Avoidance of sympathomimetics 4. Supportive therapy for hypotension, seizures, arrhythmias and dehydration
Ammonium Hydroxide (Ammonia)	Toxicity related to concentration and duration of exposure	1. Caustic burn with pain in mouth, esophagus and stomach 2. Circulatory collapse and shock 3. Complications include esophageal and gastric perforation, glottic edema, pulmonary edema, pneumonia	1. Emetics and lavage are contraindicated 2. Neutralization with water, vinegar diluted 1:4, 1% acetic acid, lemon juice 3. Further therapy as outlined under *Alkali*
Amphetamines (Benzedrine, Dexedrine Dexamyl)	Symptoms when therapeutic dose exceeded	1. Nervousness, hyperactivity, mania, psychotic-like state 2. Tachycardia, hypertension, cardiac arrhythmias 3. Convulsions and shock	1. Emesis with ipecac syrup 2. Activated charcoal 3. Control of seizures 4. Support for cardiovascular and respiratory systems 5. Hemodialysis and peritoneal dialysis 6. Chlorpromazine* (0.5–1.0 mg./kg./dose); may repeat in 4 hours (see specific antidote section in text)

TABLE 4. Treatment of Specific Poisons—*Continued*

DRUG	TOXICITY	SYMPTOMS	TREATMENT
Aniline	Cyanosis with methemoglobin levels of greater than 15%, lethargy with levels greater than 40%, potential lethal levels at greater than 70%	1. Apathy and headache 2. Cyanosis with dyspnea 3. Hypotension and convulsions 4. Circulatory and respiratory failure 5. Intravascular hemolysis	1. Emesis with ipecac syrup 2. Methylene blue intravenously as 1% solution at 1–2 mg./kg./dose. Methylene blue indicated with level of methemoglobin greater than 40% or when clinical symptoms are severe (see specific antidote section in text) 3. Oxygen 4. Removal from source of exposure 5. Hemodialysis and peritoneal dialysis
Antihistamines	Symptoms when therapeutic dose exceeded	1. Drowsiness 2. Dryness of mouth 3. Nausea 4. Headache 5. Occasionally nervousness, disorientation, hyperreflexia, seizures 6. Stupor, coma, respiratory and cardiovascular collapse	1. Emesis with ipecac syrup 2. Control of seizures 3. Support for cardiovascular and respiratory systems
Arsenic and Antimony	A dose of 5 to 50 mg. of arsenic trioxide is toxic. A dose of 2–3 mg. kg. in children may be fatal	1. Sweetish metallic taste in mouth 2. Constrictive sensation in throat 3. Diarrhea, vomiting, dehydration hyperreflexia, seizures 4. Delirium, convulsions, coma 5. Pulmonary edema	1. Emesis with ipecac syrup 2. Dimercaprol (BAL), 2.5 mg.–3 mg./kg./dose every 4 hours for 2 days, then every 12 hours for a total of 10 days; BAL treatment indicated when unknown amount ingested, with symptoms or when toxic amounts by calculation ingested (see specific antidote section in text) 3. Intravenous hydration, transfusion therapy, treatment of liver and renal decompensation
Atropine	Symptoms when therapeutic dose exceeded. Children more susceptible than adults to toxicity	1. Dry mucous membranes 2. Mydriasis 3. Hyperthermia 4. Hot, dry erythematous appearance to the skin 5. Confusion, delirium, seizures, coma 6. Circulatory and respiratory failure	1. Emesis with ipecac syrup 2. Activated charcoal 3. Control of temperature and fluid therapy 4. Barbiturates for control of seizures 5. Respiratory and circulatory support 6. Pilocarpine, 5 mg. orally, for visual disturbance, dryness of mouth, other peripheral effects
Barbiturates (Amobarbital, Secobarbital, Pentobarbital, Phenobarbital)	Potentially fatal dose 40–45 mg./kg. for short-acting barbiturates, and 65–75 mg./kg. for long-acting barbiturates. Blood levels of 4 mg./100 ml. for short-acting barbiturates, and 8 mg./100 ml. for long-acting barbiturates indicate severe ingestion	1. Drowsiness, mental confusion, coma 2. Absent reflexes, muscle flaccidity 3. Slowed respiration, hypotension 4. Cerebral edema	1. Emesis with ipecac syrup 2. Activated charcoal 3. Forced fluid diuresis 4. Alkalinization of urine for long-acting barbiturates 5. Osmotic agents and diuretics for long- and short-acting barbiturates 6. Respiratory and cardiovascular support 7. Hemodialysis and peritoneal dialysis

Boric Acid	Fatal dose is estimated at 0.1–0.5 Gm./kg.	1. Bloody diarrhea and dehydration 2. Erythroderma and exfoliation 3. Lethargy, convulsions 4. Jaundice 5. Hypotension 6. Anuria 7. Coma	1. Removal from skin 2. In case of ingestion, emesis with ipecac syrup 3. Intravenous fluids 4. Anticonvulsants for seizures 5. Peritoneal dialysis or exchange transfusion
Bromides	Blood bromide level of greater than 150 mg./100 ml. is indicative of toxicity	1. Acute ingestion causes nausea, vomiting, paralysis and coma 2. Chronic poisoning causes confusion, ataxia, slurred speech, irritability, delusions, psychotic behavior, stupor	1. Emesis with ipecac syrup 2. Sodium chloride, 5 Gm./day for 1–4 weeks (in adult), to hasten excretion 3. Hemodialysis
Camphor	Fatal dose for a 1-year-old child is approximately 1 Gm.	1. Headache 2. Burning in mouth and throat 3. Camphor odor on breath 4. Nausea and vomiting 5. Feeling of warmth, excitement, irrational behavior, muscle spasms, convulsions, coma 6. Circulatory and respiratory collapse	1. Emesis with ipecac syrup 2. Activated charcoal 3. Anticonvulsants for seizures 4. Respiratory and circulatory support 5. Hemodialysis
Carbon Monoxide	Carboxyhemoglobin concentration of 20% causes mild symptoms; 40–50%, moderate; 60–90%, death	1. Headache 2. Vertigo 3. Confusion 4. Dyspnea 5. Dilated pupils 6. Bounding pulse 7. Cherry-red color to lips and skin 8. Convulsions 9. Coma	1. Removal of patient from exposure 2. 100% oxygen by mask for 30 minutes 3. With respiratory depression, artificial respiration with 100% oxygen (see specific antidote section in text) 4. Maintain temperature and blood pressure 5. Hemodialysis
Carbon Tetrachloride	Fatal adult dose by ingestion is 3–5 ml.	1. Abdominal pain 2. Nausea and vomiting 3. Headache and confusion 4. Convulsions 5. Circulatory collapse 6. Respiratory depression 7. Coma 8. Renal and hepatic damage	1. Emesis with ipecac syrup 2. Fluid hydration 3. Avoid epinephrine and related compounds 4. Artificial respiratory support 5. Management of renal and hepatic decompensation 6. Hemodialysis
Cathartics (Mineral Oil, Ex-Lax, Phenolphthalein, Metamucil)	Generally of low toxicity	1. Irritation of gastrointestinal tract causing tenesmus, vomiting, diarrhea 2. Occasionally hypotension, collapse, coma	1. With excessive ingestion, emesis with ipecac syrup 2. Milk to decrease gastrointestinal irritation 3. If severe symptoms, hydration, treatment of shock and medication for pain

TABLE 4. Treatment of Specific Poisons–*Continued*

DRUG	TOXICITY	SYMPTOMS	TREATMENT
Chloral Hydrate	Dose greater than 50 mg./kg. causes hypnotic symptoms	1. Drowsiness 2. Mental confusion 3. Coma 4. Shock 5. Respiratory depression	1. Emesis with ipecac syrup if greater than 50 mg./kg. ingested 2. Respiratory support 3. Fluid diuresis 4. Hemodialysis
Cyanide	Severe and rapid toxicity. Survival for 4 hours associated with full recovery	1. Death in a few minutes 2. Tachycardia 3. Headache 4. Drowsiness 5. Hypotension 6. Unconsciousness 7. Convulsions	1. Immediate removal of poison by lavage or apomorphine 2. Amyl nitrate by inhalation 3. Artificial respiration with 100% oxygen 4. Sodium nitrate (3% solution) 10 ml. intravenously at a rate of 2.5–5 ml. per minute for patients greater than 25 kg. For patients less than 25 kg., 10 mg./kg. dose. This may then be repeated once at 5 mg./kg./dose 5. Sodium thiosulfate (25% solution) 50 ml. intravenously at a rate of 2.5 to 5 ml. per minute (see specific antidote section in text).
Detergents, Soaps and Cleaners	Variability of toxicity	1. Electric dishwasher and laundry granules cause caustic burns 2. Anionic detergents (Tide, Cheer, Ajax, Top Job, Comet, Windex, Mr. Clean, Lestoil, Joy, Spic'n Span, bar soap, bubble bath, household detergents) cause mild vomiting and diarrhea 3. Cationic detergents (pHisoHex, Zephiran, Diaparene) cause nausea, vomiting, convulsions, coma	Treatment of cationic detergents includes: 1. Emesis with ipecac syrup 2. Control of seizures 3. Support of respiration
Digitalis	Toxic symptoms when therapeutic dose exceeded. Single lethal dose 20 to 50 times the daily maintenance dose	1. Nausea 2. Vomiting 3. Aberrant color vision 4. Slow and irregular pulse 5. Hypotension 6. Arrhythmias due to increased myocardial irritability	1. Emesis with ipecac syrup 2. Activated charcoal 3. Adequate fluids 4. Potassium, Quinidine, Pronestyl, Xylocaine, dependent on type of arrhythmia 5. Hemodialysis and peritoneal dialysis
Ephedrine (other sympathomimetics, Epinephrine, Isuprel, Neo-Synephrine)	For ephedrine, minimal lethal dose for children is approximately 200 mg. orally	1. Nervousness 2. Tachycardia 3. Dilated pupils 4. Blurred vision 5. Convulsions, respiratory failure 6. Coma	1. Emesis with ipecac syrup 2. Control of seizures 3. Maintenance of blood pressure 4. Respiratory support

(Sansert, Ergotamine)	dose exceeded	2. Vomiting 3. Light headedness 4. Convulsions 5. Hypotension 6. Coma	2. Control of seizures 3. Respiratory and cardiovascular support 4. Vasodilators may be required 5. Peritoneal dialysis
Ethyl Alcohol	Potentially fatal dose greater than 6 ml./kg. Blood level: 0.05–0.15%, mild; 0.15–0.3%, moderate; 0.3–0.5%, severe; above 0.5%, coma	1. Initial excitement, delirium and inebriation 2. Later depression, stupor, coma 3. Alcohol odor on breath 4. Hypoglycemia 5. Slurred speech and muscle incoordination 6. Respiratory failure	1. Emesis with ipecac syrup 2. Glucose for hypoglycemia 3. Adequate hydration 4. For coma, maintenance of airway and avoidance of excessive fluids 5. Hemodialysis or peritoneal dialysis
Ferrous Sulfate	Fatal dose for a 2-year-old child estimated at 5–10 Gm.	1. Symptoms occur ½ to 2 hours postingestion 2. Vomiting, diarrhea, melena 3. Drowsiness, lethargy, pallor 4. Metabolic acidosis 5. Hepatic damage 6. Coagulation defects 7. Shock 8. Coma 9. Stricture of gastrointestinal tract	1. Emesis with ipecac syrup 2. If (a) shock and coma (b) serum iron level of greater than 500 mcg. per 100 ml. (c) overdose of unknown quantity, treat with deferoxamine, 20 mg./kg./dose every 4–6 hours intramuscularly 3. Fluid therapy and bicarbonate for acidosis 4. Hemodialysis
Fluoride	50–200 mg./kg. is the estimated fatal dose	1. Nausea, vomiting, diarrhea 2. Tremors and convulsions 3. Respiratory failure 4. Complications include jaundice, oliguria, anemia, leukopenia	1. Emesis with ipecac syrup 2. Intravenous fluids 3. Oxygen 4. Support of cardiovascular and respiratory systems 5. Calcium chloride by mouth to bind ingested fluoride (see specific antidote section in text) 6. Hemodialysis
Hormones (Enovid, Ortho-novum, Oracon, Norlestrin, Premarin)	Low toxicity	1. Nausea and vomiting 2. Fluid retention 3. Vaginal bleeding in girls	1. Emesis with ipecac syrup if more than 10 to 15 tablets have been ingested
Hydrocarbons (Kerosene, Gasoline, Mineral Spirits, Paint Thinner, Lighter Fluid, Barbecue Fluid, Dry Cleaning Fluid)	Toxic to lungs and central nervous system	1. Burning in the mouth and esophagus 2. Vomiting and diarrhea 3. Pulmonary symptoms consist of cough, fever, bloody sputum, cyanosis, rales, pulmonary infiltrates 4. Central nervous system symptoms	1. For waxes, do not induce emesis unless *very large* amounts ingested. For other, higher volatility hydrocarbons, emesis at lower amounts. Emesis is preferable to lavage 2. Activated charcoal 3. For pneumonic involvement, oxygen and antibiotics with signs of superinfection. Use of steroids is debatable 4. Supportive therapy for central nervous system involvement 5. Avoid epinephrine 6. Transfusion for methemoglobinemia

TABLE 4. Treatment of Specific Poisons—*Continued*

DRUG	TOXICITY	SYMPTOMS	TREATMENT
Insecticides (Chlorinated hydrocarbons, DDT, Dieldrin, Lindane) *Cholinesterase Inhibitors* (Parathion, Chlorthion, Bidrin, Dimetilan, Sevin)	5 Gm. of DDT will cause mild symptoms. 20 Gm. will cause severe symptoms	*Chlorinated Hydrocarbons*—vomiting, excitement, numbness, weakness, incoordination, tremors, seizures, circulatory and respiratory collapse *Cholinesterase Inhibitors* — blurred vision, sweating, miosis, tearing, salivation, papilledema, cyanosis, seizures, pulmonary edema	*Chlorinated Hydrocarbons* – Emesis with ipecac syrup. Avoidance of fats, oils, milk. Control of seizures, avoidance of sympathomimetics *Cholinesterase Inhibitors* – Emesis with ipecac syrup. Atropine sulfate, 1–4 mg. intravenously with dose repeated at intervals of 15–30 minutes. Alternate choice, the use of PAM (see section on specific antidotes in text)
Ipecac Syrup	Amounts greater than 30 ml. are toxic	1. Nausea and vomiting 2. Tachycardia, arrhythmias, hypotension 3. Dyspnea 4. Heart failure 5. Coma	1. Removal by lavage or apomorphine 2. Activated charcoal 3. Close observation for arrhythmias or heart failure
Lead	Symptoms with blood level of 40 mcg./100 ml. Danger of encephalopathy with levels greater than 80 mcg./100 ml.	1. Most lead poisoning is chronic 2. Abdominal pain, nausea, vomiting 3. Opaque lead particles on plain film of abdomen 4. Melena 5. Oliguria and anuria 6. Encephalopathy and coma	1. Emesis with ipecac syrup 2. Catharsis 3. Treatment for renal failure and encephalopathy 4. Calcium EDTA and/or BAL (see section on specific antidotes in text)
Lomotil	Toxicity when therapeutic dose exceeded	1. Lethargy 2. Hypoactive reflexes 3. Nystagmus 4. Pinpoint pupils 5. Tachycardia 6. Respiratory depression 7. Coma	1. Emesis with ipecac syrup 2. Nalline at 0.1 mg./kg./dose, Lorfan† at 0.02 mg./kg./dose or Narcan‡ at 0.01 mg./kg./dose intravenously for respiratory depression (see section on specific antidote in text)
Mercury	Mean lethal dose in adults, 1–4 Gm. Therapeutic level: blood, 20 mg./100 ml.; urine, 50 mg./100 ml.	1. Metallic taste in the mouth 2. Bloody diarrhea 3. Abdominal pain 4. Renal tubular damage and anuria 5. Respiratory failure	1. Emesis with ipecac syrup 2. Dimercaprol (BAL) intramuscularly, 2.5–3.0 mg./kg./dose given every 4 hours for 2 days and then every 12 hours for 10 days (see section on specific antidotes in text) 3. Fluid therapy, transfusion therapy and treatment of liver and renal failure 4. Hemodialysis
Methadone	80–120 mg. of methadone will cause respiratory depression. Death has been noted in a child after 80 mg. of methadone.	1. Pinpoint pupils 2. Drowsiness 3. Pale, cold skin 4. Shallow respiration 5. Coma 6. Respiratory failure	1. Emesis with ipecac syrup 2. Respiratory support and oxygen 3. Nalline, 0.1 mg./kg./dose, Lorfan† 0.02 mg./kg./dose, or Narcan‡ 0.01 mg./kg./dose intravenously for respiratory depression (see section on specific antidotes in text)

Methyl Alcohol (Wood Alcohol)	2 tsp. are toxic. Fatal dose from 2–8 oz. Toxic blood level: greater than 20 mg./100 ml. Potentially lethal blood level: greater than 50 mg./100 ml.	1. Headache, dizziness 2. Nausea and vomiting 3. Visual impairment 4. Acidosis 5. Cyanosis 6. Hypotension 7. Coma 8. Respiratory collapse	1. Emesis with ipecac syrup 2. Monitoring of acidosis, and correction using sodium bicarbonate 3. Ethyl alcohol 50% (100 proof) 0.75 ml./kg./dose (see section on specific antidotes in text) 4. Peritoneal dialysis and hemodialysis
Naphthalene (Mothballs, Repellent Cakes, Deodorizer Cakes)	Greater than 1 tsp. is toxic.	1. Nausea, vomiting, abdominal cramps 2. Convulsions 3. Coma 4. Intravascular hemolysis 5. Oliguria and anuria	1. Emesis with ipecac syrup 2. Control of seizures 3. Intravenous fluids to prevent precipitation of hemoglobin in tubules 4. Transfusion for anemia 5. Steroids for persistent severe hemolysis
Narcotic Analgesics (Morphine, Codeine, Demerol, Talwin)	Symptoms when therapeutic dose exceeded	1. Pinpoint pupils 2. Shallow respiration 3. Drowsiness progressing to coma 4. Cold skin 5. Seizure activity 6. Respiratory failure	1. Emesis with ipecac syrup, apomorphine or lavage dependent on state of consciousness 2. For respiratory failure, oxygen, artificial respiration and Nalline, 0.1 mg./kg./dose, Lorfan,† 0.02 mg./kg./dose, or Narcan,‡ 0.01 mg./kg./dose (see section on specific antidotes in text)
Nicotine	Fatal dose is about 40–60 mg. Swallowed as tobacco, nicotine is less toxic because of poor absorption from the stomach	1. Nausea and vomiting 2. Tachycardia 3. Hypertension 4. Headache 5. Sweating 6. Convulsions 7. Coma 8. Respiratory failure	1. Emesis with ipecac syrup 2. Activated charcoal 3. Control seizures 4. Respiratory support 5. Atropine for parasympathetic overstimulation
Nitrates and Nitrites	Individual susceptibility varies considerably	1. Nausea and vomiting 2. Headache 3. Flushed skin 4. Dizziness 5. Hypotension 6. Respiratory failure 7. Coma	1. Emesis with ipecac syrup 2. Oxygen 3. Blood transfusion 4. Methylene blue 1% solution intravenously at 1–2 mg./kg./dose with severe symptoms (or methemoglobin level greater than 40%) (see section on specific antidotes in text)
Polishes and Waxes (Pride, Old English, O'Cedar, Jubilee, Kleer Floor Wax, Bruce Cleaning Wax, Aerowax, Armstrong 1-Step, Pledge Furniture Polish, Stanley Furniture Cream)	Main toxicity is pulmonary, caused by aspiration. Central nervous system symptoms less prominent and are secondary to absorption from lungs	1. Burning of the mouth and esophagus 2. Vomiting and diarrhea 3. Pulmonary involvement – cough, fever, dyspnea, rales, cyanosis, pulmonary infiltrates 4. Central nervous system involvement secondary to pulmonary absorption–depression with weakness, dizziness, shallow respiration, coma	1. Do not induce emesis 2. Activated charcoal 3. For pulmonary involvement: oxygen, moisture, antibiotics when clinical course or sputum examination indicates superinfection. Use of steroids debatable. Infiltrates clear over 1–4 weeks 4. Supportive therapy for central nervous system depression

TABLE 4. Treatment of Specific Poisons–*Continued*

DRUG	TOXICITY	SYMPTOMS	TREATMENT
Psychedelic Drugs . . (LSD, Mescaline)	Duration and intensity of effect varies from drug to drug and from individual to individual	1. Dilation of pupils 2. Visual hallucinations 3. Distortion of sensory perception 4. Exaggerated sense of comprehension 5. Incoordination 6. Tachycardia 7. Mild hypertension	1. "Talking down" 2. Thorazine,* 1–2 mg./kg./dose, or Valium,§ 0.5 mg./kg./24 hours (exception: ingestion of STP [dimethoxymethyl amphetamine])
Salicylates (St. Joseph's, Bayer, Bufferin, Rexall, Empirin, Anacin, Excedrin, Congesprin)	Symptoms at 150 mg./kg. or at serum levels greater than 25–30 mg./100 ml.–50–80 mg./100 ml.: mild symptoms; 80–100 mg./100 ml.: severe symptoms; greater than 150 mg./100 ml.: potentially fatal	1. Vomiting 2. Hyperventilation 3. Fever 4. Thirst 5. Sweating 6. In small children, metabolic acidosis 7. In older children, respiratory alkalosis 8. Hypoglycemia or hyperglycemia and prolonged prothrombin times 9. Confusion, delirium, convulsions	1. Emesis with ipecac syrup 2. Activated charcoal 3. Forced fluid diuresis 4. Colloid for volume expansion 5. Glucose for hypoglycemia 6. Alkalinization of urine with bicarbonate, 2 mg./kg./dose, maintaining urine pH above 7.0. Alternate form of alkalinization includes Diamox, 5 mg./kg./dose 7. Sponging for fever 8. Vitamin K_1 for hypoprothrombinemia 9. Hemodialysis, peritoneal dialysis or exchange transfusion with (a) levels greater than 160 mg./100 ml., (b) anuria, (c) heart disease with high salicylate levels
Strychnine	Fatal dose for an adult is 15–30 mg.	1. Increased deep tendon reflexes 2. Muscle stiffening 3. Opisthotonus	1. Emesis with ipecac syrup 2. Activated charcoal by lavage tube 3. Control of seizures 4. Prevention of peripheral stimuli and enforcement of quiet
Thallium	Single doses of 8–10 mg./kg. have been fatal in children	1. Abdominal pain, vomiting, diarrhea 2. Ptosis, strabismus, mydriasis, facial palsies 3. Ataxia, tremors, choreiform movements, paresthesias 4. Diaphoresis, hyperpyrexia 5. Vomiting 6. Hypotension 7. Respiratory depression	1. Emesis with ipecac syrup 2. Potassium chloride, 5–25 Gm./day orally, will augment rate of excretion

Thyroid (Cytomel, Synthroid, Desiccated Thyroid, Choloxin)	Toxicity when therapeutic symptoms exceeded. Thyroxine is about 200 times, and triiodothyronine 800 to 1000 times, as potent as desiccated thyroid	1. Palpitations, rapid pulse 2. Headache 3. Tremors, nervousness, delirium 4. Diaphoresis, hyperpyrexia 5. Vomiting 6. Symptoms may occur up to 1 week postingestion	1. Emesis with ipecac syrup 2. No specific antidote exists
Tofranil and Related Drugs	Death has occurred in an infant with a dose of 70 mg./kg.	1. Mydriasis, blurred vision 2. Excessive sweating 3. Urinary retention 4. Dryness of the mouth 5. Drowsiness, convulsions, coma 6. Hypotension 7. Respiratory depression	1. Emesis with ipecac syrup 2. Continuous gastric lavage 3. Maintenance of blood pressure 4. Control of seizures 5. Artificial respiration for severe poisoning 6. Hemodialysis
Tranquilizers (Librium, Valium, Mellaril, Equanil, Miltown, Placidyl, Doriden, Noludar)	Toxicity when therapeutic symptoms exceeded	1. Sleepiness 2. Weakness 3. Unsteadiness 4. Incoordination 5. Hypotension 6. Cyanosis 7. Respiratory failure 8. Coma	1. Emesis with ipecac syrup 2. If comatose, lavage 3. Maintenance of an adequate airway and oxygen 4. Maintenance of blood pressure 5. Supportive therapy during coma 6. Hemodialysis and peritoneal dialysis
Turpentine and Other Volative Oils	15 ml. has caused death	1. Abdominal pain 2. Nausea 3. Vomiting 4. Diarrhea 5. Pneumonia 6. Pulmonary edema 7. Renal failure 8. Central nervous system depression progressing to coma	1. Emesis with ipecac syrup 2. Treatment of renal failure 3. Treatment of respiratory failure 4. Control of seizures
Vitamin A	Toxicity from 200,000–300,000 units	1. Fatigue 2. Anorexia 3. Vomiting 4. Bulging fontanelle 5. Increased intracranial pressure	1. Emesis with ipecac syrup with ingestion of toxic amounts
Vitamin D	Toxicity from 100,000–150,000 units	1. Elevation of serum calcium 2. Metastatic calcifications 3. Renal damage	1. Emesis with ipecac syrup with ingestion of toxic amounts

TABLE 4. Treatment of Specific Poisons—*Continued*

DRUG	TOXICITY	SYMPTOMS	TREATMENT
Warfarin	Repeated doses needed to cause symptoms. Only single ingestions that are massive in amount will cause symptoms	1. Prolonged prothrombin time and clinical bleeding occurring a few days to a few weeks following ingestion	1. Ipecac syrup following repeated ingestion or very large single ingestion 2. Monitoring of prothrombin time 3. Vitamin K (see section on specific therapy in text) 4. Occasionally transfusion therapy

* Manufacturer's precaution: Chlorpromazine (thorazine) is not recommended for children under six months of age except when lifesaving.

† Manufacturer's precaution: Lorfan is for use in treatment of significant narcotic-induced respiratory depression. Lorfan is *ineffective* against respiratory depression due to barbiturates, anesthetics and other non-narcotic agents or pathologic causes, and may increase respiratory depression in these cases.

‡ Manufacturer's precaution: Narcan is not recommended in neonates; safety in children has not been established.

§ Manufacturer's precaution: Safety and efficacy of injectable Valium in children under 12 years of age have not been established. Oral Valium is not for use in children under six months of age.

Adverse Drug Reactions – A Pharmacologic Approach

GREGORY M. CHUDZIK, PHARM.D., FRANKLIN F. DICKEY, B.S. PHARM., *and* SUMNER J. YAFFE, M.D.

The ever-increasing use of potent pharmacologic agents has been associated with an increased number of adverse reactions. The Department of Health, Education and Welfare has shown that one of seven hospital days is devoted to the care of drug toxicity, at an estimated yearly cost of three billion dollars. It has been estimated that 3 to 5 per cent of all hospital admissions are primarily for a drug reaction (Hurwitz, and Seidl et al.). The increasing potency of new drugs and the use of drug combinations will result in a greater incidence of reactions, which are both predictable and possibly preventable when the prescribing physician possesses proper pharmacologic awareness (Melmon). With this knowledge the physician may often avoid causing drug reactions; however, if they do occur, he should be able to recognize and treat them promptly.

Examination of the benefit-to-risk ratio is the initial step when an adverse drug reaction is discovered or suspected. In some instances, the need for the drug is such that one must continue the drug while using supportive therapy for the adverse reaction or side effect. Usually, however, the risk outweighs the benefits, and the use of less toxic (higher benefit-to-risk ratio) agents may be acceptable for therapy. In these cases, the offending agents must be stopped and attention devoted to the treatment of the reaction. To initiate proper treatment, the physician should be aware of the pharmacologic principles which affect the absorption, distribution, metabolism and excretion of the offending agent.

Drug reactions are often related to the lack of precise therapeutic end points and the physician's overly hopeful expectations of drug therapy. Under these circumstances the physician is tempted to increase doses until toxic levels are reached or toxicity occurs.

On the other hand, lack of an expected therapeutic effect often motivates the physician to increase the dose. Whenever a compound fails to give expected results, alteration in its absorption, metabolism, distribution or elimination should be considered and appropriate corrective steps taken. If therapeutic objectives have not been predetermined, the lack of efficacy is difficult to recognize and a useless but potentially toxic agent may continue to be administered in even higher doses.

Melmon and Morrelli have proposed a number of principles to be used in the prevention of drug reactions. Among these are the following:

1. Sound knowledge is requisite for safe therapeutics.
2. Personal experience can never substitute for judgment based on a composite of a methodically obtained fact.
3. Only when specific objectives have been established should drugs be added to an existing regimen. The benefit-to-risk ratio for each drug decreases when many are given.
4. The chemical nature of a drug may be used to predict its absorption, distribution, metabolism and excretion and, therefore, its likelihood of causing toxicity in certain disorders.
5. The use of a drug for a disorder unresponsive to it can lead to a drug overdose.
6. Continuing vigil must be maintained for unusual or changing effects produced by a drug, even though the drug has been given safely for long periods.
7. Diminution of adverse drug reaction rates requires the same knowledge that permits optimal therapeutic effects of the drug.
8. Drug effects must be continually assessed to lessen the likelihood of producing toxicity. If a drug has an adverse effect, drugs of similar chemical composition should be administered cautiously.

Let us now direct our attention to the treatment principles in the management of adverse drug reactions. It is useful to know polarity, i.e., the degree of water solubility of drugs. Highly polar compounds, such as thiazides and mercurial diuretics, are readily dissolved in water, are absorbed at a relatively slow rate and almost always depend on renal excretion. These compounds are likely to accumulate in any patient with decreased renal function.

Nonpolar compounds, such as the phenothiazines, coumarin analogues, quinidine, phenylbutazone and barbiturates, are usually well absorbed by virtue of their lipid solubility. They are highly bound to plasma proteins and in most cases require metabolism by the liver. Thus, patients receiving these agents should be monitored for hepatic function and serum protein concentrations.

It must be emphasized that not all adverse drug reactions are dose-dependent and not all occur immediately upon administration of the agent. Many are the result of long-term therapy and manifest themselves for a considerable time after administration has ceased. Therapy of this type of drug reaction is confined to symptomatic treatment. However, in those cases which are dose-dependent, familiarity with the pharmacokinetic principles and the introduction of these principles into the treatment regimen may improve the outcome.

ABSORPTION

Absorption may take place along the entire length of the gastrointestinal tract. The exact site is dependent on the physicochemical properties of the ingested substance. In most instances, absorption proceeds via passive diffusion in a manner which is similar for all biologic membranes, while specialized transport processes which require energy exist for certain other chemicals.

The physician has available to him two general approaches by which he may alter absorption of an administered agent:

1. Removal of the offending agent.
2. Retardation of the rate and degree of absorption of the agent.

Removal of the offending agent is indeed a difficult task, since the manifestation of adverse drug reactions usually denotes prior absorption of the offending agent. However, the use of techniques such as induction of emesis and gastric lavage may be helpful if the discovery of the adverse reaction comes at a time immediately following administration of further doses of the suspected drug.

Retardation of absorption may be a useful technique, provided that the physician recognizes that the nonionized form (more lipid-soluble form) of a drug will be more readily absorbed than the ionized form. Thus, acidic drugs such as aspirin, penicillin, sulfonamides and phenobarbital are more readily absorbed from the stomach where they exist in the nonionized form, while the bulk of basic drugs is absorbed from the small intestine. Theoretically, antacids, which raise the pH of the gastric contents, may be administered to delay or to inhibit the absorption of acidic drugs from the gastrointestinal tract. It is also theoretically possible that agents such as guanethidine or reserpine, which stimulate gastric acid secretion, might inhibit or delay absorption of the basic drugs.

Complexation reactions might be anticipated when cholestyramine (Cuemid, Questran) or sodium polystyrene sulfonate (Kayexalate) is being used. These resinous materials can combine with other drugs in the gastrointestinal tract and inhibit their absorption. Cholestyramine shows a higher affinity for acidic drugs but may also adsorb neutral and basic drugs to a slight extent. Perhaps the best-known physical chemical agent for adsorption of ingested material is activated charcoal. A number of studies concerning the efficacy of activated charcoal in salicylate absorption have been published. However, the effectiveness of charcoal and any adsorbent agent diminishes markedly as time from the time the drug was ingested elapses.

DISTRIBUTION

Following absorption, drugs and chemical molecules are distributed throughout the body by the vascular system. The rate at which a drug diffuses from the capillary network depends not only on the drug's concentration but also on its lipid solubility, molecular weight and state of binding to plasma proteins. Although many kinds of proteins react with drug molecules, albumin is by far the most important. A drug bound to plasma albumin is not free to diffuse to the active receptor site. It is, however, in equilibrium with a free (active) form. The fraction of bound drug decreases as the total plasma concentration of the drug increases or the concentration of protein decreases. It is possible to increase the concentration of albumin within the vascular tree by intravenous infusion and thus limit the distribution of the ingested agent. It has been demonstrated that plasma protein binding of diphenylhydantoin in an infant with hemolytic disease was markedly increased following infusion of albumin (Rane et al.). Many drugs are bound to plasma albumin, as are endogenous compounds such as steroids. In addition, acidosis, anoxia and disease states affect binding. Thus, the possibility of interaction is great, with consequent change in the amount of free drug and alteration in drug action.

It is generally recognized that three major factors govern the distribution of a drug to the various tissues of the body:

1. Blood flow to the tissues.
2. Mass of the tissue.
3. Affinity of the tissue for the drug.

Thus, just as drugs may compete with each other for plasma protein binding sites, they might also compete with each other for tissue binding sites. Saturation of specific tissue binding sites may decrease activity but increase toxicity of administered drugs, since it decreases the volume of distribution of the agent and therefore increases the circulating concentration of free or unbound drug.

METABOLISM

Foreign compounds are usually eliminated from the body only after prior metabolic conversion. This metabolic process renders the parent compound more water-soluble and thus more readily excretable. With few exceptions, the polar metabolites are considered to be less active than the parent compound, although specific information about the pharmacologic effect of drug metabolites is not often available. The principal site for the various hydroxylation, dealkylation and glucuronide conjugation steps of biotransformation is the smooth endoplasmic reticulum of the hepatic cell, also referred to as the microsomal fraction. Recent studies have shown that many drugs possess an ability to induce an increase in enzyme activity and content of the endoplasmic reticulum (Conney and Gilette). This effect, referred to as enzyme induction, acts to increase the rate of metabolism of many drugs. Phenobarbital and diphenylhydantoin have been demonstrated to be potent enzyme inducers capable of increasing the metabolism of many pharmacologic agents with resultant decrease in the magnitude and/or duration of drug effect.

EXCRETION

Elimination of compounds by urinary excretion involves three general pathways: glomerular filtration, active tubular secretion and tubular reabsorption. Glomerular filtration is a simple molecular filtration of drugs which are not bound to plasma proteins. This process may be enhanced by the displacement of highly protein-bound drugs with the addition of a second, perhaps less toxic, compound. Active tubular secretion involves transport of drug from the blood across the proximal tubular cell into the tubular urine against a concentration gradient. Enhancement of this excretion process is extremely impractical. Tubular reabsorption is a passive diffusion process by which drugs delivered into tubular urine by one of the two previously mentioned clearance methods can passively diffuse back into the blood. The urinary pH will influence the ionization of weak acids and weak bases and thus affect the extent to which these agents are reabsorbed or excreted. When a drug is in its nonionized form, it will more readily diffuse from the urine back into the blood. Therefore, for an acidic drug, a larger proportion of the drug will be in the ionized (more rapidly excreted) form in a basic urine; the converse is true for the basic drugs. We must remember that these methods of increasing renal excretion of drugs will be clinically significant only when the drug or its active metabolites are appreciably eliminated by the renal route.

CONCLUSION

The authors have attempted to identify and explain a newly recognized danger involved in drug therapy: that of the adverse drug reaction. It is evident that a number of these adverse reactions are not only predictable but possibly preventable. Thorough examination of the absorption, distribution, metabolism and excretion of drugs (and drug combinations) is essential for the welfare of the pediatric patient. If, however, an adverse drug reaction does occur, particular attention to the principles of management outlined herein may minimize the possibility of long-term iatrogenic damage.

References

Conney, A. H.: Pharmacological Implications of Microsomal Enzyme Induction. *Pharmacol. Rev.*, 19:317, 1969.

Gilette, J. R.; in Siegler, P. E., and Moyer, J. H., III (eds.): *Animal and Clinical Pharmacological Techniques in Drug Evaluation.* Chicago, Yearbook Medical Publishers, 1967, pp. 48–66.

Hurwitz, N.: Admissions to Hospital Due to Drugs. *Brit. Med. J.*, 1:539, 1969.

Melmon, K. L.: Preventable Drug Reactions–Causes and Cures. *New England J. Med.*, 284:1361, 1971.

Melmon, K. L., and Morelli, H. F. (eds.): *Clinical Pharmacology.* New York, The Macmillan Company, 1972.

Rane, A., Lunde, P. K., Yaffe, S. J., Jalling, B., and Sjoqvist, F.: Plasma Protein Binding of Diphenylhydantoin in Normal and Hyperbilirubinemic Infant Plasma. *J. Pediat.*, 78:877, 1971.

Seidl, L. G., et al.: Studies on the Epidemiology of Adverse Drug Reactions III. Reactions in Patients on a General Medical Service. *Bull. Hopkins Hosp.*, 119:299, 1966.

United States Department of Health, Education and Welfare Task Force on Prescription Drugs: Final Report. Washington, D. C., Government Printing Office, 1969.

Salicylate Intoxication

LAURENCE FINBERG, M.D.

Once the diagnosis of salicylate poisoning has been made the therapist will have to consider a number of important variables before beginning treatment. Most important among these are whether the poisoning resulted over a short period of time, such as from a large dose ingested accidentally or with suicidal intent, and the age of the patient. A lesser matter concerns the type of salicylate preparation. Most commonly the offender is aspirin (acetylsalicylate); less commonly, oil of wintergreen (methyl salicylate) may be ingested. Because oil of wintergreen is liquid, a very large dose may be easily swallowed. A level teaspoonful equals 5 Gm. of the fluid. Thus, dosage rather than any special property probably accounts for the high incidence of severe poisonings from this agent.

Salicylate preparations are efficiently and rapidly absorbed from the duodenum. On entering the blood the salicylate ion binds loosely to plasma albumin, but then rapidly diffuses throughout body water, resulting in a decrease in blood level prior to significant excretion. If the salicylate is swallowed when the stomach is empty, peak blood levels are reached in 75 to 90 minutes. About 2 hours later a plateau is reached, and then the level decreases gradually owing to excretion. After a large dose, complete excretion takes days if no assistance is given.

The major pathway of excretion is through the urine, in which the drug appears as the free salicylate ion and as two soluble conjugates formed in the liver, a glycuronide and salicuric acid (a glycine conjugate). About 90 per cent of the ingested dose eventually appears in the urine. Because the action of the liver takes place slowly, large doses of salicylate cannot be cleared rapidly by hepatic action. The excretion of free salicylate by the kidney, like that of any ion of a weak acid, is enhanced by an alkaline pH in the renal tubular fluid. In the case of salicylate, a change in urine pH from 6.5 to 7.5 (tenfold decrease in hydrogen ion) produces almost a tenfold increase in salicylate owing to inhibition of renal tubular reabsorption of the ionized form. Thus, whereas the free form is about 20 per cent of the total salicylate in an acid urine, it constitutes 80 to 95 per cent of an alkaline urine at pH values above 7.5.

The toxicity of large doses of salicylate affects the central nervous system and energy metabolism. Salicylate irritates the brain in general and in particular it stimulates the respiratory center, causing primary hyperventilation. The molecular basis for this is not known, but the effect seems to be a direct one resulting in early overbreathing with consequent reduction in the blood pCO_2. The brain irritation may result in coma or convulsions, findings usually manifest in severe toxicity.

The predominant effects of metabolism are twofold: First, there is an inhibition of two Krebs cycle enzymes, alpha-ketoglutaric dehydrogenase and succinic dehydrogenase, leading to gluconeogenesis and ketosis. A second effect results in the uncoupling of oxidative phosphorylation, causing a hypermetabolic state manifested by fever and increased oxygen consumption. Some of these effects tend to cancel each other physiologically, while others act together to augment the damage.

A particularly complicated situation arises vis-a-vis hydrogen ion metabolism and the acid-base status. The primary depression of the pCO_2 characterizes all poisoned patients. However, in the very young, from toddlers to five years of age, the most frequent victims of accidental ingestion, this phenomenon does not result, as might be expected, in a respiratory alkalemia and alkaluria. The reason derives from the rapidly developing metabolic events wherein ketoacid production results in a sharp reduction of bicarbonate ion, which at first "compensates" and, ultimately, in a few hours swamps the direct ventilatory effect on hydrogen ion level, thus resulting in acidemia. This in turn produces a vicious circle because the renal excretion of salicylate is inhibited by the resultant acid urine. Fever and diaphoresis from the hypermetabolic state join with the hyperventilation to increase water losses, a circumstance worsened by nausea, which limits water intake. The conditions described predispose to a hypernatremic type of dehydration with a metabolic acidemia plus an independently low pCO_2.

The effects of salicylate on carbohydrate metabolism may be reflected in disturbances in blood glucose levels: early hyperglycemia, and later hypoglycemic levels sometimes are seen. In animals, an ample liver glycogen store protects against salicylate poisoning. Clinical observations make it seem likely that this is true of humans as well. Additionally, over a period of a few days, salicylate depresses prothrombin production. Aspirin, but not other salicylates, seriously interferes with platelet activity and, finally, large doses of salicylate damage renal tubules. There are many other actions of salicylate, but for this discussion, those above are the pertinent ones.

ACUTE POISONING

Young children frequently present to physicians after having ingested a large dosage of salicylate over a short period of time. A dose exceeding 200 mg. per kilogram of weight invariably produces toxicity if absorbed; doses of less than 100 mg. per kilogram in a previously healthy child are not dangerous. The amounts inbetween cannot be safely predicted. Correlating these doses with blood levels shows that plateau or steady-state levels exceeding 30 mg. per 100 ml. invariably are associated with symptoms. Peak levels (at 90 minutes) may reach as high as 50 mg. per 100 ml. without symptoms, however. If the child is seen within the first 2 hours after ingestion (up to 6 hours for oil of wintergreen) either emesis should be induced or gastric lavage carried out to remove any residual drug from the stomach.

Following this step, the goals of therapy are twofold: (1) to correct the progressive physiologic disturbances of water balance, acid-base status and carbohydrate metabolism, and (2) to hasten the removal of salicylate. These aims may be accomplished simultaneously by appropriate techniques which can hydrate, cause hydrogen ion removal and remove the salicylate through the urine or, if necessary, by dialysis. Our experience with more than 600 consecutive hospitalized patients following single large ingestions, seen within 24 hours of poisoning, indicates that the renal route of excretion is satisfactory with the regimen described in the following paragraphs, since dialysis has not proved necessary for this group of patients, all of whom survived apparently undamaged.

The principles of therapy recommended here are as follows:

1. Adequate hydration with an excess of water to provide a high volume of urine.
2. Ample provision of glucose (as a 5 per cent solution) to provide excess substrate for Krebs cycle activity and to replenish liver glycogen.
3. Provision of sufficient base to correct acidosis. Some of the base should be provided as the potassium salt as soon as urine formation has been observed.
4. Provision of excess base to alkalinize the urine in conjunction with administration of carbonic anhydrase inhibitor.
5. Administration of the carbonic anhydrase inhibitor, acetazolamide, 5 mg. per kilogram of body weight subcutaneously immediately and repeated two more times at 5-hour intervals. This drug is given as a facilitator of base excretion only in conjunction with systemic alkalinization to obtain an alkaline urine without the risk of excess sodium administration. Similarly, this drug reduces risks from overvigorous implementation of step 4.

The first four steps are implemented with individual variation, depending on the state of hydration of the patient. If marked dehydration is present, emergency rehydration with replacement of deficit may be necessary. When hydration is not severely disturbed, an immediate, rapidly running, intravenous solution of ⅙ M sodium lactate, bicarbonate, succinate or acetate (the lactate is as satisfactory as the others) in 5 per cent glucose should be started. The sodium concentration of such a solution is 167 mEq. per liter, and this would be excessive if it were not possible to facilitate sodium excretion by simultaneous administration of acetazolamide.

As soon as urine is obtainable, the pH should be checked at regular intervals until it reaches 7.5 or higher. This usually takes less than an hour, frequently as little as 20 minutes. At this point, the sodium concentration of the intravenous solution should be reduced to about 40 to 50 mEq. per liter, and 20 mEq. of potassium ion per liter should be added. The anions should be about half base (lactate, bicarbonate or acetate) and half chloride. The potassium ion is important because potassium levels in serum are low in salicylate poisoning and because the acetazolamide enhances potassium loss as well as sodium loss. The rate of the infusion should be adjusted to provide water at about two to three times the ordinary maintenance allowance, e.g., at a rate of about 300 ml. per kilogram per day in a two-year-old.

In milder poisoning and when the patient presents very early following ingestion and before marked acidosis, the initial intravenous base concentration may be held to the lower (50 mEq. per liter) concentration of the sodium salt. The acetazolamide should be given promptly and potassium added when urine formation is demonstrable.

Acetazolamide without base administration would not be safe because acidosis would be worsened. This agent has been associated with the occurrence of convulsions in one author's report. We have seen this symptom a number of times prior to therapy and only rarely afterward, leaving the question of a causal relationship in doubt. We have not, in any event, seen lasting harm.

Attempts to alkalinize the urine by administration of sodium bicarbonate or other bases without the acetazolamide are not advised because of the risks of severe hypernatremia or of rapidly decreasing the cerebrospinal fluid pH through CO_2 diffusion, which occurs much faster than bicarbonate ion movement into the cerebrospinal fluid.

If no urine is formed after the initial hydration, indicating serious oliguria, either peritoneal or extracorporeal dialysis should be instituted, applying the same principles but no longer depending on the renal mechanisms to remove the salicylate. The peritoneal route, while providing a satisfactory method for correcting the physiologic disturbances, does not provide a very efficient means of salicylate removal. The addition of albumin to the dialysate helps. Extracorporeal dialysis, on the other hand, is highly efficient in both physiologic correction and removal of toxin. The hazards include anticoagulation, blood transfusion and possible blood volume or blood pressure disturbances. In our experience, only the neglected patients (three days or more) and those suffering chronic salicylism with renal damage (obviously, also patients with independent severe kidney disease) have required dialysis.

We do not recommend the use of tromethamine or exchange transfusion for acute salicylate poisoning because of hazards involved and poor efficiency of removal of the drug.

In older patients with large short-term ingestions, usually adolescents attempting suicide, management is similar except that much less base is necessary initially because there may be a primary respiratory alkalemia with alkaline urine, and there is thus considerable delay in the onset of metabolic acidosis. The rest of the management proceeds in the same way, with acetazolamide being given promptly.

CHRONIC TOXICITY

This term applies to patients who have had doses of salicylate over a period of days or weeks, usually at a high therapeutic dosage range. However, in this type of poisoning the patient may be very sick or even die with levels that are well below 30 mg. per 100 ml. Indeed, there is little correlation between illness and level in these patients, who all too often have iatrogenesis as the basis of the problem. In this group, the effects of salicylate on prothrombin production, platelets and renal tubules are more important. Vitamin K as the K_1 oxide, 5 to 10 mg. intravenously, should be administered quickly. Fresh blood transfusion is in order if bleeding is observed. The previous mode of therapy may be carried out unless oliguria becomes apparent, in which case dialysis, either peritoneal or extracorporeal, is indicated.

Acute Lead Poisoning and Asymptomatic Increased Lead Absorption

J. JULIAN CHISOLM, Jr., M.D.

Principles of Therapy. Immediate separation of the child with clinical or metabolic evidence of plumbism from high-dose sources of lead must receive first priority in any therapeutic program. Since it is often difficult to curb pica in a toddler quickly, initial emphasis is placed on separation of the child from hazardous and readily available sources, such as flaking old paint, crumbling old putty and improperly glazed pottery. Each case is reported to the local health department for identification and correction of hazardous environmental conditions. Cases are reported simultaneously to the medical-social service department (see Pica).

Chelating agents are important *adjuncts* in the management of lead poisoning; they are not a substitute for careful control of exposure. They serve to reduce dangerous increments in soft tissue lead content safely and rapidly to less toxic levels. Dosage in each case should be adjusted to the physician's estimate of the nonosseous, metabolically active fraction of the total body lead burden. According to these principles, blood lead concentrations greater than 100 micrograms of lead per 100 Gm. of whole blood and the presence of symptoms call for the highest initial dosage consistent with safety. Dosage is tapered as blood lead concentration, the amount of lead excreted in urine under the influence of chelating agents, and the metabolic indices of lead toxicity decrease toward normal. Best overall therapeutic results are probably achieved when chelation therapy is initiated in the presymptomatic or metabolic phase of lead poisoning. Although the combined use of BAL (British anti-lewisite) and Ca EDTA (edathamil calcium-disodium) therapy and fluid restriction increase the frequency of survival of patients with encephalopathy, treatment at this stage is not effective in reversing the permanent brain damage usually associated with this severe degree of acute lead poisoning. This is the major reason for instituting chelation therapy prior to the onset of obvious and severe symptoms.

Treatment of Symptomatic Cases. All symptomatic young children are treated as potential cases of acute encephalopathy. Included in this group are children with persistent vomiting and moderate to severe anemia (with the morphologic characteristics of iron deficiency), as well as those with seizures and alterations in the state of consciousness. Symptomatic patients are maintained on parenteral fluids initially. Oral fluids are withheld until symptoms abate.

Prompt institution of chelation therapy is clearly indicated in this group as soon as adequate urine flow is established. Initially, 10 per cent dextrose in water (10 to 20 ml. per kilogram of body weight) is given over a period of 1 to 2 hours. If this fails to initiate urination, mannitol* (1 to 2 Gm. per kilogram body weight) is infused intravenously in 20 per cent solution at a rate of 1 ml. per minute. As soon as urine flow is established, further intravenous fluid therapy is restricted to basal water and electrolyte requirements, to a minimal estimate of the quantities required for replacement of deficits (due to vomiting and dehydration) and to increased requirements resulting from convulsive activity or intercurrent fever. In patients with encephalopathy, proper fluid therapy is vital to survival and is best monitored by measuring the rate of urine flow. The rate of infusion is adjusted hourly until a rate is found that maintains the rate of urine flow within basal metabolic limits (0.35 to 0.5 ml. urine secreted per calorie metabolized per 24 hours). This is equivalent to a daily urinary output of 350 to 500 ml. per square meter per 24 hours. Seizures are controlled initially with Valium† and thereafter with running doses of paraldehyde during the first few days. Long-term anticonvulsive drugs (Dilantin, barbiturates) are begun toward the end of the first week of therapy while paraldehyde is being tapered off. During the acute phase, one should not await the development of frank seizures: better control can be achieved if doses of paraldehyde are given whenever there is a significant increase in muscle tone or muscle twitching. Body temperature is maintained at normal but not hypothermic levels.

Chelation therapy with BAL and Ca EDTA is given according to the dosage schedule in Table 1. The usual five-day course may be extended to seven days if severe clinical evi-

* Manufacturer's precaution: Use of mannitol in pediatric patients has not been studied comprehensively.

† Manufacturer's precaution: The safety and efficacy of injectable Valium in children under 12 years of age have not been established. Oral Valium is not to be used in children under six months of age.

dence of encephalopathy persists beyond four days. Blood lead concentrations and heme metabolites usually increase after the first course of chelation therapy, so that serial measurements should be made after the last doses of BAL and Ca EDTA and 7, 14 and 21 days thereafter. Where an initial course of BAL and Ca EDTA is not followed by D-penicillamine (Table 1), it is often necessary to give one or more subsequent courses of Ca EDTA alone. A second course of Ca EDTA is likely to be most effective if administered when the rebounding concentration reaches 80 micrograms of lead per 100 Gm. of whole blood or when erythrocyte protoporphyrin, urinary aminolevulinic acid or coproporphyrin values exceed normal by tenfold or more. Medicinal

TABLE 1. Dosage Schedule for Chelating Agents in Young Children

BAL–CA EDTA IN COMBINATION

Dosage: BAL* 4 mg./kg. body weight/dose (I.M.)
Ca EDTA† 12.5 mg./kg. body weight/dose (I.M.)

Administration: For first dose inject BAL (I.M.) only; beginning 4 hours later and q.4 hours thereafter for five to seven days, inject BAL and Ca EDTA simultaneously at separate and deep intramuscular sites; rotate injection sites.

CA EDTA ONLY

Dosage: 50 mg./kg. body weight/day in divided doses q.12 hours (I.M.)

Administration: Maximum daily dose should not exceed 1 Gm. in young children; allow two to three weeks between each three- to five-day course of therapy.

D-PENICILLAMINE‡

Dosage: 35 to 40 mg./kg. body weight/day for long-term oral therapy in divided doses.

Administration: Give on empty stomach 1½ to 2 hours prior to meals b.i.d.; contents of capsule may be mixed in a small amount of fruit or fruit juice immediately prior to administration.

*BAL. The dosage recommended for young children (4 mg./kg.) is higher on a body weight basis than that recommended by the Food and Drug Administration for adults (2.5 mg./kg.). On the basis of surface area, they are both equivalent to approximately 100 mg./m²/dose.

† Ca EDTA. Edathamil calcium-disodium (Versenate) available in 20% solution. For intramuscular use add sufficient procaine to yield a final concentration of 0.5% procaine. Intramuscular injection is more convenient in children and permits better control of intravenous fluids, a vital consideration in cases of encephalopathy. It has been used in this clinic for 20 years without untoward incident.

‡ D-Penicillamine. β,β-dimethylcysteine available as Cuprimine in 250-mg. capsules. Investigational drug; see recommendations of A.M.A. Council on Drugs for use.

iron should not be given concurrently with BAL, but it should be started immediately thereafter for correction of iron deficiency anemia, and continued until iron stores are repleted.

In symptomatic cases, no time is wasted in attempts to evacuate residual lead from the bowel by enema. Surgical decompression for relief of increased intracranial pressure is clearly contraindicated. The role of steroids in combating cerebral edema in acute lead encephalopathy is not clear.

Management of Asymptomatic Cases with Increased Lead Absorption. Prompt separation of the child from high-dose lead sources is the first step. Children with confirmed blood lead concentrations greater than 50 to 60 micrograms per 100 Gm. whole blood should be followed closely for 18 months or longer, including at least one summer during which levels remain stable or decline. Iron deficiency, if present, should be treated vigorously. Those with confirmed blood lead concentrations greater than 80 to 100 micrograms should receive BAL and Ca EDTA in combination for two to three days, followed by Ca EDTA only at the lower dosage for three additional days (Table 1). The available data are not sufficient to provide sound criteria for the use of chelating agents in children with blood lead concentrations in the 50- to 80-microgram range. We have limited chelation therapy in this group to those who also show tenfold or greater increments in (1) erythrocyte protoporphyrin and (2) daily urinary output of coproporphyrin or delta-aminolevulinic acid. We have treated children meeting these tentative criteria in a convalescent pediatric facility with oral D-penicillamine alone. Oral administration of chelating agents to outpatients should be approached with great caution: They will not counteract the effects of continued excessive intake of lead. Preliminary data suggest that serial measurements of erythrocyte protoporphyrin (and probably aminolevulinic acid dehydrase activity) may prove highly useful in follow-up and in monitoring chelation therapy.

Precautions in the Use of Chelating Agents. EDTA is not metabolized in the body, but rather is excreted unchanged by the kidney. Ca EDTA, but not BAL, must be withheld during periods of anuria. Administration of Ca EDTA at the dosage levels given must not exceed seven successive days. Untoward reactions to Ca EDTA include the following: local reactions at injection site, hypercalcemia, raised blood urea nitrogen, proteinuria, microscopic hematuria and fever. Safe administration of Ca EDTA requires the following determinations on the first, third and fifth days of each course of therapy: BUN, serum calcium, serum phosphorus and routine urinalysis. Patient receiving Ca EDTA intravenously should also be observed for irregularities of cardiac rhythm.

D-Penicillamine is contraindicated in children with a history of penicillin sensitivity. Reactions to D-penicillamine can be minimized if oral dosage is restricted to less than 40 mg. per kilogram per day. Patients who react to D-penicillamine usually do so within the first month. Proteinuria or hypersensitivity reactions (angioneurotic edema, erythematous rashes) are contraindications to its further use.

Convalescent and Long-Term Care. The aims of long-term care are to minimize recurrences, curb pica and find a safe dwelling for the child. All preschool-age housemates of index cases should be examined. All cases are reported to the medical-social service and local public health authorities. Temporary safe residence for the child should be arranged while the dwelling is being repaired according to local ordinances, especially if this entails the burning and scraping of paint. (If the home is too deteriorated to permit adequate repair, the family is assisted by the medical-social service department in finding new housing.) Once a hospitalized child is returned home, he is seen at frequent intervals, particularly during the first few months. During the first six to 12 months of convalescence, intercurrent infections may be associated with biochemical evidence of increased lead toxicity without concomitant rise in blood lead level. Such episodes may be covered by a three-day course of Ca EDTA therapy in the hospital. Serial blood lead determinations should be made monthly during the summer and at least quarterly during the winter in order to determine the trend. Blood lead values which rebound to greater than 75 to 80 micrograms per 100 Gm. whole blood probably indicate recurrent excessive ingestion of lead and call for repeat courses of Ca EDTA and repeat environmental evaluation. Phenobarbital and Dilantin are generally adequate for the control of seizures; recurrence of seizures without recurrent lead ingestion is usually indicative of a lapse in medication or failure to increase the dose in accordance with growth. For children with brain damage, plans should be made early for appropriate special placement. Where clinical evaluation and psychometric testing indicate no significant permanent injury, parents should be reassured.

References

A. M. A. Council on Drugs: A Copper Chelating Agent, Penicillamine (Cuprimine). *J.A.M.A.*, 189:847, 1964.

Chisolm, J. J., Jr.: The Use of Chelating Agents in the Treatment of Acute and Chronic Lead Intoxication in Childhood. *J. Pediat.*, 73:1–38, 1968.

Coffin, R., Phillips, J. L., Staples, W. I., and Spector, S.: Treatment of Lead Encephalopathy in Children. *J. Pediat.*, 69:198, 1966.

Foreman, H.: Toxic Side Effects of Ethylenediaminetetraacetic Acid. *J. Chron. Dis.*, 16:319, 1963.

Perlstein, M. A., and Attala, R.: Neurologic Sequelae of Plumbism in Children. *Clin. Pediat.*, 5:292–298, 1966.

Acrodynia

S. N. JAVETT, M.D.

Acrodynia is now a rare disease. As contrasted with its frequency in the years between the great wars when it was largely iatrogenic, caused by poisoning from mercury administered in teething powders, it is currently an accidental disease encountered more in adults than in children. In truth, whole generations of medical students have qualified without the opportunity of seeing a case, or for that matter even of hearing about it. Thus are they denied the erstwhile teacher's alliterative joy when expounding the main symptoms—pink hands and feet, pain, pruritus, paresthesia, photophobia, perspiration, ptyalism, papular rash, pulse and pressure raised, poor sleeping and eating.

In this light it is probable that as many cases are missed as are diagnosed, more particularly when it is realized that the characteristic pinkness of hands and feet may be missing. If poisoning is considered, an estimate of the urinary mercury becomes mandatory. The source may be found in paints and various mercury-containing ointments, the mercury being absorbed from the intact skin. Some patent medicines are not above suspicion.

Ironically, it was only toward the end of the acrodynic era that more satisfactory treatment emerged. Obviously, with the cause of the condition known, attention was turned to the elimination of mercury by chelation, initially with the use of dimercaprol (BAL), later EDTA, or the two combined. By 1960 edathamil calcium-disodium had been virtually discarded, but BAL continues to occupy an important place in treatment. It is given by intramuscular injection of a 10 per cent solution in a dose of 2.5 mg. per kilogram every 4 hours for two days: Thereafter, four more doses for one day are given, then the same dosage once or twice daily for another week. The duration of treatment is governed by the symptoms as well as by the mercury content in the urine. The pain of the injections can be eased by the prior injection of 0.5 mg. of 2 per cent procaine into the proposed site. There is little doubt that the pain attendant on injecting BAL is a deterrent to its use. Side effects are not infrequent, consisting of nausea, vomiting and fever.

The introduction in 1959 of penicillamine, which can be given orally, was more than welcome. D-Penicillamine is the D isomer of β, β-dimethylcysteine, a degradation product of penicillin having the property of chelating heavy metals due to the presence of a thiol group. It is absorbed from the gastrointestinal tract and rapidly excreted in the urine.

Side effects are uncommon. Fever, rashes, leukopenia, thrombopenia and nephrosis have been reported. The drug should be stopped until the adverse reaction subsides. Steroids may be useful in counteracting side effects. Patients sensitive to penicillin will also react to penicillamine.

The dose of penicillamine is 30 mg. per kilogram given in two or three divided doses per 24 hours. For young infants it should be dissolved in fruit juice. Treatment is continued until symptoms improve and the urinary mercury is less than 100 micrograms per liter. The average period of treatment required is three to four weeks, but in individual cases may be longer.

In a disease in which wretchedness governs the clinical picture, symptomatic treatment is important. Hydroxyzine (Atarax) and chlorpromazine* (Largactil) may be used for restlessness, and trimeprazine† for insomnia. Severe cases with marked anorexia, dehydration and weight loss may require feeding by gavage. On occasion, intravenous replacement of fluid and electrolytes has been necessary. Secondary infection, especially of urine and skin lesions, will require appropriate antibiotic treatment.

Reference

Javett, S. N., and Kaplan, B.: Acrodynia Treated with D-Penicillamine. *Am. J. Dis. Child.*, 115:71, 1968.

* Manufacturer's precaution: Chlorpromazine is not recommended for children under six months of age except when lifesaving.

† Manufacturer's precaution: Trimeprazine is not recommended for children under six months of age.

Stinging Insect Hypersensitivity

HARRY LOUIS MUELLER, M.D.

Systemic allergic reactions to stings of the Hymenoptera, which include bees, wasps, hornets, yellow jackets and stinging ants, can be life-threatening. Once such sensitivity develops it is likely to increase in severity, and the speed and degree of that increase is impossible to predict. Consequently, all patients who have had a systemic allergic reaction to one or more stings should be treated by desensitization injections. Such treatment has been protective in more than 95 per cent of the author's series of over 700 cases. Because some patients can become exquisitely sensitive and fatalities have occurred in seconds, before the victim could even take "protective medication," self-medication for emergency treatment with subsequent stings must not be relied upon.

The best available method of determining a starting dose for injection treatment of the patients is to do serial intracutaneous testing (Mueller, 1959) with graduated dilutions of whole-insect extract beginning with a dilution of 1:1,000,000. A tenfold increase in concentration can be applied every 20 minutes until an initial positive skin reaction is obtained. This should be a minimum erythema of 2 cm. plus a wheal larger than that made originally by the injected material. Testing materials of greater concentration than 1:1000 are apt to be primary irritants and may give false-positive reactions. Testing within two weeks of the acute systemic reaction is not recommended because patients may be in a refractory period with little or no available antibody to react, and may give false-negative reactions at such a time (Mueller, 1959).

Desensitization is started with a subcutaneous injection of 0.05 ml. of the dilution (of a mixture of bee, polistes wasp, hornet and yellow jacket whole-body extracts) which gave the initial positive test. The dose is increased gradually at intervals that can vary depending on how rapidly it is desirable to reach protective levels. Such increasing doses can be given twice weekly, weekly or even every two to four weeks if time allows before the next place or season of exposure is expected.

A dose of 0.05 ml. of a 1:10 concentration is equivalent in antigenic activity to the average amount of venom in one to two stings as measured by skin test titration in vitro. The maintenance protective dose should be above this level and, if tolerated, a dose of 0.25 or the equivalent of 5 to 10 stings is desirable. Table 1 is a guide to dosage increments, but each patient's treatment must be adjusted to individualized tolerance.

TABLE 1. Dosage for Treatment of Stinging Insect Hypersensitivity with Whole-Body Insect Extract

DILUTIONS ABOVE 1:100,000	DILUTIONS 1:100,000 TO 1:100	DILUTIONS 1:10
0.05 ml.	0.05 ml.	0.05 ml.
0.1 ml.	0.1 ml.	0.075 ml.
0.2 ml.	0.2 ml.	0.1 ml.
0.4 ml.	0.35 ml.	0.15 ml.
	0.5 ml.	0.2 ml.
		0.25 ml.

When the protective or maximum tolerated dose is reached, it is given as a booster at monthly intervals for a year, then every two months for the second year and every three months for the third year. It had been our practice to stop the treatment after three years and await developments with subsequent stings. A recent study of our experience over a 20-year period (Mueller et al.) has indicated that the immunity or protection is apparently retained in a little over 95 per cent of patients, but in less than 5 per cent it might wear off in from 2 to 10 years and the patient again becomes susceptible to severe and dangerous reactions to subsequent stings. In the past three years we have been giving annual booster injections to these patients, and during this time none has had systemic reactions to subsequent stings. These booster injections have been given with the full protective dose that the patient had been receiving for previous maintenance treatment.

Treated patients have been encouraged not to exert unusual effort to avoid subsequent stings and are instructed not to take any medication if stung unless definite systemic allergic symptoms occur. Protective measures are not advocated because it is valuable for both the patient and the physician to learn whether the treatment has been effective. In treated patients there is at least sufficient partial protection to allow time for protective medication to be effective in the event systemic symptoms do appear. It must be remembered that rarely, the insect's stinger may enter a capillary or venule and the antigenic venom be injected directly into the circulation. Under such circumstances the antigen-antibody reaction may be so rapid and severe that no amount of immunologic treatment will prevent anaphylaxis.

Treatment of the Acute Systemic Reaction. An acute systemic reaction to an insect sting should be treated promptly with aqueous epinephrine 1:1000 in doses consistent with the severity of the reaction, and repeated as often as indicated by the circumstances. Antihistamines by themselves will not protect against the serious results of such reactions, but they may be used in addition to epinephrine, particularly to combat urticaria and itching. Corticosteroids, by any route of administration, do not act rapidly enough to be of any value with the immediate problems of anaphylaxis, but they can be helpful as an adjunct with other supportive measures to relieve prolonged or delayed signs and symptoms. Prednisone, 30 mg. daily for three days and in diminishing doses over another four days can be helpful for persistent urticaria and angioedema. The immediate and supportive treatment of anaphylaxis from any cause is the same and is described elsewhere.

Local treatment of insect stings consisting of solutions, creams, ointments or sprays containing local anesthetics, steroids or antihistamines is of little proved value, but the application of cold is helpful to reduce discomfort, decrease circulation, slow absorption and inhibit the development of edema. Stingers (left only by bees) should be removed with tweezers or the scrape of a knife.

Emergency kits have been recommended for self-treatment of the acute reaction. The author's experience with such equipment, which relies on epinephrine and a syringe, has been unsatisfactory. When the emergency arises, the individual instructed in its use for a child is usually not available, or, in the case of self-administration, the reaction may be so sudden and severe that the patient is too ill to treat himself. Emergency medication should be provided for patients who are not desensitized or for use in the event a sting occurs before protective treatment is established. Isoproterenol sublingual tablets, 10 or 15 mg. as indicated according to age, are simple to take with no need for swallowing, but this is not effective in combating circulatory collapse. Epinephrine, 1:200 in a dispenser to use by inhalation (Medihaler-Epi) can be kept on hand to be used for obstructive respiratory symptoms and to combat circulatory collapse and shock.

Protective measures against stinging (Morse and Ghent) include the wearing of light-colored clothes, and avoidance of sweaty and other objectional odors, hair oils and perfumes when exposure is expected. In the event of an encounter with the insects, rapid evasive tactics may invite attack. These measures are not recommended as a substitute for specific desensitization treatment but only for protection in the event this specific treatment is delayed, refused or ineffective.

References

Morse, R. A., and Ghent, R. L.: Protective Measures Against Stinging Insects. *New York J. Med.*, 59: 1546, 1959.

Mueller, H. L.: Serial Intracutaneous Testing for Bee and Wasp Sensitivity. *J. Allergy*, 30:123, 1959.

Mueller, H. L., Schmid, W. H., and Rubinsztain, R.: Stinging Insect Hypersensitivity—A Twenty Year Study of Immunologic Treatment. *J. Pediat.*, in press.

Snakebite

FINDLAY E. RUSSELL, M.D., *and*
JACK WAINSCHEL, M.D.

Snake venom poisoning is an emergency requiring immediate medical attention. To be effective, treatment must include measures to retard absorption of the venom, to remove as much venom as possible from the wound, to neutralize the venom, to mitigate the effects produced by the venom and to prevent complications, including secondary infection.

Immobilization of the affected part at heart level or in a slightly dependent physiologic position with absolute rest for the victim is indicated in all cases. If the bite is on an extremity, place a constriction band above the first joint proximal to the injury. The constriction band should be made tight enough to occlude the superficial venous and lymphatic return, but not arterial flow. It should be released for 90 seconds every 10 minutes.

Longitudinal incisions 1/8 to 1/4 inch in length should be made through the fang marks, except in patients in whom there is an abnormal amount of bleeding. The incisions should be as deep as the fang penetration. In most cases the venom is ejected just beneath the skin. Suction should then be applied and continued for the first hour after the bite. To be effective, suction must be applied within the first few minutes after the bite; it is of no value if delayed for 30 minutes. Multiple incisions over the involved extremity or in advance of progressive edema are not advised. Fasciotomy should be avoided.

After the first hour, suction should be discontinued, and ice bags placed around the injured part in a manner that allows the wound to remain dry. The constriction band should be released. The ice bags should be removed when antivenin is being administered and for at least one hour thereafter. An ice bag within a towel may be placed over the wound area for 24 to 96 hours. The skin temperature should be kept between 50° and 60° F. (10° and 15° C.). Cryotherapy should be avoided.

None of the first-aid measures should be regarded as substitutes for antivenin, antibiotics and antitetanus agents; nor should they be instituted at the possible expense of delaying administration of antivenin. The amount of antivenin to be used will depend on the species and size of the snake involved and certain factors noted elsewhere (Klauber). In children, bites by rattlesnakes may require 1 to 12 vials of Antivenin (Crotalidae) Polyvalent, after appropriate skin or eye sensitivity tests. Bites by copperheads rarely require more than one or two vials.

The early administration of antivenin in children cannot be overemphasized. Whenever possible, the antivenin should be given intravenously, each vial in 10 to 30 ml. of saline. Four or five vials may be given during a 30-minute period. The initial dose should be supplemented as necessary if the swelling and edema spread, or if the other symptoms and signs persist or worsen. A measurement of the circumference of the affected part at two places above the bite taken every 15 to 30 minutes provides a good index by which to evaluate the progress of the swelling. But changes in pain, blood pressure, hemoglobin, the electrocardiogram, respiration and so forth must also be evaluated in determining the amount of additional antivenin that should be given. For bites by *Crotalus scutulatus* (the Mojave rattlesnake), particular attention must be given to the rate and type of respiratory movements.

Antivenin can be given intramuscularly distant to the wound or subcutaneously in advance of the edema, but in most cases the intravenous route is preferred. Under no circumstances should antivenin be injected into a toe or finger.

In patients sensitive to horse serum, the physician will need to weigh the risk of withholding the antivenin against the risk of death from venom poisoning. Antivenin, prepared in goats for use in patients sensitive to horse serum, is not available at this time.

An antibiotic should be given in all but trivial cases. Most clinicians recommend a broad-spectrum antibiotic. Tetanus toxoid, or tetanus antitoxin if it is indicated, should also be given. Whole blood transfusions are frequently necessary in patients in whom hemorrhage is extensive. In very severe bites in children, 250 ml. of fresh whole blood should be given on admission, if there is no serious contraindication.

Metaraminol, 0.4 mg. per kilogram, in saline or glucose (1 mg. per 25 ml.), titrated accordingly, may be indicated if shock develops. Codeine, 3 mg. per kilogram per 24 hours, may be used to alleviate pain. Oxygen should always be readily available, and after bites by *Crotalus scutulatus* and large specimens of *Crotalus adamanteus* (eastern diamondback rattlesnake), a tracheostomy set should be kept in readiness.

Corticosteroids should not be given in combination with antivenin, and probably should be avoided throughout the acute stages of the poisoning. Their use should be limited to combating the allergic manifestations provoked by the venom or the horse serum.

Often neglected, but of the utmost importance, is the follow-up care of the child. If necessary, surgical débridement should first be carried out three to five days after the bite, and physical therapy instituted immediately thereafter. Lesions should be cleansed daily with peroxide; soaked in 1:20 Burow's solution three times daily for 10 minutes; painted with an aqueous dye consisting of brilliant green 1:400 and gentian violet 1:400; and debrided as necessary. A scarlet red ointment and a polymyxin-bacitracin-neomycin preparation can be applied at bedtime. Oxygen, supplied through an improvised face mask or chamber to the involved area, is of value. The importance of physical therapy in the rehabilitation program should be stressed, and orthopedic consultation sought whenever progress is not satisfactory.

References

Ad Hoc Committee on Snakebite, National Academy of Sciences, National Research Council: Interim Statement on First-Aid Therapy for Bites by Venomous Snakes. *Toxicon,* 1:81, 1963.

Klauber, L. M.: *Rattlesnakes. Their Habits, Life Histories, and Influence on Mankind.* Berkeley, University of California Press, 1972.

Russell, F. E.: Snake Venom Poisoning; in *Cyclopedia of Medicine, Surgery and the Specialties.* Vol. II, Philadelphia, F. A. Davis Co., 1971, p. 199.

Burns

JOHN D. CRAWFORD, M.D., *and*
ALIA Y. ANTOON, M.D.

From the close of the neonatal period through the teen years, accidents kill more children than any single disease. Burns follow only automobile accidents and drowning as causes of this mortality. Two million people annually seek medical attention for burn injuries; over 100,000 are hospitalized and 50,000 are left with disfigurement. Quite in contrast to the success of preventive measures for control of infectious diseases, the injuries from burns have not abated. Nevertheless, when one considers that 80 per cent of these accidents take place within the home and that the patterns of burn injury are highly stereotyped, it becomes apparent that a significant reduction in the injury rate could be effected. The major responsibility for bringing this about lies with the pediatrician.

The vast majority of burns are the result of scalds incurred by infants six months to two years of age. As the child grows older, match play and accidents around the kitchen stove become increasingly prominent. With the beginning of the second decade a major sex difference develops, with boys predominating, the victims of injuries due to explosive ignition of flammable liquids and contact with high tension electrical wires. Burns occur when children are unattended, the kitchen injuries in the early morning hours, especially on weekends and holidays when parents are sleeping; the match play injuries in the bedroom where the child retires from sight to indulge in the forbidden activity. Homes fires, also, are more apt to occur when parents are away. Burns of all types are an increasing hazard in proportion to the number of children in the family; they are inversely related to the economic level and highly associated with marital discord.

Recently, the major focus of attention in burn prevention has been centered on the flammability and design of clothing, especially children's nightwear. However, insufficient emphasis has been placed on education. Typically, the injury consequent to ignition of clothing is compounded by the child's panic reaction. Running fans a smouldering fire even in low flammability garments and provokes a serious flame injury of the entire anterior torso, including the neck up to the ramus of the mandible. Clothing also contributes to the severity of scald burns by maintaining the hot liquid in prolonged contact with the underlying skin. The morbidity and mortality from burns will remain high until pediatricians, school authorities and public health workers mount an aggressive educational campaign based on an understanding of the epidemiology of burns, the appropriate self-help measures to be taken by the victims and the first aid required from those in the immediate vicinity.

FIRST AID

The prime consideration is to stop progressive thermal injury. No means is more rapid or effective than dousing with or immersion in cool water or other nonflammable liquid, whether the burn is due to flame, contact or scald. The panicked child who runs after ignition of clothing must be brought down, rolled on the ground and the flames smothered with an overcoat, rug or blanket—whatever is most available. This should be followed immediately by wetting with cool water or compresses to extinguish smouldering areas and reduce skin temperature to 20 to 30° C. Thereafter, burned clothing should be removed as rapidly as possible while cool compressing of the injured areas is continued. The child should be maintained supine with a free airway. Rings, bracelets, belts or any encircling, constrictive objects should be taken off before swelling occurs. The extent of local injury, pain and swelling can be much reduced by maintaining cool compresses or, if only a distal extremity is involved, immersion in water at 20 to 25° C. for up to 2 hours. Systemic hypothermia is to be avoided, however, by wrapping uninvolved areas in warm blankets and giving sips of warm liquids to patients who are alert (Epstein and Crawford).

The decision as to whether to hospitalize depends on six considerations: the extent, severity and location of the injury, the child's age and state of general health and the quality of home care available. The extent of small burns is readily estimated by remembering that the child's palm is equal to approximately 1 per cent of his surface area. At any age, patients with blistering or full thickness burns of 10 per cent or more of their body surface area should be hospitalized. Only first-degree burns result in no more than erythema, local pain and hypersensitivity to contact or pinprick. More severe, partial thickness burns rapidly blister, ooze, become indurated but remain painful and hypersensitive to touch, and continue to be erythematous and to blanch on pressure. Full thickness burns are dry, leathery and insensitive to pinprick, and pressure results in no blanching. Whereas the partial thickness burn injury has the potential to heal per primum from the deep dermal elements, the full thickness or third-degree burn never does and must be grafted if of significant extent.

Hands, face (especially the eyes) and genitalia constitute the critical areas where even relatively small second- and third-degree burns merit hospitalization. Late functional compromise to these areas is to be avoided at all costs and scars of the face and hands are much more likely than those of any other part of the body to result in long-term psychiatric disability.

For a given degree of injury, the younger the child the more important is hospitalization. The severity of injury is more difficult to judge in the thin skin of the infant; dehydration occurs much more rapidly because of the lesser fluid reserves relative to surface area and because of the propensity of infants to vomit with any serious insult; also, there is a greater susceptibility of the infant to secondary infection as compared with that of the older child. The mortality statistics for burns indicate that the prognosis is best for the 20- to 30-year-old age group; for a given degree of injury, mortality increases with declining (or advancing) age, rising sharply for the years under five.

In a burned child, the principal consideration is that of pulmonary injury. This is a complication of burns occurring indoors, especially those resulting from smokey, smouldering fires. Children with injuries sustained in such circumstances, those in whom the nasal vibrissae are burned, the voice hoarse or the tongue and posterior pharynx swollen, must be hospitalized even if the skin injuries are of small extent. This is necessary so that help will be at hand to deal with sudden compromise of the airway and the development of anoxic encephalopathy and to await a declaration of the extent of pulmonary injury. This may remain initially silent only to become manifest with dramatic suddenness at 48 or 72 hours.

Concerning the decision as to whether or not to hospitalize, the importance of the facilities available for home care requires no extended discussion for the pediatric reader.

CARE OF CHILDREN WITH SMALL BURNS

Those injuries small enough to be cared for at home should be covered, after a period of cooling and soap and water cleansing, with a wide mesh gauze having a light application of petrolatum (Xeroform). Some prefer to coat the injured area with mafenide acetate (Sulfamylon) or silver sulfadiazine (Silvadene), covering either of these creams with a sterile, nonadherent plastic-coated pad (Telfa). Unbroken blisters should generally be preserved. Once broken (it is probably better to break large very thin-walled blebs), the overlying skin should be carefully trimmed back to the edge of the bleb so that no nidus for infection is left. The area is then loosely wrapped with a bulky dressing of absorbent elastic gauze. A light splint, if necessary, may be incorporated in a final cover under an elastic wrap (Ace) for an extremity, or under an elastic adhesive tape (Elastoplast) for a portion of the trunk, shoulder or thigh. Burned extremities should be maintained in an elevated position and the dressing kept dry. If there is no oozing, odor or discomfort, the dressing can be allowed to go undisturbed for two to three days. In the late stage of healing, small moist areas can be quickly dried by application of 2 per cent merbromin solution. Systemic antibiotics are seldom indicated for children with burns suitable for care outside the hospital. If deemed important in a particular instance, low dose penicillin (200,000 units per square meter every 6 hours) or ampicillin (250 mg. every 6 hours) by mouth is suitable.

CARE OF CHILDREN WITH LARGE OR COMPLICATED BURNS REQUIRING HOSPITALIZATION

Preparations for Transfer. Children with serious burn injuries occurring at a distance from a hospital equipped for definitive care may require special measures at a smaller facility before transportation to the center. If travel of more than 2 hours' duration is necessary (and even for a shorter trip if it cannot begin without delay), certain preparations are essential. These consist of making a brief written history of the circumstance of the burn and of the past medical history. There is need also for an accurate assessment of the extent and severity of the injury with the aid of a diagram, such as that shown in Figure 1, and an appraisal of airway involvement. If airway involvement is judged a possibility, provision should at least be made for humidified oxygen during transport. If there is swelling of the pharyngeal tissues, a nasotracheal tube should be passed. Steroids are most useful in preventing pulmonary inflammation if given early and in large doses (dexamethasone, 2 to 10 mg. per square meter every 8 hours). The patient should be weighed, the stomach evacuated and a large-bore, secure intravenous line, preferably a free-running "cut down," inserted, with Ringer's lactate solution begun. This should be administered at a rate of 1 ml. per kilogram per hour, plus 1 ml. per kilogram per hour for each 10 per cent of second- and third-degree body surface burn, to a maximum of 6 ml. per kilogram per hour. A Foley catheter should be inserted and a careful record of the volume of intravenous fluids administered and of urine output commenced and maintained by a physician or well-trained attendant during transport. Minimal local care of the burned areas needs to be undertaken at this point. Usually

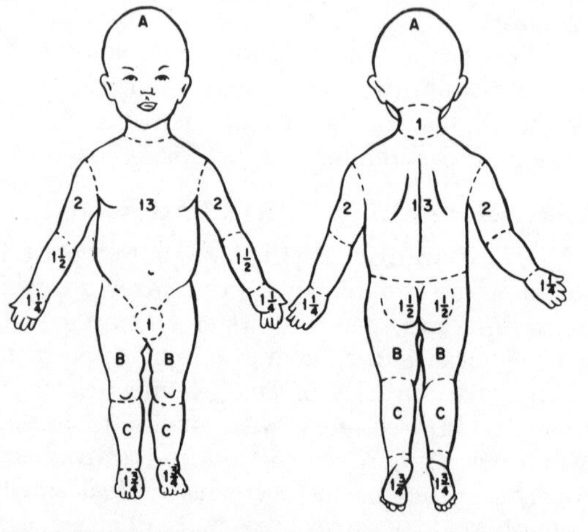

RELATIVE PERCENTAGES OF AREAS AFFECTED BY GROWTH

AREA	AGE 0	1	5
A = ½ of Head	9½	8½	6½
B = ½ of One Thigh	2¾	3¼	4
C = ½ of One Leg	2½	2½	2¾

% BURN BY AREAS

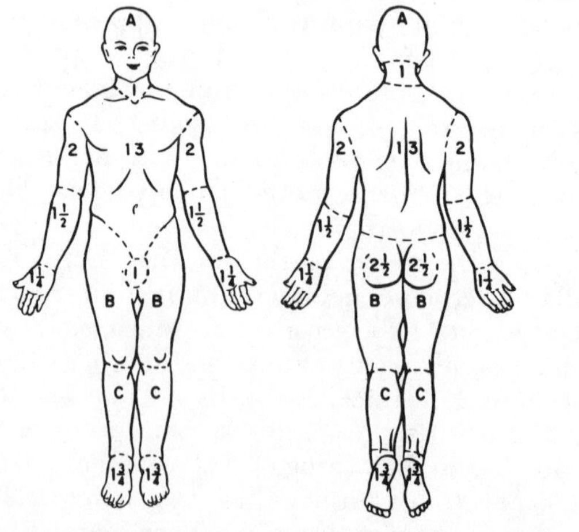

RELATIVE PERCENTAGES OF AREAS AFFECTED BY GROWTH

AREA	AGE 10	15	ADULT
A = ½ of Head	5½	4½	3½
B = ½ of One Thigh	4¼	4½	4¾
C = ½ of One Leg	3	3¼	3½

% BURNS BY AREA

FIGURE 1. Relative surface areas of various parts of the body and changes with growth. This type of diagram is helpful in mapping the areas involved by a burn, in determining their severity and for computing the percentage of the total body surface area injured. (From Einhorn, A. H.; in Barnett, H. L., and Einhorn, A. H. (eds.): *Pediatrics*. 15th ed. New York, Appleton-Century-Crofts, 1972, p. 522.)

nothing more is required than simple covering with sterile dressings. Before doing so, however, thought should be given to the need for escharotomies, because swelling under circumferential third-degree burns of an extremity can compromise its vascular supply. Paradoxically, sedation and analgesia are more often needed for the relatively superficial although very painful first- and second-degree injuries which will not need referral to a distant treatment center. Morphine (6 mg. per square meter) or meperidine (25 mg. per square meter) is suitable but should be given intravenously because absorption of agents administered subcutaneously or intramuscularly is erratic. Most children who have suffered severe third-degree burns are fully conscious; anxiety is a major component of their distress and requires constant attendance, interpretation and reassurance.

The seriously burned child has been deprived of the important thermoregulatory function of his skin and must be protected during transport from either hyper- or hypothermia.

Fluid Therapy. Enormous shifts of fluid from the intravascular to the interstitial compartment take place in the early hours following serious burn injury. Unless there is adequate fluid replacement, these shifts compromise circulation to vital organs, particularly the brain, with the development of burn encephalopathy (Antoon et al.), and the kidney, good function of which is vitally needed to excrete the large load of products of tissue catabolism (Cameron). Maintenance of an adequate circulation is also necessary to prevent progressive ischemic necrosis in damaged but still viable areas underlying tissue destroyed by the thermal insult.

The three formulas most used for calculation of fluid needs are the Evans, Brooke and Baxter recommendations (Hutcher and Haynes). A modified Baxter formula is given here because it is the simplest, it most nearly predicts the relatively larger fluid and sodium needs of children and it puts no arbitrary ceiling on the total amount of fluid administered.

First 24 Hours
Ringer's lactate, 4 ml./kg. body weight/per cent burn
One-half to be given in the first 8 hours
Second half given over the next 16 hours

Second 24 Hours
Amount of Ringer's lactate necessary to maintain serum Na normal (generally 1.5–2.5 ml./kg. per cent burn)
Plasma or equivalent, 500 ml./m^2

No formula gives more than an approximation as to what will be needed by the individual patient. Adequacy must be monitored by urine output, which should not be allowed to drop below 30 ml. per square meter per hour; by hematocrit, which should not be permitted to rise above 50 per cent; and, in large burns, by means of a central venous catheter with pressure in the superior vena cava maintained in the range of 2 to 10 cm. H_2O. Because kinins are released from the area of local injury, causing a generalized increase in capillary permeability and extravasation of albumin into interstitial spaces, most agree that colloid should be used sparingly if at all in the first 24 hours, allowing serum total protein to fall as low as 3.5 Gm. per 100 ml., as long as other parameters are satisfactory. By 48 hours the serum total protein should be boosted by plasma or albumin transfusion to 5.5 Gm. per 100 ml. and thereafter maintained at 6.0 Gm. per 100 ml. or above. In the early hours after injury and, indeed, until healing is complete, the hematocrit should be maintained at no less than 35 per cent by transfusion of packed red cells.

Pink serum or port-wine colored urine indicates hemolysis or myoglobin release from necrotic muscle, presaging possible renal shutdown from heme pigment nephropathy. If urine volume is scant, mannitol (0.5 Gm. per kilogram intravenously)* should be promptly administered and the urine alkalinized with sodium bicarbonate (0.5 mmole per kilogram). Oliguria in this circumstance or in the presence of pulmonary congestion and a rising central venous pressure requires a temporary slowing of intravenous fluid and administration of furosemide (1 to 2 mg. per kilogram).†

Fluid requirements are significantly modified by the topical therapy employed. Mafenide acetate (Sulfamylon) results in systemic acidosis due to carbonic anhydrase inhibition, and needs for alkali are increased (White and Asch). Silver nitrate wet dressings cause hypochloremic alkalosis, because absorbed nitrate is a competitive inhibitor of renal tubular chloride reabsorption and the agent results in depletion of both body sodium and chloride through surface losses in the burned areas where the silver ion forms an insoluble complex with chloride from interstitial fluid. The excess needs for sodium chloride can be computed at 3.5 mmole per 100 square cm. of

* Manufacturer's precaution: Use of mannitol in pediatric patients has not been studied comprehensively.

† Manufacturer's precaution: Furosemide should not be given to children until further experience is accumulated.

burned surface per day (100 square cm. is approximately the area of the adult's palm) (Burke et al.). The nitrate-induced alkalosis may require substitution of saline for Ringer's lactate. Silver sulfadiazine appears to provoke neither of these acid-base complications.

Topical Therapy. The three agents already mentioned are the preferred ones. Mafenide acetate, especially for children, is losing favor because of the metabolic complications already mentioned, because its adherence to the burn wound makes painful the daily removal of the old preparation before reapplication, and because eschars forming beneath the cream are very slow to separate and expose the underlying viable tissue to permit grafting.

Silver nitrate used in a 0.5 per cent solution to keep loose bulky gauze dressings constantly wet is the most effective surface treatment in terms of antibacterial action, but it is the treatment most demanding of the patient care team. One must consider not only the metabolic complications already noted but also the need to nurse the extensively burned small child in a high temperature (85° F.), high humidity (80 per cent) atmosphere to prevent chilling through evaporative heat loss. This is easily accomplished where laminar-flow, bacteria-free nursing units are available to provide an environment suitable for the child separate from that of the attendants; however, few hospitals are so equipped. Finally, the black silver chloride complex stains child, linen, attendants—indeed, virtually all surfaces contacted by the silver nitrate. This is aesthetically displeasing and has an impact on housekeeping costs.

Silver sulfadiazine cream has good antibacterial effectiveness, does not stain skin or linens and is easily removed before the required daily reapplication. It is probably the agent of choice for superficial to deep second-degree scald burns.

None of these topical agents has the ability to penetrate deeply. Thus, wet dressings or creams must be removed daily and the underlying surface debrided of all necrotic tissue easily separable from the granulating bed. Particularly when extensive leathery eschars of third-degree burns remain, care must be taken to identify, unroof and culture abscesses which have formed underneath.

These highly effective chemical agents for topical use have recently been complemented by "biologic" dressings. The latter include pig skin "xenografts," which are commercially available in lyophilized form; fresh or frozen cadaver skin "allografts"; and fresh amniotic tissue. All three have antibacterial activity superior to that of the chemical agents when used in appropriate situations. These situations include application to granulating but still infected wounds as well to deep second-degree scald burns. All reduce exudative losses and have some beneficial proteolytic action on necrotic detritus. The allografts in particular favor the spread beneath them of the patient's own epithelial elements. Removal not later than 48 hours following application is recommended. Both the allografts and xenografts tend to become vascularized and firmly adherent if left longer than this. Such behavior indicates that the granulating beds are suitable for autografting. In some centers, exploration of allografting, under immunosuppression, of skin from donors of close HL-A compatibility is being undertaken for salvage of extensively burned children.

Systemic Antibacterial Treatment. Virtually all children with burns sufficiently severe to require hospitalization should be treated with penicillin (200,000 units per square meter every 6 hours) as prophylaxis against wound invasion by beta-hemolytic streptococci. This is continued for 10 to 14 days during the period of rapid decline and more gradual recovery of the serum gamma globulin concentration. Tetanus prophylaxis in the previously immunized child consists of a 0.5 ml. booster of toxoid; if prophylaxis is indicated in a nonimmunized individual, 250 to 1500 I.U. of human tetanus immune globulin administered intramuscularly is recommended. Gas gangrene due to *Clostridium perfringens* invasion of necrotic muscle is a potential complication of electrical burns. It should be noted that muscles can be destroyed by passage of current under viable skin of an extremity between the surface burns of the entry and exit wounds. The treatment is early excision of all such devitalized deep tissues. The tendency of high voltage current in extremities to seek passage along the lowest resistance structures, the neurovascular bundles, may make amputation necessary if these have been destroyed.

Systemic antibiotic treatment should be governed by the results of frequent wound and blood cultures. One of the semisynthetic, penicillinase-resistant agents, such as cloxacillin or oxacillin, should be substituted for penicillin if a wound less than 10 days from burning is discovered to be coinfected with *Staphylococcus aureus* and group A beta-hemolytic streptococci. Pseudomonas infections of burn wounds are currently the most troublesome to eradicate and highly likely to be fatal if they become invasive with septicemia. Gentamicin, 7 to 10 mg. per kilogram per day, in four divided intramuscular doses, is the most effective treatment.

Operative excision, débridement and grafting procedures of infected wounds (infection can be assumed present in wounds four days or more after burning) are virtually certain to result in transient septicemia. Short courses (two to five days) of broad-spectrum (gentamicin plus oxacillin) antibiotics begun just prior to the procedure are helpful in protecting the seriously injured and debilitated child.

Nutrition. The burn wound sets in motion a vicious cycle of calorie and protein deficiency. Following injury, protein immediately begins to be lost by exudation from the wound and distant protein catabolism commences as a result of the body's effort to provide fuel for the abruptly elevated metabolic rate. This is mediated at least in part, by an outpouring of cortisol and norepinephrine. Energy requirements are increased because burned skin loses its intrinsic thermoregulatory function and it no longer constitutes a barrier against loss of extracellular fluid, with the result that evaporative heat losses are markedly increased. Loss of the skin's antibacterial function adds yet another component of the energy drain as infection develops to drive the vicious cycle. Yet, healing is never optimal unless the calorie balance is positive. Many hold that calorie deficit is presently the chief cause of burn mortality.

Measurements indicate that in large burns the energy requirement is twice that obtaining in the patient prior to injury. Efforts to meet this extraordinary caloric need must be instituted early, and vigorously continued until skin closure is complete. In the first few hours after burn, the gastrointestinal tract is apt to be intolerant of food, but feeding should be begun as soon as possible thereafter. Even before this, calories by the intravenous route should be instituted, adding glucose to the Ringer's lactate solution in whatever concentration is tolerated without glycosuria. A syndrome of insulinopenic, low renal threshold "pseudodiabetes" is a frequent complication in the first few days after a major burn, suppression of insulin output being secondary to the high circulating levels of norepinephrine. Insulin may be added to the intravenous fluid at a starting concentration of 1 unit per 5 grams of glucose. This should be done cautiously, for these children are apt to be exquisitely sensitive to the hormone. Subcutaneous insulin is to be avoided.

Amounts of oral feedings should be increased as rapidly as tolerated, and feedings through a nasogastric tube may be necessary in the child unable to eat by himself or to supplement the daytime oral intake by feeding through the night. A variety of liquid diet preparations are available, but a wholesome, well-balanced meal can be simply prepared for nasogastric feeding by emulsification in a blender. During postanesthetic periods and at other times, especially if diarrhea supervenes, oral intake has to be reduced and the caloric requirement met by intravenous "hyperalimentation," using one of the high carbohydrate mixtures of the type introduced by Dudrick or a fat emulsion such as Intralipid (investigational in the United States). The introduction of catheters into large central veins for infusion of the high carbohydrate mixtures elevates the risk of septicemia, especially that due to Candida organisms. The fat emulsions can be given by peripheral vein and are compatible with carbohydrate and amino acid mixtures (for example, Aminofusin) but have not yet been authorized for general use in the United States by the Food and Drug Administration.

Excision, Grafting and Anesthesia. A detailed consideration of these aspects of care of the burned child is beyond the scope of this writing. In a large burn, the anesthesiologist is an important member of the caretaking team to be assembled on admission of the child. His advice and skills are of importance in considering whether there is need to pass a nasotracheal tube or perform a tracheostomy in dealing with inflammation of the upper airway, as well as in the management of pulmonary inhalation injuries. He must be principally relied upon in the operating room for choice of an anesthetic appropriate to the planned procedure, whether it be the dissociative agent, ketamine, which allows for early resumption of oral feedings, a hypotensive regimen which reduces blood loss in major excision procedures, or one of the more classic agents such as halothane. He, too, is the person principally in charge of estimating blood losses during surgery and the replacement amounts necessary to maintain an adequate circulation and high level of tissue oxygenation.

Treatment by early excision and grafting of full-thickness burn areas is emerging as more desirable than the classic approach of allowing eschars to form and ultimately to lift off spontaneously before grafting. In small, clearly demarcated areas of full thickness injury, early excision and grafting result in shorter periods of hospitalization with less scarring and chance of contracture. A similarly aggressive approach to the very large injuries with temporary use of allografts when the victim's own donor sites are insufficient appears to be a lifesaving maneuver. Great good judgment is required to determine areas suitable for tangential excision with the Edwards's knife, thus sparing underlying fat tissue to improve the cosmetic result, as opposed to excision down to the fascia, where hemostasis is easier to achieve and there is less likelihood of septic fat necrosis under the grafts.

The orthopedic surgeon and physical therapist are also important contributors to the outcome of burns overlying joints where contractures limiting function are likely to form. Early splinting in the position of function is of vital importance, especially where burns of the hands are concerned. Skeletal fixation is well tolerated by children with burns. The risks of more than local osteomyelitis are almost negligible when other aspects of care are well attended to. Elevation of burned extremities to permit circumferential grafting and to prevent venous stasis and edema is achieved far more efficiently with skeletal fixation than with propping and external devices. Furthermore, skeletal fixation permits use of dynamic traction, physical therapy and joint motion, when desirable, to say nothing of the reduction in nursing care afforded.

Care of the Child as an Individual. Burns subject the child to a horrifying initial experience, prolonged pain, helplessness and fearful wounds open to his view during healing. Once healed and reconstructed to the best of the plastic surgeon's ability, affected areas are often permanently disfigured and attractive of unwanted attention. The child's immediate medical care may necessitate removal from home. Classically, care involves isolation from family members and all but a few attendants whose reality is disguised by gowns, masks and hair covers. Little wonder the victim's behavior tends rapidly to regress and that he refuses to eat when survival depends on high levels of nutrition. Those who do survive serious burns often fail to achieve a return to school and may even be rejected by their families. Accordingly, special efforts are required, from the essential reassurance immediately after injury through the time of full rehabilitation, in order to prevent "social death." Parents should be encouraged to visit the child frequently; modern topical antimicrobial agents and bacteria-free nursing units permit the uncovering of faces and consequent improvement of communication. Certain nurses can be freed of their most hurtful roles by organization of dressing teams made up of technicians. School teachers, play therapists, dieticians and, when necessary, surrogate mothers can play essential roles in maintaining the desire to survive. As the child's condition permits, he should be placed among others more advanced in recovery and rehabilitation. Siblings unable to visit should be prepared for the homecoming by appropriate photographs. These are also useful in preparing students and teachers for the child's return to school. Parents and teachers generally overestimate the degree of disability resulting from a healed burn injury, and all too frequently unnecessary arrangements are made for a home tutor, these being renewed in perpetuity. Such misplaced efforts carry a high risk of crowning a successful life-saving effort in the hospital with demise of the child as an individual (Caudle and Potter).

References

Antoon, A. Y., Volpe, J. J., and Crawford, J. D.: Burn Encephalopathy in Children. *Pediatrics,* 50:609, 1972.

Burke, J. F., Bondoc, C. C., and Morris, P. J.: Early Treatment of Severe Burns. Part II: Metabolism. Metabolic Effects of Topical Silver Nitrate Therapy in Burns Covering More Than Fifteen Per Cent of the Body Surface. *Ann. N. Y. Acad. Sci.,* 150(Art. 3):674, 1968.

Cameron, J. S.: Disturbances of Renal Function in Burn Patients. *Proc. Roy. Soc. Med.,* 62:49, 1968.

Caudle, P. R. K., and Potter, J.: Characteristics of Burned Children and the After Effects of the Injury. *Brit. J. Plast. Surg.,* 23:63, 1970.

Dudrick, S. J., and Rhoads, J. E.: New Horizons for Intravenous Feeding. *J.A.M.A.,* 215:939, 1971.

Epstein, M. F., and Crawford, J. D.: Cooling in the Emergency Treatment of Burns. *Pediatrics.* In press.

Hutcher, N., and Haynes, B. W., Jr.: The Evans Formula Revisited. *J. Trauma,* 12:453, 1972.

White, M. G., and Asch, M.: Acid-base Effects of Topical Mafenide Acetate in the Burned Patient. *New England J. Med.,* 284:1281, 1971.

Radiation Injury

JAMES N. YAMAZAKI, M.D.

LOW LEVEL IRRADIATION

The effects of exposure to radiation may vary greatly with age, dose, dose rate, quality of radiation and extent of the body involved. The major contributors to radiation exposure of the population continue to be natural background, with an average body dose of about 100 millirads per year, and medical application,. which now contributes comparable exposures to various tissues of the body. (See Table 1.)

TABLE 1. Estimates of Annual Whole-Body Dose Rates in the United States (1970)*

SOURCE	AVERAGE DOSE RATE† (*millirads per year*)
Environmental	
Natural	102
Global Fallout	4
Nuclear Power	0.003
Subtotal	106
Medical	
Diagnostic	72‡
Radiopharmaceuticals	1
Subtotal	73
Occupational	0.8
Miscellaneous	2
Subtotal	3
Total	182

* From the Beir report.

† The numbers shown are average values only. For given segments of the population, dose rates considerably greater than these may be experienced.

‡ Based on the abdominal dose.

Over a decade ago, considerable concern was expressed about the environmental contamination from radioactive fallout from atmospheric and surface testing of weapons. The radiation from this source continues to be small, adding about 4 millirads annually to the natural background. Now there is concern over the anticipated increase of the use of nuclear energy.* However, radiation from this source currently is minute, being about 1 per cent of natural background. Thus, by comparison, medical x-rays are by far the largest component of radiation exposure to the general population, amounting to at least 35 per cent of the total radiation dose from all sources, including natural radioactivity. Utilization of x-rays is now estimated to be increasing from 2 to 6 per cent annually, despite the fact that the United States population receives less than two-thirds of the medical radiation from medical x-rays than it did in 1964. The per capita, genetically significant doses were estimated to be 36 millirads in 1970, down from 55 millirads in 1964. The decline is attributed mainly to improved collimation (restriction of the x-ray beam to the area of the body under scrutiny). With additional new techniques, it is anticipated that the dose can be further reduced while diagnostic efficiency is increased.

The dose response to large doses of radiation at high dose rate soon after exposure has been well established in man and in animals. The pattern is true for all forms of ionizing radiation, whether it is from an external source or from internally deposited radioactive materials, or both. For example, a dose of one to several hundred rads delivered rapidly will produce within a relatively short time the "acute radiation syndrome," manifested by hematologic changes, gastrointestinal involvement and epilation. Delayed radiation effects from varying large doses of radiation have been extensively studied in laboratory animals. Such detailed information about man had been lacking until recently, when data of irradiated humans were reported. This information principally came from data accumulated over 20 years of observing the Japanese population exposed to the atomic bomb; from the observed effects on the Marshallese, who were exposed externally and internally to radioactive fallout; from the observation of patients radiated for therapeutic purposes; and from the earlier surveys of the death reports of physicians and radiologists. These data leave no doubt that ionizing radiation can induce cancer in man.

TABLE 2. Effects and Significance of Various Radiation Doses

EXPECTED EFFECT ON BIOLOGICAL SIGNIFICANCE	DOSE OF SINGLE EXPOSURE TO X- OR GAMMA-RADIATION (RADS)
Local Exposure	
Skin erythema	500–1000
Epilation	300–600
Whole-Body Exposure	
Median lethal dose	300–500
Transient disability and hematologic changes	150–200
Vomiting in 10% of people	75–125
Natural Radiation	
"Normal" weekly dose from natural radiation	0.002

Leukemia was the most frequently observed malignancy related to both partial and whole-body irradiation. The best information on the minimal carcinogenic dose in man comes

* Considering its potential magnitude and widespread distribution, a complete review of existing scientific knowledge concerning radiation exposure to human population has been made by the National Academy of Sciences and also by the United Nations Scientific Committee on the Effects of Atomic Radiation, particularly directed to the effects of low levels of ionizing radiation.

from the atomic bomb survivors. The lowest dose at which an increase in leukemia could be detected was at a dose equivalent of 32 to 85 rads. Furthermore, the dose response curve is consistent with a linear relationship, i.e., the dose effect derived from high dose and high dose rate ranges through the low dose and low dose rate ranges to zero, implying that there exists a probability that tumor induction can occur as a result of radiation injury to one or few cells. Linear nonthreshold relationships have been accepted by the National Academy of Sciences as a basis for estimating cancer risks from exposure of populations to low level exposure that is near background level, using the data from the atomic bomb survivors of Hiroshima and Nagasaki, from certain groups of patients irradiated therapeutically and from groups occupationally exposed. Attention has also been directed to information concerning the broad spectrum of the possible cellular response to varying exposure to ionizing radiation. Because there is more killing of susceptible cells at high dose and high dose rate extrapolation under these exposures, it may be postulated to underestimate the risks of irradiation at relatively low doses and low dose rates encountered in diagnostic medical x-ray exposure. Also, consider the extremely low dose rate from background radiation (approximately 0.1 rem per year), which is one-hundred million to one-hundred billion times lower than the dose rate at which effects have been observed in most irradiated populations. Such enormous differences may have important implications with respect to the production of radiation damage within cells and its repair at the molecular level.

Data on the consequences of low level irradiation at a dose level of a few milliroentgens to 50 rads utilized in current diagnostic x-ray examinations are extremely limited (Table 3). The difficulties of obtaining information at low doses are due mainly to the extremely low frequency with which effects might occur. The task of obtaining satisfactory quantitative information at low doses is handicapped by the statistical problems presented and the impracticality of designing experiments in which the probability of the demonstrable effect is in the range of one in 1000 or one in 10,000 or more. Nevertheless, such increase in incidence may be highly significant when the effects on large population groups are considered. However, injury to fetal and neonatal tissue from such low level irradiation has been demonstrated in laboratory animals. Extrapolation to human hazards must be qualified with the demonstrated differential radiosensitivity that exists between species and within species of target organs at similar developmental stages. Nevertheless, a high degree of embryologic similarity exists in man and the laboratory animal studies, particularly in early developmental stages; furthermore, experimentally induced radiation

TABLE 3. Average Skin Dose (rad) in Primary Beam (Examples)

	PER EXPOSURE		PER EXAMINATION	
	Median Value	*Range of Overdose Values*	*Median Value*	*Range of Overdose Values*
High skin dose group				
Barium swallow F	6.4[a]		8.5	
Barium meal F	4.4[a]		2.1	6–25
Barium enema F	4.9[a]		20	5–26
Pelvimetry	2	0.8–3.8	8	6–10
Lumbosacral spine	2.7	0.5–2.9	5	5–6
Cardiac catheterization			47	
Medium skin dose group				
Abdomen	0.2	0.15–1.3	1.2	1.0–1.4
Abdomen (obstetric)	2.0	0.4–3.9	3.2	2.7–3.8
Urography (descending)	1.2		3.2	1.7–5.0
Dental	0.4		2.5	1.6–3.4
Mass survey, chest	0.9		1.0	0.6–1.4
Low skin dose group				
Chest	0.02	0.006–0.09	0.14	0.07–0.15

[a]R min.$^{-1}$
F = fluoroscopy

defects are of a similar type in man. This information, therefore, must be considered carefully in the timing and use of radiation procedures in pregnant women.

Since adequate human data are not available, the estimates of genetic risks are based mainly on results of extensive laboratory experimentation, notably with mice, which leaves no doubt that irradiation is mutagenic. Any increase in genetic disease from this cause would be of vast importance, when already it is estimated that about 4 per cent live-born children suffer from various forms of genetically determined disease. Radiation-induced genetic effects have long been considered to have no threshold and are related to the total dose. However, recent studies have shown that at low dose rate there is a distinct reduction in mutation compared to that which occurs in high dose rate. Furthermore, if conception occurs after a sufficient interval following irradiation, there is further reduction of the frequency of mutation in the descendants of irradiated females, demonstrating a remarkable capacity for repair of the molecular lesion. The genetic effects among children conceived after one or both parents have been exposed to ionizing radiation have been undertaken by the Atomic Bomb Casualty Commission (ABCC)† in Hiroshima and Nagasaki. Six indicators of the genetic damage were assessed in the F_1 generation (the result of over 71,000 pregnancies). No genetic effect could be demonstrated based on increased malformation rate, on rates of stillbirths or neonatal deaths, on birthweight or on anthropometric values at 8 to 10 months in the event either mother or father were exposed. Estimates of genetic risks to man have been based on the information of radiation exposure of laboratory animals, and from the observation of human populations in Hiroshima and Nagasaki as it applies to basic human population genetics. It is now believed that the population exposure for all man-made sources of radiation other than medical should not exceed a few millirads average annual dose to the entire United States population.

AGE-DOSE FACTOR

The profound sensitivity to ionizing radiation in early life is determined by the cellular lesion, which may alter the intricate interplay of cellular proliferation, differentiation and organization following fertilization of the ovum and during subsequent growth and development of the conceptus. A broad spectrum of radiation-induced lesions may manifest themselves, depending on the stage of development of the component cell population irradiated and the radiation dose. Early in embryonic development, cell death or alteration of structure and mobility of surviving cells may result in production of developmental anomalies even with low dose radiation and, in the human, is most likely to take place in the first six to seven weeks of gestation. Later in development, alteration of cellular synthesis may prevent normal cellular differentiation. The radiosensitivity of germ cells depends on whether they are in the proliferative stage of mitosis in early embryogenesis, or in various phases of meiosis in later embryonic and postnatal life. It is well to consider that radiologic exposure during fetal or neonatal life leaves a maximal time span for the development of sequelae. Somatic radiation mutation resulting in the induction of neoplasms is profoundly altered according to the age at the time of exposure as demonstrated by the increased incidence of malignancy following irradiation of the child as compared to the adult. Furthermore, there is some evidence suggesting that the fetus is especially susceptible to radiation carcinogenesis.

When mice fetuses received 5 rads at an early stage of organogenesis comparable to the developmental stage of a human fetus at three to four weeks of gestation, an increased incidence of skeletal malformation and retardation of embryonic growth was observed. Furthermore, there was no evidence to suggest that the threshold for fetal damage occurs for values less than 5 rads. When 115 rads are administered at a similar stage of development, microphthalmia has been produced in mice. Administering 10 rads to the fetal rat can stunt the growth of neurons, and doubling this dose can alter nerve cells permanently and interfere with normal formation of the cortex. With a larger dose, gross malformation of the fetal rat brain occurs. Fractionation experiments have been conducted to simulate the clinical exposure of a pregnant patient to a low dose of ionizing radiation rather than to a single large dose. When 1 rad was administered daily to the gravid rat during gestation for a total of 20 rads, functional and behavioral disturbances were observed following an intrauterine exposure of 25 to 50 rads.

Substantial new information concerning

---

†ABCC is a cooperative research agency of the United States National Academy of Sciences and the Japanese National Institute of Health with funds provided by the United States Atomic Energy Commission and the Japanese Ministry of Health and Welfare.

the effect of intrauterine and juvenile exposure to ionizing radiation has been recently obtained. A more reliable dose estimate is now possible in regard to the possible hazard from such exposure, and particularly in regard to alteration in growth and development and carcinogenesis. By far the most informative source has been the ABCC studies. Other important contributions are from several groups of patients undergoing radiotherapy and followed for several decades, and from children exposed in utero during radiologic examination of their mothers. The earliest reports of children who developed microcephaly and mental retardation were born to mothers who during early pregnancy received pelvic radiotherapy with an estimated dose of several hundred rads. Children exposed in utero to the Hiroshima and Nagasaki bombs developed microcephaly (head circumference more than two standard deviations below the mean for sex and age) and mental retardation if the exposure occurred between the seventh to fifteenth weeks after the mother's last menstrual period. The likelihood of microcephaly was proportional to proximity to the hypocenter. Now, for the first time dose estimates resulting in the small head size place the dose between 25 and 50 rads. At maternal doses of 150 rads or more, small head circumference was often accompanied by mental retardation. Furthermore, deleterious effects were noted on body growth following in utero radiation occurring within 1500 meters from the hypocenter. With a dose estimate of 25 rads or more, subjects 17 years of age (when mature growth had been obtained) were on the average 2.25 cm. shorter, 3 kilograms lighter and 1.1 cm. smaller in head circumference.

A significant increase in fetal and infant mortality also occurred following intrauterine radiation exposure. In Nagasaki, the pregnant mothers who were within 2000 meters from the hypocenter of the atomic bomb explosion and who developed acute radiation illness reported a mortality of 45 per cent, compared with 9 per cent for those in the same distance category who had not had acute radiation sickness. Fetal mortality occurred more frequently with exposure in the first and second trimester, whereas neonatal and infant mortality occurred more frequently with exposure in the third trimester.

A cohort of 1300 survivors exposed in utero to the atomic bomb has now been observed for 24 years. Mortality increased with dose above 50 rads during the first year of life, with no increase observed during the next nine years; however, mortality again seems to have increased with dose after 10 years of age. This effect appeared only in those exposed during the third trimester. No particular cause of death was found to be related to radiation dose, except in the case of perinatal death. Most importantly, no significant decrease of cancer risk was observed from in utero radiation exposure. In contrast, several large surveys of children exposed to a few rads from diagnostic studies during their prenatal life have reported an association, with an increase in deaths from cancer in children under 10 years of age. Following such exposure, 40 to 60 per cent increase in relative risk of leukemia, cancer of the central nervous system and other cancer has been observed. The extent to which the increased risk of malignancy in the medically irradiated subject is due to radiation rather than to an association with the cause that prompted the irradiation must still be considered an open question.

There is no doubt that radiation in sufficient doses can induce cancer in man. The effect is proportionate to the dose and is in accord with data from laboratory animals. The studies from Hiroshima and Nagasaki indicate that the overall leukemogenic effect of radiation was greater in children and young people than in older persons. Among those under 10 years of age, the leukemia rate was 26 times higher if exposure was within 1500 meters of the hypocenter than when it was beyond that distance. Susceptibility to leukemia in general was three times greater when exposure occurred when the child was under 10 years of age as compared with children 10 to 19 years of age. The lowest dose response has been estimated to be a dose equivalent of about 50 rads. After a latent period of about 15 years, children (over 15,000 exposed survivors) who received radiation doses of 100 rads or more began to develop an excessive number of malignant neoplasms and now, 25 years after exposure, the accumulated increase is striking, and there is no indication that the peak has yet been reached. During the next 10 years these persons will be entering ages when ordinarily cancer rates begin to increase markedly. Although there is a total of only 19 malignant neoplasms other than leukemia, these have occurred in a group of only 1109 high dose survivors, the oldest of whom is now only 35. The cancer rate was more than six times that in children who were not in the city or who had doses estimated to be less than 10 rads.

Thyroid neoplasms can also be induced by ionizing radiation. Thyroid cancer has been observed following therapeutic radiation of the thymus in early childhood. The incidence is proportionate to dose in the range of 50 to 200 rads. Both benign and malignant thyroid neoplasm also occurred in the Marshallese children exposed to the radioactive fallout from the hydrogen bomb. The estimated dose from whole-body gamma radiation was 175 rads and the estimated thyroid dose from radioactive iodine was from 500 to 1400 rads. Two subjects who were infants at the time of exposure developed atrophy of the thyroid before puberty and manifested evidence of significant growth retardation and sluggishness of behavior. Susceptibility to induction to these tumors seems to be several times higher in children than in adults.

DOSIMETRY

Tables 1 and 3 give some perspective concerning the individual and average population exposure to irradiation. The medical x-ray exposure in Table 3 is the carefully measured energy values projected on patients undergoing x-ray examination under optimal control conditions. Depending on various exposure variables, there can be a considerable spread above the mean dose level listed in Table 3, even when good technique is utilized. Without careful control, the exposure dose can be increased greatly. For example, in a pediatric institution an analysis of their cardiac work-up revealed patients to have received as much as a total of 195 to 500 rads with repeated fluoroscopic examinations.

A more informative and precise measure of radiation exposure is the recent trend to express the dose exposure relative to the surface area or volume of exposed tissue. It is to be noted that the dose estimate in the Hiroshima population was the total of the gamma and neutron radiation. Because of their possible influence, neutrons cannot be excluded, and the low dose effect may not be directly applicable to medical x-irradiation.

CONTROL MEASURES

When optimal radiographic technique is utilized to obtain vital clinical information, the dosage involved results in an acceptable low potential risk. However, only in the fetus has the possibility of a hazard been demonstrated. The physician who uses x-ray equipment should thoroughly familiarize himself with optimal radiographic techniques in order to ensure minimal radiation exposure and should seek the guidance of his radiologist colleagues in these matters. Equipment for which the physician is responsible should be carefully monitored and its optimal exposure performance well defined and applied. Careful supervision of technical personnel is equally important. Newer developments in radiography have made it possible to reduce greatly x-ray exposure by means such as (1) the electronic system that makes possible image amplification with reduced doses through the use of television, cine-recording and magnetic tape storage, (2) improved intensifying screen materials and (3) technical developments resulting in more control and limited exposure with improvements in film speed and improvements in the design of shields and beam collimators. For example, single exposure from a single chest examination can now be reduced to 0.005 rads with Kodak RP-R type film.

Fluoroscopy, even under ideal conditions, results in excessive exposure for most routine examinations. For example, a single chest film delivers 0.02 rad to the skin. A fluoroscopic examination of the same area at the acceptably low rate of 6 rads per minute would deliver the same dose in 0.2 second, which in one minute is equivalent to the dose of 300 chest films. For this reason, routine use of fluoroscopy in pediatric offices has been discouraged by the American Academy of Pediatrics except under unusual circumstances.

To minimize radiation exposure of the very young embryo when pregnancy is unsuspected, the menstrual history should be carefully documented in order to limit exposure to the first nine or 10 days after the onset of menstruation. Exposure of the fetus should be kept at the lowest level possible, particularly during the first six weeks of pregnancy. This caution must be balanced between the careful evaluation of the need for the diagnostic x-ray procedure and the overall well-being of the mother and fetus. The clinical responsibility for requesting diagnostic x-ray procedures in women of child-bearing age remains mainly with the physician caring for the mother and with the radiologist. However, it is implicit that this responsibility be shared by the pediatrician in collaboration with the obstetrician and the radiologist.

References

Basic Radiation Protection Criteria NCRP Report No. 39. Washington, D. C., National Council on Radiation Protection and Measurements, January, 1971.

Burch, P. R. J.: Prenatal Radiation Exposure and Childhood Cancer. *Lancet,* December 5, 1970, pp. 1189.

Conference on the Pediatric Significance of Peacetime Radioactive Fallout. *Pediatrics,* 41 (Suppl.), No. 1, Part II, 1968.

Fendel, H.: Radiation Problems in Roentgen Examination of the Chest; in Kaufman, H. J., and Karger, S. (eds.): *Progress in Radiology*. New York, 1967, pp. 16–18.

Ionizing Radiation on Levels and Effects. A Report on the United Nations Scientific Committee on the Effects of Atomic Radiation to the General Assembly with Effects. Vol. I, *Levels;* Vol. II, *Effects;* United Nations, New York, 1972.

Jablon, S., Belsky, J. L., Tachikawa, K., and Steer, A.: Cancer in Japanese Exposed as Children to Atomic Bombs. *Lancet,* May 8, 1971, pp. 927–932.

Jablon, S., and Kato, H.: Childhood Cancer in Relation to Prenatal Exposure to Atomic-Bomb Radiation. *Lancet,* November 14, 1970, pp. 1000–1003.

Jablon, S., and Kato, H.: Studies of the Mortality of A-Bomb Survivors. 5. Radiation Dose and Mortality, 1950–1970. *Radiation Research,* Vol. 50, No. 3, June, 1972.

Jacobsen, L.: Low Dose X-Irradiation and Teratogenesis. Copenhagen, Munksgaard, 1968.

MacMahon, B.: Prenatal X-ray Exposure and Childhood Cancer. *J. Nat. Cancer Inst.,* 28:1173, 1962.

Miller, R. W., and Blot, J.: Small Head Size After In Utero Exposure to Atomic Radiation. *Lancet,* October 14, 1972, pp. 784–787.

Proceedings of the Symposium on the Effects of Low Radiation Doses on the Maturation of the Developing (Human) Ovum and Foetus. *Brit. J. Radiol.,* 41:714, 1968.

Reduction of Radiation on Dose in Diagnostic X-ray Procedures. Rockville, Maryland, U.S. Department of Health, Education and Welfare, Public Health Service, Food and Drug Administration, Bureau of Radiological Health, September, 1972.

Robinow, M., and Silverman, F. N.: Radiation Hazards in the Field of Pediatrics. *Pediatrics,* 20 (Suppl.): 921, 1957.

Statement on the Use of Diagnostic X-ray. Recommendations of the Committee on Radiation Hazards and the Epidemiology of Congenital Malformations. *Pediatrics,* 28:676, 1961.

Stewart, A., and Kneale, G. W.: Radiation Dose Effects in Relation to Obstetric X-rays and Childhood Cancers. *Lancet,* June 6, 1970, pp. 1185–1188.

The Effects on Populations of Exposure to Low Levels of Ionizing Radiation. Report of the Advisory Committee on The Biological Effects of Ionizing Radiations. Washington, D. C., National Academy of Sciences, National Research Council, November, 1972.

Yamazaki, J. N.: A Review of the Literature on the Radiation Dosage Required to Cause Manifest Central Nervous System Disturbances from In Utero and Postnatal Exposure. *Pediatrics,* 37 (Suppl.), No. 5, Part II, May, 1966.

Near-Drowning

(Nonfatal Submersion)

SHIRLEY A. GRAVES, M.D., *and*
JEROME H. MODELL, M.D.

Near-drowning is defined in the *Standard Nomenclature of Athletic Injuries* as "a critical aquatic predicament resolved by successful water rescue," implying that recovery is certain once the victim is removed from the water. This is not always the case, however, since some patients who have regained consciousness after near-drowning have subsequently died. To offer the victim the best chance for normal long-term survival, a plan of therapy is necessary which begins at the site of the accident and does not terminate until the patient is discharged from the hospital fully recovered.

The prime objective of emergency therapy should be to restore normal arterial blood gas and acid-base levels. Following experimental airway obstruction, the arterial oxygen tension drops to 40 mm. Hg in one minute and to 10 mm. Hg in three minutes, emphasizing the urgency for resuscitative measures. If the victim is apneic when rescued, treatment should begin in the water, if possible, with mouth-to-mouth ventilation. Although other methods of artificial ventilation have been proposed, they are inferior. The most reliable types of mechanical equipment for this purpose are the simplest, e.g., the self-inflating bag and the hand-operated oxygen valve. Pressure limited–volume variable ventilators are usually not satisfactory, since the compliance of the patient may be very low, and peak pressure is reached before an adequate volume of gas is delivered. If assisted circulation is also necessary, it is unlikely that effective ventilation will be supplied with a pressure limited device during closed chest cardiac massage.

Since hypotonic fluid is absorbed rapidly from the lung, it is useless to attempt to drain water from the lungs of a fresh water near-drowning victim. If fluid is drained, it is likely the result of emptying the stomach. After aspiration of sea water, fluid is drawn into the lung from the circulation and the proper positioning of the patient may enable the rescuer to promote drainage of fluid from the trachea without compromising artificial ventilation.

Once artificial ventilation has begun, evidence of effective circulation should be elicited. In some cases the heart may actually be beating, but because of profound hypoxia the force of contraction is so poor that a pulse cannot be palpated. If artificial ventilation is administered immediately and oxygenation of the myocardium occurs, effective circulation may be restored. If no heartbeat is detected, closed chest cardiac massage should immediately be added to the pulmonary phase of resuscitation. For many years ventricular fibrillation has been implicated as the primary cause of circulatory failure in fresh water drowning victims. Recent evidence suggests that less than 15 per cent of human fresh water drowning victims may have died as a result of ventricular fibrillation. In the majority of cases, cardiac arrest is likely to be the result of profound hypoxia. In any case, an electrocardiogram should be obtained as soon as possible to determine whether electrical defibrillation is necessary.

If the victim has not aspirated fluid and spontaneous ventilation is reestablished while effective circulation is still present, the probability of complete recovery is good. If the duration of hypoxia was short, further therapy may not be necessary. If the patient has aspirated water, however, the pulmonary lesion is not readily reversible; the prognosis is obviously less favorable and further therapy is imperative.

Since the rescuer cannot determine the state of the patient's lungs or evaluate the adequacy of arterial oxygenation at the scene of the accident, all near-drowning victims should be admitted to the hospital. During transport, all necessary resuscitative measures should be continued. Maximal oxygen concentration should be administered by inhalation, regardless of the apparent clinical condition of the patient. It must be emphasized that return of consciousness is not synonymous with recovery. One must not be led into a false sense of complacency, since delayed death from hypoxia does occur.

Initial emphasis of hospital therapy should be on intensive pulmonary care. This must begin by providing a secure airway, sufficient oxygenation and adequate ventilation. The methods vary from patient to patient, and range from simply administering oxygen to a spontaneously breathing, awake patient to establishing a patent airway with a cuffed endotracheal tube (uncuffed tube in children eight years and under), which is connected to a mechanical ventilator for continuous ventilatory support. In all cases, 100 per cent oxygen by inhalation must be continued until arterial blood gas studies verify that lesser oxygen concentrations are adequate. When it is impossible to maintain an acceptable arterial pO_2 with minimal inspired O_2 concentration, positive end-expiratory pressure (PEEP) will frequently be useful. PEEP prevents the alveoli from collapsing to a completely airless state, thus increasing functional residual capacity and allowing better ventilation-perfusion ratios. In the face of decreased blood volume, PEEP may cause a decreased venous return to the heart, which may cause a decrease in cardiac output and hypotension. This is more often the case with salt water aspiration, and it may be necessary to infuse colloid and restore the circulatory blood volume before PEEP can be used beneficially. PEEP is useful after both fresh and salt water aspiration where oxygenation at low inspired O_2 concentration is impossible. It is especially useful after fresh water near-drowning where the surface tension of the surfactant is altered and alveoli tend to collapse completely with each exhalation. Since metabolic acidosis almost invariably accompanies hypoxia in these patients, routine use of sodium bicarbonate or some other suitable buffer is indicated.

As soon as possible, the patient should be evaluated by determination of arterial pH, pO_2, pCO_2 and other variables of acid-base balance. The extent of further bicarbonate administration (mEq. of sodium bicarbonate = wt. [in kg.] × base deficit × 0.25) and ventilatory support, and the minimal inspired oxygen concentration necessary to prevent further acidosis and hypoxia will be determined by these values. If PEEP is not used, an attempt should be made to reexpand atelectatic alveoli by frequent manual hyperinflation of the lungs. Isoproterenol, given by nebulization or by careful intravenous titration, or racemic epinephrine nebulized and inhaled, may be helpful in some patients to reduce bronchospasm secondary to the aspiration of fluid. Patients with obvious pulmonary edema and froth which obstructs the airway also benefit from inhalation of an aerosol of an antifoaming agent (e.g., 20 to 30 per cent ethyl alcohol).

Since near-drowning with fluid aspiration is a form of aspiration pneumonitis, steroids and antibiotics have been recommended. Whether steroids are useful in decreasing the inflammatory reaction or whether prophylactic antibiotics are useful in preventing secondary infection remains to be documented by controlled scientific investigation. Culture of tracheal secretions should be obtained before giving antibiotics and daily thereafter. If food or other solid material has been aspirated, bronchoscopy is indicated to facilitate its removal and provide a patent airway. If gastric dilatation is present, decompression with a nasogastric tube decreases the danger of delayed aspiration and may improve ventilation by decreasing the intra-abdominal pressure.

The single most reliable laboratory test or guide in assessing the condition of the patient is the determination of arterial blood gas and acid-base status (i.e., pO_2, pCO_2, pH and base excess). Using these values and the alveolar oxygen tension, it is also possible to calculate the extent of intrapulmonary shunt present. The progression of the disease and the patient's response to therapy should be monitored frequently by repeating these tests. Other laboratory tests should be done but must be considered of secondary importance. These include serum electrolyte determinations, hemoglobin, hematocrit, plasma hemoglobin, roentgenographic examination of the chest and, in selected cases, blood volume. As stated before, changes in electrolytes and blood constituents are frequently not seen in human near-drowning victims and, when present, are not so abnormal that they represent a life-threatening emergency. Obviously, if significant electrolyte imbalance is detected by the laboratory studies, proper fluid and electrolyte solutions should be administered to correct the abnormalities.

Monitoring of the patient should include his body temperature, pulse, blood pressure, respiratory rate, intake and output, electrocardiogram and, in some cases, central venous pressure. A chest x-ray, while of value for long-range comparison, is not as useful as arterial blood gas data in treating a near-drowning victim. Patients have been reported with severe arterial hypoxemia, even when the x-ray film of the chest was within normal limits.

A large quantity of fluid can be lost into the lungs in these patients, producing a rather profound hypovolemia. These changes in blood volume are usually reflected by changes in central venous pressure. Infusion of plasma, blood or some other volume expander is indicated in such patients. The pulmonary edema seen in these patients is usually related to direct pulmonary epithelial damage or fluid shifts due to differences in electrolyte concentrations, rather than to circulatory overload and primary cardiac failure. To treat these patients with fluid restriction, such as is done for pulmonary edema secondary to congestive failure, may be ill advised.

If significant hemolysis is detected, consideration should be given to replacement of red blood cells in order to increase the patient's oxygen-carrying capacity. Osmotic diuresis should also be considered in these cases to facilitate excretion of the free plasma hemoglobin.

Consciousness usually returns in near-drowning victims when arterial oxygenation and pH are returned to normal. Occasionally, unconsciousness persists. It is in these patients that deliberate hypothermia may be considered.

The length of time that pulmonary care must be continued will vary considerably from patient to patient. In our experience, care can be terminated, on occasion, within 12 hours. However, other patients have required pulmonary support for as long as five weeks. In all cases, decisions should be based on evaluation of alveolar-arterial oxygen gradients and arterial oxygen tension rather than some simple rule-of-thumb. Care should be continued until these parameters return to normal.

Reference

Modell, J. H.: *The Pathophysiology and Treatment of Drowning and Near-Drowning*. Springfield, Illinois, Charles C Thomas, Publisher, 1971.

The Injured Child – Evaluation and Initial Management

THOMAS S. MORSE, M.D.

Remember that *saving life* comes first. *Begin* by checking ventilation and circulation.

Is the child breathing? If not, breathe for him. Tilt head well back, clear oropharynx and get air into lungs:

First–air by mouth-to-mouth.

Then–oxygen by mask.

And only then insert endotracheal tube. Select size by picking a tube that would just fit in the child's nostril. Place it deliberately and carefully. Check to see that air moves freely; if not, suction carefully down the tube. Check to see that both sides of the chest move equally. If not, is tube down too far into one bronchus; is it obstructing the other?

Check chest for:

Open wound–cover it.

Pneumothorax–insert needle into anterior axillary line on side which moves least well, followed by chest tube.

Hemothorax—insert large needle into posterior axillary line on side which moves least well, followed by chest tube.

Flail chest–abnormal movement of part of chest wall due to multiple rib fractures.

(See Thorax, below.)

Remember, oxygen doesn't cure anything. If the child needs oxygen, *find* and *treat* the *cause*.

Is the heart beating? If not, massage it *as soon as ventilation is started*. Use heel of hand over lower half of sternum, or flat surface of two fingers on infants. Ventilation *and* circulation must be accomplished *together*. It does no good to circulate anoxic blood.

Send for help and emergency equipment.

Breathe for school-age child at about 20 puffs per minute, preschool 30, infant 40 per minute. Switch to oxygen via endotracheal tube as soon as feasible.

Massage heart at 60 to 80 beats per minute. Place board under back of chest. If ventilation and massage are adequate (and started early enough), good pulse will be felt in the neck or groin with each massage, dilated pupils will constrict and peripheral circulation will improve.

Now the crisis is over. Normal beat may be restored simply by pumping oxygenated blood through the coronary arteries. Continue ventilation and circulation.

During the first five minutes of ventilation and massage:

Insert dependable intravenous needle or do cut down on a visible vein in an uninjured extremity.

Draw blood only for type and cross match.

Inject one ml. per pound of undiluted sodium bicarbonate. (This is supplied by either 44 mEq. per 50 ml., or 1 mEq. per ml.)

If bleeding is the obvious cause of arrest, pump in 10 ml. per pound of Ringer's lactate or plasma.

Dilute 1:1000 Adrenalin to 1:10,000 and inject 2 ml. intravenously.

If there is no regular beat after five minutes of good ventilation and massage, check EKG.

If EKG shows asystole, dilute 10 per cent calcium chloride to 1 per cent and give 10 ml. intravenously. Continue ventilation and massage for 2 minutes. Repeat 1 ml. per pound of undiluted sodium bicarbonate intravenously followed by 2 ml. of diluted Adrenalin and 10 ml. of diluted calcium chloride.

If EKG shows fibrillation, repeat 1 ml. per pound undiluted sodium bicarbonate and prepare to defibrillate.

Remember, the fibrillating heart does not pump blood, and anoxic heart muscle cannot be defibrillated; therefore, continue massage to the moment of defibrillation.

Shock the heart once with 150 watt-seconds. Ventilate 20 seconds; then if fibrillation persists, resume massage. After about 2 minutes, repeat 1 ml. per pound undiluted sodium bicarbonate and shock again with a higher current. Isuprel may be used instead of Adrenalin. It is supplied in 1-ml. ampules containing 0.2 mg. Dilute one to 10 and give 1 ml. diluted Isuprel in place of 2 ml. diluted Adrenalin.

If a regular beat returns but remains weak, support circulation with intravenous drip containing 2 mg. Isuprel in 500 ml.

If fibrillation persists or recurs repeatedly, inject 5 ml. 1 per cent procaine hydrochloride. (Three ml. 1 per cent Xylocaine may be better but does not yet have Food and Drug Administration approval.)

Most cases of cardiac arrest in salvageable injured children are caused by hypoxia and respond promptly to the above routine. If closed chest massage does not produce adequate circulation (palpable pulse, pupil response), decide quickly whether or not arrest is caused by exsanguination. If it is, pump rapidly 10 ml. per pound O negative low-titer uncrossmatched blood, plasma or Ringer's lactate in addition to that already given. With exsanguination ruled out or treated as above, if circulation by closed massage is still inadequate, do not hesitate to open chest.

SHOCK

In freshly injured children, shock is *almost always* caused by *blood loss* (except in burn patients). Immediately after injury, shock in injured children is practically never due to closed head injury, sepsis or heart failure (unless the heart itself has been injured). A child who has bled into shock has lost at least one-quarter of his total blood volume, or *10 ml. per pound.*

The only difference between reversible shock and irreversible shock is *time.* Work quickly.

Lay child flat with legs elevated. Stop external bleeding, usually with direct pressure over open wounds. Listen with ear to chest to be sure heart is beating. Feel peripheral pulse. If pulse is weak and rapid, extremities cool and dry, blood pressure low or absent, the child is in shock.

Insert at least one dependable intravenous needle or do cut down on visible vein in uninjured extremity; have at least one in arm if abdominal injury is suspected. Draw blood for type and cross match only (take other samples later).

Pump in 10 ml. per pound of lactated Ringer's solution, plasma or saline.

Follow with 1 ml. per pound of undiluted sodium bicarbonate. If the above treatment has restored blood pressure permanently to normal, probably no blood transfusion will be needed.

If 10 ml. per pound restores blood pressure only temporarily, type specific cross matched blood will be needed. Meanwhile, give more plasma or lactated Ringer's solution. Look for continuing blood loss under dressings, into soft tissue around major fractures or into chest or abdomen.

If 10 ml. per pound does not bring systolic pressure even temporarily to 70, consider using uncrossmatched O negative blood. Until blood is available, *keep on pumping* plasma or lactated Ringer's solution until systolic pressure is at least 70.

As soon as the emergency phase of treatment of shock is completed, insert nasogastric tube and empty stomach. Insert indwelling urethral catheter. The rate of urine output is a useful guide to adequacy of shock treatment; minimum is roughly 1 ml. per 5 pounds per hour.

After these steps, it may be helpful to insert a central venous pressure (CVP) catheter. If the child is hypotensive and the CVP is low or zero, more replacement is needed. If CVP is high and the child is still hypotensive, check chest for tension pneumothorax or cardiac tamponade. (See Thorax, below.) Stop further intravenous fluid until cause for elevated CVP is found, either in patient or equipment. (Be sure to stop assisting ventilation momentarily while measuring CVP.)

If ventilation is adequate and heart is beating, the most common treatable reason for continued hypotension is that you *still* have not given enough replacement. The other treatable reason is that a major vessel is bleeding internally. The untreatable reason is that the child got too little replacement too late.

The evaluation and management of every injured child must start in the same way, and must proceed to this point in the same orderly fashion if life is not to be lost by squandering the few precious moments during which it can be saved by restoring ventilation and circulation.

Beyond this point, the order in which the regions of the body are evaluated and treated will vary with the nature of the injury. These body regions are discussed below in a sequence which roughly parallels the descending order or urgency with which the usual injuries of children found therein must be managed.

EVALUATION

Approach every injured child with the attitude that he may have *more than one injury*. Do not let obvious surface wounds distract you from a thorough search for intra-abdominal injuries. Most life-threatening injuries which are missed on initial evaluation of an injured child are in the abdomen.

The usual intra-abdominal injuries are rupture of the spleen, liver or intestine. The former produce hidden bleeding. The latter produces peritonitis. Often more than one organ is injured.

Blood or intestinal contents in the peritoneal cavity produce pain, tenderness and spasm. If these are present initially, the following procedures are carried out:

Insert nasogastric tube, check aspirate for blood, connect to intermittent suction.

Measure and record abdominal girth. With tube working, increasing girth suggests bleeding.

Cross match whole blood, at least 20 ml. per pound of body weight.

In the absence of head injury, give Nembutal or Seconal intramuscularly, 2 mg. per pound. This will enable a tense, frightened child to relax in 20 to 30 minutes but will not mask true tenderness. If tenderness persists, explore the abdomen.

Remember: a small perforation or small tear in the spleen may not produce symptoms until hours after injury. *Check* and *check again*.

Abdominal X-rays. Obtain these as soon as initial evaluation and stabilization are completed. Take posteroanterior chest, flat and upright or decubitus films. Check for masses, evidence of free air or fluid, fractures and the position of the nasogastric tube. Small amounts of free air are best seen under the diaphragm on the *chest* film.

Serum Amylase. This is elevated in many children with blunt abdominal injury. Mild elevation is usually insignificant and returns to normal in three or four days. Elevation above four times the normal level may point to a pancreatic injury *or* to perforation of the duodenum or jejunum with leak of digestive juices into the peritoneum. Do not let an elevated amylase level deter you from exploring a tender abdomen. More than the pancreas may be injured.

Abdominal Paracentesis. This is not indicated in children with a clear-cut indication for operation, nor is it indicated in lucid, oriented children with no abdominal tenderness. It is useful, when positive, in doubtful cases, such as in children with head injuries which make evaluation of abdominal findings impossible, and also in children with pelvic fractures, rib fractures or hematuria suggesting renal injuries. These children have an obvious cause of abdominal tenderness, but may have an intra-abdominal injury as well. Use a plastic percutaneous intravenous catheter. Tap midway between the umbilicus and the mid-axillary line, first on right side and then on left side. If there is no blood, leave the catheter in place on the left side, infuse normal saline, 10 ml. per pound of body weight, and allow the fluid to run back out. This will increase accuracy of abdominal paracentesis from about 70 per cent to about 90 per cent.

Intravenous Pyelography. Every child with hematuria, i.e., any red cells at all in the urine, after an injury should be studied by pyelography. If the child has an indwelling urinary catheter, clamp it before the study begins. The best study is the infusion pyelogram. Mix sodium diatrizoate (Hypaque), 1 ml. per pound of body weight, with an equal amount of saline and infuse rapidly, i.e., all within 3 to 4 minutes. Expose the first film just as the last of the contrast material is administered, then take exposures at 5, 10, 20 and 30 minutes, including a lateral at 30 minutes. For interpretation see Kidney, below.

Cystography. Injection of contrast material via the urinary catheter into the bladder is not necessary if infusion pyelography is done as above.

Radioactive Isotope Scans. These may be very helpful on occasion, particularly if the infusion pyelogram shows no function at all on the injured side. See Kidney, below.

Selective Arteriography. In some centers, arteriography is being extensively used to evaluate kidney, liver and splenic injuries. The difficulty of performing selective arteriography on small children, and the satisfactory results of simpler diagnostic methods, limit practical application to unusual cases.

MANAGEMENT

Blood Loss. Unrecognized bleeding is the most common cause of preventable death in abdominal injury. Frequently, an obvious area of blood loss, such as a femoral fracture, is erroneously assumed to be the only area of blood loss. Injured children should not be given blood by slow intravenous drip because this makes the detection of hidden bleeding very difficult. If blood is to be given, it should be given rapidly in increments equivalent to one-eighth or one-fourth of the blood volume, i.e., increments of 5 or 10 ml. per pound of body weight. Each increment is followed by a period of observation, during which changes in pulse rate, blood pressure and hematocrit suggesting blood loss are much easier to interpret than if administration and loss of blood are going on simultaneously.

A child who is in shock following an injury has lost at least 10 ml. of blood per pound of body weight. This amount can be pumped in as fast as you can do it without fear of overloading. If this amount restores the blood pressure *permanently* to normal, no further transfusion is needed. If the blood pressure returns to normal and then slips away again, give the same amount rapidly again while making plans to handle the continuing bleeding. If 10 ml. per pound of whole blood do not restore the blood pressure even momentarily to normal, an operation to stop major hemorrhage is usually necessary. Additional blood should be given at once.

Spleen. Splenectomy is the treatment of choice at the vast majority of centers. "Conservative," i.e., nonoperative, management of a ruptured spleen is dangerous except in ideal situations, such as in trauma study units. Mortality in cases of isolated splenic rupture is very low, since diagnosis is usually easy and operation curative. About half of all deaths result from severe associated injuries. The other half occur in children with multiple injuries in whom the diagnosis of ruptured spleen is missed.

Liver. Not all liver injuries require operation, but laparotomy carries little risk and should not be withheld if bleeding persists. Hematomas are evacuated, devitalized liver tissue removed and bleeding controlled. Large lacerations are sutured; small ones are left alone. The peritoneal cavity is frequently drained, but common duct drainage by T-tube is usually *not* advisable.

Stomach. Mortality is directly related to delay in diagnosis and treatment. Careful cleaning of the peritoneal cavity, use of systemic antibiotics and simple suture of the perforation give surprisingly good results if done promptly. The usual mistake at operation is failure to look for and repair a second area of gastric perforation which is frequently present on the posterior gastric wall or lesser curvature.

Duodenum. Small blow-outs are easily closed. Large ones may tax judgment. Pancreatoduodenectomy may occasionally be necessary, but usually a simpler procedure suffices.

Small Intestine. Perforations are usually small and easily closed. These are the usual cause of persistent peritoneal irritation and smoldering leukocytosis and fever in a child whose abdomen does not contain blood. They are frequently multiple, and those at the margin of the mesentery are easily overlooked. Look carefully on *both sides.*

Avulsion of Mesentery. There are persistent localized ileus with moderate tenderness and often paracentesis suggesting a small amount of intraperitoneal blood. The bowel will usually remain intact for about 72 hours, even if completely devascularized, so early evidence of perforation is not usually found. Resection and anastomosis before perforation give good results.

Colon. Perforation of the colon causes the highest rate of mortality and morbidity of all intestinal injuries. Suture only very recent perforations or those distal to a colostomy. Exteriorize most colon perforations.

Retroperitoneal Hematoma. The pendulum is swinging toward exploration of retroperitoneal hematomas, especially those near the renal vessels, pancreas and duodenum. Leave alone distal ones, small ones and those which appear completely stable. Before approaching, plan proximal and distal vascular control and have available at least 40 ml. per pound of the freshest whole blood obtainable.

Pancreas. Most pancreatic injuries heal without treatment, but devitalized tissue should be removed. Resection of all tissue to the left of the portal vein is well tolerated. Total pancreatectomy is rarely necessary. Serum amylase elevations persisting more than 10 days after injury usually signify a complication, such as traumatic pseudocyst. These do not require complicated internal drainage. External tube drainage suffices in children.

Diaphragm. Ruptures are occasionally missed because they are uncommon. Remember to look at the diaphragm on the chest x-ray. Often the blood supply to the displaced viscera is compromised, making early operation mandatory.

Kidney. Eighty per cent of blunt kidney injuries heal without operation. These yield normal infusion pyelograms or evidence of calyceal compression. The collecting system of the injured kidney may contain less contrast material than its normal counterpart, but all dye which can be seen is in the collecting system and ureter where it belongs.

The most common indication for operation is urinary extravasation, which signifies a major laceration. This is best done two to three days after injury, when demarcation of devitalized renal tissue has taken place and bleeding from fractured parenchyma is easy to control.

The other indication for operation is vascular injury, and this must be done as an emergency if the kidney is to be salvaged. The infusion pyelogram shows no visualization at all on the injured side, the scan shows no uptake and/or the arteriogram shows no flow to the kidney.

Ureter. The ureter is rarely injured by blunt trauma but may be lacerated by a penetrating injury. The simpler the repair, the better.

Bladder. Perforation is often but not always associated with pelvic fracture. Infusion pyelogram or cystogram shows extravasation of urine. Prompt closure and suprapubic drainage is the treatment of choice.

Penetrating Injuries. Children with penetrating abdominal injuries should be surgically explored because the incidence of visceral injury is high and the risk of exploration is very low. The abdomen may be entered via any wound below the nipples.

If penetration through the peritoneum is in doubt and peritoneal irritation is not present, the skin may be closed tightly around a catheter through which 50 per cent sodium diatrizoate (Hypaque) can be injected into the wound. Children showing x-ray evidence of contrast material in the abdomen are candidates for surgical exploration. This maneuver is especially helpful in children with head injuries which make abdominal evaluation difficult.

Incision. In growing children, a long transverse incision gives good exposure and a far better cosmetic result than does a vertical incision. The latter is frequently preferable in teenagers and adults.

THORAX

The urgent thoracic injuries produce airway obstruction, tension pneumothorax, hemothorax, sucking wounds, flail chest or cardiac tamponade. The major goals in management are as follows:

To intercept exsanguination and life-threatening infections by prompt surgical closure of significant rents in the heart, major vessels, trachea, bronchi and esophagus.

To rid the pleural cavities, mediastinum and pericardium rapidly of space-occupying air, blood or fluid.

To reexpand collapsed lungs as quickly and as completely as possible.

To guard against reaccumulation of air or fluid and recurrence of pulmonary collapse.

Airway Obstruction. If blood is the cause—from pulmonary contusion, bronchial or tracheal injury or aspiration from nose or mouth—repeated gentle suction via endotracheal tube is usually adequate. If stomach contents are the cause, in addition to suction via endotracheal tube, consider bronchoscopy, hydrocortisone 100 mg. every 8 hours for two days to minimize inflammatory reaction produced by acid peptic juice, and systemic antibiotics. History and evaluation of aspirated material are important because x-ray findings may be indistinguishable from those of a pulmonary contusion.

Tension Pneumothorax. If there is embarrassed ventilation with overexpanded hemithorax, shift of trachea and bronchi to opposite side and hyperresonant hemithorax with diminished breath sounds, relieve with a needle inserted in the anterior axillary line, followed by a chest tube to underwater seal. If a large amount of air continues to flow from the tube, apply gentle suction. If the lung still cannot be expanded, perform bronchoscopic examination for major tracheal or bronchial injury. If saliva or gastric contents emerge from the chest tube, perform contrast swallow to localize esophageal perforation, which urgently requires surgical closure and mediastinal drainage. Use chest tube for all but very small pneumothoraces in children.

Hemothorax. Hemothorax varies in severity from asymptomatic to exsanguination. Major hemothorax produces a shift of mediastinal structures to the opposite side, dullness, and diminished or absent breath sounds. If bleeding into the chest alone has produced shock, urgent operation is needed to repair major vascular injury. In most other cases, bleeding subsides and exploration of the chest is not needed. Place a large chest tube in the midaxillary line to empty the chest and reexpand the lung. Follow the rate of subsequent blood loss. An hourly loss of up to 2 ml. per pound, particularly if the rate is slowing, usually will stop without operation. If loss exceeds 15 ml. per pound in the first 8 hours, and particularly if loss accelerates, early operation is indicated.

Hemopneumothorax. This is usually due to laceration of pulmonary parenchyma, most of which will heal spontaneously. If one chest tube does not handle both blood and air, insert a second tube.

Flail Chest. A segment of chest wall moves inward on inspiration and outward on expiration owing to multiple rib fractures. Treatment varies with the severity of respiratory embarrassment. Manual stabilization enables cough, which may greatly improve the child temporarily. If ventilation is not excellent, with normal blood gases following external splinting, intubate and support on respirator with positive pressure. Consider elective tracheostomy in severe forms, as positive pressure respirator may be needed for one to two weeks.

Cardiac Tamponade. Because this is infrequently seen in injured children, diagnosis is easy to overlook. It is usually but not always associated with a penetrating wound of the heart. The child gives the appearance of having both circulatory and respiratory embarrassment. The pulse is rapid and weak, pulse pressure is narrow, venous pressure is elevated and heart sounds are muffled. It may develop insidiously after initial examination has been performed. Aspirate by placing needle in xyphosternal angle and going upward, outward and backward, all at about 45 degrees to midplanes of chest. In the absence of a penetrating wound, further treatment depends on rapidity of reaccumulation. Those with rapid recurrence of tamponade, and all children with penetrating chest wound near the heart, should be promptly explored.

After assessing the chest for these urgent conditions, inspect front and back for surface wounds and palpate all over for fractures, hematomas and subcutaneous emphysema. Obtain emergency chest x-rays, portable ones if necessary. Note any deviations from expected normal and ask, "How could this abnormal finding *be explained by an injury?*" For example, could a high stomach bubble point to a ruptured diaphragm, or a widened mediastinum indicate a vascular injury rather than a preexisting enlarged thymus? Also note carefully and adjust accordingly the position of nasogastric, endotracheal, CVP or thoracostomy tubes.

NECK AND BACK

All children who complain of neck pain and all children with head injuries should be suspected of having cervical spine fracture. Move only with manual traction, with neck slightly extended.

Explore all penetrating injuries of the neck in the operating room. Do not probe neck wounds in the emergency room.

In the conscious child, check arm and leg movement. Ask for pain or paresthesias. Palpate each vertebral spinous process. Spine fractures cause pain when pressure is applied to the spinous process.

In the unconscious child, elicit withdrawal from painful stimulus; pinprick fingers and soles.

If weakness suggests spinal cord injury, give dexamethasone, 3 to 6 mg. intravenously.

Consider all spinal cord injuries *reversible,* and get emergency neurosurgical consultation.

Insert nasogastric tube and urethral catheter.

Protect anesthetic areas from pressure injury.

EXTREMITIES

The urgent problems are uncontrolled bleeding and injuries which compromise blood supply to feet and hands.

Direct pressure is usually the safest way to control bleeding. If a tourniquet is used, record the time of application, put it on tight enough to occlude arterial flow and plan prompt definitive management.

Compound fractures, dislocations and other fractures which impair blood flow require urgent treatment. Splint fractures before moving the patient.

Lacerated arteries in the distal part of leg or forearm usually may be ligated, but arterial lacerations proximal to bifurcation of brachial and popliteal arteries should be repaired if possible.

Test motor nerve function:
Axillary—abduct arm.
Brachioradialis—flex biceps.
Ulnar—spread fingers.
Median—touch thumb to little finger.
Radial—extend wrist and fingers.
Femoral—flex hip.
Sciatic—flex foot.
Check for sensory loss.

Now review findings, and try to get an accurate history of the accident. With the history in mind, go over affected areas again.

22

Unclassified Diseases

Amyloidosis

RONALD G. STRAUSS, M.D.

Amyloid is a proteinaceous material produced by reticuloendothelial cells which stains with Congo red, exhibits polarization birefringence, appears fibrillar by electron microscopy and resembles the amino-terminal variable region of immunoglobulin light chains (Glenner et al.). Familial primary amyloid syndromes may begin during childhood but are rare. Deposition of this material at this age almost invariably complicates chronic inflammatory diseases (secondary amyloidosis) (Strauss et al.).

There is no effective treatment for established amyloidosis, but suppression of inflammation in the underlying disorder may prevent or retard its production; however, it is unlikely that the lesions regress. Antimicrobial agents have practically eliminated this complication in patients with suppurative infections (Strauss et al.). Amyloidosis complicating rheumatoid arthritis is found primarily in patients with persistent disease, and inflammation should be controlled.* Although corticosteroids and immunosuppressive agents may be detrimental in experimental amyloidosis, such drugs should not be withheld if indicated for treatment of the basic disease. They do not have specific antiamyloid effects (Maxwell et al., Barth et al.).

Many organs may contain amyloid, but progressive renal failure is the major clinical problem.* If the underlying disease can be controlled and the quality of life improved, renal transplantation or chronic hemodialysis may be considered. At present, the efficacy of this treatment or the effects of immunosuppression required to control rejection in patients with amyloidosis are unknown (Cohen et al.).

* For specific management, see sections on rheumatoid arthritis and renal failure, pp. 377 and 388.

References

Barth, W. F., Willerson, J. T., Waldmann, T. A., and Decker, J. L.: Primary Amyloidosis. Clinical, Immunochemical and Immunoglobulin Metabolism Studies in Fifteen Patients. *Am. J. Med.*, 47:259, 1969.

Cohen, A. S., Bricetti, A. B., Harrington, J. T., and Mannick, J. A.: Renal Transplantation in Two Cases of Amyloidosis. *Lancet*, 2:513, 1971.

Glenner, G. G., Ein, D., and Terry, W. D.: The Immunoglobulin Origin of Amyloid. *Am. J. Med.*, 52: 141, 1972.

Maxwell, M. H., Adams, D. A., and Goldman, R.: Corticosteroid Therapy of Amyloid Nephrotic Syndrome. *Ann. Int. Med.*, 60:539, 1964.

Strauss, R. G., Schubert, W. K., and McAdams, A. J.: Amyloidosis in Childhood. *J. Pediat.*, 74:272, 1969.

Sarcoidosis

EDWIN L. KENDIG, Jr., M.D.

Since the cause of sarcoidosis is unknown, there is known specific therapy. Adrenocorticosteroids and corticotropin are the only agents available at present which can suppress the acute manifestations of sarcoidosis. These agents are used only during the acute and dangerous episodes.

Adrenocorticosteroid (or corticotropin) therapy is always indicated in patients with intrinsic ocular disease, with diffuse pulmonary lesions with alveolar-capillary block, with central nervous system lesions, with myocardial involvement, with hypersplenism and with persistent hypercalcemia. Relative indications for adrenocorticosteroid therapy include progressive or symptomatic pulmonary lesions, disfiguring cutaneous and lymph node lesions, constitutional symptoms and joint involvement, lesions of the nasal, laryngeal and bronchial mucosa and persistent facial nerve palsy.

Fresh lesions are apparently more responsive than older ones. Suppressive action is often temporary, but it is beneficial when the unremitting course of disease will produce loss of organ function. For example, adrenocorticosteroids can reduce the level of serum calcium and may thus help prevent nephrocalcinosis and renal insufficiency and possibly band keratitis. Whether adrenocorticosteroids should be used in treatment of those patients whose disease consists only of asymptomatic miliary nodules or bronchopneumonic patches in the lung fields is debatable.

In children, the initial dose of prednisone or prednisolone is 1 mg. per kilogram of body weight per day, and of triamcinolone, 0.75 mg. per kilogram of body weight per day, in four divided doses. After a few weeks the dose is gradually reduced. The course of treatment is usually about six months, but some patients require continuous maintenance therapy. Siltzbach reported the frequent occurrence of temporary relapse after discontinuation of adrenocorticosteroid therapy, but noted that improvement usually follows even if treatment is not resumed. In the management of ocular sarcoidosis, corticosteroids in the form of either ointment or drops (0.5 to 1 per cent) are utilized in conjunction with the systemic use of these agents. During the course of such local therapy the pupils are kept continuously dilated by use of an atropine ointment (1 per cent).

References

Committee on Therapy, American Thoracic Society: Treatment of Sarcoidosis. *Am. Rev. Resp. Dis.*, 103:433, 1971.

Jasper, P. L., and Denny, F. W.: Sarcoidosis in Children. *J. Pediat.*, 73:499, 1968.

Kendig, E. L., Jr.: Sarcoidosis Among Children. *J. Pediat.*, 61:269, 1962.

Siltzbach, L. E.: Sarcoidosis: Clinical Features and Management. *Med. Clin. N. Am.*, 51:483, 1967.

Familial Mediterranean Fever

(Benign Paroxysmal Peritonitis, Familial Paroxysmal Polyserositis, Armenian Disease)

ARTHUR D. SCHWABE, M.D.

Familial Mediterranean fever (FMF) is an inherited disorder of unknown etiology characterized by irregularly recurring attacks of fever and pain in the chest, abdomen or joints. The disease is most commonly seen in persons of Armenian, Jewish or Arab ethnic origin.

The clinical manifestations usually begin in childhood, occurring before the age of 10 years in 70 per cent of patients, and they represent inflammatory reactions of the peritoneal, pleural or synovial membranes. Attacks of abdominal and pleuritic chest pain usually begin suddenly and subside spontaneously within 72 hours. Symptoms of joint inflammation tend to persist longer, sometimes for several months, but rarely leave residual damage.

The white blood cell count, sedimentation rate, C-reactive protein, haptoglobins, lipoproteins and plasma fibrinogen are usually elevated during attacks, but no laboratory abnormalities specific for this disorder have been detected to date.

Principles of Treatment. Because the precise etiology of FMF is unknown, the management at present consists of symptomatic treatment of the acute attack and prophylactic measures designed to prevent or reduce the frequency of the recurring paroxysms. In selecting any therapeutic regimen for this disease, the following observations must be borne in mind:

1. Most attacks are self-limited and may be followed by prolonged, asymptomatic intervals, sometimes lasting several years.
2. Patients who have frequent attacks are particularly prone to become addicted to narcotics.
3. Agents of unproved or doubtful value, which may affect growth and development, are contraindicated in children.
4. Acute appendicitis may be difficult, if not impossible, to differentiate from FMF peritonitis manifested solely by right lower quadrant pain.
5. There is a high incidence of amyloidosis, principally involving the kidneys, in non-Ashkenazic Jews with this disease.

Treatment of the Acute Attack. Bed rest is recommended during the febrile period of each severe attack, but it is not obligatory for many mild episodes. The fever, which may rise to 104° F., and the pain usually respond to oral acetylsalicylic acid, 10 mg. per kilogram every 4 to 6 hours. When nausea, vomiting or paralytic ileus is present, the drug should be administered in suppository form.

Narcotics should be avoided unless absolutely necessary for relief of severe peritoneal inflammation. Under such circumstances a single intramuscular dose of meperidine hydrochloride (Demerol), 1.5 mg. per kilogram, may be given. Pleural effusions accompanying attacks of pleuritis are transient and require no specific therapy. Corticosteroids are not effective in preventing attacks.

Prevention. Restriction of the dietary fat intake has been a useful regimen in reducing the number of febrile paroxysms in some patients. Those with mild or infrequent attacks require no strict dietary management, but they should be advised to limit their intake of butter, cheese, ice cream and pork and to substitute low fat milk for whole milk. Patients who experience more than two attacks per month or who regularly miss three or more days of school per month should be placed on a diet containing 20 Gm. of fat or less per day. Specific instructions should be provided to patients and their parents by a dietitian.

The protein intake should be kept high by adding liberal amounts of nonfat milk, shrimp, haddock, cod or chicken breast, and a normal caloric intake should be maintained by providing unlimited amounts of fruits and vegetables. Normal weight gain and growth should not be compromised by this diet, which should be continued for at least three months before its efficacy in reducing attacks can be judged.

References

Mellinkoff, S. M., Schwabe, A. D., and Lawrence, J. S.: A Dietary Treatment for Familial Mediterranean Fever. *Arch. Int. Med.,* 108:80, 1961.

Siegal, S.: Familial Paroxysmal Polyserositis. *Am. J. Med.,* 36:893, 1964.

Sohar, E., et al.: Familial Mediterranean Fever. *Am. J. Med.,* 43:227, 1967.

23

Diseases Peculiar to the Newborn

Dysmaturity and Postmaturity

LOUIS GLUCK, M.D.

Possibly one-third of all low birth weight infants (2500 Gm. or less) are not products of premature birth but are born after gestations of 38 weeks or longer. Past confusions and polyterminology relative to such dysmaturity (e.g., small-for-dates, intrauterine growth retardation, fetal malnutrition, chronic fetal distress, pseudoprematurity, fetal growth retardation) are cleared up by considering any infant of low birth weight who is smaller than expected for his period of gestation to be dysmature. This differentiates the dysmature infant from the true prematurely born infant who also is of low birth weight but whose appropriate size suggests that fetal growth had progressed satisfactorily in utero until his gestation was interrupted some time before 36 to 37 weeks.

The dysmature infant is small for his gestational age because of abnormal fetal growth either on *an apparently malnutritional basis* secondary, for example, to maternal toxemia, placental insufficiency, maternal renal disease or multiple pregnancy; or from *a general failure to grow* owing to intrauterine infection such as rubella, to certain congenital malformations, or to genetic reasons such as trisomy.

Infants in the "fetal malnutrition" group are hypermetabolic, with high postnatal caloric requirements, and appear to grow best if their nutritional deprivation has occurred in late fetal life (manifested by low birth weight but normal length) rather than in early fetal life (manifested by low birth weight and abnormally short length for gestational age). Closely related to these, and also hypermetabolic, are the postmature infants who are retained in utero past term and who have begun, usually after 42 weeks of gestation, to show signs of significant weight loss and dehydration.

The failure-to-grow group generally is not significantly amenable to present therapy, although a major malformation may be operable and some active infections acquired in utero (e.g., toxoplasmosis) are treatable. The following discussion of therapy pertains almost entirely to "malnourished" and postmature infants.

In dysmature infants the most serious postnatal problem to anticipate is severe hypoglycemia, which may be seen within a few hours after birth; frequent monitoring of blood sugar is therefore required. The first blood sugar estimations on the infant should be made no later than 2 hours of age and hourly thereafter until stabilization of blood glucose above 40 mg. per 100 ml. Dextrostix are useful for such screening. In our experience, false results (failure to detect hypoglycemic levels) with Dextrostix estimations reading above 40 mg. per 100 ml. are rare. In the range registering less than 40 mg. per 100 ml., however, a capillary (or venous) blood sugar determination should be done, because false-negatives at 40 mg. per 100 ml. are found and because accuracy of prognosis makes it necessary to document hypoglycemia as fully as possible. Our management of the hypoglycemic infant is similar to that proposed by Cornblath, p. 336.

If the blood glucose is 20 mg. per 100 ml. or less, intravenous glucose is started immediately; a maximum of 2 ml. per kilogram of 25 per cent glucose is injected *slowly* into a peripheral vein, and peripheral intravenous infusion of 15 per cent glucose at a rate of approximately 80 to 110 ml. per kilogram per day is run continuously. By the second 24 hours, if required, this is increased to 110 to 120 ml. per kilogram per day, and 25 mEq. of sodium chloride per liter of fluid is added. If the infant is able to tolerate it, as nearly all can, oral feeding with a "breast milk simulator" (e.g., Similac, Enfamil) at 20 calories per ounce is begun by about 4 hours of age.

In the usually encountered infant, before 12 hours of age, the blood sugars are well stabilized, most often above 60 mg. per 100 ml., and the intravenous glucose is able to be tapered over a 4-hour period to 10 per cent glucose and finally to 5 per cent glucose. When it is obvious from consistent Dextrostix estimates above 40 mg. per 100 ml. that oral feedings alone will suffice, the intravenous fluids are discontinued. In calculating the infant's total fluid intake while still on intravenous infusions, the lower requirements recommended should be used if there is oral intake.

If blood glucose levels do not rise significantly and stay above the 20- to 30-mg. per 100 ml. range after 12 hours of intravenous infusion of 15 per cent glucose, ACTH may be given (7.5 units every 12 hours intramuscularly in the anterior thigh). At the outset, when hypoglycemia is detected, the physician is occasionally unable to cannulate a peripheral vein. In such an instance, glucagon, 30 micrograms per kilogram in a single injection intramuscularly, frequently will produce a transient rise in blood sugar and "buy" time to allow proper placement of an intravenous infusion.

Other concerns in management include the necessity for vigorous thermoregulation—preferably in a servo-controlled warming incubator. Presumably a lack of brown (but also white) adipose tissues in these infants contributes to their poor thermoregulatory responses. Some authors have suggested that profound hypothermia in some of these infants may in part be responsible for an undue incidence of pulmonary hemorrhage observed among dysmature infants.

It should also be appreciated as occasional sources of management problems that certain dysmature infants may have marked metabolic acidosis and elevated nonprotein nitrogen and show marked polycythemia. The acidosis and azotemia apparently result from a combination of starvation-induced cellular breakdown plus poor excretion by the placenta.

The postmature infant presents an additional problem of aspiration pneumonia, frequently involving aspiration of meconium. Where this is known in the delivery room from the meconium present at the resuscitation, aspiration (and even lavage with saline) of the trachea must be done to clear as much of the meconium as possible. The aspiration pneumonia may have associated pneumomediastinum, pneumothorax or atelectasis. When respiratory symptoms are detected, chest x-ray should be taken for evaluation. The care of infants with aspiration pneumonias includes good tracheal toilet—frequent pharyngeal catheter aspiration—with occasional suctioning of the laryngeal area under direct observation when the infant is particularly productive of mucus and seems unable to handle his secretions. It is our policy to administer parenteral antibiotics intramuscularly (anterior thigh) in a dosage of 100,000 units per kilogram of crystalline penicillin once daily, plus kanamycin, 15 mg. per kilogram per 24 hours in two divided doses, to those infants with demonstrated neonatal pneumonia.

The prognosis in postmaturity seems to be directly related to the length of gestation. Beyond a documented gestation of 43 weeks, mortality goes up sharply. Morbidity is high from the forty-second week. In the term or preterm group, mortality and morbidity seem to correlate best with the degree of retardation of both length and weight.

Birth Injuries

JAMES E. DRORBAUGH, M.D.

SKIN AND SUBCUTANEOUS TISSUE

Contusions and ecchymosis of skin and subcutaneous tissue are not uncommon and rarely cause difficulties other than possibly contributing to anemia and hyperbilirubinemia. Hematomas most frequently occur beneath the periosteum of the skull and can be quite large. They also may contribute to anemia and hyperbilirubinemia but are otherwise benign. No treatment is indicated for cephalohematomas. Even though reabsorption may take several weeks and the contours of the skull may be distorted during this time, eventual healing without residual deformity is virtually assured.

It is particularly important not to aspirate the liquid contents of cephalohematomas because infection may be introduced.

Underlying skull fracture also requires no treatment unless it is depressed. In these cases, neurologic symptoms may develop, and surgical procedures to lift up the depressed bone should be instituted.

MUSCULOSKELETAL AND NEUROMUSCULAR SYSTEMS

Injuries to muculoskeletal and neuromuscular systems occasionally occur. The well-known fractured clavicle is in this category. This injury heals without special therapy other than a figure-of-eight bandage loosely applied. One hears of nonunions, but they must be extremely rare. Fracture of the humerus also occurs and may be seen in association with paralysis of the shoulder girdle and upper extremity resulting from nerve root or brachial plexus injury. The fracture is sometimes treated by immobilization in a cast or splint; however, if paralysis is extensive, the arm is already immobilized, and healing will occur without need for immobilization. Pinning the sleeve to the shirt will suffice.

Another abnormality associated with brachial nerve injury is paralysis of the diaphragm on the affected side. At times the interference with respiration resulting from paralysis of the diaphragm may be so severe that surgical treatment is indicated.

Besides the brachial nerve injuries, one may see injuries to the peripheral facial nerve. No treatment is indicated, and eventual healing is fairly certain even though this may take four to five years.

ORGAN SYSTEMS WITHIN THE BODY

Organ systems within the body may be injured during the process of delivery. One thinks first of injuries to the brain. These injuries may result from depressed skull fractures or they may be caused by hemorrhage. Hemorrhage occurs in the subdural space, subarachnoid space, ventricular system, brain substance or a combination of these locations. These infants are apt to be extremely ill with a variety of central nervous system signs and symptoms, cyanosis, hypothermia and acidosis.

Lumbar puncture with pressure measurements and withdrawal of fluid into successive tubes is, of course, indicated for diagnostic purposes when the question of central nervous system hemorrhage arises. Some clinicians advise repeated aspiration if macroscopic blood is found in the cerebrospinal fluid, especially when pressure is increased. However, no studies are available to demonstrate the value of this procedure.

In addition to injury to the central nervous system resulting from trauma, one may encounter injuries to intra-abdominal structures. Perinephritic and periadrenal hemorrhage is sometimes encountered when vigorous resuscitation is used. Rupture of liver or spleen may occur. Unfortunately, these conditions lead to death soon after birth. The clinical condition of the infant does not warrant exploratory surgery to search for bleeding vessels or visceral lacerations. However, if time is available and if the clinical history suggests trauma to internal viscera, such surgery may be undertaken.

Resuscitation of the Newborn

BRADLEY E. SMITH, M.D.

By one minute of life, 80 per cent of newborn infants cry vigorously, display strong spontaneous muscular movements with vigorous reflex activity, have a strong cardiovascular output and may be already dispelling the slight cyanosis common at birth. In the remaining 20 per cent, varying degrees of hypoventilation, sluggishness, areflexia and other evidences of cardiovascular, respiratory and central nervous system dysfunction occur. It has been well demonstrated that these "low Apgar score babies," particularly when degree of prematurity is also considered, have an elevated incidence of mortality and both physical and neurologic morbidity (Drage and Berendes). They are most commonly characterized as "low Apgar score babies" for greater efficiency in discussion.

Low Apgar score babies require alert and thoughtful observation in the immediate neonatal minutes of life and varying degrees of resuscitative help. From 1 to 2 per cent of these infants require endotracheal resuscitation and approximately one-hundredth of one percent may require external cardiac massage (Smith).

The causes of this hypotonic condition are many (Table 1), and the resuscitating physician must attempt to diagnose the cause in order to design his therapy intelligently, for each cause has different prognostic implications. For example, moderately low Apgar scores may be caused by the effects of drugs or anesthetics alone, with no important component of hypoxemia or acidosis. However, the preponderance

TABLE 1. Etiology of Birth Depression

FETAL ASPHYXIA

- Maternal asphyxia
  - Aspiration of vomitus
  - Hypoventilation
  - Anesthestic accident
- Maternal hypotension
  - Regional anesthesia
  - Hemorrhage
  - Cardiovascular collapse
- Anemic asphyxia
  - Ethrythroblastosis
- Uterine blood flow restriction
  - Pitocin stimulation
  - "Alpha" vasoconstrictors
- Inadequate placental perfusion
  - Toxemia
  - Abruptio placentae
- Inadequate placental fetal flow
  - Nuchal cord
  - Prolapsed cord
  - Knotted cord

NEONATAL ASPHYXIA

- Blocked airway
  - Meconium aspiration
  - Mechanical upper airway obstruction
  - Congenital upper airway obstruction: web, polyp, atresia, cyst, laryngotracheal malacia, etc.
- Neonatal hypoventilation
  - Drugs
  - Anesthetics
  - Sepsis
  - CNS trauma

CENTRAL NERVOUS SYSTEM SEDATION AND AREFLEXIA

- Anesthesia
- Sedative–analgesic drugs
- Cerebral vascular accident
- Hypoxemia

of low Apgar scores results from asphyxial conditions. Therefore, low Apgar score babies can generally be expected to have hypoxemia and acidosis (Table 2).

In addition to depriving the brain, heart and other organs of much-needed oxygen, the occurrence of hypoxemia, acidosis and hypoventilation in these infants leads to poor blood flow in the lungs, decreased cardiac output, "shunting" of blood within the lungs and perpetuation of fetal type circulation. Therefore, it is essential that vigorous expansion of the lungs, either spontaneously or by intermittent positive pressure breathing techniques, be achieved as soon as possible so that this cycle can be reversed (Smith and Moya).

TABLE 2. Effects of Asphyxia on Acid-Base Status at Birth (Umbilical Artery)*

	VIGOROUS	DEPRESSED	SEVERE DEPRESSION
O_2 (mm. Hg)	18	12	6
pCO_2 (mm. Hg)	50	70	90
pH	7.20	7.00	6.80
Base deficit (mEq./liter)	6	12	18

* Representative approximate values.

Resuscitation of the newborn must be carefully planned in advance. Proper equipment and drugs must be available and tested for proper function (Table 3). The actual procedure for resuscitation must be based on a preplanned pathway relating to the etiology of the condition, the degree of hypotonia in the infant and his response to resuscitative efforts (Table 4).

TABLE 3. Equipment and Drugs

- Radiant Heater
- Suction
  - Electric suction
  - Ophthalmic bulb
  - De Lee Trap
- Ventilatory Aids
  - IPPB Device
    - Ambu type bag
    - Hustead type bag and valve
    - Kreiselman type IPPB device
    - Other automatic IPPB devices
  - Face Mask
    - Size: 0 and 1
    - Several styles
  - Oral Airway
    - Size: 00 and 0
    - Any style
  - Laryngoscope
    - Miller style
    - Size: premature and 1
  - Endotracheal Tube
    - Cole type, size: 12–18
    - Portex type, size: 2.5–4.0
    - Soft wire stylet
- Drugs
  - Calcium chloride (50 mg. I.V.)
  - *N*-allyl-normorphine (0.2 mg. I.V.)
  - Epinephrine (0.05 mg. I.V.; 0.1 mg. I.C.)
  - *No analeptics*
  - Sodium bicarbonate (See Table 5)

TABLE 4. Procedure (Primum Non Nocere)

Radiant Heat
- Dry off baby quickly
- Maintain temperature above 97° F.

Head Down, Lateral Position
- Pad behind shoulder
- Extend head and neck

Brief, Effective Suction
- Electrical suction of thin secretions
- Ophthalmic bulb for meconium and mucous

Establish Airway and Ventilation

Stimulate Baby
- Gentle flicking of soles of feet
- Gentle rubbing of back

Assist Ventilation with Oxygen if Needed
- Apgar 7-8-9-10—O_2 over face gently
- Apgar 4-5-6—O_2 over face or by IPPB mask after suction
- Apgar 0-1-2-3—O_2 by mask first, O_2 by endotracheal tube if still necessary

Endotracheal Suction and Ventilation only if Specifically Indicated

Antinarcotic and Antacid Treatment only if Specifically Indicated

Even after adequate ventilation is established, severely asphyxiated infants usually have pronounced lactic acidosis resulting from prolonged anaerobic metabolism. In order to strengthen cardiovascular and metabolic function, clinical experience has shown the efficacy of partial correction of this acidemia by the administration of sodium bicarbonate solution. The resulting dangers of iatrogenic hyperosmolarity, hypernatremia and alkalemia should not be disregarded (Table 5) (Finberg).

In the immediate postresuscitation period and for the first few days of life, severely asphyxiated newborn infants require intensive nursing and physician care. Neurologic sequelae of asphyxia, bleeding problems and respiratory distress frequently occur, particularly in asphyxiated premature infants. Respiratory infection introduced by the resuscitation procedure is rare in clinical practice. However, if indicated, prophylactic antibiotics may be administered in the usual pediatric doses.

TABLE 5. Treatment of Metabolic Acidosis and Cardiac Arrest in the Newborn (Lactic Acidosis Resulting from Asphyxia)

1. Maintain body heat at 37°–38° C.
2. Ventilate lungs well for 10 minutes
   (a) mask—IPPB oxygen
   (b) endotracheal tube IPPB oxygen
3. Evaluate effectiveness of circulation
   (a) if circulation is failing, consider sodium bicarbonate immediately, before 10 minutes have passed
4. Apgar score remains 5 or less at 10 minutes with adequate ventilation
   (a) if cause is likely to be drug, sepsis or CNS trauma *without* prolonged asphyxia, *do not* treat with emergency bicarbonate
   (b) if cause is *asphyxia,* treat with emergency sodium bicarbonate
   (c) first dose:
      i. sodium bicarbonate 4 mEq./kg.
      ii. dilute with equal volume 5% D5W

TABLE 5—*Continued*

      iii. administer over 5 minutes via umbilical vein catheter (#3 feeding tube) with I.V. catheter tip 2 cm. beyond umbilical ring
   second dose:
      iv. as drip in neonatal nursery, based on laboratory evidence of base deficit greater than 6 mEq./liter
5. Cardiac arrest
   (a) ventilate lungs 40–60/min. with mask if possible; with tube if not
   (b) commence external cardiac massage at 100–120/min. with both thumbs pressing on *middle* of sternum and fingers around thorax for posterior support
   (c) intubate trachea, continue ventilation
   (d) drugs
      i. if arrest persists, consider intracardiac epinephrine, 0.05–0.1 mg. diluted to 2 ml. with cardiac blood
      ii. consider 50 mg. intracardiac calcium chloride
      iii. (isoproterenol is *not* useful during arrest)
      iv. commence umbilical vein catheterization with #3 plastic feeding tube while maintaining external massage and ventilation
      v. sodum bicarbonate as above; however, if cardiac arrest persists, sodium bicarbonate may be repeated 2 mEq./kg. for every 5 minutes that arrest continues until 12 mEq./kg. total is reached (Note: be wary of danger of hyperosmolarity and hypernatremia)
   (e) obtain electrocardiograph monitor and prepare for intensive observation in neonatal nursery

References

Drage, J. S., and Berendes, H.: Apgar Scores and the Outcome of the Newborn, *Pediat. Clin. N. Am.,* 13:635–643, 1966.

Finberg, L.: Dangers to Infants Caused by Changes in Osmolal Concentration, *Pediatrics,* 40:1031–1034, 1967.

Smith, B. E., and Moya, F.: Resuscitation of the Depressed Newborn, *Anesthesiology,* 26:549-561, 1965.

Smith, B. E.: Ethical Dilemmas of Anesthesia and Resuscitation in 10,000 Consecutive Deliveries: Sixty-Five Ross Conference, *Ethical Dilemmas in Current Perinatal Care,* Ross Laboratories, June, 1973. In press.

Idiopathic Respiratory Distress Syndrome

WILLIAM H. TOOLEY, M.D.

Respiratory distress in the newborn infant can be caused by aspiration of meconium or blood, obstruction of the upper airway by congenital defects of the larynx, trachea or lung, pulmonary edema, pneumonia, pneumothorax, pneumomediastinum or abdominal distention. Be sure that these specific causes of respiratory distress are not present before making the diagnosis of the idiopathic respiratory distress syndrome (IRDS). There are two forms of IRDS: One is transient and usually due to the delayed absorption of lung fluid. It causes symptoms during the first day of life but resolves quickly and leaves no sequelae. The more protracted form of respiratory distress is caused by diffuse atelectasis and is the subject of this discussion.

Clinical Features. IRDS occurs in infants with immature lungs and is caused by progressive atelectasis. Infants born before 37 weeks' gestation who are asphyxiated, anemic, hypovolemic or depressed, whose mothers are diabetic, or who are born after protracted, difficult labor are most likely to develop IRDS and are said to be at "high risk."

IRDS is not a disease as such but rather the consequence of a point in development when the lung is not mature enough to support extrauterine life. It occurs in prematurely born infants because they have relatively small terminal airways, alveolar ducts and alveoli, and an unstable chest cage in combination with a deficiency of surfactant lining the alveoli. After the infant's first breath, the lungs will remain filled with gas only under the following circumstances: if the radius of the respiratory units is sufficiently large so that there is a minimal tendency to collapse at low lung volumes; if the negative intrathoracic pressure at the end of expiration (which is partly caused by the tendency of the mature chest cage to expand and tends to increase lung size) balances the alveolar surface tension (which tends to make the lung smaller); and if the surface tension at the junction of alveolar gas with the alveolar walls is small.

The diagnosis of IRDS can be made when there are no other causes of progressive respiratory insufficiency and when the infant has intercostal and sternal retractions, poor air entry noted by auscultation, expiratory grunting, arterial hypoxemia and radiographic evidence of miliary or diffuse atelectasis. Other features which are commonly present include arterial hypotension, decreased urine output, decreased intestinal motility (often with ileus), hypotonia, respiratory and metabolic acidosis, poor peripheral circulation as judged by poor vascular filling, and peripheral edema. Characteristically, the disease worsens during the first 24 to 48 hours of life, but following the third day of the disease in those infants who survive, the symptoms slowly resolve. The object of treatment is to inflate the atelectatic lungs and correct physiologic abnormalities.

Temperature. Excessive heat loss must be avoided. It would be best to treat the infant in a neutral thermal environment, i.e., that environmental temperature in which oxygen consumption is minimal, but this is not always possible. However, heat loss can be avoided during the resuscitation of infants at high risk of developing IRDS and during the treatment of infants with the disease by placing infrared heat lamps above them. Those with severe IRDS should be treated beneath radiant warmers so that there is ease of access to the patient while constant heat is provided and cooling prevented. When this is done, the axillary temperature should be maintained between 36.5° and 37.0° C. Infants with mild disease, who have fewer pieces of monitoring equipment and require less frequent manipulation, can be treated in isolation incubators with an environmental temperature appropriate for the infant's size and gestational age.

Airway. When signs of respiratory distress are first noted, the upper airway should be suctioned to remove mucus and foreign matter. If there is a history of aspiration of meconium or other particulate material, the larynx should be visualized to be sure that it is not partially occluded.

Lung Inflation. In infants at high risk of developing IRDS, and early in the course of the disease, there may be some lung units which are airless, but which can be inflated by gently distending the lung with positive pressure. Immediately after birth in "high risk" infants, an attempt should be made to expand atelectatic units with 2 to 3 minutes of positive pressure ventilation with an anesthesia bag and a face mask of appropriate size. If the infant has an endotracheal tube, the inflation should be attempted through the tube. Inflate the lungs slowly, gradually developing an airway pressure of 30 cm. H_2O over half a second. Maintain the peak pressure for

0.5 to 1 second. Attempts to inflate an atelectatic lung should be repeated every 1 to 2 hours during the first days of IRDS.

Vascular Catheters. The use of an umbilical arterial catheter permits continuous measurement of arterial blood pressure as well as the easy removal of arterial blood for analysis of pH and carbon dioxide and oxygen tensions. The frequency with which blood gas tension measurements are made depends on the severity of the infant's disease and whether his condition is changing rapidly. Blood gas tensions and pH should be measured within 15 minutes after any major change either in treatment or inspired oxygen concentration. Placement of a catheter in the aorta via an umbilical artery is a relatively simple procedure and major complications are rare if the procedure is done as described by Kitterman and associates. The catheter should be inserted to a position where the tip is in the lower abdominal aorta below the origin of the renal and inferior mesenteric arteries (L3). Early in the course of the disease, two catheters, one in the inferior vena cava and one in the aorta, are useful since hypovolemia and congestive heart failure cannot be distinguished on the basis of the systemic arterial hypotension alone. The pH and carbon dioxide tension of central venous blood are useful measures for the regulation of respiratory and metabolic acidosis. However, the oxygen tension in venous blood cannot be used to estimate the amount of inspired oxygen needed. If central vascular catheters cannot be used, peripheral arteries can be intermittently cannulated in order to obtain samples for pH and blood gas analysis. Most commonly used are the temporal, radial and dorsalis pedis arteries. When frequent arterial blood samples are needed and measurement of blood pressure is critical, a plastic catheter can be placed in one of these peripheral arteries for as long as one week.

X-Ray. A chest x-ray must always be taken when a newborn has respiratory distress in order to diagnose other correctable causes of respiratory distress like pneumothorax and diaphragmatic herniation. After an umbilical vessel has been catheterized, an abdominal x-ray should always be obtained in order to determine the location of the catheter tip.

Acidosis. Correct a metabolic acidosis (a base deficit of more than 6 mEq.) by infusing sodium bicarbonate into the aorta via the umbilical arterial catheter (with the tip below L3) or into the inferior vena cava via an umbilical vein. Do not infuse hypertonic sodium bicarbonate into an umbilical vein if its tip is in the portal sinus or vein. A concentration of 88 mEq. per 100 ml. may be used but should never be infused at a rate in excess of 1 mEq. per kilogram body weight per minute. Calculate the dose of sodium bicarbonate by multiplying the base deficit by the body weight in kilograms times 0.3. Infusions of more than 10 mEq. per kilogram body weight per 24 hours should only be used under exceptional circumstances. After correcting pH, calcium (200 mg. calcium gluconate per kilogram per day) and potassium (2 mEq. per kilogram per day) should be added to the intravascular infusion fluids, since the concentration of these electrolytes always decreases after a rapid increase in pH. If acidemia is present during initial treatment, an attempt to raise the arterial pH to 7.3 should be made by correcting both the respiratory and metabolic components. Later during the disease, only the metabolic components of the acidemia need be corrected, as long as the pH is 7.2 or above. When hypercarbia (arterial pCO_2 of over 80 mm. Hg) develops, ventilation should be assisted.

Hypovolemia and Anemia. Some "high risk" infants are hypovolemic and this may lead in part to IRDS. Whole blood (10 ml. per kilogram) or albumin (1 Gm. per kilogram) with saline should be given to such infants if they have arterial hypotension, a low or falling central hematocrit (40 ml. per 100 ml., or less) and inadequate peripheral blood flow (as indicated by pallor or slow return of color following blanching). During the course of the disease, replace blood loss due to blood sampling whenever 10 per cent of the baby's blood volume has been removed or as necessary to maintain a normal circulating blood volume with a hematocrit between 40 and 50 ml. per 100 ml. Initially, whole blood may be used to increase blood volume; later, small transfusions of packed cells are adequate. Newborn infants may maintain a normal arterial blood pressure when they are acidotic and hypovolemic. In this situation, as the pH rises, the infant's vascular capacity increases, and if he cannot quickly expand his blood volume by hemodilution, blood pressure will fall and shock will occur. For this reason, frequent measurements of arterial blood pressure during resuscitation of "high risk" infants is very important. The simultaneous measurement of central venous pressure is also valuable, since it may help to distinguish congestive heart failure from hypovolemia.

Fluids and Electrolytes. There is a difference in the volume of fluid given to infants treated in radiant warmers and that given to those in incubators. On the first day of the disease, total fluid intake (except that needed for expansion of depleted intravascular volume) should be 60 to 80 ml. per kilogram for those infants in a closed force-draft incubator, and 80 to 100 ml. per kilogram for those in radiant warmers. After the first day, infants in incubators require 100 to 125 ml. per kilogram per day, and infants in radiant warmers require 125 to 150 ml. per kilogram per day. A 10 per cent glucose solution should be used, to which the following have been added: sodium (3 mEq. per kilogram per 24 hours as sodium chloride), potassium (2 mEq. per kilogram per 24 hours as potassium chloride) and calcium (200 mg. per kilogram per 24 hours as calcium gluconate). The serum concentration of these electrolytes should be measured daily and appropriate adjustments made in the infusion solution.

Feeding. Gastric feeding should be started via an intragastric tube in all infants with IRDS no later than 48 hours of age. By the fourth day of life, most of these infants, even those with an endotracheal tube in place, accept a large enough volume of breast milk, or 20 calories per ounce of formula, to provide an intake of 100 calories per kilogram per day. Every effort should be made to provide at least 100 calories per kilogram per day by the end of the first week of life.

Irritability. Avoid unnecessary disturbance of infants who have frequent expiratory grunting. Very irritable infants may be soothed with a mild sedative, such as a whiskey nipple. Some infants on mechanical ventilators may require morphine and occasionally curare.

Vitamin K. Give 1 mg. of vitamin K oxide intramuscularly immediately after birth. This should be repeated at five days of age in those infants who receive antibiotics.

Oxygen by Hood. Place a clear plastic hood over the infant's head and flow warmed, moistened oxygen through it at the rate of 8 liters per minute. Increase the inspired oxygen concentration up to 80 to 100 per cent to maintain the arterial oxygen tension (pO_2) at 50 to 70 mm. Hg.

Continuous Positive Airway Pressure (CPAP). If, while breathing 80 to 100 per cent oxygen, the infant's arterial pO_2 is less than 50 mm. Hg, intubate the infant and apply a CPAP of 6 mm. Hg to the airway, as described by Gregory et al. If the arterial pO_2 does not rise within 10 minutes after starting CPAP, or if the infant shows signs of increasing distress, increase the CPAP by 2-mm. Hg increments until there is a sharp rise in pO_2. The maximum pressure which has been used is 16 mm. Hg. When the pO_2 rises, lower the inspired oxygen concentration by 5 to 10 per cent decrements, keeping the pO_2 between 50 and 70 mm. Hg until the inspired oxygen concentration is 40 per cent. Then, with further improvement, lower the CPAP by 1-mm. Hg decrements until atmospheric pressure is reached. When the airway pressure has been atmospheric for 4 hours, the endotracheal tube may be removed. After extubation, lower the inspired oxygen concentration as tolerated, maintaining the arterial oxygen tension between 50 and 70 mm. Hg. While CPAP is being applied, slowly inflate the infant's lungs 10 to 12 times every half hour with the anesthesia bag. The infant's chest must be percussed and his position changed every hour while CPAP is being applied. After chest percussion, irrigate the endotracheal tube and gently suction the trachea with a sterile suction tube. More detailed procedures for care of the airway are outlined elsewhere (Gregory). After extubation, chest physical therapy should be continued until the inspired oxygen is less than 30 per cent.

Ventilation with a Mechanical Ventilator. If the infant becomes apneic while on CPAP, has a pO_2 value below 30 mm. Hg or has an increasing amount of respiratory acidosis (pCO_2 above 80 mm. Hg), begin mechanical ventilation with an intermittent positive pressure ventilator (with a device to maintain a positive pressure during expiration). When the infant improves with mechanical ventilation, he can be changed to CPAP for an interval before being extubated. Intermittent negative pressure ventilators can also be used for infants with severe disease.

Summary. IRDS is a process in which many factors interact to alter homeostasis in the immature infant. While the lung matures, air spaces stabilize and atelectasis is overcome, the physician must assist ventilation and restore toward normal those physiologic variables which are affected.

References

Gregory, G. A., Kitterman, J. A., Phibbs, R. H., Tooley, W. H., and Hamilton, W. K.: Treatment of the Idiopathic Respiratory Distress Syndrome with Continuous Positive Airway Pressure. *New England J. Med.*, 284:1333, 1971.

Gregory, G. A.: Respiratory Care of Newborn Infants. *Pediat. Clin. N. Am.*, 19:311, 1972.

Kitterman, J. A., Phibbs, R. H., and Tooley, W. H.: Catheterization of Umbilical Vessels in Newborn Infants. *Pediat. Clin. N. Am.*, 17:895, 1970.

Disorders of the Umbilicus

MURDINA M. DESMOND, M.D.

The umbilicus marks the point of attachment of the umbilical cord to the abdominal wall during fetal life. With delivery these vital pathways cease to function, and the connecting structures undergo involution and separation, leaving a cicatrix marking the original insertion of the umbilical cord.

The structures of the cord include the two umbilical arteries and the vein, the urachus, remnants of the omphalomesenteric duct and Wharton's jelly, a translucent blue-white avascular substance which surrounds the vessels and is sheathed with amniotic membrane.

The cord may be stained with meconium or bilirubin. Small cords may be associated with placental insufficiency. Varicosities of the umbilical vein are not rare. These may rupture, forming a hematoma.

Cord Care. Under normal conditions the umbilical cord, like the fetus, is germ-free until passage through the birth canal and exposure to the extrauterine environment. Colonization of the cord proceeds rapidly, and with necrosis and sloughing of cord tissue an excellent environment for abundant bacterial growth is provided. The cord stump becomes colonized with the organisms in its immediate environment. Colonization of the stump by pathogens may lead to wide dissemination of the organisms within maternity and nursery units.

Umbilical cords become dry and slough within nine days after delivery. This process may be delayed in the presence of excessive environmental humidity.

Exposure of the cord directly to atmospheric air is preferable to "wet" or "closed" care. At present the best total protection is provided with the use of drying agents—either 70 per cent alcohol or triple-dye* applied daily to the cord. If umbilical catheterization is carried out as an intensive care procedure, it is important that the catheter tip be cultured for possible pathogens upon its removal.

INFECTION

Granuloma. The most common cause of delayed healing at the cord site is umbilical granuloma—a reddish area of granulation tissue remaining after sloughing of the cord. This is usually associated with infection and may be accompanied by a scant purulent discharge. Persisting granuloma has been reported following the application of talc-containing powders to the cord.

Cauterization of the site with silver nitrate is usually followed by sloughing of the granuloma and subsequent healing. If the reddened granuloma persists after two applications of silver nitrate, an umbilical polyp or a fistula should be considered (see Table 1).

Omphalitis and Cellulitis. Infection of the umbilical area may range from a simple omphalitis (redness, tenderness and edema of the periumbilical skin) to a spreading and necrotizing cellulitis. Local maceration and cellulitis may be secondary to a patent urachus or an enteric fistula. A cellulitis in the umbilical area usually implies a lymphatic spread of the infectious process locally by the superficial nodes or by deeper lymphatic vessels to the abdominal wall and lower thoracic areas. In either instance, signs of systemic infection may develop rapidly.

Infection spreads by way of the umbilical arteries to the lower abdominal wall, groin or scrotum, and by the vein to the portal system or general circulation. Treatment should be systemic. Appropriate cultures should be taken promptly (nose and throat, swab of cord, rectal, blood), as well as direct smears of any available discharge, and broad-spectrum antibiotic therapy instituted without delay. Until the organism is identified, ampicillin and either colistimethate sodium (Coly-Mycin) or kanamycin offer a good range of therapeutic efficiency. (For details see Neonatal Sepsis, p. 550).

BLEEDING

The umbilical arteries cease to pulsate within 5 minutes of delivery. Massive exsanguinating hemorrhage from the severed cord is a rapidly developing and life-threatening complication of the natal day. Because of this, it is important that methods used for umbilical cord ligation remain effective as the cord dries and becomes smaller in diameter. Effective methods for maintaining constant pressure on the cord vessels as the Wharton's jelly contracts are now available, e.g., closure with a plastic cord clamp or the banding of the cord with short lengths of latex tubing utilizing a cord bander and stretching device.

If massive bleeding from the cord occurs, the infant may suffer hypovolemic shock. Tachycardia is not common. In this emergency

* Triple-dye: acriflavine (0.114 per cent), gentian violet (0.229 per cent), brilliant green (0.229 per cent) and distilled water in sufficient quantity to make 100 ml. This agent is applied at delivery and repeated daily if the infant is kept in a humid atmosphere.

TABLE 1. Persistent Lesions of Umbilical Area

PRESENTING LESION	CLINICAL CHARACTERISTICS	LUMEN	DISCHARGE	ORIGIN	DIAGNOSIS AND MANAGEMENT
Granuloma pyogenicum	Small reddened mass, 0.5–2 cm.	None	Purulent if present	Infection at base Foreign body—talcum	Rapid response to applications of solid silver nitrate
Polyps, intestinal mucosal	Bright red, 2–10 cm.	None	Mucoid	Remnants of intestinal or gastric mucosa Sinus of omphalomesenteric duct or of peripheral area of urachus	Unaffected by astringents Histology Outlining of tract with radiopaque material introduced into lumen
Fistula, enteric	Erosive dermatitis	Yes	Gas or feces	Patent omphalomesenteric duct	Carmine red given orally is discharged at fistula opening Radiographic visualization of communication between lumen and bowel after injection of radiopaque material into lumen
Urachal lesion	Erosive dermatitis Bladder infection	Yes	Urine	Patent urachus communicating with bladder	Passage of methylene blue from lumen to voided urine and radiopaque material from lumen to bladder

we give 20 to 40 ml. of the nearest type O negative blood available (without cross matching if the emergency is great) by slow direct injection through a polyethylene catheter into the umbilical vein. Improvement is signaled by a return of color to the palms of the hands and a lessening of respiratory distress. A small amount of blood may be drawn before the administration of blood for determining hematocrit and hemoglobin levels. If the infant is not in shock, the usual typing and cross matching procedures are carried out and the blood is given slowly by intravenous drip.

CONGENITAL MALFORMATIONS

Single Umbilical Artery. A single umbilical artery occurs in 1 per cent of all deliveries (2 to 8 per cent in twin deliveries) and is associated with a higher incidence of congenital malformations. Associated anomaly is not confined to a particular area or system. The presence of a single artery alerts the physician to examine the infant more closely at delivery and at follow-up examinations.

Omphalocele. During the second and third months of fetal life the midgut extends forward into the base of the umbilical cord and returns to the developing peritoneal cavity through a process of rotation. As the midgut returns to the abdomen, the abdominal wall closes concentrically around the cord and umbilical vessels.

When this process is incomplete, a bowel-containing sac, or omphalocele, remains anterior to the fascial umbilical ring. The omphalocele is covered by a transparent membrane consisting of amnion and peritoneum and contains intestine as well as other viscera. The sac may rupture in utero, leaving exposed bowel. In this instance the bowel is often edematous and its blood supply compromised.

The defect presents a major surgical emergency and should be treated without delay. It is generally recommended that the sac be covered with saline-soaked gauze, and the infant taken directly from delivery room to operating theater.

Persistent Lesions of the Umbilicus. The most common congenital anomalies of the umbilical area involve remnants of the omphalomesenteric duct and the urachus. These commonly come to the attention of the physician as a mass or discharge at the umbilicus. The predominant clinical features are summarized in Table 1.

Umbilical Hernia. After involution of the umbilical cord has taken place, a defect (0.5 to 3 cm.) of the midline fascia of the abdominal wall may be palpable. Through this defect, peritoneum and viscera (usually small bowel) protrude into the loose skin overlying the umbilical area, forming a hernial sac 0.5 to 4 cm. in diameter. Small bowel entering the sac is easily reducible by palpation and accompanied by a gurgle.

Umbilical hernias become noticeable during the first month after delivery in a high percentage of infants, particularly the Negro race, in the prematurely born and in the presence of conditions tending to increase intra-abdominal pressure. Incarceration is rare. The majority disappear during the first year of life by centripetal contraction of the outer edge of the fascial ring. Few remain after three years. Spontaneous closure occurs up to the eighth year. Delay in closure is most frequently encountered in infants with diastasis recti. The volume of the protrusion does not diminish appreciably with contraction of the ring; rather, the hernia tends to disappear rapidly without first decreasing appreciably in size.

Strapping of the hernia appears to be of little value and is not recommended.

Surgical repair is advisable in infants with evidence of partial small bowel obstruction (herniation of bowel through a small fascial ring) and in infants with evidence of recurrent abdominal cramping. The most preferable age for elective repair in an asymptomatic patient is not clear at this time because of the high incidence of spontaneous closure, but it should probably be considered, on an individual basis, at two or three years of age.

References

Heifetz, C. J., Bilsel, Z. T., and Gaus, W. W.: Observations on the Disappearance of Umbilical Hernias of Infancy and Childhood. *Surg., Gynec. & Obstet.*, 116:469, 1963.

Nix, T. E., and Young, C. J.: Congenital Umbilical Anomalies. *Arch. Derm.*, 90:160, 1965.

The Drug-Addicted Newborn Infant

MYRON M. SOKAL, M.D.,
LUIS M. PRUDENT, M.D., *and*
L. STANLEY JAMES, M.D.

Treatment of the infant born to a mother addicted to narcotics is symptomatic rather than prophylactic. The main reason for this approach is that the symptoms of withdrawal in the infant are frequently mild and of a transitory nature. In addition, the maternal history, if obtainable, is likely to be unreliable with regard both to the time of her last dose and the quantity and purity of the drug taken.

Because the treatment is symptomatic, the physician should be thoroughly familiar with the early signs and be prepared to treat the infant if these signs progress from mild to moderate severity. The infants are often of low birth weight, premature and small for gestational age. The earliest and most commonly observed signs are those from the central nervous system. These include coarse, flapping tremors, jitteriness, irritability, hyperactivity which occasionally leads to skin abrasions, and exaggerated reflexes. Irritability is reflected in the frequent, shrill, high-pitched cry, and hyperactivity is usually associated with hungry fist sucking. The more severely affected infants will vomit their feedings and develop diarrhea; tremors and jitteriness may progress to generalized convulsions. Hyperpyrexia, frequently mentioned as part of the clinical picture, is in our experience not common; if present, the physician should be alerted to the possibility of sepsis. Dehydration may be severe and of relatively sudden onset in those infants who develop diarrhea and vomiting.

The first aspect of therapy is careful observation of all infants whose mothers are known to be addicts. In addition, because of the unreliability of maternal history, all infants who present any of the above symptoms should be regarded as potentially showing signs of drug withdrawal.

Specific drug therapy should be started only when these signs have become manifest. Several drugs have been recommended, including phenobarbital, chlorpromazine,* paregoric and methadone.† Preferences for a particular form of therapy are largely based on the physician's personal experience; there is no objective evidence which indicates the superiority of one therapeutic regimen over another. Phenobarbital, 6 to 8 mg. per kilogram per day in three to four divided doses, is usually effective in controlling the central nervous system symptoms. It should be administered orally when possible and intramuscularly if vomiting is present. In mild cases, a short course of about one week will usually suffice; for the more severely addicted infant, therapy may be necessary for a longer time. Convulsions should be treated

* Manufacturer's precaution: Chlorpromazine is not recommended for children under six months of age except when lifesaving.

† Manufacturer's precaution: Methadone is not recommended for use as an analgesic in children since documented clinical experience has been insufficient to establish a suitable dosage regimen.

with intravenous phenobarbital, 10 to 15 mg. in a single dose. If this insufficient to control the convulsions, methadone in a dose of 0.1 to 0.5 mg. per kilogram three to four times a day intramuscularly has been effective. If diarrhea is present, paregoric in a dose of 1 to 2 drops per kilogram every 4 hours may be efficacious. The dosage of this drug, as with all the others, must be individualized for each case. If the diarrhea and/or vomiting is severe, oral intake may have to be curtailed and intravenous fluids administered. It should be emphasized that the major cause of mortality in drug-addicted infants is dehydration which has been unrecognized or improperly treated. The stool should be cultured in all instances, since there have been several cases in which diarrhea was associated with enteropathic bacteria. Thus, treatment, to be effective, must be directed at both the primary signs and at the life-threatening complications.

An important aspect of care of these infants is investigation of the social situation into which they will be discharged. In many instances, both the homes and mothers may be inadequate for proper infant care. Help will be needed in establishing a proper environment. This is essential in all infants of addicted mothers whether the infants exhibit withdrawal symptoms or not.

24

Miscellaneous

Menstrual Disorders

JOSEPH L. RAUH, M.D.

The physician whose patient has a menstrual problem must answer one central question before he initiates treatment: Is there any underlying genetic or acquired organic illness which is the cause of unusually early or late menarche or some aberration in the amount, frequency, duration or pain associated with menstruation? If organic disease, i.e., either a structural defect of the ovaries and/or uterus or a systemic illness, can be ruled out, menstrual problems at adolescence are invariably related to a functional abnormality of the pituitary-ovarian axis and the delicate hormonal feedback mechanisms.

DYSMENORRHEA OR PAINFUL MENSTRUATION

Dysmenorrhea or painful menstruation is common at adolescence. It is of real consequence to the girl if it interferes with her daily routine, especially going to school. Organic disease, such as an ovarian cyst or adhesions, causing dysmenorrhea is rare. An important distinction may also be made between dysmenorrhea related to ovulation and menstrual cramps *before* the cycles are ovulatory. The former is *much* more likely to be physiologic than is the latter. Early postmenarchial dysmenorrhea may be treated with reassurance and understanding of the patient and her concerns. Medication is usually not necessary. Often the patient just needs someone to listen and be sympathetic. The girl may be mimicking the complaints of a mother or older sister.

When medication is needed for dysmenorrhea, analgesics should be tried. Narcotics are not indicated. Darvon (propoxyphene hydrochloride)* may be helpful, especially when given with aspirin. The dose of Darvon is 32 or 64 mg. every 4 to 6 hours. Heavier, more mature girls will need the larger dose of Darvon.

When analgesics are not helping and the patient is missing school or other important activities repeatedly, suppression of ovulation should be tried. A medium-estrogen dose "birth control" medication can be used effectively if the patient and her mother can emotionally and culturally tolerate the use of such medication. Enovid-E, 2.5 mg. (norethynodrel with mestranol), and Norlestin, 2.5 mg. (norethindrone acetate with ethinyl estradiol) are examples of combined estrogen-progesterone therapy. Either can be given daily for 21 days, starting on the fifth day of menstruation. Such cyclic therapy, usually effective in reducing cramps with the first period following suppression of ovulation, should be maintained for three to six months.

If combined medication is not used, Estinyl (ethinyl estradiol) is recommended. Estinyl does suppress ovulation although it is not known as a birth control drug, an advantage to a girl whose parents may be opposed to contraception. The dose is 0.05 mg. twice a day for 25 days beginning with the first day of menstruation.

OLIGOMENORRHEA

Next to dysmenorrhea, oligomenorrhea or infrequent periods constitute the most common menstrual problem at adolescence. Organic disease must be ruled out, especially diabetes, thy-

* Manufacturer's precaution: Safety of Darvon (propoxyphene hydrochloride) in children has not been established.

roid dysfunction, liver disease, malignancy, a chronic gastrointestinal problem, adrenal disease or structural ovarian or uterine pathology· like polycystic ovaries or fibroids. This is especially true if the oligomenorrhea follows ovulation, usually 18 to 24 months from menarche. Under these circumstances, experienced gynecologic consultation, examination and follow-up should be provided.

When the scanty or infrequent periods are related to anovulatory cycles and have troubled the patient for at least a year, cyclic hormone therapy to induce ovulation should be considered. An excellent regimen which avoids the psychologic implications of "birth control" therapy is the use of Premarin and Norlutate. Premarin is first given in a dosage of 0.3 to 0.625 mg. daily for 21 days starting on the fifth day after the period begins. On the seventeenth day of medication, Norlutate, 5 mg. daily, is added for five days. Withdrawal bleeding will follow cessation of therapy. Therapy should continue three to six months. This hormone regimen best mimics a natural cycle and is associated with minimal side effects.

An alternate regimen is the use of Enovid 2.5 mg. or Norlestrin 2.5 mg. daily for 21 days. These medium-estrogen-dose tablets may occasionally cause nausea, painful breasts, weight gain, headache or acne. Cyclic therapy must continue for at least three and often six months before menstruation will occur regularly without therapy. Low-estrogen-dose pills like Norinyl-1 + 50 mg. or Ortho-Novum 1/50 should not be used at adolescence because of the high incidence of breakthrough bleeding. If relapses of oligomenorrhea occur following these regimens, sequential hormone therapy using drugs like Oracon or Ortho-Novum SQ should be tried in cyclic fashion for three to six months.

MENORRHAGIA OR DYSFUNCTIONAL UTERINE BLEEDING

As with oligomenorrhea, organic disease must be excluded. Dysfunctional uterine bleeding has no structural or uterine cause. It is invariably related at adolescence to an anovulatory menstrual cycle with concomitant inadequate hormone feedback between the ovaries and the pituitary.

Excessive or prolonged menstruation may be mild, moderate or severe. When severe, the hemoglobin is often 8 Gm. per 100 ml. or lower and hospitalization for an acute bleeding problem is indicated. This situation is rare. Dilatation and curettement is indicated, and the girl should then be placed on cyclic Premarin-Norlutate therapy as outlined for oligomenorrhea. Transfusion may be necessary, as well as intensive oral iron therapy after discharge to correct the iron deficiency anemia. Ferrous sulfate, 300 mg. three times a day, is adequate iron therapy. Since iron deficiency is a fairly common cause and consequence of menorrhagia, the need for iron replacement and careful hemoglobin follow-up cannot be minimized.

Mild or moderate dysfunctional bleeding can be stopped easily and effectively with oral hormone therapy. Enovid-E, 2.5 mg., or Norlestrin 2.5 mg. twice daily for 10 days will stop the bleeding within three to five days. A normal period will ensue within two to five days after therapy is terminated or two weeks after the severe or prolonged bleeding is stopped. Then, cyclic therapy, using Premarin-Norlutate, or Enovid-E, 2.5 mg., or Norlestrin 2.5 mg., should be continued for three to six months. These regimens were described under oligomenorrhea. Supplemental oral iron therapy using ferrous sulfate, 300 mg. twice or three times a day will be needed to return the hemoglobin to normal or at least to 12 Gm. per 100 ml.

An alternate method which will induce ovulation and more normal menstruation is the use of Clomid (clomiphene citrate). Clomid is a potent ovulation-inducing agent because of its effect on the pituitary. Dysfunctional bleeding must be stopped and then ovulation induced with Clomid, 50 to 100 mg. a day, starting on the fifth day of menses and continuing for five days. This cyclic regimen is continued for three months. Clomid may be associated with such side effects as headache, pituitary enlargement, diplopia or "after image," and lower abdominal pain from ovarian swelling.

Moderate menorrhagia which must be treated more quickly than with oral therapy requires injectable medication. Premarin, 25 mg. intramuscularly every 4 hours for four doses, is recommended. This regimen will stop the bleeding in all cases except the very rare patient who requires dilatation and curettement. The regimen can be used without hospitalization in an office or emergency room setting. Following the fourth injection, Enovid, 2.5 mg., or Norlestrin 2.5 mg. twice daily for 10 days, as outlined above, should be given.

AMENORRHEA

Mean menarchial age in the United States today is 12.5 years. If menses have not begun by 14.5 years of age, the physician should be concerned. Amenorrhea may be related to organic disease. Complete absence of secondary sexual development, especially if it is associated with short stature, webbed neck or other stigmata of Turner's syndrome (ovarian agenesis), is not rare in adolescence and must be recognized and then treated with exogenous hormones. Large doses of estrogen, such as Premarin, 2.5 mg. a day, are needed for at least one year in order to produce breast and pubic hair development. Later, Enovid, 2.5 mg., or Norlestrin 2.5 mg. daily for five days beginning with the first day of the month will allow for the further development of breasts and pubic hair as well as cause moderate withdrawal bleeding. Counseling is essential for such girls so that their genetic problem is understood and their confidence in having a normal sexual life enhanced. The need and opportunity to adopt children must be explained.

Besides chromosomal aberrations, other organic diagnoses causing amenorrhea must be considered—hypothalamic lesions, tumors of the pituitary and the extrasellar region, pituitary insufficiency, disturbances of the thyroid or adrenal function including congenital adrenal hyperplasia, adrenal or ovarian tumors, polycystic ovaries, absence or anomalous development of the ovaries, uterus or vagina, imperforate hymen, testicular feminization syndrome, granulomatous endometritis, and pregnancy.

Delayed onset of menses is often due to small size and/or familial factors. If adolescence is evident physically with some breast and pubic hair development, if the patient is in good health and still growing and if there is a family history of late menarche, intensive endocrine investigation may be delayed beyond 14.5 years of age but not beyond 16.

Secondary amenorrhea may result from chronic illness (e.g., ulcerative colitis, regional enteritis, anorexia nervosa, obesity or malignancy) or from psychic factors.

VAGINAL EXAMINATION

The first vaginal examination will always be remembered by the patient. It should be pleasant, gentle and associated with careful explanation and understanding on the part of the physician. A female assistant is necessary primarily to put the patient at ease. An adequate comfortable examining table is essential with well-positioned stirrups. The size of the vaginal speculum must be carefully considered. The nulliparous, often virginal, patient is best examined with a long thin speculum which conforms to the configuration of her introitus. The Huffman speculum (V. Mueller and Co., Chicago) is ideal.

MENSTRUAL HYGIENE

Tampons or Tampax should not be discouraged at adolescence. Kotex or Modess are occasionally irritating to the perineum and vulva, spreading feces to these areas. Girls generally prefer the intravaginal absorbing agents, especially if the patient is very active and at ease with her menstruation. Young girls using tampons should be reminded to remove them. If they are forgotten, medical assistance may be needed and a "foreign body" bacterial vaginitis will ensue. Sultrin Triple Sulfa Vaginal Tablets inserted into the vagina with an applicator twice a day for 14 days is effective therapy for tampon-induced vaginitis.

Premarital Counseling for the Adolescent

JOSEPH L. RAUH, M.D.

When a single adolescent or a couple comes to the pediatrician for marital counseling, the first question which should occur to the physician is whether the girl is pregnant. Approximately one-half of all women 19 years of age and under who marry in the United States today are pregnant on their wedding day. Since almost 80 per cent of teenage marriages end in divorce, there is considerable need for immediate and comprehensive counseling at the time marriage is being considered.

If the girl is pregnant, management must first be directed toward the problems and needs of the pregnancy (see Pregnancy in Adolescence). It would be unusual for abortion or adoption to be considered if the couple intends to marry. Comprehensive prenatal care should be arranged for the girl. The physician may be asked to defer discussing the pregnancy with parents or other adults known to the couple until they are married and settled. If marriage is not going to occur, the pediatrician may be asked to help arrange for abortion or maternity home placement and eventual adoption. These arrangements will need to involve the adolescent's parents, and the doctor may have to arbitrate and referee the ensuing anger and despair caused by the difficult situation of an out-of-wedlock pregnancy.

Counseling may be considerably easier and less crisis-oriented for adolescents who intend to marry but who are not yet involved in pregnancy. The pediatrician should mention the risks of early marriage, although it will be difficult and rarely helpful for him to try to talk a boy, girl or couple out of the decision to marry.

Family planning and sexuality information are often sought. The pediatrician will usually want to refer the girl to a gynecologist for a complete pelvic examination, including a Papanicolaou smear of cervical cells for cancer screening. However, some pediatricians today, especially those working in adolescent medical programs and family planning clinics, feel competent doing visual speculum examinations of the vagina and cervix. In the absence of pelvic complaints and in the presence of a normal menstrual history and secondary sex development, this kind of vaginal examination may be entirely adequate. The doctor or doctors will want to respond to questions about family planning and the sexual concerns aroused by the boy-girl relationship. The merits, risks and side effects of each birth control method should be explained. Oral contraception works well for the relatively mature, older (18 and above) adolescent girl. Intrauterine devices will be more effective for girls who are less motivated toward contraception and who have trouble remembering to take medication every day. If pills are used, low-estrogen-dose pills (such as Norinyl-1 + 50) and sequentials should be avoided because of the risk of breakthrough menstrual bleeding and/or pregnancy if the pills are forgotten for one or more days.

Couples considering marriage should be educated concerning the need for preventive and continuous medical care. In addition to a yearly pelvic examination and Papanicolaou smear, the pediatrician should instruct the girl to perform periodic visual and manual breast self-examination for cancer. A rubella hemagglutination-inhibition antibody titer is best done, like the serologic test for syphilis, at the time of marriage before pregnancy occurs. Several states in the United States have already made this a legal requirement for marriage. Rubella vaccination would then be given along with appropriate contraception.

Pediatricians, along with general physicians, internists and obstetrician-gynecologists, are increasingly being asked to counsel couples and teach sexuality courses in senior high schools and colleges. Today's customs and modes of behavior require that traditional "premarital" information and sexuality counseling be as available to unmarried couples as to those about to be married. The physician's personal life style or code of behavior can be discussed with adolescents, but it should not be imposed on them or information withheld and alternatives not presented.

Pregnancy in Adolescence

JOSEPH L. RAUH, M.D.

Each year in the United States almost a million adolescents under the age of 20 become pregnant. Half of these pregnancies are among unmarried girls and will not result in bridal pregnancies. It is now widely known that adolescent pregnancy is associated with great risks for the mother—risk for the obstetric complications of pregnancy, prematurity, congenital defects, unplanned repeat pregnancy following a first delivery—as well as risks involving interruption of education and vocational training.

Adolescent pregnancy requires a multidisciplinary approach involving general physicians, pediatricians and obstetricians, as well as social workers, nutritionists, health educators and teachers. At the time the pregnancy is diagnosed, especially if it is out of wedlock, the girl may need crisis-intervention type counseling. The options of continuing the pregnancy or abortion should be presented and discussed in harmony with the realities of the geographic area, the cultural attitude and the personal feelings of the patient and her family. Adoption should be mentioned as an alternative to keeping the baby.

Comprehensive prenatal care is the key to reducing the risks. Regular prenatal examinations in a private practice setting or public health clinic are essential. Yet, most adolescents lack adequate health insurance for maternity care, and the financial burdens of pregnancy often jeopardize the couple's relationship as well as the girl's medical care. The Maternity and Infant Care Projects, a federally funded program, have been of particular help to young mothers. There are currently over 200 special care programs for pregnant adolescents in the United States.

The initial workup, besides a complete medical history and physical examination, should include a complete blood count, test for sickle cells (black patients), VDRL, blood typing, rubella hemagglutination-inhibition antibody titer, urinalysis, tuberculin skin test, booster immunizations for diphtheria-tetanus and polio, and individual nutrition guidance. All pregnant adolescents should be on a prenatal vitamin and mineral supplement including iron. Those patients having hemoglobins below 12 Gm. per 100 ml. should take additional iron as ferrous sulfate, 300 mg. twice a day.

An obstetrician and/or nurse-midwife should manage the obstetric aspects of prenatal care. A specially trained nurse associate or pediatrician can effectively manage the girl's general medical care, including the routine monthly examinations for episodic problems such as nausea, vomiting, headache, excessive weight gain, vaginal bleeding and so forth. The patient should be seen every month from the first trimester until 30 weeks, when visits should be biweekly until 36 weeks, and then weekly until delivery. Patients with special problems, such as a small pelvis, multiple births, diabetes, rheumatic heart disease, sickle cell anemia or previous cesarean section, should be entirely managed by an obstetrician at each visit, especially during the third trimester.

Most adolescent girls are still in school. Their education can be continued if the school district will either allow them to remain in a regular class or transfer them to a special program for pregnant girls. The special school has the advantage of permitting centralized health and sex education classes. Instruction can be provided by local health professionals from maternity programs, health departments and family planning agencies. The curriculum should include basic information about conception and human reproduction, fetal growth, prenatal care, obstetric complications, labor, delivery, the postpartum period, contraception, general medical care and infant care. The opportunity to discuss problems and feelings, either privately with a professional counselor or in groups, is essential. Such classes, along with the continuation of the regular school curriculum, have been shown to decrease all of the risks associated with adolescent pregnancy.

Family planning should be discussed with every girl during the prenatal period. Methods that have proved especially useful to high-risk adolescents, particularly the intrauterine device, should be carefully explained. Contraception should be initiated early in the postpartum period, probably at three weeks following delivery.

High Fever

ROBERT M. SMITH, M.D.

It is difficult to state at what point fever becomes sufficiently dangerous to demand specific corrective measures. Undoubtedly this will vary with the individual situation. In children who are recovering from extensive operations or who are seriously ill, any elevation of body temperature imposes a greater oxygen demand, and a fever of 101 or 102° F. may be definitely harmful.

In other, basically strong children suffering from acute febrile episodes, concern may not be felt until the temperature reaches 103 to 104° F., when the possibility of convulsions will be present. At slightly higher temperatures there may be danger of breakdown of protein molecules with permanent or fatal lesions. These situations would serve as reasonable indications for temperature-controlling measures, as would a continued fever, from any cause, of 103 to 104° F.

The specific management of children with high fever usually includes several forms of therapy. It is assumed that the diagnosis would be sought initially, and antibiotics administered if indicated. Certainly hydration and correction of acid-base disturbances should be attended to as primary aspects of treatment. Obviously, the management of each child will be varied to suit the specific occasion. In general, one should have a practical approach that can be altered as necessary. We have used the following steps in managing febrile children.

The clothing and bed clothes are removed, exposing as much of the body surface as seems suitable.

The room temperature is reduced to approximately 65° F.

If rooms are not air conditioned, fans are arranged to provide free circulation of air and evaporation of body surface moisture. Sponging of the skin is withheld until somewhat later.

A thermister is inserted in the rectum and attached to a continuously registering thermometer.

If the patient is extremely active, this exertion may promote further temperature elevation, and sedation may be instituted with pentobarbital or phenobarbital, approximately 1 mg. per pound as an initial dose if other sedatives or anticonvulsants have not already been administered. When dealing with children who may convulse, there is a dangerous tendency to oversedate the patient by adding one drug to another, until the hypoxia caused by sedative depression is far worse than that threatened by convulsions.

Aspirin is an effective and available antipyretic drug, and a good one to start initially. Administered by rectum, the dosage is variable, but may be as follows:

Infants under 1 year	150 mg. (2.5 grains)
Children 1–5 years	300 mg. (5 grains)
Children 5–10 years	600 mg. (10 grains)

These doses may be repeated three or four times at 4-hour intervals, but prolonged use may involve danger of salicylism.

Acetaminophen (Tylenol) has become more popular in recent years due to decreased gastrointestinal irritation. The suggested oral dosage is as follows (every 4 hours):

Infants under 1 year	60 mg.
Children 1–3 years	120 mg.
Children 3–6 years	180 mg.
Over 6 years	240 mg.

For maximum effect, both aspirin and acetaminophen can be used together. For this method, the dose of aspirin should be halved.

If this does not prove successful, more active methods are adopted. Here it must be emphasized that most methods of external cooling may cause shivering, which tends to increase muscular activity, increase oxygen demand and maintain or even increase the temperature. One may try sponging the skin with alcohol, but this should be stopped if shivering occurs. Chlorpromazine (Thorazine)* or one of the related phenothiazines is effective in lowering body temperature and in control of shivering, and should be used as an adjunct to active external cooling. All of these drugs have definite side effects which must be recognized. Chlorpromazine may cause hypotension, but if the blood pressure is carefully observed, the drug can be used more effectively than most of the newer and less familiar drugs. Chlorpromazine should be used by intermittent intramuscular administration in small doses. Approximately 0.2 mg. per kilogram (15 mg. for a 70-kilogram man) may be repeated at half-hour intervals until the temperature is controlled, unless hypotension interdicts further use.

After shivering has been controlled with chlorpromazine, one may proceed with sponging more actively, or if the situation is expected to be prolonged, it will be easier to use a cooling mattress. Here, an automatically circulating water mattress with adjustable temperature control is advisable, and several satisfactory models are commercially available.†

Usually such mattresses are divided into two pieces, the patient lying on one part, the other used to cover the child. Although the upper piece may be used for rapid cooling, it is seldom used to control hyperthermia. It is advisable to cover the lower mattress with a cotton sheet to prevent skin damage. The temperature of the circulating water may be started at 60 to 70° F., and then changed as necessary to maintain the desired degree of cooling. It may take several hours to gain control of a child's temperature, but subsequently it is relatively easy to keep it at the desired level, which in most cases is probably about 97° F. At this temperature the dangers of hyperthermia will be avoided without exposing the child to the disadvantages of overcooling. The child will not show mental clouding or physiologic depression, and will provide relatively few nursing problems compared to patients cooled into physiologic depression and semicoma.

Termination of cooling should be carried out slowly in order to prevent hyperthermic overreaction with warming.

* Manufacturer's precaution: Chlorpromazine (Thorazine) is not recommended in children under six months of age except when lifesaving.

† Therm-O-Rite (Therm-O-Rite Manufacturing Co., Buffalo, New York). Blanketrol (Cincinnati Sub-Zero Products, Inc., Cincinnati, Ohio).

Parenteral and Electrolyte Fluid Therapy

PHILIP L. CALCAGNO, M.D., *and*
CHARLES E. HOLLERMAN, M.D.

The primary aim of parenteral fluid therapy in the disease state is to maintain a balance of water and electrolytes within the body. In health, water stores are maintained by (1) ingestion of liquids, supplemented by water content of food which may contain 60 to 90 per cent water, and (2) metabolism of foodstuffs, yielding water of oxidation. In an ordinary mixed diet, the metabolism yields approximately 14 ml. of water for each 100 calories metabolized.

The daily water losses in normal children occur from the body in the feces, urine and saliva, and by evaporation of water from the skin and lungs. The water lost through the skin and lungs varies with the temperature, relative humidity and activity of the child. Values obtained for insensible losses by the skin and lung have been reported to be as low as 500 ml. per square meter per day in the basal state, to as high as 2300 ml. per square meter per day in the disease state (fever, hyperventilation, and so forth). An average range of 600 to 900 ml. (mean, 750 ml.) per square meter per day, or 40 to 80 ml. per 100 calories metabolized (mean, 50 ml. per 100 calories metabolized) per day, has been demonstrated in hospitalized children.

The minimal urinary water losses are dependent on renal concentrating capacity, diet, state of body hydration and integrity of the homeostatic mechanisms. The average newborn infant should be capable of maximally excreting 700 milliosmoles of solute for each liter of urinary water, or he requires 1.4 ml. of urinary water for each milliosmole excreted. Usually by two months of age, the infant should be capable of maximally excreting each milliosmole of solute with only 0.7 ml. of urinary water. Diseases affecting the renal concentrating capacity will vary these renal water requirements. Under most parenteral fluid therapy schemes, water for renal excretion of the solute load administered will range from 600 to 900 (mean, 750) ml. per square meter per day, or 40 to 80 (mean, 50) ml. per 100 calories metabolized per day.

The average stool water losses in an infant being fed formula are 100 ml. per square meter per day. With diarrhea, this value may be increased to as much as 700 ml. per square meter per day. These variations in body fluid losses make it difficult to predict with accuracy the fluid needs of each child. Accurate weight measurements are essential in calculating body fluid needs.

Regarding electrolyte losses, it will be assumed that all homeostatic mechanisms are functioning normally. Maintenance and deficit electrolyte requirements will be related to the scheme of parenteral fluid therapy. In general there are two main therapeutic regimens: (1) Maintenance and deficit needs per 100 calories metabolized, or (2) maintenance and deficit needs per square meter of body surface area.

The Per-100-Calories-Metabolized Regimen. The calorie requirements are calculated on the basis of actual weight rather than ideal weight, and are based on the following formula:

BODY WEIGHT (*kg.*)	CALORIES REQUIRED PER DAY
0–10	100 cal./kg.
10–20	1000 cal. + 50 cal. for each kg. over 10
> 20	1500 cal. + 50 cal. for each kg. over 20

Maintenance fluid and electrolytes required per 100 calories metabolized are as follows:

FLUID (*ml. per 100 calories metabolized*)	ELECTROLYTES (*mEq. per 100 calories metabolized*)		
H_2O	Na	K	Cl
100	3	2	2

Deficit therapy in the usual instance of isotonic dehydration is based on the per cent dehydration as determined by clinical estimation:

DEGREE DEHYDRATION (%)	H_2O (*ml./kg. body wt.*)	Na	K	Cl
		(*mEq./kg. body wt.*)		
5	50	4	3	3
10	100	8	6	6
15	150	12	9	9

EXAMPLE. A 12-kilogram child has a 10 per cent isotonic dehydration. His calorie requirements are 1100 calories (1000 cal. + (50 cal. × 2 kg.) = 1100 cal.). His maintenance and deficit requirements are:

	H_2O (*ml.*)	Na (*mEq.*)	K (*mEq.*)	Cl (*mEq.*)
Maintenance	1100	33	22	22
Deficit	1200	96	72	72
Total	2300	129	94	94
Per liter of solution	1000	56	40	40

The Per-Square-Meter Regimen. Calculations of surface area may be made by use of a nomogram, or may be estimated as follows:

BODY WEIGHT (*kg.*)	SURFACE AREA (*Square meters*)
0–5	0.05 × body wt. (kg.) + 0.05
6–10	0.04 × body wt. (kg.) + 0.10
11–20	0.03 × body wt. (kg.) + 0.20
21–30	0.02 × body wt. (kg.) + 0.40

The maintenance fluid and electrolyte needs are:

H_2O (*ml./m.²/day*)	Na	K	Cl
		(*mEq./m.²/day*)	
1500	52	32	32

Deficit therapy in the per-square-meter-system is based on total body water deficits, and a 10 per cent body weight loss is equivalent to a 15 per cent total body water dehydration. It is further assumed that electrolytes are lost evenly from the extracellular and intracellular fluid and, finally, that only one-half the potassium loss can be replaced in one day.

EXAMPLE. Using the same 12-kilogram child as described in the previous example, calculations based on this system are as follows:

12 kg. = 0.03 × 12 + 0.20 = 0.56 m.²
Total body water = about 70% body wt. = 8.4 liters
10% body weight dehydration = 15% × 8.4 liters = 1260 ml.

	H_2O (ml.)	Na (mEq.)	K (mEq.)	Cl (mEq.)
Maintenance	840	29	18	18
Deficit*	1260	88	3	63†
		0	50	0‡
Total	2100	117	71	81
Per liter of solution	1000	56	34	38

* 1260 = 630 extracellular fluid + 630 intracellular fluid.

† Calculation is based on normal serum value in mEq. per liter of 140 Na, 4 K and 100 Cl.

‡ Calculation is based on assumed absence of intracellular Na and Cl but with a cellular K level of 160 mEq. per liter; the K is divided by 2 for reasons previously noted.

Comment. In these examples, the two systems show little deviation from each other. Calculations would appear somewhat more simple in the per-100-calories-metabolized regimen. In both, the total 24-hour fluid therapy is calculated, which is usual in the pediatric age group. However, in a child severely dehydrated, the deficit needs could be administered over the first 8 to 12 hours, during which reevaluation of the child should be an ongoing procedure; if clinical judgment and calculations are correct, the child should be in a reasonable state of hydration at the end of that time and the maintenance needs could be administered over the next 12 to 16 hours. Should dehydration persist, reassessment of the fluid regimen is necessary.

There are commercial preparations available which in general fulfill maintenance or deficit needs. Examples are as follows:

	MAINTENANCE		DEFICIT	
	Poly-ionic Sul'n #1 (P.I.S. #1)	*E-48*	*Poly-ionic Sul'n #2 (P.I.S. #2)*	*E-75*
Sodium	30 mEq.	25 mEq.	56 mEq.	40 mEq.
Chloride	20 mEq.	22 mEq.	50 mEq.	35 mEq.
Potassium	15 mEq.	20 mEq.	25 mEq.	40 mEq.
Lactate	25 mEq.	23 mEq.	25 mEq.	20 mEq.
Phosphate	3 mEq.	3 mEq.	12 mEq.	15 mEq.
Magnesium	3 mEq.	3 mEq.	6 mEq.	–
Carbohydrate	100 Gm.	50 Gm.	100 Gm.	50 Gm.
Water	1000 ml.	1000 ml.	1000 ml.	1000 ml.

Prior to institution of fluid therapy with potassium-containing solutions, adequate renal function should be ascertained. Most frequently some degree of oliguria occurs in these patients, and raises the question as to whether the oliguria is secondary to dehydration or is a primary renal disorder. Anuria in the face of dehydration is no contraindication to fluid administration. The use of nonpotassium-continuing solutions, such as one-third normal saline (50 to 55 mEq. Na per liter, 50 to 55 mEq. Cl per liter) or one-half normal saline (75 mEq. Na per liter, 75 mEq. Cl per liter), in 5 per cent dextrose and water at a rate of 360 ml. per square meter in 45 minutes or 20 ml. per kilogram in 45 minutes, may resolve this question by rapid expansion of the plasma volume and reestablishment of renal perfusion. If the child does not void at the conclusion of this hydrating dose, the hydrating solution (i.e., without potassium) should be run at the calculated 24-hour rate until the patient voids. Occasionally, in severely dehydrated children, 4 to 5 hours may pass without the child voiding. A repeat hydrating dose (360 ml. per square meter in 45 minutes, or 20 ml. per kilogram in 45 minutes) may be administered if the child is still dehydrated and no other evidence of renal failure has been found. Most patients will void following the second trial. After the patient voids, the calculated solution may be substituted for the hydrating solution. Allowance should be made for the amount of hydrating solution used when recalculating the continued requirements.

It should be emphasized that an admission weight should be secured on all patients no matter how severely ill, since therapy is based on this parameter and subsequent daily weights and blood chemistries will aid in evaluating the adequacy of the therapeutic program.

NEWBORN AND PREMATURE INFANTS

Full-term newborn infants and premature infants must be treated differently, since greater physiologic variations occur not only from day to day, but also from infant to infant. In general, the urine flow of the newborn infant may vary from 0 to 30 ml. on the first day of life and should increase on each succeeding day. The newborn infant excretes approximately 50 per cent of a standard water load and at three weeks of age is capable of excreting 100 per cent of the water. The urinary sodium excretion in a fasting newborn infant is approximately 25 per cent of that observed in a one-month-old infant. The solute excretion increases daily with additional milk feedings; consequently, a more dilute electrolyte solution (P.I.S. #1 or E-48) is suggested for intravenous use in newborn infants. This solution is the maintenance solution for older infants and for children.

The total amount of solution administered should be less for the newborn: approximately half that given to the two-month and older child, or 750 ml. per square meter per day.

The physiologic parameters of the premature infant with regard to renal excretion extend even below those for the full-term newborn infant. The premature infants are not a homogeneous population, and a simple rule for a parenteral fluid therapy program cannot be established with any certainty. Those indices used to evaluate the multiple electrolyte fluid therapy program must be applied most rigidly to the premature infant. In general, the figure of 500 ml. per square meter per day of the dilute multiple electrolyte solution (P.I.S. #1 or E-48) has proved to be satisfactory in the premature infant after the first three days of life.

SPECIFIC CONSIDERATIONS

Hyponatremia. Hyponatremia may occur when salt losses exceed those of water, as in the adrenogenital syndrome or Addison's disease, diabetes mellitus, diarrhea, cerebral salt-wasting states, renal salt wasting states, excessive skin losses as in cystic fibrosis, chronic malnutrition, extensive tuberculosis, ileostomy or colostomy, or when there is an excess water intake such as may be seen with excessive gastric lavage with 5 per cent glucose and water, with excessive administration of 5 per cent glucose and water, with tap water enemas, in states of excessive antidiuretic hormone secretion secondary to central nervous system disease, or with increased sensitivity of the renal tubule to normal amounts of antidiuretic hormone.

In states of true sodium depletion associated with volume depletion, the children are listless, dehydrated and weak with low blood pressure, rapid thready pulse and cold clammy skin. The urine osmolality, BUN and hematocrit will be elevated. In dilutional hyponatremia without volume depletion, the children will be normally hydrated with normal blood pressure and pulse, and warm moist skin. The urine osmolality will be greater than or equal to plasma osmolality. Hyponatremia may be classified as mild, with serum sodium values of 121 to 130 mEq. per liter; as moderate, with values of 115 to 120 mEq. per liter; or as severe, with values less than 110 mEq. per liter.

In dilutional states, water restriction is the main form of therapy. If convulsions are present, hypertonic saline may be used to elevate the serum sodium level to greater than 120 mEq. per liter. In the volume-depleted states, maintenance and deficit therapy should be calculated as specified previously, and the additional sodium requirement may be approximated by use of the following formula:

Sodium desired (135 mEq./liter) − actual sodium × 0.6 − 0.7 × body weight (kg.) = mEq. sodium needed for correction.

One-third of this amount can be given as 3 per cent sodium chloride (0.5 mEq. Na per ml.) over a 2- to 4-hour period if the patient is having seizures. Blood pressure and pulmonary signs of edema should be monitored. The remainder of the sodium chloride may be given as isotonic saline.

EXAMPLE (PER-100-CALORIES-METABOLIZED REGIMEN). A 5-kilogram infant is dehydrated, with a serum sodium value of 122 mEq. per liter. Hydrating solution is followed by:

	H_2O (*ml.*)	Na (*mEq.*)	K (*mEq.*)	Cl (*mEq.*)
Maintenance	500	15	10	10
		40	30	30 proportional loss
Deficit	500	36		39 additional loss
Total	1000	91	40	79

135 − 122 × 0.6 × 5 kg. = 39 mEq. NaCl needed in addition to the proportional loss.

Hypernatremia. Hypernatremia may be seen when water losses exceed those of salt. This can occur in the following instances: (1) gastrointestinal: water deprivation, vomiting and diarrhea; (2) respiratory: hyperventilation, high altitude and high environmental temperatures; (3) skin: high environmental temperature, denudation of skin and hyperkeratosis; (4) central nervous system: sulfonamide intoxication, diabetes insipidus and fusion of the frontal lobes; (5) renal: nephrogenic diabetes insipidus, renal failure (chronic pyelonephritis, chronic nephritis), potassium deficiency and hypercalcemia; (6) excessive administration of saline in infants.

Clinical manifestations with dehydration are those of irritability, rigidity and opisthotonos with generalized convulsions. The serum sodium concentration is elevated, and an abnormal electroencephalographic tracing is usually present as well as an elevated cerebrospinal fluid protein concentration. When the serum sodium concentration is increased to disturbing levels (more than 180 mEq. per liter), the use of peritoneal dialysis has proved to be very effective in lowering the concentration. Once the diagnosis of hypernatremia has been established, a formula for correction is as follows:

Actual sodium value − desired sodium (145 mEq./liter) × 4 ml. × body weight (kg.) = ml. free water needed for correction

This should be calculated in association with the maintenance and deficit therapy for the state of dehydration.

EXAMPLE. A 5-kilogram infant is 10 per cent dehydrated, with a serum sodium value of 168 mEq. per liter. Hydrating solution is followed by:

	H_2O (*ml.*)	Na (*mEq.*)	K (*mEq.*)	Cl (*mEq.*)
Maintenance	500	15	10	10
Deficit	500	–	–	–
Total	1000	15	10	10

Free water deficit = 168 − 145 × 4 × 5 = 460 ml Therefore, in this instance the free water deficit may be considered equivalent to the dehydration deficit. In other patients this might not be true and proportional losses would also have to be calculated.

The patient corrected with glucose water alone may risk convulsions as a complicating sequela owing to rapid intracellular water shifts. The solution used may vary from P.I.S. #1 or E-48 to P.I.S. #2 or E-75. Some clinicians would use only the latter type of solutions for correction of body fluid losses. Replacement should usually be slow, over 48 to 72 hours. Associated abnormalities include hypocalcemia, with calcium levels often less than 9 mg. per 100 ml., but tetany is rare. Central nervous system complications of hemorrhage may also occur.

Potassium Deficiency. Potassium deficiency out of proportion to the usual losses caused by dehydration from gastroenteritis and starvation may require additional potassium supplementation, as may be necessary in the following conditions: renal potassium losses, adrenal-initiated potassium losses, diabetes mellitus, familial periodic paralysis, following operation with ileostomy and severe metabolic response to surgery.

The clinical manifestations are weakness, silent distention of the abdomen, dyspnea, cardiac arrhythmia and the typical electrocardiographic tracings of low potassium syndrome. Serum potassium levels are usually low, but may be normal in spite of existing potassium deficiency. Additional potassium may be given up to 100 mEq. per square meter per day if potassium therapy is required. Parenteral fluid concentrations of potassium should not exceed 40 mEq. per liter as a rule.

Pyloric Stenosis. This condition is the most frequent cause of a metabolic hypochloremic, hypokalemic alkalosis in infancy. Because this is primarily a gastric loss of potassium and chloride ions, the deficit therapy in the per-100-calories metabolized scheme is changed:

	FLUID (*ml./kg.*)	ELECTROLYTES (*mEq./kg.*)		
	H_2O	Na	K	Cl
10% dehydration	100	6	12	12

EXAMPLE. A one-month-old male infant with pyloric stenosis weighs 3.5 kilograms and has 10 per cent dehydration.

	H_2O (*ml.*)	Na (*mEq.*)	K (*mEq.*)	Cl (*mEq.*)
Maintenance	350	10.5	7	7
Deficit	350	21	42	42
Total	700	32	49	49
Per liter of solution	1000	45	70	70

The K is greater than 70 mEq. per liter and thus correction should be made slowly with solutions containing no more than 40 mEq. per liter.

Diabetes Mellitus. The child presenting for the first time with diabetes usually does so with severe acidosis and coma. The principal renal losses are water, sodium, chloride and potassium. With diabetes, the urinary losses of water may rise to 3300 ml. per square meter per day, and the urinary sodium, potassium and chloride may rise, respectively, to 220, 120 and 85 mEq. With dehydration, the glomerular filtration rate will be lowered, and as a consequence the serum concentration of potassium, urea, sulfates and phosphates will be elevated. Once urine flow and filtration are established, however, these elevated serum components will be lowered and potassium-containing solutions may be administered. With continued fluid repair, potassium deficiency may be manifest and additional potassium may be required.

There are as many fluid regimens for this condition as there are clinicians caring for these patients. Some will use normal saline; others will use P.I.S. #2 at a rate of 4000 to 6000 ml. per square meter per day for correction. If one utilizes the per-100-calories-metabolized scheme, the following is recommended:

1. Increase maintenance needs by 50 per cent, i.e., 150 ml. H_2O per 100 calories metabolized; Na-4.5, Cl-3, K-3 mEq. per 100 calories metabolized.

2. Deficit calculated per kilogram per day:

H_2O-80 ml., Na-6, K-6, Cl-5 mEq. per kilogram body weight per day.

EXAMPLE. A 10-kilogram (0.5 square meter) child is in diabetic acidosis.

1. Empirical, by 4000 to 6000 ml. per square meter per day:

5000 ml./m.^{2} = 2500 ml. of P.I.S. #2.

2. Per-100-calories-metabolized:

	H_2O (*ml.*)	Na (*mEq.*)	K (*mEq.*)	Cl (*mEq.*)
Maintenance	1500	67.5	45	45
Deficit	800	60	60	50
Total	2300	127.5	105	95
Per liter of solution	1000	56	46	41

Obviously, of utmost importance is the immediate administration of insulin in addition to fluid therapy.

Renal Failure. The administration of parenteral fluids to patients with renal failure must be accomplished after a judgment has been made concerning (1) the cause of renal failure, (2) the functional alterations present and (3) the phase of the functional renal loss.

Those etiologies related to prerenal azotemia will be differentiated and ameliorated with nonpotassium-containing solutions. The renal and postrenal etiologies will need clarification, and until such is accomplished, supplying insensible water losses plus urine flow will be a conservative and adequate approach.

The functional derangements may include glomerular and/or tubular failure. With glomerular failure of primary renal origin, dehydration deficits can be restored with nonpotassium-containing solutions and then followed with the daily insensible water losses plus urine flow. But with the administration of intravenous fluids in patients with renal insufficiency, a search for evidence of impending cardiac insufficiency should be done before and during fluid administration. Cardiac failure or pulmonary edema may easily be precipitated, and with the use of hypotonic solutions, water intoxication could be a consequence.

Problems associated with primary glomerular failure are (1) hyponatremia and (2) potassium deficiency or hyperkalemia. Hyponatremia with glomerular failure may reflect poor sodium intake, excessive gastrointestinal losses or excessive water retention. Unless the serum sodium concentration is dangerously low (120 mEq. per liter or less), sodium therapy is not indicated. If there are good reasons to suspect salt depletion associated with hyponatremia and if dilution factors can be excluded, the cautious administration of sodium may be done to a limited degree. The restriction of fluids may be the treatment of choice if expansion of the extracellular space is confirmed as the cause of hyponatremia in the face of primary glomerular failure. With hyperkalemia, reducing the hyperkalemia by known methods (such as resin administration, peritoneal dialysis and administration of glucose plus insulin) must be accomplished prior to the consideration of potassium therapy. When the urinary output is large, with hypokalemia, potassium administration may be required.

Tubular insufficiency without glomerular failure requires no special consideration, since tubular insufficiency is usually associated with losses of water and electrolytes and replacement of such may not be as hazardous with an existing normal glomerular filtration rate. However, when polyuria is present as a result of tubular failure in the face of primary glomerular failure, careful evaluation must be made before fluid therapy is administered, since excessive urine flow may reflect loss of edema fluid, and fluid administration may precipitate pulmonary edema and cardiac failure, or even renal shutdown.

Functional loss in acute renal failure has been classified into three phases: (1) oliguric, (2) diuretic and (3) recovery.

OLIGURIC PHASE. The insensible water loss decreases to approximately 300 ml. per square meter per day (or 10 ml. per kilogram per day) during this phase. Nonelectrolyte sugar solutions should be used to provide this quantity plus the urinary output. It is best to calculate the requirement on an every-8-hour basis. Daily weights should be used to determine whether the fluid intake should be increased or decreased. A loss of 100 to 200 Gm. of body weight per day is desirable.

DIURETIC PHASE. During this phase, electrolyte/sugar-containing solutions and solid food intake may be instituted. Dehydration and electrolyte depletion may occur. A determination of urinary electrolyte losses as well as serum electrolyte concentrations can be of the utmost help in preventing extreme deviations. During this phase there is a return toward normal of renal blood flow and glomerular filtration rate; the blood urea nitrogen level may rise because of back diffusion of urea.

RECOVERY PHASE. The return of glomerular and tubular function will be manifested by normal urine flow. The urinary concentrating capacity may be the last function to return and may not be complete for long periods of time. Parenteral fluids during this stage are not a problem, since the oral administration usually is adequately tolerated.

Surgery. PREOPERATIVE. It is important to note that the practice of "nothing by mouth until the A.M." will dehydrate the pediatric patient, and continuous parenteral therapy during the night could obviate the possible development of dehydration. Also, preoperative medications such as meperidine (Demerol), 100 mg. per square meter, or morphine, 10 mg. per square meter, have a depressing effect on glomerular filtration rate, renal plasma flow, urine flow and sodium excretion. These reductions may be as much as 25 to 50 per cent of control normal values. The use of intravenously administered fluids in conjunction with these drugs should be properly evaluated.

OPERATIVE. Water losses during the operative procedure under heavy drapes may be as high as 300 ml. per square meter per hour. During the administration of an anesthetic agent in surgery, metabolism may be lowered and renal function may be reduced to as much as 20 to 30 per cent of normal control values. The administration of parenteral fluids is advised in most instances merely to maintain entry into a vein. The administration of 50 ml. per square meter per hour of a carbohydrate solution should be adequate. If a prolonged operation is pending, 1/6 normal saline solution in 10 per cent carbohydrate can be substituted at the same rate. Abnormal losses may be made up with blood, plasma or a proper electrolyte solution.

POSTOPERATIVE. The principles of therapy are similar to other situations requiring parenteral fluid therapy. When urine flow is established postoperatively, potassium-containing solutions may be administered at the usual rate. Again, it should be emphasized that the use of morphine may contribute to hyponatremia and convulsions, particularly when nonelectrolyte-containing solutions are given solely. Ileostomy drainage has been shown to contain the following:

Na	100–140 mEq./liter
K	5–15 mEq./liter
Cl	90–130 mEq./liter

Patients with an ileostomy must be carefully evaluated for impending deficits. If possible, all gastrointestinal drainage should be determined for electrolyte concentrations. Gastric lavage is best done with an electrolyte-containing parenteral fluid.

Central Nervous System. Cerebral edema may be treated by giving a hypertonic urea solution (30 per cent in 10 per cent carbohydrate); 1 to 1.5 Gm. of urea per kilogram of body weight can be administered intravenously in 30 minutes. The status of the myocardium should be evaluated, and signs of impending cardiac failure during and after the infusion must be observed. These solutions and dosage may be repeated in 8 hours. Acetazolamide may be of value in water intoxication.

Mannitol* infusions may be more effective than urea. The dosage is 1 Gm. per kilogram intravenously over 15 to 30 minutes. This may be repeated three or four times in one day.

Burns. Fluid therapy with dextran or plasma is usually begun immediately to correct shock and to maintain urinary output. In the initial evaluation of the patient, these points need to be considered: (1) the extent and depth of the burn, (2) estimation of fluid requirements, (3) catheterization of the bladder, (4) determination of baseline chemistries and (5) adequacy of airway. Certain guides may be of help in estimating body surface area:

9% for each arm
18% for each leg
18% for front of torso
18% for back of torso
9% for the head and neck

The proportions of the body may vary with age, as shown:

	BODY SURFACE AREA			
	Newborn	*3 years*	*6 years*	*> 12 years*
Head	18%	15%	12%	6%
Trunk	40%	40%	40%	38%
Arms	16%	16%	16%	18%
Legs	26%	29%	32%	38%

In full-thickness (charred surface) burns, there is a linear relation between the amount of fluid lost and the percentage of body surface burned, up to 50 per cent of extracellular space volume. In burns of greater extent than 50 per cent of the body area, calculate fluid requirements as if there were only a 50 per cent burn. In general, one may give 1 ml. of plasma expander (or blood or plasma) plus 1 ml. of electrolyte solution per kilogram for each percentage of burn, plus 50 ml. per kilogram or 1500 ml. per square meter of maintenance fluid as 5 per cent glucose in water. Half the amount may be given in the first 8 hours; the remainder is given over the next 16 hours. In the second 24 hours, decrease by one-half the volume of

* Manufacturer's precaution: Use of mannitol in pediatric patients has not been studied comprehensively.

colloid and electrolyte, but use the same volume of glucose water as in the first 24 hours. The electrolyte solution used should be Ringer's lactate or a similarly constituted solution.

If the hemoglobin or hematocrat value is low, blood may be substituted for plasma as needed. Blood pressure and the rate and volume of the pulse are good indices of the adequacy of blood volume replacement therapy. Urine output should be measured with a retention catheter and should be adequate (25 per cent of fluid intake). If dehydration is suspected, 360 ml. per square meter of a carbohydrate solution can be given in 45 minutes. If oliguria persists, renal failure should be considered. Hematocrit and hemoglobin determinations should be done every 4 hours during the first 48 hours to ascertain blood, colloid or fluid needs. No single index can be used as a guide for fluid therapy; after the first 48 hours the urine volume may be adequate and yet the patient may manifest thirst and elevated serum sodium level. Oral fluids may be given in small quantities. Subsequently, high protein and high calorie feedings should be given, often by gavage (protein, 2 to 4 Gm. per kilogram of body weight per day at 50 to 100 calories per kilogram of body weight per day). Adequate vitamins and minerals are essential. By the end of the first week, most patients are able to take food by mouth.

INTRAVENOUS ALIMENTATION

The preceding sections have been concerned primarily with supplying fluid and electrolyte needs over a relatively short period of time in conditions that are usually short lived. Sustained fluid therapy in chronic catabolic states or in situations of prolonged protein and caloric deprivation require the intravenous use of nitrogen-carbohydrate-mineral mixtures (see p. 12).

References

Brucke, E., Aceto, T., and Lowe, C. U.: Intravenous Fluid Therapy for Infants and Children. *Pediatrics,* 25:496, 1960.

Filler, R. M., and Eraklis, A. J.: Care of the Critically Ill Child. Intravenous Alimentation. *Pediatrics,* 46:456, 1970.

Paine, R. S.: Emergencies of Cerebral Origin. *Pediat. Clin. N. Am.,* 9:67, 1962.

Rubin, M. I., and Calcagno, P. L.: Acute renal failure. *Pediat. Clin. N. Am.,* 9:155, 1962.

Wolferth, C. C., Jr., Peskin, G. W., and Wesche, R. W.: Fluid Therapy in Burns, Trauma, and Shock. *Pediat. Clin. N. Am.,* 11:1053, 1964.

Anesthesia: Aspects of Significance to the Pediatrician

DAVID ALLAN, M.B., Ch.B.

In a pediatric medical center there is little need for the pediatrician to know much about pediatric anesthesiology because well-trained pediatric anesthesiologists are available. In the usual community hospital environment, however, the pediatrician has a broader responsibility to the child and must assume added responsibilities in preoperative, operative and postoperative management.

In pediatric anesthesia there are few indications for local and regional anesthesia. For topical anesthesia, 4 per cent lidocaine (Xylocaine) appears to provoke fewer side reactions. If topical anesthesia is used, the dosage should be measured. Local infiltration is used extensively in emergency reception areas. It is preferable to select one agent. Lidocaine* has proved to be excellent as a local anesthetic for infiltration in a dose of 3 to 4 mg. per kilogram.

Every effort should be made to minimize the psychologic trauma during the administration of the general anesthetic. The presence of the mother during induction of anesthesia mitigates upset, and it appears that the parents should be present during the awakening process in the recovery room.

Presurgical Management. With the exceptions of trauma and infection, there are very few true emergencies in pediatric surgery. Careful preparation of the child results in optimal operative conditions. The pediatrician should be responsible for notifying the surgeon and the anesthesiologist of abnormal hemoglobin, pulse rate, blood pressure or other variants from normal for various age groups.

The drug dosage schedule in Table 1 may be used as a guide to pre-medication. Note that the dosage of atropine seems to be relatively high; the rationale is that the greatest danger during induction of anesthesia in infants and children is bradycardia. This may be due to the single or combined action of vagal reflex, overdose of anesthetic agent or hypoxia.

The pediatrician should be aware of the effect on anesthetic management of preoperative or prior medication with cortisone, promazine or reserpine.

Obviously, no child or infant should go

* Manufacturer's precaution: Experience with lidocaine (Xylocaine) in children is limited.

TABLE 1. Premedication Schedule (Intramuscular)

WEIGHT (*kg.*)	PENTAZOCINE (*Talwin*)*	ATROPINE
1.3 – 3.5		0.1 mg.
3.5 – 4.5		0.15 mg.
4.5 – 8.5		0.2 mg.
8.5 – 10.5	12 mg. (0.4 ml.)	0.3 mg.
10.5 – 13.5	15 mg. (0.5 ml.)	0.3 mg.
13.5 – 15.5	18 mg. (0.6 ml.)	0.4 mg.
15.5 – 17.5	21 mg. (0.7 ml.)	0.5 mg.
17.5 – 20	24 mg. (0.8 ml.)	0.6 mg.
20 – 22	27 mg. (0.9 ml.)	0.6 mg.
22 – 24.5	30 mg. (1.0 ml.)	0.6 mg.
24.5 – 26.5	33 mg. (1.1 ml.)	0.6 mg.
26.5 – 29	36 mg. (1.2 ml.)	0.6 mg.
29 – 31.5	39 mg. (1.3 ml.)	0.6 mg.
31.5 – 33.5	42 mg. (1.4 ml.)	0.6 mg.
33.5 – 36	45 mg. (1.5 ml.)	0.6 mg.
36 – 38	48 mg. (1.6 ml.)	0.6 mg.
38 – 40.5	51 mg. (1.7 ml.)	0.6 mg.
40.5 – 42.5	54 mg. (1.8 ml.)	0.6 mg.
42.5 – 45	57 mg. (1.9 ml.)	0.6 mg.
45 and above	60 mg. (2.0 ml.)	0.6 mg.

* Manufacturer's precaution: Because clinical experience in children under 12 years of age is limited, the use of Talwin in this age group, is not recommended.

to surgery dehydrated. Feedings need not be withheld more than 4 hours before anesthesia is given. Smaller infants should be listed first on the schedule, so that if there is a delay, there will be minimal dehydration. A sick infant should be provided with an intravenous drip to prevent dehydration during any period when oral feedings are withheld in preparation for surgery.

The anemic child is a greater operative risk. Management may be postponement of surgery with iron supplementation, immediate surgery with transfusion, or transfusion followed by surgery.

A child with a low-grade fever should not be submitted for a routine procedure. If bacteremia or viremia develops because of the handling of tissues or lowering of resistance, it may be difficult to prevent a serious complication.

Monitoring of Patients. The temperature of the child should be routinely monitored. When a nonrebreathing anesthetic circuit is employed, it is wise to warm and humidify the anesthetic gases adequately to prevent heat loss from the respiratory tract.

The patient should be continuously checked for signs of airway obstruction. A precordial stethoscope is extremely valuable in measuring respiration and diagnosing signs of obstruction. Spirometers are used for measuring ventilation. The blood pressure should be monitored using a blood pressure cuff one and one-half times the diameter of the arm. A Doppler blood pressure apparatus is useful. In more critical cases the pH, pCO_2 and pO_2 of the arterial blood should be monitored by use of a blood gas analyzer.

The greatest danger in pediatric anesthesiology is hypoventilation. Changes in the patient's color and in the vital signs are relatively late indications of hypoxia. Respiration should always be assisted or controlled.

Postoperative Management. Infants and children react differently to pain than do adolescents and adults. There are very few indications for the administration of an analgesic for postoperative pain in the infant and child. This is in direct contrast to the needs of the adolescent, who has a different threshold and reacts more intensely.

RESPIRATORY THERAPY

Respiratory therapy consists of the administration of oxygen for hypoxia, mechanical ventilation for hypoventilation, continuous positive airway pressure (CPAP) to prevent the alveoli from collapsing, humidification for a humidity deficit, mist therapy to mobilize secretions in obstructive pulmonary disease, respiratory physical therapy (postural drainage, percussion and vibration) to scavenge mobilized secretions, breathing exercises and intermittent positive pressure ventilation for abnormal breathing patterns, and aerosolized drug therapy for conditions such as bronchospasm.

Hypoxia is a broad term indicating the deprivation of oxygen regardless of etiology or site. It has a variety of causes. Since methods of treatment are closely allied to cause, the administration of oxygen infrequently corrects the basic defect. Instead, oxygen is applied as a lifesaving stop-gap until more fundamental measures can be instituted.

Therapeutic Use of Oxygen. Administration of oxygen is indicated under the following circumstances:

1. Delivery of an inadequate amount of oxygen to normal lungs.
2. Inadequate oxygenation of the blood resulting from abnormal pulmonary function, especially when hypoxia is the result of poor diffusion of oxygen across the alveolar pulmonary membrane.
3. Venous arterial shunts.
4. Inadequate arterial transport of oxygen.
5. Inadequate tissue oxygenation.

Hyperbaric oxygenation at 1 or 2 atmospheres is the choice treatment in carbon monoxide poisoning. The patient is placed in a mobile chamber, and in 20 minutes he may be awake and well. Its use in circulatory disturbances, respiratory difficulties and anaerobic and aerobic infections is still being evaluated.

In the sick child, increased physiologic shunting is frequently present in varying degrees. The shunting may be one of three types: either a portion of the cardiac output bypasses a certain area of the pulmonary capillaries, a portion of the cardiac output perfuses nonventilating alveoli (atelectasis), or a combination of both. It is impossible to predict the arterial oxygenation that can be achieved by a given inspired concentration of oxygen. The most desirable concentration of oxygen is one that allows maximal use of the oxygen-carrying capacity of arterial blood.

It is important that all equipment used in pediatric respiratory therapy be sterile. The most common method of administering oxygen to a child is by an oxygen tent. These tents can increase the oxygen in the atmosphere from 35 to 50 per cent. Oxygen should be administered only in a humidified state. If high oxygen levels are required, a mask of the Randal-Baker-Soucek type is needed along with an Ayre's valveless system or a nonrebreathing valve. Lower concentrations can be obtained with a mask of simple design with expiratory ports.

With a tracheostomy collar, and a high flow of oxygen of approximately 15 liter per minute, it is possible to obtain 80 per cent concentration of oxygen at the trachea. The concentration of oxygen in incubators can be varied from ambient to 65 per cent. Face hoods and nasal catheters have limited use in pediatric respiratory therapy. It is important that the oxygen concentration in the environment be monitored frequently with an oxygen analyzer.

The complications of oxygen administration are atelectasis, oxygen apnea, retrolental fibroplasia (the cerebral arterial pO_2 and not the inspired FiO_2 is of importance in the etiology of this disease) and bronchomalacia. (Until more is known of the last-mentioned syndrome, it would be well to give the lowest concentration of oxygen necessary for the shortest period of time.) The arterial pO_2 should not be over 100 mm. Hg.

Treatment of Inadequate Ventilation. In the treatment of inadequate ventilation, an endotracheal tube may reduce the physiologic dead space sufficiently to compensate for small degrees of hypoventilation. A hand self-inflating bag with mask may be used for the treatment of short periods of hypoventilation, but a mechanical ventilator should be employed for prolonged artificial ventilation.

Humidification and Mist Therapy. The indication for use of a humidifier is a humidity deficit in the upper airway.

It is important to realize that humidification supplies water vapor in a carrier gas, whereas mist therapy is actual particulate water suspended in a carrier gas. It is rare to have less than 100 per cent relative humidity below the carina, even in the tracheostomized patient; therefore, humidification per se can be supplied only to the upper airway. On the other hand, mist therapy can be applied to any part of the airway because the site of deposition depends largely upon particle size.

The mist must be of sufficient density that, despite heating to 98.6° F. (37° C.), 100 per cent humidification is maintained. It must also be of sufficient stability to arrive at the diseased portion of the tracheobronchial tree. In mechanically produced mists, the addition of 10 per cent propylene glycol, which decreases the vapor tension, stabilizes the mist. This is not necessary in ultrasonically produced mists, which are stable.

The humidifier of choice is one which is sterile, and disposable. The heating element should not contaminate the contents.

Respiratory Physical Therapy. When secretions are mobilized in a pathologic entity, e.g., obstructive pulmonary disease, bronchopneumonia, viral pneumonitis or bronchiolitis, the scavenging mechanisms of the body may be inadequate. In this case, respiratory physical therapy consisting of postural drainage, percussion and vibration therapy is indicated. Occasionally it is necessary to apply suction directly through a nasotracheal tube or bronchoscope.

Aerosols. Drugs may be instilled into the tracheobronchial tree in the form of aerosols with or without intermittent positive pressure breathing. Drugs commonly used in this fashion are racemic epinephrine, isopropyl norepinephrine and antimicrobials.

INTENSIVE CARE

The pediatrician should be able to respond rapidly to instances of respiratory or cardiac arrest. When a patient is found unresponsive, without pulse, blood pressure or respiration, or in a life-threatening situation, the person discovering it should first call for help and immediately start resuscitation. After the time at the start of resuscitation has been noted on the chart, the sternum should be thumped sharply once or twice (which may be enough to restart the heart) and external cardiac massage and mouth-to-mouth ventilation begun. For external cardiac massage, compress the chest with the heel of the hand at the junction of the middle and lower thirds of the sternum. The rate should be calculated in relation to the age of the patient. Adequacy of external massage is measured from the extent of the peripheral pulse. Mouth-to-mouth ventilation is conducted at a rate of 20 per minute and should be timed to occur between compressions of the chest. Adequacy of ventilation is checked by auscultation. Emergency drugs and equipment should be available, including suction equipment and a means for endotracheal intubation.

A self-inflating bag attached to a source of oxygen is employed. If one is unable to maintain an airway, endotracheal intubation should be considered. External cardiac massage should not be interrupted except for endotracheal intubation.

If no cardiac action is detected after 1 minute, inject epinephrine (1 to 4 ml. of 1:10,000 dilution) into the heart and continue the massage. The intracardiac dose is as follows: for patients less than 4 kilograms in weight, give 2 ml., for those 4 to 18 kilograms, give 3 ml. and for those more than 18 kilograms, give 4 ml. If there is no response, it is important to provide intracardiac or intravenous base buffer (sodium bicarbonate) as soon as possible to combat metabolic acidosis. Intravenous administration is instituted if resuscitation is not effective within 4 minutes.

If the electrocardiogram shows ventricular fibrillation, direct current shock should be administered as follows:

PATIENT	VOLTAGE
Small infant under 12 kg.	25/50 watt-seconds
Small child under 25 kg.	100 watt-seconds
Large child over 25 kg.	100/200 watt-seconds

If there is no response, two shocks of the same voltage in rapid succession are administered.

If ventricular standstill is present, the intracardiac epinephrine is repeated and an intravenous solution of epinephrine in a dose of 0.5 mg. per kilogram per minute is administered.

If defibrillation is unsuccessful and ventricular standstill persists, the heart may be anoxic or acidotic. Therefore, check the adequacy of ventilation and of external cardiac massage (femoral pulsations present with each cardiac massage) and provide a base buffer for metabolic acidosis. Give sodium bicarbonate intravenously rapidly (or into the heart if there is no intravenous equipment). Use 2 to 3 ml. of stock solution per kilogram (44.6 mEq. per 50 ml.), which may be repeated in 10 to 15 minutes (three or four times if needed). Search for the cause of anoxia and cardiac arrest when resuscitation is effective.

The other anesthesiologic aspects of pediatric intensive care deal primarily with the diagnosis of respiratory insufficiency, with special emphasis on long-term use of mechanical ventilators and the weaning of patients from these ventilators. Examples of disorders requiring these types of therapy are status asthmaticus, severe viral pneumonitis and bronchiolitis, and idiopathic respiratory distress syndrome of the newborn.

Genetic Disease: Diagnosis, Counseling and Prevention

MICHAEL M. KABACK, M.D., *and*
DAVID L. RIMOIN, M.D., PH.D.

The relative importance of genetic disorders to the pediatrician is increasing. Improvements in immunization programs and medical care have produced a tremendous decrease in the frequency of infectious and nutritional disease, resulting in a relative increase in morbidity and mortality due to diseases of genetic origin. Individual genetic diseases are usually rare, but when considered together they have a considerable impact on community health. It has been estimated that 6 per cent of newborn infants have a defect or will develop an illness primarily caused by genetic factors. Although the physician cannot be expected to be familiar with the clinical symptoms and genetics of each of these rare disorders, he must be knowledgeable about principles of clinical genetics and the management of patients with genetic disease. As with other forms of disease, the role of the physician in clinical genetics involves diagnosis, prognosis, treatment and prevention.

DIAGNOSIS

The first concern of the physician encountering an apparent genetic disease is to make an accurate diagnosis. Genetic counseling should *not* be attempted before a definite diagnosis is made, since an inaccurate diagnosis can lead to completely erroneous advice. A detailed family history is usually required, often accompanied by the examination of several relatives. The diagnosis may be made on purely clinical grounds, or may also require the use of specific laboratory tests, e.g., enzyme analysis and cytogenetic analysis. There are numerous pitfalls in the diagnosis of genetic disease, and an erroneous diagnosis can markedly change the recurrence risk, e.g., from zero to 50 per cent in some cases.

One common source of error in genetic counseling is genetic heterogeneity, i.e., several different disorders may result in the same clinical picture. Many diseases once thought to represent a single entity are now known to consist of several distinct diseases due to differing genetic (genocopies), chromosomal or environmental (phenocopies) causes. Recognition of the distinct cause of the clinical picture has important implications in genetic counseling. For example, a teenage boy presenting with hypogonadism may have one of a number of simply inherited diseases (e.g., the Reifenstein syndrome or isolated gonadotropin deficiency), he may have a chromosomal aberration (e.g., the Klinefelter syndrome) or he may have been exposed to a number of environmental agents (e.g., radiation or trauma). In the simply inherited diseases, the risk to his parents of having another similarly affected child is as high as 50 per cent of male births, whereas in the chromosomal or environmental disorders, the risk for recurrence is negligible.

A second difficulty in the diagnosis of genetic disorders, especially those inherited as autosomal dominant traits, is clinical variability. One member of the family may have a full-blown clinical syndrome (e.g., fractures, blue sclerae and otosclerosis in osteogenesis imperfecta), whereas an affected member of the same family may have only one of the signs (e.g., blue sclerae). This variability in the severity of the phenotype is termed *variable expressivity,* and if the effects of the mutant gene are not detectable at all, *lack of penetrance* is said to exist. Lack of penetrance, however, exists only in the eyes of the observer, for if one were able to measure the direct product of gene action (e.g., enzyme activity), one should always be able to detect the effects of the mutant. When confronted with an individual with a readily diagnosable genetic disorder and an apparently negative family history, a detailed family history and examination of pertinent relatives must be performed. For example, if the parents of a child with severe osteogenesis imperfecta are found to be completely normal, one would predict that he represented a new mutation and the chance of his parents having another affected offspring would be negligible. If, however, one of his parents was found to have the characteristic blue sclerae, he would probably have the mutant gene and the chance for recurrence in subsequent offspring would be 50 per cent. Other pitfalls in genetic counseling include nonpaternity, pseudodominant inheritance, multiple alleles with variable expression and variability in the age of onset of the clinical expression of a genetic disorder.

GENETIC COUNSELING

Prognostication in medical genetics classically involves genetic counseling, i.e., the prediction of the probability for recurrence of a hereditary disorder within a family. These risks represent a statistical chance and are determined by specific genetic laws of inheritance or from empirical observations of other affected families. In recent years the techniques of intrauterine diagnosis have allowed for the absolute detection of certain genetic diseases in the fetus. The usefulness and limitations of intrauterine diagnosis will be discussed later.

For the purpose of genetic counseling, genetic diseases can be divided into three major groups: (1) single-gene disorders, and (2) chromosomal aberrations and (3) congenital malformations and common disorders in which multiple genetic and environmental factors appear to interact.

Single-Gene Disorders

These disorders include autosomal (nonsex chromosome) and X-linked traits. Their characteristic patterns of inheritance will be briefly reviewed and recurrence risks will be discussed for selected problems. The probabilities based on the segregation of alleles during meiosis, i.e., the chance that one gene (allele) of a pair will be included in the maternal or paternal gamete, is clearly one-half.

Autosomal Dominant Disorders. Autosomal dominant traits are those which occur in the presence of only one mutant gene. In general, dominant traits usually represent defects in nonenzyme proteins, as might be found in the hemoglobinopathies and certain connective tissue disorders. The major features of autosomal dominant inheritance are vertical transmission of the trait from affected parent to affected child through two or more generations, and a 1:1 ratio of normal to affected offspring from an affected parent. Males and females are affected in equal proportions, except in rare circumstances where the trait is sex-influenced. Since most autosomal dominant traits are quite rare, almost all affected individuals can be considered to be heterozygotes.

Several problems exist in regard to genetic counseling for autosomal dominant traits. First is their tendency to be quite variable in their severity, even within members of the same family. This becomes quite important in counseling a family in whom only one patient has the full syndrome. If the child is truly the only affected individual in the family, then he most likely represents a new mutation and the chance for recurrence of this disorder in his future sibs is negligible. If one of his parents is found to be even mildly affected, then the risks for further affected siblings rises to 50 per cent. In either case, of course, the affected child will have a 50 per cent chance of passing the mutant gene on to each of his children, but the chance of his normal sibs transmitting the trait is negligible. Thus, it is extremely important to carefully examine the parents of affected individuals before giving genetic counsel. One must rule out a phenocopy or a recessive or X-linked genocopy before a new mutation can be considered.

There is, of course, no difference between individuals with a dominant syndrome who have or do not have a positive family history. In those diseases in which an affected individual is unlikely to reproduce, e.g., Apert's syndrome, most cases will be sporadic. If reproduction is only partially decreased, then a smaller proportion of individuals with the disease will be due to new mutations. For example, in achondroplasia, approximately 80 per cent of the cases have a negative family history. With the increasing social awareness of these individuals and their increasing ability to meet and mate with other dwarfs, the number of achondroplastic children born to achondroplastic parents will increase. Thus, the relative proportion of achondroplasts with positive family histories will rise, but the absolute number of new mutations will not be altered.

There is a statistical correlation between new dominant mutations and *paternal* age.

Autosomal Recessive Inheritance. Autosomal recessive traits are those which are expressed only in the presence of a double dose of mutant gene (or in rare instances in single dose, when the normal allele is deleted from the homologous chromosome). In general, autosomal recessive disorders involve enzyme-deficiency states, including almost all of the inborn errors of metabolism. They are characterized by phenotypically normal heterozygous parents with a ratio of one affected to three clinically normal offspring (of which two are carriers and one is genotypically normal). The affected individuals are usually limited to one sibship, except in cases of inbreeding, when an affected sib may marry a carrier and there would be a 50-50 chance of each of their children being affected (pseudodominant inheritance). Autosomal recessive traits are more common in the offspring of consanguineous matings, since the chance of two mates carrying the same recessive gene increases if they have inherited their genes from a common ancestor. The rarer the gene is in the population, the more often will the parents of affected individuals be related. When the frequency of the gene in the population is high (e.g., cystic fibrosis), consanguinity among the parents is not common.

Counseling for autosomal recessive traits is usually requested by the parents of an affected child. In this case, the parents are both carriers and subsequent offspring have a one in four chance of being affected. In cases of rare recessive traits, normal relatives have a very low risk of having affected children, assuming that they do not marry carriers. With common traits, however, the chance of a carrier sib marrying another carrier is relatively high, and in these instances carrier-detection programs are most important (e.g., cystic fibrosis in western Europeans and Tay-Sachs disease in Ashkenazi Jews). Carrier detection is now possible in a large number of recessive disorders, but for many traits it is still impossible and only empiric risk figures can be given.

X-linked Recessive Inheritance. X-linked recessive traits are due to genes located on the X chromosome which express themselves only in the absence of the normal allele. Since males have only one X chromosome, all males carrying the mutant gene will manifest the disease. Since females have two X chromosomes, affected females will either have a double dose of the mutant gene or have only one X chromosome (note exceptions explained by the Lyon hypothesis). In general, males are affected, the trait being transmitted by unaffected females. Maternal uncles of an affected individual are frequently also affected. Since none of the sons of an affected male receives the father's X chromosome, there is no male to male transmission. Each of the sisters of an affected male will have a 50-50 chance of being a carrier, assuming that he does not represent a new mutation. Thus, each of the sons of a sister of an affected individual has a one in four chance of being affected ($\frac{1}{2} \times \frac{1}{2}$), unless the proband is a new mutant.

Carrier detection of X-linked traits is extremely important, especially for the sisters and maternal aunts of affected males. Carrier detection is possible for certain X-linked traits, such as hemophilia, Duchenne muscular dystrophy and the Hunter syndrome. One can often detect the carrier state in a woman at risk, but one can never completely rule it out (due to the Lyon hypothesis).

When there is only one affected male in the family, the possibility of a new mutation must be considered. If the affected child is the result of a new mutation, then neither his mother nor his sisters are carriers and their chances of having affected offspring are negligible. If the mother is a carrier, then both the mother's and the sisters' future children are at risk. In those X-linked disorders in which affected individuals rarely reproduce (e.g., muscular dystrophy), approximately one-third of the sporadic cases are the result of a new mutation, and in the remaining two-thirds the mother is a carrier. In those disorders in which reproduction is only partially reduced or normal (e.g., nephrogenic diabetes insipidus and color blindness), affected males transmit the mutant X chromosome to all of their daughters, and the ratio of inherited cases to new mutant cases is much higher.

The Lyon hypothesis has important implications in counseling for X-linked traits. Briefly, this hypothesis states that in any one cell only one X chromosome is active. Thus, in a normal male (46 XY) the one X chromosome is always active, whereas in a normal female (46 XX) or in a Klinefelter's male (47 XXY), in each cell only one X chromosome is active, the other being inactivated. The decision as to which X chromosome is inactivated in each cell is made early in fetal life. All the daughter cells of each of these primordial cells have the same X chromosome inactivated. In carrier females, half of the cells on the average would have the mutant X active, and in the other half the normal X would be active. The proportion of mutant to normal X chromosomes inactivated, however, follows a normal distribution. Thus, in some cases almost all of the cells have the mutant X active; whereas at the other end of the curve, almost all of the cells have the mutant X inactivated. Those heterozygous females in whom the normal X chromosome is inactivated in almost all cells are clinically affected. Girls with only one X chromosome (45 XO Turner's syndrome) also completely express X-linked traits with only one mutant gene. Thus, a female hemophiliac could either be homozygous for the mutant, be heterozygous and have all of the normal alleles inactivated, or have Turner's syndrome as well and thus only one gene at the hemophilia locus. This random inactivation of the X chromosome in carrier females results in a mosaic phenotype in those disorders, in which the effects of the mutant can be visually identified. For example, in carriers of optic albinism, one can see a stippled fundus, the pigmented cells having the normal X active, whereas in the nonpigmented cells the mutant X is active. When dealing with carrier detection of X-linked recessive traits, one cannot completely rule out the carrier state, as an apparently normal female might, by chance, have the abnormal X inactivated in most of her cells and thus be phenotypically normal.

X-linked Dominant Inheritance. X-linked dominant traits are due to mutant genes carried on the X chromosome, which are expressed in single dose. Thus, heterozygous females, as well as hemizygous males, are clinically affected. In general, heterozygous females are less severely affected than the males. For example, in vitamin D–resistant rickets, males are usually severely affected, whereas some females may be perfectly normal except for hypophosphatemia. Among the offspring of affected males, all of the sons are normal, while all of the daughters are affected. Among the offspring of affected females, approximately half of the sons and half of the daughters are affected. In view of this marked clinical variability in heterozygous females, it is extremely important to look for minor signs of the disease.

Risks in Chromosomal Syndromes

Chromosome abnormalities are found in about 30 per cent of first-trimester spontaneous abortions, in 0.5 to 1 per cent of all newborns and in 5 to 10 per cent of the severely mentally retarded with congenital malformations. In general, they represent sporadic occurrences with a low risk for recurrence in other family members; in a few instances, such as in inherited translocations, they may be associated with higher recurrence risks.

Down's Syndrome. Down's syndrome (mongolism) is the most common chromosome disorder for which counseling is requested. The majority of patients have regular trisomy 21 with 47 chromosomes. About 5 per cent have 46 chromosomes and carry a translocation involving chromosomes of group D or group G with a no. 21 chromosome, i.e., t(D/21) or t(G/21). These translocations may be further classified as: (1) inherited, i.e., the translocation can be identified in a phenotypically normal parent, and (2) sporadic, in which the parents have normal chromosomes and it is assumed that the translocation was initially formed in one parental gamete and represents a new chromosome mutation. It is important for genetic counseling that the translocation be identified as inherited or sporadic;

inherited translocations carry an increased risk for recurrence; sporadic translocations have a low recurrence rate.

The frequency of regular trisomy 21 Down's syndrome rises sharply with increased maternal age. For example, a 21-year-old woman has a risk of about 1/1600 for having a trisomy 21 child; whereas the risk for a 40-year-old woman is approximately 1/100. Indeed, approximately one-half of Down's syndrome patients are born to women 34 years of age or older. The relative frequencies of inherited and sporadic translocations and regular trisomy are also correlated with maternal age at the time of birth of the affected child. If the child with Down's syndrome is born at a maternal age of less than 30 years, the overall probability for an inherited translocation in the affected child is about 1 in 50 (2 per cent). Among affected infants born to mothers 30 years or older, the probability is about 1 in 333 (0.3 per cent).

In families with two affected sibs, about three-quarters of these sib groups have regular trisomy and the remainder have inherited translocations or mosaicism. The explanation for recurrence of an affected child with regular trisomy is not known. In some families it may represent a random risk; in others, unknown genetic or environmental factors may be operating to cause repeated nondisjunction.

Other Autosomal Trisomy Syndromes. Recurrence risks in the trisomy 13 and 18 syndromes are small. Accurate figures are not available, but certainly the empiric risks are less than 1 per cent. Sporadic as well as inherited translocations involving the no. 18 chromosome, or the D_1 (no. 13) chromosome are described; again, insufficient data are available to determine accurate recurrence rates. They are probably low for sporadic translocations and increased for inherited translocations.

Autosomal Deletion Syndromes. The autosomal deletion syndromes, including the cat cry syndrome (partial deletion, short arm, no. 5 chromosome) and syndromes associated with deletions of the short or long arms of a no. 18 chromosome may occur as sporadic or inherited events. About 10 per cent of patients with the cat cry (cri du chat) syndromes have a parent who is a carrier of a balanced translocation. Thus, chromosome analysis of the parents is necessary to provide information for recurrence risks. The finding of normal parental karyotypes suggests a low risk; evidence that the parent carries the chromosome abnormality in a balanced form suggests a high risk.

Sex Chromosomes. Individuals with abnormal sex chromosome complements may request information on their reproductive ability, as well as on their probability of having normal children. For patients with an XO complement (Turner's syndrome) and streak gonads, sterility is almost always present. In the XXY male (Klinefelter's syndrome), sterility is usually associated with azoospermia. Females with an XXX complement have normal fertility, and with few exceptions all offspring have normal chromosome complements. Familial aggregation of all of these sex chromosome anomalies is extremely rare.

Risks in Congenital Defects and Common Diseases

Congenital malformations, nonspecific mental retardation, allergy, essential hypertension and other such anomalies represent a group of disorders in which probably polygenic as well as environmental factors play a role. Generally, an empiric risk estimate is applied to these disorders. As a general rule, the risk for a normal couple, with one affected child with any of these common congenital defects, of having a second similarly affected child ranges from 2 to 5 per cent. Undoubtedly, with some of these disorders, the apparent same disease may have different etiologies; thus, recurrence risk figures must be interpreted with caution. Affected children should be carefully examined for other malformations to rule out a simply inherited complex syndrome.

It is not enough to quote genetic risk figures to a couple without advising them of the possible courses of action they might take. Furthermore, the manner and context of the counseling must be tempered by the social, religious and psychiatric background of the family. Individuals who wish to avoid having further children after learning of their risks should be given comprehensive contraceptive and family planning guidance. Without implementing the means of prevention, counseling is wasted. Provision of information concerning adoption agencies in the community will open another alternative to those individuals who wish to raise a family. The counselor should also discuss with the parents the possibilities of institutionalizing mentally retarded children, since this will help allay guilt reactions in the parents if and when institutionalization is considered. It is also important to allay parental guilt feelings concerning the cause of the child's malformation. Mothers often think back to some accident or indiscretion during their pregnancy which they think may have caused the disorder. In this situation it is worthwhile mentioning that every couple has a 2 to 3 per cent risk of having a defective child, and the occurrence of a new mutation or the mating of two heterozygous individuals usually cannot be predicted in advance or avoided.

Although many geneticists insist that only mathematical risk figures be quoted to the parents, who then make their own decision, it is important to interpret the risk figures in terms meaningful to the counsultors and to help them reach a solution. The manner in which the risk figures are presented can certainly influence the parents' decision. For example, the parents of a phenylketonuric child may react quite differently if they are told they have a 75 per cent chance of having normal children, than if they are told there is a one in four chance of having a similarly retarded child. In many instances, the parents will approach the counselor with unfounded fears concerning the birth of a malformed child. A couple who has had one child with anencephaly may decide not to have further offspring, when in fact the risk of recurrence is only 4 per cent. The role of the counselor in reassuring such parents that the chance of having other affected children is slim is an important and rewarding task.

Carter has analyzed the results of genetic counseling in his London clinic. Of 74 females who were given a high risk of recurrence (greater than 10 per cent), 68 per cent were deterred from having further children. Carter felt that the major weakness of the counseling procedure was the failure to reassure some of the parents with low risk of recurrence (less than 10 per cent), since 25 per cent of them decided against having more offspring. These results document the value of the counseling session to parents of children with hereditary diseases and stress the importance of reassuring those parents in whom the risk of recurrence is relatively slim. The impact and accuracy of counseling significantly changes, of course, when prenatal diagnosis is available.

PREVENTION OF GENETIC DISEASE

Recognition of High-Risk Individuals. One aspect of preventive genetics is the recognition of individuals who have a high risk of developing a hereditary disorder. Prompt diagnosis will often allow for the implementation of the proper therapeutic regimen before irreversible sequelae of the disorder occur. The two major areas of importance are the antepartum or neonatal diagnosis of recessively inherited metabolic disorders, and the early recognition of those disorders in which neoplastic degeneration may be a phenotypic component.

Early diagnosis of many of the inborn errors of metabolism, such as phenylketonuria and galactosemia, will allow for the immediate institution of elimination diets which may prevent otherwise certain mental retardation. Likewise, early diagnosis and treatment of the salt-losing variety of the adrenogenital syndrome may prevent neonatal death. Parents who have had a child with a recessively inherited inborn error of metabolism must, therefore, be closely followed, and each subsequent offspring should be examined shortly after birth for evidence of the specific metabolic error.

Follow-up of high-risk individuals is also important in those genetic disorders in which malignant neoplasms may be a component, e.g., multiple polyposis of the colon, the Gardner syndrome, multiple endocrine adenomatosis and basal cell nevus syndrome. Most of the genetic disorders associated with neoplasia are inherited as autosomal dominant traits, and thus all offspring of affected individuals should be regularly examined for any stigmata of the syndrome. Furthermore, any individual with one component of a genetic syndrome known to be associated with neoplasia should be carefully examined for its other manifestations, e.g., in all individuals with multiple exostosis of the jaw and sebaceous cysts suggestive of the Gardner syndrome, sigmoidoscopy and barium enemas should be performed to rule out colonic polyposis. Early detection of these syndromes may allow for lifesaving preventive surgery.

Intrauterine Diagnosis. A major advance in the counseling and prevention of genetic disease was the development of techniques for prenatal diagnosis. By an established obstetric technique known as transabdominal amniocentesis, a small sample of amniotic fluid can be removed from the uterus at about the third to fourth month of pregnancy. From this fluid, cells which originate in the fetus can be collected and grown in the laboratory and the genetic constitution of the fetus studied. Although not all genetic parameters can be assessed by such methods, many serious genetic diseases can now be detected in the growing fetus early in pregnancy.

For families who are fearful of even attempting a pregnancy because of the high risk of having offspring with a severe genetic disease, this technique offers an important new alternative. By monitoring the pregnancy with amniocentesis and appropriate genetic study, the fetus can be evaluated with regard to certain specific genetic characteristics. If a genetically abnormal fetus is identified, one who would suffer with an untreatable and serious genetic disease, the family can elect, within the current social and legal structure in most states, to terminate the pregnancy. Where families are at high risk for such conditions in their offspring, this alternative provides a mechanism by which the couple can have its own children, without fearing the birth of an affected child. A number of severe and currently untreatable chromosomal or metabolic errors have been successfully identified in the fetus before the 20th week of gestation in this manner (Table 1).

With regard to chromosomal abnormalities like Down's syndrome, it has been well established that the risk for this disorder (and for most other chromosomal derangements as well) is greatly increased as the age of the woman increases at the time she becomes pregnant. Since the chromosomal makeup of the fetus can readily be determined by intrauterine diagnostic techniques, it has been suggested that pregnant women over 35 years of age be informed about these risks and about the alternative of intrauterine studies.

It must be strongly emphasized that this alternative be considered on a totally individual basis. For certain families this approach may be a worthwhile consideration, whereas for others it is not acceptable. We must allow for differences in individuals' beliefs and religious attitudes, both of which may strongly affect their response to such a program. In addition, it should be pointed out that the birth of a child with mongolism or some other chromosomal abnormality may not, for some families, be a tragic event. Such children can often achieve a level of happiness and love within their own families, and for this reason, the consideration of terminating a pregnancy in which such a fetus has been identified should clearly be a decision carefully considered by the family involved.

For single-gene disorders, the possibility of prospective prevention can also be raised. Certain sex-linked recessive diseases, such as the Lesch-Nyhan syndrome, can be detected by prenatal diagnostic studies. For women who carry such a sex-linked recessive gene (females in pedigrees where the disease has occurred are at increased risk of carrying the gene), the risk of having an affected son with each pregnancy (50 per cent) often prohibits such women from childbearing. Since intrauterine diagnostic studies can identify the affected male in this condition, or the male versus female fetus for other sex-linked conditions, some families have taken the alternative of prenatal diagnosis so that they can have offspring without fearing a recurrence of serious genetic disease in their child. In families in which Duchenne muscular dystrophy or classical hemophilia has occurred, females can at times be evaluated to determine whether they carry the X-linked gene for these conditions. Such women, of course, are normal, but if they do carry the gene their risk of having an affected child is as outlined previously. By carrier detection, the carrier female, once identified, can be given the alternative of fetal sex determination.

With autosomal recessive conditions, where both parents must be carriers of the same gene for there to be a risk, the problem is somewhat more complex. There are certain genetic disorders which tend to occur in certain population groups. This is because certain populations have selectively intermarried within the

TABLE 1. Genetic-Metabolic Disorders Detected Antenatally in the Midtrimester Human Fetus

DISORDER	ABNORMALITY IN AMNIOTIC FLUID CELLS
Chromosomal aberrations	abnormal karyotoype
Fabry's disease	deficient α-galactosidase activity
Galactosemia	deficient galactase-1-phosphate uridyl transferase activity
Gaucher's disease	deficient glucocerebrosidase activity
Glycogen storage disease, type II (Pompe's disease)	deficient α-1, 4-glucosidase activity
GM_1 gangliosidosis, type I (generalized gangliosidosis)	total acid β-galactosidase deficiency
Hunter's syndrome (MPS II)	abnormal kinetics of $^{35}SO_4$ incorporation
Hurler's syndrome (MPS I)	abnormal kinetics of $^{35}SO_4$ incorporation
Krabbe's disease (globoid leukodystrophy)	deficient cerebroside-β-galactosidase activity
Lesch-Nyhan syndrome	deficient hypoxanthine incorporation, deficient HGPRTase activity
Lysosomal acid phosphatase deficiency	deficient acid phosphatase activity
Maple syrup urine disease	deficient branched-chain keto acid decarboxylase activity
Metachromatic leukodystrophy	deficient aryl sulfatase-A activity
Methylmalonic aciduria	deficient methylmalonyl coenzyme A isomerase activity
Niemann-Pick disease	deficient sphingomyelinase activity
Tay-Sachs disease	deficient hexosaminidase-A activity

same population over the centuries. This results in the proliferation of certain recessive genes within the selected population. Several examples of this kind of predilection for specific genetic disorders in specific groups are well known. Sickle cell anemia in individuals of African ancestry, Tay-Sachs disease in Jews of central and eastern European origin and Thalassemia in individuals of Mediterranean background are typical examples of this phenomenon. For the most part, intrauterine diagnosis and prevention of serious genetic disease of this type is usually available only after a family has been identified as being at risk by having had an affected child. However, there are certain conditions were prospective prevention can be considered.

If a recessive genetic disease occurs predominantly in a specified population, if there is a simple, accurate and inexpensive means for detecting the individual who carries the recessive gene and if there is a means for early fetal detection of the untreatable disease, a prospective prevention approach is possible. At this time, Tay-Sachs disease meets these requirements and is the first recessive genetic disease which can be prevented in this way.

By screening individuals of child-bearing age in the at-risk population only, it should be possible to identify the infrequent couple in which both husband and wife carry the same recessive gene. These would constitute the only couples at-risk for the disease in their offspring, and they could be identified in this way even before the birth of an affected child. Since intrauterine diagnosis of Tay-Sachs disease is feasible, such couples, once identified, could be availed this alternative so that they could still reproduce without fearing the birth of a child with Tay-Sachs disease (a uniformly fatal and untreatable condition at this time).

For other recessive disorders, where intrauterine detection is not yet available, premarital screening for heterozygous carriers and follow-up counseling regarding marital and reproductive alternatives can provide an effective means of disease prevention. This is the basis for the wide-scale screening programs for sickle cell trait which have recently been established. As heterozygote screening becomes feasible for additional conditions, similar programs are likely to evolve.

Intrauterine diagnosis with selective abortion, or carrier detection with inherent restrictions of mate selection or reproduction, are both less than perfect means for preventing genetic disease. Clearly, effective treatment or even genetic cure for such conditions would be a far better alternative. These ultimate goals should maintain highest priority, with the aforementioned approaches utilized primarily as interim measures.

An understanding of basic genetic concepts, coupled with knowledge of recently developed technologies, provides important new considerations for physicians in many specialties of medicine. Certainly, the pediatrician can provide the focus for bringing a wide variety of optimal genetic services to substantial numbers of patients and their families.

References

Bergsma, D. (Ed.): Intrauterine Diagnosis and Selective Abortion. *Birth Defects: Original Article Series,* Vol. VII, No. 5, April, 1971. The National Foundation–March of Dimes.

Carter, C. O., et al.: Genetic Clinic: A Follow-up. *Lancet,* 1:281, 1971.

Harris, H. (ed.): *Early Diagnosis of Human Genetic Defects: Scientific and Ethical Considerations.* Fogarty International Center Proceedings, No. 6, Washington, D. C., U.S. Government Printing Office, 1971.

Lappe, M., et al.: Ethical and Social Issues in Screening for Genetic Disease. *New England J. Med.,* 286: 1129–1132, 1972.

McKusick, V. A.: *Human Genetics.* 2nd ed. Englewood Cliffs, New Jersey, Prentice-Hall, Inc., 1969.

Smith, D. W.: *Recognizable Patterns of Human Malformation.* Philadelphia, W. B. Saunders Company, 1970.

Stanbury, J. B., Wyngaarden, J. B., and Fredrickson, D. S.: *The Metabolic Basis of Inherited Disease.* 3rd ed. New York, The McGraw-Hill Book Company, 1972.

Drug Abuse and the Adolescent

IRA M. FRANK, M.D., *and*
J. THOMAS UNGERLEIDER, M.D.

The increasing availability of drugs means that a large number of persons will be exposed to illicit drugs, many will experiment and, of these, a small percentage will become serious users or addicts. As a result, the number of acute drug reactions is increasing accordingly. The increasing tendency toward multiple drug abuse has made diagnosis and treatment of drug reactions an even greater challenge for the physician. Moreover, acute drug reactions are often superimposed on chronic drug dependence which may lead to withdrawal symptoms during the patient's hospitalization.

IDENTIFICATION OF THE DRUG

Your patient will usually reveal what drug he has taken when you point out to him that you need the information to help him. Sometimes, however, he may not know himself what he has taken or he may believe that he has taken one drug while he has actually taken a different drug. For example, drugs which are sold as mescaline, tetrahydrocannabinol (THC) or other exotic substances are almost always found on analysis to contain LSD or LSD mixed with a stimulant such as strychnine or methedrine for an extra kick. He may have taken an impure drug or a mixture of drugs. Thus, even if your patient tells you what he thinks he has taken, he may actually have taken something else. In addition, your patient may be unable to reveal what he has taken because he is confused, disoriented or comatose.

A good medical and psychiatric history is essential, since drug abusers may suffer from malnutrition, hepatitis, abscesses, venereal disease, neuroses, schizophrenia or character disorders. Emotional stress, such as a significant loss or change in life situation, is frequently associated with suicide attempts and "unintentional overdoses."

Friends and relatives should be contacted to provide additional information. They should be there when the patient awakens. A patient who recovers from an overdose to find that he is all alone may become an even greater suicidal risk. In addition, help from friends and relatives may be invaluable in arranging a satisfactory disposition and providing for follow-up care. If the police or ambulance brings the patient to the physician, the persons involved should be questioned about the circumstances at the scene and if any pills, bottles or suicide notes were found.

DIFFERENTIAL DIAGNOSIS

Pupil signs may be helpful. LSD, amphetamines and cocaine cause dilated pupils that are responsive to light and accommodation. Barbiturates tend to produce slight constriction of the pupils, but as the degree of coma deepens the pupils dilate. Belladonna derivatives, such as Asthmador, cause fully dilated pupils which are unresponsive to light or to accommodation. Heroin, in contrast, produces pinpoint pupillary constriction. Although the patient's vital signs are not diagnostic, they are invaluable in determining the patient's initial condition and his subsequent progress. The amphetamine user, like the heroin addict, may have needle marks along his arms, thighs or abdomen, in contrast to the LSD user or the barbiturate user. This is not always reliable, however, as amphetamine "freaks," for example, frequently use barbiturates (or heroin) to "crash." (See Table 1.)

The patient's behavior is also revealing. The barbiturate user may appear "dopey," with inappropriate euphoria, wavering gait, slurred speech, confusion, disorientation and impaired memory and concentration. He will appear to be drunk but there will either be no odor of alcohol on his breath or, if he has also been drinking, the state of intoxication will be out of proportion to the odor of alcohol on his breath. The LSD user may show inappropriate behavior and conversation will sometimes be very difficult. The amphetamine user may also be talkative, hyperactive, restless, tremulous and potentially violent. He may present with a clinical picture sometimes indistinguishable from that of acute paranoid schizophrenia, with paranoid delusions, loose association, inappropriate affect and auditory and visual hallucinations. A urine sample should be analyzed, since amphetamines may be detected in the urine for up to 36 hours. His sensorium will be clear in contrast to that of the alcoholic, the barbiturate user or the heroin addict undergoing withdrawal who may present with a toxic delirium consisting of clouding of consciousness, hallucinations, tremors and convulsions.

The definitive diagnosis must often await the report of a sample of blood, urine or gastric contents. Since this usually takes hours to days, treatment often must be determined by the condition of the patient rather than by knowledge of the specific drug(s) involved. There are several exceptions in which specific treatment is available, however, such as the use of narcotic antagonists in patients who have taken an overdose of narcotics.

MARIJUANA

Marijuana smokers rarely seek medical attention. Acute anxiety attacks are usually mild and respond to psychologic support. A supportive friend or relative should remain with the patient in a quiet room and reassure him that he is having a self-limited reaction which will subside when the effects of the drug wear off. The patient should not be left alone. Valium, 10 mg. orally will help calm the patient. When marijuana is ingested, the user may become nauseated, vomit, have diarrhea or abdominal reactions; panic reactions tend to last longer and to be more intense than when marijuana is smoked, since the smoker can "titrate" his dose of marijuana to reach his optimum "high" or level of intoxication.

LSD

Although the use of LSD has markedly declined, drugs which are sold as mescaline,

TABLE 1. Intervention for Various Stages of Drug Use

ADVERSE REACTION	DIAGNOSTIC CLUES	EXPERIMENTATION	FREQUENT USE	DEPENDENCE (COMPULSIVE USE)	TREATMENT FOR ACUTE OVERDOSE
Marijuana	Anxiety, panic, distortion of time sense; conjunctival injection; tachycardia	↑	↑	—	Psychologic support
LSD	Pupils widely dilated; agitated, occasionally disoriented, confused, paranoid, assaultive	↑	↑	—	Psychologic support; avoid physical restraint if possible; Valium, 10–20 mg. P.O. or I.M. (see text), or Thorazine, 25–100 mg. P.O. or I.M.
Amphetamines and cocaine	Pupils dilated, may have needle marks, jaundice, abscesses; hyperactive, may be agitated, paranoid, potentially violent; similar to acute paranoid schizophrenia; amphetamines in urine	Preventive educational programs	Psychotherapy, family therapy, peer group therapy, drug-free residential treatment setting	Psychotherapy, drug-free residential treatment program	Same as LSD; acidification of urine
Barbiturates and sedatives	Pupils widely constricted and dilate as coma deepens; appears drunk or stuporous to comatose; may subsequently develop withdrawal syndrome	↓	↓	Withdraw very gradually, over two weeks, then psychotherapy, drug-free treatment setting	Support respiration and circulation; vasopressors, dialysis or alkalinization may be necessary; psychotherapy
Heroin	Pupils pinpoint, stuporous to comatose, needle marks, jaundice, abscesses; may subsequently develop withdrawal syndrome	↓	↓	Withdraw over one week with methadone, then psychotherapy, drug-free residential setting or methadone maintenance program	Support respiration and circulation; Nalline; drug-free residential treatment setting or methadone maintenance program

psilicybin, THC and so forth are usually found to contain LSD when analyzed. Illicit LSD today may be impure, and sometimes is mixed with methedrine, strychnine, cocaine and other drugs. Acute LSD reactions may present with varying combinations of anxiety or panic, depression, confusion and disorientation, hallucinations and paranoia. Psychologic support is essential and may be all that is required. Physical restraint should be avoided unless absolutely necessary, since this increases the patient's anxiety and paranoia. Hospitalization is sometimes necessary, although the usual LSD reaction subsides within 24 to 72 hours. Valium, 10 to 20 mg. orally or intramuscularly,* usually gives relief, although Thorazine, 25 to 100 mg. orally or intramuscularly, may be necessary. A second dose, preferably smaller than the first, may be administered in 1 hour if the patient is still very agitated.

Flashbacks are recurrences of the original LSD experience and may occur months after LSD ingestion. Usually they are brief and attenuated. They are frequently associated with psychologic stress and often with smoking marijuana. Patients should be cautioned against using other drugs, and Valium, 10 mg. orally, or Thorazine, 25 mg. orally, may be taken at the first sign of a flashback. Psychotherapy is often helpful. Occasionally an LSD reaction will precipitate a paranoid schizophrenia which may require hospitalization. This schizophrenic reaction, in contrast to flashbacks, is continuous with the LSD reaction and treated in the usual fashion.

Valium is a very safe drug to use, even though the drug(s) ingested may not be known. Since Valium and Thorazine may react synergistically with the ingested drug, the danger of hypotensive reactions must be kept in mind and the blood pressure and pulse should be taken frequently. Pressor agents, such as norepinephrine or phenylephrine, should be available (avoid epinephrine, which may produce a paradoxical hypotensive reaction).

AMPHETAMINES AND COCAINE

Acute amphetamine or cocaine intoxication may present with paranoid feelings, anxiety, agitation, hyperactivity, palpitations, possible assaultiveness, angina pectoris, headaches, nausea and abdominal cramps. It is best managed with psychologic support, physical restraint (only where absolutely necessary) and Valium or Thorazine. The doses are similar to those used in treating an LSD reaction. Acidification of the urine with ammonium chloride will greatly facilitate excretion of amphetamines. Emesis or gastric lavage, followed by a saline cathartic, will eliminate residual drugs remaining in the gastrointestinal tract. Cardiovascular and respiratory functions should be carefully monitored, and hypertension, hypotension, cardiac arrhythmia, respiratory depression or shock should be promptly treated in the usual fashion. A psychiatric evaluation is frequently indicated and hospitalization is often necessary. The chronic amphetamine abuser may also be suffering from weight loss, malnutrition, vitamin deficiencies, abscesses at the injection sites, hepatitis or venereal disease.

BARBITURATES AND SEDATIVES

The acute barbiturate or sedative overdose may present a very serious medical emergency requiring hospital facilities. Pressor agents, such as norepinephrine, should be available to manage cardiovascular collapse. Respiration may have to be assisted, a tracheostomy performed and oxygen administered. An endotracheal tube should be inflated to prevent aspiration in a comatose patient and to maintain a patent airway. The stomach should be aspirated, the initial gastric aspirate saved for analysis and a saline cathartic left in the stomach to speed the passage of substances through the gastrointestinal tract. Vital signs, blood gases, blood chemistries, chest x-rays and urine output should be closely monitored to detect possible pneumonia, atelectasis, renal failure or cardiovascular collapse. Hemodialysis, peritoneal dialysis and alkalinization of the urine with sodium bicarbonate or sodium lactate and urea may be necessary to facilitate excretion of the drug.

If a barbiturate is superimposed on a chronic barbiturate dependence, the patient may subsequently develop a severe withdrawal reaction. Within hours after the patient's sensorium has cleared from the toxic effects of the barbiturates, he may begin to feel restless, anxious, apprehensive and weak. He then develops muscle twitches, tremors, headache, insomnia, orthostatic hypotension and abdominal cramps and begins to vomit. These symptoms of central nervous system hyperirritability become very severe within the first 24 to 48 hours and frequently culminate in grand mal seizures.

* The *Physician's Desk Reference* and the package insert recommend a dosage range for Valium of 5 to 10 mg. by oral, intramuscular, or intravenous administration for treatment of moderate to severe anxiety. A maximum intravenous dose of 15 mg. is recommended for cardioversion. In our experience and in the experiences of other physicians who treat acute drug reactions, oral or intramuscular administration of up to 20 mg. is both effective and safe.

In severe untreated withdrawal from barbiturates, the patient may develop a delirium which resembles delirium tremens, with confusion, disorientation, vivid auditory, visual and tactile hallucinations, paranoid delusions and gross tremors. This delirium may last several days and culminate in severe exhaustion. Death may occur from status epilepticus, exhaustion or cardiovascular collapse.

Treatment of withdrawal symptoms consists of administering a shortacting barbiturate, such as pentobarbital, 200 to 400 mg., orally or parenterally at the first signs of a withdrawal reaction (anxiety, nervousness, nausea and tremor), usually in a hospital setting. This dose is repeated every hour until the symptoms subside and the patient is mildly intoxicated, manifesting mild ataxia, nystagmus and slurred speech. This dose of pentobarbital is then administered four times per day until the patient is stable, then reduced by not more than 100 mg. per day. If signs of withdrawal again appear, the dose is temporarily increased.

HEROIN

Acute heroin overdoses are increasingly more common and may be fatal. The heroin user may be identified by the pinpoint constriction of his pupils and the needle tracks on his arms, thighs and abdomen. Treatment is supportive, assisting respiratory and cardiovascular function whenever necessary as discussed under the treatment of acute barbiturate reaction. A narcotic-antagonist, such as Nalline, may be required; the dose may have to be repeated if the patient lapses back into respiratory depression. As with an acute reaction to barbiturates, withdrawal symptoms may appear after recovering from an overdose of heroin; these are treated with oral methadone.

Heroin addicts may be humanely and effectively withdrawn with methadone over a period of one to two weeks. This should be done (and in some states must be done) in an inpatient setting with a physician and nursing staff experienced in methadone withdrawal. The patient should then be transferred to a residential treatment setting which specializes in long-term rehabilitation. Methadone maintenance programs have proved very effective for the hardcore heroin user who has repeatedly failed in other rehabilitation efforts. "Blockading" daily doses of methadone abolish the heroin hunger and remove the "high" from injected heroin.

This type of program can eliminate the criminal activity associated with heroin addiction, so that the addict can then concentrate his efforts on taking care of himself and his family. More important, however, is that the patient is dependent on the doctors, nurses and community aides rather than the pusher. This relationship permits day-to-day contact with the patient so that any crisis can be immediately detected and the staff can intervene. It also permits close follow-up of patients and availability of rehabilitation services, such as employment assistance, family therapy, group therapy, social work intervention, educational and vocational training. Nonetheless, since methadone is a narcotic the patient will continue to be drug-dependent and addicted, and methadone maintenance should therefore be reserved for the addict who has tried to "kick" his habit repeatedly without success. It has only rarely been used in persons under 18 years of age, but some programs have lower age limits for entry, as well as requirements regarding the number of years of addiction and failures in other programs.

MEDICOLEGAL CONSIDERATIONS

We believe that the physician's primary responsibility is to his patient, and that unless the physician feels that his patient is in imminent danger of hurting himself or someone else, he is medically and ethically obligated to do nothing to harm his patient. Thus, except in unusual circumstances, we believe that the physician should make no attempt to report a patient to law enforcement officials. If, on the other hand, the police already know that the patient is being treated for a drug abuse problem, such as in cases where the patient has been brought into the hospital by the police, the physician is obligated to cooperate with the police to the extent that he makes the patient available to be interviewed, when he feels that the patient is fully oriented, alert and capable of protecting his civil rights. Statements made to the physician during the course of evaluation and treatment are protected by medical confidentiality, and the physician is neither required nor authorized to reveal this information without an informed release signed by the patient. Moreover, we believe that this umbrella of medical confidentiality extends to all medical and paramedical personnel, including ambulance attendants, nurses, aides and the hospital administration.

FOLLOW-UP CARE

Every patient who presents with an acute drug reaction should be evaluated by a psychiatrist before being discharged. The family should be contacted to provide additional information and to assist in disposition and follow-up. A sympathetic and supportive (not permissive) attitude should be encouraged. No "accidental" overdose or "suicide gesture" should be casually dismissed as "only a manipulation." Family therapy is frequently very effective. The chronic user or addict may have to be referred to a drug-free residential setting if separation from his family is indicated. The chronic heroin or barbiturate user may have to be withdrawn gradually, over a period of several weeks, in a hospital setting. The withdrawal reaction from barbiturate addiction may be especially severe, with possible convulsions, status epilepticus and, occasionally, death.

25

Roster of Drugs

A

Aarane. See *Chromolyn sodium.*

Acetaminophen (Tempra, Tylenol). Drops (15 ml.): 60 mg. per 0.6 ml. Elixir (60, 125 ml., pts.): 24 mg. per ml. Syrup (250 ml.): 24 mg. per ml. Tablets (24, 100): 300 mg. Tablets, chewable: 120 mg.

Acetazolamide (Diamox). Capsules, sustained release (30, 100): 500 mg. Tablets (100): 125, 250 mg.

Acetazolamide sodium (Diamox sodium). Vials, powder: 500 mg.

Acetest. Tablets (100, 250): sodium nitroprusside, disodium phosphate, aminoacetic acid, lactose.

Acetosulfone sodium (Promacetin). Tablets (500): 500 mg.

Acetylcysteine (Mucomyst). Vials (10, 30 ml.): 10, 20%.

Acetylpenicillamine (N-Acetyl-DL-penicillamine). Powder (1, 5 Gm.). Not available in the United States.

Acetylsalicylic acid (Aspirin). Suppositories (12): 60, 75, 125, 150, 200, 300, 600 mg. Tablets, flavored (36): 75 mg. Tablets (100): 300 mg. Tablets, enteric coated (100): 300, 600 mg.

Achromycin. See *Tetracycline hydrochloride.*

Achromycin with hydrocortisone. See *Tetracycline hydrochloride with hydrocortisone.*

Acnaveen. Cream (120 Gm.). Bar (115 Gm.). 2% sulfur, 2% salicylic acid, 1% hexachlorophene, 8% colloidal oatmeal.

Acne-Aid. Lotion (30, 60 ml.): 10% sulfur, 10% alcohol.

ACTH. Vials, powder: 25, 40 units. Vials, solution (2, 10 ml.): 20 units per ml.

ACTH gel (Depo-ACTH, HP Acthar gel). Vials (1, 5 ml.): 40, 80 units per ml.

Acthar HP gel. See *ACTH.*

Actifed. Syrup (pt.): 6 mg. pseudoephedrine hydrochloride and 0.25 mg. triprolidine hydrochloride per ml. Tablets (100): 60 mg. pseudoephedrine hydrochloride and 2.5 mg. triprolidine hydrochloride.

Actinomycin D. See *Dactinomycin.*

Activated charcoal. Powder (125 Gm., lb.).

Adenine arabinoside. Investigational.

Adrenalin hydrochloride. See *Epinephrine hydrochloride.*

Adrenalin in oil. See *Epinephrine.*

AD 3200. See *Pregestamil.*

Adriamycin (Doxorubicin). Investigational.

Adroyd. See *Oxymetholone.*

A-Fil. Cream (45 Gm.): 5% menthyl anthranilate and 5% titanium oxide. Sun stick (2 Gm.): 2.5% digalloyl trioleate.

Afrin. See *Oxymetazoline hydrochloride.*

Akineton. See *Biperiden hydrochloride.*

Akineton lactate. See *Biperiden lactate.*

Albumaid XP. Powder (2 kg.): obtained from Scientific Hospitals Supplies, Ltd., Liverpool, England.

Albumin. Vials, human, salt poor (20, 50 ml.): 25%. Solution, human, intravenous (250, 500 ml.): 5%.

Albutoin. Investigational. Flint Laboratories.

Alcohol, absolute ethyl. Ampules (2 ml.).

Alcopara. See *Bephenium hydroxynaphthoate.*

Aldactone. See *Spironolactone.*

Aldomet. See *Methyldopa.*

Aldomet ester hydrochloride. See *Methyldopate hydrochloride.*

Alidase. See *Hyaluronidase.*

Allbee. See *Vitamin B complex.*

Allopurinol (Zyloprim). Tablets (100): 100 mg.

Alma-Tar. Oil of cade (juniper tar). Lotion, bath (240 ml.): 35%. Shampoo (240 ml.): 4%.

Alpha Chymar. See *Alpha Chymotrypsin.*

Alpha-chymotrypsin (Alpha Chymar, Catarase, Zolyse). Powder, lyophilized ophthalmic: 750 units with 10 ml. special salt diluent. Powder, ophthalmic, 300 units with 2 ml. diluent.

Alpha-Keri (water-dispersible antipruritic oil). Solution (250 ml., 500 ml.). Spray (150 ml.).

Alpha-tocopherol. See *Vitamin E.*

Aluminum and magnesium hydroxides (Maalox). Suspension, oral (360 ml.): 80 mg. per ml. Tablets No. 1 (80, 100): 400 mg. Tablets No. 2 (24, 50, 100): 800 mg.

Aluminum hydroxide (Amphojel, etc.). Liquid gel (360 ml.): 65 mg. per ml. Tablets (100): 300 mg. Tablets (60): 600 mg.

Aluminum sulfate and calcium acetate. See *Domboro.*

Alupent. See *Orciprenaline sulfate.*

Amantadine hydrochloride (Symmetrel). Capsules (100): 100 mg. Syrup (pt.): 10 mg. per ml.

Ambilhar. See *Niridazole.*

Amethopterin. See *Methotrexate.*

Amethopterin sodium. See *Methotrexate sodium.*

Amicar. See *Aminocaproic acid.*

Amigen. See *Casein hydrolysate.*

Aminacrine. See *Aminoacridine hydrochloride.*

Aminosol. See *Fibrin hydrolysate.*

Ambenonium chloride (Mytelase). Tablets (100): 10, 25 mg.

Amino acids, crystalline (FreAmine). Solution (500 ml.): 8.5%, supplied with 1000-ml. bottle of dextrose 50% in water to make a 4.25% solution.

Aminoacridine hydrochloride (Vagisic Plus). Suppositories (28): 0.2%.

Aminocaproic acid (Amicar, EACA, Epsilon aminocaproic acid). Syrup (pt.): 250 mg. per ml. Tablets (100): 500 mg. Vials, intravenous (20 ml.): 250 mg. per ml.

Aminophylline. Ampules (2 ml.): 250 mg. per ml. Ampules (10 ml.): 25, 50 mg. per ml. Suppositories (12): 125, 250, 500 mg. Tablets (100): 100 mg., 200 mg.

Aminosalicylic acid (Pamisyl, PAS). Tablets (1000): 500 mg., 690 mg., 1 Gm.

Amitriptyline hydrochloride (Elavil hydrochloride). Tablets (100): 10, 25, 50 mg. Vials (10 ml.): 10 mg. per ml.

Ammoniated mercury. Ointment, ophthalmic (4 Gm.): 2.5%.

Ammonium chloride. Tablets (100): 300 mg. Tablets, enteric (100): 500 mg. and 1 Gm.

Amobarbital (Amytal). Elixir (pt.): 4, 8 mg. per ml. Tablets (100): 15, 30, 50, 100 mg.

Amobarbital sodium (Amytal sodium). Ampules, powder: 65, 125, 250, 500 mg. Capsules (100): 65, 200 mg.

Amodiaquin hydrochloride (Camoquin hydrochloride). Tablets (36): As the hydrochloride equal to 200 mg. of base.

Amphetamine sulfate (Benzedrine sulfate). Tablets (100): 5, 10 mg. Capsule, extended release (50): 15 mg.

Amphojel. See *Aluminum hydroxide.*

Amphotericin B (Fungizone). Cream (20 Gm.): 3%. Lotion (30 ml.): 3%. Ointment (20 Gm.): 3%. Vials, powder: 50 mg.

Ampicillin sodium (*Omnipen-N, Penbriten-S, Polycillin-N*). Vials, powder: 125, 250, 500 mg.; 1, 2, 4 Gm.

Ampicillin trihydrate (Omnipen, Penbritin, Polycillin). Capsules (16, 24, 100): 250, 500 mg. Suspension, oral (60, 80, 100, 150, 200 ml.) mg. per ml. Suspension (20 ml.): 100 mg. per ml. Tablets, chewable (40): 125 mg.

Amyl nitrite. Vials, fragile glass (12): 0.2, 0.3 ml.
Amytal. See *Amobarbital.*
Amytal sodium. See *Amobarbital sodium.*
Anadrol. See *Oxymetholone.*
Ancobon. See *Flucytosine.*
Anectine. See *Succinylcholine.*
Anhydrohydroxyprogesterone. See *Ethisterone.*
Ansolysen. See *Pentolinium tartrate.*
Antepar. See *Piperazine citrate.*
Anthralin. Ointment (45 Gm.): 0.1, 0.25, 0.5, 1.0%.
Antimony potassium tartrate (Tartar emetic). Injection not commercially available in United States.
Antimony sodium gluconate (Triostam). 35% antimony injection. Not commercially available in the United States.
Antiphen. See *Dichlorophen.*
Antirabies serum. Vials: 1000 units.
Antivenin, snake polyvalent. Vials (*Latrodectus mactans,* Black widow spider): one-dose vial to yield 2.5 ml. of restored horse serum. Vials (*crotalidae*): one vial to yield 10 ml. of restored horse serum.
Antrypol. See *Suramin.*
Anturane. See *Sulfinpyrazone.*
Apomorphine. Tablets, hypodermic (100): 6 mg.
Apresoline hydrochloride. See *Hydralazine hydrochloride.*
AquaMEPHYTON. See *Phytonadione.*
Aquaphor (Eucerite base). Ointment base (60 Gm., 1 lb.).
Aquasol A. See *Vitamin A.*
Aquasol E. See *Vitamin E.*
Aralen phosphate. See *Chloroquine phosphate.*
Aralen-Primaquine. See *Chloroquine-primaquine.*
Aramine bitartrate. See *Metaraminol bitartrate.*
Arasobal. See *Melarsoprol.*
Aristocort. See *Triamcinolone.*
Aristocort acetonide. See *Triamcinolone acetonide.*
Aristocort diacetate. See *Triamcinolone diacetate.*
Artane hydrochloride. See *Trihexyphenidyl hydrochloride.*
Arthropan. See *Choline salicylate.*
Artidil. See *Triprolidine.*
Artificial tears. See *Methylcellulose.*
Ascorbic acid. Ampules: 100, 500 mg. and 1 Gm. Tablets (100): 25, 50, 100, 250, 500 mg.
Aspirin. See *Acetylsalicylic acid.*
Astiban. See *Stibocaptate.*
Atabrine hydrochloride. See *Quinacrine hydrochloride.*
Atarax. See *Hydroxyzine hydrochloride.*
Atromid S. See *Clofibrate.*
Atropine sulfate. Ointment, sterile ophthalmic (4 Gm.): 0.5, 1%. Solution, sterile ophthalmic (15 ml.): 0.125, 0.25, 0.5, 1, 3%. Tablets (100): 0.3, 0.4, 0.6 mg. Vials (1, 20 ml.): 0.4 mg. per ml.
Aureomycin calcium. See *Chlortetracycline calcium.*
Aureomycin hydrochloride. See *Chlortetracycline hydrochloride.*
Aurothiglucose (Solganal). Vial (10 ml.): 50, 100 mg. per ml.
Aveeno (Colloidal oatmeal). Powder (1, 4 lb.). Packets (90 Gm.). Bar, soap-free (100 Gm.). Lotion: 180 ml.
Avenol. Bath oil (250 ml.).
Avlosulfon. See *Dapsone.*
Azathioprine (Imuran). Tablets (100): 100 mg.
Azauridine. Investigational.
Azulfidine. See *Salicylazosulfapyridine.*

B

Bacimycin. See *Bacitracin-neomycin.*
Baciquent. See *Bacitracin.*
Bacitracin (Baciquent). Ointment (15, 30 Gm.): 500 units per Gm. Ointment, ophthalmic (4 Gm.): 500 units per Gm. Vials, powder: 10,000, 50,000 units.
Bacitracin-neomycin (Bacimycin). Ointment (15 Gm.): 500 units bacitracin and 5 mg. neomycin sulfate per Gm.
BAL. See *Dimercaprol.*
Balnetar. Solution (250 ml.): tar (equivalent to 2.5% crude coal tar) in Alpha-Keri.
Banaocide. See *Diethylcarbamazine.*
Barium sulfate, micronized (Steripaque). Suspension: 100% barium sulfate. Suspension: 50% barium sulfate (Steripaque BR). Suspension: 30% barium sulfate (Steripaque V).
Basis soap. Bar (bath, toilet).
Bayer 205. See *Suramin.*
B.C.G. See *Tuberculosis vaccine.*
BCNU (bis-chloroethyl nitrosourea, Carmustine). Investigational.
Belladonna. Tincture (30 ml., pt.): approximately 40 drops per ml.
Benadryl hydrochloride. See *Diphenhydramine hydrochloride.*
Benemid. See *Probenecid.*
Benoxinate hydrochloride (Dorsacaine hydrochloride). Solution, sterile ophthalmic (15 ml.): 0.4%.
Benoxyl. See *Benzoyl peroxide.*
Bentyl. See *Dicyclomine.*
Benzalkonium chloride (Zephiran chloride). Solution, aqueous (250 ml.): 1:750. Tincture, tinted, aerosol (30, 180 ml.): 1:750.
Benzathine penicillin G (Bicillin Long-Acting). Syringes (1, 2, 4 ml.): 600,000 units per ml. Tubex (1, 2 ml.): 600,000 units per ml. Vials (10 ml.): 300,000 units per ml.
Benzedrine sulfate. See *Amphetamine sulfate.*
Benzene hexachloride (Kwell). Cream (60 ml., pt.): 1%. Lotion (60 ml., pt.): 1%. Shampoo (60 ml., pt.): 1%.
Benzethonium chloride (Phemerol). Solution, aqueous (gal.): 1:750. Tincture (gal.): 1:750.
Benzoin. Compound tincture (30, 60 ml., pt.). Spray: 360 ml. Tincture, plain (120 ml.). Spray: 310 ml.
Benzoyl peroxide (Benoxyl). Lotion (30, 60 ml.): 5, 10%.
Benztropine mesylate (Cogentin mesylate). Ampules (2 ml.): 1 mg. per ml. Talbets (100): 0.5, 1, 2 mg.
Benzyl benzoate. Lotion (pt.): 27, 50%.
Benzyl benzoate, compound (Topocide). Emulsion (125 ml., pt.): benzyl benzoate, benzocaine, chlorophenothane (DDT).
Bephenium hydroxynaphthoate (Alcopara). Granules (packets): 5 Gm. equivalent to 2.5 Gm. bephenium ion.
Betadine. See *Povidone-iodine.*
Betalin. See *Vitamin B complex.*
Betamethasone (Celestone). Cream (15, 45 Gm.): 2 mg. per Gm. Syrup (125 ml.): 0.12 mg. per ml. Tablets (30, 100): 0.6 mg. Vial (5 ml.): 6 mg. per ml.
Betamethasone 17-valerate (Valisone). Cream (5, 15, 45 Gm.): 1.2 mg. per Gm. Ointment (5, 15, 45 Gm.): 1.2 mg. per Gm. Spray (85 Gm.): 0.15%. Lotion (60 ml.): 0.1%.
Beta-sitosterol (Cytellin). Suspension (pt.): 200 mg. per ml.
Bethanechol chloride (Urecholine chloride). Ampules (1 ml.): 5 mg. per ml. Tablets (100): 5, 10, 25 mg.

Bicillin All Purpose. Vials, powder (1, 5 dose): Each 2 ml. contains 600,000 units Bicillin, 300,000 units procaine penicillin G and 300,000 units penicillin G potassium.

Bicillin C-R. Vials (10 ml.): Each ml. contains 150,000 units Bicillin and 150,000 units procaine penicillin G. Tubex (1, 2 ml.): Each ml. contains 300,000 units Bicillin and 300,000 units procaine penicillin G. Syringe (2, 4 ml.): Each ml. contains 300,000 units Bicillin and 300,000 units procaine penicillin G.

Bicillin Long-Acting. See *Benzathine penicillin G.*

Biperiden hydrochloride (Akineton). Tablets (100): 2 mg.

Biperiden lactate (Akineton lactate). Ampules (1 ml.): 5 mg. per ml.

Bisacodyl (Dulcolax). Suppositories (2, 4, 50): 100 mg. Tablets, enteric coated (24, 100): 5 mg.

Bis-chloroethyl nitrosourea. See *BCNU.*

Bishydroxycoumarin (Dicumarol). Tablets (100): 25, 50, 100 mg.

Bismuth glycolyl arsanilate. See *Glycobiarsol.*

Bis-tropamide. See *Tropicamide.*

Blenderm (surgical tape). Rolls (5 yd.): ½, 1, 1½ inches.

Bleomycin. Investigational.

Bleph 10. See *Sulfacetamide.*

Bleph 30. See *Sulfacetamide sodium.*

Blephamide. Ophthalmic liquifilm (5, 10 ml.): 0.2% prednisolone, 10% sulfacetamide, 0.12% phenylephrine hydrochloride.

Bonine. See *Meclizine hydrochloride.*

Botulism antitoxin, bivalent (types A and B, equine origin). Vials: 10,000 units of type A and type B.

Botulism antitoxin, type E. Obtainable from Communicable Disease Center, Atlanta, Georgia; Telephone 404-633-3311.

Brasivol. Aluminum oxide scrubbing particles. Base (135 Gm.). Fine (80, 165 Gm.). Medium (90, 180 Gm.). Rough (135, 195 Gm.).

Bremil. Liquid, concentrate (390 ml.). Liquid, ready to use (120 ml., qt.).

British anti-lewisite. See *Dimercaprol.*

Brompheniramine maleate (Dimetane). Ampules (1 ml.): 10 mg. per ml. Ampules (2 ml.): 100 mg. per ml. Elixir (pt.): 0.4 mg. per ml. Tablets (100): 4 mg. Tablets, sustained action (100): 8, 12 mg.

Bromsulphalein. Ampules (3, 7.5, 10 ml.).

Bronkoephrine. See *Ethylnorepinephrine.*

Bronkolixir. See *Bronkotabs.*

Bronkosol. Solution (10 ml.): 1% Dilabron brand of isoetharine hydrochloride, 0.25% phenylephrine hydrochloride, 0.1% thenyldiamine hydrochloride.

Bronkotabs. Elixir (bronkolixir) (pt.): 2.4 mg. ephedrine sulfate, 3 mg. theophylline, 0.8 mg. phenobarbital, 10 mg. glyceryl guaiacolate, 0.2 mg. chlorpheniramine maleate per ml. Tablets (100): 24 mg. ephedrine sulfate, 100 mg. theophylline, 8 mg. phenobarbital, 100 mg. glyceryl guaiacolate; 10 mg. thenyldiamine. Tablets (Bronkotabs-HAFS) (100): one-half of above potency per tablet.

Bronkotabs-HAFS. See *Bronkotabs.*

Busulfan (Myleran). Tablets (25): 2 mg.

Butabarbital sodium (Butisol sodium). Elixir (pt.): 6 mg. per ml. Tablets (100): 15, 30, 50, 100 mg. Tablets, repeat action (100): 30, 60 mg.

Butacaine sulfate (Butyn sulfate). Solution (30 ml.): 2%. Ointment, ophthalmic (4 Gm.): 2%.

Butazolindin. See *Phenylbutazone.*

Butisol sodium. See *Butabarbital sodium.*

Butyn sulfate. See *Butacaine sulfate.*

C

Cafergot. Suppositories (12): 2 mg. ergotamine tartrate and 100 mg. caffeine. Tablets (100): 1 mg. ergotamine tartrate and 100 mg. caffeine.

Calamine. Lotion (125, 250 ml.).

Calciferol (Drisdol, Vitamin D_2). Capsules (50): 50,000 units. Solution in propylene glycol (50 ml.): 250 units per drop.

Calcitonin. See *Thyrocalcitonin.*

Calcium chloride. Ampules (10 ml.): 100 mg. per ml. Solution, oral: 100 mg. per ml. (10%) prepared extemporaneously.

Calcium disodium edetate (calcium disodium versenate, EDTA). Ampules (5 ml.): 200 mg. per ml. Tablets (250): 500 mg.

Calcium disodium versenate. See *Calcium disodium edetate.*

Calcium folinate. See *Calcium leucovorin.*

Calcium gluconate. Ampules (10 ml.): 100 mg. per ml. Syrup: See *Calcium gluconogalactogluconate.* Tablets (100): 500 mg., 1 Gm.

Calcium gluconogalactogluconate (Neo-Calglucon). Ampules (10 ml.): equivalent to 10% calcium gluconate. Syrup (pt.): 260 mg. calcium per ml.

Calcium lactate. Powder (1 lb.). Tablets (100): 300, 600 mg.

Calcium leucovorin (calcium folinate, citrovorum factor, folinic acid, leucovorin). Ampules (1 ml.): 3 mg. per ml.

Camolar. See *Cycluguanil pamoate.*

Camoquin hydrochloride. See *Amodiaquin hydrochloride.*

Camphorated opium tincture. See *Paregoric.*

Candicidin (Vanobid). Ointment, vaginal (150 Gm.): 3 mg. per 5 Gm. (applicatorful). Tablets, vaginal (28): 3 mg.

Cantharidin Collodian (Cantherone). Liquid (7.5 ml.).

Cantherone. See *Cantharidin Collodian.*

Capreomycin (Caprocin). Investigational.

Caprocin. See *Capreomycin.*

Carbamazepine (Tegretol). Tablets (100): 200 mg.

Carbasone. Tablets: 250 mg.

Carbenicillin (Geoperi, Pyopen). Vials, powder: 1, 2, 5, 10 Gm.

Carbinoxamine maleate (Clistin maleate). Elixir (pt.): 0.8 mg. per ml. Tablets (100): 4 mg. Tablets, repeat action (100): 8, 12 mg.

Carbostibamide. See *Urea stibamine.*

Carmol. See *Urea.*

Carmustine. See *BCNU.*

Cascara sagrada. Aromatic fluid extract (pt.). Tablets (100): 300 mg.

Casein hydrolysate (Amigen). Solution, intravenous (500 ml.): 5%. Solution, intravenous (500 ml.): 5% with 5% dextrose.

Catarase. See *Alpha-chymotrypsin.*

Catecholdisulfonate. See *Stibophen.*

CCNU (cis-chloroethyl nitrosourea, Lomustine). Investigational.

Cedilanid. See *Lanatoside C.*

Cedilanid D. See *Deslanoside.*

Celestone. See *Betamethasone.*

Cellothyl. See *Methylcellulose.*

Cellulose filters. See *Filters, cellulose.*

Cellulose, oxidized (Oxycel, Surgicel). Pads: 3 × 3 in. Pledgets: 2 × 1 × 1 in. Strips: ½ × 5, 2 × 8, ½ × 36 in.

Celontin. See *Methsuximide.*

Cephalexin (Keflex). Capsules (24, 100): 250, 500 mg.

Suspension (60, 100 ml.): 25 mg. per ml. Suspension (10 ml.): 100 mg. per ml.

Cephaloridine (Loridine). Vials, powder: 500 mg., 1 Gm.

Cephalothin sodium (Keflin). Vials, powder (1, 2, 4 Gm.).

Cetaphil. Lotion (pt.). Ointment (1 lb.).

Cetapred. Ointment, ophthalmic (3.5 Gm.). 10% sulfacetamide sodium, 0.25% prednisolone.

Chloral hydrate (Noctec). Capsules (100): 250, 500 mg. Suppositories (12): 650 mg., 1.3 Gm. Syrup (pt.): 100 mg. per ml.

Chlorambucil (Leukeran). Tablets (50): 2 mg.

Chloramphenicol (Chloromycetin). Ampules (2 ml.): 500 mg. Capsules (100): 50, 100, 250 mg. Cream (30 Gm.): 1%. Ointment, ophthalmic (4 Gm.): 1% powder, sterile, ophthalmic (15 ml.): 25 mg. Solution, otic (15 ml.): 0.5%.

Chloramphenicol palmitate (Chloromycetin palmitate). Suspension, oral (60 ml.): 31.2 mg. per ml. of chloramphenicol.

Chloramphenicol sodium succinate (Chloromycetin sodium succinate, Mychel S). Vials, powder, intravenous: 1 Gm.

Chlordiazepoxide hydrochloride (Librium). Ampules, powder: 100 mg. Capsules (50): 5, 10, 25 mg. Tablets (Libritabs)' (50): 5, 10, 25 mg.

Chloroguanide hydrochloride (Paludrine hydrochloride, Proguanil hydrochloride). Tablets (100): 100 mg.

Chloromycetin. See *Chloramphenicol.*

Chloromycetin-hydrocortisone. Suspension, ophthalmic (5 ml.). 0.5% hydrocortisone and 0.25% chloramphenicol.

Chloromycetin palmitate. See *Chloramphenicol palmitate.*

Chloromycetin-polymyxin. Ointment, ophthalmic (4 Gm.). 1% chloramphenicol and 10,000 units polymyxin B per Gm.

Chloromycetin sodium succinate. See *Chloramphenicol sodium succinate.*

Chloroquine phosphate (Aralen phosphate). Ampules (5 ml.): 50 mg. per ml. Tablets (25): 500 mg.

Chloroquine-primaquin (Aralen-primaquin). Tablets (100): 300 mg. chloroquin base; 45 mg. primaquin base.

Chorothiazide (Diuril). Syrup (240 ml.): 50 mg. per ml. Tablets (100): 250, 500 mg.

Chlorothiazide sodium (Diuril sodium). Vials, powder, sterile: 500 mg.

Chlorpheniramine maleate (Chlor-Trimeton, Teldrin). Ampules (1 ml.): 10 mg. per ml. Capsules, sustained release (50): 8, 12 mg. Syrup (pt.): 0.5 mg. per ml. Tablets (100): 4 mg. Tablets, repeat action (100): 8, 12 mg. Vials (10 ml.): 10 mg. per ml. Vials (2 ml.): 100 mg. per ml.

Chlorpromazine (Thorazine). Suppositories (6): 25, 100 mg.

Chlorpromazine hydrochloride (Thorazine hydrochloride). Ampules (1, 2 ml.): 25 mg. per ml. Capsules, sustained release (50): 30, 75, 150, 200, 300 mg. Concentrate (120 ml.): 30 mg. per ml. Concentrate (240 ml.): 100 mg. per ml. Syrup (125 ml.): 2 mg. per ml. Tablets (100): 10, 25, 50, 100, 200 mg. Vials (10 ml.): 25 mg. per ml.

Chlorpropamide (Diabinese). Tablets (100): 100, 250 mg.

Chlortetracycline calcium (Aureomycin calcium). Syrup (125 ml., pt.): 25 mg. per ml.

Chlortetracycline hydrochloride (Aureomycin hydrochloride). Capsules (16, 100): 250 mg. Ointment (15, 30 Gm.): 3%. Ointment, ophthalmic (4 Gm.): 1%. Vial: 500 mg.

Chlorthalidone (Hygroton). Tablets (100): 50, 100 mg.

Chlor-Trimeton. See *Chlorpheniramine maleate.*

Choledyl. See *Oxtriphylline.*

Cholera vaccine (India strains). Vials (1.5 ml.): one immunization.

Cholestyramine resin (Cuemid, Questran). Packets (4 Gm.). Powder (216 Gm.).

Choline salicylate (Arthropan). Solution (250 ml., pt.): 174 mg. per ml.

Choline theophyllinate. See *Oxtriphylline.*

Choloxin. See *Sodium dextrothyroxine.*

Chorionic gonadotropin. Vials (10 ml.): 250, 500, 1000 units per ml. Vials, lyophilized powder: 5000, 10,000 and 20,000 units.

Cis-chloroethyl nitrosourea. See *CCNU.*

Citrovorum factor. See *Calcium leucovorin.*

Cleocin hydrochloride. See *Clindamycin hydrochloride.*

Cleocin palmitate. See *Clindamycin palmitate.*

Cleocin phosphate. See *Clindamycin phosphate.*

Clindamycin hydrochloride (Cleocin hydrochloride). Capsules (16, 100): 75, 150 mg.

Clindamycin palmitate (Cleocin palmitate). Suspension (80, 200 ml., pt.): 15 mg. per ml.

Clindamycin phosphate (Cleocin phosphate). Ampules (2, 4, 6 ml.): 150 mg. per ml.

Clinitest. Tablets, reagent (36, 100). Contain copper sulfate and sodium hydroxide.

Clistin maleate. See *Carbinoxamine maleate.*

Clofibrate (Atromid S). Capsules (100): 500 mg.

Clomid. See *Clomiphene citrate.*

Clomiphene citrate (Clomid). Tablets (30): 50 mg.

Cloxacillin sodium monohydrate (Tegopen). Capsules (100): 250 mg. Solution, oral (80, 150 ml.): 25 mg. per ml.

Coal tar solution (liquor carbonis detergens). Solution (90, 240 ml., pt.): 5%.

Cocaine hydrochloride. Solution, as requested.

Coccidioidin. Vials (1 ml.): 1:10, 1:100 dilution of mixed strains of *Coccidioides immitis.*

Cod liver oil. Bottles (125, 250 ml.).

Codeine phosphate. Ampules (1 ml.): 15, 30, 60 mg. per ml. Vials (20 ml.): 30, 60 mg. per ml.

Codeine sulfate. Tablets (100): 15, 30, 60 mg.

Cogentin mesylate. See *Benztropine mesylate.*

Colace. See *Dioctyl sodium sulfosuccinate.*

Colchicine. Tablets (100): 0.5, 0.6 mg. Ampules (2 ml.): 0.5 mg. per ml.

Cold cream. Cream (lb.).

Colistin sulfate (Coly-Mycin S). Suspension, otic (5, 10 ml.): 3 mg. colistin, 3.3 mg. neomycin and 10 mg. hydrocortisone per ml. Suspension, oral not absorbed (60 ml.): 5 mg. per ml.

Colistimethate sodium (Coly-Mycin M). Vials, powder: 20, 150 mg.

Colloidal oatmeal. See *Aveeno.*

Coly-Mycin M. See *Colistimethate sodium.*

Coly-Mycin S. See *Colistin sulfate.*

Combex. See *Vitamin B complex.*

Compazine. See *Prochlorperazine.*

Compazine edisylate. See *Prochlorperazine edisylate.*

Compazine maleate. See *Prochlorperazine maleate.*

Conadil. See *Ospolot.*

Congo red. Ampules (10 ml.): 1%.

Conjugated estrogenic substances (Premarin). Cream (60 Gm.): 0.625 mg. per Gm. Cream, vaginal (45 Gm.): 0.625 mg. per Gm. Lotion (60 ml.): 1 mg. per ml. Tablets (100): 0.3, 0.625, 1.25, 2.5 mg. Vials, powder, intravenous: 25 mg.

Cordran. See *Flurandrenolone.*

Cordran-N. See *Flurandrenolone with neomycin sulfate.*

Cortef. See *Hydrocortisone.*

Cortef acetate. See *Hydrocortisone acetate.*

Cortef fluid. See *Hydrocortisone cypionate.*

Corticotropin. See *ACTH.*

Cortiphate. See *Hydrocortisone phosphate.*

Cortisol succinate. See *Hydrocortisone sodium succinate.*

Cortisone acetate (Cortone acetate). Ointment, ophthalmic (3.5 Gm.): 1.5%. Tablets (50, 100): 5, 10, 25 mg. Vials (5, 10, 20 ml.): 25 mg. per ml. Vials (1, 10 ml.): 50 mg. per ml.

Cortisporin. Cream (7.5 Gm.): 0.5% hydrocortisone, neomycin, gramicidin and polymyxin. Drops, otic (5, 10 ml.): 1% hydrocortisone, neomycin, and polymyxin. Ointment (15 Gm.): 1% hydrocortisone, neomycin, zinc bacitracin and polymyxin. Ointment, ophthalmic (4 Gm.): 1% hydrocortisone, neomycin, bacitracin, and polymyxin. Suspension, ophthalmic (5 ml.): 1% hydrocortisone, neomycin and polymyxin.

Cortone acetate. See *Cortisone acetate.*

Cortril. See *Hydrocortisone.*

Cortril acetate. See *Hydrocortisone acetate.*

Cosmegen. See *Dactinomycin.*

Cotazyme. See *Pancreatin.*

Coumadin sodium. See *Warfarin sodium.*

Covermark (neutral, opaque, hypoallergenic cream). Jars, 10 shades to match skin.

Cromolyn sodium (Aarane, disodium chromoglycate, Intal). Capsules, powder for inhalation with inhaler (60): 20 mg.

Crotamitum cream (Eurax). Cream (60 Gm.): 10%. Lotion (180 ml., pt.): 10%.

Crystalline insulin. See *Insulin.*

Crystodigin. See *Digitoxin.*

Crystoids. See *Hexylresorcinol.*

Cuemid. See *Cholestyramine resin.*

Cuprimine. See *D-Penicillamine.*

Cyanide antidote package. Amyl nitrite, inhalation (12): 0.3 ml. Sodium nitrite ampules (1 × 10 ml.): 30 mg. per ml. Sodium thiosulfate ampules (2 × 50 ml.): 250 mg. per ml.

Cyanocobalamin (vitamin B_{12}). Syringe (1 ml.): 100, 1000 micrograms per ml. Tablets (100): 25, 50, 100, 250 micrograms. Vials (1, 10 ml.): 30, 50, 100, 1000 micrograms per ml.

Cyclamycin. See *Triacetyloleandomycin.*

Cycloguanil pameate (Camolar). Investigational.

Cyclogyl hydrochloride. See *Cyclopentolate hydrochoride.*

Cyclomydril. Solution, sterile, ophthalmic (2, 7.5 ml.): 0.2% cyclopentolate and 1% phenylephrine hydrochloride.

Cyclopentolate hydrochloride (Cyclogyl hydrochloride). Solution, sterile, ophthalmic (2, 15 ml.): 1%. Solution, sterile, ophthalmic (2, 7.5 ml.): 2%. Solution, sterile, ophthalmic (15 ml.): 0.5%.

Cyclophosphamide (Cytoxan). Tablets (100): 25, 50 mg. Vials: 100, 200, 500 mg.

Cycloserine (Seromycin). Capsules (40): 250 mg.

Cyproheptadine hydrochloride (Periactin hydrochloride). Syrup (pt.): 0.4 mg. per ml. Tablets (100): 4 mg.

Cytarabine. See *Cytosine arabinoside.*

Cytellin. See *Beta-sitosterol.*

Cytomel. See *Liothyronine.*

Cytosine arabinoside (Cytarabine). Vial: 100, 500 mg.

Cytoxan. See *Cyclophosphamide.*

D

Dactinomycin (Actinomycin D, Cosmegen). Vials: 0.5 mg.

DADPS. See *Dapsone.*

Dalidoine. Powder, packets (12): contains zinc sulfate, copper sulfate, and camphor for making Dalibour solution.

Dapsone (Avlosulfon, DADPS, DDS). Tablets (100): 25, 100 mg.

Daranide. See *Dichlorphenamide.*

Daraprim. See *Pyrimethamine.*

Darrow's solution (Ionosol PSL). Solution, intravenous (150, 250, 500 ml.).

Darvon. See *Propoxyphene hydrochloride.*

Darvon compound. See *Propoxyphene hydrochloride with APC.*

Daunomycin. See *Daunorubicin.*

Daunorubicin (daunomycin). Vial, powder: 20 mg.

DDS. See *Dapsone.*

Deaner. See *Seanol acetamidobenzoate.*

Deanol acetamidobenzoate (Deaner). Tablets (50, 100): 25, 100 mg.

Decadron. See *Dexamethasone.*

Decadron phosphate. See *Dexamethasone phosphate.*

Decapryn. See *Doxylamine succinate.*

Decholin. See *Dehydrocholic acid.*

Declomycin. See *Demeclocycline.*

Dehydrocholic acid (Decholin). Tablets (100): 250 mg.

Dehydroemetine. Investigational.

Delalutin. See *Hydroxyprogesterone caproate.*

Delatestryl. See *Testosterone enanthate.*

Delestrogen. See *Estradiol valerate.*

Deltasone. See *Prednisone.*

Delta-Cortef. See *Prednisolone.*

Deltra. See *Prednisone.*

Demeclocycline (Declomycin, Demethylchlortetracycline). Capsules (16, 100): 150 mg. Drops (10 ml.): 60 mg. per ml. Suspension, oral (60 ml.): 15 mg. per ml. Syrup, oral (60 ml.): 15 mg. per ml. Tablets (25): 75 mg. Tablets (16, 100): 150 mg. Tablets (12, 48): 300 mg.

Demerol hydrochloride. See *Meperidine hydrochloride.*

Demethylchlortetracycline. See *Demeclocycline.*

Dendrid. See *Idoxuridine.*

Deoxyribonuclease. See *Pancreatic dornase.*

Depo-ACTH. See *ACTH gel.*

Depo-Medrol. See *Methyl prednisolone acetate.*

Depo-Provera. See *Medroxyprogesterone acetate.*

Depo-testosterone. See *Testosterone cypionate.*

Derefil. Tablet (30, 100): 100 mg. Water soluble derivatives of chlorophyll.

Deronil. See *Dexamethasone.*

Desenex. Ointment (27, 54 Gm.): 5% undecylenic acid and 20% zinc undecylenate. Powder (45, 90 Gm.): 2% undecylenic acid and 20% zinc undecylenate. Soap. Solution (80 ml.): 10% undecylenic acid. Spray (180 Gm.).

Desferal. See *Desferoxamine.*

Desferoxamine (Desferal). Vials, powder: 500 mg.

Desitin. Ointment (30, 60, 125 Gm.): cod liver oil, zinc oxide, and talc in lanolin petrolatum base. Powder (210, 300 Gm.).

Deslanoside (Cedilanid D). Ampules (2, 4 ml.): 0.2 mg. per ml.

Desonide (Tridesilon). Cream (5, 15, 60 Gm.): 0.05%.

Desoxycorticosterone acetate (Doca, Percoten acetate). Linguets (100): 2, 5 mg. Pellets (6): 125 mg. Vials, in oil (10 ml.): 5 mg. per ml.

Desoxycorticosterone pivalate (Doca TMA, Percoten

pivalate). Vials, intramuscular (4 ml.): 25 mg. per ml.

Desoxyhydrochloride. See *Methamphetamine hydrochloride.*

Dexamethasone (Decadron, Deronil, Gammacorten, Hexadrol). Elixir (100, 240 ml.): 0.5 mg. per ml. Tablets (100): 0.25, 0.5, 0.75, 1.5, 2, 4 mg.

Dexamethasone phosphate (Decadron phosphate). Aerosol with oral attachment (12.6 Gm.). Cream (15, 30 Gm.): 0.1%. Ointment, ophthalmic (3.5 Gm.): 0.05%. Solution, ophthalmic (2.5, 5 ml.): 0.1%. Syringe (1, 2 ml.): 4 mg. per ml. Turbinaire (1% metered sprays): 0.1 mg. per spray. Vials (1, 5, 25 ml.): 4 mg. per ml.

Dexbrompheniramine maleate (Disomer). Syrup: 0.4 mg. per ml. Tablets: 2 mg. Tablets, sustain in release: 4, 6 mg.

Dexchlorpheniramine maleate (Polaramine maleate). Syrup (pt.): 0.4 mg. per ml. Tablets (100): 2 mg. Tablets, repeat action (100): 4, 6 mg.

Dexedrine sulfate. See *Dextroamphetamine sulfate.*

Dextran (Dextran 75, Gentran, Macrodex). Solution, intravenous (500 ml.): 6% in 5% dextrose. Solution, intravenous (500 ml.): 6% in isotonic sodium chloride. Solution, intravenous (500 ml.): 6% in 10% invert sugar.

Dextran LMW. See *Dextran 40.*

Dextran 40 (Dextran LMW, Rheomacrodex). Solution, intravenous (500 ml.): 10% in 5% dextrose. Solution, intravenous (500 ml.): 10% in isotonic sodium chloride.

Dextran 75. See *Dextran.*

Dextri-maltose. Powder (lb.).

Dextroamphetamine sulfate (Dexedrine sulfate). Capsules, sustained release (50): 5, 10, 15 mg. Elixir (360 ml.): 1 mg. per ml. Tablets (100): 5 mg.

Dextrose. Ampules (50 ml.): 50%. Solution, intravenous (150, 250, 500, 1000 ml.): 5% in water. Solution, intravenous (500, 1000 ml.): 5% in sodium chloride 0.9%. Solution, intravenous (500, 1000 ml.): 5% in sodium chloride 0.45%. Solution, intravenous (500 ml.): 5% in sodium chloride 0.33%. Solution, intravenous (500, 1000 ml.): 10% in water. Solution, intravenous (500 ml.): 20% in water. Solution, intravenous (500 ml.): 50% in water. Syringe (50 ml.): 50%. Vials (50 ml.): 50%.

Dextrostix. Reagent strips (25).

Diabinese. See *Chlorpropamide.*

Diamox. See *Acetazolamide.*

Diamox sodium. See *Acetazolamide.*

Dianabol. See *Methandrostenolone.*

Dianeal. See *Peritoneal dialysis.*

Diaparene. See *Methylbenzethonium chloride.*

Diapid. See *Lypressin.*

Diasone sodium. See *Sulfoxone sodium.*

Diastix. Reagent strips (25, 100): Glucose oxidase, peroxidase, and potassium iodide.

Diazepam (Valium). Ampules (2 ml.): 5 mg. per ml. Syringe (2 ml.): 5 mg. per ml. Tablets (50): 2, 5, 10 mg. Vial (10 ml.): 5 mg. per ml.

Diazoxide (Hyperstat). Ampules (20 ml.): 15 mg. per ml.

Dibenzyline. See *Phenoxybenzamine hydrochloride.*

Dibucaine (Nupercaine). Solution, ophthalmic, 0.1–0.2%.

Dichlorophen (Antiphen). Tablets (12): 500 mg. Not available in the United States.

Dichlorphenamide (Daranide). Tablets (100): 50 mg.

Dicloxacillin sodium monohydrate (Dynapen, Pathocil, Veracillin). Capsules (25, 100): 125, 250 mg. Suspension, oral (80 ml.): 12.5 mg. per ml.

Dicumarol. See *Bishydroxycoumarin.*

Dicyclomine (Bentyl). Ampules (2 ml.) 10 mg. per ml. Capsules (100): 10 mg. Syrup (pt.) 2 mg. per ml. Tablets (100): 20 mg. Vial (10 ml.): 10 mg. per ml.

Dienestrol. Cream (78 Gm.): 0.01%.

Diethylcarbamazine (Banocide, Hetrazan, Notezine). Tablets (100): 50 mg.

Diethylstilbestrol. Ampules in oil (1 ml.): 5 mg. per ml. Suppositories (6): 0.1, 0.5 mg. Tablets (100): 0.1, 0.25, 0.5, 1, 5, 25 mg.

Diethyltoluamide. See *OFF.*

Digalloyl trioleate (Sunstick, Sunswept). Cream (45 Gm.): 3.5%. Stick (4 Gm.): 2.5%.

Digitalis. Pills (100): 60, 100 mg. Tablets (100): 60, 100 mg. Tincture (120 ml.).

Digitaline Nativelle. See *Digitoxin.*

Digitoxin (Crystodigin, Digitaline Nativelle, Purodigin). Ampules (1, 2, 10 ml.): 0.2 mg. per ml. Elixir (55 ml.): 0.05 mg. per ml. Solution oral (10 ml.): 0.02 mg. per drop. Tablets (100): 0.05, 0.1, 0.15, 0.2 mg.

Digoxin (Lanoxin). Ampules, pediatric (1 ml.): 0.1 mg. per ml. Ampules (2 ml.): 0.25 mg. per ml. Elixir (60 ml.): 0.05 mg. per ml. Tablets (100): 0.125, 0.25, and 0.5 mg.

Dihydrotachysterol (Hydrocalciferol, Hytakerol, vitamin D_4). Capsules (50): 0.125 mg. Solution (15 ml.): 0.25 mg. per ml. Tablets (100): 0.2 mg.

Diiodohydroxyquin (Diodoquin, Moebiquin, Yodoxin). Tablets (25, 60): 210, 650 mg.

Dilantin. See *Diphenylhydantoin.*

Dilantin sodium. See *Diphenylhydantoin sodium.*

Dimenhydrinate (Dramamine). Ampules (1 ml.): 50 mg. Elixir (pt.): 3.1 mg. per ml. Suppositories (12): 100 mg. Tablets (100): 50 mg. Vials (5 ml.): 50 mg. per ml.

Dimercaprol (BAL, British anti-lewisite). Ampules (3 ml.): 10% in peanut oil.

Dimercaptosuccinate. See *Stibocaptate.*

Dimetane. See *Brompheniramine maleate.*

Dimetapp. Elixir (pt.): 0.8 mg. brompheniramine maleate, 1 mg. phenylephrine hydrochloride, and 1 mg. phenylpropanolamine per ml. Tablets, Extentabs (100): 12 mg. brompheniramine maleate, 15 mg. phenylephrine hydrochloride, and 15 mg. phenylpropanolamine.

Dimocillin R-T. See *Methicillin sodium.*

Dioctyl sodium sulfosuccinate (Colace). Capsules (30, 60): 50, 100 mg. Solution, oral (30 ml., pt.): 10 mg. per ml. Syrup, oral (250 ml.): 4 mg. per ml.

Diodoquin. See *Diiodohydroxyquin.*

Diphenhydramine hydrochloride (Benadryl hydrochloride). Ampules (1 ml.): 50 mg. per ml. Capsules (100): 25, 50 mg. Elixir (125 ml., pt.): 2.5 mg. per ml. Syringe (1 ml.): 50 mg. per ml. Vials (10 ml.): 10 mg. per ml.

Diphenidol (Vontrol). Ampules (2 ml.): 10 mg. per ml. Suppositories (6): 25, 50 mg. Tablets (100): 25 mg.

Diphenoxylate hydrochloride (Lomotil). Liquid, oral (60 ml.): 0.5 mg. diphenoxylate hydrochloride and 0.005 mg. atropine sulfate per ml. Tablets (100): 2.5 mg. diphenoxylate hydrochloride and 0.025 mg. atropine sulfate.

Diphenylhydantoin (Dilantin). Capsules, delayed action (100): 100 mg. Suspension, oral (250 ml.): 25 mg. per ml. Suspension, oral (250 ml.): 6 mg. per ml. Tablets, Infatabs (100): 50 mg.

Diphenylhydantoin sodium (Dilantin sodium). Capsules (100): 30, 100 mg. Vials (2, 5 ml.): 50 mg. per ml.

Diphtheria antitoxin. Vials: 1000, 10,000, 20,000 units.

Diphtheria and tetanus toxoids. Syringe (0.5 ml.). Vials, alum-precipitated (5 ml.). Vials, fluid (7.5 ml.).

Diphtheria, tetanus toxoids, and pertussis vaccine (D.P.T.). Vials, adsorbed (7.5 ml.). Vials (7.5 ml.).

Diphtheria toxin (Schick test). Vials (1): 10 tests per ml.

Diphtheria toxoid. Vial (5 ml.): Alum-precipitated. Vial (5 ml.): Aluminum phosphate adsorbed.

Disodium chromoglycate. See *Cromolyn sodium.*

Disodium edetate (disodium edetate, disodium ethylenediamine, tetra-acetic acid). Ampules (20 ml.): 150 mg. per ml.

Disodium ethylenediamine. See *Disodium edetate.*

Disomer. See *Dexbrompheniramine maleate.*

Disophrol. Tablets (100): 2 mg. dexbrompheniramine, 60 mg. isoephedrine. Tablets, sustained action (100): 6 mg. dexbrompheniramine, 120 mg. isoephedrine.

Diuril. See *Chlorothiazide.*

Diuril sodium. See *Chlorothiazide sodium.*

Doca. See *Desoxycorticosterone acetate.*

Doca TMA. See *Desoxycorticosterone pivilate.*

Dolenee. See *Propoxyphene hydrochloride.*

Dolene compound. See *Propoxyphene hydrochloride with APC.*

Dolophine. See *Methadone.*

Domeboro (aluminum sulfate and calcium acetate). Packets (12, 100). Tablets (12, 100). One packet, one tablet or one teaspoonful of powder in 1 pint of water makes a 1:20 modified Burow's solution, pH 4.2. Otic (60 ml.): 2% acetic acid in aluminum acetate solution.

Domol (skin moisturizing agent). Bath emollient (250 ml.). Lotion (250 ml.).

Donnagel-PG. Suspension, oral (180 ml.): Each 30 ml. contains 60 Gm. Kaolin, 24 mg. opium (equivalent to 6 ml. paregoric), 143 mg. pectin, 0.10 mg. hyoscyamine sulfate, 0.019 mg. atropine sulfate, and 0.006 mg. hyoscine hydrobromide.

Donnatal. Elixir (pt.): 0.02 mg. hyoscyamine sulfate, 0.001 mg. hyoscine hydrobromide, 0.004 atropine sulfate, and 3.2 mg. phenobarbital per ml. Tablets (100): 0.1 mg. hyoscyamine sulfate, 0.006 mg. hyoscine hydrobromide, 0.019 mg. atropine sulfate, and 16.2 mg. phenobarbital. Tablets, extended action (100): 0.3 mg. hyoscyamine sulfate, 0.02 mg. hyoscine hydrodromide, 0.06 mg. atropine sulfate, and 48.6 mg. phenobarbital.

Dopar. See *Levodopa.*

Doriden. See *Glutethimide.*

Dornovac. See *Pancreatic dornase.*

Dorsacaine hydrochloride. See *Benoxinate hydrochloride.*

Doxycycline (Vibramycin). Capsules (50): 50 mg. Suspension (60 ml.): 5 mg. per ml.

Doxylamine succinate (Decapryn). Syrup (pt.): 1.25 mg. per ml. Tablets (100): 12.5, 25 mg.

DPF. See *Isofluorophate.*

D.P.T. See *Diphtheria, tetanus toxoids and pertussis vaccine.*

Dramamine. See *Dimenhydrinate.*

Drisdol. See *Calciferol.*

Drixoral. Tablets, sustained action, 6 mg. dexbrompheniramine, 120 mg. isoephedrine sulfate.

DTPA. See *Diethylenetriamine.*

Dulcolax. See *Bisacodyl.*

Duovent. Tablets (100): 130 mg. theophylline, 24 mg. ephedrine, 100 mg. glyceryl guaiacolate, 8 mg. phenobarbital.

Dyclone. See *Dyclonine hydrochloride.*

Dyclonine hydrochloride (Dyclone). Solution (30 ml.): 0.5%, 1%.

Dynapen. See *Dicloxacillin sodium monohydrate.*

Dy-O-Derm. Liquid (120 ml.).

Dyphylline (Lubyllin). 71% theophylline and choline theophylline. Ampules (2 ml.): 250 mg. per ml. Elixir (pt.): 6.67 mg. per ml. Talbets (100): 100, 200 mg.

Dyrenium. See *Triamterene.*

E

EACA. See *Aminocaproic acid.*

Echothiophate iodide (Phospholine iodide). Powder with diluent (5 ml.): 0.03% (1.5 mg.); 0.06% (3 mg.); 0.125% (6.25 mg.); 0.25% (12.5 mg.); 0.06% (3 mg.).

Ectasule. Capsule, Ectasule Sr. (100): 60 mg. ephedrine sulfate, 30 mg. amobarbital. Capsule, Ectasule Jr. (100): 30 mg. ephedrine sulfate, 15 mg. amobarbital. Capsule, Ectasule Minus Sr. (100): 60 mg. ephedrine sulfate. Capsule, Ectasule Minus Jr. (100): 30 mg. ephedrine sulfate.

Edecrin. See *Ethacrynic acid.*

Edrophonium chloride (Tensilon chloride). Ampules (1 ml.): 10 mg. per ml. Vials (10 ml.): 10 mg. per ml.

EDTA. See *Calcium disodium edetate.*

Efudex. See *Fluorouracil.*

Elase. Ointment (10, 30 Gm.): 1 unit fibrinolysin and 667 units desoxyribonuclease per Gm.

Elavil hydrochloride. See *Amitriptyline hydrochloride.*

Elder red petrolatum. See *RVP.*

Eldopaque. See *Hydroquinone.*

Eldoquin. See *Hydroquinone.*

Elixophyllin. See *Theophyline.*

Elixophyllin-KI. Elixir (250 ml.): 80 mg. theophylline and 130 mg. potassium iodide per 15 ml.

Emetine hydrochloride. Ampules: 65 mg.

Emetrol. Liquid (90 ml., pt.): phosphorylated carbohydrate.

Emulave. Soap (90 Gm.): vegetable oil, or waxed lanolin, colloidal oatmeal.

Enovid. Tablets, 5 mg. (20, 100): 5 mg. norethynodrel and 0.075 mg. mestranol. Tablets, 10 mg. (50): 9.85 mg. norethynodrel and 0.15 mg. mestranol.

Enovid-E. Tablets (20, 21): 2.5 mg. norethynodrel and 0.1 mg. mestranol.

Ephedrine sulfate. Ampules (1 ml.): 25, 50 mg. Capsules (100): 25, 50 mg. Solution (30 ml.): 3%. Syrup (pt.): 4 mg. per ml.

Epinephrine (Adrenalin in oil). Ampules, oil suspension (1 ml.): 1:500 (2 mg. per ml.).

Epinephrine (Sus-Phrine). Ampules, aqueous suspension (0.5 ml.): 1:200 (5 mg. per ml.). Vials, aqueous suspension (5 ml.): 1:200 (5 mg. per ml.).

Epinephrine hydrochloride (Adrenalin hydrochloride). Ampules (1 ml.): 1 mg. per ml. Solution, inhalation (5 ml.): 10 mg. per ml. Solution, topical (30 ml.): 1 mg. per ml. Vials (30 ml.): 1 mg. per ml. Syringe (10 ml.): 1:10,000, 0.01 mg. per ml. ophthalmic.

Epsilon aminocaproic acid. See *Aminocaproic acid.*

Equanil. See *Meprobomate.*

Ergomar. See *Ergotamine tartrate.*

Ergophene. Ointment (30 Gm.): Ergot, phenol, zinc oxide, and sodium borate.

Ergotamine tartrate (Ergomar, Gynergen). Ampules (0.5, 1 ml.): 0.5 mg. per ml. Tablets, sublingual (12): 2 mg. Tablets (100): 1 mg.

Erythrocin. See *Erythromycin ethyl succinate.*

Erythrocin lactobionate. See *Erythromycin lactobionate.*

Erythrocin stearate. See *Erythromycin stearate.*

Erythromycin (Ilotycin). Ointment (15, 30 Gm.): 10

mg. per Gm. Ointment, ophthalmic (4 Gm.): 5 mg. per Gm. Tablets (24, 100): 250 mg.

Erythromycin estolate (Ilosone). Capsules (24, 100): 125, 250 mg. Drops, oral (10 ml.): 100 mg. per ml. Suspension, oral (60 ml., pt.): 25, 50 mg. per ml. Tablets (50): 500 mg. Tablets, chewable (50): 125, 250 mg.

Erythromycin ethyl succinate (Erythrocin, Pediamycin). Ampules, intramuscular (2 ml.): 50 mg. per ml. Drops (30 ml.): 40 mg. per ml. Suspension, oral (60, 100, 150, 200 ml.): 40 mg. per ml. Syringe (2 ml.): 50 mg. per ml. Tablets, chewable (50): 200 mg. Vial (10 ml.): 50 mg. per ml.

Erythromycin gluceptate (Ilotycin gluceptate). Ampules: 250, 500 mg., 1 Gm.

Erythromycin lactobionate (Erythrocin lactobionate). Vials, powder: 500 mg., 1 Gm.

Erythromycin stearate (Erythrocin stearate). Tablets (25, 100): 125, 250 mg.

Eserine. See *Physostigmine salicylate.*

Eskabarb. See *Phenobarbital.*

Estinyl. See *Ethinyl estradiol.*

Estradiol valerate (Delestrogen). Syringe (1 ml.): 20 mg. per ml. Vials (1, 5 ml.): 10 mg. per ml. Vials (5 ml.): 20, 40 mg. per ml.

Ethacrynic acid (Edecrin). Tablets (100): 25, 50 mg. Vials, lyophilized (sodium ethacrynate): 50 mg.

Ethambutol hydrochloride (Myambutol hydrochloride). Tablets (100): 100, 400 mg.

Ethinyl estradiol (Estinyl). Tablets (100): 0.02, 0.05, 0.5 mg.

Ethionamide (Trecator). Tablets (100): 250 mg.

Ethisterone (anhydrohydroxyprogesterone, Pranone). Tablets (20, 100): 5, 10, 25 mg.

Ethosuximide (Zarontin). Capsules (100): 250 mg. Syrup (250 ml.): 50 mg. per ml. (investigational).

Ethotoin (Peganone). Tablets (100): 250, 500 mg.

Ethyl hexanediol (Six-Twelve). Aerosol (210, 435 Gm.). Cream (60 Gm.). Liquid (45 ml.). Stick (30 Gm.). Towelettes (10).

Ethylstilbamine (Neostibosan). Ampules: 50, 100, 300 mg.

Etrenol. See *Hycanthone.*

Eucerin. Cream (1 lb.): equal parts Aquaphor and water.

Eucerite base. See *Aquaphor.*

Eurax. See *Crotamitum cream.*

Euresol pro capillis. See *Resorcinol monoacetate.*

F

Feosol. See *Ferrous sulfate.*

Fergon. See *Ferrous gluconate.*

Fer-In-Sol. See *Ferrous sulfate.*

Ferrous gluconate (Fergon). Elixir (pt.): 60 mg. per ml. Tablets (100): 300 mg.

Ferrous sulfate (Feosol, Fer-In-Sol). Capsules, sustained action (30): 225 mg. Drops, oral (15, 50 ml.): 125 mg. per ml. Elixir (360 ml.): 44 mg. per ml. Syrup (pt.): 30 mg. per ml. Tablets (100): 300 mg. Tablets, enteric-coated (100): 300 mg.

Fibrin hydrolysate (Aminosol). Solution, intravenous (1000 ml.): 5% with 5% dextrose. Solution, intravenous (1000 ml.): 5%.

Fibrinogen (fibrinogen human, Parenogen). Vials, powder with diluent: 1, 2 Gm.

Fibrinolysin (Thrombolysin). Vials, powder: 50,000 units.

Filters, cellulose (Millepore). Swinnex–25, type GS, 0.22 microns.

Flagyl. See *Metronidazole.*

Fleet enema (saline laxative). Disposable unit, adult: 135 ml. Disposable unit, pediatric: 68 ml.

Florinef. See *Fludrocortisone acetate.*

Florinef-S. Ointment, ophthalmic (4 Gm.): 0.1% fludrocortisone, neomycin, and gramicidin. Solution, ophthalmic (2.5 ml.): 0.1% fludrocortisone, neomycin, and gramicidin. Suspension, ophthalmic (5 ml.): 0.1% fludrocortisone, neomycin, and gramicidin with hydroxypropymethyl cellulose.

Floropryl. See *Isofluorophate.*

Flucytosine (Ancobon). Capsules (100): 250, 500 mg.

Fludrocortisone acetate (Florinef). Tablets (100): 0.1 mg.

Flumethasone pivalate (Locorten). Cream (5, 15, 60 Gm.): 0.03%.

Fluocinolone acetonide (Synalar). Cream (15, 60, 120 Gm.): 0.01, 0.025%. Cream (5, 12 Gm.): 0.2%. Ointment (15, 60 Gm.): 0.025%. Solution, squeeze bottle (20, 60 ml.): 0.01%.

Fluocinolone acetonide with neomycin sulfate (Neo-Synalar). Cream (15, 60 Gm.): 0.025% flucinolone acetonide and 0.5% neomycin sulfate.

Fluocinonide. Cream (15, 30 Gm.): 0.05%. Ointment (15, 30 Gm.): 0.05%.

Fluorescein sodium. Ampules (5 ml.): 5, 10%. Solution, sterile ophthalmic (1, 2, 15 ml.): 2%. Strips, sterile ophthalmic (200).

Fluorometholone (Oxylone). Cream (15, 60, 120 Gm.): 0.025%.

Fluoroplex. See *Fluorouracil.*

Fluorouracil (Fluoroplex, 5-fluorouracil, Efudex). Ampules (10 ml.): 50 mg. per ml. Cream (25 Gm.): 5%. Solution (10 ml.): 2, 5%.

Fluoxymesterone (Halotestin, Ultandren). Tablets (40, 50, 100): 2, 5, 10 mg.

Flurandrenolone (Cordran). Cream (30, 60 Gm.): 0.025%. Cream (7.5, 15, 60 Gm.): 0.05%. Ointment (30, 60 Gm.): 0.025%. Ointment (7.5, 15, 60 Gm.): 0.05%. Lotion (15, 60 ml.): 0.05%. Tape, roll (60 cm. × 7.5 cm. and 200 cm. × 7.5 cm.).

Flurandrenolone with neomycin sulfate (Cordran-N). Cream (7.5, 15, 60 Gm.): 0.05% flurandrenolone with 5 mg. neomycin sulfate per Gm. Ointment (7.5, 15, 60 Gm.): 0.05% flurandrenolone with 5 mg. neomycin sulfate per Gm.

Folic Acid (Folvite). Tablets (100): 0.25, 1 mg. Vials (10 ml.): 5 mg. per ml.

Folinic acid. See *Calcium leucovorin.*

Folvite. See *Folic acid.*

Formaldehyde (Formalin). Aqueous solution (100 ml.): 10%.

Formalin. See *Formaldehyde.*

Fostex. Cream (130 Gm). Soap (112 Gm.). Sulfur 2%; salicylic acid 2%.

FreAmine. See *Amino acids, crystalline.*

Frei antigen See *Lymphogranuloma venereum skin test antigen.*

Fructose. Powder (100, 500 Gm.).

Fuadin. See *Stibophen.*

Fulvicin-U/F. See *Griseofulvin.*

Fungizone. See *Amphotericin B.*

Furacin. See *Nitrofurazone.*

Furacin-E. Urethral inserts (12): 0.2% nitrofurazone, 0.008% diethyl stilbestrol, 2% diperodon.

Furadantin. See *Nitrofurantoin.*

Furadantin sodium. See *Nitrofurantoin sodium.*

Furosemide (Lasix). Ampules (2 ml.): 10 mg. per ml. Tablets (100): 40 mg.

G

Gammacorten. See *Dexamethasone.*
Gantrisin. See *Sulfisoxazole.*
Gantrisin acetyl. See *Sulfisoxazole acetyl.*
Gantrisin diethanolamine. See *Sulfisoxazole diethanolamine.*
Garamycin. See *Gentamicin sulfate.*
Gastrografin. See *Meglumine diatrizoate.*
Gelfoam. Powder, nonsterile (10 Gm.). Powder, sterile (1 Gm). Sponges: Size 12 to 13 mm. (20 × 60 × 3 mm.), size 12 to 17 mm. (20 × 60 × 7 mm.), size 50 (80 × 62.5 × 10 mm.), size 100 (80 × 125 × 10 mm.) and size 100 compressed (80 × 125 mm.).
Gemonil. See *Metharbital.*
Gentamicin sulfate (Garamycin). Cream (15 Gm.): 0.1%. Ointment, ophthalmic (4 Gm.): 0.3%. Ointment (15 Gm.): 0.1%. Vials (2 ml.): 5 mg. per ml. Vials (2 ml.): 40 mg. per ml. Solution, ophthalmic (5 ml.): 0.3%.
Gentian violet. See *Methylrosaniline chloride.*
Gentran. See *Dextran.*
Geopen. See *Carbenicillin.*
Glucagon. Ampules, powder: 1, 10 mg.
Glucatime. See *Meglumine antimonate.*
Glucola. Caronbated beverage (210 ml.): dextrose and hydrolyzable saccharides equivalent to 75 Gm. glucose.
Glutethimide (Doriden). Tablets (100): 125, 250, 500 mg.
Glycerin (glycerol). Liquid (pt.) Liquid (osmoglyn), 50% glycerin.
Glycerol. See *Glycerin.*
Glyceryl guaiacolate (Robitussin, Robitussin-DM). Syrup (125, 210 ml.): 20 mg. per ml. Syrup (125, 210 ml.): 20 mg. glyceryl guaiacolate and 3 mg. dextromethorphan per ml.
Glycobiarsol (Bismuth glycolyl arsanilate, Milibis). Suppositories (10): 250 mg. Tablets: 500 mg.
Gold sodium thiomalate (Myochristine). Ampules (1 ml.): 10, 25, 50, 100 mg. per ml. Vial (10 ml.): 50 mg. per ml.
Grifulvin V. See *Griseofulvin.*
Grisactin. See *Griseofulvin.*
Griseofulvin, micro size (Fulvicin-U/F, Grifulvin V, Grisactin). Capsules (100): 125, 250 mg. Suspension (125 ml.): 25 mg. per ml. Tablets (100): 125, 250, 500 mg.
Guanethidine sulfate (Ismelin sulfate). Tablets (100): 10, 25 mg.
Guanidine hydrochloride. Tablets (100): 125 mg.
Gynergen. See *Ergotamine tartrate.*

H

Haldol. See *Haloperidol.*
Haloperidol (Haldol). Ampules (1 ml.): 5 mg. per ml. Drops, oral concentrate (15, 120 ml.): 2 mg. per ml. (0.1 mg. per drop). Tablets (100): 0.5, 1, 2, 5 mg.
Haloprogin (Halotex). Cream (2, 10 Gm.): 1%. Solution (10, 30 ml.): 1%.
Halotestin. See *Fluoxymesterone.*
Halotex. See *Haloprogin.*
Hartmann's solution. See *Lactated Ringer's solution.*
Heparin sodium. Ampules (1 ml.): 1000, 5000, 10,000, 20,000 units per ml. Syringe, tubex (1 ml.): 1000, 5000, 7500, 10,000, 15,000, 20,000. Vials (4 ml.): 10,000 units per ml. Vials (2, 5, 10 ml.): 20,000 units per ml. Vials (10, 30 ml.): 1000 units per ml. Vials (10 ml.): 5000 units per ml.
Herpes simplex-1 vaccine, inactivated. Investigational.
Herplex. See *Idoxuridine.*
Hetrazan. See *Diethylcarbamazine.*
Hexachlorophene (pHisoHex). Emulsion (150 ml., pt.): 3%.
Hexadrol. See *Dexamethasone.*
Hexylresorcinol (Crystoids, ST-37). Pills (51): 100, 200 mg. Solution (150, 360 ml.): 0.1%.
Histadyl. See *Methapyrilene hydrochloride.*
Histoplasmin. Vial (1 ml.): histoplasma capsulation filtrate for skin test.
HMG. See *Menadotropins.*
HMS. See *Medrysone.*
Homatropine hydrobromide. Solution, sterile, ophthalmic (15 ml.): 1, 2, 5%.
HP Acthar gel. See *ACTH gel.*
Human growth hormone. N.I.H. investigational.
Human menopausal gonadotropin. See *Menadotropins.*
Humatin. See *Paromomycin.*
Hyaluronidase (Alidase, Hyazyme, Wydase). Powder, sterile (1 ml.): 150 units. Solution, stabilized (1, 10 ml.): 150 units per ml.
Hyazyme. See *Hyaluronidase.*
Hycanthone (Etrenol). Investigational.
Hydeltra. See *Prednisolone.*
Hydeltrasol. See *Prednisolone phosphate.*
Hydralazine hydrochloride (Apresoline hydrochloride). Ampule (1 ml.): 20 mg. Tablets (100): 10, 25, 50, 100 mg.
Hydriodic acid. Syrup (pt.): 14 mg. per ml. of hydrogen iodide.
Hydrocalciferol. See *Dihydrotachysterol.*
Hydrochlorothiazide (HydroDIURIL, Oretic). Tablets (100): 25, 50 mg.
Hydrocortamate (Ulcort). Ointment (15 Gm.): 0.05%.
Hydrocortisone (Cortef, Cortril, Hydrocortone, Hytone). Cream (15, 30, 125 Gm.): 0.125, 0.025, 0.5, 1%. Enema (60 ml.): 1.67 mg. per ml. Lotion (15, 30, 125 ml.): 0.25, 0.5, 1%. Suspension, oral (125 ml.): 2 mg. per ml. Tablets (50, 100): 5, 10, 20 mg. Vials, intramuscular (5 ml.): 50 mg. per ml.
Hydrocortisone acetate (Cortef acetate, Cortril acetate). Aerosol, rectal, Cortifoam: 10%. Ointment (5, 15, 30 Gm.): 1, 2.5%. Suspension, intra-articular (5 ml.): 25, 50 mg. per ml. Ointment, ophthalmic (3.5 Gm.): 1.5%. Suspension, ophthalmic (5 ml.): 2.5%.
Hydrocortisone cypionate (Cortef fluid). Suspension, oral (125 ml.): 2 mg. per ml.
Hydrocortisone phosphate (Cortiphate, Hydrocortone phosphate). Syringe (2 ml.): 50 mg. per ml. Vials (2, 10 ml.): 50 mg. per ml.
Hydrocortisone sodium succinate (Cortisol succinate, Solu-Cortef). Vial, powder: 100, 250, 500 mg., 1 Gm.
Hydrocortone. See *Hydrocortisone.*
Hydrocortone phosphate. See *Hydrocortisone phosphate.*
HydroDIURIL. See *Hydrochlorothiazide.*
Hydrogen peroxide. Solution (250 ml., pt.): 3%.
Hydronal. See *Isosorbide.*
Hydroquinone (Eldoquin, Eldopaque). Cream (15, 30 Gm.): 2%. Lotion (15 Gm.): 2%. Opaque base (15 Gm.): 2, 4%.
Hydroxyamphetamine hydrobromide (Paredrine hydrobromide). Solution, sterile ophthalmic (15 ml.): 1%.
Hydroxychloroquine sulfate (Plaquenil sulfate). Tablets (100): 200 mg.

2-Hydroxy-4 methoxy-benzophenone-5 sulfonic acid. See *Uval.*

Hydroxyprogesterone caproate (Delalutin, progesterone caproate). Syringe (1 ml.): 250 mg. per ml. Vials, in oil (2, 10 ml.): 125 mg. per ml. Vials, in oil (5 ml.): 250 mg. per ml.

Hydroxystilbamidine isethionate. Vials, powder: 225 mg.

Hydroxyzine hydrochloride (Atarax). Ampules (2 ml.): 50 mg. per ml. Syringe (1 ml.): 25, 50 mg. per ml. Syrup (pt.): 2 mg. per ml. Tablets (100): 10, 25, 50, 100 mg. Vials (10 ml.): 25, 50, mg. per ml.

Hydroxyzine pamoate (Vistaril). Capsules (100): 25, 50, 100 mg. equivalent to hydrochloride. Suspension, oral (pt.): 5 mg. per ml. equivalent to hydrochloride. Syringe (1 ml.): 25, 50 mg. per ml. Syringe (2 ml.): 50 mg. per ml. Vials (10 ml.): 25, 50 mg. per ml. as hydrochloride. Vials (2 ml.): 50 mg. per ml.

Hygroton. See *Chlorthalidone.*

Hykinone. See *Menadione sodium bisulfate.*

Hyoscine hydrobromide. See *Scopolamine hydrobromide.*

Hyparotin. See *Mumps immune globulin.*

Hyperstat. See *Diazoxide.*

Hyper-Tet. See *Tetanus immune globulin, human.*

Hypertussis. See *Pertussis immune globulin.*

Hytakerol. See *Dihydrotachysterol.*

Hy-Tet. See *Tetanus immune globulin, human.*

Hytone. See *Hydrocortisone.*

I

Idoxuridine (Dendrid, Herplex, Stoxil). Ointment. ophthalmic (4 Gm.): 0.5%. Solution, sterile ophthalmic (15 ml.): 0.1%. Injectable form investigational.

Iliotycin. See *Erythromycin.*

Ilosone. See *Erythromycin estolate.*

Ilotycin gluceptate. See *Erythromycin gluceptate.*

Imferon. See *Iron dextran.*

Imipramine hydrochloride (Tofranil). Ampules (2 ml.): 12.5 mg. per ml. Tablets (100): 10, 25, 50 mg.

Immune globulin, Rh_o (D) (Rho Gam). Vial: one dose. 1 ml. = 300 micrograms anti-D.

Immune serum globulin. Solution, 16.5%. Syringe, tubex: 1, 2 ml. Vials (2, 10 ml.).

Immu-Tet. See *Tetanus immune globulin, human.*

Imuran. See *Azathioprine.*

Inderal See *Propranolol.*

Indocin. See *Indomethacin.*

Indomethacin (Indocin). Capsules (100): 25, 50 mg.

Inflamase. See *Prednisolone phosphate.*

Inflamase forte. See *Prednisolone phosphate.*

Influenza virus vaccine (bivalent). Syringe, tubex: 0.5 ml. Vials (5 ml.).

I.N.H. See *Isoniazid.*

Inpersol. See *Peritoneal dialysis.*

Insulin (crystalline insulin). Vials: regular, beef special *or* pork (10 ml.): 40, 80, 100 units per ml.

Insulin, lente. See *Lente insulin.*

Insulin, NPH. See *Isophane insulin.*

Intal. See *Cromolyn sodium.*

Intralipid. Investigational.

Invert sugar (Travert). Solution, intravenous (150, 1000 ml.): 5% in water or saline. Solution, intravenous (250, 500, 1000 ml.): 10% in water or saline.

Iodinated glycerol (Organidin). Drops, oral (30 ml.): 50 mg. per ml. Elixir (pt.): 12 mg. per ml. Tablets (100): 30 mg.

Iodized oil (Lipiodol, Iodochloral). Ampule (5 ml.): 40%. Ampule (10 ml.): 28%, 40%. Vial (20 ml.): 28%, 40%.

Iodochloral. See *Iodized oil.*

Iodochlorhydroxyquin (Vioform). Cream (30 Gm.): 3%. Ointment (30 Gm.): 3%. Powder (15 Gm.).

Ionax. Aerosol (70 Gm.). Scrub (60 Gm.). Tube (60 Gm.). 0.2% benzalkonium chloride, polyoxyethylene ethers.

Ionil. Lotion (125, 250, 500 ml.). Salicylic acid 2%, benzalkonium chloride 0.2%, alcohol 13%.

Ionil-T. Shampoo (125, 250, 500 ml.). Salicylic acid 2%, benzalkonium chloride 0.2%, alcohol 13%.

Ionosol. See *Darrow's solution.*

Ipecac syrup. (30 ml., pt.).

Iron dextran (Imferon). Ampules, intramuscular, intravenous (2, 5 ml.): 50 mg. elemental iron per ml. Vials, intramuscular (10 ml.): 50 mg. elemental iron per ml.

Isemelin sulfate. See *Guanethidine sulfate.*

Isofluorophate (DPF, Floropryl). Ointment, ophthalmic (3.5 Gm.): 0.025%. Solution in oil, ophthalmic (5 ml.): 0.1%.

Isohist. Solution, ophthalmic (15 ml.). Chlorpheniramine, 0.1%, and phenylephrine, 0.125%.

Isolyte-M. Each 100 ml. contains: 5 Gm. dextrose, 230 mg. sodium lactate, 150 mg. potassium chloride, 130 mg. potassium phosphate, 91 mg. sodium chloride, 5 Gm. fructose.

Isoniazid (I.N.H., Nydrazid). Syrup (pt.): 10 mg. per ml. Tablets (100): 50, 100, 300 mg. Vials (10 ml.): 100 mg. per ml.

Isophane insulin (NPH insulin). Vials, regular, beef special *or* pork (10 ml.): 40, 80, 100 units per ml.

Isoproterenol hydrochloride (Isuprel hydrochloride, Proternol). Ampules (1, 5 ml.): 0.2 mg. per ml. Solution, inhalation (10 ml.): 5, 10 mg. per ml. Solution, Mistometer (300 inhalations): 125 micrograms per inhalation. Tablets, sublingual (50): 10, 15 mg. Tablets, sustained action (30): 15, 30 mg.

Isoproterenol sulfate (Medihaler-Iso, Vapo-N-Iso). Solution (300 inhalations): 75 micrograms per inhalation.

Isopto-Alkaline. See *Methylcellulose.*

Isopto-Cetamide. See *Sulfacetamide sodium.*

Isopto-Cetapred. Suspension, ophthalmic (5, 15 ml.). 10% sulfacetamide sodium, 0.25% prednisolone, 0.5% methylcellulose.

Isosorbide (Hydronal). Investigational.

Isuprel hydrochloride. See *Isoproterenol hydrochloride.*

K

Kanamycin sulfate (Kantrex). Capsules (20, 100): 500 mg. Vials (2 ml.): 37.5, 250 mg. per ml. Vials (3 ml.): 333 mg. per ml.

Kantrex. See *Kanamycin sulfate.*

Kaolin-pectin (Kaopectate). Suspension, oral (180, 300 ml.): 180 mg. kaolin and 4 mg. pectin per ml.

Kaon. See *Potassium gluconate.*

Kaopectate. See *Kaolin-pectin.*

Karaya (Sterculia). Powder (80 Gm., 1 lb.).

Kayexalate. See *Sodium polystyrene sulfonate.*

Keflex. See *Cephalexin.*

Keflin. See *Cephalothin sodium.*

Kenalog. See *Triamcinolone acetonide.*

Kenalog-S. See *Triamcinolone acetonide with neomycin sulfate.*

Keri. Lotion (225 ml.). Cream.

Ketaject. See *Ketamine hydrochloride.*

Ketalar. See *Ketamine hydrochloride.*
Ketamine hydrochloride (Ketalar, Ketaject). Vial (20, 50 ml.): 10 mg. per ml. Vial (10 ml.): 50 mg. per ml. Vial (5 ml.): 100 mg. per ml.
Ketostix. Reagent sticks (50, 100): sodium nitroprusside, sodium phosphate, glycine.
K-Lyte. Tablets, effervescent (30): 25 mEq. potassium bicarbonate.
Komed. Lotion (60 ml.): Mild 2% sodium thiosulfate, 1% salicylic acid, 1% resorcinol. Lotion (60 ml.): 8% sodium thiosulfate, 2% salicylic acid, 2% resorcinol.
Konakion. See *Phytonadione.*
Kwell. See *Benezene hexachloride.*

L

L-Arginine hydrochloride (R-Gene). Investigational.
L-Asparaginase. Vial, powder: 10,000, 50,000.
L-DOPA. See *Levodopa.*
Lacril. See *Methylcellulose.*
Lactated Ringer's solution (Hartmann's solution). Solution, intravenous (150, 250, 500, 1000 ml.).
Lactobacillus acidophilus in mineral oil. See *Neo-Cultol.*
Lanatoside C (Cedilanid). Tablets (100): 0.5 mg.
Lanoxin. See *Digoxin.*
Larodopa. See *Levodopa.*
Lasix. See *Furosemide.*
Lederplex. See *Vitamin B complex.*
Lente Iletin. See *Lente insulin.*
Lente insulin (Lente Iletin). Vials, regular, beef special, or pork (10 ml.): 40, 80 units per ml.
Leucovorin. See *Calcium leucovorin.*
Leukeran. See *Chlorambucil.*
Levallorphan tartrate (Lorfan tartrate). Ampules (1 ml.): 1 mg. per ml. Vials (10 ml.): 1 mg. per ml.
Levarterenol bitartrate (levophed bitartrate, norepinephrine bitartrate). Ampules (4 ml.): 0.2%.
Levodopa (Dopar, L-DOPA, Larodopa). Capsules (100): 100, 200, 500 mg. Tablets (100): 100, 250, 500 mg.
Levophed bitartrate. See *Levarterenol bitartrate.*
Librium. See *Chlordiazepoxide hydrochloride.*
Lidocaine hydrochloride (Xylocaine hydrochloride). Ampules (2, 5, 10 ml.): 1, 2%. Ampules (5 ml.): 4%. Jelly (30 Gm.): 2%. Ointment (35 Gm.): 2.5, 5%. Solution, topical (5, 50 ml.): 4%. Solution, viscous (100 ml.): 2%. Vials (20, 50 ml.): 0.5, 1, 2%.
Lidocaine hydrochloride with epinephrine (Xylocaine hydrochloride). Ampules (2 ml.): 2%. Vials (20, 30, 50 ml.): 0.5, 1, 2%.
Lilly M-76. See *Cyanide antidote package.*
Lincocin hydrochloride. See *Lincomycin hydrochloride.*
Lincomycin hydrochloride (Lincocin hydrochloride). Capsules (24, 100): 250, 500 mg. Syringe (2 ml.): 300 mg. per ml. Syrup (60 ml., pt.): 50 mg. per ml. Vials (2, 10 ml.): 300 mg. per ml.
Linoleic acid (Pentropin). Capsules (100).
Liothyronine (Cytomel). Tablets (100): 5, 25, 50 micrograms.
Lipiodol. See *Iodized oil.*
Liquor carbonis detergens. See *Coal tar solution.*
Liver extract. Vials, crude extract, intramuscular (10 ml.): 2, 10, 20 micrograms B_{12} acitvity per ml. Vials, purified antianemic fraction, intramuscular (10 ml.): 10, 20 micrograms B_{12} activity per ml.
Locasol. Low calcium milk substitute.
Locorten. See *Flumethasone pivalate.*
Lofenalac (special casein hydrolysate low in phenylalanine). Powder (2, 5 lb.).
Lomidine. See *Pentamidine.*
Lomotil. See *Diphenoxylate hydrochloride.*
Lomustine. See *CCNU.*
Lonalac (low sodium, high protein). Powder (1 lb.).
Lorfan tartrate. See *Levallorphan tartrate.*
Loridine. See *Cephaloridine.*
Lowila. Cake (100 Gm.): Lauryl sulfoacetate in corn dextrin base.
Luasmin. Capsules (100): 30 mg. ephedrine sulfate, 200 mg. theophylline sodium acetate, and 30 mg. phenobarbital sodium.
Lubath (dispersible cottonseed oil). Solution (250 ml., pt.).
Lubriderm. Cream (45, 120 Gm.). Lotion (125, 250 ml.). Oil, bath (250 ml.).
Lucanthone (Miracil D). Tablets (30 ml.): 200 mg.
Lufyllin. See *Dyphylline.*
Luminal. See *Phenobarbital.*
Luminal sodium. See *Phenobarbital sodium.*
Luride. See *Sodium fluoride.*
Lymphogranuloma venereum skin test antigen (Frei antigen). Vials 2 (1 ml.): 10 test antigen, 10 controls.
Lypressin (Diapid, 8 lysine vasopressin). Nasal spray (5 ml.): 50 units per ml. About 50 insufflations.
Lysine hydrochloride. Powder (10, 25, 100 Gm.).
8 Lysine vasopressin. See *Lypressin.*
Lysodren. See *Ortho-para DDD.*
Lytren (oral electrolyte formulation). Powder (250 Gm.).

M

Maalox. See *Aluminum and magnesium hydroxides.*
Macrodantin. See *Nitrofurantoin.*
Macrodex. See *Dextran.*
Mafenide (Sulfamylon). Cream (60, 120 Gm., 1 lb.): 85 mg. per Gm.
Magnesia magma. See *Magnesium hydroxide.*
Magnesium chloride. 4 Gm. provide 40 mEq. magnesium.
Magnesium citrate. 6 Gm. provide 40 mEq. magnesium.
Magnesium gluconate. Solution, extemporaneously compounded: 42 Gm. in 1000 ml. water gives 0.2 mEq. per ml.
Magnesium hydroxide (magnesia magma, milk of magnesia). Magma (pt.): 8%.
Magnesium oxide. Powder (lb.).
Magnesium sulfate. Ampules (2 ml.): 250, 500 mg. per ml. Ampules (20 ml.): 100 mg. per ml. Powder (125 Gm., 1 lb.). 50% solution provides 4 mEq. magnesium per ml.
Mandelamine. See *Methenamine mandelate.*
Mannitol. Ampules (50 ml.): 500 mg. per ml. Solution, intravenous (1000 ml.): 5, 10%. Solution, intravenous (500 ml.): 20%. Vials (50 ml.): 500 mg. per ml.
Marboran. See *Methisazone.*
Maxipen. See *Phenethicillin.*
Maxitrol. Suspension ophthalmic (5 ml.). Ointment (3.5 Gm.). Per Gm. or ml.: 0.1% dexamethasone, 3.5 mg. neomycin, 6000 units polymyxin B.
MBT. See *Meat base formula.*
MCT. See *Medium chain triglycerides.*
Measles vaccine, attenuated virus. Syringe, Edmonston

strain in chick embryo. Vials, Edmonston strain in chick embryo: one dose. Vials, Edmonston strain in canine renal tissue: one dose. Vials, Schwartz strain in chick embryo.

Meat base formula (MBT). Liquid (13 oz.).

Mebaral. See *Mephobarbital.*

Mechlorethamine hydrochloride (Mustargen hydrochloride, nitrogen mustard). Vials, sterile powder: 10 mg.

Meclizine hydrochloride (Bonine). Tablets, chewable (100): 25 mg.

Medihaler-Iso. See *Isoproterenol sulfate.*

Medium chain triglycerides (MCT, Portagen). MCT oil (gal.). Portagen powder (1 lb.): 20 calories per oz. (normal dilution) 18% protein and 22% fat.

Medrol. See *Methylprednisolone.*

Medroxyprogesterone acetate (Depo-Provera, Provera). Tablets (5, 25, 100): 2.5, 10 mg. Vials, sterile suspension (1, 5 ml.): 50, 100 mg. per ml.

Medrysone (HMS). Suspension, ophthalmic (2.5, 5, 10 ml.): 1.0%.

Meglumine antimonate (Glucantime). Investigational.

Meglumine diatrizoate (Gastrografin, Renografin). Solution (120 ml.): 76%. Vials (20, 30, 50 ml.): 30, 60, 76%.

Mel W. See *Melarsonyl potassium.*

Melarsoprol (Arsobal). Injection: 3.6% in propylene glycol. Not available in the United States.

Melarsonyl potassium (Mel W, trimelarsen). Not available in the United States.

Mellaril. See *Thioridazine.*

Meloxine. See *Methoxsalen.*

Menadiol sodium diphosphate (Synkayvite). Ampules (1 ml.): 5, 10 mg. per ml. Ampules (2 ml.): 37.5 mg. per ml. Tablets (100): 5 mg.

Menadione sodium bisulfate (Hykinone). Ampules (1 ml.): 5 mg. per ml. Ampules (1 ml.): 10 mg. per ml. Tablets (100): 5 mg.

Menadotropins (HMG, human menopausal gonadotropin, Pergonal). Ampules (2 ml.): 75 units follicle stimulating hormone (luteinizing hormone activity 75 mg.).

Menotropins. See *Pergonal.*

Mepacrine. See *Quinacrine hydrochloride.*

Meperidine hydrochloride (Demerol hydrochloride). Ampules (0.5, 1, 1.5, 2 ml.): 50 mg. per ml. Ampules (1, 2 ml.): 100 mg. per ml. Elixir (pt.): 10 mg. per ml. Syringes, disposable (1 ml.): 50, 75, 100 mg. Tablets (100): 50, 100 mg. Vials (10, 30 ml.): 50 mg. per ml. Vials (20 ml.): 100 mg. per ml.

Mephenteramine sulfate (Wyamine). Ampules (2 ml.): 15 mg. per ml. Syringe, tubex (1 ml.): 30 mg. per ml. Tablets (100): 12.5, 25 mg. Vials (1, 10 ml.): 15, 30 mg. per ml.

Mephenytoin (Mesantoin). Tablets (100): 100 mg.

Mephyton. See *Phytonadione.*

Meprobamate (Equanil, Miltown). Ampules (5 ml.): 80 mg. per ml. Capsules, sustained action (100): 200, 400 mg. Suspension, oral (125 ml.): 40 mg. per ml. Tablets (100): 200, 400 mg.

Mephobarbital (Mebaral). Tablets (100): 30, 50, 100, 200 mg.

Meralluride sodium (Mercuhydrin sodium). Ampules (1, 2 ml.): 130 mg. per ml. Vials (10 ml.): 130 mg. per ml.

Merbromin (Mercurochrome). Solution (15 ml.): 2%. Surgical solution (28, 110 ml.).

Mercaptomerin sodium (Thiomerin sodium). Syringe (1, 2 ml.): 125 mg. per ml. Vials (2, 10, 30 ml.): 125 mg. per ml. Vials, powder: 1.4 Gm.

Mercaptopurine (6-mercaptopurine, Purinthol). Tablets (25, 250): 50 mg.

Mercuhydrin sodium. See *Meralluride sodium.*

Mercuric oxide, yellow. Ointment, ophthalmic (3.5 Gm.): 1, 2%.

Mercurochrome. See *Merbromin.*

Mercury, ammoniated. Ointment, ophthalmic (4 Gm.): 2.5%.

Mesantoin. See *Mephenytoin.*

Mestinon bromide. See *Pyridostigmine bromide.*

Metamucil (psyllium hydrophilic mucilloid). Powder (210, 420 Gm.).

Metandren. See *Methyltestosterone.*

Metaproterenol sulfate. See *Orciprenaline sulfate.*

Metaraminol bitartrate (Aramine bitartrate). Ampules (1 ml.): 10 mg. per ml. Vials (10 ml.): 10 mg. per ml.

Methadone (Dolophine). Ampules (1 ml.): 10 mg. per ml. Syringe (pt.): 0.33 mg. per ml. Tablets (100): 5, 10 mg. Vials (20 ml.): 10 mg. per ml. Available only in hospital pharmacies.

Methamphetamine hydrochloride (Desoxyn hydrochloride, Methedrine hydrochloride). Tablets (100): 2.5, 5 mg. Tablets, sustained action (100): 5, 10, 15 mg.

Methandrostenolone (Dianabol). Tablets (100): 2.5, 5 mg.

Methapyrilene hydrochloride (Histadyl). Ampules (10 ml.): 20 mg. per ml. Capsules (100): 25, 50 mg. Syrup (pt.): 4 mg. per ml.

Metharbital (Gemonil). Tablets (100): 100 mg.

Methedrine hydrochloride. See *Methamphetamine hydrochloride.*

Methenamine mandelate (Mandelamine). Suspension (125 ml., pt.): 50 mg. per ml. Suspension, forte (250 ml.): 100 mg. per ml. Tablets (100): 250, 500 mg., 1 Gm.

Methicillin sodium (Dimocillin R-T, Staphcillin). Vials: 1, 4, 6 Gm.

Methi-I-Sol. See *Methylcellulose.*

Methimazole (Tapazole). Tablets (100): 5, 10 mg.

Methionine (D-L methionine). Tablets (100): 200, 500 mg.

Methisazone (Marboran). Investigational.

Methocarbamol (Robaxin). Tablets (50): 500, 750 mg. Vials (10 ml.): 100 mg. per ml.

Methotrexate (amethopterin). Tablets (100): 2.5 mg.

Methotrexate sodium (amethopterin sodium). Vials (2 ml.): 2.5, 25 mg. per ml.

Methoxamine hydrochloride (Vasoxyl). Ampules (1 ml.): 10 mg. per ml. Vials (10 ml.): 10 mg. per ml.

Methoxsalen (Meloxine, Oxsoralen). Capsules (28, 100): 10 mg. Lotion (30 ml.): 1%. Tablets (28): 10 mg.

Methoxyphenamine hydrochloride (Orthoxine hydrochloride). Syrup (pt.): 10 mg. per ml. Tablets (100): 100 mg.

Methsuximide (Celontin). Capsules (100): 150, 300 mg.

Methylbenzethonium chloride (Diaparene). Granules (250 Gm.): 6%. Lotion (150 ml.): 1:1500. Ointment (30, 60, 125 Gm.): 1:1000. Powder (125, 275 Gm.). Tablets, precrushed for diaper rinse (20).

Methylcellulose (artificial tears, Cellothyl, Isopto-Alkaline, Lacril, Meth-I-Sol, Tearisol). Solution, isotonic (15 ml.). Solution, alkaline isotonic (15 ml.): 0.45, 1%. Tablets (100): 500 mg.

Methyldopa (Aldomet). Tablets (100): 250 mg.

Methyldopate hydrochloride (Aldomet ester hydrochloride). Ampules (5 ml.): 50 mg. per ml.

Methylene blue. Ampules (1, 10 ml.): 10 mg. per ml.

Methylhydrazine. Investigational.

Methylphenidate hydrochloride (Ritalin hydrochloride). Tablets (100): 5, 10, 20 mg. Vials, powder (10 ml.): 100 mg.

Methylprednisolone (Medrol). Capsules, sustained action (30, 100): 2, 4 mg. Tablets (30, 50, 100): 2, 4, 16 mg.

Methylprednisolone acetate (Depo-Medrol). Cream (7.5, 45 Gm.): 0.25, 1%. Enema: 40 mg. Vials (1, 5 ml.): 20, 40, 80 mg. per ml.

Methylprednisolone sodium succinate (Solu-Medrol). Vials (1 ml.): 40 mg. per ml. Vial (2, 8, 16 ml.): 62.5 mg. per ml.

Methylrosaniline chloride (gentian violet). Solution (30 ml.): 1, 2%.

Methyltestosterone (Metandren, Oreton). Tablets (100): 10, 25 mg. Tablets, sublingual or buccal (100): 5, 10 mg.

Methysergide maleate (Sansert). Tablets (50): 2 mg.

Meticortelone. See *Prednisolone.*

Meticorten. See *Prednisone.*

Metimyd. Ointment, ophthalmic (3.5 Gm.): 0.5% prednisolone, 10% sodium sulfacetamide. Suspension, ophthalmic (5 ml.): 5 mg. prednisolone acetate, 100 mg. sodium sulfacetamide per ml.

Metopirone. See *Metyrapone ditartrate.*

Metronidazole (Flagyl). Inserts, vaginal (10): 500 mg. Tablets (100): 250 mg.

Metycaine. See *Piperocaine hydrochloride.*

Metyrapone ditartrate (Metopirone). Tablets (18): 250 mg. Vials (10 ml.): 100 mg. per ml.

Milibis. See *Glycobiarsol.*

Milk of magnesia. See *Magnesium hydroxide.*

Millepore. See *Filters, cellulose.*

Milotin. See *Phensuximide.*

Miltown. See *Meprobamate.*

Minocycline hydrochloride. Capsules (50): 100 mg. Syrup (60 ml.): 10 mg. per ml. Vials, powder: 100 mg.

Mintezol. See *Thiabendazole.*

Miracil D. See *Lucanthone.*

Mitotane. See *Ortho-para DDD.*

Moebiquin. See *Diiodohydroxyquin.*

Mogadon. See *Nitrazepam.*

Monopar. See *Stibazium iodide.*

Moranyl. See *Suramin.*

Morphine sulfate. Ampules (1 ml.): 8, 10, 15 mg. per ml. Syringe, tubex (1 ml.): 8, 10, 15 mg. Vials (20 ml.): 10, 15 mg. per ml.

Mucomyst. See *Acetylcysteine.*

Mull-Soy. Liquid (15.5 oz.): 20 calories per oz. (normal dilution).

Multivitamins with vitamin E (Vi-Penta). Drops, oral (15, 50, 220 ml.).

Mumps immune globulin (Hyparotin). Vials (1.5, 4.5 ml.).

Mumps skin test antigen. Vials (1 ml.): 10 tests.

Mumps vaccine, attenuated virus (Mumpsvax). Vials (2 ml.): 1 immunization.

Mumpsvax. See *Mumps vaccine, attenuated virus.*

Mustargen. See *Nitrogen mustard.*

Mustargen hydrochloride. See *Mechlorethamine.*

M.V.I. (injectable multivitamins). Ampules (10 ml.). Vials concentrate (equivalent to 10-ml. ampule (5 ml.).

Myambutol hydrochloride. See *Ethambutol hydrochloride.*

Mychel S. See *Chloramphenicol sodium succinate.*

Mycifradin. See *Neomycin sulfate.*

Myciquent. See *Neomycin sulfate.*

Mycitracin. Ointment (15, 30 Gm.) and ointment, ophthalmic (4 Gm.): 5000 units polymyxin B sulfate, 5 mg. neomycin sulfate, and 500 units bacitracin per Gm.

Mycolog. Cream or ointment (5, 15, 30, 120 Gm.): 1 mg. triamcinolone acetonide, 2.5 mg. neomycin, 0.25 mg. gramicidin, and 100,000 units nystatin per Gm.

Mycostatin. See *Nystatin.*

Mydriacyl. See *Tropicamide.*

Myleran. See *Busulfan.*

Myochristine. See *Gold sodium thiomalate.*

Mysoline. See *Primidone.*

Mytelase. See *Ambenonium chloride.*

N

Nafcillin sodium (Unipen). Capsules (24): 250 mg. Suspension, powder, oral (80 ml.): 50 mg. per ml. Vials, powder: 50 mg. 1, 2 Gm.

Nalidixic acid. Tablets: 250, 500 mg.

Nalline hydrochloride. See *Nalorphine hydrochloride.*

Nalorphine hydrochloride (Nalline hydrochloride). Ampules (1 ml.): 0.2 mg. per ml. Ampules (1, 2 ml.): 5 mg. per ml. Vials (10 ml.): 5 mg. per ml.

Naloxone (Narcan). Ampules (1 ml.): 0.4 mg. per ml. Vials (10 ml.): 0.4 mg. per ml.

Naphazoline (Vasocon). Solution, ophthalmic (15 ml.): 0.1%.

Narcan. See *Naloxone.*

Nema. See *Tetrachloroethylene.*

Nembutal sodium. See *Pentobarbital sodium.*

Neo-Aristocort. Cream (15 Gm.). Ointment (15 Gm.). Ointment, otic or ophthalmic (3.5 Gm.). 0.1% triamcinolone acetonide and 0.35% neomycin.

Neobiotic See *Neomycin sulfate.*

Neo-Calglucon. See *Calcium gluconogalactogluconate.*

Neo-Cortef. Ointment, ophthalmic or otic (3.5 Gm.): 5 or 15 mg. hydrocortisone acetate, 15 mg. neomycin sulfate per Gm. Suspension, ophthalmic or otic (2.5, 5 ml.): 5 mg. or 15 mg. hydrocortisone acetate, 5 mg. neomycin sulfate per ml.

Neo-Cultol (Lactobacillus acidophilus in mineral oil). Suspension (180 ml.).

Neo-Decadron. Cream, topical (15, 30 Gm.): 1 mg. dexamethasone and 5 mg. neomycin sulfate per Gm. Ointment, ophthalmic (4 Gm.): 0.5 mg. dexamethasone and 5 mg. neomycin sulfate per Gm. Solution, ophthalmic (2.5, 5 ml.): 1 mg. dexamethasone and 5 mg. neomycin sulfate per ml.

Neo-Delta-Cortef. Ointment, ophthalmic or otic (3.5 Gm.): 2.5 or 5.0 mg. prednisolone acetate, 5 mg. neomycin sulfate per Gm. Suspension, ophthalmic or otic (5 ml.): 2.5 mg. prednisolone acetate, 5 mg. neomycin sulfate.

Neo-Deltef. Solution, ophthalmic (2.5 ml.): 2 mg. prednisolone, 5 mg. neomycin sulfate per ml.

Neo-Hydeltrasol. Ointment, ophthalmic (3.5 Gm.): 2.5 mg. prednisolone, 5 mg. neomycin sulfate per Gm. Solution, ophthalmic (2.5, 5 ml.): 5 mg. prednisolone, 5 mg. neomycin sulfate per ml.

Neo-Medrol. Ointment, ophthalmic (4 Gm.): 0.1% methylprednisolone and 0.5% neomycin sulfate.

Neomycin sulfate (Mycifradin, Myciquent, Neobiotic). (500 mg. neomycin equivalent to 350 mg. neomycin base). Ointment, ophthalmic (4 Gm.): 5 mg. per Gm. Solution, oral (60 ml.): 25 mg. per ml. Tablets (20, 100): 500 mg. Vials, sterile powder: 500 mg.

Neo-Nysta-Cort. Ointment (15 Gm.): 10 mg. hydrocortisone, 5 mg. neomycin sulfate, and 100,000 units nystatin per Gm.

Neo-Polycin. Ointment, ophthalmic (4 Gm.): bacitracin, neomycin, and polymyxin. Ointment (15 Gm.): bacitracin, neomycin, and polymyxin. Solution, ophthalmic (10 ml.): gramicidin, neomycin, and polymyxin.

Neosone. Ointment, ophthalmic (3.5 Gm.): 15 mg. cortisone acetate and 5 mg. neomycin sulfate per Gm.

Neosporin. Cream (15 Gm.): gramicidin, neomycin, and polymyxin. Ointment (15, 30 Gm.): zinc bacitracin, neomycin, and polymyxin. Ointment, ophthalmic (4 Gm.): bacitracin, neomycin, and polymyxin. Powder (10 Gm.): polymyxin B, neomycin sulfate, and zinc bacitracin. Solution, ophthalmic (10 ml.): gramicidin, neomycin, and polymyxin. Spray, aerosol (90 Gm.): polymyxin B sulfate, neomycin sulfate, and zinc bacitracin.

Neostibosan. See *Ethylstilbamine.*

Neostigmine bromide (Prostigmine bromide). Tablets (100): 15 mg.

Neostigmine methylsulfate (Prostigmine methylsulfate). Ampules (1 ml.): 0.25, 0.5 mg. per ml. Vials (10 ml.): 0.5, 1 mg. per ml.

Neo-Synalar. See *Fluocinolone acetonide with neomycin sulfate.*

Neo-Synephrine hydrochloride. See *Phenylephrine hydrochloride.*

Nethaprin. Capsules (100): 25 mg. nethamine hydrochloride, 60 mg. butaphyllamine, and 6 mg. decapryn. Syrup (pt.): 5 mg. nethamine hydrochloride, 12 mg. butaphyllamine, and 1.2 mg. decapryn per ml.

Neutra-Phos. Dibasic sodium potassium, and monobasic sodium and potassium phosphate. 6 Gm. supply 1 Gm. phosphorus. Capsules (48): 1.25 Gm. Powder (67 Gm.).

Neutrogena. Soap, regular or unscented.

Niacin. See *Nicotinic acid.*

Niacinamide. See *Nicotinamide.*

Niclosamide (Yomesan). Investigational.

Nicotinamide (niacinamide, nicotinic acid amide). Tablets (100): 25, 50, 100 mg. Vials (5 ml.): 100 mg. per ml.

Nicotinic acid (niacin). Tablets (100): 25, 50, 100, 500 mg. Vials (10 ml.): 10 mg. per ml.

Nicotinic acid amide. See *Nicotinamide.*

Night solution. Solution, aerosol: 10% propylene glycol, 3% glycerin, and 87% water.

Nilodor. Liquid deodorant (7.5, 15 ml.).

Niridazole (Ambilhar). Tablets: 500 mg. (limited sale).

Nitrazepam. Investigational.

Nitrazine (phenaphthazine). Paper strips (100): for pH determinations within a range of 4.5 to 7.5.

Nitrofurantoin (Furadantin, Macrodantin). Capsules, macrocrystals (100): 25, 50, 100 mg. Suspension, oral (60 ml., pt.): 5 mg. per ml. Tablets (25, 100): 50, 100 mg.

Nitrofurantoin sodium (Furadantin sodium). Vials, powder: 180 mg.

Nitrofurazone (Furacin). Urethral inserts (12): 2%. Cream (14, 28 Gm.): 0.2%.

Nitrogen mustard (Mustargen). 10 mg. per vial in 20-ml. vial.

Nivea. Cream (30, 60 Gm., 1 lb.). Oil (60, 120 ml., pt.). Soap.

Nonasodium phytate See *Sodium phytate.*

Norepinephrine bitartrate. See *Levarterenol bitartrate.*

Norethindrone (Norlutin). Tablets (30): 5 mg.

Norethindrone acetate (Norlutate). Tablets (30): 5 mg.

Norinyl. Tablets (20): 1 mg. or 2 mg. norethindrone and 0.05 mg. mestranol. Tablets (21): 1 mg. norethindrone, 0.05 mg. (1/50-21) or 0.08 mg. (1/80-21) mestranol. Tablets (28): 21 tablets as above plus 7 inert tablets.

Norlestrin. Tablets (21): 1 mg. norethindrone acetate and 50 micrograms ethinyl estradiol. Tablets (28): 21 tablets as above and 7 inert tablets. Tablets (21, 100): 2.5 mg. norethindrone and 50 micrograms ethinyl estradiol.

Norlutate. See *Norethindrone acetate.*

Norlutin. See *Norethindrone.*

Normosol-M (Multiple electrolyte solution). Each 100 ml. contains 5 Gm. dextrose, 234 mg. sodium chloride, 128 mg. potassium acetate, and 21 mg. magnesium acetate.

Nor-Quen. Tablets (20): 0.08 mg. mestranol (14 white tablets), 0.08 mg. mestranol, 2 mg. norethindrone (6 blue tablets).

Notec. See *Chloral hydrate.*

Notezine. See *Diethylcarbamazine.*

Novahistine. Elixir (pt.): 0.2 mg. chlorpheniramine and 1 mg. phenylephrine per ml.

NPH insulin. See *Isophane insulin.*

Nupercaine. See *Dibucaine.*

Nutramigen (protein hydrolysate). Powder (1 lb.): 20 calories per oz. (normal dilution).

Nutraspa. Oil, bath (250 ml., pt.): oil-soluble lanolin fraction.

Nydrazid. See *Isoniazid.*

Nystaform-HC. Lotion (30 ml.): 0.5% hydrocortisone, 3% iodochlorhydroxyquin, 100,000 units per Gm. nystatin. Ointment (15 Gm.): 1% hydrocortisone, 3% iodochlorhydroxyquin, 100,000 units per Gm. nystatin.

Nystatin (Mycostatin). Cream (15 Gm.): 100,000 units per Gm. Ointment, Plastibase (15, 30 Gm.): 100,000 units per Gm. Powder (15 Gm.): 100,000 units per Gm. Suspension (60 ml.): 100,000 units per ml. Tablets (100): 500,000 units. Tablets, vaginal (15, 30): 100,000 units.

O

Oatmeal, colloidal. See *Aveeno.*

OFF (diethyl toluamide). Aerosol (195, 435 Gm.). Foam (190 Gm.). Liquid (45 ml.).

Oilatum. Cream, pH 5.5 (80 Gm.). Soap, cake (100 Gm.): neutral soap containing 7.5% free, polyunsaturated vegetable oil.

Old tuberculin (O.T.). Vials: 10 Mantoux tests.

Oleovitamin A and D (Percomorph liver oil). Capsules (100): 4000 units vitamin A and 400 units vitamin D. Drops (50 ml.): 1560 units vitamin A and 312 units vitamin D per drop. Tablets (100): 4000 units vitamin A and 400 units vitamin D.

Omnipen. See *Ampicillin trihydrate.*

Omnipen-N. See *Ampicillin sodium.*

Oncovin. See *Vincristine sulfate.*

Ophthaine. See *Proparacaine hydrochloride.*

Ophthetic. See *Proparacaine hydrochloride.*

Ophthocort. Ointment, ophthalmic (3.5 Gm.): 1% chloramphenicol, 0.5% hydrocortisone acetate, 5000 units per Gm. polymixin B.

Opium tincture, camphorated. See *Paregoric.*

Op-Thal-Zin. See *Zinc sulfate.*

Optihist. Chlorpheniramine, 0.3%, phenylephrine, 0.12%, and piperocaine 0.5%. Solution, ophthalmic (15 ml.).

Oracon. Tablets (21): 16 white containing 100 micrograms ethinyl estradiol; 5 peach containing 100 micrograms ethinyl estradiol and 25 mg. dimethisterone.

Orciprenaline sulfate (Alupent, metaproterenol sulfate). Ampules (1 ml.): 500 micrograms. Tablets: 20 mg. Not available in the United States.

Oretic. See *Hydrochlorothiazide.*

Oreton. See *Methyltestosterone.*

Oreton propionate. See *Testosterone propionate.*

Organidin. See *Iodinated glycerol.*

Orimune poliovirus vaccine. See *Poliovirus vaccine, trivalent.*

Ornade. Capsules, sustained action (50): 8 mg. chlorpheniramine maleate, 50 mg. phenylpropanolamine hydrochloride, and 2.5 mg. isopropamide iodide.

Ortho-Novum. Tablets (20): 2 mg. or 10 mg. norethindrone, 0.06 mg. mestranol. Tablets (20, 21): 1 mg. norethindrone, 0.05 mg. (1/50-21) or 0.08 mg. (1/80-21) mestranol.

Ortho-Novum SQ. Tablets (20): 14 white tablets, 0.08 mg. mestranol; 6 blue tablets, 0.08 mg. mestranol, 2 mg. norethindrone.

Ortho-para DDD (Lysodren, mitotane). Tablets: 500 mg.

Orthoxine hydrochloride. See *Methoxyphenamine hydrochloride.*

Ospolot (Conadil, Sulthiame). Investigational.

O.T. See *Old tuberculin.*

Oxacillin sodium (Prostaphlin sodium). Capsules (48, 100): 250, 500 mg. Suspension, oral (100 ml.): 50 mg. per ml. Vials, powder: 250, 500 mg., 1, 2 Gm.

Oxsoralen. See *Methoxsalen.*

Oxtriphylline (Choledyl, choline theophyllinate). 64% theophylline. Elixir (pt.) 20 mg. per ml. Tablets (100): 100, 200 mg.

Oxycel. See *Cellulose, oxidized.*

Oxylone. See *Fluorometholone.*

Oxymetazoline hydrochloride (Afrin). Solution, nasal (30 ml.): 0.5%. Spray, nasal (15 ml.): 0.5%.

Oxymetholone (Adroyd, Anadrol). Tablets (30): 2.5, 5, 10, 50 mg.

Oxytetracycline calcium (Terramycin). Drops, oral (10 ml.): 100 mg. per ml. Syrup (60 ml., pt.): 25 mg. per ml.

Oxytetracycline hydrochloride (Terramycin hydrochloride). Ampules, intramuscular (2 ml.): 50, 125 mg. per ml. Capsules (16, 100): 125, 250 mg. Ointment, ophthalmic (4 Gm.): 5 mg. oxytetracycline and 10,000 units polymixin per Gm. Solution, ophthalmic (5 ml.): 5 mg. per ml. Vials, intramuscular (10 ml.): 50 mg. per ml. Vials, powder, intravenous: 250, 500 mg.

Oxytocin (Pitocin). Ampules (0.5, 1 ml.): 10 units per ml.

Oxytocin citrate (Pitocin citrate). Tablets, buccal: 200 units.

P

P2AM. See *Pralidoxime chloride.*

Pabafilin. Gel (120 ml.): para-amino benzoic acid in ethyl alcohol 70%.

Pabanol. Solution (125 ml.): 5% para-amino benzoic acid, 70% ethyl alcohol.

Paludrine hydrochloride. See *Chloroguanide hydrochloride.*

2-PAM. See *Pralidoxime chloride.*

Pamisyl. See *Aminosalicylic acid.*

Pancreatic dornase (deoxyribonuclease, Dornovac). Vials, powder (2 ml.): 100,000 units.

Pancreatin (Cotazyme, Viokase). Capsules (100). Packets (250). Powder (125, 250 Gm.): 1.5 Gm. per teaspoon. Tablets (100, 500): 300 mg.

Panwarfin. See *Warfarin sodium.*

Papaverine. Ampules (1, 2 ml.): 30 mg. per ml. Tablets (100): 30, 60, 100, 200 mg. Vial (10 ml.): 30 mg. per ml.

Paredione. See *Paramethadione.*

Paral. See *Paraldehyde.*

Paraldehyde (Paral). Ampules (6, 12): 2, 5, 10 ml. Liquid (30 ml.). Capsules (60): 1 Gm.

Paramethadione (Paradione). Capsules (100): 150, 300 mg. Solution, oral (50 ml.): 300 mg. per ml.

Parathyroid. Vials (5 ml.): 100 units per ml.

Paredione. See *Paramethadione.*

Paredrine hydrobromide. See *Hydroxyamphetamine hydrobromide.*

Paregoric (camphorated opium tincture). Tincture (30 ml.): 0.4 mg. morphine per ml.

Parenogen. See *Fibrinogen.*

Paromomycin (Humatin.) Capsules (16): 250 mg. Syrup (60 ml.): 25 mg. per ml.

PAS. See *Aminosalicylic acid.*

Pathocil. See *Dicloxacillin sodium monohydrate.*

Pedialyte (oral electrolyte). Solution (250 ml.): hospital use only. Solution (1 qt.) 30 mEq. sodium, 20 mEq. potassium, 4 mEq. magnesium, 30 mEq. potassium, 4 mEq. magnesium, 30 mEq. chloride, 28 mEq. lactate, 50 Gm. dextrose per liter.

Pediamycin. See *Erythromycin ethyl succinate.*

Peganone. See *Ethotoin.*

Penbritin. See *Ampicillin trihydrate.*

Penbriten-S. See *Ampicillin sodium.*

D-Penicillamine (Cuprimine). Capsules (50): 250 mg.

Penicillin G potassium. 1 million units = 625 mg., 200,000 units = 125 mg., 1.68 mEq. of potassium per million units. Syrup, powder (100, 200 ml.): 40,000, 80,000 units per ml. Tablets (100): 200,000, 250,000, 400,000, 500,000, 800,000 units. Vials, powder: 200,000, 500,000, and 1, 5, 10, 20 million units.

Penicillin G, procaine. Syringes (1 ml.): 300,000 units per ml. Syringes, tubex (1 ml.): 300,000 units per ml. Syringes (1.2 ml.): 600,000 units. Syringes, tubex (1, 2, 4 ml.): 600,000 units per ml. Syringes (2 ml.): 600,000 units per ml. Vials, aqueous suspension (10 ml.): 300,000, 600,000 units per ml. Vials, suspension in oil (10 ml.): 300,000 units per ml.

Penicillin G sodium. 1.76 mEq. sodium per million units. Vials, powder: 1,000,000, 5,000,000 units.

Penicillin V. See *Phenoxymethyl penicillin.*

Penicillin VK (Phenoxymethyl penicillin potassium). Solution, oral (40, 100, 150, 200 ml.): 25 mg. (40,000 units) per ml. Solution, oral (80, 100, 150, 200 ml.): 50 mg. (80,000 units) per ml. Tablets (100): 125, 250, 500 mg. (200,000, 400,000, 800,000 units).

Pentamidine (Lomidine). Investigational.

Pentamidine isethionates. Ampules, powder: 200 mg. Obtainable from Communicable Disease Center, Atlanta, Georgia; telephone 404-633-3311.

Pentazocine. Ampules (1, 1.5, 2.0 ml.): 30 mg. per ml. Tablets (100): 50 mg. Vials (10 ml.): 30 mg. per ml.

Pentobarbital sodium (Nembutal sodium). Ampules (2, 5 ml.): 50 mg. per ml. Capsules (100): 30, 50, 100 mg. Elixir (pt.): 4 mg. per ml. Suppositories (6, 12): 30, 60, 120, 200 mg. Vials (20, 50 ml.): 50 mg. per ml.

Pentolinium tartrate (Ansolysen). Tablets (100): 20, 40, 100 mg. Vials (10 ml.): 10 mg. per ml.

Pentostam. See *Sodium stibogluconate.*

Perandren. See *Testosterone propionate.*

Percomorph liver oil. See *Oleovitamin A and D.*

Percoten acetate. See *Desoxycorticosterone acetate.*

Percoten pivalate. See *Desoxycorticosterone pivalate.*

Pergonal (Menotropins). Follicle-stimulating hormone, human. Vials (2 ml.): 75 units, luteinizing hormone activity 75 mg.

Periactin hydrochloride. See *Cyproheptadine hydrochloride.*

Peri-Colace. Capsules (30, 60): 100 mg. dioctyl sodium sulfosuccinate and 30 mg. casanthranol. Syrup (250 ml.): 4 mg. dioctyl solium sulfosuccinate and 2 mg. casanthranol per ml.

Peritoneal dialysis (Dianeal, Inpersol). Solution (1 liter): 1.5, 4.25% dextrose. Each 100 ml. contains: 140.5 mEq. sodium chloride, 3.5 mEq. calcium chloride, 1.5 mEq. magnesium chloride, and 4.45 mEq. sodium lactate.

Pernox. Cream (60 Gm.): 2% sulfur, 1.5% salicylic acid with microfine polyethylene granules.

Perphenazine (Trilafon). Ampules (1 ml.): 5 mg. per ml. Liquid, concentrate (125 ml.): 3.2 mg. per ml. Suppositories (6): 2, 4, 8, 16 mg. Syrup (125 ml.): 0.4 mg. per ml. Tablets (50): 2, 4, 8 mg. Tablets, repeat action (100): 8 mg. Vials (10 ml.): 5 mg. per ml.

Pertropin. See *Linoleic acid.*

Pertussis immune globulin (Hypertussis). Vials (1.25 ml.): equivalent to 25 ml. human hyperimmune serum.

Pertussis vaccine. See *Diphtheria.*

Phemerol. See *Benzethonium chloride.*

Phenacemide (Phenurone). Tablets (100): 500 mg.

Phenaphthazine. See *Nitrazine.*

Phenergan expectorant. Syrup (pt.): 1 mg. promethazine hydrochloride with ipecac fluidextract and potassium guaiacolate.

Phenergan hydrochloride. See *Promethazine hydrochloride.*

Phenethicillin (Maxipen). Tablets (24, 100): 250 mg.

Phenobarbital (Eskabarb, Luminal). Capsules, sustained action (100): 60, 100 mg. Elixir (pt.): 4 mg. per ml. Tablets (100): 15, 30, 60, 100 mg.

Phenobarbital sodium (Luminal sodium). Ampules, powder: 130, 300 mg. Ampules in propylene glycol (1 ml.): 130 mg.

Phenoxybenzamine hydrochloride (Dibenzyline). Capsules (100): 10 mg.

Phenoxymethyl penicillin (Penicillin V). Suspension, oral (80, 150 ml.): 36 mg. per ml. Tablets (25, 50): 125, 250, 300 mg.

Phenoxymethyl penicillin potassium. See *Penicillin VK.*

Phensuximide (Milontin). Capsules (100): 250, 500 mg. Suspension, oral (pt.): 62.5 mg. per ml.

Phentolamine hydrochloride (Regitine hydrochloride). Tablets (100): 50 mg.

Phentolamine methanesulfonate (Regitine methanesulfonate). Vials, powder: 5 mg.

Phenurone. See *Phenacemide.*

Phenylbutazone (Butazolidin). Tablets (100): 100 mg.

Phenylephrine hydrochloride (Neo-Synephrine hydrochloride). Ampules (1 ml.) 10 mg. per ml. Ampules (2 ml.): 2 mg. per ml. Elixir (pt.): 1 mg. per ml. Jelly (20 Gm.): 0.5%. Solution, nasal (30 ml.): 0.25, 0.5, 1%. Solution, nasal spray (20 ml.): 0.25, 0.5%. Solution, sterile, ophthalmic (15 ml.): 2.5%. Solution, sterile, ophthalmic (5 ml.): 10%. Solution, ophthalmic, viscous (5 ml.): 10%. Solution, nasal (15 ml.): 0.125%. Vials (5 ml.): 10 mg. per ml.

Phenylpropanolamine hydrochloride (Propadrine hydrochloride). Capsules (100): 25, 50 mg. Elixir (pt.): 4 mg. per ml.

Phenylzin. See *Zinc sulfate, 0.25%, and phenylephrine, 0.12%.*

pHisoHex. See *Hexachlorophene.*

Phospholine iodide. See *Echothiophate iodide.*

Physostigmine salicylate (Eserine). Solution, ophthalmic (15 ml.): 0.25, 0.5%.

Phytonadione (AquaMEPHYTON, Konakion, Mephyton, vitamin K_1). Ampules (0.5 ml.): 2 mg. per ml. Ampules (1 ml.): 10 mg. per ml. Tablets (100): 5 mg. Vials (2.5, 5 ml.): 10 mg. per ml.

Piperazine citrate (Antepar). Syrup (pt.): 100 mg. per ml. Tablets (100): 500 mg. Tablets, chewable (28): 500 mg.

Piperocaine hydrochloride (Metycaine). Ampules (200 ml.): 1.5%. Ampules (30 ml.): 2%. Ointment, ophthalmic (4 Gm.): 4%. Tablets (100): 150 mg.

Piromen. See *Pseudomonas polysaccharide.*

Pitocin. See *Oxytocin.*

Pitocin citrate. See *Oxytocin citrate.*

Pitressin. See *Vasopressin.*

Pitressin tannate. See *Vasopressin tannate.*

Plague vaccine, bacterial. Vials (2, 20 ml.).

Plaquenil sulfate. See *Hydroxychloroquine sulfate.*

Podophyllin resin. In benzoin tincture: 20%. Extemporaneously prepared.

Polaramine maleate. See *Dexchlorpheniramine maleate.*

Poliovirus vaccine, inactivated. Vials (10 ml.): type 1, 2, 3 purified, formalin-inactivated, prepared by the Salk method.

Poliovirus vaccine, trivalent (Orimune poliovirus vaccine). Sabin strain, types 1, 2, 3. Drops, oral (10 doses): 2 drops per dose. Pipette, disposable (single dose): 0.5 ml. Vials, oral (single dose): 0.5, 2 ml.

Polycillin. See *Ampicillin trihydrate.*

Polycillin-N. See *Ampicillin sodium.*

Polycitra. Solution (pt.): 1 Gm. citric acid, 1.5 Gm. sodium citrate, and 1.67 Gm. potassium citrate per ml.

Polymyxin B sulfate. Vials, powder: 50 mg. (500,000 units).

Polysorb hydrate. Cream (50, 425 Gm.). Lotion (125 ml.). Ointment (50 Gm.).

Polyspectrin. Solution, ophthalmic (10 ml.): 50,000 units per Gm. polymyxin B sulfate and 0.5% neomycin sulfate. Ointment, ophthalmic (3.5 Gm.): 5000 units polymyxin B sulfate, 400 units zinc bacitracin, and 5 mg. neomycin sulfate per Gm.

Polysporin. Ointment, ophthalmic (4 Gm.) and ointment, topical (15, 30 Gm.): 10,000 units polymyxin B sulfate and 500 units bacitracin per Gm.

Polytar. Oil, bath (200 ml.): vegetable and mineral tars. Soap (125 Gm.).

Pontocaine. See *Tetracaine.*

Pontocaine hydrochloride. See *Tetracaine hydrochloride.*

Portagen. See *Medium chain triglycerides.*

Posterior pituitary. Ampules, obstetric (1 ml.): 10 units per ml. Ampules, surgical (1 ml).: 20 units per ml.

Potaba. See *Potassium para-aminobenzoate.*

Potassium chloride. 75 mg. = 1 mEq. Ampules (10, 20 ml.): 2 mEq. per ml. Liquid (pt.): 0.67, 1.34, 2.68 mEq. per ml. Powder (5-Gm. packet): 20 mEq. Tablets, enteric (100): 300 mg. Vials (10, 20 ml.): 2 mEq. per ml.

Potassium gluconate (Kaon). Elixir (pt.): 1.33 mEq. potassium per ml. Tablets (100): 5 mEq. potassium.

Potassium iodide (SSKI). Solution, oral (30, 60 ml.): 1 Gm. per ml.

Potassium para-aminobenzoate (Potaba). Capsules

(240): 500 mg. Envules (50): 20 Gm. Tablets (100): 500 mg.

Potassium permanganate. Tablets (100): 300 mg. Not for oral use. One tablet in 4½ qt. water prepares 1:15,000 solution.

Potassium phosphate. Ampules (10 ml.): 3 mEq. potassium and 65 mg. phosphorus per ml. Vials (20 ml.): 2 mEq. potassium per ml.

Potassium triplex. Potassium acetate, bicarbonate, and citrate. Solution (pt.): 3 mEq. potassium per ml.

Povan. See *Pyrvinium pamoate.*

Povidone-iodine (Betadine). Ointment (30 Gm., lb.). Scrub, surgical (pt., qt.). Solution (15, 30, 250, pt., qt.).

P.P.D. See *Tuberculin, purified protein derivative.*

Pragmatar. Ointment (30 Gm.): 4% coal tar, 3% sulfur, 3% salicylic acid.

Pralidoxime chloride (Protopam chloride, 2-PAM, P2AM). Ampules, powder: 1 Gm. Tablets: 500 mg.

Pranone. See *Ethisterone.*

Prednefrin. Suspension, ophthalmic (5, 10 ml.): 0.12% (mild), 0.2% (Prednefrin-S), or 1% (forte) prednisone acetate and 0.12% phenylephrine hydrochloride.

Prednisolone (Delta-Cortef, Hydeltra, Meticortelone). Cream, meti-derm, 0.5%. Tablets (100): 1, 2.5, 5 mg. Spray, aerosol, meti-derm.

Prednisolone phosphate (Hydeltrasol Inflamase, Inflamase forte). Ointment, ophthalmic (3.5 Gm.): 0.5%. Solution, ophthalmic (5 ml.): 0.5, 0.125, 1%.

Prednisone (Deltasone, Deltra, Meticorten). Tablets (100): 1, 2.5, 5, 10, 20, 50 mg.

PreFrin-A. Solution, ophthalmic (15 ml.): pyrilamine maleate, 0.1%, and phenylephrine, 0.12%.

Pregestamil (AD3200). Powder (lb.).

Premarin. See *Conjugated estrogenic substances.*

Presun. Lotion (120 ml.): para-amino benzoic acid, 5%, and ethyl alcohol, 55%.

Primaquine phosphate. Tablets (100): 26.3 mg. (15 mg. base).

Primidone (Mysoline). Suspension, oral (250 ml.): 50 mg. per ml. Tablets (100): 50, 250 mg.

Priscoline hydrochloride. See *Tolazoline hydrochloride.*

Pro-Banthine. See *Propantheline bromide.*

Probenecid (Benemid). Tablets (100): 500 mg.

Procainamide hydrochloride (Pronestyl hydrochloride). Capsules (100): 250, 375, 500 mg. Vials (10 ml.): 100 mg. per ml.

Procaine hydrochloride. Ampules (3 ml.): 2%. Ampules (2, 6 ml.): 1%. Vials (30, 100 ml.): 1, 2%.

Prochlorperazine (Compazine). Suppositories (6): 2.5, 5, 25 mg.

Prochlorperazine edisylate (Compazine edisylate). Ampules (2 ml.): 5 mg. per ml. Concentrate (125 ml.): 10 mg. per ml. Syrup (125 ml.): 1 mg. per ml. Vials (10 ml.): 5 mg. per ml.

Prochlorperazine maleate (Compazine maleate). Capsules, sustained release (50): 10, 15, 30, 75 mg. Tablets (100): 5, 10, 25 mg.

Progesterone. Ampules in oil (1 ml.): 2.5, 10, 25, 50 mg. per ml. Vials in oil (10 ml.): 25, 50 mg. per ml.

Progesterone caproate. See *Hydroxyprogesterone caproate.*

Promacetin. See *Acetosulfone.*

Promazine (sparine). Concentrate (30, 120 ml.): 30, 100 mg. per ml. Syringe, tubex (1, 2 ml.): 25, 50 mg. per ml. Syrup (120 ml.): 2 mg. per ml. Tablets (50): 10 25, 50, 100, 200 mg. Vial (2, 10 ml.): 25, 50 mg. per ml.

Promethazine hydrochloride (Phenergan hydrochloride). Ampules (1 ml.): 25, 50 mg. per ml. Ampules, intramuscular (1 ml.): 50 mg. per ml. Suppositories (12): 25, 50 mg. Syringe, tubex (1 ml.): 25, 50 mg. per ml. Syrup (pt.): 1.25 mg. per ml. Syrup fortis (pt.): 5 mg. per ml. Tablets (100): 12.5, 25, 50 mg. Vials (10 ml.): 25, 50 mg. per ml.

Promizole. See *Thiazolsulfone.*

Pronestyl hydrochloride. See *Procainamide hydrochloride.*

Propadrine hydrochloride. See *Phenylpropanolamine.*

Propantheline bromide (Pro-Banthine). Tablets (100): 7.5, 15 mg. Vial, powder: 30 mg.

Proparacaine hydrochloride (Ophthaine, Ophthetic). Solution, ophthalmic (15 ml.): 0.5%.

Propoxyphene hydrochloride (Darvon, Dolene). Capsules (100): 32, 65 mg.

Propoxyphene hydrochloride with APC (Darvon Compound, Dolene Compound). Capsules (100): 32, 65, mg. propolyphene with aspirin, phenacetin, and caffeine.

Propranolol (Inderal). Ampules (1 ml.): 1 mg. per ml. Tablets (100): 10, 40 mg.

Propylthiouracil. Tablets (100): 50 mg.

Prostaphlin sodium. See *Oxacillin sodium.*

Prostigmine bromide. See *Neostigmine bromide.*

Prostigmine methylsulfate. See *Neostigmine methylsulfate.*

Protamine sulfate. Ampules (5, 25 ml.): 10 mg. per ml. 1 mg. neutralizes 100 units of heparin.

Protamine zinc insulin. Vials, regular, beef special, or pork (10 ml.): 40, 80, 100 units per ml.

Protapam chloride. See *Pralidoxime chloride.*

Protein hydrolysate. See *Nutramigen.*

Proternol. See *Isoproterenol hydrochloride.*

Pro-Tet. See *Tetanus immune globulin, human.*

Provera. See *Medroxyprogesterone acetate.*

Pseudoephedrine hydrochloride (Sudafed). Syrup (125 ml.): 6 mg. per ml. Tablets (100): 30, 60 mg.

Pseudomonas polysaccharide (Piromen). Vials (2, 10 ml.): 4, 10, 50 micrograms per ml.

PSL. See *Darrow's solution.*

Psyllium hydrophilic mucilloid. See *Metamucil.*

Purinthol. See *Mercaptopurine.*

Purodigin. See *Digitoxin.*

Pyopen. See *Carbenicillin.*

Pyrazinamide. See *Pyrazinoic acid amide.*

Pyrazinoic acid amide (Pyrazinamide). Tablets (500): 500 mg. (Sale restricted to hospitals only).

Pyribenzamine citrate. See *Tripelennamine citrate.*

Pyribenzamine hydrochloride. See *Tripelennamine hydrochloride.*

Pyridostigmine bromide (Mestinon bromide). Ampules (2 ml.): 5 mg. per ml. Syrup (pt.): 12 mg. per ml. Tablets (100): 60 mg. Tablets, sustained release (100): 180 mg.

Pyridoxine hydrochloride (vitamin B_6). Ampules (1 ml.): 100 mg. per ml. Tablets (100): 10, 25, 50 mg. Vials (10 ml.): 100 mg. per ml.

Pyrimethamine (Daraprim). Tablets (100): 25 mg.

Pyrimethamine isethionate. Ampules: Obtainable from Dr. George Hitchings, Burroughs Wellcome, Raleigh, North Carolina; telephone 919-549-8371.

Pyrvinium pamoate (Povan). Suspension, oral (60 ml.): 10 mg. per ml. Tablets (25): 50 mg.

Q

Quadrinal. Suspension, oral (pt.): 2.4 mg. ephedrine hydrochloride, 13 mg. theophylline calcium salicylate, 2.4 mg. phenobarbital, 30 mg. potassium iodide per ml. Tablets (100): 24 mg. ephedrine hydrochloride, 130 mg. theophylline calcium salicylate, 24 mg. phenobarbital, 300 mg. potassium iodide.

Quelicin. See *Succinylcholine.*
Questran. See *Cholestyramine resin.*
Quibron. Elixir (pt.): 10 mg. theophylline, 6 mg. glyceryl guaiacolate per ml. Capsules (100): 150 mg. theophylline, 90 mg. glyceryl guaiacolate.
Quinacrine hydrochloride (Atabrine hydrochloride, Mepacrine). Ampules, powder: 200 mg. Tablets (100): 100 mg.
Quinidine gluconate. Vials (10 ml.): 80 mg. per ml. Tablets, sustained action (30, 100): 30 mg.
Quinidine sulfate. Tablets (100): 100, 200 mg. Capsules: 200, 300 mg.
Quinine hydrochloride. Ampules (2 ml.): 300 mg. per ml. Available at most Public Health Hospitals.
Quinine sulfate. Capsules (100): 125, 200, 300 mg. Syrup (pt.): 22 mg. per ml. Tablets (100): 300 mg.

R

Rabies vaccine. Vials: one dose, duck embryo. Vials: one dose, rabbit brain and cord by Semple method.
Raudixin. See *Rauwolfia serpentina.*
Rauwolfia serpentina (Raudixin). Tablets (100): 50, 100 mg.
Regitine hydrochloride. See *Phentolamine hydrochloride.*
Regitine methanesulfonate. See *Phentolamine methanesulfonate.*
Renografin. See *Meglumine diatrizoate.*
Reserpine (Serpasil). Ampules (2 ml.): 2.5 mg. per ml. Elixir (pt.): 0.05 mg. per ml. Tablets (100): 0.1, 0.25, 1 mg. Vials (10 ml.): 2.5 mg. per ml.
Retin-A. See *Tretinoin.*
Retinoic acid. See *Tretinoin.*
Resorcinol monoacetate (Euresol Pro Capillis). Solution (30 ml.).
Restrophen. Tablets (100): 30 mg. phenobarbital, 30 mg. hyoscyamus, cypripedium, valerian and camphor.
R-Gene. See *L-Arginine hydrochloride.*
Rheomacrodex. See *Dextran 40.*
RhoGAM. See *Immune globulin, $Rh_o(D)$.*
Riboflavin. Tablets (100): 5, 10, 25 mg. Vials (10 ml.): 10, 50 mg. per ml.
Rifampin. Tablets (30, 100): 300 mg.
Ringer's solution, lactated. See *Hartmann's solution.*
Ritalin hydrochloride. See *Methylphenidate hydrochloride.*
Robaxin. See *Methocarbamol.*
Robitussin. See *Glyceryl guaiacolate.*
Robitussin-DM. See *Glyceryl guaiacolate.*
Rocky mountain spotted fever vaccine. Vials (3 ml.).
Roudec. Syrup (pt.): 0.5 mg. carbinoxamine maleate and 12 mg. pseudoephedrine per ml. Tablets, chewable (100): 2.5 mg. carbinoxamine maleate and 60 mg. pseudoephedrine.
Rovamycin. See *Spiramycin.*
RVP (Elder red petrolatum). Ointment (60 Gm., 1 lb.).
RVPaque (ultraviolet occlusive agent). Tubes (15, 37 Gm.).

S

Salbutanol. Investigational.
Salicylazosulfapyridine (Azulfidine). Tablets (100): 500 mg. Tablets, enteric (100): 500 mg.
Salicylic acid. Plaster: 40%.
Sansert. See *Methysergide maleate.*
Scarlet red. Ointment (30 Gm.): 5%.
Schick test. See *Diphtheria toxin.*
Scopolamine hydrobromide (Hyoscine hydrobromide). Ampules (1 ml.): 0.3, 0.4, 0.5, 0.6 mg. per ml. Solution, ophthalmic (5, 15 ml.): 0.25%. Vials (20 ml.): 0.5 mg. per ml.
Sebizon. See *Sulfacetamide sodium.*
Sebulex. Shampoo (125, 250 ml.): sodium sulfoacetate, kerohydric sulfur, 2%, salicylic acid, 2%.
Sebutone. Shampoo (125 ml.): Sulfur, 2%, salicylic acid, 2%.
Secobarbital (Seconal). Elixir (pt.): 4 mg. per ml.
Secobarbital sodium (Seconal sodium). Ampules, powder: 250 mg. Capsules (100): 30, 50, 100 mg. Suppositories (12): 30, 60, 125, 200 mg. Syringes (2 ml.): 50 mg. per ml. Syringes, tubex (1, 2 ml.): 50 mg. per ml. Vials (20 ml.): 50 mg. per ml.
Seconal. See *Secobarbital.*
Seconal sodium. See *Secobarbital sodium.*
Selenium sulfide (Selsun). Suspension (125 ml.): 2.5%.
Selsun. See *Selenium sulfide.*
Semi-lente Iletin. See *Semi-lente insulin.*
Semi-lente insulin (Semi-lente Iletin). Vials (10 ml.): 40, 80, 100 units per ml.
Senna concentrate. See *Senokot.*
Senokot (Senna concentrate). Granules (60, 120, 240 Gm., lb.): 450 mg. per teaspoon. Suppositories (6, 48). Syrup (60, 250 ml.). Tablets (16, 30, 100): 275 mg.
Seromycin. See *Cycloserine.*
Serpasil. See *Reserpine.*
Silvadene. *Silver sulfadiazine.*
Silver nitrate. Wax ampules, solution, ophthalmic: 1%. Stick: 75% silver nitrate, 25% potassium nitrate.
Silver sulfadiazine (Silvadene). Investigational.
Similac. Liquid (13 oz.): 20 calories per oz. (normal dilution). Liquid, bottle (120, 180, or 40 ml.). Powder (1 lb.): 20 calories per oz. (normal dilution).
Similac PM (60:40 lactalbumin-casein ratio). Powder (1 lb.): 20 calories per oz. (normal dilution).
Six-Twelve. See *Ethyl hexanediol.*
SK-SD. See *Streptokinase-streptodornase.*
Slo-phyllin. See *Theophylline.*
Smallpox vaccine. Capillary tube, avianized.
SMA/S-26 (60:40 lactalbumin-casein ratio). Powder (1 lb.): 20 calories per oz. (normal dilution).
Sobee (milk-free soya formula). Liquid (15.5 oz.): 20 calories per oz. (normal dilution). Powder (1 lb.): 20 calories per oz. (normal dilution).
Sodium antimony dimercapto succinate (Asliban, Stibocaptate). Investigational.
Sodium bicarbonate. Ampules (50 ml.): 75 mg. per ml. Syringes (10, 50 ml.): 1 mEq. per ml. Syringes (50 ml.): 0.89 mEq. per ml. Tablets (100): 300, 600 mg. Vials (50 ml.): 1 mEq. per ml.
Sodium bromide. Powder: capsules to be made extemporaneously.
Sodium chloride. Solution, intravenous (150, 250, 500, 1000 ml.).
Sodium dextrothyroxine (Choloxin). Tablets (30): 1, 2, 4, 6 mg.
Sodium fluoride (Luride). Drops, oral (40 ml.): 2.2 mg. fluoride) per 0.4 ml. (10 drops). Tablets (120): 1.1, 2.2 mg. (0.5, 1 mg. fluoride).
Sodium iodide. Ampules (10 ml.): 100 mg. per ml.
Sodium lactate. Ampules (40 ml.): molar solution. Solution, intravenous (150, 250, 500, 1000 ml.): 1/6 molar.
Sodium levothyroxine (Synthroid). Tablets (100): 0.025, 0.05, 0.1, 0.15, 0.2, 0.3, 0.5 mg. Vials, powder: 500 micrograms.

Sodium nitroprusside. Vials: prepared extemporaneously. ± 20 mg. per ml. (filter; do not autoclave; refrigerate).
Sodium phytate (Nonasodium phytate). Investigational.
Sodium polystyrene sulfonate (Kayexalate). Powder (1 lb.).
Sodium stibogluconate (Pentostam, Solustibosan). Investigational.
Sodium sulfate. Powder (1 lb.).
Soft soap (green soap). Tincture (60, 125 ml., pt.).
Solapsone (Sulphretone). Investigational.
Solbar (a broad-spectrum UV sun protectant). Lotion (75 Gm.): 3% oxybenzone and 3% dioxybenzone.
Solu-Cortef. See *Hydrocortisone sodium succinate.*
Solu-Medrol. See *Methylprednisolone sodium succinate.*
Solustibosan. See *Sodium stibogluconate.*
Sorbitol. Solution, 7% (pt.).
Soyaloid. Powder (90 Gm.): 50% colloidal soy protein, 2% polyvinylpyrrolidone.
Soyboro. Powder: aluminum acetate, boric acid, sulfate, calcium, colloidal soil complex. One packet in 1 qt. tap water.
Sparine. See *Promazine.*
Spiramycin (Rovamycine). Investigational.
Spironolactone (Aldactone). Tablets (100): 25 mg.
SSKI. See *Potassium iodide.*
ST-37. See *Hexylresorcinol.*
Staphicillin. See *Methicillin sodium.*
Staphylococcal toxoid. Vials: detoxified (5 ml.): 100, 1000 units per ml. Vials, digest modified (5 ml.): 10,000 units per ml.
Stelazine. See *Trifluoperazine.*
Sterculia. See *Karaya.*
Steripaque. See *Barium sulfate, micronized.*
Sterosan. Cream (20 Gm.): chlorquinaldol, 3%, hydrocortisone, 1%.
Stibocaptate. See *Sodium antimony dimercaptosuccinate.*
Stibophen (Catecholdisulfonate, Fuadin). Ampules (5 ml.): 6.3%.
Stilbazium iodide (Monopar). Investigational.
Stoxil. See *Idoxuridine.*
Streptokinase-streptodornase (SK-SD, Varidase.) Tablets, buccal or oral (24, 100): 10,000 units streptokinase and 2500 units streptodornase. Vials, topical: 100,000 units streptotkinase and 25,000 units streptodornase. Vials, intramuscular: 20,000 units streptokinase and 5000 units streptodornase.
Streptomycin sulfate. Powder, sterile: 1, 5 Gm. Syringes, tubex (1, 2 ml.): 500 mg. per ml. Vials 2, 10 ml.): 50 mg. per ml. Vials (2, 5, 12.5 ml.): 400 mg. per ml.
Streptozotocin. Investigational.
Succinylcholine (Anectine, Quelicin, Sucostrin). Ampules (10 ml.): 50, 100 mg. per ml. Powder, sterile flow-pack: 500, 1000 mg. Vials (10 ml.) 20 mg. per ml.
Sucostrin. See *Succinylcholine.*
Sudafed. See *Pseudoephedrine hydrochloride.*
Sulamyd sodium. See *Sulfacetamide sodium.*
Sulfacetamide sodium (Bleph 10, Bleph 30, Isopto-Cetamide, Sebizon, Sulamyd sodium). Lotion (90 Gm.): 100 mg. per Gm. Ointment, ophthalmic (4 Gm.): 10%. Solution, ophthalmic (5, 15 ml.): 10, 30%.
Sulfadiazine. Ointment, ophthalmic (4 Gm.): 5%. Suspension, oral (pt.): 100 mg. per ml. Tablets (100): 500 mg.
Sulfadiazine sodium. Ampules (10 ml.): 250 mg. per ml.
Sulfamylon. See *Mafenide.*
Sulfapyridine. Tablets (100): 500 mg.
Sulfinpyrazone (Anturane). Capsules (100): 200 mg. Tablets (100): 100 mg.
Sulfisoxazole (Gantrisin). Tablets (100): 500 mg.
Sulfisoxazole acetyl (Gantrisin acetyl). Emulsion in oil, oral (125 ml., pt.): 100 mg. per ml. Suspension, oral (125 ml., pt.): 100 mg. per ml.
Sulfisoxazole diethanolamine (Gantrisin diethanolamine). Ampules (5, 10 ml.): 400 mg. per ml. Ointment, ophthalmic (4 Gm.): 4%. Solution, ophthalmic (5 ml.): 4%.
Sulfoxone sodium (Diasone sodium). Tablets, enteric (100): 165 mg.
Sulphretone. See *Solapsone.*
Sulthiame. See *Ospolot.*
Sultrin (triple sulfa). Cream vaginal (78 Gm.): 3.42% sulfathiazole, 2.86% sulfacetamide, 3.7% sulfanilamide.
Sunstick. See *Digalloyl trioleate.*
Sunswept. See *Digalloyl trioleate.*
Suramin (Antrypol, Bayer 205, Germanin, Moranyl). Investigational.
Surgicel. See *Cellulose, oxidized.*
Sus-Phrine. See *Epinephrine.*
Symmetrel. See *Amantadine hydrochloride.*
Synalar. See *Fluocinolone acetonide.*
Synkamin (vitamin K_5). Ampules (1 ml.): 1 mg. Capsules (100): 4 mg.
Synkayvite. See *Menadiol sodium diphosphate.*
Synthroid. See *Sodium levothyroxine.*

T

Tannic acid. Powder (125 Gm.).
TAO. See *Triacetyloleandomycin.*
Tapazole. See *Methimazole.*
Tartar emetic. See *Antimony potassium tartrate.*
TAT. See *Tetanus antitoxin, horse serum.*
Tearisol. See *Methylcellulose.*
Tedral. Suspension, oral (250 ml., pt.): 2.4 mg. ephedrine hydrochloride, 13 mg. theophylline, and 0.8 mg. phenobarbital per ml. Tablets (24, 100): 24 mg, ephedrine hydrochloride, 130 mg. theophylline, and 8 mg. phenobarbital.
Tedral SA. Tablets, sustained action (100): 48 mg. ephedrine hydrochloride, 180 mg. theophylline, and 25 mg. phenobarbital.
Tegopen. See *Cloxacillin sodium monohydrate.*
Tegretol. See *Carbamazepine.*
Teldrin. See *Chlorpheniramine maleate.*
Telfa. Pads (10, 20): 1½ in. × 2 in., 2 in. × 3 in., 3 in. × 4 in.
TEM. See *Triethylene melamine.*
Temaril. See *Trimeprazine tartrate.*
Tempra. See *Acetaminophen.*
Tensilon chloride. See *Edrophonium chloride.*
Terpin hydrate and codeine. Elixir (125 ml.): 2 mg. codeine and 17 mg. terpin hydrate per ml.
Terra-Cortril. Suspension, ophthalmic or otic (5 ml.): 15 mg. hydrocortisone and 5 mg. oxytetracycline per ml.
Terramycin. See *Oxytetracycline calcium.*
Terramycin hydrochloride. See *Oxytetracycline hydrochloride.*
Tes-Tape. Package: 100 tests, glucose oxidase and glucose peroxidase.
Testosterone cypionate (Depo-Testosterone). Vials (10 ml.): 50 mg. per ml. in oil. Vials (1, 10 ml.): 100, 200 mg. per ml. in oil.
Testosterone enanthate (Delatestryl). Syringe (1 ml.): 200 mg. per ml. Vials (5 ml.): 200 mg. per ml.

Testosterone propionate (Oreton propionate, Perandren). Tablets, buccal (30, 100): 10 mg. Vials (10 ml.): 50, 100 mg. per ml.

Tetanus antitoxin, horse serum (TAT). Vials: 1500, 2000. Vials (1.5, 3 ml.): 1000 units per ml. Vials (5 ml.): 4000 units per ml.

Tetanus immune globulin, human (Hu-Tet, Hyper-Tet, Immu-Tet, Pro-Tet). Syringe: 250 units. Vials: 250 units.

Tetanus toxoid. See also *Diphtheria toxoids.* Syringe, fluid: 0.5 ml. Syringe, alum-precipitated: 0.5 ml. Vials, fluid: 1.5, 7.5 ml. Vials, alum-precipitated: 1, 5 ml.

Tetracaine (Pontocaine). Ointment, ophthalmic (4 Gm.): 0.5%.

Tetracaine hydrochloride (Pontocaine hydrochloride). Solution, sterile ophthalmic (15 ml.): 0.5%. Solution, topical (30 ml.): 2%.

Tetrachloroethylene (Nema). Capsules, veterinary (12): 0.2, 0.5, 1, 2.5, 5 ml. Used for human consumption.

Tetracycline hydrochloride (Achromycin). Capsules (100): 100, 250, 500 mg. Drops, oral (10 ml.): 100 mg. per ml. Suspension, ophthalmic, oily (4 ml.): 1%. Syrup (60 ml.): 25 mg. per ml. Vials, powder, intramuscular: 100, 250 mg. Vials, powder, intravenous: 100, 250, 500 mg.

Tetracycline hydrochloride with hydrocortisone (Achromycin with hydrocortisone). Ointment, ophthalmic.

Tetrahydrozoline hydrochloride (Visine). Solution, nasal (15, 30 ml.): 0.05%.

Tham-E. See *Tromethamine.*

Theophylline (Elixophyllin, Slo-phyllin). Capsule, sustained release (60): 125, 250 mg. Elixir (pt., qt.): 80 mg. per 15 ml. Enema, disposable unit (37 ml.): 250, 500 mg. (Fleet).

Thiabendazole (Mintezol). Suspension, oral (125 ml.): 100 mg. per ml. Tablet, chewable (36): 500 mg.

Thiamine hydrochloride (vitamin B_1). Ampules (1 ml.): 100 mg. per ml. Elixir (pt.): 0.45 mg. per ml. Syringe, tubex (1 ml.): 100 mg. per ml. Tablets (100): 10, 25, 50, 100, 250. Vials (10 ml.): 50, 100, 200 mg. per ml.

Thiazolsulfone (Promizole). Investigational.

Thioguanine. Tablets (25): 40 mg.

Thiomerin sodium. See *Mercaptomerin sodium.*

Thioridazine (Mellaril). Liquid, concentrate (120, 240 ml.): 30 mg. per ml. Tablets (100): 10, 15, 25, 50, 100, 150, 200 mg.

Thiotepa. See *Triethylenethiophosphoramide.*

Thorazine. See *Chlorpromazine.*

Thorazine hydrochloride. See *Chlorpromazine hydrochloride.*

Thrombin. Powder, topical: 1000, 5000, 10,000 units.

Thrombolysin. See *Fibrinolysin.*

Thyrocalcitonin (calcitonin). Investigational.

Thyroid. Tablets (100): 15, 30, 60, 125, 200, 300 mg. Tablets, enteric (100): 15, 30, 60, 125, 200, 300 mg.

Thyrotropic hormone. See *Thyrotropin.*

Thyrotropin (Thyrotropic hormone, Thytropar, TSH). Vials: 10 units.

Thytropar. See *Thyrotropin.*

Tigan. See *Trimethobenzamide.*

Tinactin. Cream (15 Gm.): 10 mg. tolnaftate and 5 mg. butylated hydroxytoluene per Gm. Powder (45 Gm.): 10 mg. tolnaftate per Gm. Solution (10 ml.): 10 mg. tolnaftate and 1 mg. butylated hydroxytoluene per ml. Spray, aerosol (120 Gm.): 10 mg. tolnaftate per Gm.

Tofranil. See *Imipramine hydrochloride.*

Tolazoline hydrochloride (Priscoline hydrochloride). Tablets (100): 25 mg. Tablets, Lontabs (100): 80 mg. Vials (10 ml.): 25 mg. per ml.

Topocide. See *Benzyl benzoate, compound.*

Tranexamic acid. Investigational.

Travent. See *Invert sugar.*

Trecator. See *Ethionamide.*

Tretamine. See *Triethylene melamine.*

Tretinoin (Retin-A, Retinoil acid, vitamin A acid). Solution (60 ml.): 0.05%. Swabs, saturated (30): 0.05%.

Triacetyloleandomycin (Cyclamycin, TAO). Capsules (36, 60): 250 mg. Suspension, oral (60 ml.): 25 mg. per ml.

Triamcinolone (Aristocort). Syrup (125 ml.): 0.8 mg. per ml. Tablets (30, 50): 1, 2, 4, 8, 16 mg.

Triamcinolone acetonide (Aristocort, Kenalog). Cream (15, 60, 75 Gm.): 0.025, 0.1, 0.5%. Ointment (15, 60, 75 Gm.): 0.025, 0.1%. Lotion (60 ml.): 0.025%. Lotion (15, 60 ml.): 0.1%. Paste, dental (5 Gm.): 0.1% in Orabase. Vials (1, 5 ml.): 40 mg. per ml.

Triamcinolone acetonide with neomycin sulfate (Kenalog-S). Cream (15 Gm.): 1 mg. triamcinolone acetonide, 2.5 mg. neomycin (as sulfate), 0.25 mg. gramicidin. Lotion (7.5 ml.) as above. Ointment (5, 15 Gm.), as above. Solution, ophthalmic (5 ml.) as above.

Triamcinolone diacetate (Aristocort diacetate). Vials, intralesional (5 ml.): 25 mg. per ml.

Triaminic. Concentrate (24 drops per ml.) (15 ml.): 10 mg. pyrilamine maleate, 10 mg. pheniramine maleate, and 20 mg. phenylpropanolamine hydrochloride per ml. Syrup (125 ml., pt.): 1.25 mg. pyrilamine maleate, 1.25 mg. pheniramine maleate, and 2.5 mg. phenylpropanolamine hydrochloride per ml. Tablets, timed release (100): 25 mg. pyrilamine maleate, 25 mg. pheniramine maleate and 50 mg. phenylpropanolamine hydrochloride. Tablets, Juvelets, timed release (50): 12.5 mg. pyrilamine maleate, 12.5 mg. pheniramine maleate, and 25 mg. phenylpropanolamine hydrochloride.

Triamterene (Dyrenium). Capsules (100): 100 mg.

Triclofenol piperazine. Investigational.

Tridesilon. See *Desonide.*

Tridione. See *Trimethadione.*

Triethylene melamine (TEM, tretamine). Tablets (12, 100): 5 mg.

Triethylenetetramine dihydrochloride. Investigational.

Triethylenethiophosphoramide (Thiotepa). Vials, powder: 15 mg.

Trifluoperazine (Stelazine). Concentrate (60 ml.): 10 mg. per ml. Tablets (50): 1, 2, 5, 10 mg. Vials (10 ml.): 2 mg. per ml.

Triflupromazine hydrochloride (Vesprin). Suspension high potency (125 ml.): 10 mg. per ml. Tablets (50): 10, 25, 50 mg. Vials (1 ml.): 20 mg. per ml. Vials (10 ml.): 10 mg. per ml.

Trihexyphenidyl hydrochloride (Artane hydrochloride). Capsules, sustained release (30): 5 mg. Elixir (pt.): 0.4 mg. per ml. Tablets (100): 2.5 mg.

Trilafon. See *Perphenazine.*

Trimelarsen. See *Melarsonyl potassium.*

Trimeprazine tartrate (Temaril). Capsules, sustained action (50): 5 mg. Syrup (125 ml.): 0.5 mg. per ml. Tablets (100): 2.5 mg.

Trimethadione (Tridione). Capsules (100): 300 mg. Solution, oral (pt.): 40 mg. per ml. Tablets (100): 150 mg.

Trimethobenzamide (Tigan). Ampules (2 ml.): 100 mg. per ml. Capsules (100): 100, 250 mg. Suppositories (10): 200 mg. Syringe (2 ml.): 50 mg. per ml. Vials (20 ml.): 100 mg. per ml.

Trimethylpsoralen. See *Trioxalen.*
Triostam. See *Antimony sodium gluconate.*
Trioxalen (Trimethylpsoralen, Trisoralen). Tablets (28, 100): 5 mg.
Tripelennamine citrate (Pyribenzamine citrate). Elixir (pt.): 7.5 mg. per ml. (equivalent to 5 mg. of hydrochloride.
Tripelennamine hydrochloride (Pyribenzamine hydrochloride). Ampules (1 ml.): 25 mg. per ml. Cream (30 Gm.): 2%. Ointment (30 Gm.): 2%. Tablets (100): 25, 50 mg. Tablets, sustained release (100): 50, 100 mg. Vials (10 ml.): 25 mg. per ml.
Triple dye. Formula: acriflavine 23%, brilliant green 31%, and methylrosaniline hydrochloride 46%.
Triple sulfa. See *Sultrin.*
Triple sulfonamides. See *Trisulfapyrimidines.*
Triprolidine (Actidil). Syrup (pt.): 0.25 mg. per ml. Tablets (100): 2.5 mg.
Triquin. Tablets (100): 25 mg. quinacrine hydrochloride, 65 mg. chloroquine phosphate, and 50 mg. hydroxychloroquine sulfate per tablet.
Tris buffer. See *Tromethamine.*
Trisoralen. See *Trioxalen.*
Trisulfapyrimidines (triple sulfonamides). Each 5 ml. or tablet contains: 167 mg. sulfadiazine, 167 mg. sulfamerazine, and 167 mg. salfamethazine. Suspension, oral (pt.): 100 mg. per ml. Tablets (100): 500 mg.
Tromethamine (Tham-E, tris buffer). Powder, sterile: 36 Gm.
Tropicamide (Bis-tropamide, Mydriacyl). Solution, sterile, ophthalmic (15 ml.): 0.5, 1%.
TSH. See *Thyrotropin.*
Tuberculin, purified protein derivative (P.P.D.). Stabilized solution (with tween 80). First strength (10 tests)—vial: 0.0001 mg. Intermediate strength (10 tests)—vial: 0.001 mg. Second strength (10 tests)—vial: 0.025 mg.
Tuberculosis vaccine (B.C.G.). Capillary tubes (single dose). Vial, freeze-dried powder (15 doses): 50 mg. Vial, freeze-dried powder (10 doses).
Tylenol. See *Acetaminophen.*
Typhoid vaccine. Vial (1.5, 15 ml.): 1000 million killed typhoid bacteria per ml. 0.5-ml. dose. Vials (5, 10, 20 ml.).
Typhus vaccine. Vials (1, 2, 10, 20 ml.).
Tyrosum. Solution (125 ml., pt.): Tyrothricin, 0.2 mg. per ml., isopropyl alcohol 50%.

U

Ulcort. See *Hydrocortamate.*
Ultandren. See *Fluoxymesterone.*
Ultra-lente Iletin. See *Ultra-lente insulin.*
Ultra-lente insulin (Ultra-lente Iletin). Vials (10 ml.): 40, 80, 100 units per ml.
Unibase. Cream (lb.).
Unipen. See *Nafcillin sodium.*
Urea (Carmol, Ureaphil, Urevert). Bottles, sterile powder: 40, 90 Gm. Bottles, sterile powder with diluent (93 ml.): 40 Gm. Bottles, sterile powder with diluent (210 ml.): 90 Gm. Cream (90 Gm.): 20%.
Urea stibamine (Carbostibamide). Investigational.
Ureaphil. See *Urea.*
Urecholine chloride. See *Bethanechol chloride.*
Urevert. See *Urea.*
Uridine (Uteplex). Ampules, oral (2 ml.): 1 mg. per ml.
Urokinase. Ampules: 5000 ploug units.
Uteplex. See *Uridine.*
Uval (2-hydroxy-4-methoxy-benzophenone-5-sulfonic acid). Lotion (75, 165 Gm.): 10%.

V

Vaccinia immune globulin. Distributed by American Red Cross through regional blood centers and commercially through Hyland Laboratories. Vials (5 ml.): 16.5 ml.
Vagisec Plus. See *Aminoacridine hydrochloride.*
Valisone. See *Betamethasone 17-valerate.*
Valium. See *Diazepam.*
Vancocin. See *Vancomycin HCl.*
Vancomycin hydrochloride (Vancocin). Vials, powder: 500 mg.
Vanobid. See *Candidicin.*
Vanoxide. 0.25% chlorhydroxyquinoline, 5% benzoyl peroxide. Lotion (25, 50 Gm.).
Vape-N-Iso. See *Isoproterenol.*
Varidase. See *Streptokinase-streptodornase.*
Vasocidin. Solution, ophthalmic (5, 15 ml.): 0.2% prednisolone, 10% sulfacetamide sodium, 0.125% phenylephrine.
Vasocon. *Naphazoline.*
Vasocon-A. Antazoline, 0.5%, and naphazoline, 0.05%. Solution (15 ml.): 0.05% naphazoline and 0.5% antazoline.
Vasocort. Solution (15 ml.): 0.125% phenylephrine hydrochloride, 0.02% hydrocortisone, 0.5% hydroxyamphetamine.
Vasopressin (Pitressin). Ampules (0.5, 1 ml.): 20 units per ml.
Vasopressin tannate (Pitressin tannate). Ampules (1 ml.): 5 units per ml. in oil.
Vasoxyl. See *Methoxamine hydrochloride.*
Velban. See *Vinblastine sulfate.*
Veracillin. See *Dicloxacillin sodium monohydrate.*
Verequad. Suspension (pt.): 2.4 mg. ephedrine hydrochloride, 13 mg. theophylline calcium salicylate, 0.8 mg. phenobarbital, and 10 mg. glyceryl guaiacolate per ml. Tablets (100): 24 mg. ephedrine hydrochloride, 130 mg. theophylline calcium salicylate, 8 mg. phenobarbital, and 100 mg. glyceryl guaiacolate.
Vesprin. See *Triflupromazine hydrochloride.*
Vibramycin. See *Doxycycline.*
Vinactane. See *Viomycin sulfate.*
Vinblastine sulfate (Velban). Ampules, powder: 10 mg.
Vincristine sulfate (Oncovin). Ampules, powder: 1, 5 mg.
Viocin. See *Viomycin sulfate.*
Vioform. See *Iodochlorhydroxyquin.*
Vioform with hydrocortisone. Cream (5, 20 Gm.): 1% hydrocortisone and 3% Vioform. Cream (15, 30 Gm.): 0.5% hydrocortisone and 3% Vioform. Lotion (15 ml.): 1% hydrocortisone and 3% Vioform. Ointment (5, 20 Gm.): 1% hydrocortisone and 3% Vioform. Ointment (15, 30 Gm.): 0.5% hydrocortisone and 3% Vioform.
Viokase. See *Pancreatin.*
Viomycin sulfate (Vinactane, Viocin, viomycin). Vials, powder: 1, 5 Gm. Viomycin base as sulfate.
Vi-Penta. See *Multivitamins with vitamin E.*
Visine. See *Tetrahydrozoline hydrochloride.*
Vistaril. See *Hydroxyzine pamoate.*
Vitamin A (Aquasol A). Capsules, water-miscible (100): 25,000, 50,000 units. Capsules (100): 25,000, 50,000 units. Solution, water-miscible (30 ml.): 50,000 units per ml. Vials (5 ml.): 50,000 units per ml.
Vitamin A acid. See *Tretinoin.*

Vitamin A and D-HC. Suppositories (12): 10 mg. hydrocortisone, 1500 units vitamin A, 200 units vitamin D_3 peruvian balsam, bismuth subgallate, zinc oxide.
Vitamin B complex (Allbee, Betalin, Combex, Lederplex). Contains vitamins B, B_2, and B_6, nicotinamide, and calcium pantothenate. Ampules (2 ml.). Capsules (100). Elixir. Syrup (250, 360 ml.). Tablets (100). Vials (10, 15 ml.).
Vitamin B_1. See *Thiamine hydrochloride.*
Vitamin B_6. See *Pyridoxine hydrochloride.*
Vitamin B_{12}. See *Cyanocobalamin.*
Vitamin D_2. See *Calciferol.*
Vitamin D_4. See *Dihydrotachysterol.*
Vitamin E (Alpha-tocopherol, Aquasol E). Capsules, water-miscible (100): 30, 100, 400 units. Elixir (240 ml.): 6.66 units per ml. Solution, oral (15 ml.): 50 units per ml.
Vitamin K_1. See *Phytonadione.*
Vitamin K_5. See *Synkamin.*
VolSol HC. Solution, otic (7.5 ml.): 1% hydrocortisone and 3% propanediol diacetate in propylene glycol.
Vontrol. See *Diphenidol.*

W

Warfarin sodium (Coumadin sodium, Panwarfin). Ampules, powder: 50, 75 mg. Tablets (25, 100): 2, 2.5, 5, 7.5, 10, 25 mg.
Whitfield's ointment. Ointment (30 Gm.): 12% benzoic acid, and 6% salicylic acid.
Wyamine. See *Mephenteramine sulfate.*
Wydase. See *Hyaluronidase.*

X

Xylocaine hydrochloride. See *Lidocaine hydrochloride.*

Y

Yodoxin. See *Diiodohydroxyquin.*
Yomesan. See *Niclosamide.*

Z

Zarontin. See *Ethosuximide.*
Zeasorb. Powder (60, 240 Gm.).
Zephiran chloride. See *Benzalkonium chloride.*
Zetar. Emulsion (200 ml.): 50% colloidal crude tar. Liquid (60, 200 Gm.): crude and synthetic coal tar. Liquid, decolorized (50 Gm.): synthetic coal tar. Lotion (60 ml.): 2% colloidal crude coal tar and talc. Ointment (60 Gm.): 2% colloidal crude coal tar, zinc oxide, and talc. Shampoo (200 ml.): 1% colloidal crude coal tar and 0.2% allantoin.
Zinc oxide. Ointment (30, 60 Gm.). Paste (30 Gm., 1 lb.).
Zinc peroxide. Solution (115 Gm.).
Zinc sulfate (Op-Thal-Zin, Zincate). Solution, ophthalmic (15 ml.): 0.25%. Tablets (100): 220 mg.
Zinc sulfate, 0.25%, and phenylephrine, 0.12% (Phenylzin, Zincfrin). Solution (15 ml.).
Zincate. See *Zinc sulfate.*
Zincfrin. See *Zinc sulfate, 0.25%, and phenylephrine, 0.12%.*
Zolyse. See *Alpha-chymotrypsin.*
Zoster immune globulin. Available from the Center for Disease Control, Atlanta, Georgia.
Zyloprim. See *Allopurinol.*
Zymenol. Emulsion (8, 14 oz.): 50% mineral oil with yeast culture.

Index

We invite your help to keep

CURRENT PEDIATRIC THERAPY

in tune with your needs

Use this postcard to tell us whether there is a subject you sought and failed to find, or a discussion you considered not sufficiently helpful or perhaps even out of date. We will do our best to improve the next edition.

SYDNEY S. GELLIS, M.D.

BENJAMIN M. KAGAN, M.D.

Albert E. Meier
Associate Medical Editor

Name____________________

Address____________________

City__________ State__________ ZIP__________

FIRST CLASS
PERMIT NO. 101
PHILADELPHIA, PA.

BUSINESS REPLY MAIL

NO POSTAGE STAMP NECESSARY IF MAILED IN UNITED STATES

POSTAGE WILL BE PAID BY

W. B. Saunders Company
West Washington Square
Philadelphia, Pa. 19105